THE OXFORD HANDBOOK OF

PHILOSOPHY AND PSYCHIATRY

INTERNATIONAL PERSPECTIVES IN PHILOSOPHY AND PSYCHIATRY

Series editors: Bill (K. W. M.) Fulford, Katherine Morris, John Z. Sadler, and Giovanni Stanghellini

Volumes in the series:

THE OXFORD HANDBOOK OF

PHILOSOPHY AND PSYCHIATRY

Edited by

K. W. M. FULFORD

MARTIN DAVIES

RICHARD G. T. GIPPS

GEORGE GRAHAM

JOHN Z. SADLER

GIOVANNI STANGHELLINI

and

TIM THORNTON

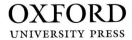

OXFORD

UNIVERSITY PRESS

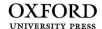
UNIVERSITY PRESS

Great Clarendon Street, Oxford, OX2 6DP,
United Kingdom

Oxford University Press is a department of the University of Oxford.
It furthers the University's objective of excellence in research, scholarship,
and education by publishing worldwide. Oxford is a registered trade mark of
Oxford University Press in the UK and in certain other countries

British Library Cataloguing in Publication Data

Data available

ISBN 978–0–19–957956–3

Printed and bound in Great Britain by
CPI Group (UK) Ltd, Croydon, CR0 4YY

Whilst every effort has been made to ensure that the contents of this work
are as complete, accurate and-up-to-date as possible at the date of writing,
Oxford University Press is not able to give any guarantee or assurance that
such is the case. Readers are urged to take appropriately qualified medical
advice in all cases. The information in this work is intended to be useful to the
general reader, but should not be used as a means of self-diagnosis or for the
prescription of medication

Links to third party websites are provided by Oxford in good faith and for
information only. Oxford disclaims any responsibility for the materials
contained in any third party website referenced in this work.

PREFACE

"Madness," the Oxford philosopher Anthony Quinton commented in a lecture to the British Academy published in 1985, "is a subject that ought to interest philosophers; but they have had surprisingly little to say about it." What a difference three decades have made! As the contributions to this book so richly illustrate, there is nowadays hardly a psychiatric stone that philosophers have left unturned. Nor is the trade one-way. If philosophers are now interested in psychiatric research and practice, so, too, are researchers and practitioners—including an increasingly vocal and effective service user community—interested in philosophy.

The Oxford Handbook of Philosophy and Psychiatry brings together what we hope is a representative cross-section of the new field. Like other Oxford Philosophy Handbooks, it is written mainly by philosophers for philosophers. In this respect it balances other contributions to the book series with which it is co-branded, the IPPP (International Perspectives in Philosophy and Psychiatry) series: *The Oxford Textbook of Philosophy and Psychiatry*, for example, is oriented more towards practice. Yet this Handbook, although primarily philosophical in focus, incorporates a number of novel features reflecting the lively dynamic between theory and practice that is such a distinctive characteristic of the new field. Thus a number of our contributors are practitioners and empirical researchers as well as philosophers; others write from first-hand experience of mental disorder; and the book as a whole is structured around the stages of the clinical encounter rather than within traditional philosophical disciplines. Nor are the Handbook's ambitions in this respect merely colligative. As we describe more fully in our introductory Chapter 1, the Handbook is supported by a website (www.oup.co.uk/companion/fulford) of narrative and other case-based materials offering what we hope will be a unique one-stop resource for philosophers entering the field.

A project as complex and ambitious as *The Oxford Handbook of Philosophy and Psychiatry* would have been impossible without the combined skills of many, and diversely talented, people. Our thanks go first to our contributors to both the book and the website: each and every one has been wonderfully generous with their time and commitment in responding to the editorial challenges of synthesis and integration across the book as a whole. Our thanks go also to the members of our International Advisory Board who made many crucial suggestions in the early stages of planning the book and have given continuing support throughout. Our two graduate researchers, Will Davies and Gemma Copsey, showed great skill and dedication and we are grateful to them for their crucial work respectively on an initial literature review and on the development of the website. George Graham was ably supported by Casey Landers. We are grateful also to David Crepaz-Keay, Jayasree Kalathil, Toby Williamson, and others at the Mental Health Foundation, a voluntary sector organization that in uniquely combining policy and service user perspectives has brought an important additional dimension to the book and its supporting website. And all of us, finally, editors and contributors alike, are grateful to the publishing team at Oxford University Press who have gone way beyond the merely professional in their commitment to the project: our thanks go particularly to Martin Baum and Peter Momtchiloff whose collaboration as commissioning editors respectively for psychiatry (and related areas) and philosophy made the book possible; to Abigail Stanley and to Beth McAllister and their respective production and marketing teams; and to Charlotte Green as project lead for her boundless energy and for her consistently good humoured and problem-solving approach.

No single volume however compendious can hope to capture, still less keep up with, every important development in this vigorously expanding field. The IPPP series will continue to publish cutting edge work. Future Oxford Handbooks in Philosophy will offer further state-of-the-art collections: the forthcoming *Oxford Handbook of Psychiatric Ethics* was conceived as a sister volume to this book; and there are clear gaps in the market for future Handbooks covering the relationships between psychopathology and such areas as phenomenology and the cognitive and neurosciences. But thirty years on from Quinton's prescient lecture our hope is that the publication of this book in what is the centenary of Karl Jaspers' *General Psychopathology* will help to secure the place of psychiatry as a subject that is and remains permanently among the interests of philosophers.

REFERENCE

Quinton, A. (1985). Madness. In A.P. Griffiths (Ed.), *Philosophy and Practice*, pp. 17–41. Cambridge: Cambridge University Press.

The Oxford Handbook of Philosophy and Psychiatry

Editors

K.W.M. Fulford
Martin Davies
Richard G.T. Gipps
George Graham
John Z. Sadler
Giovanni Stanghellini
Tim Thornton

Editorial Research Assistants

Will Davies
Gemma Copsey

International Advisory Board

Anita Avramides
Gloria Ayob
Lisa Bortolotti
Matthew Broome
Tim Bayne
John Campbell
Rachel Cooper
Thomas Fuchs
Gerrit Glas
Guy Kahane
Josef Parnas
Hanna Pickard
Nancy Potter
Matthew Ratcliffe
Johannes Roessler
Louis Sass
Julian Savulescu
Nicholas Shea
Werdie van Staden

Website

V.Y. Allison-Bolger
David Crepaz-Keay
Jayasree Kalathil
Toby Williamson

CONTENTS

SECTION III   ESTABLISHING RELATIONSHIPS

SECTION IV   SUMMONING CONCEPTS

SECTION V   DESCRIPTIVE PSYCHOPATHOLOGY

SECTION VI   ASSESSMENT AND DIAGNOSTIC CATEGORIES

SECTION VII   EXPLANATION AND UNDERSTANDING

SECTION VIII   CURE AND CARE

WEBSITE

www.oup.co.uk/companion/fulford
Timeline

Personal Narratives of Madness
  • Single narratives, autobiographies
  • Anthologies, edited collections
  • Studying/Studies on narratives

Studies of Psychotic Experience: Classic and Contemporary Accounts
  • First rank symptoms
  • Hallucinations
  • Predelusional states
  • Delusions

Contributors

V.Y. Allison-Bolger Consultant Psychiatrist, UK

Katherine Arens Department of Germanic Studies, University of Texas at Austin, Austin, TX, USA

Richard Askay University of Portland, Portland, OR, USA

Anita Avramides Faculty of Philosophy, University of Oxford, Oxford, UK

Tim Bayne Department of Philosophy, School of Social Science, University of Manchester, Manchester, UK

Michael A. Bishop Department of Philosophy, Florida State University, Tallahassee, FL, USA

Derek Bolton King's College London, Institute of Psychiatry, London, UK

Lisa Bortolotti Department of Philosophy, University of Birmingham, Birmingham, UK

Pat Bracken West Cork Mental Health Service, Bantry, Ireland

Matthew Broome Department of Psychiatry, University of Oxford, Oxford, UK; Highfield Adolescent Unit, Warneford Hospital, Oxford Health NHS Foundation Trust, Oxford, UK

John Campbell Department of Philosophy, University of California, Berkeley, CA, USA

Louis C. Charland Departments of Philosophy and Psychiatry & Faculty of Health Sciences, University of Western Ontario, London, ON, Canada

Jennifer Church Department of Philosophy, Vassar College, Poughkeepsie, NY, USA

Stephen R. L. Clark Department of Philosophy, University of Liverpool, Liverpool, UK

Giovanna Colombetti Department of Sociology, Philosophy and Anthropology, University of Exeter, Exeter, UK

Rachel Cooper Lancaster University, Lancaster, UK

Kelso Cratsley Department of Philosophy, University of Massachusetts, Boston, MA, USA

David Crepaz-Keay Mental Health Foundation, London, UK

Roger Crisp Faculty of Philosophy, University of Oxford, Oxford, UK

Larry Davidson Yale University School of Medicine, New Haven, CT, USA

Martin Davies Faculty of Philosophy and Department of Experimental Psychology, University of Oxford, Oxford, UK

Andy Egan Department of Philosophy, Rutgers University, New Brunswick, NJ, USA; Arché Philosophical Research Centre, University of St Andrews, St Andrews, Scotland

Barbara Von Eckardt Rhode Island School of Design, Providence, RI, USA

Jensen Farquhar Retired therapist and current mediator, Portland, OR, USA

Owen Flanagan Department of Philosophy, Duke University, Durham, NC, USA

Bennett Foddy Oxford Centre for Neuroethics and Oxford Uehiro Centre for Practical Ethics, Faculty of Philosophy, University of Oxford, Oxford, UK

Thomas Fuchs Psychiatric Department, University of Heidelberg, Heidelberg, Germany

K. W. M. Fulford Faculty of Philosophy, University of Oxford, Oxford, UK

Paolo Fusar-Poli Department of Psychoses Studies, Institute of Psychiatry, London, UK

Shaun Gallagher Department of Philosophy, University of Memphis, Memphis, TN, USA; School of Humanities, University of Hertfordshire, Hatfield, UK

S. Nassir Ghaemi Department of Psychiatry, Mood Disorders Program, Tufts Medical Center, Tufts University School of Medicine, Boston, MA, USA; Department of Psychiatry, Harvard Medical School, Boston, MA, USA

Grant Gillett Department of Philosophy, University of Otago, Dunedin, New Zealand

Richard G.T. Gipps Oxford University Disability Advisory Service, Oxford, UK

Gerrit Glas Institute for Mental Health, Zwolle, The Netherlands; Department of Philosophy, VU University Amsterdam, Amsterdam, The Netherlands

George Graham Department of Philosophy, Georgia State University, Birmingham, AL, USA

Thor Grünbaum Philosophy Section, Department of Media, Cognition and Communication, University of Copenhagen, Copenhagen, Denmark

Edward Harcourt Faculty of Philosophy, University of Oxford, Oxford, UK

Nick Haslam Department of Psychology, University of Melbourne, Melbourne, VIC, Australia

Rom Harré Georgetown University, Washington, DC, USA; Faculty of Philosophy, University of Oxford, Oxford, UK

R. Peter Hobson Tavistock Clinic and Behavioural and Brain Sciences Unit, Institute of Child Health, University College London, London, UK

Jim Hopkins Department of Philosophy, Kings College London, London, UK

Julian C. Hughes Northumbria Healthcare NHS Foundation Trust and the Institute for Ageing and Health, Newcastle University, Newcastle upon Tyne, UK

Daniel D. Hutto School of Humanities, University of Hertfordshire, Hatfield, UK

Terence Irwin Faculty of Philosophy, University of Oxford, Oxford, UK

David A. Jopling Department of Philosophy, Faculty of Arts, York University, Toronto, ON, Canada

Guy Kahane Oxford Uehiro Centre for Practical Ethics, Faculty of Philosophy, University of Oxford, Oxford, UK

Jayasree Kalathil Independent researcher, Survivor Research, London, UK

Elselijn Kingma Department of History and Philosophy of Science, Cambridge University, Cambridge, UK

Robert F. Krueger Department of Psychology, University of Minnesota, Minneapolis, MN, USA

Michael Lacewing Department of Philosophy, Heythrop College, University of London, London, UK

Federico Leoni Università degli Studi di Milano, Dipartimento di Filosofia, Milan, Italy

Eric Matthews Philosophy, School of Divinity, History and Philosophy, University of Aberdeen, Aberdeen, UK

Katherine J. Morris Faculty of Philosophy, University of Oxford, Oxford, UK

Christoph Mundt University of Heidelberg, Heidelberg, Germany

Dominic Murphy History and Philosophy of Science, University of Sydney, Camperdown, NSW, Australia

Marilyn Nissim-Sabat Department of Philosophy, Lewis University, Romeoville, IL, USA

Nancy Nyquist Potter Department of Philosophy, University of Louisville, Louisville, KY, USA

James Phillips Department of Psychiatry, Yale University School of Medicine, New Haven, CT, USA

Hanna Pickard Oxford Centre for Neuroethics, Faculty of Philosophy, University of Oxford, Oxford, UK

Elizabeth Pienkos Graduate School of Applied and Professional Psychology, Rutgers University, Piscataway, NJ, USA

Jeffrey Poland Department of History, Philosophy, and Social Science, Rhode Island School of Design, Providence, RI, USA; Department of Molecular Biology, Cell Biology, and Biochemistry, Brown University, Providence, RI, USA

Jennifer Radden Philosophy Department, University of Massachusetts, Boston, MA, USA

Lubomira Radoilska Faculty of Philosophy, Cambridge University, Cambridge, UK

Matthew Ratcliffe Department of Philosophy, University of Durham, Durham, UK

Daniel N. Robinson Faculty of Philosophy, University of Oxford, Oxford, UK

Johannes Roessler Philosophy Department, Warwick University, Coventry, UK

Jasna Russo Centre for Citizen Participation, Brunel University, London, UK

John Z. Sadler Division of Ethics, Department of Psychiatry, UT Southwestern, Dallas, TX, USA

Richard Samuels Department of Philosophy, Ohio State University, Columbus, OH, USA

Louis A. Sass Graduate School of Applied and Professional Psychology, Rutgers University, Piscataway, NJ, USA

Julian Savulescu Oxford Centre for Neuroethics and Oxford Uehiro Centre for Practical Ethics, Faculty of Philosophy, University of Oxford, Oxford, UK

Kenneth F. Schaffner University of Pittsburgh, Pittsburgh, PA, USA

Nicholas Shea Department of Philosophy, King's College London, London, UK

Debra Shulkes Survivor Activist and Editor, Australia/Czech Republic

Walter Sinnott-Armstrong Department of Philosophy and the Kenan Institute for Ethics at Duke University, Durham, NC, USA

Giovanni Stanghellini G. d'Annunzio University, Chieti, Italy; D. Portales University, Santiago, Chile

Fredrik Svenaeus Centre for Studies in Practical Knowledge, Department of Philosophy, Södertörn University, Huddinge, Sweden

Philip Thomas Social Science and Humanities, University of Bradford, Bradford, UK

Tim Thornton School of Health, University of Central Lancashire, Preston, UK

J. D. Trout Philosophy Department, Loyola University Chicago, Chicago, IL, USA

C. W. van Staden Division of Philosophy and Ethics of Mental Health, Department of Psychiatry, Faculty of Health Sciences, University of Pretoria, Pretoria, South Africa

Somogy Varga University of Osnabrück, Osnabrück, Germany

Lisa Ward STAR Team, Thames Valley Initiative, Oxford, UK

Toby Williamson Mental Health Foundation, London, UK

Philippe Wuyts UPC KU Leuven, Leuven, Belgium

Peter Zachar Department of Psychology, Auburn University at Montgomery, Montgomery, AL, USA

Dan Zahavi Center for Subjectivity Research, Department of Media, Cognition and Communication, University of Copenhagen, Copenhagen, Denmark

CHAPTER 1

THE NEXT HUNDRED YEARS: WATCHING OUR Ps AND Q

With the publication of this handbook in 2013, the centenary of Jaspers' *General Psychopathology*, it is natural to ask: "What comes next?" Projecting forward from the timeline shown on our website (www.oup.co.uk/companion/fulford) suggests a future of continued expansion of the field as a research-led international discipline with increasingly close connections with policy, research, and practice across all areas of mental health. Such a future is anticipated in this handbook, covering as it does a wide range of both theoretical and practical issues and with contributions from different philosophical traditions and many different parts of the world. But the timeline also contains a warning. Aside from ongoing work in phenomenology and psychoanalysis, *General Psychopathology* was followed by fifty years of silence (Fulford et al., 2003).

There are differences, of course, between Jaspers' period and our own. Notably, whereas psychiatry at the start of the twentieth century was mainly doctor-led, mental health services today are increasingly multiprofessional, and, with the growing importance of the service user voice (Williamson 2004), patient- as well as professional-led. These shifts in the model of service delivery in the early twenty-first century are reflected in this book. Like other volumes in the Oxford Handbooks in Philosophy series, *The Oxford Handbook of Philosophy and Psychiatry* is written mainly by philosophers for philosophers. But our website includes a rich and (so far as we are aware) unique collection of diverse service user narratives drawn together by the service user/survivor researchers Jayasree Kalathil, Jasna Russo and Debra Shulkes, together with the support of David Crepaz-Keay, Toby Williamson and others at the Mental Health Foundation, London; several of our contributors draw in part on personal experience of mental health difficulties; and Owen Flanagan's philosophical account of addictive disorders (Chapter 51) draws explicitly on his perspective as an "expert by experience."

There are also important similarities, however, between our two periods. Jaspers, as the first philosopher-psychiatrist, was writing at a time of rapid advances in the neurosciences so like our own that it has come to be known as psychiatry's "first biological phase." It is surely no coincidence therefore that, as the timeline indicates, cross-disciplinary work between philosophy and psychiatry should have finally taken off in a big way in the 1990s, the so-called "decade of the brain." The contemporary rise in importance of the service user voice, moreover, gives Jaspers' *General Psychopathology*, with its call for meaningful understanding as well as causal explanations in psychopathology (Stanghellini and Fuchs, in press), perhaps even greater resonance today, in psychiatry's second biological phase, than it had in its first. We return toward the end of this introduction to the significance of the service user voice for the future of psychiatric science. Our view as we will indicate is that, taken together, the twin pressures of the new neurosciences and of the service user voice make the twenty-first century potentially the best of scientific times for psychiatry. We have sought to reflect these best of scientific times in this volume with a range of topic areas covering different aspects of the sciences of the mind and brain and through the work of a number of contributors (such as Broome and Fuchs) whose research expertise straddles philosophy and key areas of contemporary neuroscience such as brain imaging.

So what can we learn from a century of philosophy and psychiatry? And where might the subject be a century hence? Clearly the details (who will do what, when, and where) remain below the horizon. There will also be much that is outside our control. The Australian psychiatrist and poet Russell Meares (2003) has pointed out that the publication of *General Psychopathology* in 1913 coincided more or less to the year with the tipping point of the "move to mechanism" which was to become the dominant European and North American zeitgeist for most of the first half of the twentieth century—small wonder therefore that Jaspers' call for meanings as well as causes in psychopathology should have gone largely unheard for so many decades. Nonetheless the past century we believe does suggest a number of conditions for flourishing that may prove helpful in guiding the future development of the field. We will look briefly at some of these, as they relate respectively to problems, products, partnership, and process, and at how we have tried to incorporate them in this book.

Problems

Of one thing at least we can be confident: by the end of the century the problems of philosophy, the "big questions" of mind and brain, of freedom and determinism, of what is and of what ought to be, will remain unresolved. In an earlier model of philosophy it would have been assumed that the role of philosophers in psychiatry is to solve problems of just this kind and thereby to provide foundations on which empirical research and practice might securely build. The search for foundations is natural enough. Consistently with the philosophy of Jaspers' time, there is something of this Philosophy-as-the-Queen-of-the-Sciences model in *General Psychopathology*: and latter day claims to having established a new philosophical foundation for psychiatry will no doubt continue to be made in years to come. But if there is a lesson from twentieth-century philosophy for psychiatry today, it is that (post-Gödel, Wittgenstein, Quine, and others) foundations are not to be had (Fulford, in press).

This is an important lesson for psychiatric science. The German historian and psychiatrist Paul Hoff (2005) has neatly summarized the history of psychiatric science as a history of repeated collapses into "single message mythologies" reflecting this or that influential school's or individual's view of the "true" nature of psychiatry. But it is an important lesson also for psychiatric practice: in psychiatry it has been the misguided conviction that this or that model provided "foundations" that has been the basis of some of the worst abuses of psychiatric care (Fulford et al. 2003).

Far from providing foundations, therefore, an important role of philosophy is to forestall premature closure on the philosophical problems by which the science and practice of psychiatry are alike characterized. In psychiatry, the lesson of history runs, big theories mean big trouble. This book, correspondingly, although including chapters by philosophers working across the full spectrum of philosophical disciplines, from ancient philosophy through value theory, phenomenology, and philosophy of mind, to core issues in the philosophy of science, offers no "foundations." Our contributors, severally and together, reflecting the lively dynamic between theory and practice that is a key characteristic of the field, offer to varying degrees new slants on their respective philosophical topics while at the same time illuminating the particular issues in contemporary mental health with which they are concerned. But there are no attempts at big theories, no claims to explaining consciousness or dissolving the problem of free will, still less to having (finally) defined mental illness.

Products

If, then, research at the interface of philosophy with psychiatry is to flourish in coming decades, it will be characterized by disciplined attention to particular well-defined problems rather than indulging in grand theory building. All of which is not to say that we should be chary of progress. To the contrary, for the field to prosper it must remain responsibly product-oriented. Our handbook indeed illustrates a number of philosophy-into-practice successes: phenomenology (Fuchs, Sass, and Pienkos; Gallagher; Grünbaum and Zahavi; Ratcliffe; Stanghellini) continues to deliver insights for both research and practice; agency (Pickard) and value theory (Fulford and van Staden) have found new applications in mental health care; and the new kid on the block, neuroethics (Foddy, Kahane, and Savulescu), is already well established as a fast growing field in its own right (Iles and Sahakian 2011).

There is though a lot packed into that word "responsibly" when it comes to being "responsibly product-oriented." For practitioners—whether patients, carers, clinicians, scientists, or indeed managers and policymakers—being responsibly product-oriented means being prepared to engage with the conceptual as well as empirical issues by which the day-to-day problems of mental health research and practice are characterized. This book as we have indicated is mainly by philosophers (some of whom are of course also practitioners) for philosophers. For those new to philosophy, there are other books in the IPPP (International Perspectives in Philosophy and Psychiatry) series, such as the *Oxford Textbook of Philosophy and Psychiatry* (Fulford et al. 2006), and the companion volume to this book, *The Oxford Handbook of Psychiatric Ethics* (Sadler et al., forthcoming), that are more practitioner-oriented. Our hope nonetheless is that, co-branded as this handbook is between the Oxford Handbooks in Philosophy and the IPPP series, it will prove a resource not only for philosophers but also for those practitioners willing and able to go deep philosophically.

For philosophers on the other hand, being responsibly product-oriented means going deep practically. On first inspection it may seem that philosophers should need little encouragement to go deep practically given the richness of the philosophical resources offered by clinical work and research in psychiatry. We have reflected this richness of resource in this book by structuring its contents around the stages of the clinical encounter rather than within conventional philosophical subject areas. The danger though is that the very richness of these philosophical resources makes psychiatry an easy prey for what might be called the "quick buck" philosopher, spinning academic publications from a superficial and often partial and unrealistic reading of their practice-based sources.

Quick buck-ism is irresponsible academically: in philosophy as in any other field we have a responsibility to put in the work necessary to get things right. When it comes to philosophical work in psychiatry though, quick buck-ism is also irresponsible clinically. This is because in psychiatry, philosophers really *can* make, and as we have indicated are *already* making, a difference. Philosophical work in psychiatry we should add hastily is not justified as such by making a difference practically. To the contrary, for the field to prosper it is we believe important that as in other areas of philosophy, its justifications remain primarily intellectual rather than (directly) practical. All the same, the fact that mental health is an area in which what philosophers say really can make a difference practically, has the unavoidable consequence that going deep is a clinical as well as academic responsibility.

PARTNERSHIP

The "responsible" in being "responsibly product-oriented" in philosophy of psychiatry thus means, equally for philosophers and for practitioners, going deep in each other's' disciplines. What this in turn implies, we believe, as a further condition for flourishing, is the need for partnership. This is essentially because so much of what either has to learn from going deep with the other is tacit and hence acquired only by working side-by-side in a shared learning experience. Expertise in health care as in other practical disciplines is defined (in part but essentially) by the skilled application of tacit knowledge: and philosophy as a whole is as much an activity based on implicit (though learnable) skills of reasoning as it is a body of explicit knowledge.

While therefore there is much that we can learn from each other working separately, going deep means working in one way or another in partnership. The qualifier in that last phrase, however, "in one way or another," is important. Exactly what form a given partnership takes will and should vary widely with the contingencies of personal and professional circumstances and according to the varying constraints of different areas of philosophy and practice.

We signaled the importance of a diversity of partnerships between philosophers and practitioners in calling this book the "The Oxford Handbook of Philosophy *and* Psychiatry." If the field is to continue to develop successfully it will need a number of philosophers *of* psychiatry, philosophers (or indeed practitioners) who self-identify as specialists in the field in the sense that most of their scholarly output is focused on the conceptual issues of research and practice at the interface between philosophy and mental health. Equally important, though, will be the perhaps much larger number of philosophers (and indeed practitioners) who as specialists in their respective scholarly fields work in part but only in part on philosophical topics in mental health. In either case, partnership, again of one kind or another will be essential. The contributors to this book illustrate some of the range of possibilities here, from individual scholarship backed by personal and practical experience, through team working of various kinds, to doubly-qualified practitioner-philosophers and philosopher-practitioners. More and different kinds of partnership (perhaps building on the additional resources offered by web-based social networking systems) will no doubt emerge in years to come. Institutional partnerships, too, will be important. There will be many difficulties: partnership even between practitioners of different kinds, presents many challenges (Wallcraft et al. 2009). But partnership of one kind or another there must surely be.

Process

As conditions for flourishing, problems, products, and partnership at and across the interface of philosophy with psychiatry are each underpinned by the need for good process. That good process presents particular challenges in a cross-disciplinary field need hardly be said. In a single-discipline field the challenges are hard enough: evidence-based medicine, for example, with a few tweaks surely the acme of good empirical process, has generated a veritable industry of practical, ethical, and indeed philosophical debate (Howick 2011). But imagine philosophy proceeding by meta-analyses of its research outputs, or, conversely, clinical trials being judged by their internal logical consistency! Clearly, good process however defined within either discipline, and although no doubt including a number of generic features (acknowledgment of sources, for example), fails to translate fully one into the other.

The twentieth-century development of philosophy of psychiatry has sought to meet the challenge of good process by adopting what amounts to an HCF (highest common factor) rather than LCD (lowest common denominator) approach: new research to the extent that it covers both fields must pass muster with the best of both. But aiming for the "best of both" of course begs the question "What is best?" The test adopted thus far has been that of twin-track but independent peer review. And peer review must surely form part of any future test of best. But peer review itself must be used in a self-reflective way if it is to avoid a degree of self-validation inimical to innovation.

Peer review and a self-reflective process have both been important in the development of this book. The original proposal for the volume went through Oxford University Press's normal processes of both independent peer and delegate committee review and we are grateful to the reviewers and delegates for the many helpful suggestions made at that stage. But we also carried out an extensive post-contract process of research and development. This process, which was strongly supported by both the Philosophy Faculty in Oxford and Oxford University Press, included a wide-ranging review of the literature (carried out mainly by Will Davies, at the time a Laces DPhil Scholar) and a workshop to which every member of our International Advisory Board generously contributed either in person or by telephone conference. The importance of partnership was particularly evident at this developmental stage of the book and became so again, as our list of contributors indicates, in the production of our supporting website.

None of which is to claim that for all our focus on process, we got all "the best": even with the generous word length of an Oxford Philosophy Handbook there were many significant contributors to the field that we were unable to include. Our aim was rather the more modest aim of examining through an open and reflective process the question of what the best might look like rather than relying (solely) on our own (albeit no doubt reasonably well-informed) views. And to the extent that the process we adopted produced much of the content and many of the distinctive features of the book (including its structuring around the stages of the clinical encounter) it proved to be nothing if not creative.

WATCHING OUR PS . . .

The importance of "watching our Ps" in coming decades if we are to avoid another fifty years of silence is well illustrated by what happened at the meeting of senior European and North American psychiatrists convened by the World Health Organization (WHO) in New York in 1959, from which, as the timeline on our website indicates, our current systems of descriptive (i.e., symptom-based) psychiatric classifications, the WHO's ICD (*International Classification of Diseases*) and the American Psychiatric Association's DSM (*Diagnostic and Statistical Manual of Mental Disorders*), are ultimately derived.

In his introduction to the mental disorders chapter of ICD-9 (the ninth edition of the ICD), Norman Sartorius, who went on to become Head of the Mental Health Section of the WHO, described a classification as providing a kind of photographic snapshot of the state of a given science at a point in time (Sartorius 1992). Two of our chapters (Poland and Von Eckhart, Chapter 44 and Sadler, Chapter 45) explore particular aspects of what by extension might be called the family photograph album of snapshots provided by successive editions of ICD and DSM. The lessons, though, for the future success of cross-disciplinary work between philosophy and psychiatry, come from understanding the precise role played by the philosopher of science, Carl Hempel, in that original New York meeting.

The received history (e.g., Kendell 1975; Sadler et al. 1994, introduction) has been one of foundations. The WHO, in its early work in the aftermath of World War II, needed reliable comparative statistics on rates of disease in different parts of the world; this in turn depended on an agreed system of classification; but in contrast with most other areas of medicine, it had proved impossible to reach international agreement on the classification of mental disorders. The New York meeting was thus convened in an attempt to reach consensus, and Hempel, as a distinguished philosopher of science, was invited to give the opening address. Drawing on the logical empiricist philosophy of science in vogue at the time, Hempel, so the story has standardly gone, argued that psychiatry was at a descriptive rather than etiological (causal theoretical) stage in its development as a science and hence should seek a common basis for its classification of mental disorders in (descriptively defined) symptoms. Hempel's analysis, the standard story has continued, was reported back to the WHO; it was adopted as the basis for a new descriptive (symptom only) glossary to ICD-8; ICD-8 with its supporting glossary achieved a high degree of international acceptance; and descriptive (symptom only) criteria went on to become the foundation for all subsequent editions of both ICD and DSM.

Hempel's role in the development of modern psychiatric classifications is rightly celebrated. Examination, however, of a transcript of the 1959 New York meeting, together with the recollections of some of those actually involved at the time, shows his role in an entirely different light (Fulford and Sartorius 2009). Hempel did indeed introduce the distinction between descriptive and etiological (causal theoretical) stages in the development of a science. But far from recommending that psychiatry should develop a descriptive classification he argued that it should continue with what he saw as its current good work in developing etiological classifications based on (the then current "big theory" in the USA) psychoanalysis. The suggestion for a descriptive classification, so the transcript of the meeting shows, came in fact not from the philosopher Hempel but from a psychiatrist, Aubrey Lewis. Adopting Hempel's terminology, Lewis proposed that:

> for the purposes of public classification we should eschew categories based on theoretical concepts and restrict ourselves to the operational, descriptive type of classification, whereas, for the purposes of certain groups, the private classification, based on a theory which seems a workable, profitable one, may be very appropriate.

At the time Lewis' proposal was not taken up. Indeed aside from qualified support from the French delegate, Dr Pichot, he was in a minority of one. A large majority of those present welcomed instead Hempel's proposal for an etiological classification and it was this (rather than a descriptive classification) that was reported back from the meeting as a recommendation to the WHO. Lewis proved, however, to be a tough minority of one. For in the event it was Lewis, working with Sartorius and others at the WHO, who went on to produce the descriptive symptom-based glossary to ICD-8 from which as noted earlier our current classifications are derived.

All the Ps are evident in this story. It is clear, first, that Lewis had a very particular problem in mind in proposing a symptom-based classification, namely the need to develop a "public" classification that was fit for the specific and well-defined purpose of collecting comparative international statistics on rates of mental disorder. It was the need to find such a classification that as we have described led to the WHO convening the New York meeting in the first place. To this extent therefore, corresponding with our second P, the meeting was by its very terms of reference product-oriented. As to being responsibly product-oriented however, the meeting failed to "go deep" in that (Lewis aside) those present simply ran with Hempel's ideas as providing (as they saw it) philosophical foundations (and hence justification) for current practice. Our third P, partnership, was the vital ingredient in "going deep" and thus producing the required classification: Hempel the philosopher was essential to the mix; but it took the psychiatrist Lewis to see the potential of Hempel's philosophy; and without the support of Sartorius as an up-and-coming WHO official, Hempel-plus-Lewis would still have equaled zero. "Good process," furthermore, our final P, had it been based on a merely mechanical application of peer review, would actually have blocked the key shift to a descriptive classification: the transcript of the New York meeting shows that as we have indicated an overwhelming majority of peers present (and they represented the great and the good of the psychiatry of the day) welcomed Hempel's support for further development of the then current etiologically-based classifications; and Lewis' proposal for a symptom-based classification failed to make it even as a minority view, either into the official summary of the meeting or into the subsequent report to the WHO.

. . . And Q

All the Ps then will be important if research at the interface of philosophy with psychiatry is to avoid the perils of failure, a brief flourishing followed as *General Psychopathology* was followed by fifty years of silence. Yet if there are perils of failure for the philosophy of psychiatry in the coming century there are perils too of success, of becoming a new orthodoxy, inward looking and ossified. This is where Q, a measure of group inter-connectedness defined by two American sociologists, Brian Uzzi and Jarrett Spiro (2005), working on the social conditions that support creativity, could be important in years to come. Research on creativity has focused mainly on the psychology of the individual. Uzzi and Spiro's work suggests that important as creative individuals undoubtedly are to the development of a new field, their creativity is to a degree dependent on the support of a group with the right balance of Q: too open a group fails to provide the necessary checks and balances to drive creativity; too closed a group seizes up for lack of new ideas.

There was Q aplenty in the run-up to the renaissance of philosophy of psychiatry. As indicated in the timeline and supporting materials on our website, many senior psychiatrists active in the 1970s and 1980s (Hill, Kendell, Kroll, Lewis, Roth, and others) wrote still influential conceptual as well as empirical research papers: and at a personal level these and others directly supported the nascent field. There was similar cross-disciplinary research and support also from the brightest and best in philosophy. In Oxford alone, Farrell, Glover, Hare, Harré, Newton-Smith, Quinton, Wilkes, and the Warnocks (Geoffrey and Mary) all contributed to the emergence of the new field either directly as authors of seminal publications and as supervisors of cross-disciplinary doctorates or indirectly through their support for the new journals, organizations and other academic infrastructure underpinning the establishment of the new field.

The philosophy of psychiatry as it has developed in recent years might be thought by some to have become somewhat too open. Certainly, as a discipline it has shown thus far a remarkable degree of collegiality, avoiding the splits into different "schools" that historically have been so much a feature of emerging fields. The HCF rather than LCD approach noted earlier has been in part an attempt to maintain the balance required for Q. Yet it has been relatively easy to remain open and collegial when we have had so little to lose. Come success, therefore, come celebrity, come the power and influence and resources of orthodoxy, and the perils of becoming too inward looking and thereby creatively sterile will be real indeed. Even in this handbook we have for all our efforts ended up being perhaps somewhat too closed with little in the way of dissenting voices (Crisp, for example, in his commentary on Fulford and van Staden, Chapter 26, is an exception). There will we hope be more dissent on our website as this is further developed; and future editors of the handbook may feel able to take more risks—a speculative 5% would go a long way to maintaining the balance required for Q.

The perils of success may seem like something of a high-class worry as things currently stand. The philosophy of psychiatry, after all, for all its recent burgeoning, remains a minnow to the neuroscience whale. Yet we need look no further than the family photograph album of psychiatric classification for a clear presentiment of success.

As we go to press new editions of both ICD (ICD-11) and DSM (DSM-5) are about to be launched. The jury is still out on how they will be received. But both have continued the excellent precedent of their predecessors in aiming for a transparent process. The American Psychiatric Association in particular anticipated the launch of the DSM revision process with a publication setting out its *Research Agenda for DSM-V* (Kupfer et al. 2002). In their introduction the editors of the Research Agenda, David Kupfer, Michael First, and Daryl Regier, who went on to become leaders of the DSM-5 review, argued that progress in the sciences of psychiatry required "an as yet unknown paradigm shift" (p. xix). True, there is no indication that it was philosophy that Kupfer and his colleagues had in mind here. All the same, the actual research issues outlined in the opening chapter of their book are all *conceptual* issues. True, also, they avoided using the word "conceptual," calling their opening chapter instead "Issues of basic nomenclature" (p. 1). But the issues outlined in their opening chapter are conceptual issues nonetheless. The particular conceptual issues they cover, moreover, show a considerable degree of overlap with the issues covered in this handbook. There is an extensive discussion of how the concept of "mental disorder" and related concepts such as "illness" and "disease" should be defined; and in just the first three pages of the chapter problems are raised respectively in the philosophy of science (core concerns include "validity" and "reliability"), in the philosophy of mind ("Cartesian dualism" is explicitly rejected), and in philosophical value theory (values being taken to differentiate what they call "sociopolitical" from "biomedical" models of disorder).

It would be straying too far into big theory building to speculate on what Kupfer, First, and Regier's anticipated new paradigm might be. The twin pressures though on contemporary psychiatry noted at the start of this introduction, of a growing service user voice and of the new neurosciences, suggest that something along the lines of Jaspers' original research agenda in *General Psychopathology*, his agenda for meanings as well as causes in psychopathology, will have to figure in some way. Philosophy at the start of the twenty-first century is of course not where it was at the start of the twentieth century. In particular, the majority of contemporary philosophers would regard it as a datum that intentional (representational) mental states (e.g., believing, wanting, seeing as) figure in causal explanations. If that is right then there are levels of description and causal explanation in which personal-level concepts figure, including phenomenological and normative concepts. Even at this level there are unresolved issues for psychopathology: Jaspers, anticipating current debates about the role of values in diagnostic concepts (Sadler, Chapter 45, this volume), resisted their inclusion in psychopathology (Stanghellini et al. 2013). But below the personal level of description and explanation, there are multiple subpersonal levels of mechanistic description and explanation, including the levels of physics, chemistry, biology, neuroscience (including computational neuroscience), and psychology (including information-processing psychology), the relationships of which to the personal level of description and explanation remain unresolved. Even leaving aside, therefore, conceptual difficulties within either level, Jaspers' agenda re-emerges in contemporary debates in philosophy and psychiatry about the relationship between the personal (as in the role of the service user voice) and the various subpersonal (as in the role of the new neurosciences) levels of description and explanation.

For these if for no other reasons, therefore, psychiatry in any new paradigm will find itself working within multiple and in some respects mutually inconsistent theoretical models and thus having to tackle research problems that are as much conceptual as empirical in nature. As such, psychiatry will have to redefine itself as a science, not as in the twentieth century trailing the traditional medical sciences of cardiology, gastroenterology and the like, but rather as a science more like theoretical physics very much at the cutting edge.

For theoretical physics, too, works within multiple and in some respects mutually inconsistent theoretical models and thus has to tackle research problems that are as much conceptual as empirical in nature. Naturally, psychiatry being a science not of particles but of people, the particular theoretical models and the particular conceptual problems with which it is concerned, will be quite different from those of physics. But the prominence afforded conceptual issues in the DSM's Research Agenda, and the range of philosophical issues evident in its opening chapter, are surely sufficient indications that any genuinely person-centered psychiatry of the future will proceed physics-like, as much by way of conceptual as of empirical research.

We should not expect a person-centered physics-like psychiatry any time soon. No less a creative genius than Max Planck, one of the founders of quantum mechanics, warned in his scientific autobiography that "new sciences aren't born, old scientists die!" (1948, p. 22, paraphrased). This is why our time frame in this introduction has been the next hundred years. Time enough then for old scientists to die and for new sciences to be born. Time enough, too, for us to face the perils not only of failure but also of success by watching our Ps and Q.

References

Fulford, K.W.M. (in press). Particular Psychopathologies: Lessons from Karl Jaspers' General Psychopathology for the new Philosophy of Psychiatry: Introduction to G. Stanghellini and T. Fuchs (Eds) *One Century of Karl Jaspers' General Psychopathology*. Oxford: Oxford University Press.

Fulford, K. W. M., Morris, K. J., Sadler, J. Z., and Stanghellini, G. (2003). Past improbable, future possible: The renaissance in philosophy and psychiatry. In K. W. M. Fulford, K. J. Morris, J. Z. Sadler, and G. Stanghellini (Eds), *Nature and Narrative: An Introduction to the New Philosophy of Psychiatry*, pp. 1–41. Oxford: Oxford University Press.

Fulford, K. W. M. and Sartorius, N. (2009). A secret history of ICD and the hidden future of DSM. In M. Broome and L. Bortolotti (Eds), *Psychiatry as Cognitive Neuroscience: Philosophical Perspectives*, pp. 29–48. Oxford: Oxford University Press.

Fulford, K. W. M., Thornton, T., and Graham, G. (2006). *Oxford Textbook of Philosophy and Psychiatry*. Oxford: Oxford University Press.

Hoff, P. (2005). Die psychopathologische Perspektive. In M. Bormuth and U. Wiesing (Eds), *Ethische Aspekte der Forschung in Psychiatrie und Psychotherapie*, pp. 71–9. Cologne: Deutscher Aerzte-Verlag.

Howick, J. (2011). *The Philosophy of Evidence-Based Medicine: A Philosophical Inquiry*. Oxford: Blackwell-Wiley.

Iles, J. and Sahakian, B. J. (Eds) (2011). *The Oxford Handbook of Neuroethics*. Oxford: Oxford University Press.

Jaspers, K. (1913). *Allgemeine Psychopathologie*. Berlin: Springer-Verlag. (Jaspers, K. (1963). *General Psychopathology* (J. Hoenig, and M.W. Hamilton, Trans.). Chicago, IL: University of Chicago Press. New edition (1997) (two volumes) with a Foreword by P. R. McHugh. Baltimore, MD: Johns Hopkins University Press.)

Kendell, R. E. (1975). *The Role of Diagnosis in Psychiatry*. Oxford: Blackwell Scientific Publications.

Kupfer, D. J., First, M. B., and Regier, D. E. (Eds) (2002). *A Research Agenda for DSM-V*. Washington, DC: American Psychiatric Association

Meares, R. (2003). Towards a psyche for psychiatry. In K. W. M. Fulford, K. J. Morris, J. Z. Sadler, and G. Stanghellini (Eds), *Nature and Narrative: An Introduction to the New Philosophy of Psychiatry*, pp. 43–56. Oxford: Oxford University Press.

Planck, M. (1948). Wissenschaftliche Selbstbiographie. Mit einem Bildnis und der von Max von Laue gehaltenen Traueransprache, p. 22. Leipzig: Johann Ambrosius Barth Verlag. (Reprinted in Planck, M. (1949/1968). *Scientific Autobiography and Other Papers* (F. Gaynor, Trans.), pp. 33–34. New York, NY: Greenwood Press.)

Sadler, J. Z., Wiggins, O. P., and Schwartz, M. A. (Eds) (1994). *Philosophical Perspectives on Psychiatric Diagnostic Classification.* Baltimore, MD: Johns Hopkins University Press.

Sadler, J. Z., van Staden, W., and Fulford, K. W. M. (Eds) (forthcoming). *The Oxford Handbook of Psychiatric Ethics.* Oxford: Oxford University Press.

Sartorius, N. (1992). Preface. In World Health Organization (Ed.), *The ICD-10 Classification of Mental and Behavioural Disorders: Clinical Descriptions and Diagnostic Guidelines*, p. vii. Geneva: World Health Organization.

Stanghellini, G., Bolton, D., and Fulford, K. W. M. (2013). Person-centred psychopathology of schizophrenia: Building on Karl Jaspers' understanding of the patient's attitude towards his illness. *Schizophrenia Bulletin, 39*(2), 287–94.

Stanghellini, G. and Fuchs, T. (Eds) (in press). *One Century of Karl Jaspers' General Psychopathology.* Oxford: Oxford University Press.

Uzzi, B. and Spiro, J. (2005) Collaboration and creativity: The small world problem. *American Journal of Sociology, 111*(2), 447–504.

Wallcraft, J., Schrank B., and Amering M. (Eds) (2009). *Handbook of Service User Involvement in Mental Health Research.* London: John Wiley & Sons Ltd.

Williamson, T. (2004) User involvement—a contemporary overview. *The Mental Health Review, 9*(1), 6–12.

SECTION I

HISTORY

CHAPTER 2

....

INTRODUCTION: HISTORY

....

Philosophy and psychiatry. "Philosophy," "psychiatry," with an "and" in the middle. But how can that be? Isn't philosophy just philosophy? Psychiatry just psychiatry? How can the former be conjoined with the latter in a fused twosome? Aren't disciplines distinct?

W. V. O. Quine (1908–2000), the distinguished Harvard philosopher and logician, once remarked that boundaries between disciplines are useful for university administrators and librarians, but should not be overestimated—as boundaries. When we carefully examine academic, scientific, and medical fields and abstract from their administrative organizations and book stack locations, we recognize that two or more disciplines often form an interactive interanimating family of intellectual and practical concerns, connected in its members, informed by mutual influence and degrees and modes of co-reliance. On which library stack or journal holdings a discipline's products are placed fails to reflect the family as a family and the internal interactions of its members.

Psychiatry and philosophy form one such family. Although psychiatry and philosophy are distinct fields or disciplines, and pull in opposite directions vis-à-vis clinical application and observation, with philosophy typically nestled in the canopy of overarching theory, and psychiatry often rooted in the soil's edge of clinical and therapeutic utility, each is bound up in the other. Each both needs and animates the other, whether all of their respective family members recognize this fact or not. Psychiatry cannot function without philosophical presupposition and reflection. Philosophy, meanwhile, is impoverished without recognizing the forms and limits of the human mind as exhibited in psychopathology and in the onset and recovery from mental illness and disorder.

The fact that each of philosophy and psychiatry is bound to and in need of the other is revealed in the pages of this handbook. In aim and effect, that is what this handbook is about, viz., the fusion of the two fields.

Intellectual history contains vivid expressions of the two fields' fusion. One important lesson of the history of mental health medicine and psychiatry, and of the roles of philosophical reflection and presupposition in the development of mental health medicine, is that many of the concerns of philosophy—especially in philosophy of mind, of science, metaphysics, ethics, and epistemology—are issues within psychiatry and mental health medicine. At the same time, many topics within psychiatry—rationality, autonomy, self-control, well-being, explanation, understanding, and numerous others—are issues that have been addressed by philosophy. The topics are proper and essential parts of the connections between philosophy and psychiatry.

To briefly mention one historically fecund example, the nature of reason and rationality, in general, and of insanity and rationality's failure, in particular, became an issue central to mental health practice 2,500 years ago with the classical Greeks. When Plato, for example, looked for a kind or type of human affliction or ill-being, madness or insanity struck him as the outstanding candidate, for madness was, alas, the most "perfect" or exemplary case of the mind's potential for dramatic imperfection. It served as a contrasting foil for his theory of human happiness and well-being. Madness exposes the rational mind as capable of falling apart and becoming profoundly ill and disordered. Plato was convinced that it unearthed the fault lines of the psyche.

The intellectual heritage bequeathed to us by the ancient Greeks is rich and resourceful indeed. But the nutritious conceptual soil from which current psychiatry grew over the course of history from Plato and through numerous other figures and periods also has produced vexing conceptual and therapeutic puzzles that have challenged successive generations of mental health practitioners and psychiatrists. It is the purpose of this first section of the handbook to offer several illustrative examinations of historical expressions or cases of the relationship between the theory and practice of mental health medicine, on the one hand, and philosophical reflection, presupposition, and analysis, on the other.

Seven chapters follow this introductory chapter in Section I. Chapter 3 by Daniel Robinson is on the roles that concepts of insanity and personal responsibility have played historically in analyses of the persons or rational agents fit for the rule of law and civil society. At a minimum, persons fit for participation in a civil society must be able to give and comprehend reasons for action, the actions of themselves and others. Robinson pays special attention to significant interactions between law and psychiatry and to the manner in which those interactions historically have been fueled by central and controversial philosophical assumptions. Robinson's chapter also examines the extent to which mental disorders in general have, over history, proven to be grounds for mitigation of personal and legal responsibility.

In Chapter 4, Terence Irwin sketches the three alternative theories of mental health and well-being of Plato, Aristotle, and the Stoics. He explores the roles that various concepts played in those theories, contrastive and comparison concepts such as reason and unreason, virtue and vice, unity and disunity of personhood. In each case he examines how such concepts and their explications produce similarities and dissimilarities in how mental illness or disorder was conceived in the Ancient World. One feature of these ancient pictures is the role that reference to a conception of a person as caring guardian or "friend" of themselves plays in each theory. This is a person, in particular, who tries to avoid conflict and internal discord. In mental health, concord and unity is sought.

Irwin's chapter is the point of departure for Chapter 5 by Edward Harcourt. Harcourt offers a series of reflections on where or how the ancients may have placed their theories of mental health and illness in the context of contemporary debates. Quite clearly some of today's attitudes would have been alien to them, but others not. Harcourt tries to sort out which is which and to explore connections with current controversies, such as debates generated by the so-called personality disorders and the anti-psychiatry movement.

Katherine Arens in Chapter 6 writes about a major figure in the history of psychiatry, a psychiatrist who exhibits just how influential philosophical assumptions may be to the theory and practice of mental health medicine. The focus of her essay is Wilhelm Griesinger (1817–1868). Griesinger was professor of psychiatry at the University of Berlin. He came to be known as the father of modern biological psychiatry. Arens describes how Griesinger worked at the juncture between medical or clinical psychology and university psychology, sought a scientific paradigm for psychiatry, and made contributions to the diagnostics and therapeutic treatment of mental illness. She focuses on Griesinger's influential masterpiece entitled *Mental Pathology and Therapeutics* (first published in 1845) and his assumption that three interactive elements are explanatorily responsible for the emergence and progression of mental disorders or illness. These are mind, body, and social–cultural environment. Besides trying to spare psychiatry the pointless task of identifying disorders in environmentally indifferent terms, Griesinger was interested in molar scale organism/environment interactions and in whether the clinical professions could develop a proper philosophical/empirical framework for distinguishing between healthy and unhealthy minds in what may be called environmentally embedded terms.

In Chapter 7, Christoph Mundt explores the background influences, immediate setting, impact, and internal content of Karl Jaspers' (1883–1969) monumental *General Psychopathology*. Jaspers' aim was to create a psychiatry balanced between emphasis on the brain and the experiences, intentions, and subjective meanings of individual persons and patients. The first aim was strictly mechanistic and impersonal; the second interpretative and person-centered. Mundt discusses a range of considerations required to understand Jaspers' work, several major figures in philosophy, psychology, and elsewhere who influenced him, and the dimensions of understanding for a mental disorder or illness that Jaspers tried to articulate and promote. Given Mundt's analysis, it is easy to see that many of Jaspers' concerns and predilections are very much alive in psychiatry today.

The French philosopher Michel Foucault (1926–1984) is the subject of Chapter 8 by Federico Leoni. Leoni examines the moral and political power concerns that inform Foucault's work on mental illness and the hidden instruments of the institutional control of human behavior that often mask themselves as medical knowledge and as forms of psychiatric language and intervention. Several of Foucault's key claims are offered for detailed inspection, including his charges that in certain respects mental institutions resemble prisons and that psychiatric labels and diagnostic practices are often fueled by financial interests and reinforced by economic incentives.

For most of western European history, depressive illness, of one form or other, has been central to the very idea of mental affliction and ill-being. The early church fathers, for example, wrote of a sin of acedia, a state of depressive despair or despondency that may take its sufferer into an emotional darkness that is beyond moral persuasion and religious ministration. In Chapter 9, Jennifer Radden and Somogy Varga argue that first-person narratives or memoirs of depression offer a kind of micro-history, a history within the life of an individual sufferer or patient, of this central form of mental disorder. Just as the history of mental illness or disorder, in general, or of the field of mental health medicine or psychiatry, requires its own historiography, its own proprietary form of interpretation, so the class or genre of illness and disability memoirs, like those written about the experience of depressive illness, requires its own interpretative framework or epistemology. So argue the authors of this chapter. They offer guidelines for the interpretation of disorder narratives or memoirs—insights into the cautionary lessons or importance of a narrative. At the core of every illness is the person with the illness. A mature conceptual synthesis of perspectives on an illness must somehow honor that core. The key is determining the proper forms and limits of that "somehow" in the case of patient narratives.

CHAPTER 3

....

THE INSANITY DEFENSE
AS A HISTORY OF
MENTAL DISORDER

....

DANIEL N. ROBINSON

The two most venerable domains of scholarship and inquiry addressed to the very nature of human nature are law and medicine. Both have passed through developmental stages as a result of advances in knowledge and alterations of perspective. Both seek practical solutions to problems arising in the actual context of lived life. At any given point in their respective developmental course, each has a more or less settled position on core precepts and accepted standards of evidence. Though different in so many respects, both—as systematic bodies of knowledge and principle—stand as sciences in the original understanding of the term. There is no corruption of language, therefore, in referring not only to medical science but also to *jural* science.

Of the several points of conflict and complementarity on which law and medicine converge, mental health has held a special place historically.[1] The history of law in the West is never indifferent to this. Note, for example, that Rome's Twelve Tables make provision for controlling the assets of one given to states of manic profligacy. Accordingly, through a study of legal history, one develops a more comprehensive understanding of how a given age addressed and, as it were, settled such philosophically vexing questions as those associated with notions of determinism and moral autonomy, contextual sources of mitigation, powers of agency, and degrees of responsibility. What history reveals is the interplay between law and science and between both of these and the philosophical foundations on which each depends for its credibility. The claims of science are said to be vindicated by evidence and proof, but both evidence and proof must satisfy criteria external to both; criteria developed through the resources of philosophical argument and analysis. The assumptions of law include centrally the proposition that persons are fit for the rule of law; that they can be held responsible and are expected to be able to give and to comprehend reasons for action.

[1] A fuller discussion of this history is the author's *Wild Beasts and Idle Humours: The Insanity Defense from Antiquity to the Present* (Robinson 1996).

All this, too, is subject to what are finally philosophical modes of evaluation. What history makes clear is that the scientific and legal conceptions of the mind and mental life have been parasitic on more fundamental philosophical assumptions, often untested and occasionally at cross purposes with the aims of law. All this is especially evident in the history of the insanity defense, the focus of this chapter.

As noted, the rule of law presupposes creatures of a special kind; viz., those able to give and to comprehend reasons for their actions; persons able to defend their actions by supplying justifications which are, after all, reasons sanctioned by law. The concept of *mens rea* is but the technical term for what is otherwise one of the core and common sense assumptions of legal responsibility and liability. Even when a legal system is silent on the particular psychological or mental powers on which such responsibility depends, the very efficacy of law arises from the possession of such powers by the public at large. Otherwise, as H. L. A. Hart noted, "no legal system could come into existence or continue to exist" (Hart 1968, p. 230).

There are, of course, many and varied legal systems. Needless to say, charting the history of the insanity defense within the ambit of a single chapter calls for severe restrictions of scope. The focus here is on Western jurisprudence as bequeathed by ancient Greek and Roman sources and on conceptions of mental disorders developed chiefly within the context of American and Anglo-European medicine.[2]

The ancient Greek world did not have written law until the archonship of Draco late in the seventh century BC. The laws were posted and, though most of them were later repealed by Solon, certain basic precepts were preserved. For example, Draco's laws make a distinction between murder and involuntary homicide (see Gagarin and Cohen 2005). Centuries before written law there were customary understandings seemingly grounded in the very nature of those fit for the rule of law itself. Proto-legal systems depend on what is taken to be the counsel of the wise as the Eleatic Stranger makes this clear to Socrates in the *Statesman*. He argues that one who must legislate "will not be able, in enacting for the general good, to provide exactly what is suitable for each particular case" and "no art whatsoever can lay down a rule which will last for all time ... (Thus) the best thing of all is not that the law should rule, but that a man should rule, supposing him to have wisdom" (Plato, *Statesman*, 294–295).

One finds an explicit recommendation for the law's treatment of the insane given in Book IX of Plato's *Laws* where the Athenian Stranger considers how the laws of Athens deal with issues of motivation and competence. He notes that laws have been enacted to deal with those who rob from the gods, who commit treasonous actions, and who manipulate the laws to their own ends. One may commit such crimes:

> in a state of madness or when affected by disease, or under the influence of extreme old age, or in a fit of childish wantonness (*hybris*), himself no better than a child. And if this be made evident to the judges ... he shall simply pay for the hurt which he may have done to another; but he shall be exempt from other penalties, unless he have slain some one and have on his

---

[2] This limitation is offset to some extent by the tendency in Islamic countries and in China to follow the rationale and often the very letter of Western law in addressing such cases. For an examination of Islamic law in this connection, see Chaleby (2001). Chapter 20 considers the insanity defense as understood in Islamic law. China's legal system is relatively young. Cases involving mental disorders have been recently discussed by Guo (2010).

hands the stain of blood. And in that case he shall go to another land and country, and there dwell for a year. (Plato, *Laws*, 864)[3]

There is no evidence in the ancient sources, however, that such philosophical reflections, any more than prevailing medical theories of insanity, yielded exculpatory consequences in the arena of adjudication. Ancient courts regarded the criminal act itself as evidence of mental capacity and saw to it that damages were compensated, crimes punished, and society protected against the deeds of the mad.

In the matter of insanity, ancient Greek law was rather more developed and explicit when considering contracts, property, and testation than when dealing with criminal offenses. One of the few detailed sources of actual judicial proceedings is Isaeus (ca. 420–350 BC). Of the many appeals he prepared for clients, 11 survive, all of them pertaining to matters of contract and testation. The mental state of relevant parties is often the grounds of challenge. For example, in the matter of the estate of Cleonymus, who died childless and whose will named relatives as beneficiaries who were, however, not next of kin, the claimants insist that Cleonymus wrote the will "in a misguided moment of passion." If, indeed, this were true, the will should be set aside on the grounds that Cleonymus was insane (*paranoian*). Again, in the matter of the estate of Menecles, whose adopted son would be beneficiary, the adoptee must argue that Menecles "was not insane or under the influence of a woman, but was in his right mind (*eu phronon*)" at the time of the adoption. In still other cases consideration is given to senility and seduction as grounds on which to overturn a will. Thus, a man who adopts a son, says Isaeus, will have the adoption invalidated if it is shown that the action was taken, "because of madness (*paranoia*) or old age or drugs or sickness, or under the influence of a woman, or compelled by force or restriction of liberty" (Isaeus 1927).[4]

In Roman law, as noted earlier, the Twelve Tables incorporated similar tests in the matter of property: "When no guardian has been appointed for an insane person, or a spendthrift, his nearest agnates, or if there are none, his other relatives, must take charge of his property."[5]

Categories of mental competence were used to partition defendants in Roman law: *non compos mentis, fanaticus, ideotus, furiosus*. These indicate the refinement of ancient law. It was common for statutes pertaining to, e.g., conditions that invalidate a contract, to refer to infants (children) and the insane in the same context. A senile and childlike father, successfully charged with insanity (*paranoia*), could be legally stripped of control of his estate by his son. The Twelve Tables identify the madman (*furiosus*) specifically, and require the nearest relatives to take over the management of his affairs if no guardian (*cura*) has been appointed. Later, at the time of the codification and promulgation of Roman law, the *Institutes* of Justinian interdict the transactions of a *prodigus* (spendthrift), though similar transactions by the *furiosus* are not thus interdicted, for "what he did was valid if he was not mad at the particular time when he did it" (*The Institutes of Justinian* 1922/1970). Prodigality, regarded

---

[3] See also Trevor Saunders' study of Plato's analysis of insanity and its medical and conceptual dimensions (Saunders 1991).

[4] For further discussion see Harrison (1968, pp. 138ff). See also the discussion of Greek law as it applied to the elderly in Garland (1990, pp. 261ff).

[5] The Twelve Tables are available online at: <http://www.fordham.edu/halsall/ancient/12tables.html>.

as something of an uncontrollable or obsessional disposition, is constrained by the laws of contract, whereas some forms of madness are taken to be episodic.

The medical practitioners of the classical world were not indifferent to these matters. The Hippocratic author writing on epilepsy rejects the "divine madness" thesis, insisting instead that:

> (F)rom the brain, and from the brain only, arise our pleasures, joys, laughter and jests, as well as our sorrows, pains, griefs and tears … It is the same things which makes us mad (*paraphronimos*) or delirious … and (causes) acts that are contrary to habit. (Hippocrates 1952, pp. vi–xx)[6]

In his *De Medicina*, Celsus (b. ca. 25 BC) summarized Greek medical theories of insanity as well as therapies that had been employed for centuries. One form, called by the Greeks *phrenesis*, is the acute insanity caused by fever. In this state, "patients are delirious and talk nonsense." In extreme cases, when the condition does not pass quickly or respond to treatments, the patient's mind comes fully under the control of illusions and imaginings ("*mens illis imaginibus addicta est*"). Additionally there are those whose insanity is expressed in the form of sadness or hilarity, violence and rebelliousness. Of the violent ones, notes Celsus, some may be impulsively harmful, others may even be "artful" (*etiam artes adhibent*), seeming to be entirely sane only to reveal their madness in mischievous acts (Celsus 1935, pp. 289ff).

There has been a long and spirited controversy surrounding the question of the continuity of Roman law in early and late medieval jurisprudence (see Radding 1988, pp. 7ff). What is clear is that, for the Canonist and Christian moralist, the issue of insanity and diminished capacity was far more complex than it was in the ancient world, and this was for reasons both practical and theoretical. First, there was the question of the validity of sacramental rites when either conducted or received by those judged to be insane or incompetent. Then there was the need to distinguish between (merely) legal offenses and those that are genuinely sinful. Bound up with this was the biblical (textual) authority for the belief that certain debilitating conditions, including insanity, are visited upon certain persons as a punishment for their sins, such that these conditions—far from conferring immunity—add further evidence of guilt. In the matter of evidence, still greater burdens were created by the need to see into the heart and soul of the defendant; into that interior life in which guilt and innocence find their wellsprings.

At least from the time of Constantine, and even with the seat of empire moved to the East, there was no frontal attack on Roman law by the Christian world. Rather, in what now must seem like a remarkably brief time, its core principles were systematically absorbed into the larger political and social objectives of the Church; so much so that, beginning with the *Corpus Juris Civilis*, it becomes difficult to identify any fully independent lines of development of Canon law, common law or, for that matter, the laws of the contemporary western democracies. However, the early Church did not catch up with this bequest immediately. There were changes of a subtle nature imposed on the older tradition. Where classical juridical reasoning and procedure tended to ignore the private recesses of conscience and belief, these were just the domains of greatest concern and interest to the Church. Accordingly,

---

[6] The treatise itself was probably composed between the fourth and third centuries BC and is fully consistent with the teachings of the Hippocratic school.

much closer attention was paid in practice to the aspects of mental life and its special vulnerabilities to which classical jurisprudence had been nearly officially aloof.

The contrast is vivid between the laws Rome had carefully crafted over the centuries and those that would arise when members of alien cultures attempted to absorb them. In 636, Rothair, the newly elected Duke of Brescia, codified customary Germanic laws. One can gauge the jurisprudence thus installed in Italy from a study of Rothair's *Edicts:* there are 338 of them. Numbers 48 to 124 record the separate penalties ("composition" for damages) assessed for assaults against specific parts of the body. Thus, (50) "On cutting off lips," (52) "Concerning the molar teeth," (69) "Concerning big toes," (70) "Concerning second toes" etc. Edict 189 is the first to mention mental illness:

> Concerning the girl who becomes a leper after her betrothal. If it happens that after a girl or woman has been betrothed she becomes leprous or mad or blind in both eyes, then her betrothed husband shall receive back his property and he shall not be required to take her to wife against his will. And he shall not be guilty in this event because it did not occur on account of his neglect *but on account of her weighty sins and resulting illness.* (Emphasis added)

As for Roman solicitude toward those judged mad, edict 323 contains both the theory of mental illness and the law's judgments:

> On madmen. If a man, because of his weighty sins, goes mad or becomes possessed and does damage to man or beast, nothing shall be required from his heirs. If the madman is killed, likewise nothing shall be required.[7]

Records from Carolingian Europe, covering the period 830–832, provide a similar picture. Lothar, judging Gerberga to be a witch, "tortured her for a long time and then executed her by the judgement of the wives of his wicked counsellors." Lothar's own passion for Waldrada was also taken to be caused by witchery. And, in order to preserve "the peace of the Church," Charles will promulgate laws in 873 that will put to the ordeal all suspected of witchcraft.[8] When Roman jurists concerned themselves with *mens rea*, the matter was more or less disposed of by the very nature of the offense. Matters are different on the assumption that one has sinned in his heart and that, "there cannot be a sin which is not voluntary" (Augustine, *Concerning the Truth of Religion*, Book XIV, ch. 27).

In the Eastern empire Christianity had preserved the teachings of Galen and the naturalistic traditions of the classical world. These influences were especially great in Byzantine medicine and would be adopted in the Islamic world of the later Middle Ages when the *bimaristan* surfaced as a veritable psychiatric hospital. In such places insanity was thoroughly "Galenized."[9] For quite some time, these same sources were rarely consulted and only partially known in the West. Even when consulted in quasi-scientific terms, there was no larger sense of how such maladies might bear upon questions of adjudication. On the whole, this situation worked a special hardship on insane or mentally retarded defendants, although St. Ambrose, St. John Chrysosthom, and St. Augustine all lent their authority to

---

[7] Quoted material is from Drew (1973). This discussion is also indebted to Dr. Drew's Introduction to the volume and to the Foreword by Edward Peters.

[8] The relevant records were kept at St. Bertin and were composed apparently by a number of chroniclers. See Nelson (1991).

[9] For detailed studies of these influences see Horden (2008).

the proposition that the insane cannot justly be punished for their actions. Augustine spoke for them all when he wrote:

> We have known certain individuals suddenly unbalanced who, with club and cudgel, stones and bites … were not found guilty because of the fact that they had done these things unknowingly and not freely, but by the impulse of some force, I know not what. For how can a man be called guilty who does not know what he has done? (Augustine, *Questions Concerning the Old and New Testament*, Question 2, cited by Pickett 1952, p. 44)

Working against this leniency, however, was the very strong *voluntarist* theory of criminal liability embraced by Christianity, thereby narrowing to some extent the range of legal defenses available to the mentally afflicted, even as the range of moral offenses constitutive of sin was enlarged. Some of these offenses were clearly tied to mental disturbances but assumed to be of the sinner's own making. Mental illness bore the heavy burdens of shame and concealment which, in the ancient world, were either muted or remarkably lacking. Theory was replacing matter-of-factness, and with mixed results.

Pope Gregory I (590–604) ruled that no cleric could be ordained if at any time he had been beset by insanity (see Pickett 1952, p. 39). But Cassian, the Egyptian monk of the fifth century, had rejected such exclusions, proposing further that the sacraments be administered every day. He and his fellow monastics were satisfied that the very existence of insanity established the reality of demons and possessions, but whose ability to possess persons could be resisted by the angelic part of human nature (Pickett 1952, p. 42). Gradually, the judgment of the instructed class began to change, aided by the introduction of long-lost texts from the classical period. Late medieval scholarship in the matter of insanity was thus classically informed and guided far less by superstition than by the now rigorous canonical principles of the Roman Catholic Church. By the conclusion of the thirteenth century, and largely as a result of the writings of St. Thomas Aquinas and the more general revival of aristotelianism, medieval theories of mental illness were increasingly naturalistic.

On such matters as the validity of sacramental rites, Thomas Aquinas carefully distinguished between insanity from birth and that occurring later in life; and between insanity without remission and that in which lucid intervals are common. It should be noted that "temporary insanity" is not a legal concept indebted to modern psychiatry, nor were medieval jurists at all reluctant to consider it. For example, in a trespass case of 1378, counsel for the defendant, Ralph Paranter, contends that, "every month between lucid intervals he was stricken with a serious sickness and thus became virtually insane during those times" (Arnold 1987, 34.23, p. 390). The point of such distinctions, so important in the context in which Thomas Aquinas wrote, is to establish the conceptual and moral dependence of sin and guilt on rationality and consent. The fineness of the requisite analysis is conveyed by his discussion of marriage covenants and insanity. He argues that, although the present mental state of a person is sufficient for the commission of mortal sin, the marriage contract calls for consent that bears on the future. Therefore, greater discretion is required. Accordingly, "man can sin mortally before he can impose upon himself some future obligation."[10] What is clearly recognized here is that there are gradations of mental status, and that incapacity as

---

[10] Thomas Aquinas, *Summa Theologiae*, Q. 43, Art. 2. It should be noted that a jurisprudential context for Thomas's own efforts was already in place at least as early as the middle of the twelfth century. In his chapter on "The age of mixed jurisprudence," Charles Radding discusses the remarkable *Expositio* of this

regards one class of thought or action may not extend to another class. It is in passages such as this that evidence is clearest of the Church's thorough absorption of classical (Roman) juridical reasoning into its own canonical context. It is worth mentioning that, to the extent the Natural Law tradition is properly identified as integral to Roman Catholicism, it is so because of this very absorption. How unsurprising, then, that Bracton borrows freely from Romanists and Canonists (e.g., Bernard of Paivia) in compiling his *De legibus Angliae* (Bracton 1915). Canon law, under the inspiration of scripture but everywhere beholden to Roman law, dealt with specific cases involving questions of mental competence. The growing canonical authority of the Pope resulted in any number of such issues being brought to Rome for settlement. The mode of settlement was adjudicative in that cases were disposed of according to carefully gathered evidence (e.g., depositions), settled law, well-established precedents, and (papal) interpretations in hard cases. R. Colin Pickett summarized a number of cases occasioned by allegations of insanity, of which the following is illustrative. A monastic priest, just before he died, declared to witnesses his intention that his earthly belongings be conveyed to the monastery, thus excluding the local church as a beneficiary. Here, then, was a conflict of interests between a bishop and an abbot. In this dispute, the Bishop of Nevers insisted that the deceased had been insane at the time he expressed his intentions and, therefore, should be regarded as having died intestate (Pickett 1949). In deciding the matter, Innocent III (1198) ruled that in such cases there is both the presumption of sanity and the resulting burden of proof imposed on those who would challenge the validity of testaments. But what of cases in which one declares himself to have been insane at some earlier time; for example, a priest seeking relief for some offense on the grounds that he had been entirely beside himself (*extra se positus*)? Again, Canon XV had long established the nullity of vows taken by the insane, but with Innocent III there is this modification: the burden of proof now shifts to the defendant, again because of the presumption of sanity. By the middle of the thirteenth century Bracton had summarized English law in this area in a phrase that could have been found in Justinian and defended by Aristotle: "For no crime is accomplished except that the desire to harm intercede" (Bracton 1915). The centuries of witch hunts and persecutions in Europe and America mark off a significant period in the evolution of legal concepts of insanity. The special nature of witchery called for alterations and even the suspension of trial procedures that had become settled features of law. In the ancient worlds of Greece and Rome, ordinary citizens readily accepted that some persons possessed exotic powers or might be chosen by the gods to be the medium for divine stratagems. It was understood that practitioners were able to perpetrate evil through a "black magic" harmful to others (*maleficium*); or that they might employ a benign "white magic" to cure illnesses and bring about good weather or a decent run of luck. Rome's Twelve Tables threatened only witches guilty of *maleficia*. As the power of ecclesiastical courts increased, along with the pronounced urbanization of European communities late in the Middle Ages, the adaptation of Roman law to Church interests was ever more vigorously pursued. Ancient distinctions between "black" and "white" magic were dissolved, all witchcraft now taken as proof of a covenant with Satan. These effects would come to be catastrophic in many European communities, but only after the merging of secular and religious thought. Given the very nature of the emerging but still undeveloped scientific outlook of the Renaissance,

---

period as evidence of the revival of jurisprudence. The work "situates the study of law into the tradition of the liberal arts" (1988, p. 129), as the expositor proceeds to list and interpret Lombard law.

it becomes less paradoxical that the greatest excesses of witch hunting would take place well into the modern era. The accusatorial procedures of early medieval law required that complaints and charges originate with the aggrieved or injured party. It was not the judge or the jurisdictional authority who prosecuted. Rather, the authorities *heard* the charges, weighed the evidence, and then ruled. Where the weight of evidence was insufficient to support a ruling, the contestants in a criminal action were called upon to face one or another *ordeal*. With the evolution of more refined (classical) procedures and the greater centralization of power, the accusatorial method was replaced by the *inquisitorial*, the judge now centrally involved in trying the case. With these developments the burdens imposed on accusers were now all but eliminated. A court finding the charges at all credible would take up the case, the officers of the court having the power to obtain and weigh the evidence, determine guilt or innocence, and set the penalties. The major gain in these procedural developments was the elimination of savage and juridically meaningless practices and their replacement by rules of evidence applied by competent jurists acting in behalf of Church or Crown. But the major liability, during the long season of the witch hunt, was that a successful prosecution for a crime such as heresy or the "white magic" of witchcraft—which often had neither victim nor eyewitness—would require the defendant's confession; a defendant no longer having the option of counter-suit. The melding of the civil offense of *maleficium* with that of heresy greatly enlarged the pool of potential suspects. Predictably the hardships wrought by these developments would be greatest for those whose medical, social, or psychological conditions resulted in signs or symptoms not readily explicable in the primitive medical idiom of the day. Epileptic seizures, various movement disorders, hysterical and neurological conditions that mar the body or modify memory, thought, and consciousness are illustrative of diseases that would prove to be especially congenial to demon-based or possession-based explanations. As for the recovered classical approach to law, the declared witch again lost out. The crime of witchcraft was the *crimen exceptum* for which standard procedures were ill-suited. Where physicians were consulted, the rationale was quite different in cases of possession and those of alleged witchcraft. D. P. Walker has noted in this connection that medical experts in witch trials were called upon to examine the accused for the devil's mark or to determine if there were supernumerary mammaries with which to nourish the demons. But doctors were not asked whether the witch was insane (see Walker 1968, p. 32). Nonetheless, in that widely adopted handbook for identifying and interrogating witches, the *Malleus Maleficarum*, necessary distinctions must be made between scientific and satanic practices and it therefore becomes important to know about each genre. The authors, Kramer and Sprenger (1486/1970), refer to information that has been gleaned by direct experience; to findings that have been reported in medical (Galenic) or naturalistic settings; to Aristotle's scientific analysis of the prophetic power of dreams—a power based on the ability of the imaginative faculty to record states of the body that might, indeed, portend disease. Further distinctions are made between healing based on mere superstition (as in believing in the power of Saturn over lead) and that based on witchcraft.

Throughout the macabre spectacle, physicians of the mind began to appear, some in the fearsome garb of inquisitor and witch-pricker, others in the long gowns of cabalistic shaman and Magus, still others in the stained and singed tunics of the herbalist, alchemist, the hermeticist; a few in the modest role of the diligent doctor. Johann Weyer's *De praestigiis daemonum et incantationibus ac veneficiis* saw six editions between 1563 and 1583 (Weyer 1991). Weyer did not deny the reality of Satan. He did not rule out the participation of demons in mental illness. Rather, he considered the weakened mind of the aged and the psychologically distressed to be something of a devil's workshop wherein all varieties of illusion may be crafted. Women tend to float, given their lighter constitution, a fact known since the time of Hippocrates. To Weyer, this was simply a fact of nature, lacking in any and all spiritual implications. He observed that drugs such as belladonna, opium, henbane, and tobacco enhanced such hallucinatory effects and could produce them in their own right. Again, forms of mental disorder did not require the participation of occult forces or beings. Those who regard themselves as possessed and admit to being witches are, he reasoned, generally suffering from melancholia. They need the attention of a physician, not an inquisitor. Inevitably Weyer's name was placed on the *Index* in Roman Catholic Europe as his book was set on fire by the Protestant faculty of Marburg.

At the time of its publication in 1563, Weyer's *De Prestigiis Daemonum* was exceptional but not entirely unique. Earlier in the sixteenth century, Paracelsus (1493–1541) wrote his brief treatise *On diseases that deprive man of health and reason*, noting in the Preface that the European clergy attribute these diseases to "ghostly beings," whereas "nature is the sole origin" of them. In this work Parcelsus argues that the loss of reason reveals itself in four principal forms: the *Lunatici* get the disease from the moon and react to its phases. The *Insani* are born with the malady, insanity being part of the family heritage. The *Vesani* suffer from toxic reactions to food, drink, or poison. The *Melancholici* become insane, losing reason in the course of a lifetime. Thus, even as approaches such as Weyer's faced hardship, the medical perspectives on insanity were growing in prominence during these very centuries.

The important trial of Hacket, Coppinger, and Arthington is illustrative. The three were charged with conspiracy, Hacket having declared himself King of Europe. In reporting the details of the case, Richard Cosin (1592/1963) set down the grounds of an insanity defense as English courts would understand this at the end of the sixteenth century. The principal categories affirmed by "the best writers" on the subject are *Furor sive Rabies*; *Dementia sive Amentia*; *Insania sive Phrenesis*; *Fatuitas, Stultia, Lethargia, & Delerium*. *Furor*, as Cosin discussed it, is the condition of the venerable *furiosus*, whose mind suffers "full blindnes or darkening of the understanding," the actor knowing not at all what he is doing or saying. *Dementia (Mente captus)* is an unremitting insanity, distinguished from *insania* in its severity. With *insania* the sufferer, though "braine-sicke, cracked-witted ... or hare-brained" is still fit for social life and is not entirely void of understanding. *Fatuitas* is the condition of the "natural fooles," though with *stultia* the victim is not included among the *Idiotes*. However, although Cosin's taxonomy is clearly informed by medical knowledge and the opinions of "the best writers," the courts at the time still hold all perpetrators responsible who are not totally mad.

By the turn of the century the naturalistic perspective had made even greater progress. As a result, courts began to consult physicians directly in ambiguous cases. Thus, when Elizabeth Jackson was tried in 1602 for bewitching Mary Glover, doctors testified in her behalf that the victim's fits were caused naturally.[11] However, even as the scientific mode of thought inaugurated by Bacon, Newton, and Galileo swept across Europe, the phenomena of the human mind remained refractory to the new methods and perspective.

---

[11] A thorough and informing study of the trial of Elizabeth Jackson, together with Edward Jorden's *Discourse* in which a decidedly psychiatric interpretation of the victim's vexations is offered, is *Witchcraft and Hysteria in Elizabethan London: Edward Jorden and the Mary Glover Case* (MacDonald 1991).

Developments in law reflected the broader influence of that classical perspective that had been embraced by the leaders of Renaissance thought. Sir Edward Coke's *Institutes of the Laws of England* appeared in 1628 and would be authoritative for the better part of two centuries. Written by one who would come to be regarded as England's greatest common lawyer, the work presents a naturalistic perspective on insanity wherever Coke addresses the matter. The perspective is an older Roman one, not at all remote from Coke's own. Coke moved the law toward secular understandings of all such matters, but more by the weight of past traditions than the light of the new science. According to the laws of England, he writes, persons of "non-sane memory" may purchase but not sell lands. But if the person then recovers, agreements entered into are "unavoydable." Coke specifies the legal sense of a diseased mind and considers the various forms of mental deficiency recognized by law: "*amens, demens, furiosus, lunaticus, fatuus, stultus.*" However, the true mark of insanity from the law's perspective is given by the phrase *pos mentis.*

Coke uses memory and understanding interchangeably in identifying the degree of psychological deficit worthy of the law's attention. Although acknowledging the exculpatory nature of a temporary insanity that is interrupted by lucid intervals, he requires of insanity itself what is essentially the total loss of cognitive prowess. The causes alluded to are all natural. The phrase he takes to be "the most sure and legall" is the one that describes one who has *no power of mind* whatever.

Sir Matthew Hale was more forward-looking than Coke and more concerned to work out the subtler aspects of insanity in relation to law. Chapter 4 of his posthumously published *The History of the Pleas of the Crown* (1680) is devoted entirely to this matter and, although not published in Hale's lifetime, it established how Britain's leading jurists were coming to regard these matters by the time of Hale's death (1676).[12] Yet, Hale's life and writings exemplify the divided nature of psychological thought even in the age of Newton. The private religious beliefs of men such as Hale still did not wander far from the authority of scripture. Witchcraft, which would find no place in Hale's discussion of legal insanity, was a topic on which he nevertheless wrote both in his unpublished papers and in briefer published tracts. In 1665, two widows appeared before him indicted for witch-craft, charged with causing children to vomit nails and see animals invisible to others. Although Hale did not speak one way or another on the matter of the actual evidence adduced against the defendants, he did direct the jury to recognize the authority of scripture as well as acts of parliament on the matter of the existence of witches. The defendants were found guilty and executed.[13]

Hale's chapter concerned with insanity begins with a classification of the defects and incapacities of mind other than infancy. In considering *dementia*, Hale delineates the usual causes ("distemper of the humours," adult cholera, melancholy, violent fevers and palsies, "a concussion or hurt of the brain, or its membranes or organs") noting that these may result in either partial or total insanity. The former is not exculpatory of capital offenses for the defendants, "are not wholly destitute of the use of reason" (Hale 1778, p. 30).

Note that the criterion remains a total want of reason. Because of this, and because *total* insanity is exculpatory, Hale alerts readers to the importance and the difficulty

[12] Matthew Hale, *The History of the Pleas of the Crown*, edition of 1778. Published from the original manuscripts by Sollom Emlyn. The first publication of Hale's papers was ordered by the House of Commons on November 29, 1680. It went through many editions.

[13] 6 *State Trials*. 687 (1665).

of assessing the degree of damage and injury caused. The criterion of 14 years is "the best measure" Hale can think of to guide jurors in difficult cases. Total insanity does not present a difficult case, for the defendant suffers from a complete alienation of mind that will be obvious to all. Partial insanity *is* difficult, for the defendant clearly is able to comprehend some things but not others. What one must ask in the latter case is whether there is sufficient rationality for the defendant to have more than a child's comprehension. It is as if Hale would take partial insanity to be more akin to *ideocy* than to perfect madness.

Hale draws a further distinction between permanent and intermittent or episodic dementia. The fixed variety he labels *phrenesis,* the latter *lunacy* "for the moon hath a great influence in all diseases of the brain, especially this kind." In such cases, the lucid intervals come between the full and the change of the moon, at which time sufferers have "at least a competent use of reason" such that, if they commit crimes while in this state, they are "subject to the same punishment, as if they had no such deficiency."

Taking out the pardonably dated references to lunar influences, Hale's brief summary of the chief causes of dementia is not only informed by the science of his day but compatible with what might even be called the modern view. He understands the several forms of dementia to be the result of a diseased brain, or biochemical (humoral) disturbances, or heredity. However, the issue at law is not one of etiology but of responsibility. The question to be settled is whether, at the time the offense was committed, the defendant was in sufficient possession of understanding to be held accountable. This question, on Hale's understanding, can be answered independently of any consideration of the defendant's brain, bile, or pedigree.

Two years after Hale had sentenced the widows to death for witchcraft, Thomas Willis's pioneering studies of the comparative anatomy of the brain were published. All of his major publications found large audiences, his *Opera Omnia* alone going through 11 editions by 1720 (see Frank 1990). The conclusions he reached after painstaking research and clinical observations establish the brain as the central organ of experience, action and emotion. Cerebral pathologies result in identifiable psychological disturbances. By the early eighteenth century, the major medical centers of Europe were given over either to essentially mechanistic or essentially chemical theories of health and disease, with all notions of "spirit" now cast chiefly in psychological and mental terms. The courts both followed and to some extent led developments along these lines.

In 1724 the Court of Common Pleas decided the case of *Rex v. Arnold.*[14] Edward Arnold was tried for felony "in maliciously and wilfully shooting at, and wounding, the Right Hon. the Lord Onslow," the defendant pleading not guilty by reason of insanity. In his charge to the jury Justice Tracy made clear that the insanity defense was a settled matter. If the defendant,

> be deprived of his reason, and consequently of his intention, he cannot be guilty …
> (However) … it is not every frantic and idle humour of a man, that will exempt him
> from justice, and the punishment of law … it must be a man that is totally deprived of his
> understanding and memory, and doth not know what he is doing, no more than an infant,
> than a brute, or a wild beast.[15]

---

[14] *Rex v. Arnold*, 16 Howell's State Trials 695 (10 George I. AD 1724).
[15] *Rex v. Arnold*, 16 Howell's State Trials 695 (10 George I. AD 1724): 754–765.

Arnold was convicted, was sentenced to be executed, and was spared through the intercession of his victim.

Tracy's instructions to the jury remain within the ambit established by Roman law and transported into Common law through Bracton, Coke, Hale, and the rest. For the insanity plea to succeed, the defendant must be insane at the time of the offense, the degree of insanity extensive enough to preclude any sensible awareness on the part of the defendant of the gravity of the action. The reasoning in criminal prosecutions was matched by the understandings of civil courts as can be seen in tests of testamentary capacity. In *Cartwright v. Cartwright* (1793)[16] Mrs. Armyne Cartwright had left a will in her own hand, leaving her not inconsiderable fortune to her brother's daughters and nothing to the issue of her father's second marriage. Her friend, Lady Macclesfield, stated in her deposition that the deceased considered her blood-brother a "much nearer and dearer relation than her brothers and sisters by the half-blood." But her physician, Dr. Battie, had instructed her nurse and other servants to keep pen and paper away from her and prevent her from writing. He went even further, informing Mrs. Cartwright that he would be a witness against any official document she might sign. However, Sir William Wynne rendered the judgment of the court, left no doubt about the grounds of his ruling:

> the deceased, by herself writing the will now before the Court, hath most plainly shewn she had a full and complete capacity to understand what was the state of her affairs and her relations.[17]

During the concluding decades of the eighteenth century the psychological maladies of George III as well as advances in medicine promoted a more humane set of attitudes toward mental illness. Medicine, too, was prepared to attach itself more firmly to objective scientific approaches to insanity. The courts, in climates of revolutionary upheaval and humanitarian reform, moved with the times. A pivotal case illustrating these developments was the trial of James Hadfield and the profoundly influential defense mounted in his behalf by Thomas Erskine (Box 3.1).[18]

The crime was that of high treason—an attempt on the life of George III—and the appointed counsel for the defense was perhaps the greatest trial lawyer in England. Erskine acknowledges before the jury that the controlling principle in England "and every other country" is:

> that it is the REASON OF MAN which makes him accountable for his actions; and that the deprivation of reason acquits him of crime.[19]

Erskine challenges this principle, dismissing ancient notions of *furious* and wild beasts as referring to entities that, even if they exist, would be unable to plan and execute a crime. He then advances, on the strength of current medical opinion, the proper legal criterion to be applied by jurors:

> *Delusion,* therefore, where there is no frenzy or raving madness, is the true character of insanity; and where it cannot be predicated of a man standing for life or death for a crime, he ought not in my opinion, be acquitted.[20]

---

[16] *Cartwright v. Cartwright*, 1 Phillimore Ecc. 90.
[17] *Cartwright v. Cartwright*, 1 Phillimore Ecc. 90, at 121.
[18] *Rex v. Hadfield*. 40 George III. AD 1800. In Howell's *State Trials*, Vol. XXVII, 1820; 1281–1356.
[19] *Rex v. Hadfield*. 40 George III. AD 1800. In Howell's *State Trials*, Vol. XXVII, 1820; 1310.
[20] *Rex v. Hadfield*. 40 George III. AD 1800. In Howell's *State Trials*, Vol. XXVII, 1820; 1310.

Box 3.1

Sir Thomas Erskine (1750–1823; Fig. 3.1) was the product of a distinguished but not prosperous family of lawyers. With the family's limited means, Erskine was unable to pursue university studies and chose to enter into military service with the Royal Navy. He rose to officer rank quickly. Indeed, in Boswell's *Life of Johnson*, we learn that Johnson met the young Erskine and was judged as conversing, "with a vivacity, fluency and precision so uncommon, that he attracted particular attention." With the encouragement of persons of influence, he retired from the army to undertake studies at Lincoln's Inn, simultaneously completing requirements for a degree from Trinity College, Cambridge.

Erskine would come to record a number of celebrated pleadings in his career as a barrister. Over a course of years he defended Lord George Gordon, Thomas Paine, and, in a case that materially altered the law's understanding of insanity, James Hadfield. His achievements gained him significant wealth and high repute. He was elected to Parliament for Portsmouth and rose to the office of Lord Chancellor in 1806. His pleadings before juries are emblems of refined and effective rhetoric, combined with a total mastery of legal procedure and precedent.

Erskine's defense of James Hadfield, who had made an attempt on the life of George III, did much to introduce what at the time was advanced thinking in medicine on the marks and measure of psychopathology. He stands as a significant figure in the rise of medical jurisprudence.

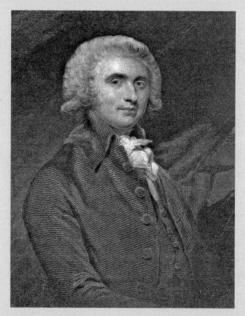

Figure 3.1 Sir Thomas Erskine. (Thomas Erskine, 1st Baron of Restormel, from 'Gallery of Portraits' (1833), English School/Private Collection/Ken Welsh/ The Bridgeman Art Library.)

Looking back over the history of the subject in 1876, Henry Maudsley would state matter of factly that, "It was at the trial of Hadfield, in 1800, for shooting at the King in Drury Lane Theatre, that Lord Hale's doctrine was first discredited, and a step forward made for the time" (Maudsley 1876, p. 91).

Difficulties arising from *Hadfield* soon made their way into both criminal and civil cases. In 1812, John Bellingham was tried and convicted of the murder of the Prime Minister, Spencer Perceval, previously Chancellor of the Exchequer. The motive was Bellingham's groundless claim that the Crown owed him money for time he had served in a Russian prison while Perceval had been Chancellor of the Exchequer. Failing to secure compensation from the Treasury, he hunted down Perceval and fired a fatal bullet at him in the lobby of the Commons House of Parliament. A plea of insanity was filed, though contested by Bellingham himself. There was no express attempt to link Bellingham's defense with that of Hadfield. Nonetheless, the odd rationale developed in *Hadfield* fostered the conclusion that actions arising from morbid delusion should be judged according to what the law would require or permit *were the contents of the delusion true*. If, indeed, James Hadfield had been commanded by God to rid the world of himself but not by taking his own life, and if he sought to obey this by having the King's defenders kill him, no English court would have found him guilty of a crime. But supposing John Bellingham's grievance to be valid, his lethal assault on Spencer Perceval would still have resulted in the law's maximum penalty.

The welter of attitudes, theories and concerns abounding in this period were crystallized, in the trial of Daniel McNaughtan in 1843.[21] Addressing the jury, counsel for the defense makes clear that one suffering from mental illness leading to "frantic imagination and ungovernable fury" cannot be punished at law and that, "to hold otherwise would be to violate every principle of justice and humanity." Determining whether the defendant qualified for such consideration resulted in the formulaton of the so-called *McNaughtan rule*. Justice Tindal expressed the "rule" thus:

> at the time of the committing of the act, the party accused was labouring under such a defect of reason, from disease of the mind, as not to know the nature and quality of the act he was doing, or, if he did know it, that he did not know he was doing what was wrong.

Tindal went on to explain that this wording is preferable to versions that cite or suggest a knowledge of the law of the land, or a general knowledge of right and wrong. The important consideration is the defendant's mental capacity as regards the specific act with which he has been charged. Problems with such a formulation were promptly recognized both in psychiatry and in law. Within two years of the verdict in McNaughtan, Griesinger's authoritative *Mental Pathology and Therapeutics* appeared, offering ample clinical data in opposition to the claim (1) that insanity invariably includes the element of delusion; (2) that the insane cannot distinguish between right and wrong; (3) that there are always irresistible motives behind the productions of madness. The one generalization he did endorse, and this on the very first page of the book is that the source of "madness" is to be found in the brain (Griesinger 1882).[22] The influential Supreme Court of New Hampshire took a leading part in the development of law as it pertains to insanity, Justice Ladd, in *State v. Jones* (1871) explicitly rejected not merely the *McNaughtan* "rule" but the very notion that matters of this sort were reducible to rules. He wrote:

---

[21] DANIEL M'NAGHTEN'S CASE, House of Lords Mews' Dig. i. 349; iv. 1112. S.C. 8 Scott N.R. 595; 1 C. and K. 130; 4 St. Tr. N.S. 847; May 26, June 19, 1843. Richard Moran was able to establish this as the correct spelling (Moran 1981).

[22] The first edition of this work (1845) was immediately accepted as authoritative.

> It is entirely obvious that a court of law undertaking to lay down an abstract general proposition, which may be given to the jury in all cases, … stands in exactly the same position as that occupied by the English judges in attempting to answer the questions propounded to them by the House of Lords in (*M'Naughten*); and whenever such an attempt is made, I think it must always be attended with failure, because it is an attempt to find what does not exist, namely, a rule of law wherewith to solve a question of fact.[23]

What the judge seeks to make clear is that a court, in propounding a legal principle, cannot thereby establish a scientific or medical fact. He takes the question of responsibility in such cases to be a medical question and thus beyond the resources of the general principles on which the rule of law depends.

Even before learning the details of *McNaughtan* Chief Justice Shaw in Massachusetts had instructed the jury in the landmark trial of Abner Rogers (1843) in such a way as to attempt to avoid the sorts of problems inherent in the "McNaughtan Rule."[24] Ample evidence attesting to the insanity of the defendant was marshaled at trial. What was special about the case, however, was Shaw's instructions to the jury which contained a new item in listing the criteria the jury must apply. Rogers was to be acquitted if the jury found that his actions were, "the result of disease."

The momentum that had been imparted as early as *Hadfield* and that increased significantly by mid century would reach its peak in American cases.[25] Again, the rationale guiding criminal cases extended to civil cases. In *Boardman v. Woodman* Justice Doe refers to Coke and Hale as men who "unfortunately copied the opinions of the medical authorities of their day on the subject of insanity," and then affirmed the principle that no crime can be committed and no will produced "by any form of mental disease, and that the indications and tests of mental disease are matters of fact."[26] In *State v. Pike* (1865) and *State v. Bartlett* (1869) the same Court corrected the "great error" of requiring defendants to prove insanity.[27] The *McNaughtan* rules were increasingly honored in the breach such that, by 1945, in *Holloway v. United States*, the "rules" are the subject of caricature. Modern science, declared the Court,

> has no place for … a separate little man in the top of one's head called reason whose function it is to guide another unruly little man called instinct, emotion or impulse in the way he should go.[28]

Nonetheless, in most jurisdictions the controlling criminal statutes well into the twentieth century in the United States and elsewhere commonly held to "right-wrong" as well as notions of the "irresistible impulses" on which Erskine had focused in *Hadfield*.

---

[23] *State v. Jones.* 50 New Hampshire 369.

[24] The complete account of this trial is found in Bigelow and Bemis (1844). Isaac Ray would discuss this trial in an article in the *Law Reporter* in 1845, reprinted in his anthology, *Contributions to Mental Pathology*. Boston, MA: Little, Brown, 1873. Ray said of this case that, "No criminal trial in this country, in which insanity was pleaded in defence, has become more widely known and been oftener cited than that of Abner Rogers" (p. 210).

[25] Henry Maudsley would remark that, although initially docilely following the lead of British jurists, recent decisions in the United States constituted a marked advance on anything that been settled to date in England (Maudsley 1876, pp. 100ff).

[26] *Boardman v. Woodman.* 47 New Hampshire 120 (1869); *State v. Jones.* 50 New Hampshire 369 (1872); p. 139.

[27] *State v. Pike.* 49 New Hampshire 399 (1872); *State v. Bartlett.* 43 New Hampshire 224.

[28] *Holloway v. United States.* 326 U.S. 687 (1945).

On the significant question of burden of proof in the matter of insanity, the US Supreme Court decided the question as early as 1895 in *Davis v. United States*. Justice Harlan noted that the controlling dicta had been laid down in *McNaughtan* and repeated often in British and American cases. But what had not been settled was whether the test to be met was one of *preponderance of evidence* or the sterner test of proof *beyond reasonable doubt*. The influential Massachusetts Supreme Court tended to impose the heavier burden on the government. The Harlan Court moved in the same direction, ruling that the defendant is entitled to acquittal if "upon all the evidence there is reasonable doubt." On the question of who bears the burden of proof, the Court ruled that it is the State's burden to prove, "that the accused, whose life it is sought to take under the forms of law, belongs to a class capable of committing crime."[29]

Harlan's rationale is that a successful insanity defense is tantamount to a finding of not guilty, whereas the failure of that defense yields a guilty verdict. As it is not a defendant's burden to prove his or her innocence, it should not be a defendant's burden to establish insanity. From 1895 until quite recently Harlan's reasoning guided Federal courts and imposed on the State the burden of adducing positive proof of sanity where the insanity defense was successfully raised. However, in the wake of the trial of John Hinckley, who was acquitted of all charges connected with his assault on President Reagan and members of the President's entourage, Congress proceeded to revamp the Federal laws pertaining to the insanity defense. In the process and building on earlier cases, the Insanity Defense Reform Act (IDRA) of 1984 established insanity as an affirmative defense to be proved by the defendant *by clear and convincing evidence*. The question of the extent to which mental disorders are mitigating has had a comparably varied history. A half-century ago great attention was given to the opinion delivered by Judge Bazelon in *Durham*, in which, following Isaac Ray, the "fallacious" nature of the right-wrong test was underscored and current legal notions of insanity duly recognized as having "little relation to the truths of mental life."[30] Judge Bazelon's opinion is as good an example of judge-made law as one is likely to find. Neither Isaac Ray nor the judge could point to actual discoveries or relevant scientific data that would rule out the right–wrong test of moral judgment as an integral aspect of "the truths of mental life." What was settled in *Durham* was that diagnostic categories such as "psychopath" and "sociopath" were acceptable for the defense of insanity, and that the traditional tests were no longer binding. In words substantially similar to those Justice Shaw had used in instructing the jury in *Rogers*, the Court in *Durham* found that "an accused is not criminally responsible if his unlawful act was the product of mental disease or mental defect." The year before *Durham*, Britain's Royal Commission on Capital Punishment had issued its own influential report, concluding that,

> The gravamen of the charge against the M'Naghten Rules is that they are not in harmony with modern medical science, which, as we have seen, is reluctant to divide the mind into separate compartments.[31]

The reasoning in *Durham* was found on further reflection to create more problems than it solved. In a number of pivotal cases Federal Appeals courts found the *Durham* principle

---

[29] *Davis v. United States*. 160 U.S. 469; 40 L. Ed. 499; 16 S. Ct. 353.
[30] *Durham v. United States*. 214 F. 2d 862 (1954).
[31] *Royal Commission on Capital Punishment Report* (Cmd. 8932), 1953; p. 113.

to be unworkable, especially in light of the wide disagreements by experts in such cases. As (then) Judge Warren Burger complained, "No rule of law can possibly be sound or workable which is dependent upon the terms of another discipline whose members are in profound disagreement about what those terms mean".[32]

The remedies for *Durham* were sought by the same Federal Appeals Court that had heard *Holloway*, *Durham*, and *Blocker*, the Court in *Brawner*[33] coming to adopt standards that had been developed by the American Law Institute (ALI) in its *Model Penal Code* and identified as the *Brawner* standard:

> A person is not responsible for criminal conduct if at the time of such conduct as a result of mental disease or defect he lacks substantial capacity either to appreciate the criminality (wrongfulness) of his conduct or to conform his conduct to the requirements of law.

Still other standards have come to modify or replace *Brawner*. The 1984 *Comprehensive Crime Control Act* recovered the very "right–wrong" test so roundly condemned by the experts of a century ago. Utah, Idaho, and Montana eliminated the insanity defense altogether, the balance of the states being roughly divided in adopting either *Brawner* or *McNaughtan*.

There have been other proposals to suspend the search for precision in specific cases and to adopt a form of categorical exemption from punishment. H. L. A. Hart concluded from the well-known failures to identify mental disorders with precision that it might be best to adopt a "coarser-grained technique" such as that which creates the class of legal infants.

The issues of exculpatory or mitigating evidence and burden of proof have raised perennial questions regarding the expert testimony and the validity of psychiatric and psychological assessments. The highest courts have moved in the direction of liberalizing the criteria to be applied to expert opinion-testimony. This is evident in the US Supreme Court ruling in *Daubert v. Merrell Dow Pharmaceuticals*.[34] Though not pertaining to insanity or to psychiatry, *Daubert* is relevant to the matter of expertise in cases of insanity because it sets guidelines for Federal courts on such central issues as who is qualified and what is to count as relevant and reliable data. In *Daubert* a lower court had based its ruling regarding expert testimony on the so-called *Frye* standard as advanced in the 1923 case of *Frye v. United States*.[35] According to this standard, scientific techniques or practices must be those that are "generally accepted" within the relevant scientific community. In *Daubert* the Court ruled that such a standard, "would be at odds with the … general approach of relaxing the traditional barriers to 'opinion' testimony."

Writing for a unanimous Court, Justice Blackman wrote:

> "Relevant evidence" is defined as that which has "any tendency to make the existence of any fact that is of consequence to the determination of the action more probable or less probable than it would be without the evidence" … The Rule's basic standard of relevance thus is a liberal one.[36]

The question of *mens rea* continues to occupy practitioners and theorists both in law and psychiatry. Some, such as Barbara Wootton, would have the concept simply "wither away."

[32] *Blocker v. United States.* 274 F. 2d 572 (1959); *Blocker v. United States.* 288 F. 2d 853 (1961).
[33] *United States v. Brawner.* 471 F. 2d 969 (1972), establishing the "Brawner" standard.
[34] 113 S. Ct. 2786, 1993.
[35] 54 App. D.C. 46, 47, 293 F. 1013, 1014.
[36] 113 S. Ct. 2786, 1993.

Or, following H. L. A. Hart, others would reserve the question to a time after conviction, and then to determine whether punishment or treatment is the proper course of action (Hart 1968; Wootton 1964). Others have argued for the defense of "Guilty but insane," now applicable in a number of jurisdictions. These questions are likely to remain unsettled at the level of psychology and psychiatry for at base they are at once juridical questions beyond the range of scientific or technical solutions and metaphysical questions perhaps beyond the range of settled knowledge itself. The history of the insanity defense displays the same oscillations found in philosophy's ageless engagement with the free will–determinism conundrum and it would be unrealistic to assume that psychiatry might offer a conclusive argument capable of settling a metaphysical dispute. It would appear that such matters, for better and for worse, are provisionally settled in the court of common sense which is guided but seldom ruled by an expertise both real and imagined.

REFERENCES

Arnold, M. (Ed.) (1987). *Select Cases of Trespass from the King's Courts 1307–1399, Vol. II*. London: The Selden Society.

Bigelow, G. T. and Bemis, G. (1844). *The Trial of Abner Rogers*. Boston, MA: Little, Brown.

Bracton, H. de (1915). *De Legibus et Consuetudinibus Angliae* (G. E. Woodbine, Ed.). New Haven, CT: Yale University Press.

Celsus. (1935). *De Medicina* (Vol. 1) (W. G. Spenser, Trans.). Cambridge, MA: Harvard University Press.

Chaleby, K. (2001). *Forensic Psychiatry in Islamic Jurisprudence*. Herndon, VA: International Institute of Islamic Thought.

Cosin, R. (1592). *Conspiracie, for pretended reformation: viz. presbyteriall discipline*, pp. 73–81. London. Excerpted in R. Hunter and I. Macalpine (Eds) (1963). *Three Hundred Years of Psychiatry*, pp. 42–5. London: Oxford University Press.

Drew, C. F. (1973). *The Lombard Laws*. Philadelphia, PA: University of Pennsylvania Press.

Frank, R. (1990). Thomas Willis and his circle: Brain and mind in seventeenth-century medicine. In G. S. Rousseau (Ed.), *The Languages of Psyche: Mind and Body in Enlightenment Thought*, pp. 107–46. Berkeley, CA: University of California Press.

Gagarin, M. and Cohen, D. (Eds) (2005). *The Cambridge Companion to Ancient Greek Law*. Cambridge: Cambridge University Press.

Garland, R. (1990). *The Greek Way of Life*. Ithaca, NY: Cornell University Press.

Griesinger, W. (1882). *Mental Pathology and Therapeutics* (C. Robertson and J. Rutherford, Trans.). New York, NY: William Wood & Co.

Guo, Z. (2010). Approaching visible justice: Procedural safeguards for mental examinations in China's capital cases. *Hastings International and Comparative Law Review, 33*, 21.

Hale, M. (1778). *The History of the Pleas of the Crown. Published from the original manuscripts by Sollom Emlyn*. London: T. Payne.

Harrison, A. R. W. (1968). *The Law of Athens, Vol. 1*. Oxford: Clarendon Press.

Hart, H. L. A. (1968). *Punishment and Responsibility*. Oxford: Oxford University Press.

Horden, P. (2008). *Hospitals and Healing from Antiquity to the Later Middle Ages*. London: Ashgate

Isaeus. (1927). *Isaeus* (E. S. Forster, Trans.). Cambridge, MA: Harvard University Press.

Kramer, H. and Sprenger, J. (1970). *Malleus Maleficarum* (M. Summers, Trans.). New York, NY: Benjamin Blom. (Original work published 1486.)

MacDonald, M. (Ed.) (1991). *Witchcraft and Hysteria in Elizabethan London: Edward Jorden and the Mary Glover Case*. London: Tavistock/Routledge.

Maudsley, H. (1876). *Responsibility in Mental Disease*. New York, NY: D. Appleton and Co.

Moran, R. (1981). *Knowing Right from Wrong: The Insanity Defense of Daniel McNaughtan*. New York, NY: Free Press.

Nelson, J. L. (Trans.) (1991). *The Annals of St-Bertin*. Manchester: University of Manchester Press.

Paracelsus (Theophrastus von Hohenheim). (1941). *The Writings of Theophrastus Paracelsus on Diseases that Deprive Man of Health and Reason* (G. Zilboorg, Trans.). In H. Sigerist (Ed.), *Four Treatises of Theophrastus von Hohenheim called Paracelsus. Vol. 1.* Baltimore, MD: Johns Hopkins University Press.

Pickett, R. C. (1949). *Roman Law and the Insane. Extract From a Thesis, Entitled "The Laws of the Church and the Insane: an Historical Synopsis of Roman and Ecclesiastical Law."* Ottawa: St. Paul's Seminary Press.

Pickett, R. C. (1952). *Mental Affliction and Church Law*. Ottawa: University of Ottawa Press.

Radding, C. M. (1988). *The Origins of Medieval Jurisprudence: Pavia and Bologna, 850–1150.* New Haven, CT: Yale University Press.

Robinson, J. N. (1996). *Wild Beasts and Idle Humours: The Insanity Defense from Antiquity to the Present*. Cambridge, MA: Harvard University Press.

Saunders, T. (1991). *Plato's Penal Code*. Oxford: Oxford University Press.

The Institutes of Justinian, Book I, Tit. XXIII (1970). (T. C. Sandars, Trans.). Westport, CT: Greenwood Press. (First published in 1922.)

Walker, N. (1968). *Crime and Insanity in England*. Edinburgh: University of Edinburgh Press.

Weyer, J. (1991). *De Praestigiis Daemonum* (J. Shea, Trans.). In G. Mora (Ed.), *Witches, Devils and Doctors in the Renaissance*. Binghampton, NY: Medieval and Renaissance Texts and Studies.

Wootton, B. (1964). *Crime and the Criminal Law*. London: Steven & Sons.

CHAPTER 4

MENTAL HEALTH AS MORAL VIRTUE: SOME ANCIENT ARGUMENTS

TERENCE IRWIN

PLATO ON MENTAL HEALTH

Plato identifies justice in the soul with mental health.[1] Just as bodily health consists in the appropriate order and relation of the different elements in the body, psychic health consists in the right order of the elements in the soul.[2] Justice is psychic health because it is the order of different psychic elements that is natural for the subject.[3] The soul contains three "parts" (or "kinds," *genê*)—the rational, the spirited, and the appetitive part that Plato has already described. These include rational desires (the rational part) and various kinds of non-rational desires (the spirited and the appetitive part). Plato argues that we need control by the rational part to produce the condition in which each part performs its proper work or function (*ergon*).

---

[1] This is the topic of Kenny (1973).

[2] "… Just and unjust in the soul are no different from healthy and unhealthy in the body … Whatever is healthy, I presume, produces health, and whatever is unhealthy produces illness…. Virtue, then, it would seem, is some sort of health, and a fine state and a good state, of soul, and vice is disease and a disfigurement (*aischos*) graceful state and weakness." (Excerpted from *Republic* 444c–e.)

[3] He gives his reason in the preceding passage: "… having prevented the kinds in his soul from doing one another's work and interfering with one another, but having put in good order what is really his own, and having mastered and ordered himself and having become a friend to himself … and having become in all respects one person from many (*pantapasin hena genomenon ek pollôn*) …" (excerpts from 443c–444a). The Greek preposition "*ek*" ("from," "out of") may refer either to the origin of a change (day came to be from night; the oak came to be from an acorn) or to an element in a compound (this book is made from paper). The genitive plural "*pollôn*" might be masculine or neuter. And so we might translate the phrase: (a) "one person instead of many people," or (b) "one person composed of many people," or (c) "one person instead of many things," or (d) as given.

Plato does not use "health" as a term of vague commendation, to indicate the condition that accords with his moral views. He has a fairly clear conception of health in mind. If the different bodily elements interacted in ways that undermined the unity and functions of the whole body, they would be sources of illness rather than health. The dominance of the non-rational parts has the same effect on a soul. To show that justice in the soul is the natural order, Plato claims that: (1) the agent "has become a friend (*philos*) to himself"; and (2) he "has become one person composed from many elements." The just soul does not cease to contain plural elements; the division between the three parts does not disappear, because they remain distinct sources of motivation. But the just person succeeds where unjust people fail, in becoming one person composed of the many. He achieves this unity because he achieves internal friendship; the plural elements are guided by the rational part, which deliberates on behalf of the whole soul.[4] Neither of the other parts can form this comprehensive view, and so neither can reach a unified plan that aims at the interest of the whole and of each part. An agent with an unjust soul is both more and less than one person in so far as he is not guided by this sort of plan. Plato takes one sort of unity in a person to result from the unity of practical reason.

His claims raise some questions: (1) Is he right to connect psychic health with psychic unity in the way he does? (2) Is he right to connect psychic unity with control by the rational part? (3) When Plato speaks of justice in the soul, he means both that the soul is well ordered and that the agent with a well-ordered soul is just in relation to other people; but is he right to connect control by the rational part with moral virtue? (4) Plato plausibly connects health and illness with different types of relations between different psychic elements. But is he right to collect these elements into "parts" of the soul? When he speaks of friendship within the parts, he seems to give them quasi-personal features. Does he treat parts as homunculi, to a degree that makes them useless for explanation, because it simply reduplicates the explanandum?

I will sketch a few answers to some of these questions. Though it would be easy to devote a whole paper on this topic to the examination of Plato, I have chosen to say more about Aristotle and the Stoics than about Plato. Aristotle is helpful because he elaborates and defends some Platonic views. The Stoics are helpful because they offer a clear alternative to Platonic and Aristotelian moral psychology, but reach the same conclusion about mental health and virtue.

What Is Plato Trying to Do?

If Plato identifies mental health and moral virtue, how is the identity to be understood? Two obvious possibilities are worth considering:

1. We may try to reduce moral virtue to mental health. We understand the character of mental health, in contrast to illness, disorder, or insanity. We explain puzzling features of the virtues by arguing that they are simply aspects of mental health (as we already understand it). If we initially take mental health to be relatively comprehensible and

---

[4] 442b6, c7.

desirable, but we are initially puzzled about virtue, we remove puzzles about virtue through this reductive account.

2. We may try to inflate mental health into moral virtue. Though we might initially suppose that mental health is a relatively comprehensible condition that demands less than moral virtue demands, further reflexion may suggest to us that we cannot maintain this division, and that the conditions for mental health are really no less demanding than those for moral virtue.

The reductive and the inflationary strategy reflect two different views about whether mental health or moral virtue is prior in our account.[5]

These two strategies may not offer either exclusive or exhaustive options. They may not be exhaustive, because we may find that neither one of mental health and virtue is prior to the other, and that each explains certain aspects of the other. They may not be mutually exclusive, because each may be prior to the other in different ways. We may roughly distinguish conceptual from explanatory priority.[6] The concept of mental health may be initially less complex than the concept of virtue, and we may find it easier to find clear examples. But to understand why these specific conditions are required for mental health we may need to understand the character of the virtues, and so the virtues may have a type of explanatory priority.

Rather than try to explain these strategies further in general, I propose to turn to some of the relevant details in Aristotle, in the hope that this specific case will clarify the main points. I have begun with Plato because he makes the comparison between moral virtue and mental health most explicit. But I turn to Aristotle because he offers a more detailed account of the virtues that allows us to see how Plato's claims might be defended. After a discussion of Aristotle, I turn to Stoic views, which offer an instructively different argument for some of Aristotle's conclusions.

Habituation and Character

Aristotle accepts Plato's division between the rational and the non-rational part of the soul, and he uses the division to explain the difference between virtue and vice. Plato recognizes two conditions: virtue is control by the rational part, and vice is control by the non-rational part.[7] Aristotle believes that we need to distinguish control of one part by another from the attitude of the controlled and the controlling parts. Hence we need to distinguish four conditions: (1) In a vicious person the rational and the non-rational parts agree in the rational pursuit of the wrong ends. (2) In an incontinent[8] person the rational and the non-rational parts disagree; the rational part pursues the right ends, but the non-rational part pursues the wrong ends, and overcomes the rational part. (3) In a continent person the rational and the non-rational parts disagree; the non-rational part pursues the wrong ends, but the rational

---

[5] Some similar questions are raised by McDowell (1998).

[6] Aristotle distinguishes priority and knowability "to us" from priority and knowability "by nature," at, e.g., *EN* 1095b2–4, *APo* 71b33–72a4. His distinction may usefully be applied to this case.

[7] Much more needs to be said about Plato. Further discussion may be found in Bobonich (2002); Irwin (1995); Lorenz (2006).

[8] Or "uncontrolled" (*akratês*).

part pursues the right ends, and overcomes the non-rational part. (4) In a virtuous person the rational and the non-rational parts agree in the rational pursuit of the right ends.[9]

This fourfold division clarifies an issue that Plato leaves obscure. We might gather from *Republic* IV that Plato identifies vice with incontinence and virtue with continence (as Aristotle conceives them). Aristotle rejects both of these identifications. The vicious person does not suffer conflict between the rational and non-rational parts. His rational part prefers unjust and intemperate (e.g.) actions over just and temperate actions, and his non-rational part shares this preference. The incontinent person is better than the vicious person because his rational judgment and desire is correct, even though his non-rational desires are strong enough to overcome his rational desire. The continent person is better than the vicious and the incontinent person, because he acts on his correct rational desires, but he is still not virtuous, because his non-rational part does not agree with these correct rational desires. The virtuous person does not simply control his non-rational part. Someone who has to control the non-rational part because it tends to mislead him needs better training until it no longer misleads him.

This training of the non-rational part is habituation (*ethismos*), which proceeds not by learning the theory of virtue but by repetition of the appropriate actions; we become just by doing just actions. First we do them without ourselves being just, but eventually we do the just actions because of the virtue of justice that we have acquired by practice. If we are to acquire the appropriate virtue, habituation must include more than repetition; we might learn to repeat an annoying military drill while hating it just as much when we have learned it perfectly, but this is not what Aristotle has in mind when he speaks of habituation. The relevant sort of habit includes the formation of the appropriate pleasures, pains, and other affective reactions.[10] The "sign" of virtue is the appropriate pleasure.[11] Virtuous people do not choose just or temperate action simply because other people will reward them, but they take pleasure in it in its own right. Vicious action offers no pleasure as great as the pleasures they gain from acting virtuously.[12]

This conception of habituation explains the difference between the virtuous person and the continent and the incontinent person. Neither of the last two has completed the appropriate habituation. Because neither of them takes the appropriate pleasure in virtuous action, their non-rational part opposes the virtuous action; in the incontinent person its opposition results in the wrong action.[13] In the virtuous person the non-rational part that agrees with reason has no appetites or spirited desires that diverge from what reason permits.

Both the incontinent and the continent person, therefore, lack internal friendship, and therefore lack the internal unity that is necessary for mental health. We do not secure internal unity if the rational part aims at the good of the whole soul, but the other parts do not accept its views, or they accept them only reluctantly. Though a non-rational part does not take the global point of view that the rational part takes, it can be trained to take pleasure in the goals that the rational part pursues. Once we achieve this harmony between the rational and non-rational parts, we have achieved internal friendship and unity. The non-rational parts favor the aims of the rational part, and by pursuing common goals they achieve unity of agency.

---

[9] The fourfold division: *EN* 1102b13–28.

[10] 1103b22–5. Aristotle insists on the training of the non-rational part at, e.g., 1095b4–13, 1179b23–31.

[11] 1104b3–8.

[12] 1153b9–14.

[13] Aristotle distinguishes obedience (*peitharchein*) to reason from listening better (*euêkoôteron*) to reason and so agreeing (*homophônein*) with reason in everything, at 1102b26–8.

MENTAL HEALTH WITHOUT VIRTUE?

Aristotle's description of these four psychic conditions explains why Plato's description of health is too simple. Plato takes health to require friendship and unity between parts of the soul, but he speaks as though control by the rational part were sufficient for both friendship and unity. Aristotle argues that control by the rational part does not ensure friendship between the parts. To have the sort of friendship and unity that marks the healthy soul, we also need agreement between the rational and non-rational parts, so that both parts do not simply go in the same direction, but also go in the same direction willingly and with enjoyment.

But Aristotle appears to depart from Plato on a still more important point. Plato maintains that virtue is health and vice is illness. Aristotle, however, seems to allow that the marks of health are found in both the virtuous and the vicious person, though not in the continent and incontinent person. We can eliminate psychic conflict and achieve psychic friendship either by virtue or by vice, since both of them imply agreement between the two parts of the soul.

This conclusion is too hasty. Plato does not simply require agreement between the parts, but also demands control by the rational part. A soul in which the rational part is inactive would not suffer from conflict between the two parts, but still would not be guided by the rational part's deliberation about the good of the whole soul. Psychic health requires this rational guidance. That is why Aristotle asks whether different agents are guided by rational decision (*prohairesis*). Decision results from wish and deliberation, and wish is the characteristic desire of the rational part. All of the four agents described by Aristotle form a rational decision, but the incontinent person does not act on it. In the continent person decision is effective, but in conflict with non-rational desire. In both the virtuous and the vicious person non-rational desires are aligned with rational decision.

And so, even if we keep in mind that psychic health requires guidance by reason, we seem to have Aristotelian reason to identify virtue with mental health. The vicious person seems to be exactly similar to the virtuous person in his relation to practical reason and non-rational desire; each of them can equally be said to follow reason. The only difference between them is that one has good ends and the other has bad ends; but this difference cannot be expressed simply by saying that one is guided by reason and the other is not.

WHAT IS WRONG WITH VICE?

Aristotle has more to say about the vicious person, however. For, while he maintains that vicious people are controlled by their rational part insofar as they act on decision, and not simply on non-rational desire, he nonetheless maintains that they follow non-rational appetite rather than reason. In the virtuous person, the non-rational part agrees with and follows the rational part, but in the vicious person this order is reversed.

Is Aristotle right about this? Is it at all plausible to claim that a cowardly or intemperate person, for instance, does not follow his rational part? In Aristotle's view, vicious people suffer from the internal conflict and self-hatred that he normally ascribes to incontinents (1166b6–13). They follow their passions, and gratify the non-rational part of the soul (1168b19–21; 1169a3–6). Only the virtuous person is free, or nearly free, of regret (1166a27–9; 1166b22–5).

We can perhaps see what Aristotle has in mind if we recall that the vicious person does not acquire his vice as a result of education and habituation that includes a process of learning to take pleasure in certain types of actions for their own sakes. In this respect vice is not symmetrical to virtue. We become vicious when vicious action becomes habitual to us. But it does not become habitual because we come to appreciate it as worth choosing for its own sake. Even Milton's Satan does not make evil his good because he is convinced that evil is better than good. He adopts it as a means to power, which he seeks in response to the humiliation of defeat and despair.[14] Less spectacular vices may result from drifting into courses of action that seem necessary to safeguard some goal that we are unwilling to give up.

In contrast to the vicious person, the virtuous person decides on the virtuous action for its own sake (1105a31–2), and because it is fine (*kalon*).[15] Virtuous people take this feature of an action to be a sufficient reason, apart from any further causal results, for choosing the action; they decide on virtuous action on principle. The vicious person, however, does not decide on vicious actions for their own sake and because they are fine. Avoiding danger is vicious if it involves betraying a worthwhile cause because of unjustified fear, but this is not why it appeals to cowards. They do not choose the cowardly action on principle. They prefer one action over another simply because it appeals to them, not because of some further conviction about its value. Their goals result from their preferences and inclinations, and they do not educate these preferences and inclinations by reflexion on what is worth pursuing.

This attitude helps to explain why Aristotle denies that vicious people have friendship between the parts of the soul. The primary type of friendship (*philia*) requires each friend to aim at the good of the other for the other's own sake, not simply as part of a strategic alliance. In a virtuous person the rational part has this sort of concern for the non-rational part. The non-rational part cannot have exactly the same attitude to the rational part, but, if it has been well trained, it can acquire an unselfish concern for the whole soul. This does not happen, according to Aristotle, in vicious people. They do not act on convictions about what deserves pursuit in its own right; hence they do not act on convictions about the good of the whole soul and its parts. They take a purely instrumental attitude to the rational part, and regard its deliberations as a mere means to the satisfaction of appetites. The parts of a vicious person's soul have a purely strategic relation to each other.

This relation makes vicious people subject to a type of regret that the virtuous person avoids. Virtuous people avoid the regret that results from blaming oneself for what one did or decided to do. This regret results from the belief that I ought to have known something, or that I ought to have decided differently in the light of what I knew. Since virtuous people care about acting on a conviction about what is best, they do not regret having acted on that conviction, and, in this respect, they are satisfied with their past action. Vicious people, however, lack this reason for satisfaction, since they do not care about acting on principle (on a conviction about what is best). The frustration of their inclinations is an undefeated reason for regret about their past actions.

Vicious people, therefore, lack the unity of agency that results from intrapersonal friendship and control by reason. Since they take their good to depend on what they want at a particular

---

[14] "So farwel Hope, and with Hope farwel Fear,/Farwel Remorse: all Good to me is lost;/Evil be thou my Good; by thee at least/Divided Empire with Heav'ns King I hold/*112:* By thee, and more then half perhaps will reigne …" (Milton, *Paradise Lost*, iv 108–12.)

[15] On the *kalon* see 1117a7–9, 1120a23–9, 1121b5–6.

time, and they do not form their desires through a conviction about what is worth choosing in its own right, they have less reason than virtuous people have to care about their future selves. Virtue of character, therefore, is necessary for friendship and unity within the self. These are the two features of psychic justice that Plato takes to be marks of mental health.

Should we agree, then, that Aristotle's claims about virtue tell us something about mental health? We might be inclined to disagree with him if we believe that mental health is good for the agent, whereas virtues of character are good for other people. Aristotle disagrees on this point; he argues that the mental features of the virtues of character are also features of a person's good. Still, his demands for unity and friendship might appear to exaggerate reasonable conditions on mental health. Admittedly, if we entirely lacked psychic cohesion, and if we always hated and repudiated every aim that we form for ourselves, our agency would have dissolved into internal conflict, dispute, recrimination, and self-loathing. But while this extreme degree of internal conflict and disunity plausibly qualifies as mental illness, we might be less convinced by Aristotle's attempt to present vice as a form of illness.

Aristotle, however, might fairly question an attempt to limit the scope of mental health to a minimal degree of internal friendship and unity. If these are elements of mental health, they are central and desirable elements of rational agency. Why, then, should we not acknowledge that greater friendship and unity produce a higher degree of mental health? Our willingness to recognize mental health in a minimal degree of friendship should make us aware of the aspects of agency that we value. We would be mistaken if we supposed that we are concerned with quite different characteristics when we think of mental health and when we think of moral virtue. The main question is not about whether we choose to confine the expression "mental health" to the minimal condition, but about what makes the minimal condition valuable. It turns out to be difficult to explain why the minimal condition is valuable without also endorsing the moralized condition.

THE STOIC ANALYSIS OF PASSIONS

This connexion between mental health and moral virtue is no less prominent in the Stoics than in Plato and Aristotle, even though it is combined with a sharply different moral psychology. They reject the Platonic and Aristotelian division between rational and non-rational parts, and revert to the Socratic identification of virtue with knowledge. The virtuous person, therefore, is the sage, who is extremely rare. Everyone who is not a sage is a fool, and all fools are mad. The knowledge that is needed to overcome this madness is exactly the same as the knowledge that we need if we are to be virtuous.[16]

At first sight, the Stoic view appears sharply different from the Platonic and Aristotelian view that we have discussed. The Platonic and Aristotelian view takes emotions, feelings, and appetites to belong to a non-rational part of the soul. Our non-rational desires arise, persist, and move us to action, contrary to our beliefs about what is best to do. The task of moral education is to harmonize the rational and non-rational parts under the control of reason. The

---

[16] The most useful collection of texts, with an informative commentary, is Long and Sedley (1987), cited as 'LS' with the section number. For further discussion of the Stoics on the passions see Nussbaum (1994); Sorabji (2000).

Stoics, however, believe that this conception of non-rational passions (*pathê*)[17] is mistaken, because a passion is a false belief, and therefore belongs to the rational part of the soul. More precisely, an "immediate" or "fresh" assent that consists in yielding to an appearance that something that is (in fact) a preferred (or non-preferred) indifferent is good (or evil).[18]

Each clause in this account relies on further Stoic doctrines. First, it identifies a passion with a type of assent (*sunkatathesis*).[19] An assent is a rational judgment about the content of an appearance (*phantasia*). If we see a stick in water that looks bent, we may assent to its being bent, and so believe that it is bent. After appropriate experience, we do not assent to its being bent, even though it still looks bent.[20] The Stoic analysis asserts that passions are constituted by evaluative beliefs. If, for instance, you resent what I have done to you, then you believe that I have inflicted some harm on you that I could reasonably have been expected to avoid. If you discover that the harm I did to you was a complete accident that I could not have been expected to avoid or foresee, your feeling toward me is not resentment.

A passion, however, is not simply an assent, but an immediate assent. This is a way of yielding (or "giving way") to an appearance, because we go along with our first impression of how things are (e.g., that the stick is bent, just as it appears). Sometimes we yield because the appearance comes on us without preparation. At other times we yield because we have not bothered to ask whether the appearance suggests the truth.[21]

The constituent belief in a passion makes the false assertion that a preferred indifferent is good, or a non-preferred indifferent is bad. According to the Stoics, virtue is the only good and vice is the only evil, because virtue is identical to happiness. What makes my life worth living cannot be sometimes good for me and sometimes bad for me; but other supposed goods apart from virtue are sometimes good for me (if I use them virtuously) and sometimes bad for me (if I fail to use them virtuously); hence they are not constituents of what makes my life worth living, and hence are not parts of happiness.[22] Since they do not matter to happiness, the Stoics call them indifferents; but since some are rationally preferable to others (e.g., health is preferable to sickness, in the right circumstances), some are preferred and others are non-preferred indifferents. A passion, therefore, is a false belief that exaggerates the importance of a preferred (or non-preferred) indifferent, because it treats it as part of what makes one's life worth living.[23,24]

Passions may conflict with reason.[25] We may form a belief on insufficient evidence, or without adding up the evidence correctly. And once we have formed it, we may stick to it because we are insensitive to counter-evidence. We think we follow our passions against our beliefs, because we do not recognize that we still believe that (say) we ought always to

[17] On the later use of "passion" see Kenny (1963); Levi (1964); James (1997).

[18] See Diogenes Laërtius vii 110–12; Cicero, *Tusculan Disputations* iv 10–15; *Academica* i 38–9; LS 65 C–D.

[19] Stobaeus, *Anthology* ii 88.1–12.

[20] Cicero, *Acad.* i 40; Diogenes Laërtius vii 177.

[21] On immediate opinions that last a long time see Cicero, *Tusc.* iii 74–5.

[22] On goods and indifferents: "The Peripatetics say that all the things they call goods contribute to living happily, whereas our school do not think the happy life is constituted by everything that deserves some value." (Cicero, *De Finibus* iii 41). See also Diogenes Laërtius vii 102–4.

[23] See the definitions of different passions in Cicero, *Tusc.* iv 14.

[24] Perhaps this point is suggested in LS 65 I.

[25] Cicero, *Off.* i 136; *Tusc.* iv 31.

avenge insults; this belief is so tenacious that, even when we think we no longer believe it, we find that we still believe it if we are insulted. We form such beliefs as we grow up, and they become ingrained in us. People who grasp the difference between goods and preferred indifferents get rid of their passions, but many people never grasp this difference, and so they are still subject to passions.

Life without passions

The Stoics believe that we ought not to harmonize our passions with reason, as Aristotle maintains; we ought to live without them altogether.[26] But we ought not to get rid of every element of a passion. We ought to avoid the mistaken assents, but we ought not to eliminate all the appearances that encourage foolish people to assent.[27] The appearance that it is bad for us to be poor, or ill, or bereaved, misleads us if we assent to its content, but it is useful if it leads us to believe truly that these things are non-preferred indifferents, and that normally we ought to avoid them. Wise people, therefore, do not try to eliminate appearances that tend to produce passions, but they interrogate and examine them, so as to draw true conclusion from them.[28]

Though Stoic sages are very rare, the rest of us can imitate their attitude to appearances. Passions tend to result from appearances that strongly suggest that something is good or bad and so encourage the immediate assent to its being good or bad. We can learn, however, to ask ourselves whether this particular object is good or bad, and we can learn to recognize when something is not good, but simply a preferred indifferent. We avoid the passion in so far as we avoid evaluative distortion.[29]

Once we recognize that the Stoics do not advise us to eliminate suggestive appearances, we might doubt whether they really advise us to eliminate passions. For if a Stoic sage in danger of shipwreck has a vivid appearance of impending death and goes pale (as the Stoics agree), is he not afraid of being shipwrecked?[30]

The Stoics answer No because they believe that when we act on our passions, our actions are voluntary, and are open to praise and blame.[31,32] This would not be true if passions were beyond our rational control. They are within our rational control to the extent that they are subject to our rational assent.[33] To the extent that we are responsible for acting on passions, we are not moved simply by suggestive appearances that are independent of our consent. Such appearances explain the goal-directed movements of non-rational animals and

---

[26] On the elimination of passions see Seneca, *Epistles*. 116.1.

[27] See Epictetus, quoted in Aulus Gellius, *Noctes Atticae* xix 1.17–18 (= Epictetus, fr. 9); Seneca, *Epistles* 71.27: "I do not remove the sage from among human beings, nor do I exclude feelings of distress (dolores) from him as from some rock that is incapable of any awareness (sensus)."

[28] On interrogation see Epictetus i 28.31; iii 8.1.

[29] Epictetus suggests that we have to be ready for the misleading suggestions that we may receive from appearances. See Epictetus i 27.6; ii 18.8–9.

[30] Augustine raises this question for the Stoics in *De Civitate Dei* ix 4.

[31] Aristotle criticizes people who try to evade responsibility for their actions by pleading that they acted on their non-rational desires (*EN* 1111a24–b3).

[32] Cicero, *Tusc.* iv 31.

[33] Cicero, *Tusc.* iv 14: Epictetus i 11.33.

of young children; hence these creatures are not responsible and have no passions, because they cannot assent to or dissent from appearances.[34] Since assent is the basis for responsibility and moral assessment, and since we are responsible for action on passion, action on passion requires assent.

We may not be convinced by the Stoic argument to show that passions are assents. It is worth comparing their view with views that distinguish passion from assent. But they are right to inquire into the relation between appearance and belief, and the feature of passions that makes them sources of responsible action. In their view, both these inquires vindicate the central place of assent in rational belief and action.

I have offered a sketch of a few elements of Stoic ethics and moral psychology. Its brevity and simplicity ignores the Stoics' arguments to show that their position is not as paradoxical as it may initially appear. But I have tried to defend the main point that is relevant to our main themes. Though the Stoics differ from Aristotle on the nature of the passions, they agree with his view that the conditions for mental health are the same as the conditions for moral virtue. We suffer from mental disorder and disturbance in so far as we suffer from delusions (cognitive error) or disordered emotions and desires (affective error). According to the Stoics, these sources of disturbance are not really distinct, because emotions are a type of cognitive error in response to an especially suggestive appearance. Like Plato and Aristotle, they have no room for a condition of mental health that falls short of moral virtue. The mentally healthy person sees the world as it is, and can act on this correct view. The Stoics claim that a correct view of the world includes a correct view of human beings and what is good for them; when we form that view and understand it, we are able to act on it, and we exercise that ability. In their view, as in the Platonic and Aristotelian view, once we understand why mental health is good for human beings, we understand why they need moral virtues.

References

Bobonich, C. (2002). *Plato's Utopia Recast*. Oxford: Oxford University Press.

Inwood, B. (1985). *Ethics and Human Action in Early Stoicism*. Oxford: Oxford University Press.

Irwin, T. H. (1995). *Plato's Ethics*. Oxford: Oxford University Press.

James, S. (1997). *Passion and Action*. Oxford: Oxford University Press.

Kenny, A. J. P. (1963). *Action, Emotion, and Will*. London: Routledge.

Kenny, A. J. P. (1973). Mental health in Plato's *Republic*. In *The Anatomy of the Soul*, pp. 1–27. Oxford: Blackwell.

Levi, A. (1964). *French Moralists*. Oxford: Oxford University Press.

Long, A. A. and Sedley, D. N. (1987). *The Hellenistic Philosophers* (2 vols). Cambridge: Cambridge University Press.

Lorenz, H. (2006). *The Brute Within*. Oxford: Oxford University Press.

McDowell, J. H. (1998). The role of *eudaimonia* in Aristotle's Ethics. In *Mind, Value, and Reality*, pp. 3–22. Cambridge, MA: Harvard University Press.

Nussbaum, M. C. (1994). *The Therapy of Desire*. Princeton, NJ: Princeton University Press.

Sorabji, R. R. K. (2000). *Emotion and Peace of Mind*. Oxford: Oxford University Press.

---

[34] Animals: Inwood (1985, ch. 3).

CHAPTER 5

....

ARISTOTLE, PLATO, AND THE ANTI-PSYCHIATRISTS: COMMENT ON IRWIN

....

EDWARD HARCOURT

Two things leap to the eye about the Platonic–Aristotelian account of mental health and mental illness Irwin sets out.[1] The first is that it is in a way very modern. For like Freud's and post-Freudian psychodynamic accounts of mental illness, it both seeks to explain mental illness in terms of conflict between parts or functions of the mind and, insofar as it does so, places the normal and the pathological on a continuum. Moreover—and now in contrast to psychodynamic accounts, many of which are allergic to any mention of morality except in a reductive or skeptical spirit—the continuum connects not only mental health and mental illness but also virtue and vice. On this view, to be maximally mentally healthy is to be virtuous, and to be maximally mentally ill, vicious. This is a controversial claim whether it is taken in (as Irwin puts it) a "reductive" or an "inflationary" direction, and in either direction it has strong echoes in modern philosophy of psychiatry. For the agenda of modern philosophy of psychiatry has to a significant extent been set by Szasz's (1962) *The Myth of Mental Illness*, one of whose signature ideas is that psychiatry misclassifies ethical problems as medical ones. If the claim is that mental illness be "inflated" to vice, Plato and Aristotle come out as robust anti-psychiatrists; if taken "reductively," on the other hand, theirs is the kind of conclusion that anti-psychiatrists object to, namely that to be morally imperfect is, after all, "only" a way of being mentally ill. At least in Aristotle—who will be my main focus in these brief remarks—there is more inflation than reduction. But even if that is so, I also suspect the Platonic–Aristotelian moral psychology which Irwin sets out does not contain the materials for a comprehensive philosophy of mental disorder.

---

[1] In what follows I shall have more to say about Aristotle than about Plato, partly because (as Irwin shows) Aristotle's theory of mental health is more subtle than Plato's, partly because to the extent that the philosophy of psychiatry has taken notice of ancient thought, it has tended to take more notice of Aristotle (see, e.g., Cooper 2007; Megone 1998, 2000; Pickard 2009, 2011a). I can excuse myself from commenting on Irwin's treatment of the Stoics only on grounds of ignorance.

One question which arises for the Platonic–Aristotelian account, and which Irwin himself raises, is whether mental health is as strongly connected to mental "unity"—that is, absence of conflict—as Plato and Aristotle say. Assuming that health is a good state for the subject to be in, it surely cannot consist *simply* in unity since, as Bradley pointed out (1876/1990), unity can be achieved by shedding desires (or loyalties, commitments, etc.), at the limit to just one, but "it is no human ideal to lead 'the life of an oyster.'" Moreover, it has been argued that the capacity to tolerate certain kinds of conflict—for example, positive and negative attitudes toward the same object—is a better state of mind than unity won at the cost of purging one or other conflicting attitude: for example, love combined with an awareness of the loved one's imperfections, or with the ability to express angry or destructive feelings toward the loved one when they arise, is a more realistic and therefore a better form of love than its idealizing counterpart (Klein 1988, p. 72). The Aristotelian might reply that a capacity for this kind of ambivalence is precisely what "unity" means in this context, but this move preserves the link between health and unity at the price of giving away the link between either and the absence of conflict—surely a fruitful topic for further discussion.

To turn now to the claim that mental illness is vice, we surely cannot identify psychiatric disorders without a conception of what counts as an emotion (or reaction, thought, etc.) that's *appropriate* to cause and context: this is the burden of Allen Horwitz's moderately anti-psychiatric critique of the *Diagnostic and Statistical Manual of Mental Disorders* (DSM)-III and -IV's almost entirely context-free, symptom-based diagnostic criteria (Horwitz 2002).[2] But of course it is Aristotle who says that "both fear and confidence and appetite and anger and pity and in general pleasure and pain may be felt both too much and too little" and that "to feel them at the right times, with reference to the right objects, towards the right people, with the right aim, and in the right way … is characteristic of excellence"—that is, of virtue (*Nicomachean Ethics* (*NE*) 1106b, Bollingen online edition, p. 1747).[3] So far so good, then, for an anti-psychiatric reading of Aristotle. But to say that schizophrenia or bipolar disorder both differ from Aristotelian virtue in respect of the appropriateness of their characteristic mental states to their causes and context falls short of saying that they lie on a continuum with virtue, and thereby also with weakness of will and vice: where on the continuum might that be? This raises the question whether Plato and Aristotle should really be credited with the claim that mental illness should be "inflated" into vice, at least in unqualified form.

Notice that Plato and Aristotle's explicit focus is on mental health, not mental illness. Now there is a way of using the term "mental health" in such a way that anyone who is not mentally healthy is mentally ill and vice versa. On the other hand, the World Health Organization (WHO) defines "health"—for better or worse—as "a state of complete physical, mental, and social well-being and not merely the absence of disease or infirmity."[4] With

---

[2] "People whose symptoms fluctuate with the emergence and dissipation of stressful social circumstances are psychologically normal."; cf. Horwitz and Wakefield (2007).

[3] In maintaining that getting it right in these respects is the work of *reason*, Aristotle is ahead of Horwitz, whose claim that to count as a mental illness it should arise "in the absence of any cause that would *expectably* give rise" to it (Horwitz 2002, p. 98, my italics) rules out far too much: what he needs is the notion of a *rational* relation to its causes.

[4] "WHO definition of Health" in Preamble to the Constitution of the World Health Organization as adopted by the International Health Conference, New York, 19–22 June, 1946; entered into force on 7 April 1948. Cited in Murphy (2009).

a multicomponent definition of "health" such as this, there may be many distinct (though possibly complementary) ways of failing to be healthy, not all of which will consist in being ill, and the same I take it goes for "mental health." Thus if what Plato and Aristotle meant was something comparable in inclusiveness to "complete mental well-being," might their account of how mental health can be compromised—in terms of degrees of defection from rational control and thereby from "unity"—not be just one of several possible complementary accounts, and therefore leave out much that we are inclined to count as mental illness?[5]

So what did they mean? Plato and Aristotle do after all talk about "madness" as well as about mental health (Plato, for example, in the *Phaedrus*, where he distinguishes between divinely inspired madness—his main topic—from madness which is "an evil" (244a); Aristotle in the *Problemata*[6]). Do these discussions reveal that they are thinking about madness, in so far as they see it as a bad thing, in terms of mental disunity (that is, as the contrary of mental health as they understand it), or as a different way of failing to be mentally healthy? In Aristotle, at least, there seems to be no simple answer. Interestingly, "madness" is mentioned in Book VII of the *Nicomachean Ethics*, in the context of Aristotle's discussion of incontinence or weak will which—as Irwin makes clear—is a topic of central importance to his account of how mental health can be compromised. In one passage, the states of being "asleep, mad or drunk" (*NE* 1147a10–23, Bollingen online edn. p. 1812) are said to exemplify the state of knowing and yet not knowing the premises of a practical syllogism which (in Aristotle's view) typifies the weak-willed, and passion is said to be a cause both of weak will and of madness. Here, then, it looks as if Aristotle is indeed thinking about madness in terms of mental disunity—i.e. in terms of the same moral psychology which underlies his account of vice and virtue. Later on in the same book, however, Aristotle describes the way in which things "not naturally pleasant ... become so through disease or madness ... as with the man who sacrificed and ate his mother, or the slave who ate the liver of his fellow" (*NE* 1148b25–30). *These* states, he says, are "beyond the limits of vice": although his main-line (dis)unity story is not completely silent about them (because these diseased tendencies can in some people be controlled, and so when such people fail to control them, we have incontinence), something further has gone wrong in such cases that isn't captured by the (dis)unity story, and this marks a gap between the "morbid or brutish wickedness" which they exemplify and ordinary wickedness, that is, the state as distant as possible from mental health on the Platonic–Aristotelian continuum which constitutes Irwin's main focus.

But now, the "slave who ate the liver of his fellow" was surely mentally ill. So it doesn't look as if everything we now call mental illness can be theorized in terms of Aristotle's (or Plato's) (dis)unity story. This is not, however, to be taken as an objection to Aristotle. On the contrary, the second *NE* passage quoted earlier is surely evidence that Aristotle *himself* did

[5] Cf. Irwin's reflections on whether vice, as well as illness, is bad for the agent rather than just bad for others: even if vice and illness do have this feature in common, it takes more to show that vice *is* illness, since there might be many ways for a state to be bad (or good) for its possessor (as the WHO definition of "health" suggests).

[6] Reprinted in Radden, J. (ed.) (2000). *The Nature of Melancholy: From Aristotle to Kristeva*, pp. 55–60. Oxford: Oxford University Press. The work may be by a follower rather than by Aristotle himself.

not intend the (dis)unity story to be a theory of everything that compromises mental health, and this is surely a virtue given the sheer diversity (Fulford et al. 2006, p. 9) of the phenomena labeled "mental disorders."[7] The passage is thus a warning both to contemporary opponents of Aristotle not to criticize him for what he doesn't say, and to contemporary friends not to try to do too much with what he does say.

Of course to say Aristotle doesn't provide a total theory of mental illness is not to say he does not provide a true partial theory, and some psychiatric conditions seem much more amenable to treatment in terms of the moral psychology underlying the (dis)unity story than others. Criteria for Cluster B personality disorders—which includes borderline and antisocial personality disorder—include impulsivity, lack of empathy, and dishonesty (Charland 2004, p. 71; Pickard 2009) that is, the absence of some central virtues (in the examples I have given, temperance and truthfulness: empathy is more complicated, in that it looks more like an underlying psychological trait that is necessary for some virtues, than like a virtue itself). Whether these absences constitute vice or, rather, incontinence presumably varies from case to case,[8] but either way a set of conditions currently classified as psychiatric disorders apparently belong squarely on the Aristotelian continuum Irwin describes.

Should the identification of mental illness with vice be taken in a reductive direction, with the implication that these personality disorders are to be seen as something to be got rid of rather than understood—as, in Bernard Williams's phrase, a set of "happenings outside one's moral self"[9]—or perhaps that those with the conditions are not responsible for their actions (Pickard 2011a)? Since the concepts of virtue and vice are so central to Aristotle's ethics, he can scarcely have intended to demonstrate their theoretical redundancy, so this reductionist view is surely not Aristotle's. Diametrically opposed to this is the view which takes the reduction in the opposite direction—that because they are moral conditions, they are not medical ones (Charland 2004, p. 64).

One neo-Aristotelian strategy for finding a middle way between these extremes is to rely on the idea, associated with Philippa Foot, that vice is a "natural defect" in humans, that is, a feature that prevents someone who has it from leading the life characteristic of creatures of its kind: night-blindness in owls is one of Foot's examples (Foot 2002). This might be thought to strengthen the connection between vice and illness without showing the theoretical redundancy of the former concept, since illnesses sound like (sometimes remediable)

---

[7] This is not to say that Aristotle had nothing to say about those aspects of mental ill-health not theorized by the structural theory. Thus in the *Physiognomics* he claims that "it is obvious that every modification of [the body] involves a modification of [the soul]. The best instance of this is to be found in manic insanity. Mania, it is generally allowed, is a condition of the soul, yet doctors cure it partly by administering purgative drugs to the body, partly by prescribing, besides these, certain courses of diet. Thus the result of proper treatment of the body is that they succeed, and that too simultaneously, not only in altering the physical condition, but also in curing the soul of mania; and the fact that the changes are simultaneous proves that the sympathetic modifications of body and soul are thoroughly concomitant," 808b11–26, Bollingen edn., p. 1242. Aristotle is talking *en psychiatre* here, but (dis)unity and the moral psychology that goes with that are nowhere to be seen.

[8] Pickard's observation that "it is likely that a borderline patient will only embark on therapy if they [believe] … that it is right to moderate and control their anger" (2009, p. 97) suggests that, at least at this stage in the evolution of their condition, the right answer is "incontinence" since there is disagreement between their rational and non-rational parts.

[9] This is the burden of Charles Taylor's objection to the "therapeutic turn" (Taylor 2007, pp. 619–21). The phrase from Williams occurs at "A Critique of Utilitarianism" (Smart and Williams 1973, p. 104).

natural defects.[10] The trouble is that it is not clear that the notion of the kind of life characteristic of human beings can be specified in such a way as to make available an account of vice in these terms that is both substantial and true. The ability to keep to agreements is arguably necessary for us to lead our characteristic kind of life, but just because it's as necessary to honest dealers as it is to confederates in an interest-rate fraud, the ability to keep agreements per se cannot be a virtue (or the absence of it a vice), but rather some more general kind of psychological capacity that underlies both some virtues and some vices. The same seems to go for the capacity to form attachments to particular others, which can undo people's lives as well as enrich them. So the characteristics necessary for our species life are less determinate than the virtues. If on the other hand "our species life" is—implausibly—defined in such a way that what's needed for it is the ability (say) to keep agreements only in so far as this is used for *good* ends, the notion of our species life is not prior to the idea of virtue, and so cannot illuminate it in the way Foot's proposal intends.[11]

However, finding a middle way need not rely on Foot's proposal. Personality disorders can be both states of a person's moral character and candidates for treatment, since there is no reason to limit the conception of "treatment" to techniques for merely getting rid of them: indeed as Hanna Pickard has argued, because it addresses problems of character, therapy for personality disorder may have much in common with the normal processes of character formation as Aristotle conceived them, including "reflection on who one would like to become."[12]

Whether or not these comments are on target, Irwin's paper brings to light the continuities between the broad themes of contemporary moral psychology and the more specialist area of philosophy of psychiatry, and suggests that anyone interested in the latter has as much reason to turn to Plato, Aristotle, and the Stoics as students of the former are already acknowledged to do.

References

Aristotle (1984). Nicomachean ethics. In J. Barnes (Ed.), *Complete Works of Aristotle, Volume 2: The Revised Oxford Translation* (Bollingen online edition), pp. 1729–867. Princeton, NJ: Princeton University Press.

Aristotle (1984). Physiognomics. In J. Barnes (Ed.), *Complete Works of Aristotle, Volume 1: The Revised Oxford Translation* (Bollingen online edition), pp. 1237–50. Princeton, NJ: Princeton University Press.

Aristotle (2000). Problemata. In J. Radden (Ed.), *The Nature of Melancholy: From Aristotle to Kristeva*, pp. 55–60. Oxford: Oxford University Press.

Bradley, F. H. (1990). *Ethical Studies*. Bristol: Thoemmes. (Original work published 1876.)

Charland, L. (2004). Moral treatment and the personality disorders. In J. Radden (Ed.), *The Philosophy of Psychiatry: A Companion*, pp. 64–77. Oxford: Oxford University Press.

---

[10] See Pickard (2011b) though Pickard differs from Foot's model in that what's under discussion is the "life worth living" rather than "species life."

[11] In fact I think the first horn of the dilemma is the correct one to embrace, though it is not helpful to Foot's proposal: see Harcourt (2012).

[12] Pickard (2009); cf. Aristotle *NE* 1128b (Bollingen online edn p. 1781), where shame is described as an appropriate emotion only for learners.

Cooper, R. (2007). *Psychiatry and Philosophy of Science.* Montreal: McGill-Queen's University Press.

Foot, P. (2002). *Natural Goodness.* Oxford: Oxford University Press.

Fulford, K. W. M., Thornton, T., and Graham, G. (Eds) (2006). *Oxford Textbook of Philosophy and Psychiatry.* Oxford: Oxford University Press.

Harcourt, E. (2012). Attachment theory, character and naturalism. In J. Peters (Ed.), *Aristotelian Ethics in Contemporary Perspective*, pp. 114–29. Routledge: London.

Horwitz, A. W. (2002). *Creating Mental Illness.* Chicago, IL: University of Chicago Press.

Horwitz, A. W. and Wakefield, J. (2007). *The Loss of Sadness.* Oxford: Oxford University Press.

Klein, M. (1988). Some theoretical conclusions regarding the emotional life of the infant. In *Envy and Gratitude*, pp. 61–93. London: Virago.

Megone, C. (1998). Aristotle's function argument and the concept of mental illness. *Philosophy, Psychiatry, & Psychology, 5*(3), 187–201.

Megone, C. (2000). Mental illness, human function, and values. *Philosophy, Psychiatry, & Psychology, 7*(1), 45–65.

Murphy, D. (2009). Concepts of disease and health. In E. N. Zalta (Ed.) *The Stanford Encyclopedia of Philosophy* (Summer 2009 Edition). [Online.] Available at: <http://plato.stanford.edu/archives/sum2009/entries/health-disease/>.

Pickard, H. (2009). Mental illness is indeed a myth. In L. Bortolotti and M. Broome (Eds), *Psychiatry as Cognitive Science: Philosophical Perspectives*, pp. 83–101. Oxford: Oxford University Press.

Pickard, H. (2011a). Responsibility without blame: empathy and the effective treatment of personality disorder. *Philosophy, Psychiatry, & Psychology, 18*(3), 209–24.

Pickard, H. (2011b). *What Aristotle Can Teach Us About Personality Disorder.* [Online.] Available at: <http://www.personalitydisorder.org.uk/2011/05/2208/>.

Szasz, T. (1962). *The Myth of Mental Illness.* London: Secker & Warburg.

Taylor, C. (2007). *A Secular Age.* Cambridge, MA: Belknap Press.

Williams, B. (1973). A critique of utilitarianism. In J. J. C. Smart and B. Williams (Eds), *Utilitarianism: For and Against*, pp. 75–150. Cambridge: Cambridge University Press.

CHAPTER 6

....

WILHELM GRIESINGER: PHILOSOPHY AS THE ORIGIN OF A NEW PSYCHIATRY

....

KATHERINE ARENS

PHYSICIAN, PSYCHIATRIST, AND PRACTICAL INNOVATOR

....

Wilhelm Griesinger (b. July 29, 1817 in Stuttgart, Germany; d. October 26, 1868 in Berlin, Germany) figures prominently in today's histories of medicine and psychiatry as an innovator whose work pointed the way to modern-day psychiatric clinical practice, to advances in neuropathology, and to modern strategies for the diagnostics of mental diseases. His institutional leadership helped to professionalize medical practice and research as he modernized clinic design and therapeutic strategies, established mental illness as a public health issue, wrote textbooks, and helped found journals and professional organizations that exist to this day.

Griesinger studied at Tübingen (a home for what is called Romantic medicine, based on speculative nature philosophy), Paris (with physiologist François Magendie), and the University of Zurich (with Johann Lukas Schönlein) before he receiving his medical degree in 1838; later study trips included Paris and Vienna. After returning to Tübingen's university medical clinic in 1843, he finished his teaching credential (*Habilitation*) and was appointed *Privatdozent* for pathology, *materia medica*, and the history of medicine. In 1845, he published the first edition of his most important work: *Mental Pathology and Therapeutics* (originally *Die Pathologie und Therapie der psychischen Krankheiten*; 1865 in French and 1867 in English), a work synthesizing psychiatry and medical pathology in ways that reformed treatment of mental illness in the west. By 1847, he was promoted to *Außerordentlicher Professor* and made editor of the *Archiv für physiologische Heilkunde*.

His growing reputation led to various leadership positions: first, as director for the university clinic in Kiel (1849), and then, in 1850, as head of the Cairo medical school (and to act as personal physician for Abbas I, Wāli of Egypt and Sudan). His two years there provided material for two important treatises on tropical diseases—*Klinische und anatomische Beobachtungen über die Krankheiten von Aegypten*, published in 1854, and *Infectionskrankheiten: Malariakrankheiten, Gelbes Fieber, Typhus, Pest, Cholera*, in 1857. By 1854, he was appointed professor (*Ordinarius*) of clinical medicine and head of the Tübingen clinic; in 1859, he moved on to head the *Heil- und Erziehungsanstalt Mariaberg bei Gammertingen* (Württemberg), one of the first institutions for children and youth with mental disabilities. Starting in 1860, when he was appointed to the Zurich clinic in the division for internal medicine, he was involved in planning Zurich's Burghölzli mental hospital, which opened in 1865. By that time, he had already moved to Berlin as director of the Polyclinic, the *Charité I*, when this mental institution (now named after him) was modernized to include positions in neurology. His chair for psychiatry and neurology (starting in 1865) was the first of its kind in Germany. Just before his premature death in 1868 of perityphlitis and diphtheria, he founded two important journals for psychiatry: *Medicinisch-psychologische Gesellschaft* (1867) and the *Archiv für Psychiatrie und Nervenkrankheiten* (1867), editing the first volume of the latter himself before his death.

Griesinger in the History of Medicine

The history of medicine remembers Griesinger's eminent career for his reforms to the treatment of mental illness and of the asylum system. He theorized that the mentally ill needed to be reintegrated into society and so limited their hospitalization and worked instead in developing other support systems to continue their care. He also integrated psychiatry as a practice with physiology and medicine, decisively redefining it as a science rather than a moral therapeutics. Thus his work echoes the latter nineteenth-century program of characterizing the symptomology of mental diseases and improving diagnostics by correlating theories about disease with empiricist observation (as was characteristic of Vienna's medical school)—first, with observation of the brain and nervous system, but then also of social behavior, acknowledging how diseases presented themselves in multiple forms.

Earlier histories present him more as a synthesizer than an innovator, a situation explained by Otto M. Marx in "Wilhelm Griesinger and the history of psychiatry: A reassessment" (1972). His study of the historical accounts of Griesinger's work, especially the necrologies, showed how Griesinger's premature death left his image open and subject to editing. Many of these texts attest that, by his death, Griesinger was beginning to look anachronistic because he was not an experimentalist in the modern sense using laboratory experiments on the body/mind interface.[1] Late in the nineteenth century, Richard Freiherr von Krafft-Ebing identified him only as a neuropathologist and empirical psychologist, thus solidifying his reputation as a clinician of diseases of the brain, without much further claim to relevance for psychology or philosophy (although decisive in redefining psychiatry as more than moral practice).

---

[1] For an example of how a psychological laboratory functioned in the era, see Andreas Mayer, *Mikroskopie der Psyche: Die Anfänge der Psychoanalyse im Hypnose-Labor* (2002).

Griesinger's twentieth-century reputation did not improve. He was, for instance, left out of Edwin G. Boring's influential standard *A History of Experimental Psychology* (1929/1950), a text that defined experimentalism as laboratory-based, not based on clinical observation. A "renaissance" set in after 1985 with Henri Ellenberger's *The Discovery of the Unconscious* (1970) and its brief, mainly biographical note that goes to the other extreme, slighting Griesinger's clinical reputation and stressing instead how he integrated neurology into psychology and psychiatry. Klaus Doerner's influential *Madman and the Bourgeoisie: A Social History of Insanity and Psychiatry* (1969/1981) recaptures Griesinger's innovation in a socio-political dimension, tying his work into the general climate of social unrest and change of the mid century in Europe as part of the era's work of "practical change" (p. 273), in his rewrite of asylum practice as humane. Like Ellenberger, Doerner slights Griesinger's work in neuropathology and neurology, dismissing it as "medical" work without pursuing the question of how it integrated with social psychology (p. 273). Still, it was Doerner's Griesinger who turned psychiatry into both a science and a social science, mixing theory and practice in integrating a modern materialism (empiricism) into a new asylum practice heretofore heavily influenced by notions of moral improvement as defined in England.

The assessment of Griesinger's work and impact improved dramatically in the 1980s. Bettina Wahrig-Schmidt, in *Der junge Wilhelm Griesinger im Spannungsfeld zwischen Philosophie und Physiologie* (1985) and an article from *Klassiker der Medizin* (1987), places Griesinger more firmly within the era's intellectual life by tracing his personal and intellectual biographies as keys to his professional engagement, and then by outlining his systematic approach to mental illness as indeed scientific. Other contributions that originated in theses or dissertations, most notably by Hedwig Gisela Engels (1983), Gerald Detlafs (1993), and Kai Sammet (1997), reclaim Griesinger's practical contributions to social psychiatry. They show how radical he was considered to be as he battled the political climates that resisted more humane and palliative-developmental approaches to treatment and socialization of disturbed individuals, working against the restraint and punishment strategies used in moral-based asylum cultures. Katherine Arens (1996) recast Griesinger's model of mind as existing in the philosophical tradition out of which psychology originated, extending from Kant, Herder, and Hegel into the twentieth century; she argues his work as more modern than Freud and as anticipating Jacques Lacan.

In *Psychiatry in an Anthropological and Biomedical Context* (1980/1985), Gerlof Verwey most significantly recasts Griesinger's contribution to the philosophy of medicine at the time by showing how he redefined medicine's institutional position, placing it next to the sciences rather than considering it a kind of moral-social practice. Verwey's Griesinger rejected Lotze and Herbart's extreme cognitivist positions (known as the *Psychiker*) because they overemphasized the mind's contribution in their psychological models, privileging consciousness as the seat of identity and knowledge rather than the body or society. At the same time, the Young Hegelian left was concerned about Kant's identification of science with materialism or empiricism (his purported "somaticism" (Verwey 1980/1985, p. 41)), which would render psychiatry almost completely subservient to scientific medicine.

In his later book, *Wilhelm Griesinger: Psychiatrie als ärztlicher Humanismus* (2004), Verwey brings his Griesinger story a chapter further, moving far beyond Doerner in valorizing Griesinger's asylum practice and providing an elegant, magisterial overview of this work as appropriate to a liberal Biedermeier intellectual engaged in all facets of public life. This Griesinger appears as a multifaceted medical professional whose theoretical work culminates in the 1861 second edition of his textbook, when he engages in a second intense period of clinical psychiatric research. That text stresses the symptomology of mental illness recovered by means of a "methdologicial naturalism" rather than experimentalism (Verwey 2004, p. 18), with diagnoses that respect anatomy and neuropathology as well as personal situation. In this reading, Griesinger's physician has an important role as a scientist and as an observer of the patient, looking for therapy and cure in social rehabilitation rather than in English-style moral treatment. Critically, this Griesinger moved beyond the era's attempt to find a uniform, rigid treatment for mental diseases (seen as themselves uniform, as *Einheitspsychose* (p. 44)), and toward the recognition that observable symptoms might actually derive from a variety of somatic causes. He moved away from formulaics and traced mental diseases as stemming from individuals' experiences and their facility in making representations (much as Freud redefined the study of dreams). Thus Griesinger (cited by Freud[2]) turns to therapy and reform in social context and correlates the soma to mental illness. In this framing, the material world (including such social institutions as religion (p. 73)) produces illness in individuals, and so it may require critique as disease-producing.

Overall these assessments are still marked by twentieth- and twenty-first-century assumptions about what science meant in the nineteenth century. They undervalue the influence of a central institutional fact: that psychology was still part of philosophy in Griesinger's era (see Arens 1989), making it virtually impossible to locate scholars' rigidly defined *Somatiker* and *Psychiker*—theorists espousing respectively bodily and mental origins for mental disease—within any contemporaneous medical or practical contexts. Today, it is more productive to understand the philosophical bases for Griesinger's work in early twentieth-century traditions more familiar from the work of Marburg Neokantians like Ernst Cassirer, who saw mind as both making determinate contributions to knowledge and as situated empirically and historically within social networks. This Griesinger emerges more overtly as a Left Hegelian in his politics and as a professional wedding theory and praxis in recovering the politics of historical experience in the formation of the individual subject.

Griesinger's generation was sensitized to tensions between "speculative philosophy" and "scientific empiricism," and accommodated both poles, which led his work to be rejected by the Nazis and classified as philosophy (Doerner 1969/1981, p. 275). This rejection clearly stemmed from Griesinger's insistence on a healthy environment for mental wellness, which would weaken claims for eugenics. Similarly, Binswanger stated that Griesinger's work represented the "psychology of the understanding," but refused to acknowledge how central Griesinger's historical sociology or anthropology was to psychological models of the day.

Reclaiming Griesinger for Philosophy

Following a broader history of philosophy and science allows us to situate Griesinger within German Idealism and tie him more closely to philosophy through his influential masterpiece, *Mental Pathology and Therapeutics*, arguably the era's most famous psychiatric

---

[2] Freud cites Griesinger explicitly as late as 1911, in his "Formulations on the Two Principles of Mental Functioning." Freud's teacher, Meynert, was known to have admired Griesinger's work. See also O. M. Marx, Nineteenth-century medical psychology (1970).

textbook. Despite disagreements about the degree of their relevance, Immanuel Kant, Johann Friedrich Herbart, and Georg W. F. Hegel are generally acknowledged among Griesinger's sources. Their contributions need to be seen as grounding various facets of Griesinger's enterprise.

Despite Kant's reputation as a transcendental idealist based on his three *Critiques* (*Critique of Pure Reason* (1781/1787/1998), *Critique of Practical Reason* (1787/1996), and *Critique of Judgment* (1790/2000)), his work extends into the practical sphere, as well, demonstrating how the mind yields knowledge in historical contexts.[3] For instance, Kant offers a practical psychology of individual experience in his *Anthropology from a Pragmatic Point of View* (a set of university lectures first delivered in the academic year 1772–1773). His anthropology traces how historically observable human behavior affects the mind's basic operations. In so doing, Kant rejected the eighteenth-century "faculty psychology" that organized the capacities of the mind topographically and structurally, each area of the mind having a fixed and discrete task in producing human knowledge and behavior. Kant stressed instead how the mind's fundamental capacities rest on a biological substrate in the brain that functions as an a priori for all mental acts, yet also how each individual mind will nonetheless adapt and change as it is influenced by history, culture, and environment.

Kant's redefinition of mind also makes the human mind social in its essence, since minds interact with each other and pass on cultural legacies every bit as determining as nature. Not only do the capacities of an individual mind and body affect how knowledge is generated, group experience, culture, and history also influence mind and its products. Human cognitive capacities evolve synchronically, as a set of relationships to context conditioned by appetite and aversion (*Lust und Unlust*), and to volition (*Begehrungsvermögen*), as supported by the individual's contact with the group (Kant 1980, pp. 10–11). Mind and body also evolve diachronically, as the group's experiences from its cultural locus change across time, forcing their minds and bodies to adapt. Knowledge is thus not just transcendental (as cognitivist Kantians would assume), but also contingent on the subject's position in history. Each individual mind develops synchronically as it interacts with its environment (natural and cultural) and diachronically as it interacts with its past (both personal and cultural-historical). Kant's model of the mind is thus also dynamic rather than structural-static, as the individual evolves an inner sense of experience and self, affected by intellect and physical experience: "Inner sense is not pure apperception, a consciousness of what man *does*, for this belongs to the capacity for thinking; but rather [a consciousness] of that which he *undergoes*, as far as he is affected by his own play of thoughts" (Kant 1980, p. 31). The psychology that grew out of it accounts for acts of cognition and those of volition exercised by mind in the world, thus tying an individual's mind and physical organism to the surrounding group, as well.

Fifty years before Griesinger, Johann Friedrich Herbart (1776–1841), a dissenter to Kantianism who assumed his academic chair in Königsberg, nonetheless picked up the central tenets of Kant's model to innovate in another dimension. Not only did Herbart explore how the mind reacted to historical and social contexts as it evolved its sense of self and cognitive abilities, he also pursued a practical pedagogy that could foster this evolution. Herbart's

---

[3] The recent translations by a team headed by Paul Guyer should now be considered the editions of record: *Critique of Pure Reason* (Kant 1998), "Critique of practical reason," included in *Practical Philosophy* (Kant 1996), and the newly renamed *Critique of the Power of Judgment* (Kant 2000).

work modeled how physiological and psychological *training* (not only experience) could contribute to an individual's psyche, as that individual's mind and self are conditioned by its body's physical restrictions and capacities: what an individual knows will relate to what that individual's body can perceive. Herbart used a physiological-mathematical approach to how mind constructs knowledge and self, explicated in two important books: the *Textbook of Psychology* (*Lehrbuch der Psychologie*) (1816/1834) and *Psychology as a Science* (*Psychologie als Wissenschaft*) (1824). This model of mind stresses its dynamic and affective responses, based on both memory and current sense data, under the constraints of individual physiology and environmental input (cultural and historical).

Herbart models the mind as a system seeking equilibrium and the maintenance of identity through automatized cognitive, affective, and physiological responses (Herbart 1964a, p. 374). Thus for Herbart as for Kant, the study of mind becomes not only a study of the brain, but also of ego, the *ich* (Herbart 1964b, p. 251), and of how a community reinforces individuals' psychological traits. At the same time, Herbart's educational psychology highlights the significance of the body: well-balanced minds are healthy, but their continued equilibria will depend on their physical dispositions and their affective responses to experience and learning, as well. The teacher must work with the students' minds on their own terms rather than imposing a normative path towards learning. Anticipating Montessori methods, Herbart's pedagogues strive through experience to increase students' facility in the association of ideas, and thus their flexibility in mental function.

The third of Griesinger's philosophical progenitors was Hegel, who generalized how individual minds come to consciousness and knowledge of the world, in a dialectical confrontation between the individual's psyche and new experience. As the mind confronts its environment, a culture's past becomes present as the mind confronts its own new present experiences. For the 1848 generation of which Griesinger was a member, Hegel's model of history represented everyday life as a series of such confrontations. In them, an individual mind strives towards liberation within the group and control over the knowledge of history, seeking expression for new experiences within the framework of inherited knowledge and individual ability. Finding such expression means that the mind has achieved a synthesis and avoided being "unhappy," transcending its boundedness and its subjection to incoming experience and freeing itself to move forward in consciousness, as Hegel outlined in the *Phenomenology of Mind*. Hegel's work led Griesinger (as it would Marx) to a model of how individual mind is determined by its environment, its own past, and (in mediated form) the past of its own culture. In the healthy individual mind, each such confrontation forces a synthesis and changes the equilibrium of the mind, learning from experience and mastering it.

This Herbartian reading of Hegel goes further than Hegel did in pursuing individual psychology, while Herbart's focus on the individual occluded the political implications of ongoing confrontations with history, as Hegel stressed. It was left to Wilhelm Griesinger to take up these threads and join them in his reformation of medical treatment for the mentally ill. He took not only the humanistic and political impulses of his generation into the asylum, but a new image of mind as a balance between history and the present, between new experience and inherited and established habit—an innovation for which Sigmund Freud is usually given credit. Yet where Freud would see that confrontation as a confrontation between a determinate organic individual and the culture limiting him (the id and the superego in conflict, to be resolved by the emergence of a functional ego-identity), Griesinger values both the individual and the role of community in creating an individual's identity and mental stability.

Griesinger's Psychiatry: A New Philosophy of Disease

Griesinger's most influential work, his textbook *Mental Pathology and Therapeutics*,[4] was from the first acknowledged as standing at the junction of medicine and philosophy. His translators call his work "medico-metaphysics" in their foreword: a scientific metaphysics of the mind combined with a practical, empirically tested medical therapeutics. Griesinger's own introduction situates his work at the juncture between clinical or medical psychology (aimed at improving clinical therapeutics) and university psychology (then, a more speculative field, too often associated with an abstract reading of Hegel, associated with "that fantastical bombast, sounding of the spiritual world, which is still sometimes apparent in psychological literature" rather than medical observation (Griesinger 1882, p. vi).

Medical history remembers Griesinger's eloquence in linking the brain and mental disease. Yet his own argumentation reaches beyond mechanical models correlating disease with physical damage or malfunction. Nor does he localize mental powers like the will in any specific brain structure, as physiologically based theories would. Instead, Griesinger reads brain structure in terms of function, acknowledging that certain areas of the brain are most active in *processing* of certain types of stimuli yet not localizing processing in any one area. "Higher-order functions of mind" like will and memory do not exist structurally, but only as heuristics for complex combinations of simple brain functions. Empirically, one can ascertain only what sections of the brain are at work in processing stimuli, but not what type of work is actually being done. Consequently, an individual brain may be active in the same regions while willing or evincing moral sense, but that observation does not exhaust what else might be going on in the brain: "While we are forced by facts to refer understanding and will to the brain, still, however, nothing can be assumed as to the relation existing between these mental acts and the brain, the relation of soul to material" (Griesinger 1882, p. 4). Mental acts and mental illness, will and reason, correlate with organic function, but are not identical with the organism's structure alone.

Griesinger thus attributes to mind a significant complexity, upholding Hegel's premise of knowledge being a product of an interaction between mind and environment, as well as Herbart's emphasis on the plasticity of mind, which assumes that the brain and body limit the mind organically and as part of a historical locus, but do not constrain it. Griesinger has thus recast the mind/brain problem in more than mechanical or structural terms; anatomy cannot answer "unanswerable questions" about "imponderables" (Griesinger 1882, p. 5). To be sure, anatomy is a necessary starting point for descriptions of mental diseases, but not a sufficient source for diagnostics in the modern sense. All brain diseases, after all, do not manifest as mental pathology or illness; some have physical ailments as their symptoms. At the same time, some brain diseases do affect mind function and cause mental pathologies.

---

[4] Cited here in the 1882 edition of the 1867 translation from the second German edition.

In outlining the etiology of individual mental illnesses, Griesinger pursues how mental disease can be caused by an individual's soul (his term for the interior life of an individual), as that soul is constructed and challenged in a confrontation with culture and experience (Griesinger 1882, p. 5). In his approach to diagnostics, the mind stands in a dynamic relationship with the brain and also in dialectical relationships with the world and its own past experience (cultural and personal). He finds in the various external signs of such relationships evidence of the mind's negotiations between the self (a preserved mass of older experience) and current experience. Medical judgments about that mind's wellness or illness, in turn, rest on the physician's observations of the individual's negotiations with environmental stimuli (be they natural or social in origin). Mental illness is a state of persistent failure in such negotiations, a persistent inability of the individual to function normally within the observable parameters of the group.

Griesinger will expand that notion of function far beyond a mechanical model, and especially beyond moralistic approaches to mental illness. Using normative moral standards to judge behavior as signs of mental illness will be particularly ineffective in coming to a proper diagnosis, he feels, since morality is an abstract concept imposed by culture inadequate to capturing and evaluating an individual's inner consciousness and mental function. Moral judgments about behaviors do not illuminate the individual mind in context, as it grapples with new stimuli. Instead, mental illness is better described as a state when an individual's overall ability to function within the group is disturbed. Mental pathology emerges when an individual's biological endowment and personal store of experience is disturbed in its confrontation with culture and new experiential data, and when, in consequence, the mind's functional equilibrium is damaged or abandoned, leaving the individual with lessened ability to negotiate between the personal states of mind and identity and new or external stimuli.

The critical result is that Griesinger abandons any absolute standard for identifying mental illness or its etiology as he espouses a model of embodied mind. A physician can establish a diagnosis of mental disease by determining what the individual's normal function is, as indexed against that individual's cultural situation and physical constitution. Normal function finds the two poles of this relationship in an equilibrium defining the individual's behavioral norm—an empirically observable baseline for behavior, to be considered in conjunction with physical and cultural endowments. The disease will then be modeled and understood as a dialectic of experience badly engaged, a derangement of dynamic and ongoing dialectical relationships between the self and the external world. A diagnosis, then, starts from a dual empirical baseline (physiological and behavioral) for evidence of mental pathology, not from a priori assumptions that specific diseases are signaled by behaviors or organic dysfunctions (Griesinger 1882, p. 14). To equate mental diseases with either brain function or behavior alone is again scientific reductionism, no matter that the brain is the seat of organic reflexes which ground mind, record individual history, and contribute to behavior (Griesinger 1882, p. 19). Griesinger stresses that "psychical life" evolves, interposing itself between sensory input and individual action, creating a "third element" within the mind:

> It forms, as it were, an accessory sphere which treads midway between sensation and motor impulse, and, as it grows, acquires richness and extent; it becomes gradually a powerful, and in itself a complex centre which rules in many relations sensation and movement, and

within which moves the whole mental life of the man. This sphere is that of the intelligence. (Griesinger 1882, p. 19)

In one sense, this definition of mind as intelligence reflects the era's prejudices that mental illness is mental weakness. Yet Griesinger is more precise: motor life belongs to the body, sensations are impressions registered in the brain, and intelligence (as individual mind, or the ego) synthesizes the input from both. This synthetic psychic life thus is the amalgam grounding individual behavior; it reflects but extends Kant's distinction between apperception, understanding, and reason in human intelligence, as in the *Critique of Pure Reason*, as three different moments in producing knowledge, and in Hegel's definition of mind as developing in history.

Griesinger turns to speech as more specific evidence of how psychic function, motor relationships, and outside experience produce individual behavior patterns (Griesinger 1882, p. 20–21). Language is evidence of how outer senses relate to the inner sense of intelligence; it documents how experience and learning have been shaped into concepts by the individual and used (§ 18). These ideas are assimilated into the intelligence's equilibrium, reproduced, and operated upon (§ 19). Even more critically, the production and reproduction of concepts as words and phrases is accompanied by affects facilitating or blocking processing and behavior: "Mental pain may be occasioned by all that disturbs the normal course and combination of the ideas which represent the *I* and which therefore limits its freedom" (p. 25). An individual experiences as normal those data that are familiar parts of intelligence; discrepancies will elicit affective reactions and motor impulses, hopefully to be synthesized into new concepts: "The mixing of the intuitions of movement with our perceptions is the intermediate process through which every manifestation of our intellectual life must pass" (p. 28). This mixing of perception and movement (physical and mental) also implicates culture, as the mind's equilibrium of relatively stable reference points learned and preserved predisposes the individual towards certain reactions (p. 29).

A persistent equilibrium of ideas definitive of a particular mind produces behavioral patterns that emerge as that mind's will, especially as resisting change in its equilibrium, to preserve the identity formed: "Originally the individual is in no respects free; he becomes so, first, by being possessed of a mass of well-ordered and easily-evoked perceptions, out of which there is formed a strong kernel, the *I*" (Griesinger 1882, p. 31). Thus the *I*, the ego, again is defined as a synthetic product of processed impressions, based on the individual's soma, history, and experience—a definition Griesinger acknowledges as deriving in part from Herbart's description of how individuals learn, and one that Freud would borrow decades later. Concomitantly, the individual will be identified as ill when either organic dysfunction sets in or when mental equilibrium is distorted to the point of decentering (p. 33).

Griesinger's model for mental wellness and illness underscores language and behavior as cues to the individual mind's norm as established by past experience and culture and to its illness in the case of deviance. His synthesis builds on his philosophical predecessors yet takes them into the solid plane of medical practice and social pragmatics—the legacy of Left Hegelian social and political criticism integrated with the period's vanguard standard for diagnostics based on material evidence. Mental disease always has two faces (one individual, and one cultural) and is grounded in an individual's history and ability to adapt over time to new experience (or not). In consequence, in later sections of *Mental Pathology*, as Griesinger turns to elaborate on the etiology of more specific mental diseases, he will describe each both developmentally and dialectically, accounting for stages of a disease in terms of stress and response over time, as well as into the organic and behavioral evidence for it.

THE ETIOLOGY AND SYMPTOMOLOGY
OF MENTAL DISEASE

In the fourth chapter of *Mental Pathology*, Griesinger begins to evolve his diagnostic manual, a description of various mental diseases in terms of their origins and symptomatic behaviors. He begins by outlining the etiology of mental diseases, arising when an individual's ego loses its internal equilibrium due to either physiological or environmental factors, and thus as it ceases to be able to confront and freely process incoming stimuli as experience and integrate them with existing knowledge. Even "Elementary Disorders" of the mind are best understood as produced by improper relationships between the ego and environmental input. Critically, they do not emerge spontaneously but rather develop over the long term, and they will manifest in both willed behavior and the body.

Griesinger uses this logic to describe all mental illnesses as anomalies of states of being, as minds moving into and becoming fixed in conditions outside of the norm. Some of these anomalies originate within the individual mind, when an individual mental equilibrium blocks receptivity to new data: anomalies of sentiment (Griesinger 1882, p. 45), anomalies of thought (slow, fast, or odd thought processes which can yield delusions (p. 47)), and anomalies of the will (where the inner life forces itself onto the outer life, such as, a "morbidly increased feeling of self" (p. 53)). This class of diseases manifests itself in exaltation or delusion.

Another class of anomaly originates in an individual's loss of mental equilibrium and hence of the center of his identity: "disorders of sensation," in which physical sensation overwhelms the prior knowledge comprising the mind and identity. These diseases are tied to the senses, but are by no means solely organic in origin. Instead, they document a disjunction between sensation and mind, when mental mistakes and inappropriate behaviors emerge because incoming stimuli are not processed in customary fashion—when the customary self and its equilibrium is lost:

> The chief point is invariably this—that, in the great majority of cases, there appears with the mental disease a change in the mental disposition of the patient in his sentiments, desires, habits, conduct, and opinions. He is no more the same; his former *I* becomes changed, he becomes estranged to himself (alienated). (Griesinger 1882, p. 81)

Such processing problems can, over the long term, lead to serious mental illness when the patient despairs. Insanity proper (the topic of chapter 5) is not caused by the body, but physical problems help predispose individuals to such processing disjunctions. These illnesses must thus be diagnosed behaviorally, rather than as states of being. In consequence, evidence for the patient's loss of self must be collected as part of a patient's medical history: change in habits are keys to the individual's maladaptive alienation, "the suspected exaggeration of certain phases of his [the patient's] individuality" (Griesinger 1882, p. 81). One clue to a patient's diagnosis can be found when his mood does not change in response to changes in outer circumstance (p. 92).

When Griesinger transposes this model into practical contexts, his plans for mental institutions thus cast them as both behavioral laboratories and therapy units, testing and helping to recalibrate patients' equilibria toward their functional norm. In this approach to therapy, he emerges also as more socially progressive than Freud, because he accounts for environmental, as well as internal, stressors. The experiences of Anna O. or Dora were causes of their diseases, but Griesinger would add that their environments were as well—factors that Freud more or less ignored. Griesinger explicitly sees predisposing causes of mental disease in the patient's social and national groups (and thus shared by many). In this sense, a diagnosis should consider that certain groups (cultures, nations, classes, regions) have higher concentrations of the insane (Griesinger 1882, p. 95), since civilization and social mores may contribute to insanity.

Thus, in the "Cause and Mode of Origin of Mental Disease," for instance, Griesinger insists that the physician know the patient's history *ab ovo*, to uncover the disease's etiology (Griesinger 1882, p. 90). Organic disease will also play into this history, as a trigger for the onset of mental disease, as it can cause a breakdown or a permanent debilitation inhibiting mental processing ("insanity" may have both a mental and a physical component). Nonetheless, Griesinger stresses that the *reported* onset of an illness is often not its *actual* one, given that disease is a long-term development of a pattern of interaction, growing toward a time when the mind can no longer function normally, can no longer respond to nature or culture, given that a cultural mental pattern is at the base of an individual one.[5] Professions, the seasons, social position, heredity, and education all affect mental disease as well, but they are never sufficient causes. The physiological dimension of mental illness will also play in, as well (chapter 3): "irritation of the brain," physical, or psychical shock can disturb the individual's equilibrium and ability to process data. Most critically, what have been assumed to be purely physical causes of mental illness, such as "hyperæmias within the cranium," may actually be the result of long-term imbalances, behaviors and habits, not their causes (p. 116).

With this, Griesinger has provided a modern model for the etiology of mental illness amalgamating philosophical models of mind with medical-empirical evidence, both organic and behavioral. He casts mental illness not as a state, but a process or transaction that has become unbalanced, and shows how it must be diagnosed through observation of behavior as well as physiologically. Moreover, mental illness is not "caused," it develops in historical time; and it is not inevitable—he avoids both cultural and physical determinism. This etiology is Griesinger's foundation for the diagnostic manual and the therapeutic models for which he is most famous.

The large part 3 of Griesinger's treatise, the "Forms of Mental Disease," expands his model into a diagnostic manual, with each disease described as a correlation between behavioral and physical symptoms with problems in mental processing. Taking then-familiar disease nomenclature as his point of departure (terms such as melancholia and hypochondria), Griesinger models each disease as a discrete failure in the dialectics between mental content and experience, as a particular form of misalignment between mind and body that can condition mental disease.

---

[5] See Gaw (1993) for a contemporary view on mental illness incorporating these viewpoints.

Depressions, for example, are diseases that evolve when the body or mind feels wrong to the individual. Etiologically, the individual's growing sense of wrongness causes odd behavior, when the individual tries to compensate or cover up, then reacts emotionally to sense a loss of will or control, often under pressure of bodily or cultural threat. The illness sets in when the individual begins to favor the wrong or injured part of the self and avoids using it (like favoring an injured leg long after it has healed), most often by withdrawing from contact with those parts of the environment that would challenge the affected (weak, depressed) part of the self. In the worst cases, mind and body begin to disassociate, eschewing the synthesis of new data into their identities and manifesting symptoms like feeble health, illogical delusions, or longings and nostalgia, relying on memory instead of the present. The depressed individual withdraws from any active dialectic with the world, and often also from a dialectic between mind and body, favoring the mind as it is caught in its past, and unable to process incoming environmental data. Depression for Griesinger is a disease stemming from a failed mental dialectic, in which the patient's current self is overpowered by the weight of data from the past or the environment.

Mental exaltations and manias are diseases that invert this relationship between mind and body, as the mind gradually overpowers the body and the world. Where a depressed individual withdraws from contact with the environment, a manic individual has an unhealthy and overdone self-confidence and will, often accompanied by mood swings and ceaseless motion or stimulation, playing out hyper-exaggerated connections between mind and body, often suppressing new sense input and even masking organic disease. The body or mind of such an individual can even be burnt out through over-stimulation, indirectly causing death, or he can totally withdraw into a fantasy world of monomaniac delusion. The manic disease thus is characterized by a self overpowering external input.

Other "States of Mental Weakness" (chapter 3) can also grow into diseases when the ego or self eschews or avoids the confrontation of inner and outer worlds—when the mental equilibrium of the intellect refuses to assimilate new information. In such cases, the patient is unable to create a congruity between inner and outer life, and the attendant sense of self gradually unravels, as the individual allows the ego to disintegrate rather than enter into conflict. Dementia and chronic mania are such diseases of non-synthesis. Sufferers of these diseases appear normal and well adjusted to the newcomer, yet the physician who knows their histories will see that they have replaced their earlier, lively mental life by a new, non-conflicted, and usually much duller or simpler mental one. They prefer peace and physical health, surviving by assuming a delusional normalcy that suppresses individual will and attendant conflicts between body, intellect, and environment (Griesinger 1882, p. 238).

These two examples are typical for Griesinger's taxonomy of mental disease: each is described in terms of dialectical confrontations or interactions between the mind and experience. This confrontation, when deviating from the norm, can allow sense data to enslave the mind's imagination, or the mind to remain fixed in the past or withdraw from the present rather than internalizing new information. Even as Griesinger correlates these dialectics between mind and experience to "The Pathological Anatomy of Mental Disease," he stresses that not only the brain, but also other organs, may be implicated in the feedback loop between mind, body, and world, as social pressure and physiology evolve into a full-blown mental disease, marking the body by means of mental stress, and revealing itself behaviorally. Not surprisingly, then, Griesinger stresses dialectical rehabilitation in his approach to therapeutics and asylum practice, outlined in the fifth part of the *Mental Therapeutics*. The physician will institutionalize the patient to take control of his physical and mental being, to move toward a cure by restoring the lost mental equilibrium of mind and experience. That is done by a retraining of the mind, body, and social interface together, with both physical and mental care involved. The patient's prognosis will depend on how far the disease has progressed and on whether mental disequilibrium has altered anatomy irreversibly.

Griesinger's approach to disease and therapy thus accommodates both the cognitive and social individual. The physician must, first, isolate and diagnose illness on the basis of the patient's personal and cultural history, then treat physical ailments, and then finally treat the mind "morally," in terms of the social norms and individual circumstance in which the individual is to function. The goal is reeducation and consciousness raising about the dysfunctional mental patterns that destroy mental equilibria between mind and body, history, and the present. Abnormal behavior should not be attacked, but gradually transformed, so that the mind's equilibrium can be reestablished at the individual's functional norm within the environment and culture. This transformation must not be seen as superficial resocialization, since it aims at reprogramming the individual's agency in establishing environmental, physical, and moral interfaces with his world, and thus in rebuilding a balanced and functional ego. The therapist who deals with a patient nonetheless has a choice of strategies to remediate interfaces, just as the pedagogue may teach his students using a variety of strategies. Most critically, the physician may intervene in *any* of three realms to help a patient regain wellness—to heal the body as a physician, the mind as a cultural critic, or the ego as a facilitator of an individual's wishes and teacher enabling his or her growth vis-à-vis the past.

Griesinger's *Mental Pathology* thus synthesizes principles drawn from his era's philosophical vanguard with pragmatic, empirical medical practice. His physician must rely heavily on empirical observation, a patient's individual symptomology, medical and social history, and medical diagnosis of the body. At the same time, that physician must respect the individual's position within the environment. A disease's etiology can only be understood as implicating physiology, individual history, and behavior, and in light of the goal of an evolving personal identity that can survive test confrontations with reality, and that can easily be skewed through shock, cultural incompatibility, or problems with individual will. He honors the individual while recognizing how fragile the equilibrium of self—Freud's *ich*—is in times of transformation, stress, and political pressure. Griesinger's mental patient remains an individual who needs to communicate with the present and the community, a social being able to assert his agency and individual will as a normal part of society and history. That individual may, over time, be forced into mental illness if circumstances (personal, historical, physiological) overwhelm the learning and habit that has to that point enabled him.

Griesinger as a Reader of Idealism

Remembering Griesinger as a physician and psychiatrist obscures how close psychology and philosophy lay in the nineteenth century, in an era where normal science considered theory and practice to be mutually informing. Philosophy was the theoretical enterprise, while disciplines like psychology, medicine, and pedagogy took its principles and sought contexts of praxis that would realize them in human history and development. The traditions summarized in today's philosophy under the rubric of German Idealism undervalue that link, obscuring real contemporaneous links between points of theory and practice, such as those between Kant and Herbart, Hegel and the practical politics of the Left Hegelians.

Wilhelm Griesinger's work underscores the need for revised histories of philosophy and medicine (especially psychology and psychiatric medicine). His work is evidence for a politically activist and scientifically empiricist reading of the idealist traditions, as he created the therapeutics of modern medical practice by integrating the most modern advances in science (including pathology, neurology, anatomy, and medical chemistry) with the kind of Left Hegelian demands on praxis that will emerge in Marx's work. In a real sense, Griesinger's psychiatry reveals readings of both Kant and Hegel alive in the mid-nineteenth century but since lost—readings of idealism stressing nurture, social transformation, and somatic knowledge rather than cognitivism. Griesinger has found in the idealist traditions not a too-simple dichotomy between mind and body, but a paradigm that unites mind, body, and social-historical communities. Academic philosophy of the latter nineteenth century and beyond has preferred apriorist readings of idealism and reduced dialectics to Hegel's historical principle, leaving aside its cognitive value for individuals and groups changing over time. Griesinger also provides practical evidence of an evolving paradigm for normal science in the era, one that accommodates induction from material evidence as well as deduction from premises.

References

Arens, K. (1989). *Structures of Knowing: Psychologies of the Nineteenth Century.* Boston Studies in the Philosophy of Science, Vol. 113. Dordrecht: Reidel.

Arens, K. (1996). Wilhelm Griesinger: Psychiatry between philosophy and praxis. *Philosophy, Psychiatry, & Psychology, 3*(3) 147–63.

Boring, E. G. (1950). *A History of Experimental Psychology* (2nd edn). New York, NY: Appleton-Century-Crofts. (1st edn published 1929.)

Ellenberger, H. F. (1970). *The Discovery of the Unconscious: The History and Evolution of Dynamic Psychiatry.* New York, NY: Basic Books.

Detlafs, G. (1993). *Wilhelm Griesingers Ansätze zur Psychiatriereform.* Pfaffenweiler: Centruarus Verlagegesellschaft.

Doerner, K. (1981). *Madmen and the Bourgeoisie: A Social History of Insanity and Psychiatry* (J. Neugroschel and J. Steinberg, Trans.). Oxford: Basil Blackwell. (Original work published in 1969 in German.)

Engels, H. G. (1983). *Wilhelm Griesinger's Innovations in Treatment of the Insane.* MA Thesis, University of Calgary, Canada.

Gaw, A. C. (Ed.) (1993). *Culture, Ethnicity, and Mental Illness.* Washington, DC: American Psychiatric Press.

Griesinger, W. (1845). *Pathologie und Therapie der psychischen Krankheiten für Ärzte und Studierende.* Stuttgart: Adolph Krabbe. (2nd rev. edn 1861; 3rd edn 1871: Braunschweig: Friedrich Wreden.)

Griesinger, W. (1854). Klinische und anatomische Beobachtungen über die Krankheiten von Aegypten. *Archiv für physiologische Heilkunde* (Stuttgart), *13*, 528–75.

Griesinger, W. (1857). *Infectionskrankheiten: Malariakrankheiten, Gelbes Fieber, Typhus, Pest, Cholera.* Erlangen: Enke, Erlangen.

Griesinger, W. (1865). *Traité des Maladies Mentales: Pathologie et Thérapeutique.* Paris: Delahaye.

Griesinger, W. (1882). *Mental Pathology and Therapeutics* (C. L. Robertson and J. Rutherford, Trans. from the 2nd German edn). New York, NY: William Wood & Co. (London: New Sydenham Society, 1867; Facsimile reprint, 1989: Birmingham, AL: Classics of Psychiatry & Behavioral Sciences Library.)

Herbart, J. F. (1964a). *Lehrbuch zur Psychologie. Sämtliche Werke*, Bd. 4 (K. Kehrbach and O. Flügel, Eds). Aalen: Scientia Verlag.

Herbart, J. F. (1964b). *Psychologie als Wissenschaft neu gegründet auf Erfahrung: Erster synthetischer Theil and Zweiter analytischer Theil. Sämtliche Werke*, Bd. 5 & 6. Aalen: Scientia Verlag.

Kant, I. (1980). *Anthropologie in pragmatischer Hinsicht* (7th edn). Hamburg: Felix Meiner. (*Anthropology from a Pragmatic Point of View* (M. J. Gregor, Trans.), 1974. The Hague: Nijhoff.)

Kant, I. (1996). *Practical Philosophy* (M.J. Gregor, Ed. and trans). Cambridge: Cambridge University Press.

Kant, I. (1998). *Critique of Pure Reason* (P. Guyer and A. W. Wood, Eds. and Trans.). Cambridge: Cambridge University Press.

Kant, I. (2000). *Critique of the Power of Judgment* (P. Guyer and E. Matthers, Eds. and Trans.). Cambridge: Cambridge University Press.

Marx, O. M. (1970). Nineteenth-century medical psychology: Theoretical problems in the work of Griesinger, Meynert, and Wernicke. *Isis, 61*, 355–70.

Marx, O. M. (1972). Wilhelm Griesinger and the history of psychiatry: A Reassessment. *Bulletin of the History of Medicine, XLVI*(6), 519–44.

Mayer, A. (2002). *Mikroskopie der Psyche: Die Anfänge der Psychoanalyse im Hypnose-Labor.* Göttingen: Wallstein Verlag.

Sammet, K. (1997). *"Ueber Irrenanstalten und deren Weiterentwicklung in Deutschland": Wilhelm Griesinger im Streit mit der konservativen Anstaltspsychiatrie 1865–1868* (Dissertation Hamburg). Münster: LIT Verlag.

Verwey, G. (1985). *Psychiatry in an Anthropological and Biomedical Context: Philosophical Presuppositions and Implications of German Psychiatry, 1820–1870* (L. Richards with P. Hyams and J. Staargaard, Trans.). Dordrecht: Reidel/Kluwer Academic Publishers. (Original work published in 1980 in Dutch.)

Verwey, G. (2004). *Wilhelm Griesinger: Psychiatrie als ärztlicher Humanismus.* Nijmegen: Arts & Boeve.

Wahrig-Schmidt, B. (1985). *Der junge Wilhelm Griesinger im Spannungsfeld zwischen Philosophie und Physiologie.* Tübingen: Gunter Narr.

Wahrig-Schmidt, B. (1987). Wilhelm Griesinger 1817–1868. In D. van Engelhardt and F. Hartmann (Eds), *Klassiker der Medizin*, pp. 172–89. München: Beck.

CHAPTER 7

THE PHILOSOPHICAL ROOTS OF KARL JASPERS' *GENERAL PSYCHOPATHOLOGY*

CHRISTOPH MUNDT

INTRODUCTORY REMARKS

Karl Jaspers' epochal work *Allgemeine Psychopathologie* (referred to as AP; English translation *General Psychopathology* (1959) referred to as GP) represented a "fresh start" event of psychopathological methodology at that time. Its point of departure in the first edition was psychology, at that time much more than today a non-medical discipline close to both the empirical and the conceptual approaches. Philosophy was as prevalent and esteemed as experimental psychology. In contrast, the basic concepts of mental illness the young Jaspers was confronted with before 1913 were characterized by two essential features: Firstly, they more or less arbitrarily picked up disease models from medical, to a lesser degree from psychological or common sense, domains with very heterogeneous ways of access to mental life and without broad reflection on the methodology of how to get access to it. Secondly, from the mid-nineteenth century biological paradigms were much more favored for pathogenetic theories and classification in psychiatry than psychological models.

After Pinel's and Esquirol's teaching of mono-manias and dream as models of incapacitated mental function, the detection of the pathogenesis of progressive paralysis provoked a sway to medical paradigms of dysfunction and classification of mental illness. Lombroso emphasized the genetic endowment for explaining and—much worse—prognosis of forensic patients. In 1845, Griesinger resumed the model of dementia for psychotic illness and its course, and in 1911, when Jaspers started working on AP, Bleuler highlighted its potentially less devastative course than earlier presumed. However, his renaming of dementia praecox to schizophrenia was again inspired by a neurological paradigm: the dissociation of single mental functions found with the cerebral anatomy of the speech centers in the 1870s.

Jaspers' intention was to go to the very roots of the apprehension of psychic phenomena, i.e., how do we manage to get access to them? What are the implications for the type of knowledge we gain by different ways of access? What can we know at all and at best about the mental condition and functioning of another person? What is methodologically adequate to encompass the complex amalgamation of psycho-pathological symptoms comprised of mental, physical, social, and spiritual influences? What can be said about the causation of mental symptoms given the open-system nature of man with his ability to transcend?

METHODOLOGICAL PROCEDURE

The fourth edition of *Allgemeine Psychopathologie* (AP) is considered to be the first one of the nine which unfolds the methodological awareness of fundamentally different approaches to biological and psychological phenomena. This awareness also necessarily implies different categories of causation. Therefore the distinction was introduced between determined causation—the model of physics—versus developmental evolution—the model of historiography. Later, transcendence was considered as a third category out of reach of the science of psychopathology. For man, to Jaspers, is an inexhaustible "open system" with self-reflection, self-molding, longing for, and mostly confessing to meaning beyond oneself.

In her critical evaluation and comparison of the different editions of AP, Kirkbright (2008) mentions that Jaspers' publisher urged him to write the second edition only four months after the publication of the first. The difference to the fourth edition is the most decisive one—it was entirely rewritten during Jaspers' enforced retirement and interdiction to teach under the Nazi regime in 1941/1942. In a letter to his father, Jaspers wrote that a philosophical work was intended with an open perspective beyond the empirical approach. A new chapter on "The Whole of Existence" was intended to deepen psychopathology to the existential roots of man. A particular note was dedicated to the critique on Freud. Jaspers called Freud's theories pseudo-science. The fourth edition presented the intricate consideration of Dilthey's and Max Weber's work for a sound methodological foundation of the access to mental phenomena.

For our purpose the eighth edition of AP (1965) was the best available and usable. The philosophical quotations from the list of references were looked up in the text and registered according to the roughly thirty philosophers quoted. The place of context, the argument, and content to be introduced by the quotation was registered and described respectively. There are about 250 quotations from about thirty philosophers. Many of the quotations are referred to over long text passages or are scattered over many disconnected passages of AP. Only a selection of them can be used to unfold the most basic conceptual foundations of AP that were influenced through them and pertaining up to now. The sequence of dealing with the most influential philosophers in AP follows two principles: (1) basic methodological foundations of the structure of AP—the influence of Windelband, Dilthey, and

Weber; and (2) the steps from very basic methodological to more detailed specific aspects of psychopathology.

Methodological Dualism: Windelband, Dilthey, and Weber

One of the earliest and most influential essays on the methodological distinction between historiography and natural sciences was laid out in Wilhelm Windelband's introductory lecture as rector of the University of Strasbourg (Windelband 1900). Although Windelband was not quoted by Jaspers, he is noteworthy due to his indirect influence on Jaspers' thinking. Setting off from Locke's and Descartes' distinction of sensation and reflection (given their different notion on ideas being acquired for Locke, being partly inborn for Descartes), Windelband differentiates "in all its crudity" methodological rules that are adequate to deal with something which happens versus those rules adequate to phenomena of imagination. The aim of the former being the evidenced, empirically based apodictic contention, the aim of the latter the singular descriptive assessment and judgment. The former follows laws to be found by empirical methods, the latter refers to the characterization of events of unique quality. Both share experience as the basis of expertise. Knowledge of rules allows intervention. However, all judgment and valuing merely and entirely applies to the singular and unique. An analytic dissection of causative elements of history down to its deepest roots is impossible. Hence history conveys a notion of freedom and incommensurability. Science will never be able to bridge this methodological gap.

Windelband's inauguration lecture guides us to Dilthey (1952, 1955, 1958), the most influential philosopher for Jaspers after Max Weber. Dilthey says in his volume on "The Understanding of Other Persons and Their Life Manifestations" (1952) that understanding evolves from interests in daily living. One has to know what the other person intends, feels, wishes, apprehends. Dilthey differentiates terms, judgments, more extended thought contexts as one class; acting, expression of perceptions, and feelings as another one. In this latter realm of phenomena there is no right or wrong but instead sincerity or deception. Under extreme conditions there is an elementary understanding of the expression of acting or gestures beyond deception. Dilthey refers to the "objective mind" ("*objektiver Geist*") referring to Hegel's idea that the multitude of communicating minds merges to a collective mind which can be considered as objective in their terms. For Hegel it is a metaphysical process structuring the historical development. In the objective mind the consensual collective meaning of living actions and communication is met by the individual. In Dilthey's view this is brought about by the vast knowledge of common-sense meanings and an inner core reality emerging from a core communality connecting the individuals of a cultural unity. The more distance there is between plain and complex contents, the more insecurity of interpretation and understanding ensues. Dilthey develops a complex set of intellectual and perceptual tools to refine and sharpen common-sense meanings without neglecting their basic deficits of consensual definition. The visitor to a theater play is used as a paradigm for the dialectics inside the individual as dialectics happen between the members of society: the visitor's mind may be captured by the play as long as he attends it. Only afterward does sufficient detachment from the immediate impression by the play enable the visitor to reflect upon the content of the play and join the elaboration of congruity with others. Interesting, Dilthey's tone and argument stay defensive in justifying the methods of the humanities and in particular historiography—so important a paradigm for understanding patients' life histories. Hence natural sciences' challenge of superiority seems still stingy to him. According to Dilthey, the perpetuated dialectics between the expressing and the expressed, between the causing action and the effected situation "unfold the realm of the individual." A certain order of this repetitive process may emerge in forming a typology of cognitive patterns which allow cognitive economization. This view refers to Max Weber's construct of the "ideal types."

Another important attempt of Dilthey to clarify and strengthen the methodology of the humanities is excellently transferable to psychiatric case histories: the concept of putting oneself into the perspective of another person, forming the inner world of the respective person in the perceiving person by feeling how it is to use this person's perspective. Dilthey uses the example of a poem for explanation. It may be difficult to understand first hand but by rereading it molds more and more a Gestalt of reception. This Gestalt may not be congruent with all other readers' perception but very likely joins one of several possible patterns of interpretation.

In the "Introduction to the Humanities," volume 1, Dilthey (1955) attacks the natural sciences because they do not pervade to holistic perception and interpretation of the nature, the "coherence and conditions of nature." The isolated consideration of nature, he says is a monism, an arrangement not representing the object as it appears. He also criticizes Kant because of his unhistorical stance: the subject was conceived as a paradigmatic universal one, static without historicity. This was particularly pronounced in "Kritik der theoretischen Vernunft": "The abstractions which the history of metaphysics has left behind are not yet completely done away with" (Dilthey 1926).

In "Structure of the Historical World in the Humanities" (1958), Dilthey emphasizes the dialectic nature of the realm of meanings. "Whenever and wherever the mind (Geist) manifests it contains a joint I and you," we may add: and a joint me. It constitutes the "objective mind," the structure of meaning of the language. There has to be an ascendance from the socially joint meaning to the individual understanding. There is a relation of an individual's own identity to partial identities in others which is partly joint identity and partly opens the perspective for participating and identifying with others by means of communality with them. This perspective may entail a very personal notion with regard to the "historical situation" when Jaspers came across Dilthey's philosophy.

Although Dilthey is only quoted once in GP, with other authors (Wach, Droysen; Roscher and Knies; in the Second Part "Meaningful Psychic Connections: Psychology of Meaning—Verstehende Psychology"; AP 8th edn, p. 250; GP, p. 301) it is deeply permeated by Dilthey's thoughts. The passages about understanding and explaining, understanding and interpretation, and the passages about limits of understanding rest greatly with Dilthey's statements as does the section on pseudo-understanding.

Dilthey's influence on Jaspers' concept of the methodologically dualistic psychopathological access to psychic phenomena cannot be captured without his appreciation, even admiration for Max Weber (1995). He got four entries of quotations in AP (pp. 6, 173, 250, 469; GP, pp. 144, 476, 848), the really significant ones on p. 250 (GP p. 476) where Jaspers delivers his appreciation of and gratitude to Dilthey and Weber for their Psychology of Meaning

(Understanding) and Weber's construct of the "Ideal Types." Jaspers considers their work as an indispensable tool for producing some degree of evidence in the humanities, especially in history and in particular for "meaningful psychology" to be applied to the biographical history of psychiatric patients.

Peter-Ulrich Merz (1990) has summarized Max Weber's and Heinrich Rickert's foundation of "meaningful understanding of sociology." Rickert, a neo-Kantian philosopher, suggested separating subjects and objects in historiography and doing away with hermeneutics. There must be no mingling of logical and psychological elements, he claimed. The aim was to overcome the differentiation of the fact proper and its appearance. The latter is considered as the ultimately recognizable product of logic and its process of examination in historiography. This debate obviously is essential for evaluating the validity of biographical anamnesis in psychiatry.

Being principally in consent with Rickert, Max Weber nevertheless goes further by merging fact proper and its appearance with his model of tentative or probe-intention. The aim is an approximation to ever more stringent characterization of a historical process, event, situation, or character. Typifying the historical process is different from applying or finding strict rules or laws as in physics. Weber discerns between humanities and culture-related sciences. The former allow fairly strict rules to constitute classes whereas the latter only allow "characterization." The "meaningful understanding" of sociology belongs to the latter discipline. However, the approximation process by probing intention as mentioned earlier produces more stringency than mere empathy or "meaningful" sociology. The Ideal Type formation has turned out to become a widely used tool for this approximation process of classification. The tool of the Ideal Type is meant to bridge the gap between empirical historiography and value- or meaning-based characterization of historical phenomena. Hence the Ideal Type is an abstraction of something individual, unrepeatable, unique. And yet it is an abstraction of characteristics such as psychopathological narratives which are immediately plausible even though a singular manifestation of the type may not even show one of its particular characteristics at all. In this case the common feature is the perspective to be realized, to be striving for.

Constituting an Ideal Type requires a construct sufficiently plausible to our fantasy, objectively possible, and adequate to our nomological knowledge. Merz considers this concept of "individual causality" as originated by Rickert and adopted by Weber.

The construct of the Ideal Type suggests causality being attributable to it since the type does not manifest in a singular quality but in particulars of thinking, sensing, judgment, and their presentation in many different situations and at different times.

A threefold integration is needed for understanding motives by interpretation: purportedly presented motifs have to be separated from sincere ones; the acting usually happens to a great extent spontaneously without deep reflexion and only "half-knowledge" of the real motifs; the interpreting historian needs to understand the historical person better than he himself. Max Weber emphasized that the statistically defined "average type" is definitely distinct from the Ideal Type.

There is some ambiguity in Jaspers' quoting and evaluating of ideas of these authors he obviously respected very highly: they are only briefly mentioned but are very influential on his work for perspective taking. There is such a notion with Dilthey and Weber, and also with Husserl. The latter obviously was not much interested in contact and hence was difficult for Jaspers to approach. Max Weber, however, was revered by Jaspers as a scientist and for his personality and character. Jaspers (1946) wrote an essay on him: "Max Weber. Politician, Researcher, Philosopher." In this book he acknowledges in particular Weber's sincerity and authenticity, and also his prime objective to yield truth with his science. He probably shared his feeling of being rebuffed by the modern technical epoch. Jaspers appreciated the freedom of his perspective, the courage to put up with unperfected work since no science can ever be perfected, and his rejection in taking guidance, to be master and model. He also appreciated the essayistic nature of his work by saying that the extraordinary fragment gains more weight than the seemingly comprehensive opus magnum never exhaustive by the nature of philosophy. He reproached Heidegger for the latter.

Uncovering the Unconscious: Freud, Nietzsche, and Kierkegaard

In contrast to the revered philosophers Dilthey and Weber who were only quoted once and four times respectively, one of Jaspers' main adversaries, Sigmund Freud, received about 30 quite lengthy and harsh quotations throughout the large volume. Nietzsche and Freud shared an interest in unmasking self-deception of man. We start with Freud to direct attention to what Jaspers virtually despised and what he appreciated.

Jaspers' critical attitude against psychoanalysis sharpened in focus over the years from partial acknowledgment in the first edition of AP up to the sharp, even polemic attacks against the institutionalization of psychoanalysis at the University of Heidelberg after World War II. Bormuth (2004) divides his essay on Jaspers' "Critique of Psychoanalysis" into three parts: the perspectives of psychopathology, existential philosophy, and the eventual "radical" critique.

The critique from a psychopathological perspective: Jaspers' critique from the perspective of psychopathology focuses on the lack of reliability of discovering content and influence of unconscious mechanisms. However, considering just what he called the "unnoticed" takes into account but one part of Freud's concept which lacks the revolutionary component of his theory: namely uncovering the disguised wish and covered intention which is discrepant to the conscious contents. Jaspers' methodological scrutiny, otherwise so meticulous, is missing in this instance. The rather global rejection of dream interpretation should not have prevented doing justice to other writings of Freud as case histories which more convincingly suggest the possible pervasiveness of the unconscious. Jaspers himself had probably no experience with long-term psychotherapeutic treatments, which allow a very intimate perception of shame-inflicted topics which are difficult to get access to with a psychopathological focus without the trust of long-lasting psychotherapeutic care for the relationship. Certainly correct is the skepticism toward an overextended interpretation without empirical basis. Not refutable suppositions do in fact discredit psychoanalysis. Jaspers found an asylum in Max Scheler's philosophy, in particular the sections on psychic development by molding and sublimating the forces of instinctual drives (AP, p. 270).

The critique from the perspective of existential philosophy: Bormuth hinges Jaspers' existential philosophical perspective on psychoanalysis from the point of view of existential philosophy on the confrontation of the state versus individual, humanity versus technical progress, freedom to individual self-determination versus subordination under manipulated state mass organizations. Jaspers distrusts Marxism, "genetic hygiene" of populations, and psychoanalysis as unable to improve civilization. Lining up psychoanalysis in this sequence certainly does not do justice to it looking at its historical reception since then. We may confer Thomas Mann's high appreciation of psychoanalysis as an act of belated enlightenment expressing the attitude of many scientist and artists. A side motif appears in Bormuth's detailed essay when he mentions Jaspers' repudiation of the liberation of sexual love as destructive for the retreat in privacy as the ultimate authenticity of existence.

The radicalized critique of psychoanalysis: Under this heading Bormuth summarizes Jaspers' polemic controversies after World War II on the institutionalization of psychoanalysis at the University of Heidelberg and in particular the inauguration of the mandatory teaching analysis (Bormuth 2008). Jaspers' canny comparison of the teaching analysis with the exercitations of Jesuits is fully justified. Nevertheless he could not put up with the great success of psychoanalysis and its anticlerical component accepted at least for two generations in Europe and the USA as a modern enlightenment of feeling, relating, and emancipating from authorities.

It is interesting otherwise how warm and accepting Jaspers' tone is delivering Nietzsche's ability to cover up the truth behind the façade (Jaspers 1981). The danger of truth being the defined knowledge for sure; instead truth is the knowledge of its sham nature, pretence, fake, life being deeply sunk in untruth. Jaspers quotes passages (pp. 262ff.) where Nietzsche comes very close to Freud: Who is curious enough to go to the ground would be confronted with the greedy, murderous, cruel, never satiable as the very basic nature of man. Truth would be a destructive element for human life, in particular for the developing person. The basic instincts are stronger than any feelings of values. Truth would be the annihilation of illusion and thus self -destruction of mankind. Jaspers emphasizes Nietzsche's questioning of any mode of continuity, stability, tenacity as prone to complacency, compliance with self-corruption, losing the openness.

It is perhaps a reference to Jaspers' preoccupation with the validity of the psychopathological examination that he was attracted by Nietzsche's fatalistic view: all knowledge of the world is interpretation, and science is interpretation of the interpreted. Knowledge about the world is never a safe asset but a limited term. Understanding without valuing merely expresses ambivalence (p. 258). The aim of philosophy: to become aware of oneself. Other quotations of Nietzsche are even closer to Freud, for example, on repression, subliming, as if copied. And yet repeatedly Jaspers intersperses derogatory remarks about Freud. Another topic taken over from Nietzsche is the characterization of man as the not fixed animal that means not rooted, anchored, set (AP, p. 647), addressing the topic of free will, decision, and responsibility.

Under the perspective of Jaspers' psychopathological work and given his embittered opposition to Freud's psychoanalysis, his warm hearted and yet unexpected sympathy with Nietzsche appears as a diverted integration of psychoanalytic findings. Embedding the phenomena in philosophy instead of a medical discipline with scholars, regularities of tuition, teaching analysis, etc. may be better suited to his philosophical approach. His competence rested with philosophy not with psychotherapeutic long-term treatments and the elaboration of therapeutic relationships. He confessed to the asymmetry of therapeutic relationships. In particular, the psychotherapist's resonance of transference and counter-transference was alien to him. Jaspers' successor, the hermeneutic Gadamer, later said: "Both psychotherapist and patient conclude their dialog as changed persons." It is the opposite of Jaspers' concept of an asymmetric therapeutic relationship with authority and superiority of knowledge on the side of the therapist and a subordinated scholar-like recipient attitude of the patient.

Summing up his confessions about the replacement of Freud by Nietzsche, Jaspers concludes with the statement that the foundation of psychiatry as a profession cannot be brought about with Freud, Adler, and Jung but with the Greek philosophers, Augustine, Kant, Kierkegaard, Hegel, and Nietzsche (AP, p. 681).

Kierkegaard is quoted fifteen times in GP almost exclusively in conjunction with Nietzsche and without more detailed content of his writings. Most of the passages deal with bashing Freud and psychoanalysis stating that Nietzsche and Kierkegaard are the "two really great" who uncovered the hidden depth underneath our conscious mind, Freud being a concretistic epigone. Therefore, for this purpose we treat Nietzsche and Kierkegaard as a unity in the context of the anti-Freudian passages in AP. Nevertheless some remarks about Jaspers' reverence of Kierkegaard seem appropriate. He considers him with Nietzsche together as the "greatest of self-reflecting, self-interpreting, self-understanding psychologists." Jaspers regards him as having delivered a schema of self-reflection which never comes to a standstill but remains an everlasting dialectic process, a "continually prodding spur." If it is authentic self-understanding, it ensues as a process not as a state. And "revelation comes in being oneself" (GP, p. 350 GP; AP, p. 290). Kierkegaard makes self-revelation visible, Jaspers says. It is wrong to strive for concluded knowledge, for completed, exhausted insight. Any fixation, the fact that any standstill means missing the truth. Jaspers cannot but deplore that Freud prevented by his writings the immediate direct impact of the two great philosophers Nietzsche and Kierkegaard on psychiatry. Existence, he says, is untouchable by psychopathology (GP, p. 356).

A special aspect of Kierkegaard's philosophy to Jaspers is the point of absurdity in religious faith. Jaspers himself confirms that faith is characterized by absurdity, otherwise the step into faith does not make sense. He quotes Tertullian, emphasized by Kierkegaard, including his own stance to faith: "credo quia absurdum." Jaspers holds that in Luther's time religious belief rejected reason with a tendency to promote the absurd. In contrast, Catholicism, since Thomas Aquinas, had denied that the content of faith was absurd. Rather a distinction should be made between that what was beyond understanding as the content of revelation and that what was contrary to reason: the absurd (GP, p. 731; AP, p. 613). Guilt (or "guilt feelings" as in psychopathological states of depression, for example) has been a major topic in Kierkegaard's mental condition. Destiny, pre-emption, and the "language of the deity" play a role for Kierkegaard's mental condition and suffering.

To sum up Jaspers' dealing with Kierkegaard: Most of the quotations refer to Kierkegaard in conjunction with Nietzsche. In the few passages where Kierkegaard is focused on solely, two elements of interest prevail in his way of dealing with him: Firstly, the replacement of the atheist Freud's dealing with the "shadowed ground" of the psyche by a believing Christian philosopher; and religion as transcendental component of philosophy and also of psychopathology. Secondly, Kierkegaard becomes a sort of armament against Freud whose work on the unconscious was received in public at the turn of the prudish late nineteenth century as a second and specific sort of enlightenment. So Kierkegaard delivered the ammunition for the defense of transcendence with the topics of religious belief and guilt for Jaspers' unobtrusive yet tenacious resistance against Freud.

Ontology and Phenomenology: Static Versus Developmental?

Martin Heidegger is referred to by Jaspers mainly in the context with Kierkegaard and Nietzsche leaving the differentiation of phenomenology and ontology aside. In GP, Jaspers quotes Heidegger's main work *Sein und Zeit* under the heading of ontology and psychological teaching of structure: In the stream of philosophy highlighting existence since Kierkegaard and Nietzsche, Heidegger has attempted to create a conclusive body of knowledge: Fundamental ontology branching out in "existentialia." They are meant to characterize a fundamental "being-in-the-world" with its emotional tone, anxiety, concern, destiny to die. The existentialia precondition all human existence and conduct and determine them. Jaspers comments on them: "The concrete illustrations are valuable but I consider Heidegger's attempt to be a philosophical error in principle because it does not lead the student on to philosophise in his turn but offers him a total schema of human life as if it were knowledge" (GP, p. 776). Heidegger's analysis of being-in-the-world is meant to characterize both "the ontic," i.e., the basis of how we experience and behave in daily living, as well as the ontological, i.e., the deeply rooted authenticity of existence. It should be noted that Heidegger's use of the term "ontological" does not refer to the science of the ontic but specifically to the "authentic being." The being according to the determinants of existence means to be authentic ("*eigentlich*"). The covered, diluted, derived, imitated way of being is considered as "the average way of being," i.e., the general, the impersonal "one," the generalized everybody. Since this philosophy does not lead the reader to philosophize himself it remains sterile as a closed teaching, according to Jaspers. It will not be a means to improve and sustain practical living but is itself just another means of disguise of existence. This would be even more devastating since Heidegger's teaching purports a language of the greatest affinity to existential philosophy and yet misses its core purpose to enlighten existence to a degree that it cannot be taken seriously, Jaspers says. Such a teaching cannot claim to open an avenue viable to permeate and elucidate the structure and psychopathology of man (GP, p. 649). His philosophy of the "absolute," he says, casts fog over existence as a perpetuated process of enlightening (GP, p. 649). Such a harsh criticism of a highly esteemed philosopher, an amply and intensively revered authority, was unusual even for Jaspers. It may be interpreted on the background of Heidegger's indulgence with national socialism in 1933 to 1935 when he was appointed rector of the University of Freiburg and thereafter. After World War II Jaspers was called upon by the allied administration as a moral authority to guide the reestablishment of Heidelberg University. The correspondence between the two philosophers on this occasion is remarkably dry but evading in tone with regard to the past. All affect remains encapsulated in their philosophies and their references to each other (Mundt 2009).

PHENOMENOLOGY

When defining the term "phenomenology" Jaspers declares that he wants to use this term in a more restricted sense than Hegel. He will not cover "the whole field of mental phenomena as revealed in consciousness, history, and conceptual thought" (GP, p. 55; AP, p. 47). Jaspers will only use it for the narrower field of individual psychic experience. It is closer to Husserl's early use of the term in the sense of descriptive psychology in connection with the phenomenon of consciousness. Jaspers rejects the term in the sense that Husserl later used it: "The Appearance of Things" ("*Wesensschau*") is brought about by eidetic reduction which in turn needs an exclusion of unspecific, disturbing perceptions. This procedure requires the attitude of "bracketing" (epoché). We do not pursue this any further here, writes Jaspers. He emphasizes the empirical nature of phenomenology in his definition. He sticks to a purely empirical enquiry maintained from the patient's communication. However, unlike the natural sciences it rests with just the mental representation by the investigator. The logical principle, though, is not different to the natural sciences. The quality of the information gained depends on systematic categories, well-done formulations, contrasting comparisons, recording of similar phenomena, definition of order and classes of phenomena which appear conjointly, in clusters or transitions. Hence Wiggins' and Schwartz's (1997) attempt to trace Husserl's method of bracketing in Jaspers' approach of understanding contains a misperception: representing the patient's report in the investigator's mind is equaled with bracketing. Jaspers clearly states that only information reported by the patient can be the subject of content-related findings.

In different contexts (GP, pp. 262, 285) Jaspers refers again to Hegel, stating that he is the most and actually only systematic phenomenologist. Referring to the very basic role of dialectics in his work, he says that Hegel is helpful for understanding contrasts and oppositional attitudes in psychic life which seemingly are not to be reconciled. Dialectics may also be particularly helpful for coping with limit situations, a central topic in Jaspers' work. Limit situations are related to maturation, self-finding, defining one's self (cf. Mundt, in press). They demonstrate the flow character of psychic states and attitudes, Jaspers says. Hence Hegel's dialectics are indispensable for understanding the psyche. "Life has become a concept of the whole as in the philosophy of the young Hegel or in the life philosophies of the romantic and later periods" (GP, p. 532; AP, p. 446). Jaspers' high esteem, respect, and appreciation of Hegel are expressed in a statement when he says:

> A human image wants to be gained from an anthropology nurtured on Greek philosophy, on Augustine and Kierkegaard, Kant, Hegel and Nietzsche. The human image should only be defined by the greatest of the human beings and only they should coin the modes of speech to be used in talking of the psyche. It is from them we can learn to use the concepts which will help the individual to illuminate himself. (GP, p. 821; AP, p. 686, AP)

Jaspers' relationship with Husserl appears as somewhat unhappy at the beginning on the personal level, and critical on the side of Jaspers later. His reminiscences of the first personal encounter when Jaspers was still a young, hardly known postgraduate student convey a notion of disappointment that there was no deeper interest and engagement to be elicited from Husserl. It remains open whether disappointment due to the lack of interest and resonance from Husserl has made it difficult for Jaspers to sympathize with his philosophy or whether factual reasons were predominant. In any case, Jaspers was skeptical about whether grasping the essences by completely dismantling perceptions from accidental attributions could be done reliably and reproducibly. Instead Jaspers stipulated that the information about the patient's mental state must be based entirely on the patient's own personal statement. Everything else is neither sufficiently valid nor reliable. The technique of bracketing requires an uncontrollable introspective procedure which is not safely reproducible. However, Jaspers' adoption of the eidetic approach taken from Max Weber and his claim of fairly reproducible empathy and understanding seem to be not too far away from the systematized bracketing suggested by Husserl.

As a consequence, Jaspers was very critical about phenomenologists who applied the concept of dismantling psychic phenomena to their very core essences by "*Wesens-Schau.*" Their philosophical roots were Husserl's phenomenology mainly with the technique of "bracketing," Heidegger, Merleau-Ponty, Bergson, and others. In the chapter on German and French psychiatrists-phenomenologists (Erwin Straus, Victor v. Gebsattel, Kunz, Storch, Ludwig Binswanger), so influential in German and French psychiatry in the 1950s through 1960s, Jaspers criticizes in particular the uniformity of the claimed pathogenetic hypotheses: the main point in his view is the speculative interpretative character of the hypotheses and their lack of differentiation between different disease entities. Metaphoric descriptive phrases turn to scientific definitions of disease entities claiming a phenomenological essence of the nature of the disease. Examples taken from statements on "endogenous" depression are "disturbance of vital events" (GP, pp. 540–541), or the "elementary obstruction on becoming," "standstill in the flow of personal becoming," the "inhibition of the personally molded urge to become." Jaspers quotes passages of the writings of von Gebsattel on the phenomenology of obsessive-compulsive disorders (GP, p. 451) which contain formulations like "standing water stagnates" or the interpretation of the symptoms that "the purpose of obsession is to ward off magical meaning."

Obviously, the speculative, interpretative nature of this approach was suspect to Jaspers. He rejected this approach determinedly to the great disappointment of the philosopher psychiatrists, contending that it produces neither proper psychopathology nor proper philosophy: "The amazement of the observer is not a sufficient solicitation of discovery." Jaspers holds on to a strict separation of empirical and transcendental focus of research and thinking. He summarizes his critique on phenomenology in five paragraphs: (1) Anthropological phenomenology strives to "go beyond all knowledgeable." Totality and origin of man cannot be an objective of empirical research. (2) Claims of a "basic disturbance" remain ill defined and ambiguous. (3) Empirical evidence of the "Inhibition of Becoming" is impossible. (4) It is highly questionable to draw conclusions from the concept of a "basic disturbance" since it is ill defined and unspecific. (5) Verification or refutation of pathogenetic findings by phenomenology is impossible. Hence phenomenology produces pseudo-knowledge.

Jaspers goes even further with his critique toward polemic when he says that Wernicke was "thinking from outside to the inner world of man, Freud from the inner world to the outside manifestation" (AP, p. 458). Both were disciples of Meynert, he said, both limited in their scope of man. He concludes with a phrase otherwise unfamiliar to him: "Both exert a spirit of absurdity and inhumanity" (AP, p. 458). With the latter statement Jaspers is in sharp contrast to Thomas Mann's warm homage to Freud on behalf of his eightieth birthday when he expressed that Freud had contributed to a more enlightened and humane civilization. He considered both humanism and humanity as the predominant features to have emanated from Freud's teachings.

Positive resonance to phenomenological viewing by Jaspers is rare. Therefore one quotation (AP, p. 237) should be mentioned which demonstrates that, like others, Jaspers, too, has preferences beyond strict principles. The phenomenologist von Baeyer's subtle analyses of schizophrenic delusion received a positive connotation from Jaspers. He agreed that the inner world of a person with schizophrenia will better unfold and be better opened for empathy by exploring and knowing the details of the patient's delusion. Von Baeyer was a phenomenologist in his own rights with original work on the change of the schizophrenic patient's world. The special cognitive, affective, mental, and somatic retardation in melancholia was described by von Baeyer and other authors as "Vital Inhibition" (retardation). This naming, however, was turned down by Jaspers as a concretism of the "existence which is the historic sincerity of the unconditional." A positive mentioning was also given to the work of Bachofen for his research on symbols (AP, p. 278) with the qualification that this is "sober and industrious" work. It inspired Jung who in turn was attributed briskness by Jaspers. While French phenomenologists like Minkowski and Bergson got away with a brief positive mention on their research on time experience in melancholia (AP, p. 70), Binswanger was worth more than ten quotations with harsh devaluing comments: "Interesting descriptions but as a whole genetically not understandable"; the treatise on "flight of ideas" was called superficial by Jaspers, it does not contribute "anything substantial" (AP, pp. 240–241).

Psychosomatic medicine rose in Germany after World War II due to the writings and pervasive personality of Viktor von Weizsäcker. In the 1960s, Alexander Mitscherlich managed to found the first chair of psychosomatic medicine at the University of Heidelberg. Von Weizsäcker was quoted in AP once (AP, p. 567) in a basically friendly and acknowledging tone but which was critical toward von Weizsäcker's interpretation that Hegel died of cholera just when (and because) he learned of the French revolution.

To sum up the section on phenomenology, it can be stated that Jaspers, by and large, did not appreciate this direction of psychopathology at all: "Neither proper psychopathology nor proper philosophy results from it." His rejection was in contrast to the great success of this field in the 1950s and 1960s. It is revitalized today by the interest of neuropsychologists for interpreting their results. The wholistic approach of phenomenology criticized by Jaspers is more or less useless for defining disease entities of the standardized and operationalized diagnostic manuals. However, neurocognitive research has rediscovered phenomenology as being extremely helpful for interpreting their findings and framing them by theories. It appears that bridging the gap from the highly focused experiment on the neuronal level to more complex patterns of function is often amazingly well done by phenomenology. Examples are mirror neuron research and intercorporality, Theory of Mind and the diversifying phenomenology of intersubjectivity, or the prefrontal neuronal structures of executive control and Husserl's intentionality (Mundt and Weisbrod 2004).

THE VERY FOUNDATIONS OF PHILOSOPHY

The roots of Western philosophy in Greece and the philosophy of the Middle Ages are treated and used by Jaspers in the same pragmatic way as he deals with the contemporary philosophical authors: utility is decisive for the quotation no matter which topic is concerned and which century the quoted author originated from. In addition, these citations are scattered over the whole book demonstrating that there is no systematic elaboration of a philosophical foundation of psychopathology. Instead, Jaspers follows a pragmatic adoption of philosophers from any period of time if their work can contribute to clarify basic assumptions of the nature of man and their implications for understanding psychopathology. Even more so if they can be used to corroborate an argument of Jaspers' methodological position or else setting the limits of what we can know at all about man´s psychic nature. This way of approaching philosophy in a rather sober way according to pragmatic reasons of utility is refreshing for the readership since it does so without distracting adoration of philosophers. The latter often restricts bold application in case it does not really dare examine the utility of a specific philosophy let alone its appropriation and application to a defined instance. This natural, pragmatic attitude has another valuable side effect: it dismantles intricate theories and suppositions to their core assumptions, to be used to open a perspective for further discussion. Jaspers' citation of Aristotle in one instance may serve as an example. Jaspers wants to confirm that a person's perception and conception of the world deeply depends on the mode of his movements. Jaspers finds this assertion in writings of Aristotle and applies it to findings of Trendelenburg (AP, p. 170) on anomalies of movements in Korsakow patients. He also relates subsiding vital drives in this state and the tendency to stick to one Gestalt to the retardation of imagination and the belated conclusion of Gestalt. This in turn, he claims, relates to the forthcoming of hallucinations.

Similar to the quotations of Aristotle, Augustine is also mentioned exclusively in context with other philosophers, mainly Kierkegaard and Nietzsche. Jaspers uses these quotations to corroborate the argument against Freud that only "the greatest of mankind's minds are entitled to coin the interpretation of man." Descartes, whose thinking is actually close to Jaspers' dualistic methodological position, is quoted just once (AP, p. 190) for his "incredibly empty hypothesis" of the pineal gland, conceived by Descartes as the horseman riding the horse, i.e., the soul. From Aristotle through Thomas Aquinas, Jaspers says, the unity of the physical and spiritual nature of man was agreed to be a unity. Descartes was the first to separate them into two distinct entities. Jaspers holds against this schism that one hypothesis is as wrong as the other. Only one of these two natures of man can be grasped at a time. Taken as a whole they elapse. Coincidence of body and mind may happen though (AP, p. 613). Jaspers also mentions Thomas Aquinas' distinction between what is beyond comprehension: the content of revelation; and what is contrary to reason: the absurd (GP, p. 731; AP, p. 613).

Transcendence

This part of Jaspers' *General Psychopathology* determinedly goes beyond scientific knowledge and perhaps even beyond reason toward confession. It asks for the essence of man in its entirety. The term which is meant to cover this comprehensive wholistic perspective on man is "existence." This term is declared to be a philosophical idea not something concrete to be materialized or possibly object of empirical research. Illumining existence is possible to a certain degree by transcendence. To Jaspers, the essence of man is his open nature, i.e., his anticipation of and longing for a more comprehensive context beyond our perception and our ability to conceive but with a certainty founded in ourselves even if it ultimately needs faith. Including faith as an element of a scientific textbook may occur strange at first but certainly is necessary to reflect upon given that there is not any one culture without religion. Hence one may consider human beings' search for the openness of human existence as an intrinsic essence of their mind. Taking this statement as a fact it necessarily becomes an essential part of general psychopathology.

Intriguingly, Jaspers uses a sort of vague language when he writes about transcendence. Given his sharp definitions otherwise this cannot but be taken as specific wording signifying the openness and inconclusiveness of man's search for meaning beyond existence. There is always something beyond psychopathology in the mind of a patient. Jaspers says: "We want to keep our awareness of the inexhaustibility and the enigmatic character of every individual mental patient even in the apparently most commonplace case" (GP, p. 767; AP, p. 640). The incompleteness of man makes existence a continued search and striving, a struggling with oneself given the openness of man's nature. Any finality, any limitation of existence, any temporality is abhorrent to man. Jaspers' attempt to capture the very nature of the Human Being says: firstly man is determined by spanning from the empirical reality of what we know scientifically and yet reaches in the essence of his nature to god; secondly in the different forms of the Encompassing man illumines himself from his origins; thirdly, searching in the world and failing he becomes aware of where he comes from and where he goes. Only in the first category man is accessible to scientific research.

Hence Jaspers emphasizes that existence is nothing concrete but an immaterial encompassing condition from which mental objects only emerge by the subject–object division. Philosophy does not mean these concrete mental objects as such but transcending beyond grasps the Encompassing. The empirical sciences are a step stone for transcendence since just the excellence of science makes us feel the gap to the Encompassing.

Recent research may object in this instance since certain degrees of freedom are brought about in many biological systems by generating incidental events or material, for example, antibodies generated by the immune system which in turn allow specificity to segregate foreign molecules according to utility. Although those mechanisms are far away from what Jaspers addresses with transcendence, it may be objected that the open-system nature as ultimate background is inherent in nature generally.

In a section on "philosophical confusion" by unnoticed, disguised, or unobtrusive philosophy, Jaspers says that instead of real illumining of existence psychological self-mirroring ensues with purposes in the material world. "If this movement is converted in objective assertions and prescriptions, directions and declared goals, then our thought about life itself may become a characterless sophistry" (GP, p. 772; AP, p. 645). This section is followed by a reaffirmation of the disapproval of psychoanalysis as a way of looking at the world, a "*Weltanschauung*" disguised as science or psychology and made resistant against critique by making psychoanalysis itself a weapon against the critics. The pathos of sincerity was experienced deeper, more convincingly, Jaspers claims, with the "great enlighteners," Nietzsche and Kierkegaard.

Jaspers discriminates soul, mind, and body. Mind represents the content the soul refers to. The body is its Being. Like the body is animated by the soul so is the mind bound to the soul and borne by it (AP, p. 259). However, the soul withdraws. Instead, we achieve only the superficial, expression, contents and the conditional, the body, existence. The status of the soul in between existence and transcendence leaves us unable to come to a conclusion with self-understanding. Hence all psychology which is based on interpreting intrinsically remains inconclusive.

Conclusion

Karl Jaspers' book *General Psychopathology* is a monument of continued reflection, integration of sciences and humanities, delineating and separating the non-matching erroneous side tracks of an assembly of disciplines which mirror the complexity of man by the multitude of their facets and their heterogeneity. Although he left psychiatry as his field of daily work early, he kept in touch with it throughout his lifetime by complementing, enlarging, and focusing AP up to the eighth edition. The most decisive step of developing AP was the introduction of methodological dualism in the fourth edition based on the concepts of Windelband, Dilthey, and Max Weber. Accepting the two realms of empirical and interpretative sciences as given due to the nature of man meant cutting the Gordian knot as simple as it may appear in retrospect. This approach overcame the medical model as the sole option for psychopathology, long predominant since the 1820s when the pathogenesis of progressive paralysis was understood.

The introduction of transcendence as a sort of third methodological column was surprisingly disregarded by many recipients of the book. It appears as revolutionary at its time and until today to integrate this into a scientific textbook like the acceptance of the methodological dualism as something inevitably given. This third realm of access to human mental life concerns spiritual mental life. Jaspers allocated it the heading of transcendence. Transcendence signifies both the method to practice spirituality and signifying the state the successfully transcending person arrives at. Jaspers does not elude terms as soul, faith, God. Transcendence is meant to signify human nature as open, as able to go beyond itself in conceiving, behaving, socializing, in short the being of the mind as a whole. An essential aspect of the condition of transcendence is its indeterminacy. This is conveyed in any sentence of the passages dealing with it and it contrasts the sharp definitions of terms otherwise.

This topic of AP was particularly neglected in the positivistic approaches of psychiatry after the change of paradigms in the 1970s. It may be revitalized by recent developments in the neurocognitive sciences. Generating incidental events inside living organisms has been shown to be a biological tool enabling a sort of acting which comes close to free will assertion. It is as essential to the immune system as it is to the hare, whose dodging has been shown to be irregular otherwise it would not survive. If we consider the biological systems' ability to generate incidental events as entrance to something close to free will, transcendence may be considered as a sort of second-order freedom essential to man and distinct from the body and mind categories.

Jaspers' evaluation of both psychiatric and philosophical authors was very frank throughout the decades irrespective of their reputation. The arch-enemy was Sigmund Freud, closely followed by the lot of phenomenologists. Much of Jaspers' criticisms of Freud are certainly valid, in particular that he uses concretisms of mental phenomena and their structural and functional character. Even more detrimental to Freud's scientific heritage was the attempt to indoctrinate disciples. This is alien to any sincere science. Jaspers fought against Alexander Mitscherlich when he was founding the first psychoanalytic chair of psychosomatic medicine in Germany after World War II in Heidelberg. He urged him, in vain, to skip the teaching analysis at least. Nevertheless, the gist of psychoanalysis without its concretisms has merged nowadays with the variegated mainstream of scientific psychotherapy. Jaspers was a bit narrow in this respect not to acknowledge the valid core of psychoanalysis as a psychology of the unconscious if it is liberated from its ideological ballast.

In contrast, phenomenologists were not accused of being too focused but of too general, undifferentiated, interpretative, shallow statements of psychopathology. We do not agree with Wiggins and Schwartz (1997) that Jaspers took over from Husserl his notion of presuppositionlessness and intuition. This certainly would have been incompatible with Dilthey's and Max Weber's methodological foundations. Jaspers determinedly rejected epoché as not reliable. Apart from Viktor von Weizsäcker, French and German psychiatrist-phenomenologists were criticized by Jaspers for their vague impressionistic way of characterizing psychopathology, resembling a piece of art rather than one of science.

However, the psychopathology of delusion is an example that Jaspers' "objective" view from "outside" in the sense of a "process" opposite to "development" falls short of phenomenological interpretation, for example, taking the criterion of "false belief." Blankenburg's view on delusion was an existential one that actually could have been appealing to Jaspers: delusion, Blankenburg says, is a pre-predicative statement, pseudo-denominative. In fact the patient transports an utterance about his state of mind. The delusion of persecution thus conveys a message about the self being crunched and crumbled, alienated. Diffuse feelings emerge, not predicative, emanating, like music to be heard intoning an existential feeling. It is an interpretation which turned out to be extremely helpful for psychotherapy with deluded schizophrenia patients (Mundt, 1996).

It may be considered as an irony of scientific history in the context of AP that just the experimental neurosciences are so fond of phenomenology. The empirical scientific focus on minute neural functions has joined the discipline with the most wholesome, atmospheric approach of the widest aperture for a very ingenuous cooperation.

What are the most intriguing lessons we can learn from Jaspers? Tolerating and sustaining the tension between paradigms instead of fighting them, putting up with contradictions inevitably given and getting different paradigms and disciplines in touch. It is amazing that even after one hundred years Jaspers' work is still needed for orientation and clarification of methodological positions and the interpretation of findings.

ACKNOWLEDGMENTS

I am very grateful to Chiara Cigognini, Heidelberg, for her support of this work with the literature search and checking.

REFERENCES

Bormuth, M. (2004). Die Psychoanalysekritik von Karl Jaspers als Weltanschauungskritik. In B. Weidmann (Ed.), *Existenz in Kommunikation. Zur philosophischen Ethik von Karl Jaspers*, pp. 215–20. Würzburg: Königshausen & Neumann.

Bormuth, M. (2008). Selbstreflexion bei Jaspers im Blick auf das psychiatrische Werk. In S. Rinofer-Kreidl and H. Wiltsche (Eds), *Karl Jaspers' Allgemeine Psychopathologie zwischen Wissenschaft, Philosophie und Praxis*, pp. 109–26. Würzburg: Königshausen & Neumann.

Dilthey, W. (1952). *Das Verstehen anderer Personen und ihrer Lebensäußerungen.* Stuttgart: B. G. Teubner Verlagsgesellschaft.

Dilthey, W. (1955). *Gesammelte Schriften, 1. Band: Einleitung in die Geisteswissenschaften. Versuch einer Grundlegung für das Studium der Gesellschaft und der Geschichte.* Stuttgart: B. G. Teubner Verlagsgesellschaft.

Dilthey, W. (1958). *Der Aufbau der geschichtlichen Welt in den Geisteswissenschaften.* Stuttgart: B.G. Teubner-Verlagsgesellschaft.

Jaspers, K. (1946). *Max Weber. Politiker Forscher Philosoph.* Bremen: Joh. Strohm Verlag.

Jaspers, K. (1959). *General Psychopathology, Volume One* (J. Hoenig and M. W. Hamilton (Trans). Baltimore, MD: Johns Hopkins University Press.

Jaspers, K. (1959). *General Psychopathology, Volume Two* (J. Hoenig and M. W. Hamilton (Trans). Baltimore, MD: Johns Hopkins University Press.

Jaspers, K. (1965). *Allgemeine Psychopathologie* (8th edn). Berlin: Springer-Verlag.

Jaspers, K. (1981). *Nietzsche. Einführung in das Verständnis seines Philosophierens* (4th edn). Berlin: Walter de Gruyter.

Kirkbright, S. (2008). Ein kritischer Vergleich zwischen den verschiedenen Ausgaben von Karl Jaspers Allgemeiner Psychopathologie. In S. Rinofer-Kreidl and H. Wiltsche (Eds), *Karl Jaspers' Allgemeine Psychopathologie zwischen Wissenschaft, Philosophie und Praxis,* pp. 21–9. Würzburg: Königshausen & Neumann.

Merz, P. -U. (1990). *Max Weber und Heinrich Rickert. Die erkenntnistheoretischen Grundlagen der verstehenden Soziologie.* Würzburg: Königshausen & Neumann.

Mundt, C. (1996). Zur Psychotherapie des Wahns. *Nervenarzt, 67,* 515–23.

Mundt, C. (2009). Geleitwort. In D. Engelhardt, H.-J. von, Gerigk (Eds), *Karl Jaspers im Schnittpunkt von Zeitgeschichte, Psychopathologie, Literatur und Film, V-X.* Heidelberg: Mattes.

Mundt, C. (in press). Jaspers' concept of limit situation: Extensions and clinical application. In T. Breyer, T. Fuchs, and C. Mundt (Eds), *Karl Jaspers' Psychopathology and Philosophy.* New York: Springer.

Mundt, C. and Weisbrod, M. (2004). Neuropsychologische Entsprechungen und therapeutische Konsequenzen des strukturdynamischen Modells. [Neuropsychological equivalences and therapeutic consequences of the dynamic structural model]. *Fortschritte Neurologie Psychiatie, 72*(Suppl 1), 14–22.

Weber, M. (1995). *Schriften zur Soziologie.* Stuttgart: Philipp Reclam Jun.

Wiggins, O. P. and Schwartz, M. S. (1997). Edmund Husserl's influence on Karl Jaspers' phenomenology. *Philosophy, Psychiatry, & Psychology, 4*(1), 15–36.

Wiggins, O. P., Schwartz, M. A., Spitzer, M. (1992). Phenomenological/descriptive psychiatry: The methods of Edmund Husserl and Karl Jaspers. In M Spitzer, F. Uehlein, M. A. Schwartz, and C. Mundt (Eds), *Phenomenology, Language, and Schizophrenia,* pp. 46–69. New York, NY: Springer.

Windelband, W. (1900). *Geschichte und Naturwissenschaft. Rede zum Antritt des Rectorats der Kaiser-Wilhelm-Universität Straßburg.* Strasbourg: J. H. Ed. Heitz (Heitz & Mündel).

....

CHAPTER 8

FROM MADNESS TO MENTAL ILLNESS: PSYCHIATRY AND BIOPOLITICS IN MICHEL FOUCAULT

....

FEDERICO LEONI

Madmen, Criminals, Sinners

....

The list of Foucault's interests and fields of research spans a quite unusual variety of topics and issues, including crime, madness, epidemics, health, hunger, punishment, wars and strategies, pleasure and asceticism, masturbation and chastity, military life and hermaphroditism, schools, mental hospitals, prisons, barracks, factories, and companies. Foucault's style of inquiry typically lies halfway between, on the one hand, history and philosophy and, on the other, epistemology of the human sciences and genealogy of the main social, political, and economic institutions of modernity.

The list would be as long as that of the disciplines whose function it is to address the same topics with a descriptive, prescriptive, contemplative, or administrative approach. Such a function is the object of Foucault's archaeological and genealogical inquiry, an inquiry into the historical process which gradually led to the emergence of numerous practices and disciplines which radically contributed to the framing of what we optimistically call "man": psychiatry, physiology, medicine, economics, human sciences, penitentiary architecture, *Polizeiwissenshaft*, jurisprudence, practices of state administration, contemporary and modern biopolitics, ancient forms of wisdom, monastic life and early-Christian moral precepts, the grammar of Port-Royal, and so on.

It is a strange quasi-Borgesian list. However, upon closer scrutiny, behind the sequence of these quite surrealistic *trouvailles* one detects both a continuity and a thin web of connections extending from one context to another and influencing the course of Foucault's research and production—from *History of Madness* (1961)[1] to *The Birth of the Clinic* (1963), *Words and Things* (1966), *Discipline and Punish* (1975), *The Will to Knowledge* (1976), *The Cure of the Self* (1984), and *The Usage of Pleasures* (1984). Each time, Foucault focuses on the other (hidden) side of a given phenomenon, and attempts to explain the visible side through this concealed side, the clean and reassuring surface through the secret life of an apparently anonymous depth. Tell me how you deal with madness—he seems to imply—and I will tell you what your beliefs about reason are, what kind of "rational" subjects your disciplines and practices produce. Tell me how you deal with crime, how you build your prisons, what use you make of your spies and laws, your guards and judges, your doctors and nurses, and I'll tell you who you want to be, and what you think "being" means.

In a mental hospital, one is sometimes isolated and chained, freed or judged, healed or made ill. The closer we look, the thinner the boundaries between the science of police and the science of madness, the architecture of prisons and the architecture of schools, the madman and the criminal, the healthy and the ill, the normal and the abnormal, the child and the savage start to appear. Here, again, the web of archaeological and genealogical connections becomes visible. Depending on the circumstances, illness can be seen in different ways: as a kind of pathology or deviance, as an anomaly waiting to be cured or a guilt deserving punishment, as an eccentricity to hide, as a sin to confess or as a possession to exorcise. Illness is everywhere and nowhere—and so are crime, normality, justice, and, on the other side, the sick person, the criminal, the child. Everywhere we look, we find imperceptible relationships, derivations, interruptions, and recommencements. Kant wrote that the goal of every philosophical quest is to answer the question: "What is man?" However, according to Foucault's archaeology, "man" is the most emblematic and illusory of modern inventions; it is the concept, the grandest one, and the most pregnant with manifold and disturbing consequences. It is not incidental that *History of Madness*, written as a doctoral thesis, was then complemented by another thesis dedicated to Kant's anthropology (it was a rule of the French academia that a doctoral dissertation should be accompanied by a second one). The modern invention of the human sciences, conceived not only as descriptive but also, and even more so, as prescriptive sciences, would thereafter occupy a key position within Foucault's work (Foucault 2008).

LOOK, LIBERATION, SUBJUGATION

One section in *History of Madness* (Foucault 1961) is of particular interest here. Foucault focuses on Philippe Pinel, the French psychiatrist who marked a turn in the history of the treatments of mental illness. In Paris, during the French Revolution, Pinel finally broke the chains that still confined the madman in the dungeons of the Bastille. Against the violence of the iron fetters and the practice of abandoning the "senseless" people (*les insensés*) to a destiny of dark meaninglessness, Pinel opposed a totally different vision of alienistic medicine. Madness, far from being senseless darkness, entails a meaning on which to shed light: it has become a "moral illness," and it is on the moral level that it should be treated. Pinel was a liberator.

---

[1] All dates in brackets refer to the original date of publication of Foucault's works. Quotations are then referenced directly in the text following the author–date style.

Foucault, however, looks at the other side of this "liberation." In this kind of humanistic or humanitarian psychiatry, he finds all the evidence for a new and different paradigm of subjugation (*assujetissement*). What is Pinel's "moral treatment" about? Foucault answers by pointing to three figures of rare effectiveness. The first is that of "silence." An old priest, suffering from delusions of grandeur, thinks he must re-live the Passion of Christ. Pinel orders him to be freed from his shackles, but forbids anyone to talk to him: "This rigorously observed prohibition had a more tangible effect on this man so imbued with himself than either the irons or his cell; he felt humiliated by the abandonment, and by this new form of isolation within his full liberty" (Pinel, quoted in Foucault 2006, p. 496). The shame resulting from being exposed to the gaze of other people and the silence filling his days become his new way of relating to others. The result of this change, in turn, is a new relationship with himself.

The second figure is called "recognition by mirror." Three madmen believe they are kings. A guard, properly instructed, suggests to one of them that disputing with the other two is a waste of time, since they are evidently crazy. Madness, argues Foucault, is invited to look at itself using the other person as a mirror. But a further step shifts the focus of such revelation: "One day when he was less agitated the guard approached him and asked him if he was king, why didn't he bring his detention to an end" (Foucault 2006, p. 498). He finally sees the contradiction and, fifteen days later, gives up his royal title and his delirium and returns to his family and usual life. Again, madness has seen itself. This time, however, it has done so not by looking at the others, but by looking directly at itself. Faced with its own reflection, madness feels shame, confesses its waywardness, and turns into an object of confession, complaint and evaluation (Foucault 2006, pp. 498–500).

The third figure is that of the "perpetual judgment." Thanks to this new mirror effect, madness is relentlessly invited to judge itself; yet it is also continuously judged from the outside, and not by a moral and/or scientific conscience, but rather before a sort of invisible and permanently active jury. When the "alienated patient" takes a bath, Pinel explains referring to a female patient, "the fault that has been committed or the omission of the important duty is recalled," and suddenly a jet of ice-cold water is thrown on her; the patient "is made to understand that it is for her good and that recourse is regretfully made to measures of such violence" (Pinel, quoted in Foucault 2006, p. 501).

At the end of the eighteenth century, Foucault concludes, no liberation of the mentally ill took place, but, rather, what emerged was an objectification of the concept of their freedom—which does not mean this was simply a false liberation. If this were the case, it would be enough to achieve a "real" and true liberation, which in turn would mean that the results of Foucault's archaeology are quite poor. Rather, what Foucault implies is that every liberation, precisely because it is a "real" liberation, is at the same time a form of subjugation, and overlaps perfectly with its opposite: the other side of any liberation is the threat of being subjected. Over the course of his following works, Foucault would dedicate further reflections to such mysterious coincidences of opposites.

SUBJECT AND DEVICE

The triple articulation of the "moral treatment" is a good example of what, in the following years, Foucault would define more and more as a kind of "device." A device is, in this case, a specific articulated space. There would be no need to free the madmen if they did not already inhabit the space of a "great confinement," according to the definition in *History of Madness*: walls, corridors, large common rooms and tiny isolated cells, and then also the particular disposition of doors, windows, slits and passageways. But no mental institution or penitentiary may exist without a certain society, a certain urban planning, and a certain set of laws. These forms of organization are connected to executive powers, habits and, ultimately, to countless functions, attendants, and tricks which work as guarantors of such space and its effectiveness.

Thus the device is a space, a set of things, a web of relationships, and a constellation of bodies; it is the madman looking at the other madmen, and vice versa. It is the madman's word amidst the confusion of the other madmen's words, but also the attendant's word which sets him free and subjects him at the same time, isolating him from the buzz of his mates by according him an inner silent voice and an instrument of complaint and confession, of liberation, and further condemnation. In these passages from *History of Madness*, we find the prefiguration of Foucault's future interests in Christian confession as forerunner of psychoanalytic talk, which will be developed in *The Will to Knowledge* of 1976. The device is all and none of this at the same time: it is not something that can be defined or grasped as such. It is the functioning and the objective effectiveness of a number of elements which no intentionality predisposed or set in motion. It is an uninterrupted genesis of structures, potential differences, resistances, and getaways. Some empty space becomes available and is immediately filled, and a certain matter shows itself malleable to the action of opposite forces. Various forms of organization are built or destroyed. The issue of subjectivity compacts itself around certain points in this field of structures. At the same time it splits along certain lines of fracture appearing in the field. We are what we can be; we think what we must think.

Disciplined Bodies, Souls at Work

Years after the publication of *History of Madness*, Foucault shifts the object of his inquiry from mental hospitals to prisons. The results of such inquiry appear in the middle of the 1970s in a book entitled *Discipline and Punish* (1975). The shift is worth mentioning, considering that Foucault would return to the topic of madness with a radically different perspective in a series of lectures on *The Psychiatric Power* held at the Collège de France in the years 1973–1974 (the transcripts have been published under the same title in 2003, long after Foucault's death).

Let us begin with *Discipline and Punish*. This time Foucault's goal is to study the complex juridical, police, and penitentiary devices. He believes that, in order to reconstruct the history of modern subjectivity, it is necessary to analyze the practices surrounding and regulating a context which is by definition peripheral to the political apparatuses, and to the great discourses of reason. Again, Foucault shows that the center is shaped at the periphery. "Man" is defined where the devices concern themselves with "almost-human" or "non-human" figures such as criminals, those who have been convicted, sentenced, and tortured.

In *Discipline and Punish*, Foucault examines the two extremes of the functioning of the juridical-penitentiary device. The first is characterized by the practice of public executions. The book starts with a dazzling description, both for the virtuosity of Foucault's rhetoric and the disturbing content of the scene. It is the description of the execution of a certain

Damien, his hands and feet tied to four horses pulling in four diverging directions, quartering the body of the unfortunate before the eyes of an enchanted crowd. The public torment, Foucault notes, is designed as a perverse and somehow grandiose show, offered to the crowd as simultaneously both a warning and a feast thrown by a sovereign who is the personification of power and the final target of any crime, whatever its seriousness. Each punishment means the reaffirmation of an absolute sovereignty, a power which invisibly rules and judges, but also carves in the most visible and showy way the insignia of its overwhelming force in the bodies of its subjects, and in the theater of the public square.

At the other extreme from the seventeenth-century absolutist monarchies, we have the nineteenth-century ascending bourgeoisie and incipient industrialization. At this stage, the juridical and penitentiary device undergoes a profound transformation. The value of each operand has changed: the judgment has now become public and the trial is a debate taking place, at least in theory, before everyone's eyes. The punishment, instead, is hidden, even invisible, and is usually inflicted within prisons located at the extreme periphery of towns: nothing spectacular and no trace of quick, intense, and disturbing actions targeting the body of the condemned. On the contrary, what we have is a slow and meticulous work which acts on the body only to reach the soul, forcibly disciplining the inmate's gestures in order to build a new person. Each time the bodies and souls are shaped by the devices. The spectacular torment had molded bodies in a specific manner, creating an object that did not exist before: it had provided both women and men with a body which would serve as a public stage or as a document into which the power was to carve its prerogatives. Two centuries later, the prison molds "disciplined bodies" (as Foucault puts it) which are transformed to fit the narrow spaces of the cells, and made to adapt to the fine web of limits and passageways which either block their passage, or through which they slither. The intentions of these bodies are shaped by the piercing look which scans them continuously from a hidden and invisible point of view. This way, the condition of the prisoner is a permanent and inescapable visibility.

Thus, looking becomes an anonymous and impersonal function, a force that unfolds independently of the presence or the absence of an observer and an observed. Even if the guard were not there, the inmate would believe he is being watched. In the end, he would watch himself, having incorporated that anonymous look which inspected him and anatomized the most common of his gestures. This process generates a new kind of subject and/or object, a subject which coincides completely with this procedure of self-control. All of its actions are inscribed in the space of this conformity. This subject continuously works on itself. Or, better still, the "subject" here becomes nothing but the name of this relentless inspection and rectification of behaviors and intentions. This leads to a condition in which the work of optimization, and the optimization of work, become the two inseparable faces of the disciplined subject—of the "docile bodies," as Foucault puts it in *Discipline and Punish*.

THE DEPOSITION OF SOVEREIGNTY AND THE INSTAURATION OF THE "PSY-FUNCTION"

In his lectures on *Psychiatric Power*, Foucault develops two theses which are of particular interest here. The first relies on the analysis of a famous episode, mentioned by many scholars after Foucault to explain the shift from sovereign power to disciplinary power. As we will see, psychiatry plays a decisive role in this shift.

The episode is the madness of King George III (Foucault 2003, lecture of November 14, 1973). The king has gone insane and, following the diagnosis of the psychiatrist Francis Willis, is deprived of his entire authority. It is a sort of "upside down consecration," writes Foucault. George III is forced to live the rest of his life in a surveyed isolation, not so different, apart from its distinguished luxury, from that of any other "mad" Englishman of his time. Psychiatric power is the new sovereign, the new holder of a power that no longer works in accordance with the schemes of sovereignty.

Foucault uses this episode as an emblem, and in this emblem we must read a metaphor and a synecdoche at the same time. First the metaphor: the king is taken to a padded room, but it is the entire traditional device which is dissolving, undermined by an anonymous, multiform power embodied by grey functionaries instead of the representatives of an ancient war-like prestige. The scene takes place away from indiscreet eyes, in that silent privacy which is the key setting of the disciplinary power. The king deprived of his powers is not abandoned to the will of an enemy ruler who has defied and crushed him on the battlefield. He is left to a number of attendants and procedures that will help him contain the explosion of his madness, channeling his disordered energies into a peaceful administrative routine. Now the synecdoche: the psychiatrist has become one of the many functionaries of the new power, insofar as psychiatry has become one of the many disciplines configuring its new paradigm. At the same time, psychiatry and the psychiatrist stand for the whole system of these new disciplines: they give shape to the spirit, the techniques, and the tools which every other disciplinary power will adopt in order to exercise its minute and invisible control over bodies, gestures, and intentions.

The second thesis brings us much closer to our time and enables us to understand the position psychiatry occupies in it (lecture of November 7, 1973). Psychiatry crossed a very important threshold between the early modern age (including the seventeenth century) and the liberal age (nineteenth century). This threshold concerns the criteria for recognition of mental illness and, consequently, the position and function of psychiatry with respect to the mentally ill person. In the age of Descartes, madness was conceived as a mistake of judgment or as a wrong representation of oneself and the world. To suffer from delusions meant to believe in something "wrong," which bore the imprint of alienation from the realm of founded beliefs, immediately verifiable by comparing the madman's views with the real world. Thus, the experience of madness, and the intervention of those who had to deal with it, occurred within the context of knowledge and representation. At the beginning of the nineteenth century, however, a new standard of identification and perhaps, at a deeper level, a new function of psychiatry start to emerge. Psychiatry deals no longer with the problem of recognition of madness, but rather with that of managing its consequences. According to this epistemologically and practically changed scenario, the madman becomes, above all, a man or a woman who is the victim of a force he or she cannot master.

The writings of Philippe Pinel and other psychiatrists mentioned by Foucault leave no doubt about this. The passions of the mad person are not controllable, the ideas that inhabit his delirious mind are not wrong so much as violent, and even dangerous to himself and to others. The psychiatrist is faced with a new field of phenomena wherein he finds new objects worthy of inspection, because something new and different has attracted his attention. Now it is the force, not the mistake, which stands out in that field, and the goal of the psychiatrist is the control of a force, not the identification of a mistake. By concentrating its efforts on the handling of a force which is primarily seen as excessive and incoherent, psychiatry turns into a key element within the set of disciplinary knowledge and techniques. In the age of liberalism and mass industrialization, where an embryonic globalization of markets is emerging, each discipline has to conceive of man as a bundle of forces in need of regimentation, of continuous supervision, and of scrupulous adjustment to a certain standard prescribing the "good use" of such forces. Once again psychiatry, according to Foucault, appears both as part of the disciplinary system and as the whole system itself. Together with the legion of different professionals who would join his cause during the nineteenth and the twentieth century (psychologists, psychoanalysts, pedagogues, and social workers), the psychiatrist becomes the purest expression of a function whose final goal is the public order and the individual's most efficient performance in interaction with other individuals.

In one of his most intense lectures on *Psychiatric Power* (held on November 28, 1973), Foucault calls this phenomenon the "psy-function." At this stage, madness has become yet another object: no longer a mistake, nor a violent, overwhelming power. Rather, it is seen as a kind of white noise, a lack of efficiency, or wasteful expenditure of the energy the individual should have been able to perfectly coordinate with the other forces forming what we usually call "society." The psy-function aims at restoring the efficiency of the individual and of the collective performance. Its role is to reduce people's bodies, behaviors, and physical and psychological performances to a certain standard and economy of forces, which in turn liberalism considers as the goal and proper good of society, or as the ground on which society spontaneously tends to organize itself (Foucault would study the developments of disciplinary powers into another paradigm of power, called "biopower," in a later period of his teaching: see the courses on *Security, Territory, Population* (1977–1978), and *Birth of Biopolitics* (1978–1979)).

This way, psychiatry takes on a unique aspect amongst the medical sciences, to which it nevertheless refers more and more often during the nineteenth century, especially since the neurological dimension has become a significant part of its language. A famous French surgeon cited by Georges Canguilhem (2002, p. 90) once said that health is that precarious condition which never looks promising and always turns into disease. If this is true, we could say that the goal of psychiatry as a psy-function is not so much that of healing and restoring mental health, but rather that of managing an uncertain condition which fluctuates between pathology and non-pathology, without belonging to either field. This kind of "grey zone"— neither health nor illness—is in fact the only source of the variability of a parameter which, in the end, has nothing to do with the individual's illness or well-being, because it is concerned only with the quality and nature of the control exercised by psychiatry on some of the behavioral performances of such individual.

THE INVENTION OF HUMAN CAPITAL

In his course on *Psychiatric Power*, Foucault points out that all this implies a "confiscation" of everyone's body, time, and life (lecture of November 21, 1973). One could argue that before the emergence of the psy-function, things such as a virgin body, time, and life never existed. The specific performance of the sovereign's power was to display the body of the condemned as a place for exemplary and showy punishments. The specific performance of today's disciplinary power is the constant exploration and optimization of a set of behavioral performances: rather than the confiscation of a certain resource or skill, this means, simultaneously, the invention, promotion, and exploitation of a new resource. Thus, the new paradigm of the liberal age invents, promotes, and exploits a new resource: the time and life of people considered as a mass, as a social organism, and as an organic whole.

This is one of the points Foucault would elaborate with increasing clarity over the following years. We find it, plainly stated, throughout *The Will to Knowledge* (1976). Power does not move from the center to the periphery, from the top to the bottom, nor from the instance which denies or censors to the force which is diminished or annihilated. Rather, its functioning is more articulated, for power positions itself horizontally and proceeds by means of alliances, complicities, and co-options. It completes and promotes its counterpart, urges and triggers the forces upon which it works, and channels and empowers the energies it wants to administrate. To govern—once the symbolic threshold of the deposition of George III is crossed—does not mean to say no, nor does it mean to kill an enemy: it means to say yes, to sign alliances, to orient and to enrich a potential. Foucault's psy-function operates in the same way, and prepares new functions which will further promote this subtle art of optimization and exploitation of individual and collective performances. The result is that, on the one hand, European societies become "psychiatrized," and, on the other, the psy-function becomes "sociologized." In other words, the psy-function becomes the science of society itself, the main instrument of theoretical analysis and of practical intervention on the social organism, and the key paradigm for the optimization and empowerment of its global performances.

In this context, the practice of writing, verbalization, data collection, and the art of statistics play a key role (Foucault 2004a; on Foucault 2004a, see Redaelli 2011, pp. 134–173). Schools, barracks, hospitals, but also police stations, courts of justice, prisons, and mental hospitals, become places where behaviors and exceptions to the rules are constantly catalogued and monitored. The continuous examination typical of the disciplinary power grows stronger with the diffusion of such filing systems and techniques of recording, extraction, and confrontation of data. What Foucault had defined as "disciplined bodies" have now become a general stock of "life" reduced to long data strings, recorded in neat charts where every measure is set in relation to a reference value, and exemplified in schemes that sum up differentials which are ever-changing and in constant need of updating and correction. The intervention of such a power does not consist in the exceptional and spectacular punishment of an extraordinary crime, but rather in the restless process of assessment and correction of the tiniest flaws and the less perceptible performances. The key instruments of this kind of power are statistics, the careful management of data variability, and the identification of arithmetic laws and techniques which allow for the management of aleatory factors. The actions of children and elderly people, workers and housewives, insane patients, sick people, and criminals have become more and more traceable and targetable. The effect of the whole device is the unprecedented possibility of optimizing a given resource, and the definition of that particular object of administration which is the human performance: the "human resource" in its totality.

Indirectly, this change reshapes the nature of the individual as it emerged from the practices of disciplinary power of the eighteenth and nineteenth century. The individual itself is now conceivable only as a resource to administrate and optimize, as an anonymous and generic sum of behavioral potentialities. A new paradigm takes the place of the disciplinary power. The twentieth century begins under the sign of the so-called "biopower." This is the main thesis of the course taught by Foucault in the years 1978–1979, entitled *Birth of Biopolitics* (Foucault 2004b). The target of biopower is that new field of objectivity represented by the life of a population, and that new system of variables represented by the vital performance of a society. This kind of resource becomes visible and manageable only under particular conditions, that is, only when it is watched and governed from far away, not with the eyes of the guard watching a line of cells, but with the detached and synoptical look of the statistical researcher, the demographer, the epidemiologist, and the economist. These are, in fact, the "new" sciences or, better, the new devices which emerged between the eighteenth and the twentieth century: their nature and their role in shaping a society which is still, in many ways, our society, form the object of Foucault's research (Foucault 2004a, 2004b).

In the age of biopower, the management of such new forms of objectivity represented by the "vitality" of a population has become the main goal of power, which aims to promote its quality, intensity, and duration. These are guaranteed through different initiatives such as mass education, vocational training, and the national welfare state. Among the resources whose highest profitability must be guaranteed by the individual we find: personal behavior, the sum of competences and skills (including, in some cases, even the biological competences of the body), exposure to certain forms of sickness and the capacity for recovery, genetic patrimony and the promises and threats inscribed in the genes. In terms of anonymous performative efficiency, the general and statistic vitality of the population finds its precise equivalent in the individual. There is in fact nothing individual in these "individual" resources, but rather a certain quantity of forces, a certain supply of competences, a certain capital of capabilities (behavioral or biological) whose expression must be developed and optimized. The individual has become conceivable and manageable only as a "human capital" (Foucault 2004b, lecture held on March 14, 1979).

From one point of view, this shift was not hard to predict. Its premonitory symptoms could be easily spotted in the features of the already-mentioned psy-function. The idea of madness being a force to tame and a chaotic energy to measure and organize anticipated this outcome: the individual becomes a capital of competences and possibilities, waiting to be regimented and brought to full expression. From another point of view, this displacement takes place only by the end of the nineteenth and in the first half of the twentieth century, when the psy-function and the disciplinary powers adopt new tools and a new logic. In particular, this happens when the path of the psy-function overlaps with that of the statistical approaches to those new fields of objectivity, which are the social body as a whole and the collective efficiency as a general flux and capital.

Logic of Optimization

The liberal man, who exchanges goods according to the principle of utilitarianism, the comparability of values, and the equity and equilibrium of transactions, is now eclipsed by the neoliberal man, shaped by the values of an almost Darwinian struggle. Such values consist in producing the same goods with lesser resources, in reaching the highest productive efficiency compared to market averages, in exploiting every resource (human and non-human) to obtain the highest standard of performances, and so on. The result is not equilibrium, but disequilibrium—not equality, but inequality, and struggle for life (Foucault 2004b, lecture of November 7, 1979).

The "value of life," so often mentioned in the age of neoliberalism, seems almost invariably destined to turn into this kind of strictly economical evaluation and re-evaluation of a set of biological and behavioral capabilities. What we are dealing with here are, in fact, strictly non-individual and non-subjective sets of capabilities: the pure manual ability for certain physical work, the simple conversation skills necessary for working in a call center, the people skills required by management positions, and, finally, a general willingness to pursue an education which is sufficiently differentiated to meet the needs of a certain productive mechanism and, on the other hand, undifferentiated enough to meet those of a totally different one. The worker has become entirely unspecific, amenable to forming and re-forming, being trained and trained again, and not opposing resistance to any of the incoming work opportunities. Therefore, the final result of the total transcription of the disciplined body into the malleable and optimized categories of the management of human resources is the "vitality" of such a completely de-individualized individual. Moreover, it is not out of place, in this case, to talk of mere "vitality," because, in this new context, there is no longer any difference between behavioral performance and cognitive performance, between biological performance and intellectual performance, and between relational performance and productive performance. All has become "resource," and all that biopower needs to do is to design and provide the conditions for its highest profitability, maximizing the profitability of that capital with respect to its performance.

"Optimization," then, becomes a sort of keyword for this reading and planning of individual behavior and society, which works almost exclusively in arithmetical and economical terms. The distinction between means and ends, as such, loses meaning. Nothing in this scenario can be considered "worthy," nothing here is a goal or an end. It can only be computable as a step along the path leading to a further step. Any attempt to establish a link between points A and B will result only in the planning of a better way to multiply the resources amassed at point A, in order to create other resources to be amassed at point B. Then, another identical operation will multiply and amass the resources of point B at another point C. The individual itself will survive only as the empty space where means and ends coincide: the perfectly indifferent space where the capital to be exploited, and the instance that promotes its exploitation, completely overlap. While the individual designed by the disciplinary power controlled and punished itself, the human resource designed by the biopolitical device promotes and exploits itself. And it promotes and exploits itself in order to promote and exploit itself again and again, more and more deeply, without any trace of what classical metaphysics would have called *telos*.

DSM and Insurance Companies

At this point we might ask what place psychiatry occupies within this new paradigm. In many ways, psychiatry lay at the beginning of the path that leads to it. Such a paradigm, however, absorbs psychiatry and assigns a new function to it.

The most widespread model for psychiatry in the Western world is represented by the *Diagnostic and Statistical Manual of Mental Disorders* (DSM). The DSM has become a key device of our time, a point where the three separate paths described by Foucault meet in an increasingly systematic convergence.

Let us briefly recall these three paths: firstly, the establishment of the psy-function as a general function of enunciation and regulation of disciplinary powers, together with some key aspects of biopower; secondly, the establishment of writing as a means of objectification, schematization, constant evaluation and re-evaluation of the variables targeted by disciplinary powers and biopowers; thirdly, the emergence of a particular approach, based on what might be named an "insurance logic," meaning a logic that is profoundly consubstantial to the logic of the financial enterprise.

We can start from the last point—a point only briefly mentioned by Foucault's analysis, but which lies at the core of *L'état providence*, written by François Ewald, a pupil of Foucault's, now arguably one of the leading scholars of French insurance economy. The logic of the enterprise is, for reasons that are far from incidental, based on risk. The way an enterprise works is the way of the bet. The entrepreneur invests money today, foreseeing a possible profit tomorrow. There is more: the businessman invests a capital which will be fully available only at a later time, if everything goes according to his plans. This is the reason why, at the beginning, the modern enterprise presupposed what Marx called "primary accumulation," whose function was later taken over by the resources lent by the banking system. In an entrepreneurial system, wealth is produced through debts, and every debt becomes a resource only in the sense that it is the postponement of a present vacuum to a future one.

From another point of view, each debt can be postponed to the future and finally solved only at the cost of a risk which is entailed by it: the risk of insolvency. The answer, in this case, can only be one: the multiplication and systematization of all those procedures which deal with risk insurance, whether it concerns monetary capital, a set of means of production, material wealth, a certain stock of relational skills or personal resources, or a certain package of cognitive and behavioral capabilities (both individual and collective). Now that an enterprise is more often than not an individual enterprise, and the individual is increasingly described and "planned" as the entrepreneur of himself (Foucault 2004b, lecture of November 14, 1979), insuring one's skills and resources has become crucially important: the purpose is to guarantee and preserve such fragile resources for the entire course of one's life, from the education of souls to the training of the bodies, from the preservation of health and physical efficiency to the management of aging, illness, or death.

Thus, an increasing share of the contemporary insurance device concerns the insurance of the human capital which lies in the cognitive, behavioral, affective, or relational skills of an individual who has become the entrepreneur of himself (*entrepreneur de soi-meme*). But this is precisely the point where the path of the insurance device intersects with the other two paths mentioned earlier, generating a grid within which the management of health and the management of human capital broadly overlap. It is in this context that we must recognize—in Foucaultian terms—the relevance of the DSM as a device. On the one hand, in fact, the role of the psy-function, and more generally of all biomedical knowledges, is to evaluate the individual's cognitive and behavioral capabilities each time, and, in a broader sense, to assess the "vitality" of that same individual, together with the set of biological resources available to him or her. The point is to identify which typologies and levels of risk are linked to those resources, so that the insurance company may define its own system of warranties, calculating the probabilities that a certain risk may occur, the amount of the premium paid by the insured client, and the indemnity remitted by the insurance company. Here, the biomedical knowledge is already governed by biopower, and its business is not therapy, but the administration both of a capital and of the risks connected to the future exploitation of such capital.

On the other hand, after two centuries of waiting, the device of writing has finally allowed the psy-function and the insurance function to speak the same language. More precisely, the writing device shaped the psy-function and the insurance function from their very origin: the result is that now they completely concur on a certain standard of objectivity, translate and confront jointly defined symptoms, calculate with the very same tools the inefficiencies and the probabilities of recovery from certain diseases, and, finally, they identify which individuals society, conceived as an enterprise, should or should not make its bet on. In brief, the optimization of the biomedical administration of wealth goes hand in hand with the biopolitical optimization of human capital.

Mental Illness and Neoliberal Reason

Every tool prescribes the rules of its own use. It is also true that those rules always allow a margin of freedom, in the sense that somehow we can apply to that same tool the rules of another tool and use it differently. However, the roots of the DSM lie in an insurance-oriented mentality, and this clearly affects the kind of psychiatric model such tool suggests and, inevitably, prescribes to those who adopt it.

It is well known that the DSM was elaborated in the USA as an answer to a number of clearly disciplinary needs, in a Foucaultian sense. On the one hand, it has military origins; it is a tool designed for the psychological and behavioral screening of groups, based on the model of other similar tools already in use by other branches of military medicine. On the other hand, the reasons that led to its formulation are extremely rational and simple, in the sense of that organizational rationality and constant optimization of processes which are the essential form and content of neoliberal reason.

In fact, the whole US health care system follows a private insurance-like policy. In the USA the insurance function is not performed by the government (as it is in Europe with the welfare state), but by private companies tied to an openly entrepreneurial logic. Such a situation, by the way, reveals and uncovers an intrinsic component of European public welfare, which is in fact quickly evolving toward a privatized model. Given these circumstances, it should come as no surprise that the need for standardized tools for quantifying the biological damage suffered by a certain individual emerged in the United States much earlier than it did in other countries. Such measurements take into account the past conditions of the individual as a possible cause of such damage, and the costs of both the therapy and the other means necessary to sustain the individual in the event of an incomplete recovery. The DSM is, from this point of view, nothing more and nothing less than the accomplishment of a purely medical insurance-oriented need, within the specificity of the psy-context or function.

This means two things. On the one hand, the DSM should be considered a collateral effect of a broader phenomenon, which consists in the fact that medical sciences have grown in the direction of the logic of insurance companies, carrying psychiatry along in the process, and transmitting to it their need for, so to speak, informatized and economically optimized diagnoses and prognoses. The information written in the medical records must be as simple as possible, easy to exchange and compare, constantly updated, and immediately translatable into other languages—above all, into the language of enterprises and insurance companies. Such language is influenced by the logic of statistics and risk management, which expresses the relationship between the costs of a therapy, its individual benefits, and its collective consequences. On the other hand, it is precisely biomedical knowledge and the public or private insurance logic which were originally shaped in accordance with the procedures of control and restoration of performance efficiency, developed for the first time in the history of European societies by psychiatry and the Foucaultian psy-function.

However, the biomedical paradigm seems to incorporate the "psy" paradigm. The cognitive and behavioral (and affective, and intersubjective, etc.) functions described and transformed by the DSM into something computable are defined in total analogy with the damages and the biological functions verifiable inside any biomedical laboratory. As we have seen, it is the biopolitical paradigm which produces a general flattening of physical, cognitive, behavioral, affective, and relational performance. In each of these cases, the question is simply to calculate the profitability of a certain set of resources, belonging not so much to an individual, but to the "vitality" of a group or population. On its part, the psy-paradigm dictates to the biomedical sciences a kind of clinical approach in which the diagnosis is not entirely therapeutically oriented (recovery from a disease), but aims at handling certain inefficiencies in view of their sustainability and their statistical, epidemiological, and economic significance. The list of these resources must include not only physical strength and the ability to carry on heavy tasks (which were paramount when production was mainly industrial and grounded in the assembly line), but also the relational and cognitive, affective and hermeneutical skills needed to fill the increasing demand for the organizational professions which characterize our society—including a capability which classical metaphysics considered specific to mankind and exquisitely spiritual: language. Just consider how much of our lives as consumers and/or producers is based on the use of *logos*, that is, on the human ability to exercise a linguistic or in general a semiotic function, to interact in a world of signs and to be oriented by, or led by, a jungle of images or a web of spectacular functions.

Thus, psy-device, biomedical device, and insurance device converge in the definition and production of man as a bundle of economically relevant performances, as a web of abilities and resources which might be damaged, restored, organized, and optimized. From this point of view, the DSM represents the exact reverse of those business manuals used in the departments of economics as well as in personnel departments. Such manuals imposed the theme of organizational efficiency, thereby promoting a restless activity of corporate training focused on the definition and promotion of certain behaviors. The optimum of those behaviors could be defined, first, in terms of adaptive efficiency to the enterprise organism, then, in terms of the capability of an individual to interiorize that same entrepreneurship, and finally, as the almost automatic coordination of the individual self-entrepreneur monads. Management manuals, from this point of view, optimistically develop the *pars construens* of a certain human type, whose deconstruction is carried out in a perfectly specular manner by the DSM. In other words, if in Descartes' time madness was defined as *déraison*, in the time of organizing reason, of the insurance-like management of resources and of biopolitical performance optimization, madness can only be regarded as mental illness. Mental illness, in turn, can be conceived only as behavioral inefficiency, lack of relational skills, inadequate cognitive or affective proficiency—that is, as a human capital waiting to be restored, and as a biological capital waiting to be optimized.

References

Canguilhem, G. (2002). *Ecrits sur la médecine*. Paris: Seuil.

Ewald, F. (1986). *L'État providence*. Paris: Grasset.

Foucault, M. (1961). *Histoire de la folie à l'age Classique*. Paris: Gallimard.

Foucault, M. (1963). *Naissance de la clinique. Une archéologie du regard medical*. Paris: Presses Universitaires de France.

Foucault, M. (1966). *Les mots et les choses. Une archéologie des sciences humaines*. Paris: Gallimard.

Foucault, M. (1975). *Surveiller et punir. Naissance de la prison*. Paris: Gallimard.

Foucault, M. (1976). *La volonté de savoir (Histoire de la sexualité, Vol. 1)*. Paris: Gallimard.

Foucault, M. (1984a). *Le souci de soi (Histoire de la sexualité, Vol. 2)*. Paris: Gallimard.

Foucault, M. (1984b). *The Usage of Pleasures (Histoire de la sexualité, Vol. 3)*. Paris: Gallimard.

Foucault, M. (2003). *Le pouvoir psychiatrique*. Paris: Seuil.

Foucault, M. (2004a). *Sécurité, Territoire, Population*. Paris: Seuil.

Foucault, M. (2004b). *Naissance de la biopolitique*. Paris: Seuil.

Foucault, M. (2006). *History of Madness*. London: Routledge.

Foucault, M. (2008). *Introduction à l'anthropologie de Kant*. Paris: Vrin.

Redaelli, E. (2011). *L'incanto del dispositivo*. Pisa: ETS.

CHAPTER 9

THE EPISTEMOLOGICAL VALUE OF DEPRESSION MEMOIRS: A META-ANALYSIS

JENNIFER RADDEN AND SOMOGY VARGA

The psychological symptoms of melancholia were from ancient times elaborated in medical lore as well as more literary and philosophical writing. Since before the early modern era, when Burton was famously both sufferer and chronicler of melancholy states, these accounts have been supplemented by autobiographical descriptions. The best of such personal documents are unmatched in their narrative force, helping us understand the experience of disorder in ways that even the most detailed and careful clinical third-person description cannot do.

Until the nineteenth century brought new scientific models of disorder, medical practitioners attended closely to the subjective experience and such narratives of illness, placing them within the patient's life and life story (Bury 2001). With the rise of the modern clinic and the possibilities that modern laboratories offered, however, the patient's subjective experience and understanding of the disorder in her life has become less important (Bury 2001; Lawrence 1994). Over time, the focus of the doctor changed to gathering reliable information about symptoms that could be linked to specific biological states. Not surprisingly, the success and expansion of medical and pharmaceutical possibilities has also meant that subjective accounts of the experience of disorder have become increasingly less important, or even irrelevant.

The last two decades have witnessed a movement countering this tendency as illness narratives of all kinds entered public discourse.[1] Autobiographical writing on physical illnesses and disability has dominated the field, yet in recent years there has also been an impressive

---

[1] These personal accounts have entered public discourse with the simultaneous decline in medical authority, explosion of available information about disorders, and self-help groups fostering and spreading that information. A new vocabulary has been provided for personal narratives of illness by non-experts, giving voice to the experience of being ill, and focusing on the whole person often ignored

boom in autobiographical writing about mental illness.[2] Importantly, such autobiographical writing is beginning to "work back" and inform medical understanding itself, both within medicine more generally, and within medical psychiatry. There is a growing acceptance of personal narratives in medical scholarship used for illustrative effect, and the prospect of research that builds on such narratives in more substantive ways.

While research attention to autobiographical testimony must be welcomed, it also presents a special challenge and raises epistemological issues that need to be addressed. This is because the memoirs invite approach as *veritable sources of rich description of experience*, rather than as particular texts representing a literary genre. Yet they are apparently both— and, as we demonstrate here, it is due to their ambiguous status as both that these personal narratives belie easy or conclusive interpretation.

This matter of the *epistemological status* of depression memoirs is the subject of the following discussion. Viewed as symptom descriptions and reports of inner states, the value of these accounts must be questioned. This is not because they are entirely fictive, as some theories would have it. It is because *what* they are remains unresolved. Depression memoirs may tell us more about the discourse on depression within the medium of literature than about the concrete and "raw" experience of depression itself. Just what they tell us, however, remains indeterminate. Thus our claim here is the epistemological one—that the extent to which these descriptions illuminate the true nature of depressive experience, rather than reflecting a literary genre and cultural meanings, *cannot be discerned*. We do not wish to deny that there are facts of the matter about such experiences that some autobiographical writing may quite accurately describe, but if there are, memoirs will not provide us with an easy way of discovering those facts.

Complicating our thesis, memoirs of any kind possess a degree of this sort of opacity, due to both the nature of the literary conventions governing their writing, and the nature of autobiographical memory. In this respect depression memoirs are not distinctive. Yet—as the sustained example of attitudes about self-identity is used here to illustrate—additional and special indeterminacy affects our interpretation of depression memoirs. And these more general and more particular ambiguities each affect what we can learn from such accounts. Not only particular literary conventions, cultural meanings, and cognitive deficits affecting memory, we show, but the characteristic and constitutive *moods* associated with depression, impede efforts to assign depression memoirs a place on the spectrum between reports of immediate experience and cultural or fictive artifacts. Their ambiguous status is reason to employ caution in drawing conclusions from them.

Depression memoirs invite this analysis for several reasons. First, they are numerous, and as long as we count pre-twentieth-century narratives of states of melancholia among

in the medical sphere (Hawkins 1993). Moreover, the recursive and self-reflective work involved in telling autobiographical stories is now considered as a means to repair and order experience after a disruptive disorder (Becker 1997; Frank 2000; Kleinman 1988; Nelson 2001, Smorti et al. 2010). The recounting of one's story is thought to restore a sense of agency, and in some cases, patients not only actively engage with their experience of disorder, but this upsetting experience is described as an important source for the restoration of a sense of self. The narrative repair of the sense of self after an episode of disorder is specifically pertinent to autobiographical work on mental disorders, because in these cases the sense of self is so regularly and profoundly affected.

  [2] By one count there have been at least one hundred autobiographies centered on first-person accounts of mental disorder (Sommer et al. 1998). See also Hornstein (2002).

their number, they go back a very long way. Second, they are characterized by description of experience that is richly phenomenal—emotions, feelings, and moods, not merely beliefs or behavioral responses. They involve states and conditions that resist reductive behavioral or neurobiological analysis. Independent of depression's neurochemical makeup, and of whatever cultural elements frame its description, there is *something it is like* to be depressed.[3]

The argument will proceed in three parts. At the outset, depression memoirs are contextualized within the genre of autobiography as well as the subgenre of illness and disability memoir or "autopathography," and we stress the ambiguities common to all autobiographical writing: the constraints imposed by its genre, on the one hand, and the nature of autobiographical memory, on the other. In the second part we then describe sources of ambiguity distinctive to depression memoirs, some illustrated by examples from first-person descriptions of melancholia and depression and others tied to the status of depressive states as moods. The focus of these examples is the depiction of self inasmuch as this reveals *proprietary relations* about the ownership of experience ("my," "mine"), that, in occurring as part of conscious thought, involves *reflective self-awareness*. In the third part of the chapter, some empirical corroboration for these claims of indeterminacy is introduced—in research showing that depression affects autobiographical memory and writing style in ways that will influence the structure and content of the narrative. Concluding the discussion, implications for research are noted. The indeterminacy identified here is not a reason to dismiss depression memoirs so much as to employ caution in using them—which in turn calls for sensitivity to the context of that use.

Autobiographical Writing and "Indeterminacy"

As a significant literary genre in the Western world by the eighteenth century, autobiography was intrinsically linked to the rise of a cultural outlook, viz., that we are individuals with unique personal identities that evolve over the course of a lifetime, and can be retrospectively made sense of (Anderson 2001; Eakin 1992; Gusdorf 1956). Changing literary standards and practices influence autobiographical writing, but there are a few fairly stable characteristics. First, autobiographical writing combines narration of significant life episodes with reflection upon their significance for the person's identity, disclosing a self-image that intertwines aspects of who one takes oneself to be and who one wishes to be (Eakin 1992; Wright 2006).[4] Second, a tacit "contract" between author and reader involves an agreement that the author, the protagonist (who undergoes the events that the author recalls), and the narrator, are one (Lejeune 1982). Within such identity there is a polyphony of voices: the protagonist who undergoes the events that the author recalls, the narrator who reflects on

---

[3] By putting it this way, we do not mean to suggest that there is complete commonality among the experiences of depression sufferers. It seems more likely that depressive feelings bear at most a Wittgensteinian family resemblance to one another.

[4] Indeed, the very formation of a self-conception requires an interpretation of our pasts and ourselves as individual subjects with an ongoing history (Schechtman 1994).

these experiences, and the author who—by way of protagonist and narrator—chooses to publicly present significant aspects of his identity.

As a genre, autobiography gives rise to many theoretical challenges, including the matter of its truth-value, i.e., the degree of faithfulness of the author regarding the recalled experiences, and the extent to which such a text lends itself to a "realist" reading (as closer to a report of fact than a work of fiction).[5] Whether autobiography is closer to fact or fiction is itself contested by theorists, moreover, it has been argued that the status of autobiography as belonging either to the realm of truth or the realm of fiction is not only unresolved but irresolvable (Anderson 2001; Wright 2006).

Depression memoirs find their place then, within a genre whose fundamental status as a source of evidentiary support is contested. If for this reason alone, such memoirs must be problematic and ambiguous, their meanings remaining, as we shall put it henceforth, *indeterminate*. Adding to this uncertain status and indeterminacy are first, the specific literary medium of autobiography (see "Law of the genre") and second, the processes of co-construction in autobiographical memory (see "Co-construction in autobiographical memory").

"Law of the genre"

First, there is what—echoing Jacques Derrida (1980)—can be called "the law of the genre." All autobiographical writing entails a set of recognizable conventions and literary forms that establish tacit principles, limits, and norms, according to Derrida, many of which are shared with fiction. So autobiographical writing entails an act of personal self-shaping that springs from ordering experience *within* specific literary laws of closure and coherence, dramatic, and rhetorical devices and conventions. This is why autobiographical writing has been described as a "cultural act" (Spengemann and Lundquist 1965), in which individuals' views of themselves are shaped by adherence to the law of the genre.

This aspect of autobiographical writing indicates some of the difficulty involved in its interpretation. But importantly, the acknowledgment of these features of autobiographical writing (such as the elements that are shared with fictional works) does not seem to us to in itself warrant the attribution of fictionality. Our point is not that the literary medium is something like a meaning-generating entity by itself ("defacing" any subject with its codes and tropes, as poststructuralism would have it). It is merely that what autobiography

---

[5] Analyzing autobiographical discourse, more traditional approaches have opted for grouping autobiography with biography and history, presupposing a correspondence theory of reference. According to such a view, it is both possible and preferable in autobiographical writing to offer an exact, unfiltered and unmediated recreation of an event or experience. However, in the course of the last five decades, there has been growing acceptance of the presence of fictive features and specifically literary techniques in autobiographical writing. The entrance of poststructuralist thought into literary theory, and the influential work of Paul De Man, Roland Barthes, and Jacques Derrida, marked a radical reorientation: not only has the correspondence theory of reference been rejected, but autobiography became acknowledged as a particular kind of fiction (De Man 1979). In this position, autobiographical discourse does not really entail a reference to something outside the text, and it does not recount, but rather creates the realities it invokes. The autobiographical subject is disfigured and "defaced," as De Man puts it, through text, i.e., the text reshapes and alters the subjective content of whatever is said.

ostensibly describes, the "raw" particular experiences, may not be reliable. Rather, in a much more complex manner, it reveals how such experiences can be made sense of, and how they can be organized and narrated for a specific literary context so as to achieve a coherent self-representation. Thus, even besides obvious factors (conscious and unconscious omissions, voluntarily and involuntarily misrepresentations by authors to convince their audience, a desire for uniqueness and dramatic effect, and external editorial intervention, for example) the manner in which autobiographical writing involves self-disclosure will reflect the particular literary medium within which it is situated, and should prompt us to use caution in interpreting its content.

Co-construction in autobiographical memory

In all its forms, self-reflection from a distance, or autobiographical memory, involves the co-construction of what is recalled, establishing a link of the present self of the author with a set of past experiences, but in a loop-like, dynamic way: what is recollected influences our self-concepts, yet it is itself influenced and altered on the basis of current self-conceptions (Sutton 2003; Wilson and Ross 2003).[6]

The retrospective position of the author in autobiographical writing adds to the text's ambiguity because a gap opens up between the perspectives of the author as external, retrospective narrator, and the author himself as the protagonist. Due to this gap, readers witness both what the experience of the protagonist was like at the earlier, remembered time, but at the same time also something more, viz., the reflection of the author about the episode, with which the description is entwined. Drawing on Peter Goldie's work, we can say that this meta-level of reflection renders the meaning of autobiographical writing additionally indeterminate in at least three ways corresponding to the three different gaps the story must accommodate.[7] An *epistemic* gap will create indeterminacy because the author is now in possession of relevant information that was not available then, which may change what is remembered. There may be an *evaluative* gap resulting in indeterminacy, because the author now evaluates the experience differently, which may interfere with the content remembered. Finally, an *emotional* gap can interfere because the author now feels differently about what happened may add further indeterminacy. Thus, the experience that the author may struggle to recount unavoidably gets "infected" (Goldie 2011, p. 129), not only by the looping effects of autobiographical memory, but additionally by the complex ambiguity of the authorial position.

So far we have invoked reasons why the epistemological value of experiences recounted in any autobiographical writing should be approached carefully, since its meaning will likely be more opaque than it at first seems. Before turning to the particular indeterminacies

---

6 See also Neisser and Fivush (1994).

7 Goldie uses the term "ironic" in the sense of dramatic irony, and speaks of the ironic position adopted in remembering, where a gap (but one that is closed through narrativity) separates several perspectives: "The gap can be triply ironic: it can be ironic epistemically—now I know what I did not know then; it can be ironic evaluatively—I now evaluate what happened in a way that I did not at the time; and it can be ironic emotionally—I now feel differently about what happened from the way that I felt at the time.... In autobiographical memory, and more generally in narrative thinking about one's past, these internal and external perspectives can become intertwined" (Goldie 2011, p. 129).

associated with depression memoirs, however, we also need to consider them as examples of the subgenre of illness and disability memoirs.

Illness memoirs: Autopathography

The illness memoir or autopathography is a highly popular kind of autobiographical writing. Organized around an experience of illness or disability, it usually comprises a personal reconstruction of the experiential dimension of the condition as well as reflection on its meaning and place in the life of the author (Frank 2000; Hawkins 1993; Wiltshire 2000). It provides insight into a life in the disquieting absence of order, showing ruptures of the self and life history and coherence in a world that has collapsed (Conway 2007, p. 9).

Like the genre of autobiography, this subgenre also has its own particular rules, functions, and norms that shape the content. Thus, compared to much other autobiographical writing, the function of the autopathography is likely to be more complex and ambitious: the task of its author not only to describe, but often also to restore to coherence by finding new meaning to bind remembered experiences together, even establishing a new personal identity (Bury 2001; Hawkins 1993, p. 3).[8]

Also, in autopathography, the "laws" are pervasively influenced, and constrained, by the social or cultural meanings characterizing illnesses and disabilities.[9] In memoirs of stigmatized illnesses such as sexually transmitted diseases (or mental disorder, to which we will come presently), authors must struggle with prevalent harmful metaphors and negative attitudes in order to cast the relevant experiences in a way that can yield a coherent narrative of a life worth telling and living. Accounts of illness and particularly of experience with physical disability, regularly demonstrate binary ideas and metaphors, it has been pointed out: the self is represented as transcending the ailing or deficient body (Leder 1990; Lindgren 2004; Wendel 1996); there are tropes of illness and disability as enemy, battled and vanquished by the sufferer (Bury 2001; Kelly and Dickinson 1997);[10] and a "logic of exclusion" casts disease as "an alien invader within the self" (Hawkins 1993, p. 148).

The extent to which such attitudes exhibited in accounts of physical disease and disability find parallels in memoirs of more psychological disorder such as depression, however, requires investigation; it is explored in the section entitled "Indeterminacy particular to depression memoirs".

Summing up, autopathography will exhibit the ambiguity and "indeterminacy" it shares with any autobiographical writing. It will also challenge the reader inasmuch as its meanings

---

[8] Hyden (1997) uses the term "regeneration" to underscore this twofold process undergoing a severe life crisis and the emergence of a new personal identity.

[9] Susan Sontag (1989) has famously demonstrated how cancer is understood in the frame of warfare and military metaphors (effortlessly fitting the "narrative of triumph"), while AIDS had the connotations of transgression, hedonist excess, and perverse sexuality.

[10] The subgenre autopathography has been seen to have inherited—and been limited by—some of the narrative patterns of the earlier autobiographical subgenre of religious conversion, where a "sinner" upon an encounter with God undergoes a change and eventually embraces a spiritual life (Hawkins 1993). Other tropes include the "narrative of triumph" (Conway 1997), and the "quest narrative" (Frank 1995) which both explain a disintegrating experience and conveys that in given circumstances the ill can actively confront their illness in a "battle."

will be constrained by its complex function as an attempt to link elements in an often deeply disrupted story, by the limits of its narrative schemas, and by the normatively loaded cultural meanings within which it is constructed. Together, these aspects must have a decisive impact on the way the illness is experienced, how it can be told, and how it can be integrated into a coherent narrative. Thus, the reportorial accuracy of autopathographies and the epistemological status of experiences recounted cannot be presupposed with confidence. This will be true of all autobiographical writing, but additional skepticism will often be warranted with memoirs filtered through the lens of experiences with illness (and disability).

INDETERMINACY PARTICULAR TO
DEPRESSION MEMOIRS

Some of the distinctive indeterminacy attaching to depression memoirs is illustrated here using the sustained example of depictions of self-identity. Today's identity politics and unprecedented emphasis on personal identity make some description of the relationship between self and illness, or self and symptoms almost de rigueur in contemporary first-person accounts. Our focus, then, is what appear to be typical attitudes toward one's experiences, symptoms, and disorder, attitudes that are *proprietary*. Thus, phrases such as "my symptoms," "my illness," "my mood states," "the despair I felt," are claims about one's subjective states that either explicitly employ the ownership language of possessives (mine, my), or strongly imply a proprietary relation linking self and depressive states or experiences. An example is Andrew Solomon's remark that "To regret my depression now would be to regret *the most fundamental part of myself*" (Solomon 2001, p. 440 emphasis added).

Our claim is not that all depression memoirs exhibit these proprietary attitudes; some don't, and others engage with the question in ways that render this an over-simplified characterization.[11] But many do, and those examples are useful to illustrate the indeterminacy that impedes efforts to establish an unambiguous reading of such texts.

The examples under discussion here spring from reflection and forms of reflective rather than non-reflective self-awareness.[12] This level of description of what we can call the *proprietary relations of reflective self-awareness*, remains uncommitted on the more basic contrast between higher-order monitoring approaches that separate as logically distinct the state from its monitoring, and same-order approaches that see the one as constitutive of the other.[13]

---

[11] See, for instance, Tracy Thompson's reflection on this relationship: "I could say 'There is something wrong with my brain.' That was different from saying 'There is something wrong with me.' ... So I was sick. But this was my brain I was talking about, not my gallbladder or my kidneys .... It produced behavior, the sum total of which was somehow me" (Thompson 1995, pp. 189–190).

[12] For a review of non-reflective self-awareness, see Varga (2012).

[13] Even narrowed to representations of self-identity this way, these are complex and multifaceted depictions. Depression memoirs exhibit a range of different descriptions, from apparent reports of immediate phenomenal experience to all manner of conclusions about experiences of depressive episodes. Feeling states and frames of mind from discrete, remembered moments are often depicted, but particular depressive experiences are also the basis for judgments, sometimes explicit, at other times

In contrasting personal accounts of mental disorder, more and less symptom-integrating and symptom-alienating depictions of the relationships between self and symptoms are identifiable (Radden 2008).[14] *Symptom-alienating* descriptions employ distancing metaphors, where symptom and disorder are represented as alienable from, rather than integral to, the self. The illness and its symptoms, it is suggested, are at most a peripheral aspect of the whole person; recovery is identified with the absence ("remission") of all symptoms; and emphasis is on striving to live, "outside" the illness, taking back an identity hitherto reduced to these symptoms. Here, the symptoms are conceived as little more than by-products of inherent, biological disorder with no intrinsic interest, meaning, or relevance to the person from whose dysfunctional brain they emanate, and are often spoken of as apt for being controlled or "managed."[15] Symptom alienating metaphors are seen in Kay Jamison's observation that however blocked within her mind the dimness (of depression) became, "it almost always seemed an *outside force* that was at war with my natural self" (Jamison 1995, p. 15).

By contrast, some memoirs reveal more *symptom-integrating* language—depicting states and traits as central to, and constitutive of, the identity of the person, and as part, and sometimes a central part, of the self. Instead of alienated, they are embraced, even valorized.[16] Rather than inconsequential effects of a diseased brain, they are represented as meaningful aspects of experience and identity. Thus we get remarks such as Solomon's, quoted earlier, that to afterward regret his depression would be to regret a fundamental part of himself.

The cultural legacy

The history of melancholia and depression provides one obvious source for representations of self-identity to be found in depression narratives, seeming to explain symptom-integrating descriptions when they occur. Glamorous associations long attached to the notion of melancholia, and in the afterglow of the tradition in which melancholy bespoke brilliance, creativity, and inspiration, the drawbacks of depressive moods are not unalloyed. These are admired and desirable attributes, likely to be identified with—how could one resist? That said, the cultural meaning of "depression" is itself unsettled, with strands that are less attractive. In the everyday meaning of "depression" at least two differing connotations reverberate: those more positive "heroic" ones, and an interpretation depicting sufferers as deficient and overly sensitive poseurs and lacking firm will, or womanly in their abject passivity.[17] The author of a depression memoir must navigate between these different meanings and place herself in relation to these contradictory associations.

able to be inferred, about the more general relation between self identity and depression—whether understood as particular symptoms, as a disease entity, or as something else again.

  [14] Others have noted different contrasts among such memoirs. Westerbeek and Mutaers (2008) separate these works into person-oriented and problem-oriented narratives, for example.

  [15] Rhetoric from the "recovery" movement echoes, likely grows out of, and also nourishes this set of assumptions in first-person narratives.

  [16] "I have been addicted to despair" Meri Nana-Ama Danquah writes of her depression: "Most times, in its most superficial and seductive sense, it is rich and enticing" (Danquah 2003, pp. 151, 155).

  [17] See Kristeva (1989), Radden (2000, pp. 39–47), and Ussher (2011).

Another aspect of the cultural legacy emphasizes the links uniting melancholy and depression with self.[18] In other psychiatric disorders the sufferer often posits the focus of his trouble in the world outside himself—as menacing and malevolent, for example, in the case of paranoia, or as otherwise out of joint. *By contrast*, whether personal, medical, literary, or theoretical, accounts of the symptoms of melancholia (and later of depression) persistently emphasize themes of self-consciousness and self-focus; experience linked to its subject. Extreme self-consciousness, for example, was long believed a prominent symptom of melancholia. Some reference to this occurs in earlier writing, but it becomes very evident in the era when Burton and others defined and elaborated on the traits accompanying feelings of melancholy. The melancholy man is recognized to be self-centered, self-conscious, and self-absorbed.[19] Confusingly, Burton's era saw a blurring between the traits associated with melancholy and those depicted and valorized in literary representations, which also included heightened self focus of these kinds (Greenblatt 1980). As a defining aspect of the influential literary and philosophical selves that came with modern individualism, this way of seeing and fashioning ourselves, whether as authors, citizens, patients, or autobiographers, was inescapable. Yet reference to these traits as evidence of something closer to pathology can also be found in work such as Burton's. The melancholic is *overly, excessively*, and *dysfunctionally* self-focused.

Also linking depressive states and self-identity is a trend that becomes most evident during the late nineteenth century, where we find stress on the negative self-assessments associated with melancholy and depression. Freud's complex analysis of melancholia is entirely focused on the self and tied to his account of narcissism.[20] And among psychodynamic explanations of depression, this analysis changed little during the subsequent century.

Factors likely influencing how the self and its symptoms are construed include another set of cultural meanings—broad theoretical and philosophical ideas about the nature of the self and self-identity.[21] Such theories may be expected to affect self-construction regardless of the disorder depicted. But more specific to mood disorders are the tenets of psychiatric lore itself in its depictions of depression. Of the increased use of diagnostic manuals by patients, Serife Tekin notes, "In this sense, the DSM organizes not only how patients' mood disorders are therapeutically addressed, but also how these patients make sense of their lived experiences, i.e., to understand their mental disorders and to understand themselves, their interpersonal relationships and other important components of their lives" (Tekin in press). Moreover, homage to earlier memoirs is also evident in contemporary writing.[22]

---

[18] Because the causes of mental disorder are little understood, they have been deemed likely to implicate the sufferer's character taken as a whole, rather than some particular bodily part (Sontag 1989). And this too might indicate more symptom-integrating descriptions.

[19] The melancholic man "dare not come in company for feare hee should be misused, disgraced, overshoot himselfe in gesture or speeches... he thinkes every man observes him" (Burton 1989, p. 395).

[20] On analogy with grief, Freud traces the cause of melancholia to the loss of a loved object, now shifted, as the result of the splitting of the self, to the patient's own ego (Freud 1957).

[21] See, for instance, recent attention to various forms of "neurochemical selves" (Rose 2007), self-fashioned and not (Dumit 2003). See also Tekin (2011).

[22] Examples of such self-reference include Susannah Kaysen's *Girl, Interrupted* (1993), with its echoes of *The Yellow Wallpaper* (Gilman 1980), and Sally Brampton's references to Solomon's writing (Brampton 2008).

In short, cultural meanings suggest innumerable ways to link melancholy and depressive states with the self and self-identity. But the general point can be made with the two examples elaborated earlier—its link to glamorous associations, and its tie to self-identity, self-centeredness, and self-awareness. If some depression memoirs exhibit a more symptom-integrating style than other memoirs of mental disorder, much within their cultural context can readily explain why.

Once we seek explanations for depictions of self-identity in depression memoirs, other aspects of the phenomena are implicated. Depressive symptoms seem to have echoes in more normal and normative states: versions of many depression symptoms are common and even proper responses to life's vicissitudes. To the range of sad, dejected mood states we associate with bereavement and depression alike, can be added comparable responses—to marital dissolution, or status loss, for example (Horwitz and Wakefield 2006, pp. 30–38). Because of this "normalizing" context, and parallel with what Horwitz and Wakefield call normal sadnesses, the inclination to identify with the dejected moods that occur as symptoms of depression seems likely to be strong and unthinking. They are part of a set of traits accepted, by ourselves and by those around us, as not only common human responses, but normal and fitting ones.

A related aspect likely to affect attitudes toward symptoms in the depression sufferer is that reasoning, judgment, and particularly interpersonal communication are not as immediately and observably compromised by depression as by some other disorders (such as schizophrenia).[23] Moods of despair and sadness will be easier to integrate, both by their sufferer and by those around her, than the jarring and disruptive intrusion of symptoms such as inner voices, delusions, and the confused sequencing of thought disorder. The subtler effects of depressive moods on judgment are not inconsiderable; moreover, severe psychotic depression also occurs. Nonetheless, even many severe depressions have barely perceptible effects on these capabilities.

Arguably, both this assessment and the observation that depression echoes more normal and normative states are distorted by today's loose diagnostic category of depression, whose margins may extend further into normality than do the margins of other diagnostic types.[24] Even as it is presently identified, however, depression is primarily a disorder affecting mood rather than more cognitive capabilities, leaving many aspects of reasoning, judgment, and communication apparently unaffected. And we turn now to the other feature of depressive states requiring attention here—their status as moods.

Depression as constituted by moods

Common responses, attitudes, and emotions associated with milder and more serious depression include: feeling sad, miserable, dispirited, listless, bored, dull, world weary, oppressed, and disgusted with oneself; being inclined to disparaging self-assessments

---

[23] See Oyebode's assessment that "There is a dearth of good descriptions of psychotic experience compared with descriptions of mood disturbance. This difference is perhaps understandable given the effects of schizophrenia on motivation, drive and use of language" (Oyebode 2003, p. 268).

[24] This is the claim put forward by Horwitz and Wakefield, who wish to reduce the class of true depressive disorders by more stringently separating it from "normal sadnesses."

(I am worthless, incompetent, sinful, the most guilty person in the whole world, and so on). Depressive states apparently comprise at least two broad kinds, these examples show, separable conceptually into feeling and cognitive or belief elements. These elements interpenetrate, of course: belief states emerge from and seemingly give rise to, inchoate feelings; moreover from a phenomenological perspective, these characteristically discouraged attitudes and beliefs are co-mingled with the feelings states. Although in varying mixes, many and perhaps most depressive states combine elements of each sort.[25] The more belief-like of these states (the conviction that I am worthless, for example) are often distinguished as *emotions*; in contrast to more amorphous and pervasive *mood* states, e.g., a sense of disinterested listlessness.[26] Thus, emotions, it has been said, are about particulars, or particulars generalized, while moods are about nothing in particular, or sometimes they are about our world as a whole (Solomon 1993, p. 112).[27] (As the case of listlessness suggests, moods include bodily sensations, a point often confirmed in depression memoirs.[28])

It seems apparent that the amorphous side of mood states will be implicated in the unresolved and indeterminate quality of depression memoirs. Thus, although many authors of published autopathographies are gifted writers, they often emphasize that depressive experience almost eludes expression.[29] If not beyond the capabilities of language, they insist, depressive suffering is exceptionally challenging to put into words. All autobiographical writing involves the co-construction of retrospective states, as we have seen, because the remembered is dynamically altered on the basis of current self-conceptions through the looping effects of autobiographical memory. If the experience itself is of an imprecise and quasi-incomprehensible nature, then so much the greater must be the co-constructive efforts of the rememberer in embellishing and redrawing boundaries to depict it.

We earlier employed the example of proprietary attitudes of reflective self-awareness to illustrate the way elements of culture might account for the presence of symptom-integrating

---

[25] See Goldie (2010).

[26] One of the most compelling descriptions of the pervasiveness of moods is by Mill: of a dull state of nerves, he wrote, "one of those moods when what is pleasure at other times, becomes insipid or indifferent" (Mill 1873/1989, p. 112).

[27] Heidegger (1962) makes the same distinction: moods are non-intentional (or pre-intentional, because they are not about anything particular, but the world as such), while emotions are intentional.

[28] See, for example, this observation about the experience of depression: "My body became inert, heavy and burdensome. Every gesture was hard … My existence was pared away almost to nothing, except for the self-contempt that bruised my eye sockets and throat, that turned my stomach and made my tongue into some large, coarse creature in my mouth" (Shaw 1997, pp. 26–27, in Oyebode 2003, p. 266).

[29] See Wolpert "My current, rather bitter view, is that if you can describe your severe depression you have not really had one" (Wolpert 2003b, p. 270; 2003a). Smith (1999), Solomon (2001), Styron (1990), and Wurtzel (1995) all note the inadequacy of ordinary language in face of the quasi-incomprehensible disruptive experience of depression (see also Stern 2003; Westerbeek and Mutsaers 2008). Styron (1990, p. 83) describes depressive experience as "beyond expression," while Solomon (2001) maintains that it may only be captured in metaphorical or allegoric language. Kristeva too, speaks of "non-communicable grief" that defies narration, arguing that the disruptive experience of depression is antithetical to narrative codification into a meaningful and coherent plot. (Kristeva 1989; Stone 2004). Such claims have been made about describing other kinds of disorder as well, so we do not mean to suggest that depression is exclusively difficult in this respect.

style in depression memoirs. The same example can now be used as we consider the relationship of the self to its depressive moods.

Moods are affections, and are unbounded in their psychological effects, coloring and framing experience in its (momentary) totality.[30] Two features relevant to the relation between selves and their moods deserve attention here. First, at the time it is experienced the mood seems to interfere with our adopting a standpoint from where its appraisal could be made, for any such assessment will likely succumb to the influence of the mood. We cannot easily distance ourselves from a mood by doubting or disbelieving, rather than embracing, it. We are either in the mood—or not. (Matthew Ratcliffe makes this point when he says moods do not feature in our phenomenology *as states of subjects* (Ratcliffe 2008, p. 48).) Moreover, we find ourselves passive recipients of moods, as powerless in our apprehension of them as we are our unbidden thoughts, or our perceptions. Moods *assail us*, is the way Heidegger puts it. Combining these two features, we can see why, at least while they last, their status as *pervasive affections* seems to render moods an inescapable part of our selves and who we are.

By contrast, the cognitive or belief states making up depression (such as the self-denigrating assessment that "I am worthless"), are more readily alienated from the subject even when, with the self as their objects, they are directed toward it. My belief that I am worthless can be criticized as an overgeneralization, as contradicted by the facts, as inconsistent with my other beliefs, and so on. It is those states that cognitive therapy is able to work on revising, apparently quite effectively.[31] As also for other beliefs (as well as belief-like states such as hoping, wishing, regretting, etc.) cognitive states can be held at some distance and considered—in terms of their causes, their grounding, their likely truth or falsity, and their fit with the person's, or others', beliefs, and with other aspects of the subject's affective-conative composition. In this respect my mental states exemplify the familiar intentionalist model of the mental and consciousness. And as the objects of mental agency, these beliefs can be summoned, examined, affirmed, and doubted.

Depression memoirs are not usually (in fact are rarely), completed during episodes of disorder. And when we write or speak of our moods after the fact it is with full agency, and at some later time. Subsequent framing or reframing come with the control and distance that are absent in the moody moment. Despite these differences between experiencing and later describing or recalling the mood state, we still see some hint of the attributes noted earlier. When the low moods of depression are depicted, such reframing often takes the form of "That (person) was not me" rather than "That mood was not mine." In contrast is the sort of reframing that often seems to occur after episodes of other kinds of disorder. A now-relinquished delusional belief is depicted as "I was [then] subject to nonsensical and unreasonable delusions," to quote from George Trosse's memoir (Trosse 1982, p. 32)—not "That (person) was not me."

The suggestion here, then, is that symptom-integrating depictions found in some depression memoirs may reflect the prevalence of non-cognitive feeling states among the subjective symptoms of depression.

---

[30] Heidegger puts this by calling moods *existential orientations*, rather than subjective states.
[31] See Beck and Alford (2009) and Beck et al. (1979).

Empirical Evidence

Employing the extended example of proprietary attitudes of reflective self-awareness, we have explored some of the likely sources of the ambiguities in depression memoirs that will limit our ability to place them on the continuum between reports of inner states and experiences and entirely fictive works. A number of these sources, we saw, involve literary conventions; others are elements of cultural meaning. By contrast their status as moods (which includes the challenge they pose for subjects describing them) apparently reflects something closer to a constitutive feature of the depression itself. Also closer to constitutive of depression may be aspects of the autobiographical memory of depression sufferers that have been identified through empirical research.

Among a variety of cognitive deficits that accompany depression, studies have revealed several sorts of memory impairment (Burt et al. 1995). One robustly confirmed finding in depressed patients is a deficient recall pattern affecting autobiographical memory (Kuyken and Dalgleish 1995; Puffet et al. 1991). The impairment with regard to specific memories is often referred to as *over-general memory*: instead of retrieving a particular occurrence that took place at a certain time, patients tend to recall a larger interval of their life and respond not so much to any particular event as to a whole class of related events. What is of particular interest in our context is that even after clinical improvement, this over-general remembering, together with deficient access to emotional and positive memories, remain (Mackinger et al. 2000; Nandrino et al. 2002). By contrast, several other kinds of memory performance of depressed patients have been shown to improve, or alter, with recovery (Burt et al. 1995). Moreover, in a very different, qualitative study designed to show the healing effect of autobiographical writing, the patients' writing style changed with their clinical improvement (Smorti et al. 2010).[32]

A lingering inability to recall emotional and positive memories, and the tendency toward overgeneralized autobiographical remembering can all be expected to influence the depression memoir. It has been proposed that rather than a function of acute depressive symptomatology, these deficiencies of autobiographical memory represent a stable marker in depression sufferers, perhaps related to other deficiencies (Kuyken and Dalgleish 1995). Whether narrowly or more globally construed however, the point remains: such deficits in remembering seem likely to affect the co-construction of remembering. Similarly, stylistic alterations from the time of depressive episodes to the time of recovery suggest an instability that must add to the indeterminacies affecting our reading of depression memoirs. And further to our general conclusion, such memory deficiencies and stylistic changes will have implications for the reportorial status of depression memoirs, limiting our ability to assign such memoirs a place on the continuum between fact and fiction.

---

[32] Text analysis showed that later narratives employed different terms, and verbs in conjunctive form, for example—results taken to suggest movement towards the present and the "world of possibility" (Smorti et al. 2010, p. 569).

CONCLUSION

First-person memoirs are a rich resource, yet they must be approached with sensitivity to the context in and purposes for which they are employed. An inextricable fusion of phenomenal experience, more and less intrinsic attributes, and cultural meanings, is what we understand by normal subjective experience, and find in all memoirs, which have been rightly recognized to be works of "faction" (Bury 2001). This fusion is a given in many everyday contexts and, particularly, the context of care where, it has been pointed out, personal narrative is the level of concern, and is nothing less than—the "ordinary forms through which we attempt to order the sense and meaning of our actions, experiences, and beliefs" (Stanghellini 2011, p. 26). As an extension of these essential forms of communication, in treatment as in everyday life, memoirs of depression will always have value.

Research and philosophical contexts impose different and more stringent demands, however. In drawing on autobiographical accounts of depression, whether employing them in conceptual analysis, as the basis for developing theoretical models, or even quoting them for illustrative purposes, caution is called for. The ambiguities surrounding first-person accounting of experience, particularly notable in written memoirs, *should* be of concern to the researcher.

REFERENCES

Anderson, L. (2001). *Autobiography*. London: Routledge.

Barthes, R. (1989). The death of the author. In P. Rice and P. Waugh (Eds), *Modern Literary Theory: A Reader*, pp. 114–18. London: Edward Arnold.

Beck, A. T. and Alford, B. A. (2009). *Depression: Causes and Treatment*. Philadelphia, PA: University of Pennsylvania Press.

Beck, A. T., Rush, A. J., Shaw, B. F., and Emery, G. (1979). *Cognitive Therapy of Depression*. New York, NY: Guilford Press.

Becker, G. (1997). *Disrupted Lives: How People Create Meaning in a Chaotic World*. Berkeley, CA: University of California Press.

Brampton, S. (2008). *Shoot the Damn Dog: A Memoir of Depression*. New York, NY: W. W. Norton & Company.

Burt, D. B., Zembar, M. J., and Niederehe, G. (1995). Depression and memory impairment: A meta-analysis of the association, its pattern and specificity. *Psychological Bulletin, 117*, 285–305.

Burton, R. (1989). *The Anatomy of Melancholy* (T. Faulkner, N. Kiessling, and R. Blair, Eds). Oxford: Clarendon Press.

Bury, M. (2001). Illness narratives: fact or fiction? *Sociology of Health and Illness, 23*(3), 263–85.

Clifford, J. S., Norcross, J. C., and Sommer, R. (1999). Autobiographies of mental health clients: Psychologists' uses and recommendations. *Professional Psychology: Research and Practice, 30*, 56–9.

Conway, K. (2007). *Illness and the Limits of Expression*. Ann Arbor, MI: The University of Michigan Press.

Danquah, M. N. -A. (2003). *Willow Weep for Me.* Reprinted in R. Shannonhouse (Ed.), *Out of Her Mind*, pp. 151–5. New York, NY: Modern Library.

De Man, P. (1979). Autobiograpy as de-facement. *Modern Language Notes, 94,* 919–30.

Derrida, J. (1980). The law of genre. *Critical Inquiry, 7*(1), 55–81.

Dumit, J. (2003). Is it me or my brain? Depression and neuroscientific facts. *Journal of Medical Humanities, 24,* 35–47.

Eakin, J. P. (1992). *Touching the World: Reference in Autobiography.* Princeton, NJ: Princeton University Press.

Frank, A. W. (1995). *The Wounded Storyteller: Body, Illness and Ethics.* Chicago, IL: Chicago University Press.

Frank, A. W. (2000). Illness and autobiographical work: dialogue as narrative destabilisation. *Qualitative Sociology, 23*(1), 135–56.

Freud, S. (1957). Mourning and melancholia. In *Collected Papers* (Vol. 4, authorized translation under the supervision of J. Rivière), pp. 152–70. London: Hogarth Press.

Gilman, C. P. (1980). *The Yellow Wallpaper.* Reprinted in A. Lane (Ed.), *Charlotte Perkins Gilman Reader*, pp. 3–19. New York, NY: Vintage.

Greenblatt, S. (1980). *Renaissance Self-Fashioning: From More to Shakespeare.* Chicago, IL: University of Chicago Press.

Gusdorf, G. (1956). *Conditions and Limits of Autobiography.* Princeton, NJ: Princeton University Press.

Goldie, P. (Ed.) (2010). *The Oxford Handbook of Philosophy of the Emotions.* Oxford: Oxford University Press.

Goldie, P. (2011). Grief: A narrative account. *Ratio, XXIV,* 119–37.

Hawkins, A. H. (1993). *Reconstructing Illness: Studies in Pathography.* West Lafayette, IN: Purdue University Press.

Heidegger, M. (1962). *Being and Time* (J. Macquarrie and E. Robinson, Trans.). New York, NY: Harper & Row, Publishers.

Hornstein, G. (2002). Narratives of madness, as told from within. *Chronicle of Higher Education, January 25,* B7–10.

Horwitz, A. and Wakefield, J. (2006). *The Loss of Sadness: How Psychiatry Transformed Normal Sorrow into Depressive Disorder.* New York, NY: Oxford University Press.

Hyden, L.-C. (1997). Illness and narrative. *Sociology of Health and Illness, 19,* 48–69.

Jamison, K. (1995). *An Unquiet Mind: A Memoir of Moods and Madness.* New York, NY: Knopf.

Kaysen, S. (1993). *Girl, Interrupted.* New York, NY: Vintage Books.

Kelly, M. P. and Dickinson, H. (1997). The narrative self in autobiographical accounts of illness. *The Sociological Review, 45*(2), 254–78.

Kleinman, A. (1988). *The Illness Narratives: Suffering, Healing and the Human Condition.* New York, NY: Basic Books.

Kristeva, J. (1989). *Black Sun: Depression and Melancholy* (L. Roudiez, Trans.). New York, NY: Columbia University Press.

Kuyken, W. and Dalgleish, T. (1995). Autobiographical memory and depression. *British Journal of Clinical Psychology, 34,* 89–92.

Lawrence, C. (1994). *Medicine in the Making of Modern Britain, 1700–1920.* London: Routledge.

Leder, D. (1990). *The Absent Body.* Chicago, IL: Chicago University Press.

Lejeune, P. (1982). The autobiographical contract. In T. Todorov (Ed.), *French Literary Theory Today*, pp. 192–207. Cambridge, Cambridge University Press.

Lindgren, K. (2004). Bodies in trouble: Identity, embodiment and disability. In B. Smith and B. Hutchinson (Eds), *Gendering Disability*, pp. 145–65. Rutgers, NJ: Rutgers University Press.

Mackinger, H. F., Pachinger, M. M., Leibetseder, M. M., and Fartacek, R. R. (2000). Autobiographical memories in women remitted from major depression. *Journal of Abnormal Psychology*, 109(2), 331–4.

Mill, J. S. (1989). *Autobiography* (J. M. Robson, Ed.). London: Penguin. (Original work published 1873.)

Nandrino, J.-L., Pezard, L., Posté, A., Revéillère, C., and Beaune, D. (2002). Autobiographical memory in major depression: A comparison between first-episode and recurrent patients. *Psychopathology*, 35, 335–40.

Neisser, U. and Fivush, R. (Eds) (1994). *The Remembering Self*. Cambridge: Cambridge University Press.

Nelson, H. L. (2001). *Damaged Identities, Narrative Repair*. Ithaca, NY: Cornell University Press.

Oyebode, F. (2003). Autobiographical narrative and psychiatry. *Advances in Psychiatric Treatment*, 9, 265–70.

Puffet, A., Jehin-Marchot, D., Timsit-Berthier, M., and Timsit, M. (1991). Autobiographical memory and major depressive states. *European Psychiatry*, 6, 141–5.

Radden, J. (Ed.) (2000). *The Nature of Melancholy*. Oxford: Oxford University Press.

Radden, J. (2008). My symptoms, myself: Reading mental illness memoirs for identity assumptions. In H. Clark (Ed.), *Depression and Narrative: Telling the Dark*, pp. 15–28. New York, NY: SUNY Press.

Ratcliffe, M. (2008). *Feelings of Being: Phenomenology, Psychiatry and the Sense of Reality*. Oxford: Oxford University Press.

Rose, N. (2007). *The Politics of Life Itself: Biomedicine, Power and Subjectivity in the Twenty First Century*. Princeton, NJ: Princeton University Press.

Schechtman, M. (1994). The truth about memory. *Philosophical Psychology*, 7, 3–18.

Shaw, F. (1997). *Out of Me*. London: Penguin.

Smith, J. (1999). *Where the Roots Reach for Water: A Personal and Natural History of Melancholia*. New York, NY: North Point Press.

Smorti, A., Pananti, B., and Rizzo, A. (2010). Autobiography as tool to improve lifestyle, well being, and self-narrative in patients with mental disorders. *Journal of Nervous & Mental Disease*, 198(8), 564–71.

Solomon, A. (2001). *The Noonday Demon: An Atlas of Depression*. New York, NY: Scribner.

Solomon, R. (1993). *The Passions*. New York, NY: Doubleday.

Sommer, R., Clifford, J. S., and Norcross, J. C. (1998). A bibliography of mental patients' autobiographies: An update and classification system. *American Journal of Psychiatry*, 155, 1261–4.

Sontag, S. (1989). *Illness as Metaphor and AIDS and Its Metaphors*. New York, NY: Anchor.

Spengemann, W. C. and Lundquist, L. R. (1965). Autobiography and American myth. *American Quarterly*, 17, 501–19.

Stanghellini, G. (2011). Clinical phenomenology: A method for care? *Philosophy, Pyschiatry, & Psychology*, 18, 25–9.

Stern, T. (2003). Border narratives: Three first-person accounts of depression. *Studies in the Literary Imagination*, 36(2), 91–107.

Stone, B. (2004). Towards a writing without power: Notes on the narration of madness. *Auto/Biography*, 12, 16–33.

Styron, W. (1990). *Darkness Visible: A Memoir of Madness*. New York, NY: Random House.

Sutton, J. (2003). Memory. In E. N. Zalta (Ed.), *The Stanford Encyclopedia of Philosophy*. [Online.] Available at: <http://plato.stanford.edu/entries/memory>.

Tekin, S. (2011). Self-concept through the diagnostic looking glass: Narratives and mental disorder. *Philosophical Psychology*, 24(3), 357–80.

Tekin, S. (in press). Self-insight in the time of mood disorders: After the diagnosis, beyond the treatment. *Philosophy, Psychiatry, & Psychology*.

Thompson, T. (1995). *The Beast: A Reckoning with Depression*. New York, NY: G. P. Putnam's Sons.

Trosse, G. (1982). *Life of the Reverend Mr George Trosse: Written by Himself, and Published Posthumously According to His Order in 1714*. Reprinted in D. Peterson (Ed.), *A Mad People's History of Madness*, pp. 27–38. Pittsburgh, PA: Pittsburgh University Press.

Ussher, J. M. (2011). *The Madness of Women: Myth and Experience*. London: Routledge.

Varga, S. (2012). Non-reflective self-awareness and psychopathology. Do we need a situated account? *Journal of Consciousness Studies*, 19, 164–93.

Wendell, S. (1996). *The Rejected Body*. New York, NY: Routledge.

Westerbeek, J. and Mutsaers, K. (2008). Depression narratives: How the self became a problem. *Literature and Medicine*, 27(1), 25–55.

Wilson, A. E. and Ross, M. (2003). The identity function of autobiographical memory: Time is on our side. *Memory*, 11, 137–49.

Wiltshire, J. (2000) Biography, pathography, and the recovery of meaning. *Cambridge Quarterly*, 29, 409–22.

Wolpert, L. (1999). *Malignant Sadness: The Anatomy of Depression*. New York, NY: Free Press.

Wolpert, L. (2003a). Stigma of depression—a personal view. *British Medical Bulletin*, 57(1), 221–4.

Wolpert, L. (2003b). Invited commentary on autobiographical narrative and psychiatry. *Advances in Psychiatric Treatment*, 9, 265–70.

Wright, J. L. (2006). *The Philosopher's I: Autobiography and the Search for the Self*. Albany, NY: State University of New York Press.

Wurtzel, E. (1995). *Prozac Nation: Young and Depressed in America*. New York, NY: Riverhead.

SECTION II

CONTEXTS OF CARE

CHAPTER 10

INTRODUCTION: CONTEXTS OF CARE

All works within the contemporary and past philosophy of psychiatry are critical in the sense of providing insightful analysis and description of psychiatric phenomena, uncovering metaphysical and other kinds of assumptions, and making meaningful distinctions about core concepts and procedures. Such is the work of philosophy broadly conceived. However, the philosophy of psychiatry has always had a strand of scholarship which was critical in the social–political sense as well. That is, this path in the philosophy of psychiatry explores the social, cultural, and political contexts of psychiatry, mental health care, and service systems. In this sense of philosophy-as-criticism, psychiatric concepts, procedures, and systems are analyzed not just to deepen intellectual understanding of the field, but also to embrace a kind of utilitarian interest that seeks sociopolitical revision, reform, or revolution. The philosophy of psychiatry as social criticism does not simply analyze psychiatry as it is; it points toward what psychiatry could, and should, be. This tradition extends historically from the late-medieval and Enlightenment eras, when elite intellectuals such as Johann Weyer, John Locke, Teresa of Avila, and Immanuel Kant questioned the traditional assumptions about madness as spiritual or occult phenomena. Instead, these thought leaders began the reformulation of madness as disease, as medical phenomena, which in turn demanded analysis of such concepts as rationality, affection, and conation. This emerging "modern" concept of madness/insanity/mental disorder has certainly prevailed into the present day, at least among most educated peoples around the world, but the Enlightenment victory was then, and now, only partial. Many cultures and subcultures still experience madness within, to use Edwin R. Wallace's (1994) coinage, magico-religious frameworks and cosmologies. Mental disorder is still open to interpretation from many different sets of metaphysical assumptions, and such metaphysical assumptions can, as our authors in this section illustrate, be liberating or imprisoning, and, sometimes, both at once. Moreover, the philosophy of psychiatry has raised questions about the adequacy of Enlightenment accounts of madness. Our authors in this section challenge today's, post-Enlightenment, assumptions about psychiatry and mental health, revisiting our metaphysical assumptions as well as our ethics. Not satisfied with psychiatry and the mental health system as they are, these authors point to what psychiatry and the mental health system can and should be.

The critique offered by Pat Bracken and Phil Thomas in Chapter 11 takes up the post-Enlightenment, "modernist" metaphysical assumptions directly, identifying three core assumptions of contemporary mental health care: (1) That mental illness is related to mechanistic failures, whether biological, psychological, or related to social systems. (2) These mechanisms or processes are "modeled in causal terms" which can and are abstracted away from the full context of the phenomena. (3) Mental illness should be addressed through technological tools and procedures, again abstracted away from everyday human concerns like "opinions, values, relationships, or priorities." For Bracken and Thomas, these modes of thinking frame the terms of engagement with the mentally ill for all—clinician, policymaker, citizen. They argue that these modes of thinking set up and maintain power relationships for the mental health system that are self-interested and self-maintaining, disempowering the people whom the system is aiming to "help"—the mental health service user. They frame contemporary acknowledgments of the role of the patient as "partner" as little more than offering patients a handmaiden role to the larger mental health service system. Their vision for a "postpsychiatry" involves rediscovery of a different set of metaphysical assumptions about mental health and illness, a reinstatement of the ethical primacy of service users' opinions, values, relationships, or priorities, and the reduction of the social power of psychiatrists in rendering assistance to those with mental distress.

In her essay about the legacy of racism and sexism in psychiatry and mental health (Chapter 12), Marilyn Nissim-Sabat considers four sets of theoretical accounts, each with their own metaphysical assumptions and methodological framework. Professor Nissim-Sabat is concerned that not only have racist/sexist trends in the field been inadequately addressed, but the intellectual tools in addressing the issues have been inadequately set. In her analysis of ontological naturalism and methodological naturalism, Nissim-Sabat notes that a tendency to "biologize" race and gender differences presupposes a universality to biodifference which is neither argued for nor established. Nissim-Sabat frames her discussion of social constructionism, her second theoretical account, as a tension between realism and anti-realist metaphysical accounts. She explores this tension from the standpoint of Ron Mallon's *A Field Guide to Social Construction*, finding that Mallon smuggles in a form of realist naturalism in the form of cognitive predispositions towards categorizing objects and people.

In her third theoretical exploration vis-à-vis sex and gender, Nissim-Sabat provides a transparent exposition of the self-refuting radical relativism (e.g., everything is relative, including this statement) over against her preferred brand of relativism, "relativity-to," which she argues is neither self-refuting nor a true metaphysical relativism. This analysis is then applied to ordinary-language discourse on bigotry, then to Erik Gillett's work on social construction of truth-claims in psychoanalysis. Nissim-Sabat finds Gillett's approach wanting in that Gillett is never able to provide a non-relativistic account of culture and history to ground psychoanalytic truth-claims.

What is needed, for Nissim-Sabat, is an epistemic framework that does not posit essences as "material entities" but rather posits essences as "intentional objects of consciousness" that are subject to affirmation or rejection by philosophical evidence. Husserlian phenomenology provides such an epistemic framework. Phenomenological method avoids the metaphysical trap of failing to account for assumptions, a trap that the phenomenological method of *epoche*, suspending presuppositions, explicitly addresses. Such a method is not just relevant to exploration of race and gender, but conditions a methodological openness of mind that is incompatible with prejudice and discrimination.

In his essay on psychiatry and medicalization, Louis Charland (Chapter 13), turns the usual public decrying of medicalization upside down and instead concludes that medicalization is dangerous to psychiatry as a profession and field. Criticized by the anti-psychiatrists as problematic in defining too many human problems as medical problems, psychiatry appears to have partnered, historically to the present, with the pharmaceutical industry to find increasing kinds of human problems as psychopathological and demanding drug therapy. The gist of Charland's argument centers on the "unbridled commercialization of psychopharmacology," which threatens to trivialize psychiatry as a discipline, as understanding and demand for treatment moves out of the consulting room and into Internet social media and your home TV set's direct-to-consumer advertising. Even diagnosis, a raison d'être of psychiatric training and expertise, has been dismantled and appropriated by Internet-based chat rooms, blogs, and interest groups who make their own decisions about what is, and is not, a legitimate disorder. Charland develops his perspective through a historical analysis of the development of psychopharmacological science and its appropriation by the pharmaceutical industry.

In discussing the relationship between psychiatry and technology, James Phillips (Chapter 14) frames technology in terms of three "faces": The first involving technology as a practical tool in addressing the goals of medicine, most prominently, medication treatments. The second face of technology concerns technology as a means of apprehending or "seeing" things that otherwise psychiatrists wouldn't. Technology supplies us instruments, from psychological tests to magnetic resonance imaging scanners, which allow us to see new things, as well as marginalize other facets of our experience in the process. The third face takes a more explicitly metaphysical turn: technology also transforms how we think and our life choices, through what Phillips calls "instrumental reason." Phillips then systematically explores the meaning and significance of these three technological faces in relation to psychiatry as a profession and practice. What is crucial to his analysis is how technology, through its ubiquity and ultimately, banality in our lives, comes to change how we conduct ourselves and what we think is important. His examples are many and vivid; a paradigm example is the National Institute of Mental Health's Research Domain Criteria, a new "diagnostic" system for psychiatry that is divorced from ordinary experience and built upon highly abstract theoretical entities, themselves only accessible through instruments, scales, and neuroscientific measurements. In the second half of his chapter, Phillips places these trends into the history of philosophy, finding the roots of instrumental reason in Aristotle and elaborated by Enlightenment rationalism. In the concluding pages of his essay he evaluates these technological changes in psychiatry, and explores what a "right balance" in our attitudes and use of technologies might mean.

If Phillips explored the meaning of rating scales, abstract neuroscientific concepts, and technogadgetry for psychiatry, Larry Davidson, in Chapter 15, returns us to the nitty-gritty of fundamental concepts of illness: cure and recovery. He uses a semantic analysis of these two words to reveal the second-person/objective character of "cure," and the first-person/subjective character of "recovery." A doctor may "cure" you, but she doesn't "recover" you. Echoing the concerns of Bracken and Thomas in the beginning of this section, Davidson explores the historical roots of this unilateralism in psychiatric practice, where the patient is a passive recipient of physician ministrations. In the context of this historical review, Davidson challenges the prognostic and therapeutic nihilism of received views of schizophrenia, and suggests that Kraepelin and the Bleulers themselves may have not believed that the ultimate fate of people with dementia praecox was as uniformly grim as thought today. In his contrasting of Pinel's and Pussin's patient-empowering moral treatment approach, he explores the self-fulfilling prophesies of poor outcome through the provision of squalid hospital conditions and treatments that impoverish morale, rather than enhance it. From this historical context Davidson then presents a contemporary model of recovery from mental illness; one not based upon cure but rather aiming to enhance functioning and quality of life, showing that the gratifications of work and employment, demonstrated by supported-employment studies of chronically ill persons, is a key to improving functioning. In this regard, the progress in "treatment" of schizophrenia has primarily occurred through the enhancement of functioning rather than the refinements of psychopharmacology treatments discovered in the mid-twentieth century. Davidson's message is that to cure schizophrenia is misguided—and to aid in recovery should be our new direction.

CHAPTER 11

CHALLENGES TO THE MODERNIST IDENTITY OF PSYCHIATRY: USER EMPOWERMENT AND RECOVERY

PAT BRACKEN AND PHILIP THOMAS

INTRODUCTION

In this chapter, we shall seek: (1) to demonstrate that psychiatry is, and always has been, a quintessentially modernist[1] enterprise and (2) to show that this identity is deeply problematic and at odds with the sort of medical engagement that is required in the field of mental health.

A modernist approach is one that is guided by a technological[2] understanding of the issues at hand. It involves the following assumptions:

1. The problems to be addressed have to do with faulty *mechanisms or processes* of some sort. These are most often understood as being biological in nature, but

---

[1] We will elaborate on our use of the terms "modernity" and "modernism" at the beginning of the next section ("Modernity, technical expertise, and psychiatry").

[2] Our use of the terms "technical" and "technological" are close to Phillips' (2009) definition of "technical reason" in the introduction to his edited volume titled *Philosophical Perspectives on Technology and Psychiatry*: "With the use of technical reason knowledge is structured in an instrumental, means/ends manner. For any problem there is a stock of knowledge that can be ordered in formulaic fashion so that once the problem is presented, the correct solution (the means) can be applied to fix (the end) the problem. A particular problem is always an instance of a general type, and for the type there is a typical solution. The formula in medicine goes: if the patient has condition A, apply treatment B. The currently popular evidence-based medicine and treatment algorithms, as well as manualized treatment primers, are examples of this kind of technical thinking" (p. 9).

technological versions of psychology provide descriptions of "faulty cognitive or emotional processing," for example.

2. It is assumed that the mechanism or process can be *modeled in causal terms*, i.e., described in a way that is universal, a way that works regardless of the context.

3. Technological interventions are *instrumental*. They have nothing to do with opinions, values, relationships, or priorities.

The modernist approach is usually seen as promoting a liberation from "myths" about mental illness that led to stigma and oppression in the past. Many anti-stigma campaigns are actually premised on a strong presentation of this modernist, technological orientation. Mental illness is not a spiritual or moral issue but a technical one, due to a faulty biological or psychological mechanism. States of mental distress are characterized in terms of "symptoms" and it is generally assumed that a medical framework and vocabulary can capture the essential nature of such problems. Diseases of the body are the subject matter of pathology; those of the mind are the domain of psychopathology. Mental problems can be scientifically investigated and modeled. They can be measured and counted. Experts exist who can organize treatments and interventions. Progress is to be understood in terms of new scientific discoveries in neuroscience, psychology, or psychopharmacology. Such discoveries happen in university departments and research laboratories.

The modernist framework does not ignore non-technical issues to do with relationships, meanings, or values, but these are understood as being of secondary importance only. Likewise, service user organizations are not dismissed; but they are seen only as helpful collaborators in terms of fund-raising, identifying patients for research projects, and testifying to the benefits of various expert interventions. They are also understood to provide peer support for individuals who suffer from conditions that have been identified and mapped by psychiatry and its allied disciplines. Modernist psychiatry is happy to consult with such organizations but only if they are willing to accept the medical framing of their experiences. Individuals and organizations that fail to conform to this are regarded as being problematic: they are often simply dismissed as being unscientific, ideological, or simply anti-psychiatry.

The modernist, technological approach works to separate our discourse about mental distress from background contextual issues. It systematically seeks to sideline non-technological aspects of mental health and privileges those aspects such as biological factors that are the domain of the expert. This move promotes the gaze of the expert doctor who is trained to understand distress in terms of psychopathology.[3] In media discussions of mental health issues, in government determinations of research and service priorities, in the shaping of mental health policies and laws, nationally and internationally, the technological approach has universal dominance. While service users are increasingly spoken about as "partners," in the end (in all these domains) the pronouncements of experts of one sort or another are what count.

---

[3] While psychopathology is currently the dominant way of framing and understanding states of mental distress, it is not the only technical approach to mental health problems. Many psychological approaches, while critical of the "medical model," nevertheless approach mental distress primarily as a technical problem to be modeled and measured. They also present a set of interventions based on the logic of their model. All of this is organized and presented in a particular vocabulary that is developed over time by experts.

As this move empowers the doctor, it works to disempower the service user. Service users are not the ones who develop the concepts, plan the research, or set the service priorities. Controlling the discourse through which we discuss mental health issues works to privilege the role of the professional. Across the world, mental health laws systematically position mental patients as subject to the power of medical professionals. Such laws are premised on the idea that these professionals possess a scientific expertise about mental distress. In other words, the modernist, technical framing of mental health problems underscores professional power. And, as in any situation where there is a major imbalance of power between two groups, abuses have resulted from this. It is worth remembering that it was eugenic theories endorsed by psychiatrists and adopted by politicians that led to the mass killing of mental patients during the Nazi era in Germany.[4]

Our essential argument is that the modernist agenda that shapes current thinking and practice in psychiatry serves to disempower patients, while justifying professional authority. Thus, there is a need for a fundamental rethink of psychiatric theory and practice if we are genuine about a move to "user-centered" or "recovery-orientated" services. There is also a need to rethink our approach to campaigns that aim to reduce the stigma surrounding mental health issues.

In this chapter we shall first discuss modernism and show that psychiatry is a modernist project. We will argue that psychiatry would not have been possible outside the post-Enlightenment cultural preoccupation with reason, science, and technology. The modernist focus of psychiatry was in evidence when psychoanalytic thought was prominent but this focus has been intensified in the most recent swing toward neuroscience. We will then look at recent developments in the service user movement and show how this represents a direct challenge to the technological framing of mental health problems. We will finish by arguing that if psychiatry is to engage productively with this movement, if it is to take user empowerment seriously, if it is to genuinely embrace a "recovery" philosophy, it will have to imagine an alternative way of bringing medicine and mental illness together.

We have proposed the concept of "postpsychiatry" as a way of thinking about how we might move away from the modernist orientation that currently shapes psychiatric thinking (Bracken and Thomas 2005). Postpsychiatry represents an attempt to imagine a different sort of medical engagement with states of madness, distress, and alienation. It is not anti-medical or anti-psychiatry. But in its challenge to the dominant modernist, technological version of psychiatry, postpsychiatry seeks to diminish the power and authority assumed by the profession. It is hoped that this will assist in the creation of conditions wherein the voices of service users are no longer silenced. Only service users can empower themselves, but by systematically critiquing the philosophical assumptions that underpin current psychiatry as

---

[4] Dorothea S. Buck-Zerchin, who experienced 70 years in the German psychiatric system, including forced treatment and sterilization, wrote in 2007: "According to the latest research results submitted by the historian Professor Hans-Walter Schmuhl nearly 300,000 asylum and nursing care home patients were gassed, poisoned and starved to death. 80,000 of these came from Polish, French and Soviet institutions. Considering that our politicians, psychiatrists and theologians have nearly completely repressed this most drastic kind of compulsory treatment in the form of killing people whose lives were considered 'devoid of value,' it is mostly left up to us users and survivors of psychiatry to preserve the memory of those murdered in the name of psychiatry in our hearts" (Buck-Zerchin, 2007, p. 23). Psychiatry is one discourse where philosophical assumptions about the nature of mental functioning can have devastating consequences.

well as the empirical evidence used to justify its theories and practices, postpsychiatry seeks to be an ally in this endeavor.

Intellectually, postpsychiatry draws on a number of sources including: the literature of "recovery" that has emerged from within the service user movement; critical analyses of the science of psychiatric classification, explanation, and treatment; and philosophical insights into the nature of modernism. The latter have emerged mainly through the discourses of phenomenology and postmodernist thought.

Modernity, Technical Expertise, and Psychiatry

Modernity and technology

The words "modern," "modernism," and "modernity" are used in different ways by different writers. They mean different things in different contexts. They defy any easy definition. In addition, the history of culture and ideas is not linear or straightforward. We use these words to indicate a certain view of the world and our place in it. This is one associated with the European Enlightenment and the shift from religious revelation to human reason as the path to truth that this movement invoked. Bradley Lewis (2006, p. 65) writes:

> For the Enlightenment philosophers, "premodern" life (as I will call it) was rife with superstition and mythical fancy that were holding back human advancement. The Enlightenment dream was that through the liberation of reason and experience, knowledge would progress. With better knowledge would come advancement in human life through better control of the world.

The "world" here came to include the human world. The growth of the human sciences (psychology, sociology, anthropology, linguistics, etc.) from the nineteenth century was very much a product of this quest for human advancement through the application of scientific reason.

We see modernity as that period, post Enlightenment, when science became the road to progress and religion became of lesser importance. We use the term modernism to indicate a faith that our problems (including human problems in the territory of relationships, conflicts, and power) can be framed scientifically. This faith extends to a belief that technical, not moral, religious, or political interventions should be at the forefront of our quest to deal with human pain and suffering.

For us, modernity is defined by this technological focus. In his book, *The Technological Society*, Jacques Ellul (1964) traced the development of technology into the twentieth century. Ellul argued that technology is not just an "add on" to our modern society, something we could imagine living without. Rather, he describes a totalizing effect of technology. It dominates and shapes our culture in a profound way. Technology is to modernity what Catholicism was to the European Middle Ages. Understanding both the natural world and the world of human problems becomes primarily a scientific challenge in the modern era. While we still respond to the world through art and still acknowledge an ethical dimension to human problems, the technological imperative supersedes all others.

Many sociologists have mapped the extent to which we are a society shaped according to a technological imperative. Thirty-five years ago, in his book *Limits to Medicine. Medical Nemesis: The Expropriation of Health*, Ivan Illich (1976) put forward the idea of "cultural iatrogenesis." By this he meant that the technology of modern medicine has come to dominate our lives to the extent that it has actually undermined our own (individual and community) capacity to heal and help ourselves. He argued that modern medicine was actually destructive of health, which he defined as "the autonomous power to cope." Illich (1976, p. 42) wrote:

> the so-called health professions have an ever deeper, culturally health-denying effect in so far as they destroy the potential of people to deal with their human weakness, vulnerability, and uniqueness in a personal and autonomous way. The patient in the grip of contemporary medicine is but one instance of mankind in the grip of its pernicious techniques.

In his exploration of cultural iatrogenesis, Illich describes how death has been understood, responded to, and represented in different societies across the ages. In the modern era, death has become first and foremost a technical challenge. He writes:

> In its extreme form 'natural death' is now that point at which the human organism refuses any further input of treatment. People die when the electro-encephalogram indicates that their brain waves have flattened out: they do not take a last breath, or die because their heart stops. (Illich 1976, p. 209)

Illich, like most other sociologists writing on this subject, presents a very negative view of the growing dominance of technology. Perhaps he is too harsh. Anyone whose life has been saved by a modern medical intervention might well beg to differ! However, he is surely correct in his analysis of how profoundly we are now orientated according to a technological understanding of health and healing. Some may celebrate this move; others bemoan it. What is clear is that whether we conceive of technology as a blessing or a curse, there is no getting away from the fact that technology now shapes our lives in very profound ways.

The sociologist Anthony Giddens has written a great deal about the dynamics of modernity. Giddens speaks about the "separation of time and space" in modernity. In premodern societies, he argues, most people lived their lives in local communities that were bound together by living in a particular locality. Their understanding of the dimensions of the world was given to them by their experience of their own locality. This locality also provided the means whereby people experienced the passage of time. For example, the seasons shaped the pattern of agriculture which, in turn, shaped the activities of the community over time. Prior to clocks and maps, people experienced space and time in a way that was profoundly shaped by the local context. With the move to a culture of modernity, Giddens argues that there has been a "disembedding" of social institutions. There are a number of aspects to this but what interests us here is how Giddens (1991, p. 18) describes the rise of technicalized expertise:

> Expert systems bracket time and space through deploying modes of technical expertise which have validity independent of the practitioners and clients who make use of them. Such systems penetrate virtually all aspects of social life in conditions of modernity—in respects of the food we eat, the medicines we take, the buildings we inhabit, the forms of transport we use and a multiplicity of other phenomena. Expert systems are not confined to areas of technological expertise. They extend to social relations themselves and to the intimacies of the

self. The doctor, counselor and therapist are as central to the expert systems of modernity as the scientist, technician or engineer.

So, one central aspect of modernity is the major role given to experts and their systems of knowledge in shaping how we understand ourselves and how we live our lives.

Psychiatry as a product of the enlightenment

In its quest to develop a predictive science of the human "mind" and its problems, psychiatry has always been on the side of reason and order. We have theorized (Bracken and Thomas 2005, p. 7) that psychiatry itself is very much a product of the European Enlightenment. Without the focus on the individual subject and the increasing orientation toward reason and rationality that came with the Enlightenment, psychiatry could never have been born.

This focus on the individual can be seen in a number of domains. In the humanities, the vicissitudes of the individual's journey through life became increasingly important in art forms such as poetry, the novel, and drama. In law, the idea of "human rights" that are attached to individuals came into being. In philosophy, the nineteenth century saw the emergence of a number of movements such as phenomenology which were concerned with the nature of individual experience. This concern with the interior, with the nature of the mind, and the processes underscoring individual experience were all reflected in the emergence of psychoanalysis at the end of the nineteenth century. In this chapter, we shall not explore this particular connection between psychiatry and the Enlightenment further. We will concentrate instead on the role of reason and rationality in the generation of the discipline.

Reason and the asylum

First, the Enlightenment gave rise to a cultural sensibility in which irrational behaviour became deeply problematic. In the end, it became an issue that could not be left to families to manage but was something that required the full attention of the state. In post-Enlightenment society the mad were a source of scandal. They became the "other"; a threatening presence in need of removal. The historian Roy Porter (2002, p. 122) writes:

> Not least, the asylum idea reflected the long-term cultural shift from religion to scientific secularism. In traditional Christendom, it was the distinction between believers and heretics, saints and sinners, which had been crucial—that between the sane and the crazy had counted for little. This changed, and the great divide, since the 'age of reason', became that between the rational and the rest, demarcated and enforced at bottom by the asylum walls. The keys of St Peter had been replaced by the keys of psychiatry. The instituting of the asylum set up a cordon sanitaire delineating the 'normal' from the 'mad', which underlined the Otherhood of the insane and carved out a managerial milieu in which that alienness could be handled.

Porter and other historians are often at pains to point out that the institutionalization of madness was not something organized by doctors, let alone psychiatrists. It was not a medical act but a form of social engineering in which individuals who were seen as difficult were to be excluded. In turn, the asylum, by bringing together large numbers of "mad" people and placing them in the care of asylum doctors, provided the material for a new discourse to emerge. Prior to the asylum era, there was no real organized body of knowledge called "psychiatry." There were various disparate medical theories about madness and the emotions but no unified profession as such. For example, Porter (2002, p. 135) writes:

> Esquirol's transformation of the classification and diagnosis of mental disorder was made possible by the abundance of data provided by asylums, enabling diagnosticians to build up clearly defined profiles of psychiatric diseases capable of being identified by their symptoms. Observation of asylum patients led to more precise differentiations in theory and practice—epileptics, for instance, became standardly distinguished from the insane.

Thus the origins of psychiatry as a discrete discipline, with an identity separate from the rest of medicine, were in the asylums of the nineteenth century. Psychiatry came into being on the back of an original act of social exclusion. But asylum doctors were nevertheless very keen to maintain their specifically medical identity. As the century progressed they fought to assert their technical expertise in the field of madness. For example, in the courts, psychiatrists claimed to be able to distinguish criminality from insanity and did so in the language of medicine.

Psychiatry and the rise of technical expertise

The Enlightenment also led to the promotion of scientific approaches to investigating and solving problems that would previously have been the domain of religion. This led to the growth of psychology and the other human sciences. Psychoanalysis was very much a product of this quest to "map" the mind in a scientific fashion. Freud was primarily a doctor and sought to develop psychoanalysis as a legitimate medical intervention. One of his greatest insights was into the important role played by human relationships both in generating mental health problems and in helping individuals recover from such problems. However, as a "scientist," his instinct was to provide models and to "technicalize" the territory of such relationships. The therapeutic relationship itself came to be formulated, not in a language of care, but in terms of transference and counter-transference. While some later analysts have used these concepts in non-medical, non-technical ways, Freud was very clear that his new creation was intended to be a branch of the natural sciences. In fact, he was dismissive of approaches to psychology that were put forward by proponents of the *Geisteswissenschaften* movement. Grünbaum (1984) argues that Freud was at pains to establish the natural science credentials of psychoanalysis and quotes him from 1933:

> the intellect and the mind are objects for scientific research in exactly the same way as any non-human things. Psycho-analysis has a special right to speak for the scientific *Weltanschauung* .... If ... the investigation of the intellectual and emotional functions of men (and of animals) is included in science, then it will be seen that ... no new sources of knowledge or methods of research have come into being. (Freud, quoted in Grünbaum, 1984, p. 2)

Furthermore, Grünbaum makes the point that it was his "clinical theory of personality and therapy" that Freud was most at pains to establish as scientific. The forms of psychoanalysis that were influential within psychiatry through much of the twentieth century followed this modernist agenda, and presented analysis as a form of technical expertise. Of course, other, more hermeneutic and less-technological forms of psychoanalytic discourse have also emerged.

In recent years biological approaches to understanding human distress have come to dominate within psychiatry. Academic departments of psychiatry have become centers of neuroscience. This is sometimes called the "new psychiatry." Bradley Lewis (2006, p. 61) writes:

> The new psychiatry compulsively repeats more than it changes. Indeed, using a broader historical sweep, the new psychiatry's shift from a psychoanalytic rhetoric to a neuroscience rhetoric is not so much a change as a hardening and further modernist expansion of the worst aspects of the psychoanalytic science that preceded it.

This takes many forms but in relation to psychiatry we see it in three major developments: the almost obsessive quest to develop a comprehensive classification system, the search to provide causal explanatory models (genetic, neurological, and psychological) of mental problems and the attempt to structure our understanding of mental health interventions according to the logic of evidence-based medicine.

Since its origins in the asylums, psychiatry has endorsed the Enlightenment goal of ordering the world according to reason. Its territory was that of madness and its aim has always been to map this territory accurately, provide scientific explanations and models, and develop a set of technical interventions. All of this was proposed in the language of medicine. To be a "doctor of the mind," the psychiatrist would have to be able to diagnose, classify, and explain madness just as the endocrinologist accounted for the disorders of the hormonal system. Furthermore, the psychiatrist would have to develop treatments and provide accurate prognoses just as other doctors did. The goal was not primarily care, understanding, or comfort, so words such as "kindness," "respect," "empowerment," and "solidarity" have never figured centrally in any major psychiatric text.

THE SERVICE USER MOVEMENT AND THE STRUGGLE TO REDEFINE EXPERTISE

Foucault famously wrote that the history of psychiatry is the history of a "monologue of reason about unreason" (Foucault 1971, pp. xii–xiii). By this, we believe he meant that the professionalized discourse about mental illness has effectively excluded and denied the voices of patients and silenced their attempts to define themselves and the nature of their problems. Even critical discourses about psychiatry (including most of what is called anti-psychiatry) have been dominated by the voices of professionals and academics. However, in recent years, the rise of the user movement has opened the possibility of genuine dialogue. Although mental patients were collectively pursuing their goals as far back as the seventeenth century (Campbell 2009), it was really not until the 1980s that effective user organizations began to emerge. Since then the rise of the movement has been rapid. In the UK alone, it is now estimated that there are at least 300 groups with an approximate membership of 9000 (Wallcraft et al. 2003). In this section, we will examine how user organizations are beginning to question the dominance of technicalized expertise in the field of mental health. Such organizations seek not to impose a new model or paradigm but simply to open the field to a different ways of understanding and framing mental health problems. By demonstrating that real and meaningful support can be organized and delivered to people struggling with states of madness and distress in a non-technological idiom, such groups undermine the modernist claim that there is only one legitimate way of framing and understanding such experiences.

The user movement is now a worldwide phenomenon. It is growing from strength to strength. Organizations set up by service users are now consulted by national governments, the World Health Organization, the United Nations, and even the World Psychiatric Association.[5]

However, it is clear that while many service users share certain concerns, there is a very wide range of opinions within the movement and diverse priorities and agendas. Some service users are happy to define themselves and their problems through the concepts made available to them by psychiatry. In other words, they accept that getting a "diagnosis" is important and that this can only be produced by a trained psychiatrist. While they may be unhappy with the organization of services and the attitudes of staff, nevertheless they accept the fundamentals of the medical model and are happy to use the language of psychopathology in discussions of their difficulties. Such individuals and organizations are happy to work with professional organizations on research projects, campaigns to improve services, and to end stigma, etc. From the other side, professional organizations are always quick to point to their work with such individuals and organizations when challenged about the extent to which they are prepared to cooperate with consumers of services.

Because of their support for the medical framing of mental health problems, some of these groups have been supported financially by the pharmaceutical industry. The European-wide organization GAMIAN Europe (Global Alliance of Mental Illness Advocacy) was actually set up by the pharmaceutical company Bristol-Myers Squibb (Herxheimer 2003, p. 1209). In the USA, the organization NAMI (National Alliance for the Mentally Ill), has literally received millions of dollars in funding from the pharmaceutical industry (Herxheimer 2003).

However, there are also many people who have used services who are unhappy with the psychopathological framework. They sometimes refer to themselves as "survivors" of the system as they maintain that psychiatry and mental health services are most often toxic to those who use them and count themselves lucky to have survived. Such groups and individuals hold different views themselves but are generally united by a rejection of the technological framework and the way it defines mental health problems through an expert vocabulary and logic. This is essentially a *critical* service user movement. One of its main objectives is to show up the assumptions that guide traditional psychiatry and to demonstrate that these assumptions are not necessarily valid. It seeks to show how mental health problems can be understood in different ways and that different ways of intervening, other than the traditional menu of drugs and/or therapy, can provide solid paths along which people can recover.

For example, the Icarus Project is a support organization in the USA, set up in 2002 by young people with a diagnosis of "bipolar disorder." This organization has sought to rethink "bipolar experience" and remove it from the category of pathology. They stress the creativity that often comes with the experiences of hypomania and even depression. They argue that it makes more sense to them to regard their experiences as "dangerous gifts," parts of themselves that ask to be "cultivated and taken care of," rather than as a disease or disorder

---

[5] <http://www.mindfreedom.org/campaign/global/wpa-meets-with-movement>

to be "cured" or "eliminated." The organization works to provide a sense of community for people who feel "isolated from and alienated by traditional approaches to mental health." Importantly, members of the Icarus Project reject the dominance of psychopathology and seek to assert their own definitions of what happens to them and what helps them:

> For us, a key component of our work is reclaiming our right to self-definition, choosing how we each reckon and work with our madness. That said, many of us have found that when we cease to see our psychic pain and sensitivities as diseases, that labels like "madness" and "crazy" suddenly become imbued with new, more positive nuances. Instead of serving to further remind us of our difference and thus sickness, we can reclaim these words and make them terms of endearment or even of positive identification, much like the gay pride movement has adopted the word "queer." (Mitchell-Brody 2007, p. 141)

The Icarus approach resonates with that of the loosely connected Mad Pride movement. This is made up of groups in different parts of the world who organize events (usually involving music, food, and fun) that celebrate the contributions made by people who experience episodes of madness and distress. Mad Pride models itself on the Gay Pride marches and festivals that are now a regular feature in many countries across the world. The idea is to shift from a negative to a positive discourse about mental health. Mad Pride insists that the experiences that we commonly label "mental illness," while often very painful, are not without meaning and under different social and cultural circumstances could have the potential to be transformative and helpful.

Similar ideas are put forward by the Hearing Voices Network (HVN). This emerged in the Netherlands in the late 1980s and, although it was initiated by a psychiatrist, Professor Marius Romme (Romme and Escher 1993), it has been developed largely through the efforts of people who hear voices themselves across Europe and America. The HVN is not only a peer-support organization but it offers a completely different way of understanding and responding to voice hearing. It challenges one of the fundamental assumptions of psychopathology: that the experience of hearing voices (when no one is speaking) is simply a symptom, a meaningless indicator of an underlying disease process, something to be eliminated with medication. Romme and Escher (2007, p. 134) write:

> Accepting voices and making sense of them is an approach in which voices are seen as signals of problems in life. Therefore it does not make much sense to treat them as a symptom of an illness, nor try to cure a disease that is supposed to produce these voices. Suppressing these voices is not the right learning experience for coping with them and the problems that lay at their roots. Suppressing these problems does not help solve these problems. The traditional line of thinking in psychiatry where voices are seen as a symptom of an illness and as resulting from a disease, is not only incorrect, but also harmful, because it alienates voice hearers from their experiences, makes them powerless and often turns voice hearing into a chronic problem.

Other organizations (such as the Paranoia Network and Evolving Minds in the UK) also aim not just to be support groups (important as this may be) but to also develop and present challenges to the dominant psychopathology framework. They seek to reframe experiences of madness, distress, and alienation and turn them into human, rather than technical, problems. Of central importance here is the move to question the professional expertise that is given credibility and underscored by the technological approach. Groups like Icarus and HVN do not accept the medical framing of their experiences and thus do not accept that doctors hold the "truth" of what they struggle with. Rather, they seek to explore an alternate sort of expertise: one that is built up over time by such groups themselves. This is based on peer support, critical reflection on the nature of their problems, and a refusal of the current power structures in the mental health field.

They have come to regard the technological approach as deeply disempowering. By framing their problems (bipolar experience, voices) simply as symptoms to be targeted with medication, this approach says to the service user: "you will not be able to deal with this problem without expert medical/technical knowledge." It has the tendency to render the service-user passive in the face of their experiences and creates a dependency on the professional for a way of moving forward.

In their book *Alternatives Beyond Psychiatry*, Peter Stastny and Peter Lehmann (2007a) bring together accounts of various initiatives from around the world that all present an alternative way of understanding and responding to madness and distress. Some of these initiatives are small and in the process of getting organized, others are well established and strong. Many of them involve collaborations between professionals and service users. However, the professional perspective does not dominate and they all work with an openness to diverse ways of framing and responding to states of madness, distress, and alienation.

Rethinking the Role of Professionals in Mental Health Work

Organization like HMV, Icarus, Mad Pride, and Mind Freedom have been arguing against the dominance of the medical framework for some time. The contributors to the *Alternatives Beyond Psychiatry* book are activists, people who have made a decision to group together to struggle for alternatives. Psychiatry has often dismissed their views as unrepresentative of the majority of psychiatric patients. As Stastny and Lehmann (2007b, p. 407) write:

> Psychiatry still turns a cold shoulder to the movement of (ex-) users and survivors of psychiatry and its supporters, scorning its proposals for reform along with the important knowledge it has generated; without political pressure, we can only find the occasional application of protective paternalism.

We have already acknowledged that some patients are happy to accept the technical approach and, at least in the short term, find the medical framing of their problems to be helpful. However, there is also evidence that very many patients who are not active in the service user movement nevertheless find psychiatric interventions problematic and sometimes harmful. In their important book *Experiencing Psychiatry: Users' Views of Services*, Rogers, Pilgrim, and Lacey reported the results of a major survey of users' experiences of psychiatric care. They point to a substantial discrepancy between the ways in which service users understood their problems and the way in which these problems were framed by the professionals involved in their care:

> The typical psychiatric formulation of personal problems tended to be construed in bio-medical terms (as indicated by the type of diagnosis and treatment given). In contrast, it

was evident that contact with health services resulted, in the eyes of patients, from a complexity of cumulative personal and domestic events. Particular, precipitating or "triggering" factors were often difficult to identify as a unitary cause of a "breakdown." People seem to experience mental distress as a continuum of everyday life, without an easily identifiable genesis. (Rogers et al. 1993, p. 175)

Furthermore, this study revealed that many service users did not really value a technicalized form of expertise in their professionals. They were more focused on the human aspects of their encounters with staff: Were they treated with dignity, kindness, and respect? Were their views listened to and accepted? Were the professionals able to understand their priorities and take them seriously? In other words, did the professionals' training properly equip them to encounter the worlds of their patients in a way that was empowering and supportive or were they trained in a way that meant such encounters were often undermining for the service user?

> High levels of "skill" and "expertise," whether in psychological therapies, medicine or nursing, run counter to the emphasis on *deskilling*, which is implied by what users identify as being beneficial: that is, if professionals were to approximate to the conception preferred by users, they would have to shed most or all of their pretensions towards specialized knowledge. (Rogers et al. 1993, p. 178)

In recent years, evidence has been accumulating that many psychiatric interventions work, but not because they "fix" any particular biological or psychological deficit. For example, a series of meta-analyses of antidepressant drug trials have shown that most of the benefits of these drugs can be explained by the very strong placebo response in the treatment of states of depression. Turner et al.'s (2008) meta-analysis of Food and Drug Administration (FDA) data (which had access to unpublished as well as published research results) concluded that although antidepressants were generally superior to placebo, most of the benefit from these drugs could be explained by the placebo effect. Kirsch et al.'s (2008) examination of FDA data found that over 80% of the improvement seen in the drug groups was duplicated in the placebo groups. Using the National Institute for Health and Clinical Excellence criterion for judging clinical effectiveness, these authors concluded that the additional benefit of antidepressants over placebo was not clinically significant.

The placebo effect essentially involves the patient unconsciously mustering up the energy and motivation to get better. It is generated by non-specific aspects of the treatment encounter and involves an increase in hope associated with taking a treatment, trust in the practitioner who prescribed it, and a sense of meaning brought about by negotiating an understandable and acceptable explanation for one's suffering (Moerman 2002).

Psychotherapy has also proven to be effective in the treatment of depression. Currently the most often prescribed form of psychotherapy is cognitive behavioral therapy (CBT). This is usually thought to work by modifying faults in cognitive content and processing that are said to be specific to depression. Its proponents, including its founder, regard it as a specific technology targeted at specific psychological "faults" (Beck 1993). However, several studies have shown that most of the specific features of CBT can be dispensed with without adversely affecting outcomes (Jacobson et al. 1996). In a comprehensive review of studies of the different components of CBT, Longmore and Worrell (2007, p. 173) concluded that there is "little evidence that specific cognitive interventions significantly increase the effectiveness of the therapy."

What is clear from this brief look at treatments for depression is that they work, not by fixing a set of specific technical faults in the patient's biology or psychology, but through the generation of meaning, trust, and hope. This perspective is one that resonates with the growing literature on recovery in mental health. The word "recovery" is often used in discussions about physical health to indicate a situation where the patient has become free of illness. When we say that someone is "in recovery" we mean that they have recovered their health. The disease is gone. In the area of mental health, the situation is more complicated. Here the word "recovery" has two different sets of connotations. As Mike Slade writes (2009), it is "one word, two meanings." The first corresponds to the way it is used, as shown earlier, in discussions of physical health. This has to do with someone being "cured" of their illness, their mental symptoms have all disappeared. We might say that this is the "clinical" use of the term. However, in recent years, the word has also come to mean something different in mental health circles. This usage has emerged from within the service user movement. A number of people who had been informed that they were suffering from lifelong psychiatric conditions managed to find paths that led them to a reality of personal recovery. They then wrote about their journeys in an attempt to provide inspiration for others. While some of these paths involved mental health services, many did not. Some reported that traditional mental health services had worked to impede their recovery and some reported that they had been damaged by the way psychiatry framed their problems and intervened in their lives.

A large literature centered on these personal accounts of recovery from serious mental health problems has now emerged.[6] This literature moves the discussion about mental problems away from the medical and technical focus on issues such as diagnosis, assessment, classification, prognosis, and treatment. Instead, this recovery literature highlights the central importance of the non-technical, non-specific aspects of care. The recovery literature prioritizes questions such as: how hope is generated and sustained, how dignity can be maintained even in the midst of crisis, and how a sense of personal empowerment is often the driving force behind an individual's journey toward health.

This recovery literature resonates with the findings of a series of empirical studies of what service users say about their experiences both of mental illness itself and of the services set up to help them. These also highlight the *primary* importance of the non-technical aspects of mental health. For example, the *Strategies for Living Project* (Faulkner and Layzell 2000), organized by the London-based Mental Health Foundation, involved consumer-led research exploring what service users wanted from mental health services. The priorities of service-users were:

- acceptance
- shared experience and shared identity (i.e., meeting with others who have had similar experiences)
- emotional support
- a reason for living
- finding meaning and purpose in life
- peace of mind, relaxation

---

[6] The American psychologist Gail Hornstein has been collecting such narratives for many years. See her 2002 paper, "Narratives of madness, as told from within."

- taking control and having choices
- security and safety
- pleasure.

When we use the term "recovery orientation" we are talking about developing a focus on these priorities and learning from both the empirical evidence produced by service users and the messages that have emerged from the recovery literature.

In a recovery-orientated service, the technical expertise of the professional is not ignored but it is rendered of *secondary* importance. In such a service, there is an emphasis on relationships and an understanding that mental health problems are very rarely "fixed" with some sort of technical intervention. Instead, it is accepted that working with the patient and their own understanding of what is happening is important. Care is taken not to silence this understanding and replace it with the technical framework of the professional expert.

As Mike Slade (2009, p. 42) says:

> In a service focused on personal recovery, disagreement with a clinical model simply does not matter—what is important is that the person finds their own meaning, which makes some sense of their experience and provides hope for the future. Why? Because suffering with meaning is bearable—meaningless suffering is what drives you mad. Finding meaning *is* moving on. By contrast, in a mental health service focused on clinical recovery, lack of insight is always to be avoided, because it is a symptom of illness and symptoms are, by definition, undesirable.

Conclusion

In this chapter, we have argued that psychiatry is very much a modernist enterprise, focused on framing mental problems as technical challenges and responding to these with expert-prescribed interventions. It has sought to bring medicine to bear on mental distress and madness in a way that replicates the authority that doctors hold in other branches of medicine. To do this it has had to ignore the conceptual and ethical differences between the world of the "mental" and that of the "body" and treat the former as though it could be understood through exactly the same scientific approach as has been developed in the rest of medicine. In this move, problems with our thoughts, emotions, relationships, and behaviors are encountered in the same way that we encounter problems with our kidneys, lungs, and nervous systems. Psychopathology parallels bodily pathology and interventions are framed as treatments. While this was true in the form of psychoanalysis that impacted on psychiatry in the first half of the twentieth century, it has been deepened in the era of neuroscience.

We have argued elsewhere that this framing of medicine's relation to madness in a modernist idiom is profoundly mistaken (Bracken and Thomas 2005). We believe that a very different relationship is possible and needed if medicine is going to be of genuine value to patients with mental problems. The growing service user movement challenges head-on this modernist agenda of psychiatry. It denies the truth of the psychopathology framework and demands that its alternative understanding of madness and distress be heard. As we write, the voice of modernist psychiatry is louder. Everyday, we hear promises of breakthroughs and we read increasingly desperate assertions of the wonders of neuroscience.

But the contradiction between the views of service users and the empirical evidence about how treatments work on one side and the pronouncements of psychiatric experts on the other grows starker.

Postpsychiatry represents the belief that a different sort of medical engagement with madness is possible. This approach does not seek or claim to hold the "truth" about mental problems. It seeks to put "ethics before technology." By this we mean that the non-technical aspects of mental health problems should have priority over the technical aspects. We mean that our mental health discourse should begin with care and kindness, dignity, and respect, and work with service users to keep these to the fore. From this discourse, as a secondary event, specific technical questions will arise and will require a response. These can be approached through collaborations between service users and professionals. This approach would be in keeping with insights from the current recovery literature and with the demands of organizations such as the Icarus Project and Hearing Voices Network.

References

Beck, A. T. (1993). Cognitive therapy: past, present, and future. *Journal of Consulting and Clinical Psychology*, 61, 194–8.

Bracken, P. and Thomas, P. (2005). *Postpsychiatry: Mental Health in a Postmodern World*. Oxford: Oxford University Press.

Buck-Zerchin, D. (2007). Seventy years of coercion in psychiatric institutions, experienced and witnessed. In P. Stastny and P. Lehmann (Eds), *Alternatives Beyond Psychiatry*, pp. 19–28. Berlin: Peter Lehmann Publishing.

Campbell, P. (2009). The service user/survivor movement. In J. Reynolds, R. Muston, T. Heller, J. Leach, M. McCormick, J. Wallcraft, *et al.* (Eds), *Mental Health Still Matters*, pp. 46–52. Milton Keynes: Open University/Palgrave Macmillan.

Ellul, J. (1964). *The Technological Society*. New York, NY: Vintage Books.

Faulkner, A. and Layzell, S. (2000). *Strategies for Living: A Report of User-Led Research into People's Strategies for Living with Mental Distress*. London: Mental Health Foundation.

Foucault, M. (1971). *Madness and Civilization: A History of Insanity in the Age of Reason*. London: Tavistock.

Freud, S. (1933). The structure of the unconscious. In *New Introductory Lectures on Psychoanalysis* (W. J. H. Sprott, Trans.), pp. 104–5, 105–7, 108–12. New York, NY: Norton.

Giddens, A. (1991). *Modernity and Self-Identity. Self and Society in the Late Modern Age*. Cambridge: Polity Press.

Grünbaum, A. (1984). *The Foundations of Psychoanalysis: A Philosophical Critique*. Berkeley, CA: University of California Press.

Herxheimer, A. (2003). Relationships between the pharmaceutical industry and patients' organizations. *British Medical Journal*, 326, 1208–10.

Hornstein, G. (2002). Narratives of madness, as told from within. *Chronicle of Higher Education*, January 25, B7–10.

Illich, I. (1976). *Limits to Medicine. Medical Nemesis: The Expropriation of Health*. Harmondsworth: Penguin.

Jacobson, N. S., Dobson, K. S., Truax, P. A., Addis, M., Koerner, K., Gollan, J. K., *et al.* (1996). A component analysis of cognitive-behavioural treatment for depression. *Journal of Consulting and Clinical Psychology*, 64, 295–304.

Kirsch, I., Deacon, B. J., Huedo-Medina, T. B., Scoboria, A., Moore, T. J., and Johnson, B. T. (2008). Initial severity and antidepressant benefits: a meta-analysis of data submitted to the Food and Drug Administration. *Public Library of Science: Medicine*, 5, e45.

Lewis, B. (2006). *Moving Beyond Prozac, DSM, and the New Psychiatry. The Birth of Postpsychiatry*. Ann Arbor, MI: University of Michigan Press.

Longmore, R. J. and Worrell, M. (2007). Do we need to challenge thoughts in cognitive behaviour therapy? *Clinical Psychology Review*, 27, 173–87.

Mitchell-Brody, M. (2007). The Icarus Project: dangerous gifts, iridescent visions and mad community. In P. Stastny and P. Lehmann (Eds), *Alternatives Beyond Psychiatry*, pp. 137–45. Berlin: Peter Lehmann Publishing.

Moerman, D. (2002). *Meaning, Medicine and the 'Placebo Effect'*. Cambridge: Cambridge University Press.

Phillips, J. (2009). Introduction. In J. Phillips (Ed.), *Philosophical Perspectives on Technology and Psychiatry*, pp. 1–19. Oxford: Oxford University Press.

Porter, R. (2002). *Madness: A Brief History*. Oxford: Oxford University Press.

Rogers, A., Pilgrim, D., and Lacey, R. (1993). *Experiencing Psychiatry: Users' Views of Services*. Basingstoke: MacMillan Press.

Romme, M. and Escher, S. (1993). *Accepting Voices*. London: MIND Publications.

Romme, M. and Escher, S. (2007). INTERVOICE: Accepting and making sense of voices. In P. Stastny and P. Lehmann (Eds), *Alternatives Beyond Psychiatry*, pp. 131–6. Berlin: Peter Lehmann Publishing.

Slade, M. (2009). *Personal Recovery and Mental Illness*. Cambridge: Cambridge University Press.

Stastny, P. and Lehmann, P. (2007a). *Alternatives Beyond Psychiatry*. Berlin: Peter Lehmann Publishing.

Stastny, P. and Lehmann, P. (2007b). Reforms or alternatives? A better psychiatry or better alternatives? In P. Stastny and P. Lehmann (Eds), *Alternatives Beyond Psychiatry*, pp. 402–12. Berlin: Peter Lehmann Publishing.

Turner, E.H. and Rosenthal, R. (2008). Efficacy of antidepressants. Is not an absolute measure, and it depends on how clinical significance is defined. *British Medical Journal*, 336, 516–17.

Wallcraft, J., Read, J., and Sweeney, A. (2003). *On Our Own Terms: Users and Survivors of Mental Health Services Working Together for Support and Change*. London: Sainsbury Centre for Mental Health.

CHAPTER 12

RACE AND GENDER IN PHILOSOPHY OF PSYCHIATRY: SCIENCE, RELATIVISM, AND PHENOMENOLOGY

MARILYN NISSIM-SABAT

INTRODUCTION

A preponderance of evidence shows that psychiatry has been imbued with racism and sexism throughout its history. "Racism" and "sexism" denote prejudices against groups and individual members of them such that differences are marked as inferiority and those so marked are often viewed as less than human. Groups that have been so marked include people of African and Native American descent living in North America and Europe, ethnic minorities, e.g., the Roma in Europe, the Turks in Germany, the Senegalese in France, and, all over the world, Jews, homosexuals, and women. Given the scope and accessibility of the evidence, the shameful history of racism and sexism in psychiatry and other mental health disciplines is incontestable. For this reason, though important sources are cited,[1] no attempt will be made in this chapter to rehearse or augment that evidence. Rather than this, the focus here will be on a critical analysis of particular theoretical frameworks in their interplay with issues of race and gender. The purpose of this approach is to show that theoretical perspective is one of the most important factors in play in working toward the goal of eliminating

[1] Many of the most important studies documenting racism and sexism in psychiatry are referenced in two chapters of Radden (2004). These are: Potter, pp. 237–243, and Nissim-Sabat, pp. 244–257. See also Nissim-Sabat (2001, pp. 44–59). An additional more recent and excellent reference that is relevant to both racism and sexism in psychiatry is Metzl (2009). This book contains numerous references to articles and reports that document racism and sexism in the history of psychiatry.

racism and sexism from psychiatry and psychology. Though in the final section of this chapter Husserlian phenomenology is proposed as a philosophical perspective that is conducive to overcoming bias in theory, this is not intended to override the main goal of this chapter, which is to show the relevance of theory to the goal of eliminating racism and sexism from psychiatry.

A case in point is the ongoing debate as to whether or not eliminating the category of race from medicine, psychology, and psychiatry will negatively affect treatment. Some maintain that "race" is a genetic variable and, therefore, can be used without generating or implying racial discrimination, for example, in the form of racial profiling.[2] Others maintain that this is not possible because the concept of race is so heavily laden with racism that the two are inseparable.[3]

Much of the literature of this debate involves studies and critiques of studies of pharmacological agents for treating many diseases, including, of course, ever increasing use of psychotropic drugs to treat symptoms of mental disorders, e.g., depression, anxiety, schizophrenia, bipolar disorder, and so on.[4] An important issue concerns the advisability of construing biomedical research and drug policy as if they can be isolated from psychosocial development, culture, and the social, including economic, forces impinging on patients. For some critics, so to isolate research is to allow one's work to be skewed by an ideology, naturalism,[5] and to that extent to be unscientific. This alleged ideology is reflected also in the medical model of disease that is still dominant in psychiatry.[6] Indeed, naturalism and various interpretations of its relation or non-relation to racism and sexism is at the heart of the controversy regarding use of the concept of race in psychiatry: Is naturalism a stance that yields scientific objectivity and thus transcends racism, or is it part of the problem, reductive in a manner that simply sidesteps or dismisses racism and thus enables it to remain in play, or even collusively fosters it?

Another case in point regarding the interplay of race and gender and theoretical frameworks in philosophy of psychiatry concerns numerous studies that detail the ways in which prejudice against women has pervaded the history of psychiatry. Maleness has historically been seen as superior to femaleness, which itself has often been seen—by Freud, for example—as a mark of inferiority (see Freud 1966). Various psychiatric diagnoses (such as

---

[2] In this chapter, the terms "racial profiling" and "gender profiling" will be used strictly in the pejorative sense to mean *unwarranted* use of race, gender, or ethnicity as a factor in deciding on diagnosis, treatment, or behavior toward an individual or group.

[3] An extraordinarily rich mine of profusely documented articles by leading researchers representing all significant points of view on the issues of race, genetics, and biomedical research can be found on the web forum, *Is Race "Real"?*. This blog is a web forum sponsored by the Social Sciences Research Council and can be found at <http://www.raceandgenomics.ssrc.org>. Additionally, the key issues are discussed in Outram and Ellison (2010, pp. 92–123), and Whitmarsh and Jones (2010).

[4] Moncrieff (2008, p. 235) documents increasing use of psychiatric drugs: "Use of psychiatric drugs has risen dramatically. In the UK, for example, prescriptions for antidepressants rose by 235% in the ten years up to 2002 (National Institute for Clinical Excellence, 2004). In the USA, 11% of women and 5% of men now take an antidepressant drug" (Stagnitti, 2005).

[5] Good overviews and analyses of the problematic status of naturalism in psychiatry can be found in Thornton (2004), and Patil and Giordano (2010).

[6] A critique of the medical model in psychiatry can be found in Schwartz and Wiggins (1985). A philosophically sophisticated explanation, defense, and critique of the medical model in psychiatry can be found in Patil and Giordano (2010).

"hysteria" and "borderline personality disorder") have been reserved for females,[7] just as various diagnoses (schizophrenia, for example) were and are assigned to black people in a disproportionately higher frequency than they are assigned to white people (Metzl 2009). Feminist thinkers in psychiatry have attempted to show that the very idea of sexism is a construct indicative of either ignorance or denial of the social construction of gender, indeed denial that gendered behavior is profoundly affected, even determined, by the environmental milieu in which human development occurs. Various versions of this philosophical perspective fall under the rubric of social construction.

Naturalism and social construction(ism)[8] are philosophical perspectives; they are stances, attitudes, or explanatory models that purportedly offer means of comprehending the relevant phenomena. They are deeply implicated in attempts to understand and correct the continued tendency toward racism and sexism in biomedical research, psychiatry, psychology, and psychoanalysis. To show this, first I will prepare the ground with initial working definitions of naturalism and constructionism (also called constructivism) and the philosophical presuppositions linked with them: realism and antirealism. The explanations of these concepts given here are merely schematic and do not reflect the many extant interpretations and philosophical usages of them. They should be considered working definitions to facilitate discussion and thought.

Naturalism is usually discussed under two rubrics: ontological (or metaphysical) naturalism and methodological naturalism. Ontological naturalism is concerned with what does and does not exist. It holds that nature is all there is, and all basic truths are truths of nature. This perspective is generally associated with philosophical realism:

> A realist about a subject-matter S may hold (i) that the kinds of things described by S exist; (ii) that their existence is independent of us, or not an artifact of our minds, or our language or conceptual scheme … ; (iv) that the statements we make in S have truth conditions, being straightforward descriptions of aspects of the world and made true or false by facts in the world. (Blackburn 2008, p. 308)

Among the kinds of things cited by Blackburn that may be the focus of realism is "the external world" (p. 308). Thus, ontological naturalism is a perspective on the external world viewed as "nature"; it is the view that the external world, or, more precisely, nature, exists and is a mind-independent reality. This is to be differentiated from Platonic realism, according to which universals exist, or are real, independent of things, or of nature (p. 374).

Methodological, or scientific, naturalism focuses on epistemology: How can we gain trustworthy knowledge of the natural world? It is concerned with practical methods for acquiring knowledge independently of one's metaphysical or religious views, and requires that hypotheses be explained and tested only by reference to natural causes and events. Methodological naturalism is not necessarily linked with realism; presumably, it is held independently of one's metaphysical or religious views.[9] Yet, if it is claimed that methodological naturalism

---

[7] Elaine Showalter's (1987) magisterial study, *The Female Malady*, and her subsequent writings on gender and mental disorder are the recognized starting point for studying sexism in psychiatry. A more recent treatment is Hirshbein (2010). See also Wirth-Cauchon (2000).

[8] In this chapter, the terms social construction(ism) and constructivism will be used interchangeably and in conformity with the usages of authors cited.

[9] See <http://www.ask.com/wiki/Scientificnaturalism?qsrc=3044> (retrieved February 2011).

is concerned with acquiring knowledge of "the natural world," whether or not ontological naturalism is held will be determined, it would seem, by whether or not the methodological naturalist holds a realist view of nature.

Constructionism is also used in several senses. Some of these are outlined in Ron Mallon's (2007) article, to be discussed at length, "A Field Guide to Social Construction." Mallon points out that:

> Social constructionists are particularly interested in phenomena that are contingent upon human culture and human decisions—contingent upon the theories, texts, conventions, practices, and conceptual schemes of particular individuals and groups of people in particular places and times .... Thinking of constructionism in this general way allows us to recognize the affinity of explicitly "constructionist" accounts with a wide range of work in the social sciences and humanities that abjures the label "social construction"—for example Foucault's talk of "discursive formations," Ian Hacking's discussions of "historical ontology," Arnold Davidson's work on "historical epistemology," and a host of titles that discuss "inventing," "creating," or "making up," various phenomena. (Mallon 2007, p. 94)

Constructionism is generally associated with antirealism, according to which entities of any or all kinds do not have "objective" reality, that is, they have no mind-independent existence:

> The term anti-realism is used to describe any position involving either the denial of an objective reality of entities of a certain type or the denial that verification-transcendent statements about a type of entity are either true or false. This latter construal is sometimes expressed by saying "there is no fact of the matter as to whether or not P." (Retrieved from http://wikipedia.org/wiki/Anti-realism, February 15, 2011)

In view of this, realists often claim that antirealists reject the notion of objective truth.

To set the stage for a critique of both naturalism and constructionism, as well as an attempt to delineate a third way, it is important to see exactly how naturalism and constructionism on one hand, and, on the other hand, the encounter with racism and sexism play out in contemporary research in the mental health disciplines. An analysis of two recent articles in which all of these factors are in play will facilitate this process.

NATURALISM

The article to be discussed here is "Beyond Inclusion, Beyond Difference: The Biopolitics of Health" by Steven Epstein (2010). Epstein begins with a description of the reform movement that arose "in the early to mid-1980s in the United States" when "an eclectic group began to demand new ways of attending to identity and difference in the domain of biomedical research." Epstein points out that Bernadine Healy, first female director of the National Institutes of Health in the US, wrote in 2003 that "the orthodoxy of sameness ... often impairs our attitude toward clinical research ... we tended to want to reduce the human to ... [the] white male ... and make that the normative standard ..." According to Epstein, "Reformers opposed this false universalism and argued for the inclusion of more women, people of color, children, and the elderly as research subjects ..." (p. 64). He then brings home his point: "The presumption—one which merits scrutiny—was that the relevant categories of identity politics were also the relevant categories of medical differentiation. On the basis of this presumption, reformers called for the measurement of medical differences by categorical identity." (p. 65). Epstein refers to this view as the "inclusion-and-difference paradigm" owing to the dual mandate to include underrepresented groups in medical research, e.g., women and racial and ethnic minorities, and, at the same time, to acknowledge difference by refusing to assume that findings from any one group can be extrapolated to others, and to do this through "the measurement of medical differences by categorical identity." By "categorical identity" Epstein means category of social group identity.

However progressive its intention, Epstein shows that and how the inclusion-and-difference model led, not only to racial profiling, but to gender profiling as well. Indeed, as we shall see, Epstein's findings, as well as the limitations of his perspective as a means of comprehending the results, point toward the necessity for a more philosophically engaged analysis than his, especially in regard to the issue of the nature and role of universals. As noted earlier, Epstein characterized what Healey referred to as "the orthodoxy of sameness," i.e., the use of the white male as the one-size-fits-all standard, as a "false universalism" (p. 64) and thus implied that there is or may be a universalism that is not false. Epstein, however, elides this issue entirely. Yet, it is a pivotal philosophical issue in race and gender studies: Are there human universals that are nevertheless not exclusionary, and, if not, in what other way can relativism be transcended? This question will be discussed in the context of the problem of relativism.

Pursuing his critique of the "advocates of the inclusion-and-difference paradigm," Epstein points out that they:

> repudiated ... the notion that humanity could be standardized at the level of the species ... But, at the same time, these skeptics of universalism did not ... [embrace] ... total particularity.... Though they ... invoked the rhetoric of 'individualized therapy' ... advocates proposed that the working units of biomedical knowledge making could be *social groups*: women, children, the elderly, Asian Americans, and so on. The inclusion-and-difference paradigm therefore enshrines ... *niche standardization*: a general way of transforming human populations into standardized objects available for scientific scrutiny, political administration, marketing, or other purposes that rejects both universalism and individualism and instead standardizes at the level of the categorical social group—one standard for men, another for women; one standard for blacks, another for whites; ... and so on. (Epstein 2010, p. 70; Epstein's emphases)

Thus, the inclusion-and-difference paradigm, astutely characterized by Epstein as rejecting "both universalism and individualism" (though, as noted, he does not in his article discuss universals as such,) has the striking consequence of actually "flattening" differences, i.e., creating "a sort of generalized difference." If difference is not associated with individuals, or with some notion of human universality, or with some mediation of these, with what other than a "generalized difference" can it be associated? Epstein explains this through a discussion of the "relation between race and sex in debates about biology and health." He points out that "race differences and sex differences are different differences, and cannot be conflated" (p. 73), as, he avers, they are so conflated in a generalized difference model that is based on categorical social groups.

Epstein notes that "even while asserting the incommensurability of differences," for example, the differences attributed to race and those attributed to sex, or some differences between males and females, "we should also pay careful attention to the broadly *similar* processes by which scientific and political actors seek to naturalize differences *of whatever sort* and to ground them in human biology" (Epstein's italics) (p. 74). Here Epstein links naturalism with the grounding of difference in biology, though he does not equate them. Naturalism, he seems to think, consists in reifying biologized categories. Such reification occurs, for example, when all differences are automatically attributed to biological or genetic differences, while at the same time ruling out other sources of difference or challenges to the biological grounding of differences. The example Epstein gives is this: it is assumed that women have smaller rib cages then men and that this difference is genetically marked; however, this phenomenon ought not to be attributed to a genetic difference inasmuch as rib cage size fluctuates statistically, i.e., some women have larger rib cages than many men. Just so, many of the differences between African Americans and Caucasian Americans ought not to be attributed to genetics in that they, too, fluctuate statistically.

On this account, if all differences, including those that fluctuate statistically as well as behavioral differences, are held to be biologically based, then the types of differences attributed to race and those attributed to gender, which, since they vary independently of one another, are incommensurable, are rendered the same: they are all held to be biological phenomena. Such biologization of all differences lends itself to reification to accommodate politicized categories. The inclusion-and-difference model has this result in that it accommodates both biology and politics and is then hospitable to the naturalization, the reification, of these categories of standardized social objects inasmuch as differences among and within them are flattened. This leads further to decisions and actions based on differences that have been thus naturalistically insulated from any sort of cross-checking or revision. As objectified, or reified, then, "standard social objects" are treated as realities.

Epstein goes on to cite many studies and interpretations of data to show that there are very real and very pronounced biomedical differences between men and women. Is Epstein, in citing these studies, proffering the view that we need to accept that there are categorical differences reflecting the identity politics movement as it has been incarnated in policy and science? No, he is not proffering this view precisely because it developed under the influence of naturalizing tendencies endemic to the science/politics interface which in turn led to the flattening of differences. What Epstein does show is that, while the categorical model has allowed for an attack on the profiling of black people by arguing that many allegedly biological differences with non-black people are statistical fluctuations and not genetic variables, the same has not occurred for women. It is assumed that all differences between men and women are biologically constituted and thus, when these differences are taken into consideration, there is no question of profiling of women. That is, women cannot be profiled, this view assumes, because they really are genetically different from men. Epstein's point is, however, that when naturalistically biologized gender differences are then insulated from any possible revision. He asks, "To what extent, if any, is the case of biological differences by sex or gender analogous to that of biological differences by race and ethnicity? What does it mean that racial profiling in medicine has become an intellectual battleground, while sex profiling has not?" (p. 77). Further, he writes that "It appears that many critics of racial profiling in medicine have engaged in boundary work, erecting a wall between sex and race to designate the study of sex differences as good science and the study of race differences as bad science" (p. 77). Epstein then points out that while some genetic, sex-linked traits may, and probably do, demarcate women and men, in fact "most of the claims about sex differences are ... statements about differences between averages," as he indicated in the example of rib cage size noted earlier. Epstein's fundamental critique of the inclusion-and-difference model is then that naturalizing difference does not mean just that there are categorical, biologically based differences among groups; additionally, naturalization means that these categories are taken to be all-encompassing, leaving no possibility of showing that certain traits that are different in men and women are in fact not a consequence of biology but rather of social and cultural forces impinging on men and women. Thus, naturalization is not just saying that, yes, biology is determinative for categories of people, e.g., men and women. Rather, the problem is that when gender differences are naturalized or reified, researchers become ideologically motivated to exclude certain possibilities that ought not to be excluded. It is for this reason that feminists, for example, have condemned biological explanations of behavior as "essentialist," which means that the biological factor is seen to be functioning as a master controlling essence.

It should be clear at this point that Epstein is descrying the failure of science and society to protect individuals from the naturalizing processes in play in scientific and political models. He writes that, "In both cases [race and gender], an over eagerness to assume and naturalize difference may ... get in the way of addressing the serious racial and gender disparities in health outcomes." We should ask: "What happens to our ability to address social inequalities when we assume that differential health outcomes are simply a consequence of biological differences between groups?" (p. 80). This trenchant question is one that the mental health disciplines must ask.

Clearly then, Epstein is a critic of naturalization in biomedical science. He points out the collusion of science and politics in the form of the assumption that biomedical categories are the same as political categories or identifiers and vice versa. Though he does not discuss this explicitly, his critical framework, like that of many others in this field, has been influenced by Foucault's work on biopolitical power. The term biopolitics is one of the chief markers of reference to the work of Foucault.[10] However, Epstein does not proffer an alternative to naturalism. He sees it as harmful to both society and individuals, but he has no explicit discussion of an alternative philosophical framework for psychiatry and biomedical research. Thus, while Epstein's analysis of the serious deficiencies of the inclusion-and-difference model is important, his article lacks critical and philosophical acuity in that, even after invoking universals, it fails to explain their potential to counteract the tendency toward naturalizing difference.

SOCIAL CONSTRUCTIONISM

The article to be examined here is Mallon's "A Field Guide to Social Construction" (2007). He begins his article by pointing out that:

> An enormous amount of work in the humanities and social sciences is organized around the idea that phenomena are "socially constructed." Things as diverse as quarks and wife abuse are said to be socially constructed, and constructionist positions figure prominently in discussions

[10] Epstein references Michel Foucault (1979, 1980). The influence of Foucault's work on all of the social and behavioral sciences, as well as the humanities, is incalculable.

of race, gender, sexual orientation, emotions, and mental illness.... Many academics associate
"social constructionism" with the so-called "science wars" in which social constructionism
is identified with some sort of radical anti-realism about reality ... If this were all there is to
constructionism, then this enormous body of work might have little to offer the philosophical
naturalist that looks to science as a central ... way of knowing the world. But the move to
radical anti-realism is only one way to develop the central idea of constructionism ... and
much of this work remains interesting and provocative within a broadly naturalist and realist
framework. (Mallon 2007, p. 93)

What then is the distinction that Mallon is making between antirealism and radical antirealism? He avers that social constructionism is a form of antirealism, but need not be a
form of radical antirealism, as it need not be constituted as the belief that there is nothing
at all that exists as ontologically independent of our conceptual schemas, that is, that reality is socially constructed. The non-radically antirealist constructionist then could accept
that certain things relevant to human beings might or do exist as ontologically independent of our conceptual schemas, e.g., that biological entities are not socially constructed. His
point is that social constructionism can be compatible with realism. What is most interesting here is the way in which he explicates his stance, i.e., his belief that "a broadly naturalist
and realist framework" is compatible with constructionism in the context of mental health,
race, and gender. To see this, it is first necessary to examine additional distinctions made by
Mallon.

He differentiates types of social constructionism using Hacking's distinction between
the construction of "ideas" and "objects" (Hacking, 1999, 21ff.; Mallon 2007, p. 95), or, in
Mallon's terms, social construction of theories and social construction of "human kinds."
He further differentiates the latter into construction by individuation, by social dependence, and by social role (Mallon 2007, p. 97). Mallon's views, expressed particularly in his
discussion of social role constructionism, psychology, and race and gender are germane
to the issues under discussion here. Those who maintain that theories are socially constructed, "typically defend particular views of what (rather than facts or data) determines
the content of accepted theories." Mallon, however, stresses the social construction of
human kinds:

If the social construction of theories is primarily identified with the 'science wars, claims about
the social construction of human kinds are primarily identified with what we might call the
"human nature wars ... " Cast in Manichean terms, on one side of the dispute are defenders
of human nature who insist on a central role for innate human biology and psychology in
explaining human traits, including dispositions and behaviors. And on the other side are
human kind constructionists who argue that culture and human decision fundamentally
shape the human kinds to which we belong. These global positions are powerful in that they
guide research programs in more specific domains, domains like morality, the emotions,
sexual difference, racial classification, and so forth. (Mallon 2007, p. 97)

It is, however, in his discussion of social role constructionism that Mallon attempts to
bolster his view that constructionism and naturalism are compatible. He begins by citing
a study that "explains differences in the professional achievement of men and women by
offering a host of evidence suggesting that cognitive schemas for gender categories systematically alter the social situations of men and women, biasing our interpretations of
their performances in ways that subtly but systematically disadvantage women over time"

(p. 102). Mallon then discusses an example of a constructionist account of how social role models operate:

> And in the philosophy of psychology and psychiatry, social role accounts of emotions ... or social role explanations of multiple personality disorder ... have been offered. In each case the central idea is that the theory of a kind of person structures the situation or developmental environment of a person in ways that offer alternate explanations of the person's features.... At the extreme, social role models suggest that culture acts as a kind of script that tightly controls behavior and that can be altered as a way of transforming behavior. For example, Hacking documents the ways in which changes in the widely held conception of multiple personality disorder throughout the 1980's resulted in behavioral changes among diagnosed multiples— result in, for example, the proliferation of more and more "personalities" within each patient. (Mallon 2007, p. 102)

It is at this point that Mallon clarifies his ideas through discussion of race in order to show the relevance of both naturalism and non-radically antirealist constructionism.

He writes that:

> recent work on racial categorization in cognitive and evolutionary psychology has, like constructionism about racial theories, begun with the falsity of biological theories of race. But in contrast to constructionists' emphasis on cultural determinants of folk racial theories, these psychologists posit a role for innate psychological propensities to categorize persons in particular ways ... Such accounts might hold that psychological predispositions contribute to the formation of racial social roles that have played an important role in racial oppression .... If we follow Valian in allowing that the world we face offers systematically different circumstances to males and females due to the gendered cognitive schemas that we all use to understand and interact with the world, we have all the resources we need to offer a constructionist explanation of many explananda whether or not we think biology produces gender differences more generally. To pursue the constructionist explanation we need only deny that biological sex offers a complete explanation of some particular explananda. We need not insist that there is no effect of biological sex whatsoever. (Mallon 2007, p. 103)

Thus, Mallon points out that if the research on cognitive schemata is accurate, then a naturalistic account of race is quite compatible with a constructionist account. He views cognitive schemata as material entities, most likely as some sort of brain wiring, as a material aspect of the person. So, while agreeing that race is not at all a biological phenomenon as such, a theory which posits the existence of human kinds known as races is a consequence, for Mallon, at least in part, of a psychological predisposition to categorize people in certain ways. This psychological predisposition, then contributes to the formation of racial social roles that have played an important role in racial oppression. Mallon implies that the disposition to form the cognitive category of racial social roles in some important way is innate in human beings and that it contributes significantly to the occurrence of antiblack racism.

Noteworthy here is Mallon's concurrence with virtually all theoretical work being done today in psychiatry, natural science, social science, and the humanities that the meaning of innateness means innate in human beings in the sense that it is a biological substrate within us. This notion of innateness, though it has been prevalent for at least several decades, is the antithesis of the notion of innateness that runs through the entire history of philosophy until contemporary thought, particularly postmodernism, emerged. A good touchstone for this discussion is Descartes. A philosopher in the rationalist tradition inaugurated by

Socrates/Plato, Descartes posited innate ideas within us in that we are res cogitans, thinking things, in radical contrast with res extensa, extended things. So, for him, as in the tradition, innateness vis-à-vis human beings meant precisely non-material, i.e., not extended (in space) "things" or "substances." Today, innateness has come to mean the opposite of this, to wit, a biological, material element or substrate within us that is determinative of our minds and behavior. Thus, when Mallon speaks of innateness, as, for example, predispositions to categorize people, he is taking a realist stance: these innate things, he implies, exist in a manner ontologically independent of culture, language, and so on, i.e., they are extended substances or things.

Mallon's argument regarding race then seems to be that this innate psychological predisposition is one of the materially determined and determinate factors that is important in the formation of race prejudice and oppression, and these are factors that constructionism that is not radically antirealist can enlighten us about. Thus, each perspective, naturalist and constructionist, contributes to our understanding of racism.

The notion of a predisposition in the human mind to categorize people into different types has a high degree of plausibility. Many questions however can be raised about this formulation. For example: How do we come by this predisposition? Is it known how psychic or mental predispositions, including one as fundamental as the categorization of kinds in the world, are formed? The field of evolutionary biology is in great flux regarding this and other questions relevant to human development (Keller 2010). Thus, to state that such psychological predispositions satisfy the naturalist's realist requirement that they exist ontologically independently of culture, history, language, and so on is not prima facie demonstrable. Since Mallon's argument here is a realist one, a Kantian argument such that categorization is an a priori condition for the possibility of thought is not relevant, nor is physicalist reduction of mind to brain compatible with a Kantian perspective. Nevertheless, whether or not it is demonstrable and therefore correct, is Mallon on the mark to claim that this predisposition somehow figures importantly in the development of racism and oppression? And, if not, what could motivate such a view?

The question is, why are people categorized into groups, for example, racial and gender groups that are oppressed or disparaged? In the first place, isn't it at least as plausible to aver that there exists a predisposition to categorize all of the things in the world into groups? Why single out the categorization of human beings? Isn't the categorization of human beings into natural kinds,[11] i.e., human kinds, just a subset of categorization of things in general? Moreover, certainly the categorization of human beings is morally unexceptionable—it is not as such discriminatory or oppressive to so categorize people. Rather, racism and oppression arise when differences are marked as inferiority. Thus, since Mallon begins by rejecting the view that race as such is a genetic variable, it is difficult to understand what he thinks is the contribution to racism and oppression of the innate (biological) predisposition to categorize people. Its bare existence may be necessary, but certainly is not sufficient; but then, the bare existence of life is necessary, but not sufficient, to be a human being. Thus, Mallon's claim that biologically construed cognitive predispositions are materially important for the formation of racism is trivial, not merely because it is one of a multitude of biological factors; it is trivial in addition because it is construed by Mallon as in isolation from all other

---

[11] "A believer in natural kinds holds that nature is itself divided into different kinds and species, and that our predicates and classifications must coincide with these divisions." (Blackburn 2008, p. 245).

factors in the genesis of racism and oppression, e.g., historical, cultural, political, economic, and social factors. There is evidence as well that cognitive functions and brain states and functioning, can be formed and influenced by all of these factors (Keller 2010). Most importantly, racism and sexism are a matter of a failure of human responsibility and justice.

The distinction that Mallon attempts to establish between antirealism and what he terms radical antirealism is correlative to another distinction often made in discussions of social constructionism, and that is a distinction between relativism and radical relativism. Mallon claims that what he calls radical antirealism is, as noted earlier, the social constructionist view that there is nothing at all that exists as ontologically independent of our conceptual schemas, that is, that reality is socially constructed. The notion that reality is entirely socially constructed is equivalent to the notion that reality is entirely relative to our beliefs about it, a form of relativism. As will be discussed in the next section, the problem of relativism is profoundly relevant to understanding how it is that racism and sexism have not yet been eliminated from theory construction in psychiatry.

Relativism

Relativism, then, is an issue that bears directly on the ways in which race and gender are intertwined in theory in the social sciences, mental health disciplines, and the humanities as well, including critical race and gender studies. Indeed, the question of relativism is crucially determinative regarding whether or not racism and sexism can be grasped for what they are, i.e., unjust stigmatizations of groups of people as inferior, and whether or not these distortions can be purged from theory. Moreover, the most frequently mounted charge against social constructionism (or constructivism) is that of relativism, a charge which, if correct, would vitiate all claims. In order to proceed, it is necessary first to stipulate how the term "relativism" and associated terms are conceptualized and used in this chapter.

The term "relativism" in this chapter denotes the notion that everything is relative to something else. There is, across a wide field of disciplines, a large consensus that, since it posits a principle that is itself excluded from the universal relativism (everything is relative except the principle of relativism itself), this notion of relativism is self-refuting and therefore fails on logical grounds. For this reason, and to their credit, researchers and writers in psychiatry and the social sciences are at great pains to show that their work is not relativistic in the given sense of relativism. Most importantly, however, this notion of relativism will, in this chapter, be differentiated from and counterposed to another notion, that of what is termed here "*relativity-to*" (with the linking hyphen). In this chapter, "relativity-to" means that something, "a," is relative to something else, "b," that is not itself relative, i.e., something that is in some sense held to be non-relative or "absolute," e.g., a transhistorical universal, or an essence. While the distinction made here between relativism and relativity-to can be found in the vast literature on relativism, often both terms are discussed under the rubric of "relativism" as if they are two different kinds of relativism. From the point of view of this chapter, relativity-to is held to be, *in some sense non-relative*. Indeed, if one accepts that relativism as such is an incoherent notion, it is difficult to see any stance other than "relativity-to" that could be a viable alternative perspective. This problematic will be explored and illustrated next.

Regarding psychiatry in general and psychoanalysis in particular, relativism is often construed as having two modes: (1) so-called radical relativism, also construed as "anything-goes" relativism, which corresponds to the notion of relativism explained above (and to Mallon's category of "radical antirealism"); and (2) a form of relativism that is allegedly not "radical" and is held to be logically tenable and a viable stance within the social-constructionism paradigm (and, in Mallon's view, a form of antirealism that is nevertheless compatible with biological realism). The aim here is to show that what is construed as "radical relativism" is, logically, that is philosophically, the only mode of relativism as such, and to show further that what is construed as non-radical relativism is either relativism as such, or an entirely different state of affairs, namely relativity-to which, it is averred here, is no form of relativism at all. I will maintain, moreover, that the confusion or conflation of relativity-to with relativism has obfuscated theory in the mental health disciplines.

In order to show the importance of this problematic, let us just initially lay out some plausible implications of the distinction between relativism and relativity-to in the context of racism and sexism. Racists and sexists might argue that, since everything is relative and therefore no stance can be privileged over any other stance, their view, i.e., that black people and women as groups and as individuals in those groups are inferior to white people in general and white males in particular is just as valid as any other view, even its opposite. However, often those who hold such relativistic views do not admit to doing so and may or may not be aware of the self-contradictory aspect of such relativism. Indeed, bigots often claim that their views are in fact true and can be justified. More often that not, however, the evidence cited and the arguments made can be shown to be illogical and counterfactual. Nevertheless, even in the face of such refutation, the bigots cling to their views. Thus, they are revealed to be "closet" relativists who believe that they are right just because this is what they believe, i.e., that their views are valid just because they are their views.[12] Given this scenario, we can see how crucially important it is, in the struggle against racism and sexism, that theory, which impacts on practice, be clear on just what does and doesn't constitute self-refuting relativism, and what a viable alternative to it might be.

Additionally, we will see in this chapter that the failure clearly to differentiate relativism from relativity-to has had the unfortunate effect of enabling contemporary thought to move from the notion, or meaning, of essences as universals or transhistorical phenomena not reducible to any material substrate, to the notion of essences as biological givens. This move has in particular crippled thought by prohibiting reflection on the possibility of human universals, or essences, that are not genetic variables, biological entities, or any type of material entity, but nevertheless could provide the basis, as we shall see, for a decisive theoretical repudiation of racism and sexism.

The problem of relativism has intensely preoccupied psychoanalytic theory throughout its history, and especially in the last 20 years, or so. This problem is endemic to any field of study that is inhabited by constructionist theories, for example, literary theory, all of the

---

[12]   A good example or model of this type of bigot is Creon, the King of Thebes, in Sophocles' renowned play, *Antigone*. Creon's dialogues with all of the other characters in the play show him to harbor an extreme form of sexism expressed quite overtly. Yet his rationale for all of his views is identical to that of Thrasymachus in Book I of Plato's *Republic*, namely that might makes right. If this is so, then all views are relative to the will of the most powerful. If might makes right, then right does not make right, and "right" then has no rational grounding and is entirely relative in the sense of relativism.

social sciences, and critical race theory and gender theory, and so on. However, it has been a most vexing problem for psychoanalysis in particular in that psychoanalysis is both theory and practice. If theories are shown to be relativistic in the sense of relativism, how can they be applied to or reflected in practice? How can we determine, for example, what aspect or aspects of psychoanalysis, or any other treatment modality, are mutative in the sense of contributing to or facilitating patients' improvement? An important and often cited dialogue on social constructionism and relativism is Eric Gillett's (1998) "Relativism and the Social-Constructivist Paradigm." Gillett's article is followed by two critical commentaries and a response from Gillett.[13]

Gillett singles out for criticism psychoanalytic theorists who avow some version of constructionism and deny that they are anything-goes relativists. Gillett's primary critical foil is the well-known psychoanalytical theorist Irwin Hoffman, author of *Ritual and Spontaneity in Psychoanalysis* (published in 1998, the same year as Gillett's article and not referenced by Gillett) and several extremely influential papers. Gillett argues that Hoffman makes contradictory claims: on one hand, he espouses what Gillett refers to as non-controversial constructionist relativism or NCR, i.e., a form of relativism that is not anything-goes, but on the other hand his views reflect CCR or controversial constructionist relativism—or anything-goes relativism. CCR is anything-goes relativism; NCR, which Gillett endorses, is a form of relativism that is not "radical" and is therefore acceptable relativism (for Mallon, a form of antirealism compatible with biologism). Gillett explains the meaning of both non-controversial constructivism and controversial constructivism in this way:

> It is non controversial that beliefs influence reality via their effects on a person's actions. Controversial constructivism, however, asserts that beliefs have a direct influence on their referents and, in fact, "construct" these referents. Mount Everest exists because people believe it exists. (Gillett 1998, p. 39)

As this statement clearly implies, Gillett maintains that CCR is an antirealist position, whereas, by implication, NCR is compatible with realism. I will show that what Gillett refers to as non-controversial relativism or NCR is an incoherent notion, and is so because Gillett fails to draw the necessary distinction between relativism and relativity-to.

Gillett focuses his discussion of Hoffman on the latter's analysis of how the theory of transference in psychoanalysis has evolved from a positivist to a post-positivist, constructivist (constructionist) one. Since the transference, the unconscious aspect of the patient's relation with the analyst, is, to this day, one of the defining postulates of psychoanalysis, how it is understood is a matter of great significance. Hoffman discusses contemporary critiques of Freud's "blank screen" notion of the stance of the psychoanalyst vis-à-vis with the patient. According to this blank screen notion as viewed in classical psychoanalysis, the analyst gives no hint or clue to the patient regarding her, the analyst's, inner life, thoughts, and feelings. She is a screen on which the patient projects his, the patient's, fantasies. Hoffman maintains that there are "conservative" and "radical" critiques of this classical blank screen notion of transference. Gillett explains Hoffman's distinction in this way: "Conservative critics

---

[13] In fairness to Gillett, it should be noted that in order to focus on my critique of his views, and given space limitations, I have not included some of his arguments and formulations. Gillett's article is extremely well written and well conceived and readers interested in these issues should read his entire article, the responses to it, and his response to his critics.

[of the blank screen notion of transference] give more careful attention [than classical ana-lysts do] to realistic aspects of the patient's experience [of the analyst], but retain the concept of 'transference distortion'" (Gillett 1998, p. 42). For Hoffman, Gillett points out, "conserva-tive critics of the blank screen fallacy always end up perpetuating that very fallacy" (quoted by Gillett, p. 42). To explain the radical critiques of Freud favored by Hoffman, Gillett quotes Hoffman: "The radical critic of the blank screen model denies that there is any aspect of the patient's experience that pertains to the therapist's inner motives that can be unequivo-cally designated as distorting of reality" (quoted by Gillett, p. 42). Hoffman adds that noth-ing in the patient's experience can be designated as faithful to reality either, and continues: "The radical critic is a relativist ... [T]he perspective that the patient brings to bear ... is one among many ... each of which highlights different facets of the analyst's involvement. This amounts to a different paradigm ...." (quoted by Gillett, p. 42, my ellipses). Hoffman calls this new paradigm for psychoanalysis "social constructivist" (quoted by Gillett, p. 42), but denies that it is a form of anything-goes or radical relativism, despite the fact that it implies that no aspect of the patient's experience of the analyst is privileged or more, or less, attuned to reality than any other aspect. Gillett points out that, in his writings Hoffmann has passages, like these reflecting Hoffman's view of the transference, that, Gillett maintains, endorse anything-goes relativism, which Gillett calls CCR or controversial constructivist relativism, as well as some passages that seemingly reject CCR and instead endorse NCR or non-controversial relativism. So, one of Gillett's critiques of Hoffman is that the latter confuses or conflates CCR and NCR (p. 47). The point of my critique of both Gillett and Hoffman is that, as I shall show, the tendency to conflate the two perspectives is a function of the circumstance that there are not two such perspectives as Gillett avers, but only one; Hoffman, on the other hand, denies that he is proposing CCR, and does not see that he is proposing CCR because, like Gillett, he does not see that one is either a radical relativist or no relativist at all.

This can be shown through an analysis of Gillett's explanation of NCR and his repeated statements that everyone believes in NCR and that no one would reject it. Here is Gillett's explanation of NCR which purportedly can be clearly differentiated from CCR:

> The central thesis of this paper is that most versions of ... constructivism fall into two categories which I call "non controversial" versus "controversial." The former holds that beliefs about reality are constructed by the mind and are relative to various frameworks: history, culture, and individual circumstances. Controversial relativism holds, by contrast, that truth itself is constructed by the mind and is relative to various frameworks, including those Kuhn (1970) calls "paradigms." (Gillett 1998, p. 37)

Thus, Gillett maintains that Hoffman implies strongly that "truth" is created in the analytic setting, since there is no way to determine which of the many "aspects" of the relation-ship reflects the reality of that relationship. But, what exactly does Gillett mean when he states that NCR, the correct perspective, means that "beliefs about reality ... are relative to ... history, culture and individual circumstances"? Are history, culture, and individual circumstances, to which our beliefs about reality are held to be relative, then understood by Gillett to be, or to have elements that are not themselves relative to anything at all? Gillett does not assert this. Since Gillett believes that there is a relation between our beliefs about reality and the truth of what reality is, then he needs to clarify his conception of the relativity of beliefs to, e.g., culture. For, unless the phenomena to which our beliefs are said to be relative, e.g., culture, are in some sense non-relative, non-controversial construction-ist relativism is just as relativistic as controversial constructionist relativism. The reason for this is that if culture is construed, as it generally is, to be a phenomenon of meaning, and if one construes meaning itself as entirely relative with no relation to any universality, then all meanings are relative to all other meanings and there are no non-relative meanings. The upshot of this is that truth claims or beliefs about reality could not be justified because all other truth claims, including contradictory ones, would be posited as equally justifiable. On what basis would one decide which claims to test or otherwise attempt to justify? And, on what basis could one maintain that there is a non-trivial relation between beliefs about reality and what reality is?

Cultural constructionists, the anthropologist Ruth Benedict, for example, one of the orig-inal architects of cultural relativism, maintained, in her famous book *Patterns of Culture* (1959), that there is nothing non-relative in human culture, including its ethical dimension, and that cultural forms are all just accommodations to biological needs in a given material environment. The example of Benedict's advocacy of both cultural and ethical relativism, on one hand, and biologism on the other hand, shows that in fact relativism and biologism, that is, relativism and ontological realism, are not at all incompatible. If Gillett does think that there is something non-relative in human culture, or history, or individual circumstances, to which our beliefs are said by him to be relative, he never indicates that he thinks so or offers any recognition that this is a problem or a question. It is for this reason, I believe, that Lou Fourcher, one of the commentators on Gillett's paper, wrote that:

> In the following remarks on Dr. Gillett's stimulating paper, I will contend that his disagreement with Hoffman and constructivism is better understood as a vehicle for promoting physicalist realism in psychology and psychoanalysis based on the idea that science has an exclusive access to truth. (Fourcher 1998, p. 49)

This is indeed the strong impression conveyed by Gillett's views in his paper and his cri-tique of Hoffman.

Gillett's goal was to show that there is a form of relativism that is not anything-goes relativism. I have maintained that he failed in this endeavor, nor did he express the view that there is an element in all of the historical and cultural factors that he admits influence beliefs that is not relative—i.e., that is grounded in something alleged to be transhistori-cal, essential, or universal. I contend that the only logically sound way to constitute a non relativist, i.e., non-anything-goes perspective, is to show that beliefs are relative-to social, cultural, linguistic, or historical phenomena, i.e., relative in the sense that some dimensions or moments of these phenomena are universals, i.e., certain values, and thus are not them-selves relative to anything at all. This conforms to the notion of universality that is embed-ded in the history of philosophy: universals are non-relative factors in human existence that are not reducible to a mind independent materiality—e.g., not "essences" in the contempo-rary sense of "essentialism"—biological or physical entities. Gillett points out that science is the quest for truth based on belief in its attainability. For Gillett, this notion of truth entails a knowable, mind-independent "reality"; this is the stance of physicalist reductionism. However, "truth" need not entail this. For the phenomenologist, as will be elaborated later, universals (in Husserl's terms, eide or essences) exist, not as material entities but rather as intentional objects of consciousness[14] and they are subject to evidential criteria of truth and falsity (Hopkins 2010, p. 7). If universals do not exist in this sense, then either radical relativism, i.e., relativism as such, or biological, physicalist reductionism, or both, hold sway; yet, the former is not an option because it is self-refuting, and biological reductionism entails realism, an ontological stance that is not demonstrable and is not incompatible with radical relativism, as seen for example in the work of Benedict and many other social scientists and psychologists, for example, the psychiatrist and philosopher Edwin R. Wallace (1985).[15] Husserlian phenomenology, to be elaborated in the "Phenomenology" section, begins with the insight that neither ontological realism nor ontological antirealism is demonstrable. This is so because we can only know what exists in virtue of our minds, our consciousness, and therefore in principle we cannot know whether or not anything exists independent of our minds.

The point is, then, that in order to transcend the tendency to fall into anything-goes relativism and, at the same time, to credibly reject biological reductionism, or naturalism, one must constitute an epistemological stance that will obviate this Scylla and Charybdis by showing that there are universals embedded, or, in Husserl's terms, sedimented, in human existence that are neither biologistic essences (essentialism) nor relativistically meaningless. As we shall see, Husserlian phenomenology is just such an epistemological stance.[16] I maintain as well that obviating this Scylla and Charybdis dilemma is the way that very well might preclude racism, sexism, and other prejudices from deforming theory and practice in psychiatry.

Phenomenology[17]

The purpose of this section is to propose an alternate philosophical stance that would transcend the false dichotomy of relativism or reductionism, which as I have attempted to show,

[14] The phenomenological notion of the intentionality of consciousness means as follows: Since there is no consciousness without an object, consciousness is "consciousness-of" either an "outer" or physical object, or an "inner" object, e.g., a concept. Thus, consciousness "intends" its objects, that is, it constitutes them as they give themselves to consciousness. "Constitutes" does not mean that consciousness creates its objects ab nova; it means rather that objects can be grasped and explicated through explication of the sedimentation of sense that is embedded in their givenness to consciousness just as they are.

[15] An analysis of Wallace's views in the context of the issue sexism in psychiatry can be found in Nissim-Sabat (2009).

[16] In this I follow Soffer (1991), who wrote that "Phenomenology itself cannot be employed to derive a totalizing relativism, a relativism which everywhere forsakes or denies the universal. Rather, the relativist denial of all universals is only the reverse side of the dogmatic, *un*philosophical absolutism characteristic of objectivism" (p. 203). Clearly, Soffer here is implying the notion of "relativity-to" that I introduced earlier to denote a "relativism" (*sic!*) that nowhere "forsakes or denies" the universal.

[17] The evaluation of the Husserlian challenge to relativism in this chapter is in broad agreement with the evaluation in Gail Soffer's (1991) magisterial treatment in her *Husserl and the Question of Relativism*. Our views, both Soffer's and my own, are encompassed within the phenomenological tradition usually described as a philosophical stance within Continental Philosophy. However, chapter 1 of Soffer's book (pp. 1–27) takes up the challenge to phenomenology of many major philosophers of the Anglo-American or Analytic tradition in philosophy, including Putnam, Goodman, McCallagh, Okrent, Barnes and Bloor, and others. Elsewhere in the book, Soffer also discusses Wittgenstein's notion of "family resemblances."

does not offer a theoretical stance that poses a challenge to the racism and sexism that continue to be accommodated in psychiatry. The material is not intended to be viewed as more than an outline that hopefully will lead readers to become more interested in Husserlian phenomenology as a potential theoretical framework for psychiatry.

The phenomenological method, as propounded by Edmund Husserl, is initiated by performance of a new attitude such that all ontological commitments are suspended. This act is motivated by awareness that the ultimate ontology of the world is in principle unknowable.[18] Like methodological realism, phenomenology establishes the scientificity of the disciplines by showing that their findings are grounded in evidence. However, since methodological realism does not begin with an act of suspending ontological commitments, it leaves the door open to such commitments. For this reason, the evidence cited by methodological realism is compromised by its openness to one or another ontological stance. On the other hand, given that phenomenological evidence, unlike that correlated with methodological realism, is methodologically and in principle shorn of presupposed ontological commitments, it is evidential in a completely new way. The method of phenomenology enables investigation of the world as phenomenon, just as it gives itself to consciousness, to the mind.

In his last work, *The Crisis of European Sciences and Transcendental Phenomenology* (1970), Husserl directly engaged the distinction between relativism and relativity-to, as well as the compatibility of relativism and naturalistic reductionism. In the *Crisis*, Husserl wrote, regarding "the one world that is common to all," that

> precisely this world and everything that happens in it, used as needed for scientific and other ends, bears, on the other hand, for every natural scientist in his thematic orientation toward its "objective truth," the stamp "merely subjective and relative." .... This "subjective-relative" is supposed to be overcome; one can and should correlate it with a hypothetical being-in-itself, a substrate for logical-mathematical "truths-in-themselves" that one can approximate. (Husserl 1970, p. 126)

And so, that which Gillett refers to as anything-goes relativism, or controversial constructivism that implies that reality is or can be subjectively created, is designated by Husserl as "the subjective-relative," as that which as such, for the natural scientist, has no truth value and therefore must be "overcome" by research that presupposes an underlying "being-in-itself," i.e., ontological realism. Thus, owing to a prior commitment to naturalistic reduction, naturalistic science views all that is actually experienced in consciousness as *merely* subjective-relative, that is, as subjectivistic, as lacking objectivity or any relation to the scientist's quest for knowledge of an objective reality.

Husserl refers to the immediate givenness of the experienced world as the "life-world," the one world in which we always already do and must find ourselves, scientists and non-scientists alike, that is the source of all phenomenological evidence. Writing about the motive of phenomenology itself to seek "truth-in-itself," Husserl wrote that,

> When we set up this objectivity as a goal ... we make a set of hypotheses through which the pure life-world is surpassed. We have precluded this "surpassing" through the first epoche [suspension] (that which concerns the objective sciences), and now we have the

---

[18] Heidegger and his followers have severely criticized and rejected Husserl's notion that phenomenology must begin with the phenomenological reduction. This critique is discussed at length in Heidegger (1975).

embarrassment of wondering what else can be undertaken scientifically, as something that can be established once and for all and for everyone. But this sort of embarrassment disappears as soon as we consider that the life-world does have, in all its relative features, a general structure. This general structure, to which everything that exists relatively is bound, is not itself relative. (Husserl 1970, p. 139)

Here, Husserl clearly writes that the "relative features" of the life-world are not a "subjective-relative" as they are for the naturalistic scientist, and thus to be dismissed. Rather than this, the "relative features" of the life-world are themselves relative-to something that is not itself relative. Husserl then explains that the non-relative, general structure of the life-world is the correlate of "a universal a priori which is itself prior, precisely as that of the pure life-world. Only through recourse to this a priori to be unfolded in an a priori science of its own, can our a priori science, the objective-logical ones, achieve a truly radical, a seriously scientific, grounding, which, under the circumstance, they absolutely require" (Husserl 1970, p. 141).

For Husserl, then, the problem of relativism exists only in that the reductive natural sciences fail to grasp that their a priori presuppositions are inexplicable unless understood to be grounded in a prior a priori, an a priori of the life-world itself, which all science presupposes. Thus, for Husserl, the subjective-relative emerges only where the apriority of the life-world is hidden, as it was by Galileo, the "discovering and concealing genius" (Husserl 1970, p. 52). For Husserl, Galileo constituted natural science as naturalistic (pp. 23–59). Husserl shows that rather than relativistic, as conferring equal validity on all opinions, the evidence experienced in our encounter with the life world is always relative-to the infinite a priori that is transcendental intersubjectivity.

In this context, Husserl makes remarks that suggest an originating factor that could generate sexism and racism. This factor emerges, as Epstein suggested, when difference is naturalized, when differences are construed as "facts" and thus as fixed objects for judgment. In the *Crisis*, Husserl wrote that, "when we are thrown into an alien social sphere, that of the Negroes in the Congo, Chinese peasants, etc. we discover that their truths, the facts that for them are fixed … are by no means the same as ours. But if we set up the goal of a truth about the objects which is unconditionally valid for all subjects …. we make a set of hypotheses through which the pure life-world is surpassed" (Husserl 1970, p. 139). But for Husserl, this surpassing is not toward a reductive realism but rather toward an a priori of the life-world, of the possibilities to be and become human. Awareness and recognition of such openness to the universal and infinite possibilities to be human would then be an attitude of mind that would preclude judgments of inferiority that are tantamount to denials of the humanity of those so stigmatized. Moreover, the phenomenological meaning of evidence as givenness within an attitude of suspension of all presuppositions would enable critique of evidence alleged to demonstrate the inferiority of certain individuals and groups.

Husserlian phenomenology, then, exposes as no other philosophical perspective has yet achieved, the difference between relativism and relativity-to, the necessity for science to surpass relativism, and the ultimate grounding of science in the relativity of the life-world to the universals that inhere in the a priori of our humanness.

Finally, in the *Crisis*, Husserl elaborated "the way into phenomenology through psychology," (pp. 191–257), and spoke of psychology, including "the recent depth psychology" (p. 237) as "the *truly decisive field*" (p. 208, Husserl's emphasis) of phenomenological research. Thus, ridding psychiatry of racism and sexism is a goal that would be of immense benefit to humanity and would stand as a model for all human endeavors.

References

Benedict, R. (1959). *Patterns of Culture*. Boston, MA: Houghton Mifflin.

Blackburn, S. (2008). *Oxford Dictionary of Philosophy* (2nd edn, rev.). Oxford: Oxford University Press.

Epstein, S. (2010). Beyond inclusion, beyond difference: The biopolitics of health. In I. Whitmarsh and D. S. Jones (Eds), *What's the Use of Race? Modern Governance and the Biology of Difference*, pp. 63–123. Cambridge, MA: MIT Press.

Foucault, M. (1979). *Discipline and Punish: The Birth of the Prison*. New York, NY: Vintage Books.

Foucault, M. (1980). *The History of Sexuality, Volume I* (R. Hurley, Trans.). New York, NY: Vintage Books.

Fourcher, L. (1998). Commentary on "Relativism and the social constructivist paradigm". *Philosophy, Psychology & Psychiatry*, 5(1), 49–51.

Freud, S. (1966). On femininity. In *The Complete Introductory Lectures on Psychoanalysis* (L. Strachey, Trans.), pp. 576–99. New York, NY: Norton.

Gillett, E. (1998). Relativism and the social-constructivist paradigm. *Philosophy, Psychology & Psychiatry*, 5(1), 37–48.

Hacking, I. (1999). *The Social Construction of What?* Cambridge, MA: Harvard University Press.

Heidegger, M. (1975). Introduction. In *Basic Problems in Phenomenology*, pp. 1–23. Bloomington, IN: Indiana University Press.

Hirshbein, L. (2010). Sex and gender in psychiatry: A view from history. *Journal of Medical Humanities*, 32(2), 155–70.

Hoffman, I. Z. (1998). *Ritual and Spontaneity in Psychoanalysis: A Dialectical-Constructivist View*. Hillside, NJ: Analytic Press.

Hopkins, B. C. (2010). *The Philosophy of Husserl*. Montreal: McGill-Queen's University Press.

Husserl, E. (1970). *The Crisis of European Sciences and Transcendental Phenomenology* (D. Carr, Trans.). Evanston, IL: Northwestern University Press.

Keller, E. F. (2010). *The Mirage of a Space Between Nature and Nurture*. Durham, NC: Duke University Press.

Mallon, R. (2007). A field guide to social construction. *Philosophy Compass*, 2(1), 93–108.

Metzl, J. (2009). *The Protest Psychosis: How Schizophrenia Became a Black Disease*. Boston, MA: Beacon Press.

Moncrieff, J. (2008). Neoliberalism and biopsychiatry: A marriage of convenience. In C.I. Cohen and S. Timimi (Eds), *Liberatory Psychiatry: Philosophy, politics, and mental Health*, pp. 234–55. Cambridge: Cambridge University Press.

Nissim-Sabat, M. (2001). Philosophy, psychiatry, and race. *Philosophy, Psychiatry, & Psychology*, 8, 44–59.

Nissim-Sabat, M. (2004). Race and culture. In J. Radden (Ed.), *The Philosophy of Psychiatry: A Companion*, pp. 244–57. Oxford: Oxford University Press.

Nissim-Sabat, M. (2009). *Neither Victim nor Survivor: Thinking Toward a New Humanity*. Lanham, MD: Lexington Books.

Outram, S. M. and Ellison, G. T. H. (2010). Arguments against the use of racialized categories as genetic variables in biomedical research: What are they and why are they being ignored? In I. Whitmarsh and D. S. Jones (Eds), *What's the Use of Race? Modern Governance and the Biology of Difference*, pp. 92–123. Cambridge, MA: MIT Press.

Patil, T. and Giordano, J. (2010). On the ontological assumptions of the medical model of psychiatry: philosophical considerations and pragmatic tasks. *Philosophy, Ethics, and Humanities in Medicine*, 5, 3.

Potter, N. (2004). Gender. In J. Radden (Ed.), *The Philosophy of Psychiatry: A Companion*, pp. 237–43. Oxford: Oxford University Press.

Radden, J. (Ed.) (2004). *The Philosophy of Psychiatry: A Companion*. Oxford: Oxford University Press.

Showalter, E. (1985). *The Female Malady: Women, Madness, and English Culture, 1830–1980*. New York, NY: Pantheon.

Social Sciences Research Council Web Forum. *Is Race "Real"?* Available at: <http://www.raceandgenomics.ssrc.org>. (Retrieved February 2011.)

Soffer, G. (1991). *Husserl and the Question of Relativism*. Dordrecht: Kluwer Academic Publishers.

Thornton, T. (2004). Reductionism/antireductionism. In J. Radden (Ed.), *The Philosophy of Psychiatry: A Companion*, pp. 191–204. Oxford: Oxford University Press.

Wallace, E. R., IV. (1985). *Historiography and Causation in Psychoanalysis*. Hillsdale, NJ: Analytic Press.

Wirth-Cauchon, J. (2000). *Women and Borderline Personality Disorder*. New Brunswick, NJ: Rutgers University Press.

CHAPTER 13

WHY PSYCHIATRY SHOULD FEAR MEDICALIZATION

LOUIS C. CHARLAND

Somehow, the field has lost its grip over diagnosis and therapeutics.

Edward Shorter, *Before Prozac: The Troubled History of Mood Disorders in Psychiatry* (2009)

I think that psychiatrists have now got to show what they're made of.

Michael Shepherd, *Pharmacology: Specific and Non-Specific* (1998)

PSYCHIATRY UNDER ATTACK

Insofar as it aspires to be a genuine branch of medical science, it would seem that psychiatry should welcome medicalization. After all, historically, medicalization has been the indispensable ally of psychiatry in its march to become a legitimate branch of medical science. Certainly, a psychiatry without any medical terms and concepts cannot qualify as a medical discipline or subspecialty. Yet paradoxically, we appear to have reached a stage where psychiatry should fear, rather than welcome, medicalization. The reason is that medicalization is not what it was. The old ally appears to have turned into an enemy. At least in some quarters.

Of course, psychiatry already has enemies. Under the banner of "anti-psychiatry," former consumers of psychiatric services—"survivors"—as well as social activists of all stripes, have mounted a formidable campaign against the psychiatric establishment. This "anti-psychiatry" movement has its intellectual heroes, philosophers and social thinkers like Michael Foucault, Ivan Illich, Thomas Scheff, and others (Foucault 1972; Illich 1973; Scheff 1966). A notable feature of these attacks on psychiatry is that they usually come from the outside, from individuals who are not themselves psychiatrists or otherwise allied with psychiatry. This perhaps may help explain why, despite their popularity, these attacks appear to have had relatively little impact on the actual theory and practice of psychiatry. At least insofar as medicalization is concerned.

More recently, psychiatry has had to face a new kind of enemy. But this one has been attacking from the inside. Indeed, psychiatry is now facing open revolt in its own ranks. Thomas Szasz and Ronald Laing are perhaps the first and best known leaders of this new insurgence (Laing 1967; Szasz 1961, 2010). Peter Breggin, the Judas of modern psychiatry, is probably the most infamous (Breggin 1991). There is also David Healy, the current *enfant terrible* of the psychiatric establishment (Healy 2004). Healy is rather unique in that his views arguably have had a real impact on psychiatric theory and practice. However, he is no anti-psychiatrist. Along with Marcia Angell (2004), Nassir Ghaemi (2003), Alfred Freedman (2010), Joanna Moncrieff (2009), and others, he is part of a growing consortium of established psychiatrists with serious concerns about the scientific integrity of the profession and the ethical consequences of this for consumers of psychiatric services and society at large.

Psychiatry is therefore under attack, both from inside and outside. But who truly is the enemy, the proper target, of these attacks? This, of course, is a complex interpretative question, since specific motives and objectives tend to vary among anti-psychiatrists and their new "allies" in the psychiatric establishment. Nonetheless, there is a common theme—a common locus of concern—that seems to unite all these parties. This is medicalization. The worry is that there is something scientifically inappropriate, and also ethically objectionable, about both the scope and the nature of medicalization in contemporary psychiatry. The roots of the problem lie especially in the domain of psychopharmacology, which can be defined as "the scientific discipline which deals with detection of psychopathologic symptoms and syndromes, and the identification of nosological entities, which are affected by psychotropic drugs" (Ban 2010, p. 705). "Neuropsychopharmacology," in turn, can be defined as the scientific discipline that "studies the relationship between neuronal and mental events with centrally acting drugs" (Ban 2011, p. 229). For ease of exposition, we will refer to "psychopharmacology" in what follows, even though "neuropsychopharmacology is also usually directly implicated.

The central argument of this chapter is that we appear to have reached a stage in the evolution of psychopharmacology where it is not only anti-psychiatrists who ought to worry about medicalization. Psychiatry also has an important stake in the question. But not the one that is typically supposed—which is to *defend* medicalization. Quite the contrary. Medicalization is no longer simply the professed enemy of anti-psychiatry and its supporters. It is now also an enemy of psychiatry. Consequently, some of the battle lines between psychiatry and anti-psychiatry need to be redrawn.

DEFINING MEDICALIZATION

Let us define "medicalization" as the process by which aspects of thinking, feeling, and behavior, that were previously described without medical terms and concepts, are re-described using such terms and concepts. In the words of Peter Conrad: "'medicalisation' describes a process by which non-medical problems become defined and treated as medical problems, usually in terms of illness and disorders" (Conrad 2007, p. 4). Note that medicalization in this sense is not only an objective social process on a grand scale, with numerous economic and political antecedents and implications. It is also a highly personal subjective matter that affects how individuals understand and label themselves, a core feature of their sense of identity (Charland 2004a, 2004b).

As a sociolinguistic phenomenon, medicalization can be defined as the redescription, in medical terms, of phenomena that were not previously described in medical terms. De-medicalization, then, is the redescription, in non-medical terms, of phenomena that were previously described in medical terms. Re-medicalization, in turn, is the redescription, in new medical terms, of phenomena previously described in older medical terms. Note that this definition and its derivatives remain neutral on the question of whether medicalization is good or bad. It is neutral on the question of whether medicalization is a mark of scientific progress that contributes to human freedom, or, say, an oppressive sign of the increasing iatrogenic colonization of the human mind by the pharmaceutical industry— "pharmageddon" (Social Audit 2007). Such evaluative conclusions require separate, additional, arguments of their own.

The problem with this definition of medicalization, of course, is that, like any definition, it relies on the definition of other terms. In this case, the key term is "medical." This kind of circularity is an easy trap to fall into where medicalization is concerned. But once forewarned, it is easy to avoid. For example, Thomas Szasz tells us that "the concept of 'medicalization' rests on the assumption that some phenomena belong in the domain of medicine, and some do not" (Szasz 2007, p. xiii). However, commendably, he then goes on to point out that "unless we agree on some clearly defined criteria that define the class called 'disease' or 'medical problem' it is fruitless to debate whether any particular act of medicalization is 'valid' or not" (p. xiii). Precisely.

Probably the best solution to this semantic quandary is to grant that there is a problem, and solve it, when it arises, by stipulating what counts as "medical" in a specific context. Very likely, there is no one particular definition of "medical" that is going to cover all branches of medical science. Terminological boundaries and usage are also likely to shift as medical science progresses or retreats, adding new theoretical terms, or removing old ones. Let us then simply stipulate that "medical," in the context of medicalization in psychiatry, begins with the official published lexicon and accepted theoretical terms of art of the psychiatric profession in North America and Europe. This lexicon can be found in the *Diagnostic and Statistical Manual of Mental Disorders* (DSM) of the American Psychiatric Association (APA), and its European counterpart, the "Mental and Behavioral Disorders" section of the *International Classification of Diseases* (APA 2004; World Health Organization 2007). Note that this descriptive solution does not solve the prescriptive problem of when a term, concept, or intervention, should count as "medical" in the context of psychiatry. But it does provide a relatively stable starting point for engaging such debates.

A notable feature about the anti-psychiatry diatribe on medicalization in psychiatry is how ineffective it has been in slowing the growth of medicalization there. Indeed, it is ironic that every successive edition of the DSM seems to add more disorders to the list of mental ills that can afflict us (Caplan 1995), a process that is not only compounded, but also greatly complicated, by globalization (Waters 2010). Along the way, common everyday features of subjective experience and bodily functioning are transformed into auspicious signs and symptoms of mental illness and disorder (Shorter 1992). Current indications are that the new version of the DSM—namely, DSM-5—will contain not only a more complex and erudite theoretical medical nomenclature, now based on a dimensional conceptualization of mental disorder, but also probably more permutations of disorders and their diagnostic criteria than previous versions (APA 2011). Thus, compared with earlier times, when the official nomenclature of psychiatry consisted of less than a half-dozen mental disorders, we may be entering an era of hyper-medicalization, which, on a social level, is increasingly reflected in a parallel "hyper-narrativity" that is emerging among consumers of psychiatric services.

In order to understand the inexorable growth of medicalization in modern psychiatry, it is necessary to look more closely at the internal workings of medicalization as a social process. The reference to "process" in this definition is important. However, speaking of medicalization as "a" process is potentially misleading, since medicalization is not a single, uniform, process, but rather the cumulative sum of many different processes. To date, these various processes have all been contributing to the growth of medicalization, like individual tributaries merging into a larger waterway. As the nature and scope of medicalization in psychiatry has evolved overtime, new tributaries have appeared and old ones have disappeared. The new tributaries have altered the shape and course of existing waterways.

Let us consider this metaphor in more concrete terms. The new tributaries alluded to in the metaphor are meant to represent new scientific, social, economic, and political forces in the evolution of medicalization in psychiatry. The shifting waterways are the theory and practice of psychiatry. There are two new major forces ("tributaries") that impact on the theory and practice of psychiatry today that will concern us. They are especially relevant to the new, antagonistic, relationship that has emerged between medicalization and psychiatry. The first has to do with the manner in which commercialization has infected medicalization in the area of psychopharmacology. The second has to do with the manner in which social media like the Internet have altered both the scope and the nature of medicalization, including the distribution of power among major stakeholders, which now include consumers. With the advent of these two new forces, medicalization in psychiatry has taken a new turn. The purpose of the present chapter is to explore these new developments and their consequences for the relationship between medicalization and psychiatry.

Before we begin, an important word of caution is in order. Since these are topics that usually arouse a lot of passion, it is important to dispel any doubts or worries about hidden agendas at the very start. So let us be clear. This chapter is not intended as a contribution to, or defense of, anti-psychiatry. In fact, the aim is precisely the opposite. It is a call to arms to protect the scientific and ethical integrity of psychiatry from a new enemy: profligate, industry-driven, commercial medicalization, and its more nefarious social consequences. This, arguably, is the true and proper enemy of anti-psychiatry. Or at least one of them. The argument of this chapter is that it is now also the enemy of psychiatry. Therefore this is no ideological or political romantic threnody in defense of a utopia without medical terms and concepts, or a psychiatry that can aspire to pure science without any abuses of power or commercial interests. Instead, this is a pragmatic philosophical reassessment of psychiatry today, an attempt to understand a medical discipline in trouble, at serious risk of losing its original scientific and ethical sense of purpose. Our allegiance, then, is ultimately to psychiatry, the branch of medicine that Philippe Pinel and other like-minded pioneers of the Enlightenment sought to establish (Pinel 1809). Appropriately, it is Pinel, an arch defender of the scientific method in psychiatry, who wrote: "It is an art of no little importance to administer medicines properly: but it is an art of much greater and difficult acquisition to know when to suspend or altogether omit them" (Hickish et al. 2008, p. xiii).

Subterfuge in Psychopharmacology

Anti-psychiatrists and other critics of psychiatry often argue that contemporary psychiatry has been co-opted by the pharmaceutical and other allied forces of "industry" (Elliott 2011; Moynihan and Cassels 2009; Whitaker 2010). The problem has reached a point where even leading psychiatrists openly recognize and discuss these dangers (Angell 2004; Ghaemi 2003; Healy 2004; Kassirer 2005; Moncrieff 2009). Notably, there have been calls by such leaders in the field to revise psychiatric ethics accordingly (Freedman 2010; see also APA 2010; Baciu et al. 2007). Despite all this foment within psychiatry, for the most part, the philosophy of psychiatry and psychiatric ethics have remained largely silent on these issues. This in spite of the fact that there is already an important philosophical recognition that psychiatric theory and practice are clearly not simply based on "fact" but are also heavily dependent on "value" (Fulford 1989; Sadler 2003). The major worry that needs to be addressed in this case is that psychiatry is now no longer sufficiently autonomous to fulfill its scientific medical mandate. It is far too closely allied with the goals and objectives of the pharmaceutical industry. Psychopharmacology is the area of psychiatry where these kinds of issues are presently of most concern. It is in this quarter of psychiatry, especially, that the charge of a possible subterfuge and hijacking of psychiatry by industry is most plausible and disturbing. Note that these concerns regarding issues of value in psychopharmacology cannot be circumvented or explained away on the grounds that they are merely restricted to what philosophers and historians of science call the "context of discovery," namely, processes of hypothesis formation (Popper 1935/2002, pp. 6–10). They are also integral to the "context of justification" and lie at the heart of scientific method and how hypotheses are tested in psychopharmacology.

By way of prelude, it is worth reminding ourselves that, as a form of independent professional scientific inquiry, psychiatry existed long before the advent of anything like the modern pharmaceutical industrial complex (Libenau 1987; Porter 2002; Sneader 1990). Medical professionals interested in "mental science" usually published their own theories and classifications, subject, of course, to the vicissitudes of current scientific fashion, local politics, and general intellectual trends. While drugs and tonics were often prescribed, as a rule, the guilds and individuals responsible for those products had little or no direct power over the medical professionals that administered the products, even less over the theories that governed their use (Healy 1997, pp. 7–21). Suffice it to say that things have changed dramatically. While it is no doubt true that there have always been commercial factors and interests at play in the history of psychiatry, we have reached a point where the nature, scope, and magnitude of commercialization involved has no comparable analogue to earlier times.

One of the most important elements behind the commercialization of medicalization in psychopharmacology today is the randomized clinical trial (Ghaemi 2003; Healy 2008; Shorter 2009). Now the accepted gold standard for just about all psychiatric research in the area of psychopharmacology, the randomized controlled trial normally trumps all other forms of evidence (but see Healy 2008, p. 131; Shorter 2009, pp. 6–9). Sample sizes for the desired levels of statistical power and significance in contemporary drug testing and evaluation mean that clinical trials are very large (Ban 2011, pp. 234–235; Ghaemi 2003, pp. 251–264). If randomized controlled trials were conducted according to accepted standards of scientific research, such as transparency and access to all relevant data and evidence, there might be no problem. But this precisely is the problem. Patent law and the proprietary secrecy of industry with respect to transparency and unfettered access to clinical trial data undermine the open kind of scrutiny and verification that is the hallmark of Western science (Freedman 2010; Healy 2004). Some argue that the problem is even larger than this and goes to the very roots of what is considered scientific method in psychopharmacology in psychiatry. It is the clinical trial that is the Trojan horse in this subterfuge. Not, of course, the clinical trial in itself. But rather the manner in which it has been put to use in this particular context: psychopharmacology.

Ironically, once the weapon of choice for debunking fashionable "therapeutic bandwagons," some critics argue that clinical trials are now used to launch such drugs (Healy 2008, pp. 129–134, 217). Put bluntly, the charge is that "industry has commandeered the RCT for marketing purposes" (Healy 2008, p. 134). The main problem, in this case, is that contemporary clinical trials for many psychotropic drugs often show very minimal therapeutic effects, and deliver drugs of questionable efficacy (Moncrieff 2009). Minimal drug effects are attributed to the drugs when in fact it is equally plausible to trace them to non-specific contributions of the placebo effect (Kirsh 2009). As a result, many randomized clinical trials in contemporary psychopharmacology tend to require constant reassessment and re-evaluation by highly complex and controversial meta-analyses, sometimes leading to remarkably divergent recommendations for public health policy (see, e.g., Ban 2008; Sartorius et al. 2007).

Consider a standard bar chart representation plotting response rates for all drug versus placebo antidepressant trials undertaken by the Food and Drug Administration over a given period (Healy 2008, p. 130, fig. 4.1). One column indicates a 50% response rate for the active drug, and the second column indicates a 40% response rate for the placebo. The chart represents the finding that "on average, antidepressants or mood stabilizers have effects in 50% of patients in trials, whereas the placebo has comparable effect in 40%" (Healy 2008, p. 129). What proponents in favor of a drug or class of drugs will usually "see" and reason here, is that there is a slight superiority of the active drug over placebo. Many will reason that the drug therefore "works." Skeptics, however, will "see" and reason that the difference between the drug and placebo is so small that it shows the drug doesn't truly "work" (but see Ban 2006, pp. 437–438). The former group concludes that the drugs should be prescribed, while the latter group concludes that—all things being equal—it is probably the placebo that should be prescribed. This is somewhat reminiscent of the famous duck–rabbit illusion, where a traced figure can appear both as a duck or a rabbit depending on how one "sees" it.

Behind this interesting divergence of interpretation is the oft forgotten fact that, historically, clinical trials "were not designed to show that treatments worked" (Healy 2008, p. 116; see also Shepherd 1998). As noted earlier, originally, randomized clinical trials "were aimed at identifying unsuccessful therapeutic interventions and bring bandwagons to a stop" (Healy 2008, p. 116). The fallacy involved is apparently as easy to commit as it is easy to miss. It can be summarized as follows:

Philosophically, RCTs are constructed on the basis of a null hypothesis. When the null hypothesis is refuted, it means that it is not right to say that the treatment has no effect. This is not the same as saying that the treatment "works" and therefore should be given (Healy 2008, p. 128).

The problem, then, is that randomized clinical trials in psychopharmacology—and indeed elsewhere—have been commandeered by industry to do something they were not originally designed to do. They have been engineered to show that drugs work, when instead they were originally designed to test the null hypothesis (Shepherd 1998, p. 255). One odd fact that emerges from randomized trials when placebos are employed is connected to the non-specificity and heterogeneity of treatment response. In the example we are considering, this becomes clear when we look at individual responses to the prescribed treatments under investigation. The problem in our example is that, in actual fact, in any group of ten patients, there are five that do not respond to either the drug or the placebo, meaning that "one responds to the drug while nine do not" (Healy 2008, p. 131; see also, e.g., Davis et al. 1993; Klerman and Cole 1965). Under these conditions, why give the drug to all patients? Advocates of the drugs see one in two patients responding to the drug. In contrast, every two out of five seem to respond to placebo. Adding side effects to the equation, it can be argued on this basis that prescribing the placebo is probably best, safest, and most cost-effective, course (Kirsch 2009).

Obviously, this analysis can be debated. Nevertheless, for us, it is the existence of genuine debate in the relevant peer-reviewed literature that counts. If the skeptic's argument is sound then, in a case like this one, prescribing the drug and developing new ones is the more risky and costly alternative. We should be aiming, rather, to prescribe the placebo and enhance the placebo response. Verifying that a treatment works in the case of antidepressant drugs in psychiatry, then, is very different from verifying that a drug like penicillin works in general medicine (Healy 2008, p. 131). In the case of penicillin and its influence, say, on pulmonary pneumonia, treatment effects are directly observable and normally it is unnecessary to invoke clinical trials to resolve questions of uncertainty. In the case of many psychoactive drugs for psychiatric conditions, however, the situation is vastly different. There is much uncertainty over treatment effects, which are often not directly observable, but based on self-reports structured by rating-scales. Moreover, the uncertainty over whether and to what "specific" extent apparent treatment effects derive from the influence of the active ingredients in drugs themselves, makes psychiatry vulnerable to highly complex debates and staggering differences of opinion that simply do not arise in the case of drugs like penicillin (Healy 2008, p. 130; see also Elliott 2003, pp. 288–303). Moreover, the professed specificity of many of the alleged treatments we currently have is something of an illusion, especially when those treatments are also prescribed—off-label—for other indications, and when robust side effects are factored in. The kind of polypharmacy that ensues from all this has led some experts to openly advocate for a new version of the Hippocratic injunction to do no harm, but this one specially tailored to psychopharmacology. Thus, psychiatrist Nassir Ghaemi—certainly no "anti-psychiatrist"—tells us we should adopt a "Hippocratic Psychopharmacology" that adheres to two rules. The first is "Holmes' Rule," which states that "medications are guilty until proven innocent" (Ghaemi 2007, p. 55). The second is "Osler's Rule," which states that we should "treat diseases not symptoms" (p. 55). Clearly, Healy is no longer alone. There are now other, equally prestigious, psychiatrists who share his worries and have worries of their own.

To sum up, with commercial interests largely in charge of medicalization in psychopharmacology, psychiatry is courting scientific trivialization. Much drug development today amounts to little more than minor molecular manipulations on existing compounds that are then marketed for new specially created conditions (Moynihan and Cassels 2005). The randomized clinical trial has become a mechanism for generating "me-too" drugs that have little advantage over existing drugs (Shorter 1993, p. 255). Moreover, clinical trials today are invariably used to produce drugs for uniform application across populations and little attention is paid to exploring the reasons for heterogeneity in treatment response within specified nosological groups (Ban 1987). The goal is no longer so much to "carve nature at the joints," but instead provide "one-size-fits-all" drugs and diagnostic categories (Shorter 2009, pp. 163–168, 203–214). Rampant off-label prescribing only serves to complicate these problems, since numerous psychiatric drugs are now prescribed for conditions they were never originally indicated or approved for, often leading to extravagant polypharmacy (Ghaemi 2002). To make matters worse, there is a veritable litany of ongoing lawsuits and methodological disputes over the safety and efficacy of major classes of drugs, which regularly command headline attention (see, e.g., Harris 2004; Wilson 2010). Finally, the pernicious and pervasive practice of "ghostwriting" and other regulatory anomalies in the manner in which new psychiatric drugs are approved and promoted is often decidedly unethical and contrary to accepted standards of academic research and authorship (Elliott 2011; Lemmens 2004; McHenry and Juriedini 2008).

Evidently, in the area of psychopharmacology at least, psychiatry is in quite a quandary. There is a growing malaise that, in this area, psychiatry has steered perilously off course. It bears repeating that this is not simply the opinion of a small group of fanatical anti-psychiatrists, or irate "survivors," but also now the considered opinion of leading figures in the field. It is disheartening that even some of the most successful pioneers in the application of randomized clinical trials to psychiatry share in this disillusionment. For example, in a telling interview toward the end of his career, Michael Shepherd, reminisces about the legacy of randomized clinical trials in psychopharmacology, with considerable cynicism. He says:

> The real issue is that these topics have a scientific core and if you look at scientific side of them there is only one way to proceed and that is to put forward the hypothesis and refute it, and if you fail you've got something positive which you can then build on etc. That's true in every branch of science. But these topics have spin-offs—like money, reputation, fraud and publicity and 101 other things, which you can take out of the issue and make your own without ever actually getting involved in the scientific issues concerned... [T]his sort of thing goes on and on and it's part of the process. You must recognize that it exists, that it has always existed and that it will always exist and if you don't separate from that the fundamental scientific issues, you just get lost and the whole thing gets degraded. That's happened, sadly. (Shepherd 1998, pp. 255–256)

In conclusion, the developments we have reviewed suggest that medicalization in psychopharmacology is compromised by unbridled commercialization. As a result, psychiatry is courting scientific trivialization as tonics for known conditions multiply and additional ones for new conditions are produced. The original goals and aims of psychiatry as a medical science are increasingly threatened and marginal (Ghaemi 2003). The quest to discover and develop cures for mental diseases, of "carving nature at the joints," seems remote indeed. Admittedly, there may be very few, or even no, "magic bullets" to be had (Healy 1997, pp. 20–21, 87–95). However, this in no way entails giving up on the need for a psychopharmacology with scientific and ethical integrity (see, e.g., Ghaemi 2007; Healy 2009). Which, in part, means designing clinical trials designed to investigate the reasons for heterogeneity in treatment response (Ban 1987). The key here was and still is the identification of *pharmacologically homogeneous* populations within the *pharmacologically heterogeneous* psychiatric diagnoses (Ban 1987, 2006). To be sure, the goals and objectives of psychiatry may change, but wanton commercial trivialization remains undesirable at any time, both scientifically and ethically.

Admittedly, there is nothing inherently wrong with "tonics," polyvalent compounds that are more or less indiscriminately, but hopefully safely, applied to try and alleviate symptoms of mental distress. The problem has to with the manner in which the "manifest image" of psychiatry in this case fails to correspond with its true "scientific image" (van Frassen 1980). The "manifest image" of psychopharmacology which psychiatry tries to project is that it is in the business of finding magic bullets, or at least cures, for specific mental disorders, or diseases. On its side, the public is led to believe that they are being prescribed treatments for such diseases, medications that correct the "chemical imbalances" that cause those conditions. On their side, health professionals of all stripes are also sold this picture of psychopharmacology and psychiatry. However, in actual scientific fact, this is not what psychopharmacology in psychiatry is doing at all. Scientifically, it is mostly in the business of producing interchangeable polyvalent compounds of questionable efficacy that might alleviate symptoms but typically do not target or cure diseases. This discrepancy between the manifest and scientific image of psychiatry in the area of psychopharmacology is tantamount to deception. It has widespread nefarious social and personal consequences for consumers, to which we now turn.

New Looping Effect of Kinds

The immediate social consequence of unbridled commercialization in psychopharmacology is a steady accumulation of new symptom clusters that qualify as mental disorders, all of which are normally said to require treatment by pharmacological means. There is nothing in current consensus-based nosological classifications to prevent such an accumulation. And so, in direct contravention of William of Ockham's famous dictum—"Ockham's Razor"—mental disorders and their subtypes are multiplied in the name of commercial objectives, beyond all reasonable scientific necessity. Rampant cross-pollination—"comorbidity"—occurs at both the diagnostic and treatment level, creating a fertile marketing environment where experimentation and polypharmacy is usually the rule (Ghaemi 2002, p. 8). Over time, as one classification of mental disorder succeeds another, some disorders are added, some are modified, and others are removed. Hence the need for a definition of medicalization that recognizes "medicalization," de-medicalization," and "re-medicalization."

Insufficient attention has been paid to the clinical and ethical implications of this sea of change for consumers of psychiatric services. There are both clinical and ethical issues involved, usually a combination of both. Changes in psychiatric diagnostic categories or "labels" may sometimes be accompanied by changes in behavior and self-conception on the part of those who are labeled (Charland 2004a; Elliott 2003; Hacking 1995; Sass 2007). Obviously, there are important ethical questions regarding the possibility of iatrogenic harm that need to be raised in such cases. The language of "social construction" is often invoked in these contexts, typically to reflect the fact that psychiatric labels are social constructs that are created to suit social purposes. The prominent role that social media have come to play in the social dissemination of such labels and their adoption by consumers of psychiatric services is just starting to be recognized. However, the picture that emerges is paradoxical.

On the one hand, the promotion and marketing of new diagnostic labels and their alleged pharmacological treatments to consumers and health professionals alike is more pervasive and insidious than ever. Yet, on the other hand, the same social media that act as vehicles for this relentless campaign of dissemination can also be used to combat it. Indeed, never before have consumers exercised so much power over the psychiatric establishment. At the same time, never before have they been so vulnerable (Charland 2004b). The hypothesis of the "looping effects of kinds" plays a pivotal role in understanding how and why the addition of social media to the social forces that shape medicalization have played such a pivotal role in changing both the scope, and indeed the nature, of the social processes involved.

Late nineteenth-century photographic records and artistic depictions of hysterical patients at the Salpêtrière Hospital in Paris provide a striking historical record of the manner in which signs and symptoms of psychiatric disorder can be shaped by local medical culture and fashion (Didi-Hubermann 1982). Examining the complex lavish poses of patients of the famous Dr Charcot during this period, there can be little doubt that the behaviors displayed by those patients are not a natural consequence of their neurotic condition, but rather carefully choreographed medical scripts learned and reinforced through interaction with the medical system. This "looping effect" of psychiatric labels—or "human kinds"—is very well described by philosopher Ian Hacking in his historical studies on the emergence of multiple personality disorder and dissociative fugue (Hacking 1995, 1998, 1999). Additional studies by illustrious social scientists such as Thomas Scheff and Irving Goffman provide valuable additional evidence that can be enlisted in defense this hypothesis of the "looping effect of kinds" (Goffman 1963; Scheff 1966).

In his work on the looping effect of kinds, Hacking makes an important addition to the historiography and philosophical understanding of the transient nature of mental disorders such as fugue and hysteria. He invokes the biological metaphor of an "ecological niche" to explain how it is that a particular disorder seems to appear at a particular place and time but not elsewhere. This biological metaphor of a "niche" is supplemented by explanatory principles that are likened to "vectors"; namely, medical taxonomy, cultural polarity, observability, and release (Hacking 1999, pp. 82–83). This is not the place to review the details of Hacking's ingenious and very interesting theory of transient mental disorders. The relevant point is that the appearance of specific disorders at a given place and time is made possible by a specific configuration of historical factors and social forces that make the existence of that disorder "possible" in precisely that circumstance. A second feature of this account is that once a disorder appears, it can, as it were, spread and take on a life of its own. As individuals are labeled with the chosen nosological term or category for a disorder, they often come to adopt the disorder as their own, a feature of themselves. Through a process of internalization and reinforcement, the disorder and its particular set of signs and symptoms become linked to self-identity, sometimes permanently. In this manner, a person labeled with the psychiatric diagnostic label "hysteria" may start to conceive of themselves as a hysteric. The label has become a key feature of the "kind" of person they *are*, who they take themselves to *be* (Charland 2004a; Elliott 2003, esp. pp. 100–129, 208–237; Sass 2007; Tan et al. 2007).

Hacking's theory of the ecological niche and the looping effect of kinds is lacking in one important respect. It ignores the role of social media like the Internet in the social construction of transient mental disorders (Comstock 2011; Giles 2011; Jutel 2011; Leibing 2009; Parsell 2008; Vandereycken 2011). But in fact these social media represent a new and distinct vector in the ecological niche that makes transient mental disorders possible. The looping effect of kinds hypothesis therefore needs to be supplemented and altered accordingly. This is why in the present chapter it is referred to in modified form, as the "new looping effect of kinds."

Hacking's own account of the rise and fall of multiple personality requires but omits the mention of such a social media vector (Hacking 1995). When, with the publication of DSM-IV, the DSM-III "multiple personality disorder" label was dropped and replaced by "dissociative identity disorder," consumer groups and advocates of the old label rallied and protested—largely on the Internet (Charland 2004a). Some consumer advocate organizations that represented persons diagnosed with multiple personality disorder simply refused to adopt the new dissociative label and openly defied the nosological edicts of the new DSM. This defiance took place openly and brazenly, on the Internet. Another example of this kind of phenomenon is the existence of pro-anorexia Internet sites where consumers tout and praise the virtues of anorexia as a lifestyle and deny its seriousness a disease (Fox et al. 2005; Gavin et al. 2008). Finally, there is also the curious case of the apotemnophiles ("amputee wannabees"), who apparently originally met through Internet chat rooms and then proceeded to mobilize support, again through the Internet, to the point where they have now lobbied the APA to grant disease status to their condition (Elliott 2003, pp. 208–236).

Putting aside for the moment the question of whether these changes are good or bad, the relevant point is that probably none of these exercises of consumer power would have been possible without the Internet. The particular organized social forms that these acts of defiance represent all involve a mobilization of individuals into groups in a shared public forum provided by a network of linked Internet websites and chat rooms. Note that this defiance largely takes place beyond the reach of the forces of establishment psychiatry and industry. The reality of this new kind of social forum for consumer mobilization and expression is evident in the fact that both psychiatry and the pharmaceutical industry have had to create their own Internet sites and resources in order to have a voice in the new order of things—in order to further and defend their interests and exercise what power they can.

Recent studies unequivocally show that the looping effect of kinds and its impact on self-identity is a very real and robust phenomenon. For example, anorexic patients will often refuse treatment on the grounds that anorexia is a core feature of who they are (Tan et al. 2007). There are also compelling personal narratives of how even psychiatric labels and diagnostic categories such as "schizophrenia" can become so entrenched in a person's sense of their own identity that they will fear and refuse the news that they have been misdiagnosed, rather than welcome it (Charland 2004a; see also Sass 2007). Special websites and chat rooms organized by various psychiatric patient consumer groups amply illustrate the hold and fascination that psychiatric labels can have on persons who accept those labels as their own. Apparently, new social media have dramatically expanded the scope and depth of the manner in which the looping effect of kinds can subjectively bind persons to psychiatric labels and build communities of like-minded sufferers.

These phenomena are relatively new and obviously require further study. Yet their implications for the relationship between psychiatry and medicalization are already quite clear. Psychiatry is losing control over the manner in which psychiatric labels are publicly disseminated and understood by consumers. Never before have consumers of psychiatric services been able to so brazenly and successfully challenge the nosological edicts of the psychiatric establishment. Easy access to social media is the prime social factor—the new "vector"— that is responsible for this remarkable new social phenomenon. There is, however, another, darker, side to the social forces unleashed by the Internet. The reverse side of this new consumer power is an increased risk of vulnerability to manipulation and control by the pharmaceutical industrial complex, which has also adapted social media to its profiteering ends. There is also the risk of self-harm through self-medicalization, cases where consumers stand to suffer on account of their allegiance to a label and self-conception or lifestyle that is not ultimately in their best interest. The new vector, therefore, can cut several ways. It can serve the aims of consumer freedom and empowerment, or the ends of psychiatry and industry, or the ends of consumers who wish to promote or adopt harmful or inappropriate labels and behaviors. All of these new manifestations of medicalization are developments that psychiatry ought to fear. One thing is sure, however. It is that neither psychiatry nor industry is the only voice in the "manufacture of madness" anymore. Consumers also now have a voice of their own. Sometimes, consumers even have the last word, as the tale of the de-medicalization of homosexuality nicely illustrates (Spitzer 1981).

Conclusion and Postscript:
Another Enemy

The introduction of the randomized controlled trial into psychopharmacology, and the manner in which it has been co-opted for commercial purposes, has turned medicalization in psychiatry from a friendly asset into a treacherous liability. As a result of this subterfuge, psychopharmacology, psychopathology, and nosology are courting trivialization and the ethical and scientific integrity of psychiatry is at risk. The pernicious social consequences of these developments have been greatly amplified by a new form of the looping effect of kinds, due to the wide availability and access to social media like the Internet. As a result, consumers have more power than ever in how they respond to medicalization. At the same time, consumers of psychiatric services are at increased risk of iatrogenic harm resulting from unnecessary medicalization, re-medicalization, and de-medicalization, as well as increased risk of self-harm because of the largely unregulated nature of the Internet.

In order to avoid falling into triviality and safeguard its scientific and ethical integrity, psychiatry must rally its forces and vigorously, but meticulously, engage the rampant commercialization that has infected medicalization in contemporary psychopharmacology. This will be difficult as the enemy—the randomized controlled trial—now lies within. Perhaps this is the best place to begin the task of scientific and ethical reform in psychiatry. However, the randomized clinical trial is not the only enemy psychiatry must contend with as it seeks to rehabilitate itself. Commercial medicalization has another, equally insidious, face. There is another enemy, an accomplice, which also has its own supporting professional and commercial motives and industry. This is the rating scale.

The origins of the rating scale in psychiatry are coterminous with the introduction of clinical trials (Ban 2011, pp. 234–235; Healy 1997, pp. 98–104). Now the pride and joy of the psychological establishment, the rating scale is a *sine qua non* of just about all clinical trials research. Of course, like the clinical trial, the rating scale can be put to legitimate scientific use, or overstated and scientifically corrupted in the pursuit of questionable aims. What is seldom recognized is that, in the present commercial orientation of medicalization in psychopharmacology, its dehumanizing powers and their social consequences are possibly even more pervasive and pernicious than those that accompany the trivialization of psychopharmacology (Healy 2008, pp. 127–134).

Worries about the present status and use of rating scales in psychopharmacology are complex and hard to summarize. Abstraction from the clinical encounter and consequent reduction and loss of information are one important factor (Berrios and Villarasa 1990). Observations or confounding clinical data that fall outside the specific factors that are isolated and encoded with scales might be overlooked (Berrios and Markova 2002). However, it is really the manner in which ratings scales are currently integrated with a specific application of clinical trials methodology in psychopharmacology that makes rating scales problematic for psychiatry. Thomas Ban describes the issues this way:

> Rating scales can be sensitized by the omission of psychopathological symptoms, relevant to psychiatric nosology, which are not influenced by treatment, or by retaining only those items (variables) of a scale, which show the largest changes. While the use of sensitive scales helps to demonstrate therapeutic effectiveness in the shortest possible time in the smallest number of patients, the omission of relevant psychopathological symptoms to psychiatric nosology precludes the possibility of finding by meta-analyses any relevant information for the identification of treatment-responsive forms of illness in the data collected in efficacy studies with psychotropic drugs. Since one of the essential prerequisites for the development of neuropsychopharmacology is the identification of a treatment responsive form of illness, consensus-based classifications and sensitized rating scales blocked the development of the combined discipline. By interfering with the development of neuropsychopharmacology, they also precluded the possibility of using psychotropic drugs meaningfully in biological research in psychiatry. (Ban 2006, p. 425)

There are important consequences for psychopathology inherent in these developments. Perhaps the most important is the pharmacological heterogeneity within psychiatric diagnoses and resulting shift of attention away from psychotropic drugs that selectively target specific mental pathologies, to general tonics with variable effects across multiple diagnostic nosological groups. Ban explains:

> As the use of psychotropic drugs developed with this methodology increased, psychopathology was gradually replaced by psychiatric rating scale variables and psychiatric nosology gave way to consensus-based diagnostic algorithms. This led to an enlargement of the psychiatric populations within diagnostic groups and an extension of the scope of psychiatry to include, in addition to pathologies in mental processing, also behavioral anomalies with compromised social functioning. Simultaneously, treatment in psychiatry became evidence-based, albeit the evidence for demonstrated efficacy that was stipulated by regulatory authorities has made drugs available for clinical use even if only 1 in 4 patients was expected to respond favorably. As the pharmacological heterogeneity within psychiatric diagnoses precluded the linking of pharmacodynamic action of drugs to their effect on mental pathology, in the selection from drugs for treatment the primary consideration was their differential propensity for inducing side effects. (Ban 2010, p. 9)

No doubt, there is room for debate on these matters and Ban's interpretation of these developments can be challenged. Beliefs and assumptions about the proper aims and nature of psychopathology in psychiatry, and its relation to psychopharmacology, are sure to play an important part in such debates. Clearly it is impossible to settle these questions in a single chapter. Suffice it to say that in its efforts to regain scientific and ethical integrity, psychiatry cannot simply rest content with revisiting its relationship with clinical trial methodology. It will also have to revisit the terms of its long-standing, but uneasy, alliance with psychology and the rating scale. Remember also that these are not simply abstruse methodological matters for specialists. Through the new looping effect of kinds, they can have widespread and dramatic social consequences for consumers of psychiatric services and society as a whole.

ACKNOWLEDGMENTS

I would like to thank David Healy, Richard Gipps, Walter Glannon, Abraham Rudnick, Duff Waring, Christian Perring, and Peter Zachar, for very helpful comments on previous drafts of this chapter. Thanks also to Tom Ban for his encouragement, some very challenging discussions, and early access to the volumes of his *Oral History of Neuropsychopharmacology, The First 50 Years, Peer Interviews* (now published).

REFERENCES

American Psychiatric Association. (2004). *Diagnostic and Statistical Manual of Mental Disorders-IV-TR*. Washington DC: American Psychiatric Association.

American Psychiatric Association (2010). *Policies and Procedures to be Developed and Followed in all APA Organizational Relationships*. Available at: <http://www.psych.org/Resources/Governance/Disclosure-of-Interests-and-Affiliations/APA-Code-of-Conduct.aspx>.

American Psychiatric Association. (2011). *DSM-5 Development*. Available at: <http://www.dsm5.org/Pages/Default.aspx> (retrieved June 26, 2011).

Angell, M. (2004). *The Truth About Drug Companies*. New York, NY: Random House.

Baciu, A., Stratton, K., and Burke, S. P. (Eds) (2007). *Committee on the Assessment of the US Drug Safety System. The Future of Drug Safety: Promoting and Protecting the Health of the Public*. Washington, DC: National Academic Press.

Ban, T. A. (1987). Prolegomenon to the clinical prerequisite: Psychopharmacology and the classification of mental disorders. *Progress in Neuro-Psychopharmacology and Biological Psychiatry*, 11(5), 527–80.

Ban, T. A. (2006). Academic psychiatry and the pharmaceutical industry. *Progress in Neuro-Psychopharmacology and Biological Psychiatry*, 30, 429–41.

Ban, T. A. (2008). Comment on: 'Antidepressant medications and other treatments of depressive disorders: A CINP Task Force Report based on a review of evidence'. *International Journal of Neuropsychopharmacology*, 11(4), 583–5.

Ban, T. A. (2010). Neuropsychopharmacology and the history of pharmacotherapy in psychiatry: A review of developments in the 20th century. In T. A. Ban, D. Healy, and E. Shorter (Eds), *Reflections on Twentieth Century Pharmacology* (Vol. 4, 2nd edn), pp. 697–726. The History of Psychopharmacology and the CNIP (Collegium Internationale Neuro-Psychopharmacologicum), as told in Autobiography. East Kilrbride: Animula, CNIP.

Ban, T. A. (2011). *An Oral History of Neuropsychopharmacology, The First Fifty Years, Peer Interviews* (10 vols). Brentwood, TN: American College of Neuropsychopharmacology, Amazon.

Ban, T. A., Healy, D., and Edward Shorter (Eds) (2010). *Reflections on Twentieth Century Pharmacology* (Vol. 4, 2nd edn). The History of Psychopharmacology and the CNIP (Collegium Internationale Neuro-Psychopharmacologicum), as told in Autobiography. East Kilrbride: Animula, CNIP. Available at: <http://cinp.org/fileadmin/documents/history/books/VOL4_opt.pdf>.

Berrios, G. E. and Bulbena-Villarasa, A. (1990). The Hamilton Depression Scale and the Numerical Description of the Symptoms of Depression. *Psychopharmacology Series*, 9, 80–92.

Berrios, G. E. and Markova, I. S. (2002). Conceptual issues. In H. D'haenen, J. A. den Boer, and P. Willner (Eds), *Biological Psychiatry* (Vol. 1), pp. 3–25. New York, NY: Wiley.

Breggin, P. (1991). *Toxic Psychiatry*. New York, NY: St. Martin's Press.

Caplan, P. (1995). *They Say You're Crazy: How the World's Most Powerful Psychiatrists Decide Who's Normal*. Reading, MA: Perseus Books.

Charland, L. C. (2004a). A madness for identity: Psychiatric labels, consumer autonomy, and the perils of the internet. *Philosophy, Psychiatry, & Psychology*, 11(4), 335–49.

Charland, L. C. (2004b). As autonomy heads into harm's way. *Philosophy, Psychiatry, & Psychology*, 11(4), 361–3.

Comstock, E. J. (2011). The end of drugging children: Toward the genealogy of the ADHD subject. *Journal of the History of the Behavioral Sciences*, 47(1), 44–69.

Conrad, P. (2007). *The Medicalisation of Society: On the Transformation of Human Conditions into Treatable Disorders*. Baltimore, MD: Johns Hopkins University Press.

Davis, J. M., Wang, Z., and Janicak, P. G. (1993). A quantitative analysis of clinical drug trials for the treatment of affective disorders. *Psychopharmacological Bulletin*, 29, 175–81.

Didi-Hubermann, G. (1982). *Invention de l'hystérie. Charcot et l'Iconographie photographique de la Salpêtrière, sur l'École de la Salpêtrière*. Paris: Macula.

Elliott, C. (2003). *Better Than Well: American Medicine Meets the American Dream*. New York, NY: Norton.

Elliott, C. (2011). *White Cat, Black Hat: Adventures on the Dark Side of Medicine*. Boston, MA: Beacon Press.

Foucault, M. (1972). *Histoire de la folie à l'âge classique*. Paris: Gallimard.

Freedman, A. M. (2010). Ethics and neuropsychopharmacology. In T. A. Ban, D. Healy, and E. Shorter (Eds), *Reflections on Twentieth Century Pharmacology* (Vol. 4, 2nd edn), pp. 673–80. (The History of Psychopharmacology and the CNIP (Collegium Internationale Neuro-Psychopharmacologicum), as told in Autobiography.) East Kilrbride: Animula, CNIP.

Fox, N., Ward, K., and O'Rourke, A. (2005). Pro-anorexia, weight-loss drugs and the internet: An 'anti-recovery' explanatory model of anorexia. *Sociology of Health & Illness*, 27(7), 944–71.

Fulford, K. W. M. (1989). *Moral Theory and Medical Practice*. Cambridge: Cambridge University Press.

Gavin, J., Rodham, K., and Poyer, H. (2008). The presentation of "pro-anorexia" in online group interactions. *Qualitative Health Research*, 18, 325–34.

Ghaemi, N. (2002). All the worse for the fishes: Conceptual and historical background of polypharmacy in psychiatry. In N. Ghaemi (Ed.), *Polypharmacy in Psychiatry*, pp. 1–32. New York, NY: Marcel Dekker Inc.

Ghaemi, N. (2003). *The Concepts of Psychiatry: A Pluralistic Approach to the Mind and Mental Illness*. Baltimore, MD: Johns Hopkins University Press.

Ghaemi, N. (2007). *Mood Disorders: A Practical Guide*. Philadelphia, PA: Lippincott, Williams & Wilkins.

Giles, D. C. (2011). Self- and other-diagnosis in user-led mental health online communities. *Qualitative Health Research*, 21(3), 419–28.

Goffman, I. (1963). *Stigma: Notes on the Management of a Spoiled Identity*. New York, NY: Simon & Shuster.

Hacking, I. (1995). *Rewriting the Soul: Multiple Personality and the Sciences of Memory*. Princeton, NJ: Princeton University Press.

Hacking, I. (1998). *Mad Travelers: Reflections on the Reality of Transient Mental Illnesses*. Charlottesville, VA: University of Press of Virginia.

Hacking, I. (1999). *The Social Construction of What?* Cambridge, MA: Harvard University Press.

Harris, G. (2004). FDA panel urges stronger warning on antidepressants. *New York Times*, September 15, A1, A19.

Healy, D. (1997). *The Antidepressant Era*. Cambridge, MA: Harvard University Press.

Healy, D. (Ed.) (1998). *The Psychopharmacologists, Vol. II*. London: Altman.

Healy, D. (2004). *Let Them Eat Prozac: The Unhealthy Relationship Between the Pharmaceutical Industry and Depression*. New York, NY: New York University Press.

Healy, D. (2008). *Mania: A Short History of Bipolar Disorder*. Baltimore, MD: Johns Hopkins University Press.

Healy, D. (2009). *Psychiatric Drugs Explained* (5th edn). Edinburgh: Churchill Livingstone, Elsevier.

Illich, I. (1973). *Medical Nemesis: The Expropriation of Health*. London: Marlon Boyars.

Jutel, A. G. (2011). *Putting a Name To It: Diagnosis in Contemporary Society*. Baltimore, MD: Johns Hopkins University Press.

Kassirer, J. (2005). *On The Take: How Medicine's Complicity with Big Business Can Endanger Your Health*. New York, NY: Oxford University Press.

Kirsh, I. (2009). *The Emperor's New Drugs: Exploding the Anti-Depressant Myth*. London: The Bodley Head.

Klerman, G. L. and Cole J. O. (1965). Clinical pharmacology of imipramine and related antidepressant compounds. *Pharmacological Reviews*, 17, 101–41.

Laing, R. (1967). *The Politics of Experience*. New York, NY: Pantheon Books.

Leibing, A. (2009). Lessening the evils, online: Embodied molecules and the politics of hope in Parkinson's disease. *Science Studies*, 22(2), 80–101.

Lemmens, T. (2004). Leopards in the temple: Restoring scientific integrity to the commercialized research scene. *Journal of Law Medical Ethics*, 32, 641–57.

Libenau, J. (1987). *Medical Science and the Medical Industry*. Basingstoke: Macmillan.

McHenry, L. B. and Jureidini, J. N. (2008). Industry-sponsored ghostwriting in clinical trial reporting: A case study. *Accountability in Research*, 15, 152–67.

Moncrieff, J. (2009). *The Myth of the Chemical Cure: A Critique of Psychiatric Drug Treatment*. Basingstoke: Palgrave Macmillan.

Moynihan, R. and Cassels, A. (2009). *Selling Sickness: How the World's Biggest Pharmaceutical Companies Are Turning Us All Into Patients*. New York, NY: Nation Books.

Parsell, M. (2008). Pernicious virtual communities: identity, polarisation, and the web. *Ethics and Information Technology*, 10(1), 41–56.

Pinel, P. (2008). *Medico-Philosophical Treatise on Mental Alienation. Second Edition, Entirely Reworked and Extensively Expanded* (G. Hickish, D. Healy, and L. C. Charland, Trans.). Chippenham: Wiley-Blackwell. (Original work published 1809.) Available at: <www.interscience.wiley.com>.

Popper, K. (2002). *The Logic of Scientific Discovery*. New York, NY: Routledge. (Original work published 1935.)

Porter, R. (2002). *A Brief History of Madness*. Oxford: Oxford University Press.

Sadler, J. Z. (2003). *Values and Psychiatric Diagnosis*. Oxford: Oxford University Press.

Sartorius, N., Baghai, T. C., Baldwin, D. S., Barrett, B., Brand, U., Fleischhacker, W., et al. (2007). Antidepressant medications and other treatments of depressive disorders: A CINP Task Force Report based on a review of evidence. *International Journal of Neuropsychopharmacology*, *10*(Suppl. 1), S1–207.

Sass, L. A. (2007). 'Schizophrenic person' or 'person with schizophrenia'? An essay on illness and the self. *Theory & Psychology*, *17*(3), 395–420.

Scheff, T. J. (1966). *Being Mentally Ill: A Sociological Theory*. Chicago, IL: Aldine.

Shepherd, M. (1998). Pharmacology: Specific and non-specific. In D. Healy (Ed.), *The Psychopharmacologists, Vol. II*, pp. 237–58. New York, NY: Altman.

Shorter, E. (1992). *From Paralysis to Fatigue: A History of Psychosomatic Illness in the Modern Era*. New York, NY: The Free Press.

Shorter, E. (1993). *A Short History of Psychiatry: From the Era of the Asylum to the Age of Prozac*. New York, NY: Wiley.

Shorter, E. (2009). *Before Prozac: The Troubled History of Mood Disorders in Psychiatry*. Oxford: Oxford University Press.

Sneader, W. (1990). The prehistory of psychotherapeutic agents. *Journal of Psychopharmacology*, *4*(3), 115–19.

Social Audit (2007). *Pharmageddon? References and notes*. [Online.] Available at: <http://www.socialaudit.org.uk/6070716-%20REFS-NOTES.htm#Pharmageddon?>.

Spitzer, R. L. (1981). The diagnostic status of homosexuality in DSM-III: a reformulation of the issues. *American Journal of Psychiatry*, *138*, 210–15.

Szasz, T. S. (1961). *The Myth of Mental Illness: Foundations of a Theory of Personal Conduct*. New York, NY: Harper.

Szasz, T. S. (2007). *The Medicalisation of Everyday Life*. Syracuse, NY: Syracuse University Press.

Tan, J. O. A., Hope, P. T., Stewart, D. A., and Fitzpatrick, P. R (2007). Competence to make treatment decisions in anorexia nervosa: thinking processes and values. *Philosophy, Psychiatry & Psychology*, *13*(4), 267–82.

Vandereycken, W. (2011). Media hype, diagnostic fad or genuine disorder? Professionals' opinions about night eating syndrome, orthorexia, muscle dysmorphia, and emetophobia. *Eating Disorders*, *19*, 145–55.

Van Frassen, B. (1980). *The Scientific Image*. New York, NY: Oxford University Press.

Waters, E. (2010). *Crazy Like Us: The Globalization of the American Psyche*. New York, NY: Free Press.

Whitaker, R. (2010). *Anatomy of an Epidemic: Magic Bullets, Psychiatric Drugs, and the Astonishing Rise of Mental Illness in America*. New York, NY: Random House.

Wilson, D. (2010). Antipsychotic drugs—side effects may include lawsuits. *New York Times*, October 2.

World Health Organization. (2007). *International Classification of Diseases and Related Health Problems 10th Revision*. Available at: <http://www.who.int/classifications/icd/en/>.

CHAPTER 14

TECHNOLOGY AND PSYCHIATRY

JAMES PHILLIPS

INTRODUCTION

Let's begin with an ordinary clinical experience. The patient has made an appointment and is in my office for the first time. We do the usual formalities, take our seats, and I ask the patient what is going on and why she is here. She describes symptoms of depression; and, when prompted, puts them in their historical and current context. We begin the treatment.

From the perspective of medical treatment, this situation is ambiguous. First, the patient is describing primarily emotional and "mental" symptoms rather than somatic symptoms; she is not describing symptoms of possible heart disease, diabetes, or joint disease; and for that reason we typically do not proceed to a physical examination or further medical evaluation. The question now arises: What is she expecting and what am I offering? Is she expecting some form of talk therapy, or rather medication that will eliminate the symptoms, or both? If we begin with a preliminary understanding of technology as the development and use of physical tools to aid in our mastery of the world—medication is a technology in a way that talk therapy is not—we can see that my patient and I are now at some kind of crossroads of technology and psychiatry. We will each bring to the clinical encounter our respective attitudes regarding the role of technology in psychiatry, and she and I will have to clarify those attitudes.

I intend with this simple clinical vignette to underline the ambiguous role of technology in the mental health field. But this ambiguity reflects a larger one in our culture. As citizens of the twenty-first century our lives are dominated by technology. We live with and through its achievements, and for immediate examples I need look no further than the computer on which I am writing this text, the Internet through which I will send it out, and (to revert to older technology) the worldwide postal system through which I will convey a hard copy. What is true of the rest of life is of course true of medicine. Beyond a certain age, most of us owe our existence and our continued vigor to some achievement of medical technology. And what is true in a major way of general medicine is to a significant degree true of psychiatry.

Newer medications have continued to expand our armamentarium of psychotropic agents; and while the decade of the brain, the 1990s, did not fulfill its promises of neuroscientific breakthroughs, neuroscience continues to promise ever more technological advances for the field.

As I suggested earlier, the role of technology, when thought of as a set of physical tools, remains highly ambiguous in the field of psychiatry. We continue to do a lot of old-fashioned talking in our clinical work, but we also prescribe pharmacologic agents—and we debate the merits of each. If your bias is on the side of psychotherapy, the fact that our arsenal of technical tools is pretty scant compared to the rest of medicine is not a problem. But if you emphasize technological advancement, you may experience the field as suffering from a deficiency state—an inferiority complex in relation to the rest of medicine. Other doctors have magnetic resonance images, colonoscopes, surgery, radiation, and countless other physical instruments, while all we can offer as technical instruments are medication and occasional electroconvulsive therapy (ECT). The tension then becomes whether to make the field more technological, or to see the urgency to increase our technology as a betrayal of the humanistic dimension of our specialty.

In this chapter I shall address in our field what others address on a more global scale: how to benefit from the technological order that defines modern society without turning ourselves into technological beings.

Technology in psychiatry has in fact several sides or faces, of which I will emphasize three: technology as tools of treatment, technology as method of investigation, and finally technology as a way of thinking, the technical attitude.

The first face of technology in psychiatry is that of its tools (physical tools of treatment as in the earlier given preliminary definition, but also tools in a broader sense of both diagnosis and treatment). The primary physical tool of psychiatry is psychotropic medication, and this brings us into the familiar territory of technological products as they pervade contemporary life in our conquest of air, earth, and illness. This aspect of technology most obviously reflects the view of technology as dominating our lives and our sense of ourselves (Ellul 1964; Marcuse 1968; Winner 1986). For a critical perspective on the conquests of technology I rely on the work of philosopher Albert Borgmann, who describes the tendency of these conquests to mutate into commodities, as well as the way in which technological advance moves toward a picture of our lives *as lived* by commodities, as dominated by an endless quest (indeed, greed) for ever more technological *things*. Such analysis leads to further description of how the commodities begin to redefine our sense of ourselves. Prozac in this sense is not just a technological advance; it becomes a commodity which we cannot do without.

A second face of technology has to do with reality as it is revealed by technological instruments of investigation. With this dimension of technology the real becomes that which is made visible through the lens of technology. With our advancing imaging technology we probe ever deeper into the structures of the brain. To state it rather simply, the disordered brain circuit as revealed with the instruments of neuroscience becomes the *real* in psychiatry. But even at a more superficial level, the psychiatrically real becomes that which can be seen, the symptom, and especially that which can be measured. Disorders and treatments are reduced to what can be defined by diagnostic criteria and what can be mapped out on a scale. At this level, data are the real in psychiatry. Philosopher Don Ihde is our guide in this section.

With the final face of technology in psychiatry, I take a step back from the first two aspects of psychiatric technology and approach technology more broadly as a way of thinking, a way that is inherent in the technological approach to life—what I call technical reason and what has also been called instrumental reason. For a sense of technical reason you need only think of Francis Bacon's naïve and optimistic conviction that the modern era would witness the mastery of the material world through the wonders of technological inventions.

The technical attitude, or technical reason, is very pervasive in psychiatry. In view of psychiatry's limited results in these other two areas—technological products and technologically acquired information—it's not surprising that the field has emphasized this core aspect of technology, technical or technological thinking. If we don't have that many treatment tools and not much to show for our neuroscientific research, we can at least claim to think and work technologically in our scientific and clinical interventions.

For the analysis in this section I turn back to Aristotle and forward to his contemporary heirs, Stephen Toulmin and Hans-Georg Gadamer (the latter taking off from his mentor Heidegger's analysis of technology), to supply a philosophical background to our understanding of the technical way of thinking.

In the final section of the chapter I try to integrate the accomplishments of technology into the humanistic core of our discipline. We should be able to benefit from the achievements of technology without turning our field into a toolbox of technological products.

TECHNOLOGICAL TOOLS IN PSYCHIATRY

A first face of technology in psychiatry is that of technological achievements. Although official psychiatry continues to promise technological advances in therapeutics (Insel and Cuthbert 2009; Miller 2010; National Institutes of Mental Health (NIMH) 2008, 2010a, 2010b), our technological toolbox remains rather threadbare, especially when compared to the rest of medicine. While general medicine can claim coronary bypass, organ transplants, in vitro fertilization, and countless other interventions, we are reduced to a modest list that includes psychotropic medications and ECT, somewhat experimental modalities like repetitive transcranial magnetic stimulation (rTMS), vagus nerve stimulation, deep brain stimulation, and finally the computer-enhanced modalities such as computerized therapy and long-distance therapy. Certainly at this time our main technological accomplishment is psychopharmacology, and for that reason I begin this discussion with psychiatric medications. Since Albert Borgmann has provided the philosophical critique of technology most applicable to psychopharmacology, I focus on his analysis in this section.

Psychopharmacology and the device paradigm

In his first contribution to the philosophy of technology, *Technology and the Character of Contemporary Life* (Borgmann 1984), Albert Borgmann introduced the concept of the device paradigm, understood broadly to describe the way in which our contact with the natural world has been altered by the technological devices that mediate and facilitate our control of the world. For Borgmann these devices are inherently ambiguous: on the one hand they assist our control of a recalcitrant physical world; on the other hand they stand between us and a direct contact with the world. The concept is best understood through examples, which are readily available. We have replaced the function of heating our houses through open hearths with a thermostat, which controls an out-of-sight furnace. We have replaced the procurement of water from a well with the spigot, which produces water from heaven knows where with the turn of the hand. The CD replaces a direct contact with music, and the microwaving of frozen dinners replaces the experience of preparing the food (not to speak of the experience of growing it).

Other features characterize the device paradigm. We are interested in the product, not the process that generates it. Further, the process—the device—becomes both invisible and incomprehensible. If the house is cold, we flick the thermostat, with no thought or aware-ness of the mechanical process taking place behind the scenes to produce the heat. And if asked about that process, most of us will have only the crudest understanding of how the heat production actually works. Borgmann summarizes these features with the notion of *commodity*. Heat, water, food, music become commodities which we expect technological machines to provide for us.

We now question how well the device paradigm assists us in understanding the technol-ogy of psychopharmacology. Can we understand Prozac from the perspective of the device paradigm? To what degree can we analyze Prozac the way we analyze a thermostat?

First, we can agree on the obvious point that pharmacology is a technology, a technologi-cal tool. Prozac is a product of applied science to achieve an end. The end, we say, is the relief of depression or anxiety. To state the procedure in the crudest fashion, we say, take the pill and you'll feel better. The commodity here is well-being, relief of depression. The device is the pill. When the patient (or the doctor) is working under this paradigm, relieving depres-sion with Prozac is like making the house warmer through adjusting the thermostat. In both cases, the device is invisible or hidden. The average homeowner doesn't see or know how the heat is produced (except through a vague idea of furnaces burning oil), and the patient doesn't know how the Prozac works to relieve depression (except at times though vague, imaginary notions of serotonin deficiency). We need to add with regard to this latter point that in the case of Prozac the experts share the ignorance of the patient. Although they know more neuroscience that the patient, they also don't understand exactly how antidepressants work.

For Borgmann, the problematic effect of the device paradigm is that it changes one's rela-tion to the natural world, and in doing so alters one's sense of oneself. Something similar, albeit much more complex, may happen with psychotropic agents. Namely, they also may alter our sense of ourselves. Of course, if one is depressed it is perfectly reasonable to see oneself as a biological organism whose depression will be ameliorated with the technologi-cal product, Prozac, just as a diabetic will benefit from an appropriate pharmacologic treat-ment. The problem occurs if one stops seeing oneself as a whole, embodied human being with a problem for which part of the treatment is the pharmacologic agent, and instead starts to see oneself as a malfunctioning technology machine whose malfunction (symptoms) can be fixed with the right technological intervention. In that scenario, the patient presents as a broken object (or broken, mindless organism), and the psychiatrist takes out the psychiat-ric repair manual and applies the technical, pharmacologic fix. This is of course stating the problem overly starkly, but in clinical practice we see do patients treating their psychologi-cal distress in this manner all too frequently.

In his effort to find a corrective for the problems of the device paradigm, Borgmann develops his notion of "focal things," experiences such as walking and running, gardening, and preparing family meals, all of which put us back into contact with the natural world. They are all experiences that are not mediated by technological devices. For Borgmann, this is a way of balancing the benefits of technology with activities that keep us in touch with the unmechanized, natural world.

The application of "focal things" to psychiatry is again complex. It certainly involves resisting the tendency to view ourselves only as technological things or mindless organisms, in need of the technological fix or the happiness-commodity provided by the pharmacological agent. It includes a complex awareness by both patient and psychiatrist of the patient as a person who is both mind and body—a unity that we by no means fully understand—and for whom psychotropic agents work through the body to assist the mind, and regarding whom, finally, the use of such agents does not define him or her as a mechanical or biological thing.

More concretely, one obvious application of Borgmann's "focal things" to psychiatry is psychotherapy. The combination of psychotherapy and psychopharmacology represents an integration of technology and the humanistic dimension of psychiatry. The use of the two treatment modalities together bespeaks at attitude on the part of both clinician and patient that the latter is a complex unity of mind and body—and embodied mind, or more simply, a person. Other examples of "focal things" in the treatment context would be group and occupational therapy, as well as the non-verbal therapies such as art therapy, movement therapy, and meditation—all designed to help the patient become re-engaged in the world, as opposed to seeing himself as a depressed, inert blob waiting to be fixed with the magic pill.

Other somatic treatments

Among somatic treatments other than psychotropic medications, ECT has the longest history and the biggest track record of therapeutic success; rTMS, vagus nerve stimulation, and deep brain stimulation are newer physical modalities with limited evidence for efficacy and uncertain futures. What is notable about these therapeutic modalities is that they are used for patients with severe degrees of psychiatric illness for whom psychotherapy is of minimal benefit (at least in that stage of their illness), and that, in addition, their use in any event would often render the patient unable to engage in psychotherapy. In the context of this discussion, then, they represent situations in which the somatic, technological intervention is doing most of the therapeutic work. I say "most" because, as in any serious medical treatment, there is always an important role for the clinicians and other professional staff to support the patient through the treatment.

With these somatic treatments we leave Borgmann and the device paradigm behind. Patients requiring ECT or another of the somatic treatments are usually depressed to a point that reflecting on the treatment as a device paradigm and the patient as a consumer of commodities doesn't make much sense.

Information technology and electronic communication

In this discussion of technological products, we need finally to consider the developing role of information technology and electronic products in psychiatry. The list of computer-assisted and electronic tools for diagnosis and treatment is rapidly expanding, with both technologically assisted diagnosis and treatment as well as multiple tools for online self-diagnosis and treatment, self-help groups, and psycho-education (Carey 2010; Cavanaugh and Shapiro 2004; Iseminger and Theobald 2009; Kobak et al. 1997; Kruger 2009; Newman et al. 1999; Proudfoot 2004; Rothbaum et al. 1995; Wright and Wright 1997). With this emergence of electronic and computer technologies, we should also keep in mind older non-computer-based technologies such as psychological and neuropsychological testing, as well as other non-electronic diagnostic assessment tools.

One of the striking features of the current literature on technologically implemented diagnostic and therapeutic instruments is that the news is all positive. In a representative statement, showing both the enthusiasm for a computerized diagnostic instrument, as well as the ambiguities surrounding use of the instrument, Kobak writes:

> In the current study patients were more willing to admit symptoms of certain psychiatric disorders to the computer than to the primary care physicians. Rates of alcohol abuse in primary care patients were twice as high on the computer as rates obtained by either the clinician administering the SCID or the primary care physician conducting the PRIME-MD; rates of obsessive-compulsive disorder were 3 times as high on the computer as rates obtained by the primary care physician. (Kobak et al. 1997, p. 910).

He then goes on to write:

> Whether this reflects clinician underdiagnosis of these disorders or an overdiagnosis of these disorders by computer cannot be determined from our data. However, low rates of clinician detection of these disorders has traditionally been a problem. The sensitivity, specificity, and positive predictive value of the computer for these disorders were high, indicating a high level of accuracy. Clearly, the computer offers a way to identify disorders that would have been missed in routine practice. On the other hand, computer rates of panic disorder were half of the rates obtained by the primary care physician and one fourth of those obtained by the SCID. Reasons for this discrepancy is (*sic*) not apparent, and requires further investigation. (Kobak et al. 1997, p. 910).

The statement is interesting and revealing in that the author persists in his enthusiasm and advocacy for the diagnostic instrument despite the fact that the study itself imposes serious questions as to its accuracy and worth. Should we, for instance, conclude that the instrument works well for obsessive-compulsive disorder (OCD) but poorly for panic disorder, or should we conclude rather that the dramatic discrepancy between OCD and panic disorder poses larger questions about the use of the instrument until we have understood and corrected the obvious flaws in the instrument? In general, we can conclude that such instruments offer much potential but require much more research. Some will certainly have a place in the psychiatry of the future, but which instruments they will be, and what will be their place, is at this time all quite unclear.

In concluding this section on computer technology in psychiatry, I wish to give special attention to direct communication, with both voice and video, through the computer. Through the use of Skype and other similar technologies, clinicians can conduct live therapy (and of course supervision or any other communication) over any distance. In the case of Skype therapy we are not talking about a research modality whose efficacy is being studied and evaluated; rather, we are talking about a technological modality that is being used with an increasing frequency (Hoffman 2011). Certainly the most dramatic use of this technology is the China American Psychoanalytic Alliance (CAPA n.d.; Osnos 2011; Wan 2010). The program is an effort to introduce psychoanalysis and psychoanalytically oriented therapy, as well as training in psychoanalytically oriented therapy, to a Chinese professional audience that has not had the opportunity for any serious exposure to psychoanalytic theory and practice. In this program, full psychoanalyses and intensive therapies are conducted by American psychoanalysts and analytically oriented therapists on Chinese patients in China. The program also includes Skype supervision and educational courses for Chinese therapists.

The advantages of Skype communication are obvious. One significant advantage is that it allows basic psychiatric treatment at a distance, and thus the potential for reaching individuals with no access to psychiatric care. Another advantage is that it is not vulnerable to many of the objections and drawbacks to computerized treatment. That is, the patient is in the "presence" of a real clinician and not talking to a robot. Finally, from a philosophic perspective, Skype communication, unlike many other electronic modalities, does not drive treatment to focus on the symptom; the therapist can integrate symptom and meaning in the same manner she does in the office encounter.

These advantages stated, questions remain, and as in the case of other computerized modalities, research is needed (Cartriene et al. 2010). Obvious questions requiring research are, on the one hand, how successfully does distance psychotherapy replicate face-to-face treatment, and on the other hand, what are the clinical and ethical limitations in treating a disturbed patient with long-distance treatment when the treatment includes medications as well as psychotherapy?

Technology as Investigative Tool in Psychiatry

A second face of technology has to do with reality as it is revealed by technological instruments. With this dimension of technology the real becomes that which is made visible through the lens of technology. In psychiatry, we experience the technological lens at a variety of levels. At a surface level, the psychiatrically real becomes that which can be seen, the symptom, and especially that which can be measured. Disorders and treatments are reduced to what can be defined by diagnostic criteria and or can be mapped out on a scale. Once again we witness the orientation of technology to the symptom. On a completely different level, with our advancing imaging technology, we probe ever deeper into the structures of the brain, and in this psychiatry of the future, the psychiatrically real becomes what is revealed by neuroscience.

The philosopher who has worked most intensively on this aspect of technology is Don Ihde, and in this section I invoke his work (Ihde 1990, 1991, 1993). In contrast to Heidegger (1976), who interpreted technology globally as the way in which being is disclosed in the modern era, Ihde focuses on particular technological artifacts as making possible particular aspects of world-disclosure (Verbeek 2001, p. 123). The telescope, to take a simple example, is not just an exemplar of technology as the modern self-disclosure of being; it is a technological instrument that allows us to see aspects of the world previously unavailable to our natural vision.

Starting from the core question of the phenomenological tradition in philosophy—the subject–object, or human–world, relationship—Ihde studies the mediating role of technology, or technological instruments, in that relationship. In wearing my eyeglasses, for instance, I still have a visual, perceptual relationship to my world, but it is mediated—and enhanced—through the use of my glasses.

Ihde distinguishes different forms of technological mediation. The most straightforward kind of mediation—exemplified in the earlier example of eye glasses—is the *embodiment relation*: "*embodiment relations* are uses of technologies which enhance (and non-neutrally *transform*) our perceptual-bodily experience of an environment or world" (Ihde 1993, p. 111). In this form of technological mediation I am relating to my world in the usual way, e.g., seeing, but with the aid of the instrument. A more complex level of mediation is the *hermeneutic relation*. In this form the instrument does not simply enhance my usual relation to the world. The instrument is not obvious or transparent, as in a pair of eyeglasses. Rather, the instrument provides a representation of the world that must be interpreted. The world is not perceived through the instrument but by means of it. A simple example is the thermostat, which we have invoked in another context. I do not experience heat in the thermostat; I interpret numbers and switches on the thermostat in their relation to the heating of my house. Again, my relationship to the world is mediated, but not in the straightforward manner of eyeglasses. "The object is still being referred to, but is now translated into a dial reading which indicates some more abstract (and thus more reduced) aspect of the object, such as weight or heat. And the process requires a special reading skill which knows how the instrument refers" (Ibid, 112). Finally, Ihde moves from these straightforward forms of technological mediation to a third level in which technology mediates the entire background of our life-world (Ihde 1990). At this level he recognizes a concordance with Borgmann's notion of living our life through technological commodities.

Surface instruments of investigation

It is easy to find psychiatric examples of the first two mediating instruments. A psychiatric equivalent of the embodiment relation, the eyeglasses, is the interview format and symptom checklist that I have trained myself to use. I see the patient and speak with the patient, but what I see emerges from a dialectic of question and response, all somewhat controlled by the psychiatric lens I bring to the encounter. My vision is attuned to the symptom checklist, and my questions (and the patient's responses) follow from that.

Another variation on this kind of mediation is the DSM (*Diagnostic and Statistical Manual of Mental Disorders*) diagnoses and criteria lists—and of course the manualized interview formats directed toward making the correct DSM diagnosis. Again, these instruments direct the interviewer toward asking appropriate symptom-related questions that lead to a DSM diagnosis. The psychiatrically real becomes what is listed in the manual and what is revealed in and through the diagnostic criteria to warrant one of the official diagnoses. The manual with its criteria both assist in making the diagnosis but at the same time determine what will count *as* a diagnosis (Phillips 2002; Sadler 2005).

For a straightforward example of the hermeneutic relation, we can go to the symptom inventories, such as depression, anxiety, and psychosis inventories, that result in a score. The score is like a dial; a higher score represents, for example, a more severe case of depression.

Let us bear in mind that the efficacy of pharmaceuticals—and therefore one of the foundations of evidence-based psychiatry—is based on these inventories. The routine for proving the efficacy of, say, a new antidepressant is to administer an inventory such as the Hamilton Depression Rating Scale (HAM-D) or Beck Depression Inventory (BDI) at the onset and later points of the randomized controlled trial and to show that the scores of the new medication separate off from either placebo or other known antidepressants. The entire process depends on the interpretation of the inventory scores as an accurate reflection of the patient's degree of depression. In Ihde's terms, those scores now hermeneutically "represent" the depression. Thus the hermeneutic relation. It would technically be more accurate to report that the candidate antidepressant has successfully lowered subjects' inventory scores, as opposed to reporting that it demonstrated efficacy as an antidepressant (Geddes and Harrison 1997; Sacket 1997).

Finally, we have a dramatic example of hermeneutic mediation in the proposed incorporation of dimensional measures into DSM-5. The measures will take a number of forms: severity scales for individual disorders, complicated measures for the personality disorders, and "cross-cutting" measures that cut across disorders. Regarding the importance of these measures, Regier and colleagues have written:

> The single most important precondition for moving forward to improve the clinical and scientific utility of DSM-5 will be the incorporation of simple dimensional measures for assessing syndromes within broad diagnostic categories and supraordinate dimensions that cross current diagnostic boundaries. Thus, we have decided that one, if not the major, difference between DSM-IV and DSM-5 will be the more prominent use of dimensional measures in DSM-5. (Regier et al. 2009)

Here we certainly have a triumph of Idhe's hermeneutic technological mediation in the new DSM.

Deep instruments of investigation

For examples of Ihde's third level of technological mediation, we move to the deeper level of scientific understanding of psychiatric phenomena through the evolving fields of genetics and neuroscience. It is a given of this work that, as in the rest of medicine, further understanding involves biological science, in this case brain science, and that, for instance, we won't achieve scientific understanding of psychiatric disorders if we limit ourselves to a discipline such as psychology. Predictably, this will drive us again to an understanding in terms of symptoms and behavioral manifestations of psychiatric disorders, as opposed to understanding in terms of meaning structures.

A starting point for this discussion is the recognition that, following two decades and more of intense investigation in genetics and neuroscience, we have little to show for our efforts, leaving us with the conclusion that psychiatric entities are far more complicated than we anticipated. They are, after all, intimately connected to the brain, which is by far the most complicated organ of the body. Thus the 1990s, the decade of the brain, did not fulfill its expectations, and a decade later we are still trying to approach those expectations.

In a recent article in *Science*, "The future of psychiatric research: Genomes and neural circuits" (Akil et al. 2010), Akil and colleagues reviewed the current state of psychiatric research and proposed a working plan for the future. They note both the enormous burden—in terms of suffering and cost—of psychiatric illnesses, as well as the fact that "there have been no major breakthroughs in the treatment of schizophrenia in the last 50 years and no major breakthroughs in the treatment of depression in the last 20 years" (p. 1580). They attribute this lack of progress to the complexity of the brain and argue that this situation "calls for a new perspective and a combination of novel tools and analytical methods" (p. 1580).

The authors note that psychiatric disorders are likely the result of disruptions of neural circuits that may happen in many ways. Further, these disruptions are in turn caused at least in part by thousands of genes working and malfunctioning in a great variety of ways. The consequence of this complexity is that we should not expect to discover, for instance, that a condition such as schizophrenia will exhibit one pattern of disordered circuitry caused by one simple genetic pattern. Rather, we should expect that the psychiatric condition—the phenotype—will be the end point of a great variety of genetic and neural circuit combinations. The authors hasten to add that "This does not mean, however, that these diseases are not genetically based and transmitted, nor does it suggest that the search for genetic causes will be fruitless" (Akil et al. 2010, p. 1580). After all, there is family aggregation of psychiatric illnesses, schizophrenia showing an identical-twin concordance of 50% and autism 80%. On the other hand, we have to expect that one family's genetic mutational profile may be different from another's, and that further, one family's—or one patient's—dysregulated circuitry may be different from another's. There will then not be one phenotype for schizophrenia, but many, consistent with the phenotypic heterogeneity we actually see.

For the future, the authors foresee progress coming from the use of two powerful sets of tools. On the one hand we are able to sequence the complete genomes of afflicted families and individuals at increasingly lower cost. On the other hand we have already located areas of neural circuitry dysregulation for a number of psychiatric conditions, and we have increasingly sophisticated tools for studying such circuits. The use of these two sets of tools together, in both animal models and humans, should significantly advance our understanding of major psychiatric disorders. The authors estimate a cost of a billion dollars to analyze 100,000 personal genomes over the next ten years, and an equivalent amount for analysis of the neural circuitry. They conclude that "Two hundred million dollars a year, the sum of monies that will be needed, is a very small price to pay to reduce or eliminate the awful misery and burden to society caused by mental illness" (Akil et al. 2010, p. 1581).

The program proposed by Akil et al. is in fact being launched by the National Institutes of Mental Health in the USA (NIMH 2008, 2010a, 2010b; see also Cuthbert and Insel 2010; Hyman 2007; Insel et al. 2010) in its Research Domain Criteria (RDoC) project. The group has tentatively identified five "constructs" or "domains of function," each chosen because of existing evidence that the domain is bound by a particular neural circuitry.

The RDoC research framework can be considered as a matrix whose rows correspond to specified dimensions of function; these are explicitly termed "Constructs," i.e., a concept summarizing data about a specified functional dimension of behavior (and implementing genes and circuits) that is subject to continual refinement with advances in science. Constructs represent the fundamental unit of analysis in this system, and it is anticipated that most studies would focus on one construct (or perhaps compare two constructs on relevant measures).

Related constructs are grouped into major Domains of functioning, reflecting contemporary thinking about major aspects of motivation, cognition, and social behavior; the five domains are Negative Affect (aka Negative Emotionality or Negative Arousal), Positive Affect, Cognition, Social Behavior, and Arousal/Regulatory systems. The columns of the matrix represent different classes of variables (or units of analysis) used to study the domains/constructs. Six such classes have been specified; these are genes, molecules, cells, neural circuits, behaviors, and self-reports. Circuits represent the core aspect of these classes of variables—both because they are central to the various biological and behavioral levels of analysis, and because they are used to constrain the number of constructs that are defined. Investigators can select any level of analysis to be the independent variable for classification (or multiple levels in some cases, e.g., behavioral functioning stratified by a genetic polymorphism), and dependent variables can be selected from multiple columns. (National 2010a, p. 2)

In the context of this chapter, we need to bear in mind that the entire RDoC project is premised on a thoroughly biological model of psychiatry that views psychiatric disorders in terms of brain dysfunction. As Insel and the NIMH group write:

RDoC classification rests on three assumptions. First, the RDoC framework conceptualizes mental illnesses as brain disorders. In contrast to neurological disorders with identifiable lesions, mental disorders can be addressed as disorders of brain circuits. Second, RDoC classification assumes that the dysfunction in neural circuits can be identified with the tools of clinical neuroscience, including electrophysiology, functional neuroimaging, and new methods for quantifying connections *in vivo*. Third, the RDoC framework assumes that data from genetics and clinical neuroscience will yield biosignatures that will augment clinical symptoms and signs for clinical management. Examples where clinically relevant models of circuitry-behavior relationships augur future clinical use include fear/extinction, reward, executive function, and impulse control. For example, the practitioner of the future could supplement a clinical evaluation of what we now call an "anxiety disorder" with data from functional or structural imaging, genomic sequencing, and laboratory-based evaluations of fear conditioning and extinction to determine prognosis and appropriate treatment, analogous to what is done routinely today in many other areas of medicine. (Insel et al. 2010, p. 749)

If RDoC represents the psychiatry of the future, we are indeed moving toward a notion of the psychiatrically real as that which can be revealed by the technological instruments available to us.

TECHNICAL REASON IN PSYCHIATRY

Technical reason is not the technology of treatment tools like medications, and not a technology of discovery as in neuroscience, but rather the way of thinking that is inherent in the technological approach to life. We should note that the technical attitude pervades the two faces of technology described earlier. For instance, the tendency of both medications and neuroscientific findings to focus on symptoms and reduce the patient to a fixable thing is a prime example of the work of technical reason. Analysis of technical reason (also referred to as instrumental reason) has a long history beginning with Aristotle, and for that reason I will briefly review the tradition of analysis that begins with him.

Technical reason

What, then, is technical reason? The technical perspective is rather simple to understand.

To get an immediate grasp on it you simply have to imagine the technology of any artifact—washing machine, automobile, computer—in our everyday material world. We start with a body of generalized knowledge that includes an explanation of how the artifact works and directions for fixing it when it is not working properly. In this arrangement the individual problem is always an example of a general problem, not a unique problem that requires a unique, highly individualized intervention. A malfunctioning spark plug is simply a malfunctioning spark plug; the solution is to clean it or replace it. From this point of view, knowledge is essentially instrumental, organized into means/ends structures; any problem can be analyzed in a way that allows for a means/ends formulation and a formulaic solution. The competent technician is the person who can diagnose the type of problem and apply the appropriate remedy. Issues like the personality of the technician drop out of this equation.

It is not difficult to grasp the application of this approach to medicine and psychiatry. The patient's problem is an example of condition A, which requires the application of treatment B. The physician is the technician whose skill is in recognizing the patient's presenting symptoms as examples of condition A and in knowing how to apply treatment B. In this model of the physician, his or her job is not that different from technicians of other fields. It's a short step to viewing medical care from the metaphor of the repair manual (Phillips 2002, p. 77).

Three aspects of this technical approach to diagnosis and treatment in psychiatry need to be emphasized, the first relating to the treatment situation, the second to the treater, and the third to the patient. Regarding the first, the technical approach places emphasis on the general type of problem, not on its particular instantiation; the emphasis is on the diagnostic category and not on the individual patient. We focus on questions like, how do I diagnose and treat schizophrenia, as opposed to, how do I think about and treat this patient as more than an instance of a type. In the terminology of the instrumentalist formula, the end is the diagnosis and treatment of schizophrenia; the means is the treatment modality that works for this general disorder. Variations among individual schizophrenic patients are accorded importance only to the extent that they can be aggregated into subgroups of the general type.

A second aspect of the technical approach is that the generalized, instrumentalist approach to treatment reduces the individuality of the treater, who is now a technician applying the appropriate treatment principles. We now have the generic psychiatrist doing generic treatment, in the same manner that a generic physician can treat a case of pneumonia with the appropriate antibiotic and accomplish the treatment goal. Examples of generic psychiatry abound. In psychopharmacology we have treatment algorithms to direct the "evidence-based" treatment of whatever condition. For the talking therapies we have treatment manuals for the competing treatment approaches. Such modalities as cognitive behavior therapy (CBT), dialectical behavior therapy, and interpersonal psychotherapy are favored because they are readily manualized, but there are also manuals for the more traditional psychodynamic therapies. Of course the fact that these manuals offer competing approaches to treat the same conditions represents a crack in the technical paradigm, which would dictate one technically correct treatment approach for each psychiatric disorder.

The third aspect of the technical approach has to do with the identity of the patient. Who, indeed, *is* the patient of such technically based treatment? The patient is a bearer of symptoms, something simpler and more objectified than a person with a unique, individual history, whose symptoms are seen in a complex, narrative web of that history. If we allow all the complexity of the individual history into our account, it becomes difficult to view the patient through a simple technical lens and difficult to apply a generalized treatment (Phillips 2003).

When the technical attitude prevails, the patient is thus seen as an aggregate of symptoms and behaviors. The principle of coherence is simply the tendency of symptoms and behaviors to aggregate together, often in the clusters described in the diagnostic manual. In medicine this is the so-called syndrome. Philosophically, this is psychiatry at its most nominalist. The disorder is simply whatever fits a particular symptom criteria set. If a deeper law of coherence is sought than that of symptom aggregation, it is that of the patient as organism, of the psychiatric disorder as a biological condition expressing itself in external manifestations in the way the measles virus expresses itself in the typical rash.

Contemporary medicine and psychiatry provide us with a vivid illustration of all three aspects of technical reason, namely the highly popular evidence-based medicine (EBM—or EBP, evidence-based psychiatry) (Cooper 2003; Geddes and Harrison 1997; Maier 2006; Sackett et al. 1996; Williams and Garner 2002). In the context of this discussion, EBP illustrates all the aspects of a technical, instrumentalist approach as described earlier. It targets the general problem, e.g., depression, not the patient in his or her individuality; it turns the clinician into a technician, the generic psychiatrist treating the generic patient; and it reduces the patient—the person—to a cluster of symptoms in need of a fix. EBP points to both the advantages and the limitations of a technically based approach to treatment. In general it proceeds in a straightforward manner. Frame your questions carefully and then use available evidence to answer the questions. Evidence is sought in randomized controlled trials (RCTs), and the greater the number of RTCs on which a clinical decision or treatment modality is based, the more reliable is that decision or treatment modality. In this treatment paradigm, meta-analyses of RCTs are at the summit of high-quality evidence, and the opinion of the individual practitioner at the bottom.

The argument for EBP is obvious: make decisions based on the best available evidence. What then are the arguments against it? They are never that it is invalid, only that it is limited and overvalued. To begin with, EBP requires validity of psychiatric diagnoses and works best when making basic psychopharmacological decisions: What is the best medication for this diagnostic condition? But proponents of EBP tend to overestimate the validity of psychiatric diagnoses and underestimate the complexity of those supposedly simple questions. For instance, for most psychiatric conditions requiring pharmacologic treatment, we have a great variety of choices—choices of both class of medication and of which medication from within the class. At times the choice of medication is straightforward, but at other times, as with the refractory patient, the choice is quite complex. In these latter situations the treatment algorithms offer only very limited guidance, and the (hopefully experienced) practitioner makes a decision how to proceed in this particular case. Thus the treatment decision falls to the person at the bottom of the EBP scale, the practitioner. It is not surprising that experienced clinicians take the treatment algorithms of EBP with a grain of salt. They are aware that the algorithms offer basic guidance and protect against egregious mistakes, but they are also aware that the algorithms will often fail them in the trenches of clinical practice.

Philosophical analysis of technical reason

I begin the philosophical analysis of technical reason with Aristotle and carry his analysis into the present with two of his contemporary students, Stephen Toulmin, working out of the analytic tradition, and Hans-Georg Gadamer, working out of the phenomenological tradition. Each of these contemporary philosophers follows Aristotle in contrasting technical reason with practical reason. In this chapter I will focus mainly on Toulmin's analysis.

In the *Nichomachean Ethics* Aristotle distinguishes: (1) technical knowledge, *techné*, which is concerned with the process of making something, *poïesis* and (2) practical knowledge, *phronēsis*, which is concerned with action and living well, *praxis*. The master of a technique has a firm idea of the thing to be made and is able to work from this clearly held idea to the production of the object. The idea of the completed object can be understood separately from the means, the *techné*, of producing it. Aristotle's model for *techné* and *poïesis* is the skilled craftsman, who possesses expertise in the principles governing his particular area of production, such as house-building. This is an expertise that has a strong theoretical component—a knowledge of cause and effect in the particular area—and that can be taught to other potential craftsmen.

Practical knowledge or *phronēsis* is sharply contrasted with the theory-laden expertise of *techné*. Concerned with action and the question of how to live well, practical knowledge is bound to the particular situation and the unique challenges it poses. The particular situation is an area in which unvarying universal principles are not available that will dictate what is to be done. The general principle is there for guidance, but in each circumstance it will be applied—and indeed understood—somewhat differently. Practical knowledge cannot be simply taught—or learned from a manual; it is learned through experience, for which there is no substitute. Aristotle writes:

> Practical wisdom on the other hand is concerned with things human and things about which it is possible to deliberate; for we say this is above all the work of the man of practical wisdom, to deliberate well … Nor is practical wisdom concerned with universals only—it must also recognize the particulars; for it is practical, and practice is concerned with particulars. This is why some who do not know, and especially those who have experience, are more practical than others who know. (Aristotle 1941, 1141b, pp. 1028–1029)

It is of interest that Aristotle's frequent example of practical knowledge is medicine. For him the physician does not work with fixed, invariable, universal truths but must modify the general principle always to fit the particular clinical situation (Gadamer 1993/1996).

Aristotle's distinction between technical and practical knowledge was at the origin of all future discussion of the distinction between theory and practice, or theory and experience. With the transformation of knowledge and epistemology in the seventeenth century, a transformation we associate with the names of Descartes and Galileo, Aristotle's technical knowledge was assimilated into modern rationalism (and what I am calling technical reason), and the role of practical knowledge or experience was devalued into the category of unreliable subjective opinion.

We have had to wait until the twentieth century for a full rehabilitation of Aristotle's practical knowledge. In the analytic tradition the origins of technical reason have been traced by Stephen Toulmin. In *Cosmopolis* (Toulmin 1990) and especially *Return to Reason* (Toulmin 2001) Toulmin describes the early decades of the seventeenth century as a pivotal period in which, for a variety of historical and social reasons (the Thirty Years' War being prominent among them), the thinking public reacted strongly against the broad humanism and skepticism of the sixteenth century and longed for a kind of knowledge that would be certain and reliable. Galileo supplied a method and Descartes gave it a full philosophical articulation. Through the use of geometric and mathematical analysis, nature could be understood with the rigor of mathematical certainty.

As Toulmin traces this intellectual history, seventeenth-century rationalism abrogated the distinction between "rationality" and "reasonableness," two forms of thinking or argumentation with which thinking people were comfortable in previous times. Certain methods of inquiry and subjects were seen as philosophically serious or "rational" in a way that others were not. As a result, authority came to attach particularly to scientific and technical inquiries that put those methods to use. Instead of a free-for-all of ideas and speculation—a competition for attention across all realms of inquiry—there was a hierarchy of prestige, so that investigations and activities were ordered with an eye to certain intellectual demands. Beside the *rationality* of astronomy and geometry, the *reasonableness* of narratives came to seem a soft-centered notion, lacking a solid basis in philosophical theory, let alone substantive scientific support. Issues of formal consistency and deductive proof thus came to have a special prestige, and achieved a kind of *certainty* that other kinds of opinions could never share. As time went on, academic philosophers came to see literary authors like Michel de Montaigne—an essayist who had little use for "disciplines" and put equally little reliance on formal logic—as not being philosophers at all, let alone scientists (Toulmin 2001, p. 15).

Toulmin traces this discussion back to Aristotle and to the subsequent fate of his ideas. On the one hand the development of modern science required a rejection of Aristotelian science (the Copernican revolution in astronomy and Galileo's analysis of motion are the two immediate examples). On the other hand, seventeenth-century rationalism also, and without warrant, dismissed Aristotle's distinction between theoretical and practical knowledge, his forerunners of Toulmin's rationality and reasonableness. For Aristotle, different subject matters require different styles of thinking. While mathematics allows for universal, context-free principles, questions about how to live require practical knowledge (*phronēsis*). Practical knowledge involves generalities or "universals," but these are always context-dependent and subject to reformulation to fit the particular occasion. In dealing with human behavior we use generalities of the sort: "in this kind of situation, people will usually act in such-and-such a manner." As Toulmin reminds us, "in real-life situations, many universals hold generally rather than invariably. So, in medicine and other human disciplines, we must remember the difference between the general factual assumptions that support 'reasonable' arguments in the practical arts, and the 'rational' deductions that are the stock-in-trade of mathematically formulated theories" (Toulmin 2001, p. 111).

For Toulmin, the legacy of seventeenth-century rationalism is thus a general disparagement of Aristotelian practical knowledge. "The idea that all the practical arts owe a debt to the skills Aristotle calls *phronēsis* was not especially welcome to rational-minded thinkers in the modern period" (p. 114). Toulmin is clear that medicine is one of the "practical arts" that fit into Aristotle's category of practical knowledge (following Aristotle's own of medicine to that category). It certainly makes sense to include psychiatry with general medicine as a practical art. The conclusion from this analysis is that medicine (and psychiatry) are left with two choices: accept the debased status of the other practical arts, or switch categories and try to demonstrate your status as a full science. In this chapter I have tried to show psychiatry's effort to gain scientific respectability through its adoption of the standards of scientific, technical thinking. The treatment algorithms and manuals that should be useful *aids* in practice are inflated into the *science* of practice, and the consequence is a dumbed-down psychiatry with a patina of science.

Without drawing it out in detail, I end this section by pointing out that an analysis similar to that of Toulmin has been carried out in the Continental tradition, by Hans-Georg Gadamer, following the analysis of modern technology by his mentor, Martin Heidegger. Heidegger initiated a major interpretation of the history of technology with his argument that modern technology is not simply the technical application of science but rather a mind-set that precedes modern science and that views the world as a storehouse of materials for human use (Heidegger 1976). His student Hans-Georg Gadamer made the connection of the Heideggerian analysis of technology as technical reason with Aristotles' analysis of theoretical and practical knowledge and carried out an analysis of modern rationality similar to that of Toulmin. Working in an entirely different tradition, Gadamer develops an extensive analysis of hermeneutics as the unique method of the "human sciences" (the *Geisteswissenschaften*) as opposed to the methodology of the "natural sciences" (the *Naturwissenschaften*). He associates Aristotelian *phronēsis* with hermeneutics, and he makes the same connection as does Toulmin between practical knowledge and medical illness and treatment (Gadamer 1960/1975, 1993/1996; see also Dunne 1993; Phillips 2002a, 2002b).

The Role of Technology in Psychiatry

The cardinal theme of this chapter is the role of technology in psychiatry, and with that the balance between technological and non-technological aspects of the field. I have analyzed the role of technology from three perspectives—technology as tools of diagnosis and treatment, technology as instruments of investigation, and technology as a way of thinking. In each perspective we have noted the tendency of technology to drive psychiatry toward an identity as a brain-based science and practice, with an emphasis on symptoms, symptom clusters, and technically based somatic treatments. The exceptions to this generalization regarding treatment are, on the one hand, treatments that are technically based but not somatic (e.g., CBT and manualized psychotherapy), and treatments in which technology may actually facilitate a mind-based treatment modality (e.g., Skype psychotherapy).

A number of related forces have come together to promote the technical hegemony in psychiatry. These include the resurgence of the medical model with a biomedical understanding of psychiatric disorders, the rise and dominance of neuroscience, the recent successes of psychopharmacology, the pressures from governmental and insurance agencies to view psychiatric conditions as technically and pharmacologically fixable illnesses, and finally the prominence of the DSMs as technically oriented classification systems (Phillips 2002). The combined effect of all these forces is to view psychiatric disorders as biologically based symptom clusters which are sensitive to technical, primarily pharmacologic, interventions, and to view the patient as the mindless symptom cluster as described earlier (Eisenberg 1986).

What we are searching for is a balance in which we can benefit from the achievements of technology without reducing our specialty to an exclusively technical enterprise, with a cadre of psychiatric mechanics fixing a population of broken patients. The earlier discussed effort to associate medicine and psychiatry with Aristotelian practical knowledge represented the search for an older tradition in which the technological and the non-technological dimensions of psychiatry could be properly balanced. In the concluding paragraphs I will approach the question of balance of two ongoing discussions in psychiatry: the first involving how we understand the concepts of mind and brain, the second how we view the roles of psychological and somatic treatments. Of course brain and somatic treatments lend themselves to understanding in the terminology of technology, while mind and psychology veer toward a non-technological understanding.

Regarding the first discussion, the tendency of technology to drive psychiatry toward an identity as a symptom-based, biological, brain science and practice is illustrated in the title of a report in *Science* on the RDoC: "Beyond DSM: Seeking a brain-based classification of mental illness" (Miller 2010). This title accurately reflects the statement quoted earlier by the NIMH group that "RDoC classification rests on three assumptions. First, the RDoC framework conceptualizes mental illnesses as brain disorders" (Insel et al. 2010, p. 749). This position is hardly new. In a 1989 article entitled "Biological psychiatry: Is there any other kind?" (Guze 1989), Guze argued strongly for a biological psychiatry:

> The nature and development of mental functions is the centre of psychiatric interest, just as the nature and development of bodily functions generally are the centre of medical interest. Psychiatry is a branch of medicine, which in turn is a form of applied biology. It follows, therefore, that biological science, broadly defined, is the foundation of medical science and hence of medical practice. The other disciplines can and must make their contributions, but they cannot displace biology from its critical role. (p. 319)

Although Guze argues for a clear grounding of psychiatry in the biological sciences, he does find a place for psychotherapy. It is, however, supportive and rehabilitative psychotherapy, not different from the psychotherapy that has a place in the treatment of any medical condition. He remains skeptical about psychological therapies premised on notions of psychological causes of psychiatric illness.

Similar views can be found in others arguing strongly for psychiatry as a biological science, on par with other medical sciences (Detre 1987; Detre and McDonald 1997; Kandel 1998, 1999). As with the newer generation of biological psychiatrists espousing the RDoC project, it is difficult to know what these researchers mean when they speak of letting psychology and psychotherapy in through the back door of biological psychiatry.

These writers keep their focus on the brain, as that keeps them squarely in the territory of biology. For an example of a biologically oriented psychiatrist who is comfortable talking about mind, I invoke Nancy Andreasen, who writes:

> Psychiatry is the medical specialty that studies and treats a variety of disorders that affect the mind—mental illnesses. Because our minds create our humanity and our sense of self, our specialty cares for illnesses that affect the core of our existence. The common theme that unites all mental illnesses is that they are expressed in signs and symptoms that reflect the activity of mind—memory, mood and emotion, fear and anxiety, sensory perception, attention, impulse control, pleasure, appetitive drives, willed actions, executive functions, ability to think in representations, language, creativity and imagination, consciousness, introspection, and a host of other mental activities. Our science explores the mechanisms of these activities of the mind and the way their disruption leads to mental illnesses. When disruption occurs

in syndromal patterns in these multiple systems of the mind, we observe disorders that we diagnose as dementias, schizophrenias, mood disorders, anxiety disorders, or other mental illnesses. Our specialty is defined by our patients, our science, and our history, not by the form of treatment provided (e.g., psychotherapy, medications), nor by the presence or absence of known mechanisms of illness. Psychiatry is defined by its province: the mind. We are fortunate to have chosen to explore such interesting territory. If psychiatry deals with diseases of the mind, does it also deal with diseases of the brain? Unequivocally, yes. What we call "mind" is the expression of the activity of the brain. "Mind" is our abstract term that refers to mental functions such as memory or mood, while "brain" is the neural assembly of molecules, cells, and circuits that produce those functions. (Andreasen 1997a, p. 592)

While Andreasen does not—understandably—answer the larger philosophical questions of the relation of mind and brain, what she does accomplish is to invoke the mind–brain distinction to point to mind as the distinctive province of psychiatry. Treating depression is different from treating pneumonia or amyotrophic lateral sclerosis. Psychiatry is not general medicine, and it is not neurology—although it will overlap with both in countless ways. This chapter is not the place to engage the vast topic of mind and brain, although it is worth pointing out that the current "embodied mind" research is pushing that discussion forward (see, e.g., Damasio 1994; Thompson 2007). In the context of this chapter, however, we can agree that technology partners better with brain than with mind.

The question of mind and brain as conflicting and complementary foci for psychiatric attention leads naturally into the further question of the respective roles of psychotherapy and somatic treatments. In overly simple terms, pharmacotherapy is on the side of a brain and technology based psychiatry, and psychotherapy is on the side of a mind-based, non-technology based psychiatry. The goal we are striving for is of course a reasonable, patient-based combination of the two—a psychiatry that is, in Leon Eisenberg's terms, neither mindless nor brainless (1986).

Psychotherapy is interesting in that, despite the many efforts to transform it into a technology, it resists such efforts and at its core remains a treatment modality that stubbornly resists the dictates of technical reason. In this it is exemplary of Aristotelian practical knowledge, with a persistent focus on the individual patient. Whatever the differences among the many different psychotherapies, the most basic feature they share in common is that all involve a meeting of at least two individuals and the capacity of the one to have a therapeutic effect on the other. In psychotherapy the patient does have an interior life that is like that of no other. There is no alternative but to treat him or her as the individual he or she is. What makes psychotherapy so insistently a form of practical knowledge is that the clinician cannot treat the patient merely as a type without destroying the therapy itself.

We don't really know why and how psychotherapy works. We are able to identify ingredients of the psychotherapy process, ingredients such as understanding, sympathy, suggestion, authority, positive regard, interpretation, insight. Probably most psychotherapies involve some combination of all of these, and any particular psychotherapy will involve more of one than another. Part of psychiatry or psychotherapy as practical knowledge will be the experienced expertise in knowing when to apply more of one ingredient and when more of another—when, for instance, understanding is important and when a show of authority might be helpful (cf. Shedler 2006 for a contemporary review of this process).

But if psychotherapy is not a technology, it should not be brainless. Whatever we mean by mind and brain, we are both; and psychiatric treatment very commonly involves both psychotherapy and pharmacotherapy. With the latter, the treatment assumes a technological dimension; and in good treatment there is no conflict between the technological and non-technological dimensions.

Conclusion

The subject of this chapter has been the place of technology in psychiatry, and the challenge has been to delineate the current role and effects of technology in our field—both present and future. To say the obvious, we neither want a psychiatry that is nothing but technology, nor a psychiatry that does not take advantage of what technology can offer. Our goal remains that of finding the right balance.

As has been evident in this chapter, the binary of the technological and non-technology in psychiatry can be mapped onto binaries: biology and psychology, mind and brain, medication and psychotherapy, diagnosis and patient, theory and instantiation, general and individual, technical and practical reason. These binaries are not precisely isomorphic with each other, but all contribute to evaluating the role of technology in psychiatry, both in the present and in the desired future.

References

Akil, H., Brenner, S., Kandel, E. R., Kendler, K. S., King, M.-C., Scolnick, E., *et al.* (2010). The future of psychiatric research: genomes and neural circuits. *Science*, *327*, 1580–1.

Andreasen, N. (1997a). Editorial: What is psychiatry? *American Journal of Psychiatry*, *154*, 591–3.

Aristotle (1941). Nichomachean ethics. In R. McKeon (Ed. and Trans.), *The Basic Works of Aristotle*, pp. 927–1112. New York, NY: Random House.

Borgmann, A. (1984). *Technology and the Character of Contemporary Life: A Philosophical Inquiry.* Chicago, IL: The University of Chicago Press.

Carey, B. (2010). In cybertherapy, avatars assist with healing. *The New York Times*, November 22.

Cartriene, J. A., Ahern, D. K., and Locke, S. E. (2010). A roadmap to computer-based psychotherapy in the United States. *Harvard Review of Psychiatry*, *18*(2), 80–95.

Cavanaugh, K. and Shapiro, D. (2004). Computer treatment for common mental health problems. *Journal of Clinical Psychology*, *60*(3), 239–51.

China American Psychoanalytic Alliance (CAPA). (n.d.). [Website.] Available at: <http://www.capachina.org/CAPA/Home.html>.

Cooper, B. (2003). Evidence-based mental health policy: a critical appraisal. *British Journal of Psychiatry*, *183*, 105–13.

Cuthbert, B. and Insel, T. (2010). The data of diagnosis: New approaches to psychiatric classification. *Psychiatry*, *73*(4), 311–14.

Damasio, A. (1994). *Descartes' Error: Emotion, Reason, and the Human Brain.* New York, NY: Penguin Putnam.

Detre, T. (1987). The future of psychiatry. *American Journal of Psychiatry*, *144*, 621–5.

Detre, T. and McDonald, M. C. (1997). Managed care and the future of psychiatry. *Archives of General Psychiatry*, *54*, 201–4.

Dunne, J. (1993). *Back to the Rough Ground: 'Phronesis' and 'Techne' in Modern Philosophy and in Aristotle*. Notre Dame, IN: University of Notre Dame Press.

Eisenberg, L. (1986). Mindlessness and brainlessness in psychiatry. *British Journal of Psychiatry*, *148*, 497–508.

Ellul, J. (1964). *The Technological Society*. New York, NY: Vintage Books.

Gadamer, H. -G. (1975). *Truth and Method* (J. C. B. Mohr, Trans.). New York, NY: Continuum Press. (Original work published 1960.)

Gadamer, H. -G. (1996). *The Enigma of Health: The Art of Healing in a Scientific Age* (J. Gaiger and N. Walker, Trans.). Stanford, CA: Stanford University Press. (Original work published 1993.)

Geddes, J. R. and Harrison, P. J. (1997). Closing the gap between research and practice. *The British Journal of Psychiatry*, *171*(9), 220–5.

Guze, S. B. (1989). Biological psychiatry: Is there any other kind? *Psychological Medicine*, *19*, 315–23.

Heidegger, M. (1976). The question concerning technology. In D. Krell (Ed.), *Martin Heidegger: Basic Writings*, pp. 283–318. New York, NY: Harper & Roe.

Hoffman, J. (2011). When your therapist is only a click away. *New York Times*, September 23.

Hyman, S. E. (2007). Can neuroscience be integrated into the DSM-V? *Nature Reviews Neuroscience*, *8*, 725–32.

Ihde, D. (1990). *Technology and the Lifeworld: From Garden to Earth*. Bloomington, IN: Indiana University Press.

Ihde, D. (1991). *Instrumental Reason: The Interface between Philosophy of Science and Philosophy of Technology*. Bloomington, IN: Indiana University Press.

Ihde, D. (1993). *Philosophy of Technology: An Introduction*. New York, NY: Paragon House.

Insel, T. and Cuthbert, B. (2009). Endophenotypes: bridging genomic complexity and disorder heterogeneity. *Biological Psychiatry*, *66*(11), 988–9.

Insel, T., Cuthbert, B., Garvey, M., Heinssen, R., Kozak, M., Pine, D. S., *et al.* (2010). Research domain criteria (RDoC): Toward a new classification framework for research on mental disorders. *American Journal of Psychiatry*, *167*(7), 748–51.

Iseminger, K. and Theobald, D. (2009). Philosophical considerations of an Internet-enabled telephone and computer psychiatric symptom monitoring system: Maintaining the balance between subjectivity and objectivity. In J. Phillips (Ed.), *Philosophical Perspectives on Technology and Psychiatry*, pp. 215–30. Oxford: Oxford University Press.

Kandel, E. (1998). A new intellectual framework for psychiatry. *American Journal of Psychiatry*, *155*(4), 457–69.

Kandel, E. (1999). Biology and the future of psychoanalysis: A new intellectual framework for psychiatry revisited. *American Journal of Psychiatry*, *156*(4), 505–25.

Kobak, K. A., Taylor, L. H., Dottl, S. L., Greist, J. H., Jefferson, J. W., Burroughs, D., *et al.* (1997). A computer-administered telephone interview to identify mental disorders. *Journal of the American Medical Association*, *278*(11), 905–10.

Kruger, R. (2009). The assessment of emotional awareness: Can technology make a contribution? In J. Phillips (Ed.), *Philosophical Perspectives on Technology and Psychiatry*, pp. 249–62. Oxford: Oxford University Press.

Maier, T. (2006). Evidence-based psychiatry: Understanding the limitations of a method. *Journal of Evaluation in Clinical Practice*, *12*, 325–9.

Marcuse, H. (1968). *One Dimensional Man*. Boston, MA: Beacon Press.

Miller, G. (2010). Beyond DSM: seeking a brain-based classification of mental illness. *Science*, *327*, 1437.

National Institutes of Mental Health (2008). *National Institute of Mental Health Strategic Plan. U.S. Department of Health & Human Services, NIH Publication No. 08-6368*. Bethesda, MD: National Institutes of Mental Health.

National Institutes of Mental Health (2010a). *From Discovery to Cure: Accelerating the Development of New and Personalized Interventions for Mental Illnesses. Report of the National Advisory Mental Health Council's Workshop: 31.* Bethesda, MD: National Institutes of Mental Health.

National Institutes of Mental Health (2010b). *NIMH Research Domain Criteria (RDoC)*, pp. 1–5. Bethesda, MD: National Institutes of Mental Health.

Newman, M. G., Andres, J. C., and Taylor, C. B. (1999). Palmtop computer program for the treatment of generalized anxiety disorder. *Behavior Modification, 23*, 597–619.

Osnos, E. (2011). Meet Dr. Freud: Does psychoanalysis have a future in an authoritarian state? *The New Yorker*, January 10, 54–63.

Phillips, J. (2002). Managed care's reconstruction of human existence: The triumph of technical reason. *Theoretical Medicine, 23*, 339–58.

Phillips, J. (2002). Technical reason in the DSM-IV: An unacknowledged value. In J. Z. Sadler (Ed.), *Descriptions & Prescriptions: Values, Mental Disorders, and the DSMs*, pp. 76–95. Baltimore, MD: Johns Hopkins University Press.

Phillips, J. (2003). Psychopathology and the narrative self. *Philosophy, Psychiatry, & Psychology, 10*, 313–28.

Proudfoot, J. G. (2004). Computer-based treatment for anxiety and depression: Is it feasible? Is it effective? *Neuroscience and Biobehavioral Reviews, 28*, 353–63.

Regier, D. A., Narrow, W. E., Kuhl, E. A., and Kupfer, D. J. (2009). The conceptual development of DSM-V. *American Journal of Psychiatry, 166*(6), 645–50.

Rothbaum, B. O., Hodges, L. F., Kooper, R., Opdyke, D., Williford, J. S., and North, M. (1995). Effectiveness of computer-generated (virtual reality) graded exposure in the treatment of acrophobia. *American Journal of Psychiatry, 152*(4), 626–8.

Sacket, D. L. (1997). Evidence-based medicine. *Seminars in Perinatology, 21*, 3–5.

Sackett, D. L., Rosenberg, W., Gray, J. A., Haynes, R. B., and Richardson, W. S. (1996). Evidence based medicine: What it is and what it isn't: It's about integrating individual clinical expertise and the best external evidence. *British Medical Journal, 312*, 71–2.

Sadler, J. (2005). Technology. In *Values and Psychiatric Diagnosis*, pp. 327–58. Oxford: Oxford University Press.

Shedler, J. (2006). *That was then, this is now: An introduction to contemporary psychodynamic therapy.* Available at: <http://www.psychsystems.net/Publications/Shedler/Shedler%20%282006%29%20That%20was%20then,%20this%20is%20now%20R8.pdf>.

Thompson, E. (2007). *Mind in Life: Biology, Phenomenology, and the Sciences of Mind.* Cambridge, MA: Harvard University Press.

Toulmin, S. (1990). *Cosmopolis: The Hidden Agenda of Modernity.* Chicago, IL: University of Chicago Press.

Toulmin, S. (2001). *Return to Reason.* Cambridge, MA: Harvard University Press.

Verbeek, P.-P. (2001). Don Ihde: The technological lifeworld. In H. Achterhuis (Ed.), *American Philosophy of Technology: The Empirical Turn*, pp. 119–46. Bloomington, IN: Indiana University Press.

Wan, W. (2010). Freud coming into fashion in China. *The Washington Post*, October 11.

Williams, D. and Garner, J. (2002). The case against the 'evidence': A different perspective on evidence-based medicine. *British Journal of Psychiatry, 180*, 8–12.

Winner, L. (1986). *The Whale and the Reactor.* Chicago, IL: University of Chicago Press.

Wright, J. and Wright, A. (1997). Computer-assisted psychotherapy. *Journal of Psychotherapy Practice and Research, 6*(4), 315–29.

CHAPTER 15

··

CURE AND RECOVERY

··

LARRY DAVIDSON

> Medical books … those monuments to nature's fragility and the power of science
> which make us tremble when they treat even the slightest indisposition by indi-
> cating these can bring death in their train, but which accord us complete security
> when they speak of the virtue of the remedies as if we were immortal!
>
> Montesquieu

This quip of Montesquieu is unfortunately just as relevant today as it was when he wrote it
over two hundred years ago. Especially in psychiatry, there has been a history of viewing
serious mental illnesses as pervasive and permanent, and as leading at least to chronic disability if not to premature dementia and death. At the same time, there has been a consistent
search for the single treatment, the "magic bullet," which will make the disorder go away, the
miracle cure that will end the person's and their family's suffering and restore everything to
normalcy, or at least to some appearance of reason. But, as Montesquieu had wryly foreseen,
and as the last decade has provided persuasive evidence of, our science has been relatively
impotent in the face of serious mental illness while nature has proved not to be so fragile.
Following this line of reasoning, I will suggest in this chapter that the field's preoccupation
with finding a cure has blinded it to the reality of recovery in the lives of our patients.

By making such a statement, I am obviously arguing for a meaningful distinction between
the two concepts of cure and recovery.[1] As a noun, "cure" refers to a means of healing or
restoring to health; a remedy; a method or course of remedial treatment; a restoration to
health; or a means of correcting or relieving anything that is troublesome or detrimental.
As a verb, "to cure" means to restore to health or to relieve or rid a person of something
detrimental, like an illness. As a noun, "recovery" refers similarly to restoration or return to
health from sickness, and in this case the two concepts are synonymous. But "recovery" also
means the regaining of something lost or taken away or restoration or return to any former
and better state or condition, and in this sense is a broader term than cure.

For our present purposes, though, it is in their uses as verbs that the more salient differences between the two concepts emerge. As a verb, "to recover" may refer to regaining
health after being sick, wounded, or otherwise detrimentally affected, and in this way appear
to resemble "to cure." But the agent, the source of action, in each case is different. "To cure"

---

[1] All definitions are derived from <http://dictionary.reference.com>.

is something that I can do to or for you. It typically refers to what health care practitioners do to or for their patients. It would be an uncommon expression to say that I cure myself. In contrast, "to recover" typically refers to what the person who has been ill or wounded does himself or herself. I do not "recover" you, but you recover from whatever has happened to you. This shift in the origin of the action of the verb also is evident in the other definitions of "to recover" that include getting back or regaining something lost or taken away; regaining one's strength, composure, or balance; or regaining a former and better state or condition.

What this brief review of definitions suggests is that curing serious mental illnesses is a process in which one person—in this case a doctor—can engage for the benefit of another person—the patient—who then is understood to be restored to a healthy state following the onset of an illness or other troublesome or detrimental condition or event. Recovery, on the other hand, is a process in which one person—in this case a person with a serious mental illness—can engage to regain something lost or taken away, regain a former and better state or condition, or regain his or her strength, composure, or balance. In addition to the difference in agency pointed out earlier, the notion of cure is most commonly applied to cases of medical illnesses while the notion of recovery can be applied across a broader range of phenomena including, but not limited to, such illnesses. Although this chapter will not deal in depth with the philosophical and theoretical issues involved in determining whether or not, or in what ways, serious mental illnesses are in fact medical illnesses, it is important for our present purposes nonetheless to emphasize that for a person to be in recovery does not require him or her to view the condition he or she is recovering from to be an illness.

With this framework established, this chapter will suggest that psychiatry has focused on what psychiatrists can do to cure serious mental illnesses, to a large degree to the exclusion of considering what people with serious mental illnesses can do to recover from the fate that has befallen them. To justify this conjecture, and explore its implications for our understanding and treatment of serious mental illness, we turn to key intellectual figures in the history of psychiatry to discuss what they observed about the nature of these disorders and the various outcomes associated with them. In exploring their perspectives, we identify an intriguing discrepancy that they appear to have stumbled across without either acknowledging or resolving. The discrepancy is this: while we have yet to discover a cure for serious mental illness, many people nonetheless recover from it. In bringing the chapter to a close, we consider the implications of this unresolved discrepancy for future theory, research, and practice.

While somewhat out of chronological order, we begin with the work of Emil Kraepelin and the Bleulers, Eugen and Manfred, prior to returning to their predecessors in Philippe Pinel and Jean Baptiste Pussin. From the moral treatment era of Pinel we then return to our present-day situation. We begin with Kraepelin because his appears to be the most influential legacy in promoting a view of serious mental illnesses as pervasive, permanent, and incurable conditions in the face of which the afflicted individual can do little, if anything, for him- or herself. We begin here in the hope of laying the conceptual foundations for a decidedly post-Kraepelinian psychiatry; a psychiatry which has appeared only in glimpses both prior to and following Kraepelin's publication of his *Textbook of Clinical Psychiatry* at the turn of the twentieth century. Returning to the earlier vision of Pinel, and following the lead of Manfred Bleuler and others, we argue for a psychiatry in which the person's own efforts toward recovery are encouraged and supported while we continue to attempt to understand the nature of these disorders and to search for a cure.

WAS "DEMENTIA PRAECOX"
EVER PREMATURE DEMENTIA?

> Experience shows that [incurable mental infirmity] is by far the most frequent result of dementia praecox. The importance of our diagnosis would therefore consist in this: that we are now able, at the very beginning of the illness, to predict its resulting in a characteristic state of feebleness. (Kraepelin 1904, p. 28)

As appears to be justified by the passage quoted, Kraepelin is credited both with coining the term "dementia praecox" for the condition we now refer to as schizophrenia and with asserting that a prognosis of "incurable mental infirmity" could be established upon an initial diagnosis of this condition. For much of the one hundred years since, and in most quarters of clinical psychiatry, practitioners have followed Kraepelin's lead. As a result, generations of individuals experiencing an episode of psychosis have been told that they will have this illness for the remainder of their lives, that they will need to take psychiatric medications for the same duration, and that they should give up any hopes of ever working, returning to or completing school, marrying, having children, or having any vestiges of a "normal" life (e.g., Deegan 1993; North 1987). Their families, in turn, have been told to grieve the loss of their loved one who would not be returning, either from the distant state hospital to which he or she had been confined or, more recently, from the ravages of this all-pervasive illness that is assumed to result in premature dementia or "feebleness" (Atkinson 1994; Kuipers et al. 1992).

But was this ever actually the case, even with the diagnosis of dementia praecox? In the earlier passage, for instance, note that Kraepelin describes "incurable mental infirmity" as "by far the most frequent result" of dementia praecox. He does not say, that is, that it is the only or inevitable result, as his diagnostic framework would seem to require. After all, it was the presumptive inevitability of the downward course of the disorder that was the primary criterion by which schizophrenia was to be distinguished from manic depression (and which gave it the name of "premature dementia"). This view was asserted unequivocally by Kraepelin at times, as when he used such terms as "invariable" and "permanent," as in the following:

> The complete loss of mental activity, and of interest in particular, and the failure of every impulse to energy, are such characteristic and fundamental indications that they give a very definite stamp to the condition in both cases. Together with the weakness of judgment, they are invariable and permanent fundamental features of dementia praecox, accompanying the whole evolution of the disease. (Kraepelin 1904, p. 26)

But then in the very same paragraph from which the opening passage in this section was taken, he continues:

> The prognosis, however, is really by no means simple. Whether dementia praecox is susceptible of a complete and permanent recovery answering to the strict demands of science is still very doubtful, if not impossible to decide. But improvements are not at all unusual, which in practice may be considered equivalent to cures. (1904, pp. 28–29)

If improvements to such a degree that they may be "considered equivalent to cures" are "not at all unusual," how can the same illness be described as permanent and incurable? This is a contradiction that appears neither to be acknowledged nor to be resolved in Kraepelin's writings. We are left to make sense of it ourselves, and in doing so can consider at least two possibilities.

The first possibility is suggested by the very opening sentences of the chapter on dementia praecox in his *Textbook of Clinical Psychiatry*. There we read:

> Dementia praecox is the name provisionally applied to a large group of cases which are characterized in common by a pronounced tendency to mental deterioration ...
>
> Dementia fortunately does not occur in all cases, but it is so prominent a feature that the name dementia praecox is best retained until the symptom group is better understood. (1907, p. 219)

In this view, dementia praecox is introduced temporarily as a provisional term that is useful in characterizing "a large group," perhaps a majority, of cases of this previously unnamed disease. Even though the name does not appear to apply to all cases of the disease—because there are in fact a smaller number of cases in which people recover—these cases are still to be included under this provisional label until a better understanding of the illness in question can be achieved. What this view does not explain is what important features the incurable cases have in common with the recovered cases that would argue for their sharing a common label in the first place. If, in fact, the defining feature of the illness is that it inevitably leads to premature dementia, then how can cases of recovery be counted as instances of this same illness? The only other features of this illness that Kraepelin describes are features that are also shared by other psychiatric conditions, such as manic depression. If it is the progressive deterioration resulting in premature dementia that differentiates schizophrenia from manic depression, then people who recover should not be counted as having schizophrenia.

Based on this logic, generations of practitioners have since insisted that if people do indeed recover, then they must have been misdiagnosed to begin with. But the possibility of recovery was already acknowledged at the time of the original conceptualization of the diagnosis, as we saw earlier. In his descriptions of the subtypes of dementia praecox, Kraepelin again appeared to contradict his own premise in this way. He writes, for example, that in 8% of the cases of the hebephrenic subtype of dementia praecox "the symptoms of the disease entirely disappear, leaving the patients apparently in their normal condition" (1907, p. 241), while the percentage of full recovery in the case of the catatonic subtype is 13% (1907, p. 256). In the case of the paranoid subtype, he at first insists that "the outcome is always deterioration" (1907, p. 264), but then on the next page we read:

> In some cases the delusions gradually fade, are never expressed, are forgotten or wholly denied, and at the same time there appears some insight ... Or the delusions and hallucinations may be retained, while the patients become quite indifferent to them, and rarely complain of persecutions or show agitation. They are usually capable of employment, and sometimes are even industrious, the "Pope" becoming a trusted farm-hand, and the "queen" a good seamstress. (1907, p. 265)

Nowhere does Kraepelin himself suggest that such people, who appear to recover and return to a normal life, were misdiagnosed with dementia praecox and instead suffered from manic depression or some other disease. Rather, his suggestion appears to be that there are

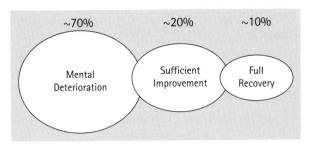

FIGURE 15.1 Various outcomes of dementia praecox as defined by Kraepelin.

"a large number of cases" of what he terms dementia praecox that have a prominent, pronounced tendency to mental deterioration, but that there also are a smaller number of such cases in which full recovery occurs. In addition—and to complicate matters more—there appear to be a larger number of cases which do not suffer mental deterioration but in which a lesser degree of recovery occurs, as when he writes that: "very many patients improve sufficiently so that they are able to return to their homes or to their full liberty" (1907, p. 274). With this further disclaimer, we are left with the picture of the various outcomes of dementia praecox as shown in Fig. 15.1.

If such a wide range of outcomes were possible, why, then, characterize the disease as premature dementia, even if as a provisional label? The second explanation that would have to be added to the first is that whatever important (yet unarticulated) features all of these cases have in common (that allow all of them to be included under the same label), these features must be permanent or lifelong, even if they are not expressed or obvious at any given time. Even when people appear to be recovered, they may still be suffering from dementia praecox without showing any outward signs or symptoms. For example, in the paragraph quoted earlier, following his statement that "very many patients improve sufficiently ..." Kraepelin continues: "But in advising this [i.e., that patients go home or be restored to liberty], one must not overlook the possibility of exacerbations" (1907, p. 274). Similarly, while declaring that the outcome of the paranoid subtype is always deterioration, Kraepelin allows that "remissions in symptoms may occur" (1907, p. 264). How is it that the symptoms can go into remission but the outcome of the illness nonetheless remains one of deterioration? It must be that the illness process itself continues on, even in the absence of symptoms or despite the presence of functional improvements that Kraepelin acknowledged may be "considered equivalent to cures."

At this point, it may strike the reader that we are merely discovering the obvious. We now know schizophrenia to be a chronic condition that may have periodic exacerbations or relapses, do we not? Is not the figure quoted of the various outcomes of dementia praecox consistent with current understandings of the "heterogeneity" in outcome in schizophrenia that has been accepted over the last twenty or so years (e.g., Carpenter and Kirkpatrick 1988)? But to make these simple associations is to miss the point I am trying to make, which is that these accepted truths, these conventional wisdoms, come down to us directly from Kraepelin's interpretations of his observations. By returning to the source, I am raising the question of the validity of these highly influential interpretations. They may seem obvious now, after a century of their practical application, but it is just as possible that these interpretations created the reality we now see in practice as were derived from it.

The question remains: If the person no longer shows any signs or symptoms of the disorder, what makes us think that the disorder is still present? If the person leaves the hospital, lives independently, takes up a job successfully, and no longer appears to be experiencing the detrimental effects of the illness, what justifies the inference that the illness is still there, perhaps being held at bay but nonetheless smoldering under the surface? As Groucho Marx once said: "If it looks like a duck, quacks like a duck, and waddles like a duck, it's probably a duck." What does it take for functional improvements that may be "considered equivalent to cures" to actually be cures? Or, in other words, when does "remission" constitute "recovery"? While this was an issue that Kraepelin apparently was not pressured to resolve, it has since emerged, a century later, as an issue with which clinical research must now come to grips (Andreasen et al. 2005).

The Bleulers

> As the disease needs not progress as far as dementia and does not always appear praecociter, i.e., during puberty or soon after, I prefer the name schizophrenia. (E. Bleuler 1924, p. 373)
>
> On the courses of schizophrenias over many years or decades, only a very one-sided concept was possible, and it was principally inferred from experiences with patients who were permanently hospitalized or who were rehospitalized after intermittent remissions. But nothing was really known about the fates of the great numbers of patients with whom, after their release, the doctor lost contact. (M. Bleuler 1978, p. 412)

And so we turn at this juncture to the work of the Bleulers: Eugen Bleuler, who rejected the term dementia praecox precisely for the reasons given earlier and replaced it with the term schizophrenia, and his son Manfred, who both provides useful perspective on his father's career while also adding his own observations on the courses and outcomes of schizophrenia in people who he, for the first time in the history of psychiatry, purposely and rigorously followed over a significant period of time.

Even though he eventually rejected the term dementia praecox for the reasons given earlier in this chapter, Eugen Bleuler nonetheless continued Kraepelin's legacy of viewing the disease he came to rename as schizophrenia as being a lifelong condition. So, while in discussing the rationale for rejecting dementia praecox, Eugen Bleuler acknowledged that: "This disease may come to a standstill at every stage and many of its symptoms may clear up very much or altogether" (1924, p. 373), he still remained skeptical of the notion of a cure. On this topic he wrote: "A small part is 'cured' to such extent that only a very careful inspection shows any sign of the disease ... Nevertheless there are a great many 'social cures'" (1924, p. 435). In other words, even people who appear to be totally cured will, upon "a very careful inspection," still show some subtle signs of the ongoing presence of the disease (signs which, like Kraepelin's common features, were never articulated).

On the surface, however, many people appeared to be able to function well and no longer demonstrated the more obvious signs or symptoms of the illness. Yet, as with Kraepelin, the fairly common appearance of such people who had attained "social cures" (similar to Kraepelin's "sufficient improvement") did not dissuade Eugen Bleuler from viewing the underlying illness itself to be chronic. The problem here, as it was earlier, was determination of what exactly constituted this underlying chronicity. As Bleuler acknowledged, we do not yet know what it is that is chronic, and even when we think we might have determined a person's course to be chronic based on years of observation, surprises still occur:

> Actual chronic conditions are capable of little improvement; only we do not always know what is chronic. There are patients who for many years are at the same stage of excitement but still give the impression, more or less, of being acute and are then again surprisingly capable of improvements; after ten or twenty years in rarer cases, apparently entirely unsocial patients may be discharged as again capable of work. (1924, pp. 440–441).

Rather than changing the prognosis associated with this condition from which many people seemed to have recovered, Eugen Bleuler came to the somewhat surprising conclusion from his observations of such surprising turnarounds in the course of what he thought to be a chronic illness that there appeared to be very little that practitioners could do to actually treat the condition. While exacerbations, relapses, and remissions might appear to occur in relation to events going on in the person's life (or not), they appeared to have little to do with the action or interventions of the doctor. For this reason, he came to the conclusion that:

> Most schizophrenics [sic] are not to be treated at all, or at any rate outside of asylums. They belong in asylums only when there are special indications … and then especially temporarily for purposes of training. They should be discharged as soon as possible, because later they are gotten rid of much less easily. (1924, p. 443).

By "gotten rid of," Bleuler was commenting on the remarkable speed with which both the patient and his or her loved ones became accommodated to the structure of the asylum, making discharge and return to the family increasingly difficult the longer the person remained confined. Beyond the safety and containment it provided, the asylum was therefore seen as primarily destructive in its influences on the person and the course of his or her illness.

What Eugen Bleuler recommended instead was that the person remain as much as possible in the natural settings in which he or she lived prior to onset, being provided with whatever "training" might be required to function satisfactorily within these settings. As he wrote: "The supreme remedy which in the majority of cases still accomplishes very much and sometimes everything that can be desired is training for work under conditions that are as normal as possible" (1924, p. 443). What facilitated improvement, and at times even (social) cure, was to keep the person engaged in community life and to provide the instruction and guidance he or she needed in order to participate in these activities in a normal manner. Little, if anything, could be done to address the underlying illness, but if something could be done to help the person lead a more normal life despite this, this might nevertheless accomplish "everything that can be desired."

For Eugen Bleuler, then, schizophrenia appeared to be a chronic condition for which no real treatments had been found and for which the influence of the asylum was regressive. Yet many people with this condition appeared to recover from it, some so fully that it required the close inspection of an expert to detect the lingering presence of the condition, and many to the point of achieving social cures which enabled them to function more or less as healthy adults (e.g., living independently, working, etc.). Finally, the best thing that practitioners could do to promote social cures—or, in fewer cases, full recovery—was to provide training in the everyday life activities in which the person engaged in the natural settings where these activities normally occurred.

Given the definitions with which we began this chapter, it is unclear why Bleuler referred to people who experienced significant improvements as representing "social cures." He was convinced that no effective treatments for this condition yet existed and that the only helpful thing practitioners could do was to provide "training" in employment and everyday life activities. It does not appear that practitioners were offering anything that could be considered a "cure," yet many people nonetheless were recovering. At the same time, Bleuler appears for the most part to have continued to believe in the presence of a chronic illness that persisted in the absence of signs or symptoms of the disorder; an illness for which practitioners nonetheless remained the primary responsible party, despite the fact that there was really very little they could do in the way of a cure. In this way, Bleuler appears to have embodied Montesquieu's particular form of folly: attributing fragility to nature, and omnipotence to medicine, when neither were warranted by the facts.

One reason that might account, in part, for why Eugen Bleuler continued this same unjustified tendency that characterized Kraepelin's work has been offered by his son. Himself an observant psychiatrist, Manfred Bleuler noted both the origin and the impact of his father's Kraepelinian expectations of his patients with schizophrenia. He writes:

> From 1886 to 1898, E. Bleuler dedicated himself completely to his community of schizophrenics [sic] as director of the remote psychiatric clinic of Rheinau ... Two decades later, during and after the First World War, he went back to Rheinau to visit about once a year ... His former schizophrenic patients always greeted him warmly and enthusiastically. Much as these greetings pleased him, he usually made the painful observation, "Most of them did seem to have deteriorated." Then, depressed, he would ask, "Is there really nothing that can stop this disease?" If he spent all his life wrestling with the question whether there was an "organic process" at the basis of schizophrenia, it was mainly because of experiences like the above. But E. Bleuler did not know how many improved patients were out for their Sunday walks during his visits, and certainly not how many had been released and were living at home, recovered. (1978, p. 413)

The phenomenon Manfred Bleuler had identified in his father's experience, as well as in "a number of generations of clinical psychiatrists [who] had experiences similar to his" (1978, p. 413), has since come to be described as "the clinician's illusion" (Cohen and Cohen 1984). The clinician's illusion refers to the fact that people who work in clinical settings, such as Eugen Bleuler, tend to see people who are ill when they are most ill and often only when they are ill. They do not have the same exposure to people who are, or *when* they are, well. And if they only see the people who are ill, or only see people when they are ill, they tend to assume that all people with that condition are always sick. What Manfred Bleuler noticed in his father and in the generations of psychiatrists preceding and contemporaneous with him, was that they did not stop to consider that perhaps they were not seeing people who had had that condition but who were well because they were, in fact, doing well (and therefore not in treatment).

Should this be the case, it suggests that the estimates Kraepelin and Bleuler made of the percent of full recoveries and of sufficient improvements/social cures would be underestimates of the true rates of recovery in the broader population of individuals with schizophrenia. For example, Kraepelin might have been prompted to caution us that we "must not overlook the possibility of exacerbations" in patients who had been discharged due to his experiences of some patients being readmitted to his hospital despite what appeared to be "sufficient improvements." But the readmission of a few patients would need to be compared to the number of discharged patients who did not return in a deteriorated state; a figure neither Kraepelin nor Eugen Bleuler ever reported.

It was to begin to get at these kinds of numbers that Manfred Bleuler conducted his own prospective cohort study of 208 people diagnosed with schizophrenia over a span of 27 years. The first study of its kind in the history of the field, Manfred Bleuler's findings provide a stark contrast to those of his father's generation. The findings of this study have since been replicated by numerous investigators in numerous countries across the globe, and have established a very different picture of the course and outcome of schizophrenia from that developed by Kraepelin and ambivalently accepted by Eugen Bleuler.

What did Manfred Bleuler find? In a nutshell, he found that: "after a five-year duration of the illness, schizophrenics [sic] do not generally deteriorate any further. Instead, from then on, tendencies for improvement prevail over tendencies for deterioration" (1978, p. 497). In other words, more people recover from the disorder over time than not, with Kraepelin's end state of mental deterioration being more the exception than the norm. Writes Manfred Bleuler:

> Easily half to three-quarters of all schizophrenics [sic] about ten or more years after onset, attain reasonably stable states that last for many years. Such states then undergo no more dramatic changes … Some two-thirds to three-fourths of schizophrenias are benign, and only about one-third or less are malignant … About one fourth to one third of the 'end states' are long-term recoveries, and about one-tenth to one-fifth are the severe chronic psychoses. (1978, p. 414).

Less than one-third of people diagnosed with schizophrenia will show the classic Kraepelinian course, while the other two-thirds to three-fourths will experience significant improvements over time, many recovering fully. Given that the classic Kraepelinian course was actually only found by Kraepelin himself in a majority, but not in all, cases, we can use these findings to revise the picture we presented in Fig. 15.1 as shown in Fig. 15.2. As mentioned earlier, these findings have since been replicated by numerous investigators in numerous countries, with John Strauss (e.g., Strauss and Carpenter, 1972; Strauss et al. 1985), Courtenay Harding (e.g., Harding et al 1987), and Luc Ciompi (e.g., 1980) being some of the better known.

Having reconsidered Kraepelin's actual observations of the heterogeneity in course and outcome that resulted in Fig. 15.1, we might suggest that Manfred Bleuler's research led simply to revisions in his estimates for the different categories, ranging from severe chronic to full recovery, as depicted in Fig. 15.2. But in the early 1970s, when these data were first

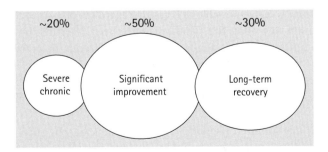

FIGURE 15.2 Various outcomes of schizophrenia as found by Manfred Bleuler.

published, they were viewed against the backdrop of the pervasive set of beliefs and attitudes that had resulted from select sections of Kraepelin's prose rather than from a full appreciation of the richness of his observations. As we showed earlier, patients diagnosed with either dementia praecox or schizophrenia were assumed to have a lifelong illness that would eventually result in mental deterioration—despite the fact that this illness was never fully described and many of these people appeared, at least on the surface, to be functioning well. In the face of this set of beliefs and associated attitudes, it struck Manfred Bleuler that his findings represented more of a "revolution" rather than merely a revision. He wrote that his findings:

> seem revolutionary when compared with the schizophrenic theory of a continuous regressive process toward a state of idiocy. Fortunately this theory has outlived its blossom; although now, as then, it exerts its paralyzing influence on therapeutic initiative, and in its own secretive, insidious way, promotes hopelessness and resignation among doctors, nurses, families, and among the patients themselves. (M. Bleuler 1978, p. 413)

It is worth noting that these findings were being published only a decade or so after the first large wave of deinstitutionalization, during which tens of thousands of former long-stay inpatients were being afforded the opportunity to live on their own in the community, and coincident with the birth of the mental health ex-patient/consumer/survivor movement. Since then, these revolutionary findings have been accepted in some quarters as providing the scientific foundation for a social and political "recovery movement" that is now influencing mental health policy across the globe. Since the beginning of the twenty-first century, an increasing number of countries have embraced the vision of recovery and, in the words of the American policy mandate, "a life in the community for everyone" with a serious mental illness (SAMHSA 2007). This vision has the potential to counteract the effects of the Kraepelinian legacy, thawing and mobilizing previously frozen therapeutic initiative and promoting a more hopeful and determined attitude among practitioners, patients, and their families.

But skepticism remains; the theory of a continuous process in schizophrenia has yet to fully "outlive its blossom." After all, even Manfred Bleuler, despite his own revolutionary findings, continued to refer to his patients as "schizophrenics," suggesting that this condition defined, from the time of diagnosis to the time of their eventual demise, who these people were as people. While many investigators will now concede that schizophrenia does not lead to progressive deterioration resulting in "incurable mental infirmity" in all cases (as the data clearly do not bear this out), they nonetheless still seem to accept Kraepelin's belief that he had identified a disease entity that was life-long in nature and from which it simply was not possible to recover. Regardless of how well the person may appear, regardless of how long the symptoms have been in remission and the person has been able to function, once diagnosed with schizophrenia the person will have that condition for the remainder of his or her life; he or she will remain "a schizophrenic" rather than a person who has recovered from schizophrenia. To the degree to which this belief persists, the revolution Manfred Bleuler believed he was initiating remains to be achieved.

The hypothesis that Manfred Bleuler offered to account for why such a revolution was required was based on a sampling bias which resulted in Kraepelin and his father only seeing patients who had remained in hospitals for long periods of time and/or were repeatedly readmitted with intermittent episodes of disorder, thereby having little to no opportunity to see people who were recovering or had recovered from the disorder. Should this hypothesis be correct, we would expect to find a higher rate of recovery in samples that were not subjected to prolonged hospitalization. These are the samples found post institutionalization, such as in those studies conducted by Strauss and Harding, but we would also expect to find such samples in the era prior to institutionalization, which began in the mid 1800s. It is to this earlier period that we now turn.

Pinel, Pussin, and *"Le Traitement Moral"*

> To consider madness as a usually incurable illness is to assert a vague proposition that is constantly refuted by the most authentic facts. (Philippe Pinel, in his 1794 Address to the Society for Natural History, cited in Weiner 1992, p. 730)

The era that paved the way for the advent of long-term institutionalization has been known as the "moral treatment" era, and its history is relevant to our discussion in two ways.

First of all, and as conveyed in the earlier quote from Pinel, moral treatment clinicians did indeed find a higher recovery rate than Kraepelin or Eugen Bleuler. In fact, they reported a rate of recovery even higher than that found by Manfred Bleuler and more recent studies, with up to 80–90% of persons admitted with what we would now consider a psychotic disorder demonstrating substantial to full recovery (e.g., Bockoven 1956). These numbers have at times been discredited, if not dismissed, by critics who claim that they were inflated and based on misleading methods such as counting each episode as a full recovery even when the person was readmitted at a later time. Such a misrepresentation may have accompanied the marketing of the "lunacy trade" once private retreat and asylum owners began to focus on potential profit margins (Parry-Jones 1972; Scull 1981), but were unlikely to characterize the earlier efforts of the founders of moral treatment. Pinel, in particular, was dedicated to close observation and accurate documentation of his patients' condition, and reports these observations in fastidious detail in the second edition of his *Treatise*. Here he reported that: "there is a probability of 93% that the treatment adopted at the Salpêtrière will be successful if the alienation is recent and has not been treated anywhere else" (1809/2008, p. 167).

Pinel's disclaimer in this estimate of the probability of recovery brings us to the second way in which the moral treatment era is relevant to our present discussion. Note that Pinel is confident of the likelihood of recovery if the onset is recent and the person had not already been treated elsewhere. The issue of recent onset makes intuitive sense, as the shorter the duration of the illness prior to treatment, the more likely is a rapid and full recovery. This intuition of Pinel's has since been supported by a body of research on the duration of untreated psychosis, confirming his suspicion that the longer the illness had been established prior to the person's receiving care the poorer the outcome (e.g., Marshall et al. 2005; Perkins et al. 2005).

But what of his second condition, that the person had not already been treated elsewhere? This was based on Pinel's experience of other asylums and hospitals, which at the time were mostly violent and dehumanizing settings for confinement which, in his opinion, made the illness worse rather than better. As he wrote:

> Public asylums for maniacs have been regarded as places of confinement for such of its member as are become dangerous to the peace of society. The managers of those institutions, who are frequently men of little knowledge and less humanity, have been permitted to exercise toward their innocent prisoners a most arbitrary system of cruelty and violence. (1809/2008, p. 4).

Not surprisingly, what resulted from such cruel and violent treatment in Pinel's opinion were dramatically worse outcomes and an associated belief in the incurability of madness, which asylum managers could then use to justify their system. Contrasting the outcomes produced by such means with those of the moral treatment he espoused, he wrote:

> Prejudice and negligence have led most hospices to accept as a principle the complete incurability of all deranged patients. To achieve this, infallible steps are taken: close confinement, acts of harshness and violence, and the use of chains. In a very small number of properly run hospices it is agreed that this illness can be cured; and, what is better, repeated experience proves this. (1809/2008, p. 154)

Pinel's caution in accepting patients from other hospitals adds a new and important dimension to Manfred Bleuler's insight into the clinician's illusion. Manfred Bleuler had suggested that once mental hospitals had been built and psychiatrists had taken them over, the vast majority of their observations of mental illness came from their experiences within the hospital setting. But once inside of hospitals, practitioners not only primarily saw people who were ill, but they also, and importantly, saw them in environments which only worsened their conditions rather than alleviated their suffering. This was why Eugen Bleuler recommended that people with schizophrenia not be treated in hospital settings unless absolutely necessary, and then for as short a period as possible. In addition to the fact that he followed people after they left the hospital, Manfred Bleuler suggested that another reason why his research documented much better recovery rates than that of his father was because his participants had been fortunate in their "avoidance of ineffective measures" (1978, p. 415). People are more likely to recover if they have only had the illness for a short time *and* if they have not been further compromised by damaging treatment they have received at the hands of others. Even in hospitals that tried to provide the kind of training prescribed by Eugen Bleuler, the assumptions and expectations of chronicity and disability, and resulting culture of despair and hopelessness, were sure to influence how patients envisioned their prospects for, and the degree to which they actively pursued, recovery.

What kind of treatment did Pinel provide in contrast to that of his contemporaries? The medical historian Dora Weiner argues that "it is important to point out" that Pinel's term for his approach, and that of Jean Baptiste Pussin who had been the governor of the Bicetre before his arrival—"*le traitement moral*"—"meant psychological treatment, in contrast to physical treatment … The term should not be translated into the English 'moral' with its connotation of moralizing," she continues, "which the French does not convey" (1979, p. 727). Pinel had not found the somatic treatments of his day to be effective, nor did he believe that any evidence had been provided to establish that mental illnesses were due to irreparable lesions in the brain, which was the conventional wisdom of the day. What he found when he arrived at the Bicetre was an entirely different approach practiced by Pussin and his wife, an approach that stressed non-somatic methods which Pinel described as "prudent management" (cited in Weiner 1992, p. 729). When asked by Pinel to describe what he had found to work best in promoting recovery among the asylum patients, Pussin responded:

> My experience has shown, and shows daily, that to further the cure of these unfortunates one must treat them with as much kindness as possible, dominate them without mistreatment, gain their confidence, fight the cause of their illness, and make them envision a happier future. I have always fought this illness by psychological means and thus known the happiness of some favorable results. (Cited in Weiner, 1979, p. 1133)

In addition to the principles described, the other concrete strategy that Pussin had found most effective was that of engaging the patients in meaningful work. He continued:

> Work, among other things, seems to me almost necessary, not only because it provides for exercise but also because it offers distraction. Work, in fact, belongs to the category of psychological remedies on which I especially insist. (Cited in Weiner 1992, p. 1133)

It is interesting to recall here Eugen Bleuler's comment that the only treatment that appeared to be effective for his patients with schizophrenia was "training for work under conditions that are as normal as possible." It is also interesting to note that even Kraepelin had made a similar observation with regard to patients who did not seem to show improvement otherwise, suggesting that: "An essential feature of the care of these mental shipwrecks is healthful employment, preferably out of doors" (1907, p. 272). There is an impressive degree of consistency between these observations that span centuries about what appears to be useful in enabling people with schizophrenia to experience sufficient improvements in functioning and to achieve social cures. What did not remain consistent over time were expectations of chronicity and the role of the asylum. Pinel and Pussin viewed their prudent management strategies (i.e., non-somatic "treatments") as leading to cures and considered their discharged patients to have recovered. Kraepelin and Eugen Bleuler, on the other hand, viewed their own, primarily somatic, interventions to be largely ineffective and considered their discharged patients as having a chronic and incurable illness, even when no signs of illness or impairment remained.

To see where things stand now, we return to the present day and review what we think we have learned about the nature of serious mental illnesses, their treatment, and recovery over the last half-century.

FROM CURE TO RECOVERY

> Treatments do not "cure" schizophrenia or fully ameliorate symptoms and problems for the majority of affected individuals. (Kreyenbuhl et al. 2010, p. 101)

This conclusion was taken from the overview provided by the team of distinguished investigators who recently completed an update of the PORT (Patient Outcomes Research Team) recommendations for evidence-based treatment of schizophrenia. Having exhaustively reviewed all of the treatment studies published since their last update five years earlier, the authors determined that newer antipsychotic medications are not that much better than the older ones, and that their side effects, while different, are still onerous. Only about 70% of people with schizophrenia will derive any relief from these medications, and their benefits are limited to only one domain of symptoms—i.e., primarily the so-called positive symptoms of hallucinations and delusions—and have little to no impact on the more disabling aspects of the disease (i.e., negative symptoms and cognitive impairments). Psychotherapeutic approaches, while promising, thus far only show an increase in the rate of reduction of the same positive symptoms, from 41% with medications alone to 59% with therapy (Kingdon and Turkington 2005; Zimmermann et al. 2005), having little to no effect on other domains.

Yet, despite the fact that there continues to be no cure, many people with schizophrenia recover. Interventions that have elaborated on Eugen Bleuler's notion of training, which do not aim to cure the illness but rather to enhance functioning, have been shown to have more robust effect sizes and more impact on people's everyday lives than those that aim to cure. Supported employment, for example—which represents our current-day version of facilitating a person's access to meaningful work outside of hospital settings—has been shown to have an average effect size of around 0.85, which is considered to fall in the "large" range of effect sizes and is higher than that for antipsychotic medications (Becker et al. 2007). In five recent investigations that compared supported employment to conventional rehabilitation services, over half of participants in supported employment programs worked competitively versus 18% of those in the comparison groups (weighted mean effect size was 0.79). Those participating in supported employment were about four times more likely than comparison participants to obtain competitive work (Bond et al., 2001). The 0.85 effect size was derived from quasi-experimental studies of converting day treatment to supported employment, in which between 40% and 60% of participants enrolled in supported employment obtained competitive work as compared to less than 20% of those not enrolled (Becker et al. 2007). This kind of "training" remains the most effective intervention for improving functioning in schizophrenia.

These data suggest that the only real breakthrough in the treatment of schizophrenia since the accidental discovery of chlorpromazine in the 1950s—the only real progress that has been made in the last half-century of scientific investigation—has been in finding ways to improve the functioning, and the lives, of people with the disorder. No progress has been made toward finding a cause or a cure, and the interventions that have been shown to work best cannot actually be considered "treatment" at all. Ordinarily considered to fall under the label of psychiatric rehabilitation, the provision of in vivo support that forms the core of all of these interventions may be best considered a prosthesis or a tool that the person with the disorder may use to compensate for impaired domains of functioning. As with a crutch or a wheelchair, this prosthesis may be needed for a shorter or longer period of time, depending on the severity of the illness, the quality of the person–environment fit, and the availability of other strengths and assets that may be used for this purpose. What is clear, though, is that some sizeable percentage of people who have this disorder will recover from it over time. They may be aided in their recovery by the provision of such supports by other people, but also may be impeded in their recovery by the actions and expectations of others who treat them as hopeless cases or "mental shipwrecks." Regardless, while we continue to search for a cause and a cure it is clear that many people recover from this condition without, or even despite, us.

Conclusion

As long as we recognize in the schizophrenic [*sic*] a fellow sufferer and comrade-in-arms, he remains one of us. But when we see in him someone whom a pathological heritage or a degenerate brain has rendered inaccessible, inhuman, different, or strange, we involuntarily turn away from him.—Yet it is so very beneficial to the schizophrenic [*sic*] for us to stay close to him! (M. Bleuler 1978, p. 502)

As long as the causes and cures of serious mental illnesses elude our science, it appears that we are most effective in helping people to live the best lives they can in the face of the illness, rather than in insisting that the illness go away. We have not been successful in our attempts to rid our patients of these illnesses, and, for the roughly one hundred-year period of institutionalization, these efforts resulted only in our society getting rid of the patients instead. It was during this regrettable period that the field became convinced of the incurability of the illness, but, as we have seen, the poor outcomes that were observed had as much to do with the treatments provided as with the illness itself. A question remains as to why, after two centuries of research consistently documenting recovery, this notion of incurability persists.

Manfred Bleuler reminds us that the first, essential step toward being helpful to people with serious mental illnesses is to remain convinced that the person is a "fellow sufferer," that he or she is still "one of us." Attitudes and approaches that view the person with a serious mental illness as somehow qualitatively and permanently other than us have been, and will continue to be, very destructive. Putative discoveries of irreparable organic etiologies have been misguided and misleading, and continue to be contradicted by outcome data. Overcoming this Kraepelinian legacy will require more than the discovery of better medications. It will require expanding our theoretical models, and the scope of our practice, to include the active role people play in truly recovering from the disorder. The only real heroes in the historical review of psychiatry that I have offered here have been the patients themselves. A post-Kraepelinian psychiatry will be more likely to be of use to them if it shifts its focus from what doctors do to the processes of recovery in which they have been engaged, largely on their own, for at least the last two hundred years.

References

Andreasen, N.C., Carpenter, W. T., Kane J. M., Lasser, R. A., Marder, S. R., and Weinberger, D. R. (2005). Remission in schizophrenia: Proposed criteria and rationale for consensus. *American Journal of Psychiatry*, 162, 441–9.

Atkinson, S. (1994). Grieving and loss in parents with a schizophrenic child. *American Journal of Psychiatry*, 151, 1137–9.

Becker, D., Whitley, R., Bailey, E. L., and Drake, R. E. (2007). Long-term employment trajectories among participants with severe mental illness in supported employment. *Psychiatric Services*, 58, 922–8.

Bleuler, E. (1924). *Textbook of Psychiatry* (A. A. Brill, Trans.). New York, NY: The MacMillan Company.

Bleuler, M. (1978). *The Schizophrenic Disorders: Long-Term Patient and Family Studies* (S. M. Clemens, Trans.). New Haven, CT: Yale University Press.

Bockoven, J. S. (1956). Moral treatment in American psychiatry. *Journal of Nervous and Mental Disease, 124,* 292–321.

Carpenter, W. T. and Kirkpatrick, B. (1988). The heterogeneity of the long-term course of schizophrenia. *Schizophrenia Bulletin, 14,* 645–52.

Ciompi, L. (1980). The natural history of schizophrenia in the long-term. *British Journal of Psychiatry, 136,* 413–20.

Cohen, P. and Cohen, J. (1984). The clinician's illusion. *Archives of General Psychiatry, 41,* 1178–82.

Deegan, P. (1993). Recovering our sense of value after being labeled mentally ill. *Journal of Psychosocial Nursing, 31*(4), 7–11.

Harding, C. M., Zubin, J., and Strauss, J. S. (1987). Chronicity in schizophrenia: Fact, partial fact, or artifact? *Hospital and Community Psychiatry, 38,* 477–86.

Kingdon, D. G., and Turkington, D. (2005). *Cognitive Therapy of Schizophrenia.* New York, NY: Guilford Press.

Kraepelin, E. (1904). *Lectures on Clinical Psychiatry* (T. Johnstone, Ed.). New York, NY: William Wood & Company.

Kraepelin, E. (1907). *Clinical Psychiatry: A Textbook for Students and Physicians* (A. R. Diefendorf, Trans.). New York, NY: The MacMillan Company.

Kreyenbuhl, J., Buchanan, R., Kelley, D., Noel, J. M., Boggs, D. L., Fischer, B. A., *et al.* (2010). The 2009 schizophrenia PORT psychopharmacological treatment recommendations and summary statements. *Schizophrenia Bulletin, 36,* 71–93.

Kuipers, E., Leff, J., and Lamb, D. (1992). *Family Work for Schizophrenia: A Practical Guide.* London: Royal College of Psychiatrists.

Marshall, M., Lewis, S., Lockwood, A., Drake, R., Jones, P., and Croudace T. (2005). Association between duration of untreated psychosis and in cohorts of first-episode outcome patients: a systematic review. *Archives of General Psychiatry, 62,* 975–83.

North, C. (1987). *Welcome Silence.* New York, NY: Simon & Schuster.

Parry-Jones, W. L. (1972). *The Trade in Lunacy: A Study of Private Madhouses in England in the eighteenth and nineteenth centuries.* London: Routledge & K. Paul.

Perkins, D. O., Gu, H., Boteva, K., and Lieberman, J. A. (2005). Relationship between duration of untreated psychosis and outcome in first-episode schizophrenia: a critical review and meta-analysis. *American Journal of Psychiatry, 162*(10), 1785–804.

Pinel, P. (2008). *Medico-Philosophical Treatise on Mental Alienation* (G. Hickish, D. Healy, and L. C. Chardland, Trans.) (2nd edn). Oxford: Wiley-Blackwell. (Original work published 1809.)

SAMHSA. (2007). *National Consensus Statement on Mental Health Recovery.* Rockville, MD: US Department of Health and Human Services.

Scull, A. (1981). *Madhouses, Mad-Doctors, and Madmen: The Social History of Psychiatry in the Victorian Era.* Philadelphia, PA: University of Pennsylvania Press.

Strauss, J. S. and Carpenter, W. T., Jr. (1972). Prediction of outcome in schizophrenia: I. Characteristics of outcome. *Archives of General Psychiatry, 27,* 739–46.

Strauss, J. S., Hafez, H., Lieberman, P., and Harding, C. M. (1985). The course of psychiatric disorder: III. Longitudinal principles. *American Journal of Psychiatry, 142*(3), 289–96.

Weiner, D. B. (1979). The apprenticeship of Philippe Pine: A new document, "Observations of Citizen Pussin on the Insane." *American Journal of Psychiatry, 36*(9), 1128–34.

Weiner, D. B. (1992). Pinel's "Memoir on Madness" of December 11, 1794: A fundamental text of modern psychiatry. *American Journal of Psychiatry, 149,* 725–32.

Zimmermann, G., Favrod, J., Trieu, V. H., and Pomini, V. (2005). The effect of cognitive behavioral treatment on the positive symptoms of schizophrenia spectrum disorders: A meta-analysis. *Schizophrenia Research, 77,* 1–9.

SECTION III

ESTABLISHING RELATIONSHIPS

CHAPTER 16

....

INTRODUCTION:
ESTABLISHING
RELATIONSHIPS

....

A cross-disciplinary discussion of the basis of interpersonal relating is of interest to philosophers and psychiatrists for several reasons. The first, and perhaps most important reason, is that psychiatry is chiefly about establishing therapeutic relationship and understanding other forms of life. The history of psychiatry is disseminated with errors, sometimes catastrophic ones, involving forgetting this elementary ethical as well as methodological principle. Diagnostic assessment and therapeutic prescription, the two columns of psychiatric practice, presuppose the clinician's capacity to encounter the patient and to make sense of his experiences, emotions, cognitions and actions. Psychiatric practice without establishing relationship and without attempting to understand the other's mind is not only ineffective—it is iatrogenic.

A second reason for the importance of a philosophical discussion of interpersonal relating is that the development of successful clinical practice may depend, at least partly, on having an accurate understanding of the basic character of unimpaired interpersonal relating because such understanding can shed light on the nature and source of its disturbed forms. How we think about the basis of "mind minding" competencies influences how we think about the prognosis and possible treatment of dysfunctional interpersonal relating.

A third reason is that philosophical frameworks influence the way we think about and evaluate possible psychiatric disorders. Philosophical discussions may be of direct practical importance to psychiatry given that different theories of other-awareness suggest different potential ways of devising therapies. The issue of other-awareness is closely related to self-awareness. This notion is notoriously ambiguous. Chapter 17 ("Varieties of Self-Awareness") by Grünbaum and Zahavi is about self-awareness.

In everyday life, self-awareness is often thought to be a matter of a person thinking about herself. But even that apparently simple definition can cover a variety of very different accomplishments. Consider for instance, the difference between introspectively scrutinizing one's occurrent experience, thinking about one's past performance, anxiously appraising how others perceive one or taking pride in one's ability to fulfil a chosen social role. Grünbaum and Zahavi venture into this theoretical debate, and help us to make sense of the philosophical, psychological, psychiatric, and neuroscientific literature filled with competing, conflicting, and complementary definitions. In their chapter, they argue that explicit (reflective) self-conscious thinking is founded on an implicit (pre-reflective) form of self-awareness built into the very structure of phenomenal consciousness. Their argument is that a theory denying the existence of pre-reflective or minimal self-awareness has difficulties explaining a number of essential features of explicit first-person self-reference, and that this will impede a proper understanding of certain types of psychopathology.

How we think about the basis of "mind minding" competencies—as Dan Hutto argues in his chapter on "Interpersonal Relating" (Chapter 18)—influences how we think about the prognosis and possible treatment of dysfunctional interpersonal relating. Another reason is that philosophical frameworks influence the way we think about and evaluate possible psychiatric disorders and philosophical discussions may be of direct practical importance to psychiatry given that different theories suggest different potential ways of devising therapies. Hutto's chapter is divided into five parts. The first one highlights some basic facts about the complexity and multifaceted character of interpersonal relating and some of its most prominent dysfunctions. The second introduces popular "mind minding" hypotheses which claim that the dysfunctions in question are rooted in impaired capacities for attending to and attributing mental states to others. Part three summarizes recent evidence from cognitive psychology and neuroscience with which these "mind minding" hypotheses must be made compatible. The fourth highlights the important differences between two main philosophical frameworks—frameworks that offer opposing ways of understanding the nature of mind minding capacities. Focusing on these differences, the final part highlights how adoption of these philosophical frameworks matters to thinking about the prognosis and strategies for the treatment of certain mental disorders.

Shaun Gallagher develops some of these issues in his chapter on "Intersubjectivity and Psychopathology" (Chapter 19). He first reviews and discusses mainstream theories of social cognition, namely theory of mind, which characterizes intersubjective relations in terms of the cognitive practice of mindreading. He then introduces so-called "interaction theory" (IT) which involves a shift away from defining the problem of social cognition in terms of mental states hidden away in the mind of the other. This phenomenology-based approach, which borrows from developmental studies of primary and secondary intersubjectivity, emphasizes perceived social affordances and the engaged interactions taking place in our shared, intersubjective world. In developing the basic tenets of IT he clearly explains the concept of "primary intersubjectivity," which refers to perceptual and motor processes that allow newborns to engage with others from birth, and the processes of "secondary intersubjectivity," starting around nine months of age, whereby infants begin to enter into contexts of shared attention and tie actions to pragmatic and social contexts in which they learn what things mean and what they are for. Following the pioneering work of Colwyn Trevarthen, Gallagher explains that in joint attention and joint actions the child looks to the body and the expressive movement of the other to discern the intention of the person or to find the meaning of some object. Children begin to see that another's movements and expressions often depend on meaningful and pragmatic contexts and are mediated by the surrounding world. Others are not given primarily as minds that we encounter cognitively. We perceive them as agents whose actions are framed in pragmatic and socially defined contexts.

Anita Avramides and Nancy Potter further develop the theme of intersubjectivity in their chapters (Chapters 20 and 21). In Chapter 20, "Other Minds, Autism, and Depth in Human Interaction," Avramides suggests that, when considering the problem of other minds, we need to distinguish between "thick" and "thin" versions of it. The "thick" version corresponds to the question, "How do I know that I am not the only mind?" The "thin" one raises the question, "How do I know what another is thinking or feeling?" She discusses Dretske's position, which while acknowledging the thick problem, proposes a perceptual model of our knowledge of other minds that addresses only the thin version. She then considers the "quality" of our interactions with others and, following Wittgenstein, suggests that where individuals share a nature their interactions exhibit a quality that she calls "depth." She concludes that where that nature is not, or is only partially, shared, one might expect to find the quality of the interaction between persons disturbed—as it is the case with child autism.

Nancy Potter explores the "Empathic Foundations of Clinical Knowledge" in Chapter 21. Assuming that clinicians need a rich understanding of empathy, she treats empathy not just as an understanding attitude toward others, but as a moral and epistemic virtue. The reasoning necessary for empathy as a virtue is not abstract and detached; instead, it requires that we think about context, feelings, and social relations in a psychologically rich way—a way that attends to the full subjectivity of others—so as to determine the rightness or wrongness of particular actions. She argues that without empathy the moral agent is unable fully to grasp the moral features of certain situations. Treating empathy as a moral and epistemic virtue commits us to the view that empathetic responses are, at least to some degree, under our control. Following Hodges and Wegner she also distinguishes two kinds of empathies, "automatic" and "controlled" empathy. This clinical characterization of automatic empathy—through which we can take another's viewpoint and experience that person's world with no effort at all—is probably the equivalent to "natural virtue" in Aristotle's sense. But people can also consciously and intentionally produce empathy. This may be called "controlled empathy," matching up with the full virtue in the Aristotelian sense.

Grant Gillett and Rom Harré, in their "Discourse and Diseases of the Psyche" (Chapter 22), discuss (next to empathy) the second column of intersubjectivity. Seeing the human being as a situated individual in relation to others they argue that first and foremost it is "discourse" that creates meaning. They explain that in psychiatry, as elsewhere, meaning depends on the way we pick out events and what is part of them, on how we differentiate the networks in which they make sense, and reconstitute connections between events that show how they engender one another. How we paint the picture of a phenomenon (say, a disorder) shapes our understanding of it. They suggest that a discursive analysis of the subjective body as it is framed in discourse is likely to help us make sense of a wide range of human phenomena as they cause distress and present to a clinic. As examples of this, they take anorexia and hysteria: both can be seen as quasi-moral and interpersonal responses to life events creating insecurity about identity and the possibility of a life lived on your own terms. We can and do address them in terms of developing life skills that equip a person to face challenges that they currently find overwhelming and unable to be met. Following Kristeva and Levinas, they argue that each malady of the soul is unique or particular to a situated person such that the suffering patient, like every other human being, is an enigma. As enigma, every psychiatric patient is the product of a unique history in which are embodied the many and diverse traces of our dealings with him or her and a flesh and blood answer to the question, "Who am I?"

Finally, Giovanni Stanghellini develops these issues, and particularly empathy and the discursive approaches in the clinical context, in Chapter 23, "Philosophical Resources for the Psychiatric Interview." Stanghellini first reviews the basic tenets of mainstream psychiatric interviewing techniques—the so-called technical approach—highlighting their main draw-backs and limitations. Since the psychiatric interview is, first and foremost, a search for symptoms, he then spends considerable time analyzing the different ways of conceptualizing symptoms in the bio-medical, psychodynamic, and phenomenological–hermeneutical paradigms. Then, he describes the *family of dispositives* in use during the interview, that is the first- (subjective), second- (dialogical), and third-person (objective) mode of interviewing. A short history of the discipline of psychopathology, the basic science for psychiatric assessment, introduces three levels of the psychopathological inquiry: descriptive psychopathology, whose main purpose is to systematically study conscious experiences, order and classify them, and create valid and reliable terminology; clinical psychopathology, which is a pragmatic tool for bridging relevant symptoms to diagnostic categories; and structural psychopathology, which assumes that the manifold of phenomena of a given mental disorder are a meaningful whole and searches for meaningful units. The chapter concludes with a phenomenologically- and hermeneutically-informed flowchart for the psychiatric interview.

CHAPTER 17

....

VARIETIES OF
SELF-AWARENESS

....

THOR GRÜNBAUM AND DAN ZAHAVI

INTRODUCTION

....

The notion of "self-awareness" (or "self-consciousness") is notoriously ambiguous.[1] In everyday life, self-awareness is often thought to be a matter of a person thinking about herself. But even that apparently simple definition can cover a variety of very different cognitive accomplishments. Consider, for instance, the difference between introspectively scrutinizing one's occurrent experience, thinking about one's past performance, anxiously appraising how others perceive one, or taking pride in one's ability to fulfill a chosen social role. If one ventures into the theoretical debate, the complexity only multiplies, since the philosophical, psychological, psychiatric, and neuroscientific literature is filled with competing, conflicting, and complementary definitions.

To mention just a few important theories: In developmental and social psychology, prominent theories understand self-awareness as an explicit act of recognizing oneself as a physical and socially embodied individual. Lewis (2003) has, for example, argued that the so-called mirror-recognition task is the decisive test for self-consciousness. And Mead (1962) argued that self-consciousness is a matter of becoming an object to oneself in virtue of one's social relations to others. In psychopathology, it has occasionally been argued by psychologists and psychiatrists that self-awareness requires that one has a theory of mind which one can apply to oneself. For instance, Baron-Cohen and Frith and Happé have all argued that one can test the presence of self-awareness in persons with autism by using classical theory of mind tasks, such as the false-belief task or the appearance-reality task (Baron-Cohen 1989, pp, 581, 591; Frith and Happé 1999, pp. 1, 5).

In philosophy, there seems to be general agreement that we must distinguish between, on the one hand, self-awareness as a form of recognition or identification building on perceptual or testimonial evidence and, on the other hand, non-recognitional and

---

[1] In the following we will be using both concepts synonymously.

non-identificatory forms of self-awareness. Philosophers disagree, however, about how to understand this distinction and what is required for a form of self-awareness to be non-recognitional and non-identificatory. Some argue that in order to be in possession of self-consciousness, one must be able to think of oneself *as* oneself. That is, one must be able to *conceptualize* the distinction between self and non-self (Baker 2000, pp. 67–68). Others argue that for a creature to be self-conscious it is not sufficient that the creature in question is able to self-ascribe experiences on an individual basis without recognizing the identity of that to which the experiences are ascribed. Rather, the creature must be capable of thinking of the self-ascribed experiences as belonging to one and the same self (cf. Cassam 1997).

Another vexed issue in contemporary philosophical discussions is how to understand the relationship between self-conscious thinking (thinking about oneself with a first-person concept) and first-order conscious experience. Again philosophers disagree. Some think that self-conscious thinking requires that there is a minimal (implicit) form of self-awareness built into the first-order conscious experience (cf. Burge 1998; Kriegel 2009; Zahavi 1999); whereas others deny the existence of minimal self-awareness (e.g., Tye 2009, pp. 4–8).

All these issues and discussions about the nature of self-awareness have broader theoretical implications, for example, for our understanding of certain psychopathological phenomena. A number of contemporary debates about psychopathological disorders and symptoms rely on some understanding of ownership and awareness of oneself. In particular, different theories of self-awareness lead us to understand the notion of ownership (of a mental state or conscious experience) in different ways, and, as we will see, this has implications for how to understand a phenomenon like thought insertion. It is our hope that this chapter can contribute to a clarification of the meaning of the fundamental notions of ownership, self-awareness, and self-reference by placing them within a broader philosophical discussion about the nature of consciousness and self-consciousness.

In this chapter, we argue that explicit (reflective) self-conscious thinking is founded on an implicit (pre-reflective) form of self-awareness built into the very structure of phenomenal consciousness. In broad strokes, our argument is that a theory denying the existence of pre-reflective or minimal self-awareness has difficulties explaining a number of essential features of explicit first-person self-reference, and that this will impede a proper understanding of certain types of psychopathology.

REFLECTIVE SELF-AWARENESS:
TWO FORMS OF OWNERSHIP

Paradigmatically, the phenomenon of self-awareness is manifest when we think thoughts that concern ourselves or have beliefs or conceptions of ourselves. Such reflective thoughts and beliefs can vary in many dimensions. Let us here focus on the kind of self-awareness that manifests itself in self-conscious judgments of the form "I am ...," "I think ...," "I see ...," etc.

A person is thinking a self-conscious thought or making self-conscious judgment when she consciously thinks or judges that some property or activity belongs to herself. Some notion of "belonging to the self" or "ownership" is therefore central to a proper understanding of self-conscious thinking and self-awareness in general. In contemporary philosophical literature, we find at least two different notions of ownership being used to describe self-conscious thinking.

The first notion of ownership concerns a particular class of self-conscious thoughts, namely, those made on the basis of information "from the inside," for example, on the basis of introspection. By contrast, a judgment is made "from the outside" if it is based on exteroceptive perception or testimony. Self-conscious judgments "from the inside" are often said to be epistemically incorrigible, in particular they are usually thought to be immune to the error from misidentification (McGinn 1983). By the notion of immunity to error from misidentification (IEM), philosophers have been explaining the fact that when it comes to judgments or avowals like "I am looking at a cup" or "I believe that CO_2 reduction is important," it does not make much sense for the subject of these thoughts to engage in asking who the subject of seeing the tree or believing something about CO_2 really is (Coliva 2006; Evans 1982; Pryor 1999; Shoemaker 1968—but see our discussion of thought insertion). A common explanation of this peculiar form of incorrigibility is to say that when a person does not base her self-conscious judgment on her perceptual or testimonial knowledge of the instantiation of some property in the world, but rather bases it on some immediate familiarity with her own experience or thinking, then her judgment does not involve any identificatory step. Consequently, if the subject is wrong in self-ascribing some property, there will be no possibility of retreating to some initial knowledge of the property being instantiated in some other individual in the world.

The second notion of ownership characterizing self-conscious thinking can be said to be more fundamental. Rather than characterizing only judgments made "from the inside," the second notion concerns all self-conscious thoughts, i.e., thoughts referring to oneself by the use of the first-person concept "I." All judgments making use of the first-person concept share important features (we will return to these features later). Crucially, they are all guaranteed success in actually referring to the subject of thinking (Castañeda 1968). It is impossible to be thinking an I-thought and not be referring to oneself. I can be radically deluded in my self-ascription ("I am the ruler of the universe" or "I am Napoleon") but I am still ascribing the property to myself. If I am thinking that my hand is bleeding or that I am courageous, then there is no possible situation where I could end up actually referring to someone else. I could, of course, come to realize that I am in fact not the person who is bleeding (the bleeding hand belongs to someone else) or the one who is courageous, and I should consequently stop thinking of myself as having the property in question. However, insofar as I am thinking of myself with an "I"-concept I am immune to reference failure.

It is important to distinguish between the notion of ownership characterized by IEM and the notion of ownership involved in the phenomenon of immunity to reference failure. Regardless of whether or not her self-conscious judgment is IEM, the person is referring to herself—the object—in a way that has at least the following constant feature: when a person refers to herself in thinking by an "I"-concept, she knows she is referring to herself and this knowledge makes whatever she is ascribing to herself stand out as something which is significant to her. Just think of the enormous difference there is for a subject between thinking "My hand is bleeding" and "That guy's hand is bleeding," even though in both cases the judgment is grounded on identification on the basis of observational evidence. So, there is something important about the ability to refer to oneself with an "I"-concept which is not captured when talking about IEM.

But what are then the distinctive and necessary features characterizing the second notion of ownership involved in self-conscious thinking (i.e., in thinking "I"-thoughts)? A first point to mention is the crucial difference between referring to oneself with a first-person concept (*I am bleeding from my hand*) and referring to oneself with third-person concept, here defined as everything which is not a first-person concept (e.g., *that guy is bleeding from his hand*—thought when looking in a mirror without realizing that I am looking at myself). We can mark this distinction as one between first-person self-reference and third-person self-reference. Two important things distinguish first-person self-reference from its third-person counterpart.

Firstly, there are epistemic differences. A person cannot think an "I"-thought without understanding and knowing that she is thinking something about herself. When thinking an "I"-thought she is not only necessarily guaranteed success in referring to the right object, she also knows and understands that she is referring to herself and that she could not be referring to anyone else. By contrast, when referring to myself in the third-person mode (by a name, a perceptual demonstrative, or a definite description) there is always the danger that I am in fact referring to someone else or that I do not realize that I am in fact referring to myself (Castañeda 1967; Perry 1977). Thus even in the case where I am referring to myself by some definite description or name, it is possible that I could be thinking about myself without knowing and understanding that I am doing so. By contrast, if you can show that a person who is allegedly thinking an "I"-thought is in fact referring to someone else by her "I" or that she does not realize that she is in fact referring to herself, then you have simply shown that she was not thinking an "I"-thought at all.

Secondly, as already hinted at, there are important motivational differences between first-person self-reference and third-person self-reference in thinking. If I overhear people at work talking about some individual as being "obnoxious, pompous, and a miser," it might not mean much to me and I might not care. But if it dawns on me that they are talking about me and that I am the individual who is "obnoxious, pompous, and a miser," then it should matter a great deal to me and I would care. Ascribing some property to oneself by first-person self-reference thus relates the subject to the property in a special motivational way: in a way that matters to her emotional feeling, thinking, and practical reasoning. This was one of the facts Perry (1979) brought out with his famous example of himself in the supermarket suddenly realizing he was the person leaving behind a trail of sugar.

Drawing a distinction between the fact that *certain forms* of self-conscious thinking are immune to failure from misidentification and the fact that *all forms* of self-conscious thoughts are immune to reference failure, and consequently between two forms of ownership, is important to ongoing discussions of schizophrenia, and in particular of the phenomenon of thought insertion.

Thought insertion is a theoretically puzzling phenomenon. On the one hand, the schizophrenic subject's own thinking becomes alien to her to such a degree that she experiences her own thoughts as not being hers. On the other hand, she can report having the experience of inserted thought and thus have no problem of making first-person self-reference. A quick glance at the literature on thought insertion demonstrates the importance of the two forms of ownership and the distinctive features of self-conscious thinking for a proper understanding of the kind of self-alienation we find in thought insertion.

In an influential 1999 paper on thought insertion, Campbell made the following observation:

> The thought inserted into the subject's mind is indeed in some sense his, just because it has been successfully inserted into his mind; it has some special relation to him. He has, for example, some especially direct knowledge of it. On the other hand, there is, the patient insists, a sense in which the thought is not his, a sense in which the thought is someone else's, and not just in that someone else originated the thought and communicated it to the subject. (Campbell 1999, p. 610)

Not unlike us, Campbell is making a distinction between two forms of ownership of thought. One form of ownership has to do with a thought simply appearing in "my stream of consciousness" (Campbell 1999, p. 621); it is one of which I have "immediate introspective knowledge" (p. 615). This form of ownership refers to the fact that the experiences I am living through are given differently to me than to anybody else. The other form of ownership has to do with whether or not the thinker of the thought "recognize himself to be the agent" (p. 619) or causal origin of the thought. It is in this other sense of ownership (which might also be termed *authorship*) that Campbell thinks that a schizophrenic patient can hold that his thoughts are alien and thought by someone else. According to Campbell, for a schizophrenic person suffering from a delusion of inserted thought, her own thinking can stop being immune to error from misidentification. That is, for such an individual, it makes sense to wonder whether she is really the person thinking this thought (but see Coliva 2002).

Many contributions to the discussion of thought insertion following in the wake of Campbell's (1999) paper have largely accepted his distinction between two forms of ownership. There are, however, what appears to be substantial disagreements about how to understand Campbell's second form of ownership. Broadly speaking, there seems to be three general trends in accounting for the second form, i.e., the type of authorship that is somehow missing in inserted thoughts. One tendency is to think that authorship should be understood in terms of agency or causal source. Some authors consequently think that the lack of authorship in the case of thought insertion should be explained in terms of the breakdown of a particular type of action-control mechanism responsible for the feeling of agency (Gallagher 2000, 2004; Proust 2006). The second trend is to think that the absence of authorship should be explained as a rational reaction to strange thoughts that seem out of sync with the subject's background beliefs and values (Campbell 1999; Stephens and Graham 1994; Vosgerau and Newen 2007). Finally, a third trend has been to understand thought insertion as a kind of withdrawal and utter disengagement from one's own thinking (Hoerl 2001; Young 2006). A further open question is whether the notion of ownership as authorship corresponds to our first form of ownership (characterized by IEM) or is a new form of its own.

Glossing over these disagreements, we can say that there is a way in which the subject's experience and thinking become so alien to the subject that her self-conscious judgments about her own experience and thinking start to resemble judgments based on information from the "outside" (perception or testimony). However, even in cases of extreme alienation vis-à-vis her own experience and thinking, the subject's self-conscious judgments have, however, not lost their distinctive epistemic and motivational features.

We do not need to get further involved in this debate here. The important point concerns our initial distinction between two forms of ownership. Despite various other disagreements, most participants in the current debate (Campbell included) agree that the fundamental kind of ownership is not lost in the case of inserted thoughts. The patient complaining that his thoughts feel alien to her is still making a successful first-personal self-reference.

What Makes First-Person
Self-Reference Possible?

An important and central question for theories of self-awareness is what makes first-person self-reference in thinking possible. That is, what enables a person to think self-conscious thoughts? What enables her to be reflectively self-aware? When asking such a question we are interested in which capacities a person must possess in order to be able to engage in self-conscious thinking (capacities which are not lost even in delusions of inserted thought).

We are of course not interested in the total set of necessary capacities. We can, in the present context, exclude general capacities necessary for being able to think, and focus exclusively on what is needed for a person to be able to think first-person thoughts. This is in itself a very complex issue. Recent debates have highlighted different necessary conditions for self-conscious thinking (reflective self-awareness). Some have argued that the thinker must be able to conceive of herself as a spatiotemporal object which traces a route through the world, in order to be able to refer to herself (Campbell 1994; Cassam 1997; Strawson 1966). Others have focused on the question of which meta-cognitive abilities a subject must necessarily have in order to take herself as an object of thinking, i.e., to reflect in thought on her own thinking, experience, and action (Proust 2010). Third, self-conscious thinking has been seen as a specific expression of the subject's conscious perspective on the world (McGinn 1983, pp. 17, 105, 139). On the latter account, a necessary condition for reflective self-awareness is consequently that first-order experience must have a certain structure. It is this last condition which we will focus on in the remainder of the article.

Consciousness and Minimal Self-Awareness

How must a subject's conscious experience be structured if she is to be able to engage in reflective self-awareness? One suggestion is that reflection does not produce its theme ex nihilo, but that it, on the contrary, draws and builds on a certain tacit self-familiarity that is built into the very stream of consciousness. Indeed a number of philosophers have been arguing that reflective self-awareness presupposes a primitive pre-reflective self-awareness as its condition of possibility, and that this primitive form is simply a matter of the ongoing first-personal character of experiential life.

One way to get at this minimal or pre-reflective form of self-awareness is to raise the question regarding first-person authority. When I say "my arm hurts," or "I thought you had forgotten our appointment," or "I plan to work at home tomorrow" it is customary to say that I make such statements with first-person authority. This is not to say that I am infallible, but if people disbelieve me, it is generally because they think that I am insincere rather than mistaken (Finkelstein 2003, p. 9). On what is such first-person authority based? As Finkelstein has rightly stressed, we only speak with first-person authority about our *conscious* mental states. We do not speak with such authority about our un- or non-conscious mental states, even though we might know about them through various indirect means, say, through long conversations with a psychoanalyst or cognitive psychologist. Of course, insofar as we come to know about the states, they are to some extent something of which we become conscious, but that does not make them conscious in the relevant intransitive sense of the term. No, in order for us to speak with first-person authority about a mental state, the mental state must be one we *consciously* live through (Finkelstein 2003, p. 116).

What is gained by adding the adverb "consciously"? What is the difference between those mental states that remain non-conscious and those that make us consciously aware of objects? A decisive difference is that there is something it is like to consciously perceive, imagine, or remember x. Now, on a standard conception of phenomenal consciousness, a mental state is phenomenally conscious if there is something it is like for the subject to be in it (Nagel 1974; Searle 1992). But this arguably requires the subject to have some awareness of the state in question, although this doesn't have to entail that the subject must be aware of the state in the sense of noticing or attending to or thinking about the state (Block 2007; Burge 2006; Zahavi 1999). Furthermore, one reason why phenomenal experiences are frequently said to be subjective is because they are characterized by a subjective mode of existence in the sense that they necessarily feel like something *for someone*. As it is sometimes phrased, all experiences are implicitly characterized by a certain *mineness or for-me-ness* (Zahavi 1999, 2005).

Related views have recently been defended by both Levine and Kriegel. According to Levine, there are three features that are distinctive of mental phenomena: rationality, intentionality, and consciousness (experience) (Levine 2001, p. 4). When analyzing experience, however, we need to realize that there is more to it than its qualitative character, i.e., the fact that the experience is reddish or greenish or painful or pleasurable. Rather, we also need to bear in mind that the experience in question is like something for me, and that conscious experience consequently involves an experiential perspective or point of view (Levine 2001, p. 7). Along very similar lines, Kriegel has argued that phenomenal character involves both qualitative character, e.g., the bluish component, and subjective character, i.e., the for-me component (Kriegel 2009, p. 8). He further describes the subjective character as that which remains invariant across all phenomenal characters, and argues that a phenomenally conscious state's qualitative character is what makes it the phenomenally conscious state it is, while its subjective character is what makes it a phenomenally conscious state at all (Kriegel 2009, pp. 2, 58).

A possible objection to this view is that it is simply phenomenologically unwarranted to insist on the pervasive experiential reality of self-consciousness. There are different ways of articulating this kind of concern. Consider first the criticism that Dainton has directed against the proposal that there should be some unique phenomenal feature that is present in all experiences belonging to the same subject and which marks them out as mine and mine alone (Dainton 2008, p, 150). In rejecting this claim—it just isn't phenomenologically convincing to claim that each and every one of my experiences possess the same phenomenal property, a stamp or label that clearly and unequivocally identifies them as mine (Dainton 2004, p.380)—Dainton also takes himself to be rejecting the proposal that all experiences are characterized by mineness or for-me-ness (Dainton 2008, p. 242). Likewise, Schear has argued that to claim that experience is always characterized by pre-reflective self-awareness is to fall prey to the so-called refrigerator fallacy, i.e., thinking that the light is always on, simply because it is always on whenever we open the door of the refrigerator. In short, we should avoid conflating the presence of a *capacity* for self-consciousness with the *actualization* of that capacity: "Accordingly, self-consciousness is more justly construed, on phenomenological grounds, as a potentiality—generally unactualized, but always actualizable—of the world-immersed experience of someone capable of first-person thought" (Schear 2009, p. 99). Thus, according to Schear, self-consciousness is a capacity that is only exercised or actualized on special occasions, namely whenever we reflect. Moreover, this can only happen if we possess the capacity for first-person thoughts.

To argue that our experiential life is as such characterized by mineness and for-me-ness is, however, not to deny that we need to recognize a diversity of qualitatively different kinds of self-experiences. There is indeed an experiential difference between being absorbed in a movie; being humiliated by your peers; laboriously trying to decipher a menu written in a language you hardly know; being suddenly hit in the face by a snowball; trying to convince yourself to jump from the ten-meter diving board. To deny that these different experiences exemplify different types of self-awareness is indeed to distort phenomenology. But this recognition is quite compatible with the view that there is also something that this diversity has in common. To speak of the mineness or for-me-ness of experience is not meant to suggest that a subject owns the experiences in a way that is even remotely similar to the way it might possess external objects of various sorts (a car, a pair of trousers, or a house in Sweden). Nor is the point to refer to an abiding quality or datum of experience on a par with, say, the scent of crushed mint leaves. The for-me-ness or mineness doesn't refer to a specific experiential content, to a specific *what*, say, a vivid sense of one's own unmistakable personality, nor does it refer to the diachronic or synchronic sum of such content, or to some other relation that might obtain between the contents in question. Rather, the for-me-ness or mineness refers to the distinct manner or *how* of experiencing. It refers to the first-personal presence of experience, it refers to the fact that the experiences I am living through present themselves differently (but not necessarily better) to me than to anybody else. Indeed, to stress the intimate link between consciousness and self-awareness as we have been doing is simply to take the subjectivity of experience seriously. It could consequently be claimed that anybody who denies the for-me-ness or mineness of experience simply fails to recognize an essential constitutive aspect of experience. It would entail the view that my own mind prior to reflection is either not given to me at all—I would be mind- or self-blind—or present to me in exactly the same way as the minds of others.

A view like the one we are endorsing has a clear phenomenological ancestry, in that it was a view that most thinkers in the phenomenological tradition defended (cf. Zahavi 1999, 2005). But the view has also found many advocates in analytical philosophy of mind. As Goldman writes,

> [Consider] the case of thinking about *x* or attending to *x*. In the process of thinking about *x* there is already an implicit awareness that one is thinking about *x*. There is no need for reflection here, for taking a step back from thinking about *x* in order to examine it ... When we are thinking about *x*, the mind is focused on *x*, not on our thinking of *x*. Nevertheless, the process of thinking about *x* carries with it a non-reflective self-awareness. (Goldman 1970, p. 96)

Related views have been defended by Owen Flanagan, who not only argues that consciousness involves self-consciousness in the weak sense that there is something it is like for the subject to have the experience, but has also spoken of the low-level self-consciousness involved in experiencing my experiences as *mine* (Flanagan 1992, p. 194). Picking up on a recent suggestion of Uriah Kriegel's, it might here be helpful to distinguish two types of self-consciousness, a transitive and an intransitive. We might say that a subject is in possession of transitive self-consciousness when "she is conscious of her thought that p or conscious of her perception of x" and in possession of intransitive self-consciousness when "she is consciously thinking that p or consciously perceiving x." What is the difference between the two types of self-consciousness? Kriegel lists four differences, and claims that whereas the first type is introspective, rare, voluntary and effortful, the second is none of these (Kriegel 2003, p. 104). According to Kriegel, the latter type of self-consciousness, intransitive self-consciousness, captures one of the important senses of consciousness. Indeed, intransitive self-consciousness can be seen as a necessary condition for, and constitutive feature of, phenomenal consciousness. Or to put it differently, a mental state that lacks intransitive self-consciousness is a non-conscious state (Kriegel 2003, pp. 103–106, 2009, ch. 4).

If one accepts this line of reasoning, one has a ready answer to the question regarding the basis of first-person authority. I can be first-person authoritative with respect to the mental states I consciously live through because these mental states are characterized by a subjective presence. Now, the claim is not that first-personal givenness in and by itself amounts to authoritative first-person knowledge (or critical self-deliberation), nor is the suggestion that we should obliterate the difference between the two, but the suggestion is that the former provides an experiential grounding of any subsequent self-ascription, reflective appropriation, and thematic self-identification.

Does an endorsement of pre-reflective self-awareness commit one to a form of *detectivism*, to use the label coined by Finkelstein? No. The suggestion is not that first-person authority is to be explained by means of a kind of inward observation or introspection that allows us to detect or discover the content of our own mind (Finkelstein 2003, p. 2). The claim is not that experiences are things we perceive or observe and that the relation between an experience and its first-personal character (subjective presence) is to be cashed out in terms of an act–object structure. The point is rather that experiential processes are intrinsically self-revealing. This is also why it is better to say that we see, hear, or feel *consciously*, instead of saying that there is a perception of an object, and in addition an awareness of the perception. The decisive advantage of the adverbial phrasing is that it avoids interpreting the secondary awareness as a form of object-consciousness. This temptation remains as long as we talk of experiential episodes as episodes *of* which we are conscious. This is also why we are following the phenomenological tradition in calling the basic type of self-awareness "pre-reflective." By doing so, we wish to emphasize that it does not involve an additional second-order mental state that in some way is directed in an explicit manner towards the experience in question. Rather, the minimal self-awareness must be understood as an intrinsic feature of the primary experience. Moreover, it is not thematic, attentive, or voluntarily brought about; rather it is tacit, non-observational (that is, it is not a kind of introspective observation of myself), and non-objectifying (that is, it does not turn my experience into an object of attention). I can, of course, reflect on and attend to my experience; I can make it the theme or object of my attention, but prior to reflecting on it, I was not "mindblind." The experience was already present to me, it was already something *for me*, and in that sense it counts as being pre-reflectively conscious.

Now, what is the relation between minimal or pre-reflective self-awareness and reflective self-awareness or self-conscious thinking? Are there any reasons to think that a theory of minimal self-awareness has anything substantial to contribute to our understanding of self-conscious thinking? Some have objected that even if something like non-objectifying self-consciousness is possible, it will be far too weak and vague to allow for or to explain the distinctive character of our first-person thinking (Caston 2006, p. 4; Thomasson 2006, p. 6). This, however, seems a somewhat puzzling objection. We can readily agree that pre-reflective self-consciousness does not amount to self-conscious thinking. In order to obtain knowledge about one's experiences something more than pre-reflective self-consciousness is needed. But from the fact that pre-reflective self-consciousness is not sufficient for first-person thinking, one can obviously not conclude that it is therefore also unnecessary if such thinking is to be possible. Even if the situations where we explicitly designate our own experiences as our own are the exceptions, we still need to understand how such situations are possible, and as the argument goes, it would be impossible to account for these explicit forms of self-ascription, where we recognize an experience as being our own, if it was not for the fact that our experiential life is fundamentally characterized by for-me-ness, and by the primitive and minimal form of self-reference it entails. To put it differently, a minimal or thin form of self-experience is a condition of possibility for the more articulated forms of conceptual self-consciousness that we incontestably enjoy from time to time. Had our experiences been completely anonymous or impersonal when originally lived through, any subsequent appropriation would be inexplicable.

But is this really true? Is it really true that minimal self-awareness, the for-me-ness aspect, is a necessary feature of conscious experience without which something like reflective self-awareness would be utterly inexplicable? One way to answer such questions is by taking a further look at theories of consciousness that deny the existence of minimal self-awareness and ask how they fare in explaining our ability to make first-person self-reference in thinking.

Anonymity Theory of Consciousness

In what follows, we will call any theory denying the existence of minimal self-awareness an *anonymity theory of phenomenal consciousness* (anonymity theory for short). One way to grasp the anonymity theory is in the following way. According to the theory of minimal self-awareness, conscious experience does not only involve conscious representation or presentation of something (things, events, or facts in the world), it also involves a conscious manifestation for a subject. Conscious experience is, as McGinn once remarked, Janus-faced: It has a world-directed aspect, it presents the world in a certain way, but at the same time, it also involves presence to the subject, and hence a subjective point of view. In short, it is of something other than the subject and it is like something for the subject (1991, p. 29). According to the minimal self-awareness theory, this for-me-ness aspect of conscious experience is part of what is consciously experienced. The for-me-ness is a phenomenal feature of the conscious experience. It is exactly this idea which is denied by the anonymity theory. The latter is not denying that experience, or more generally mental states and events occur to or belong to subjects. The fact that experience necessarily happens to a subject and in that sense belong to the subject is a conceptual and/or metaphysical fact. Rather the objection is that ownership of experience, rather than being a feature internal to experience, is a purely external metaphysical relation (Searle 2005; Tye 1995, pp. 10–12).

In contemporary philosophy of mind, people defending so-called strong intentionalism seem to endorse a version of the anonymity theory. Strong intentionalism can be defined as the view which endorses the following two claims: (1) all states that are phenomenally conscious are intentional states (mental states with representational content); and (2) the phenomenal character of conscious states is identical to or supervenes on the state's intentional content (for discussion, see Crane 2009). To see the intuitive appeal of this position, take the case of vision. When I open my eyes and enjoy visual experiences (i.e., look around), the world seems to present itself to me. I do not see representations of the world or fleeting phenomenal data—I see the objects themselves as they are located there in front of me (say, on my desk). Capitalizing on this basic fact, we might say that all that is phenomenally present to me in a visual experience is the world as it is presented to me. The phenomenal properties that I experience are thus experienced as being properties of the objects that I am seeing. This becomes obvious, according to proponents of strong intentionalism, when I turn my attention introspectively to what it is like for me to have the experience. Every time I attend to features of my experience or its particular character I end up attending to features of the objects I am looking at. The experience is, in this sense, said to be transparent (Dretske 1995, 2003a; Tye 1995, 2003).

Strong intentionalism is not merely a theory about visual experience. It purports to be a general theory of consciousness. The strategy proposed by the strong intentionalist is therefore to generalize the account of visual experience to all forms of conscious experience. Consequently, strong intentionalism is not the (weaker) view that all phenomenal states are intentional (Crane 2003). This kind of weak intentionalism could allow for phenomenal properties that are not identical to or supervene on properties of the content. For example, weak intentionalism would be consistent with the existence of phenomenal properties which are properties of the experience (for example, non-representational properties characterizing an experience as a visual experience, a recollection, or an imagining—in other words, characterizing the attitude and not the content). By contrast, the strong intentionalist claims that the phenomenal character of all forms of conscious state is identical to or supervenes on the state's intentional content. This means that conscious experience does not provide the subject with any direct knowledge of the experience (its type and character) simply in virtue of living through the experience in question. Hence, knowledge of being engaged in the conscious act of seeing (rather than imagining) has to be inferred from the way in which the world is being represented (Byrne 2005, 2010; Dretske 1999, 2003b).

One way to understand the entailed idea of the completely anonymous or impersonal character of experience is by analogy with cinematic representation. In his famous paper on imagination, Bernard Williams (1966/1973, p. 37) pointed out that there are two ways in which we can understand perspective in cinematic representation. What is filmed is filmed from a location in space. The representation has lines of vision pointing back and converging in the perspectival location of the camera, and as a consequence things will be represented as appearing to the left, to the right, in the centre, in front of, being partly occluded, etc., with respect to this perspectival location or origin. Sometimes this perspectival origin is presented as belonging to a character in the represented world. If that is the case, then if the character scratches her nose, we will see her hand entering the picture, getting nearer the centre, and growing bigger in characteristic ways. Most often, however, the perspective is relative to no one. It does not belong to the camera, or to the director, or to me as a member of the audience. It belongs to neither of these since neither of these are part of the represented world. When we see two lovers kiss in a movie, often neither the camera, nor the director, nor the audience are parts of the world of the lovers. There is a perspective, but it is impersonal. There is nothing inherently different in the representational character or content with respect to the two forms of cinematic representation. In the first form of cinematic perspective, the perspective belongs to a character in the represented world by way of conventional signs. But in fact, both forms of cinematic perspective are equally impersonal.

If experience is strictly impersonal in this sense, then conscious experience does not in itself involve or imply any self-awareness or for-me-ness. For the same reason, conscious experience does not in itself ground self-knowledge: it provides the subject with immediate knowledge of the world, but not of her own conscious life. By contrast, according to the minimal self-awareness theory, experience not only presents the world but in a minimal, pre-reflective way the experience also presents itself to the subject. The experience itself can be thought to directly provide the material needed for a self-conscious judgment like "*I am looking* at a tree" in the sense that experience is providing an element which is necessary for our ability to make first-person self-reference in thinking. Not so for the anonymity theory. On the completely impersonal account of phenomenal consciousness, the phenomenal content of experience does not by itself provide the subject with any such element. The experience provides the subject with information about the world and only derivatively (and given some additional assumptions) with information about the experience (Dretske 2003b). But if we assume that it is an important task for a philosophical account of self-awareness to be able to explain a person's ability to refer to herself with a first-person concept, the worry is that the anonymity theory has no way of explaining this ability.

It might be replied that there are at least two ways in which the anonymity theory can explain first-person self-reference in self-conscious thinking. The first way concerns the perspectival nature of perceptual experience and the second way the general semantic rules governing the use of "I." Let us first have a look at the perspectival character of perception. Maybe the anonymity theory could use the perspectival nature of perceptual content as a form of uniquely self-specifying knowledge. In perception, things appear as located in space, to the right, to the left, in front, behind, within reach, out of reach, all with respect to my embodied point of view. Perceptual content thus has an implicit "back-reference" to the perceiving subject. If it did not, perception could not directly control action. The idea is not that the reference is fixed by what I am perceptually attending to (as with demonstratives) but rather by the indexical "back-reference" to the perceiver. James J. Gibson's ecological optics and his notion of affordances might be exploited to substantiate this idea.

One option would be to say that the implicit "self-reference" of perceptual content is what grounds our ability to think first-personal thoughts. The "I"-concept is a singular referring concept, and as such it might be thought that the use of it in self-conscious thinking requires that the thinker is in possession of knowledge that uniquely specifies the referent. The background assumption here could be that singular reference requires that the thinker knows which object she is referring to (Evans 1982, ch. 6; Strawson 1959; cf. Anscombe 1975; O'Brien 2007, ch. 2). The perspectival structure of perceptual content provides the perceiver with knowledge of a unique object: the self. This self-knowledge is what grounds the ability to refer to oneself in the first-person way. The indexical nature of the content of perception is what fixes the reference of the "I" and grounds our ability to think "I"-thoughts (Bermúdez 1998).

There are good reasons for thinking that this proposal does not work. Remember that first-person self-reference in self-conscious thinking is such that a person cannot think an "I"-thought without knowing and understanding that she is referring to herself in the first-person way. On the account under consideration now, this knowing and understanding is explained by the perspectival nature of perceptual content. The problem for this idea is that we can imagine a person who loses this knowledge without losing her ability to first-person self-refer.

Recall that the nature of the perceptual experience is supposedly impersonal in the sense that the cinematic representation is impersonal: it is referring back to some perspectival origin but the identity of the origin is left undetermined. The identity is picked out by the logical equivalent of a definite description: the perceiver of this perceptual presentation. As with any definite description, we can imagine a situation where the thinker is referring to herself without knowing that this is what she is doing (Perry 1979). We can thus imagine a person enjoying or suffering some visual presentation (seeing a tree) who begins to wonder who the perceiver actually is (i.e., who actually fills out the perspectival "origin-slot"). Such a subject might become convinced that it is in fact not her who is seeing the tree but someone else (perhaps this chap Chris) who then flashes the perceptual presentations on to the subject's mind as images on a screen. Paraphrasing a now famous statement by a patient reported by Frith (1992, p. 66), this subject might think *I am being visually presented with a tree but I am not really the one seeing it; this chap Chris is.* If something like this is possible, it goes to show that perceptual content cannot fix the reference of the "I" by providing the thinker with the necessary form of self-knowledge. The point is that if visual experience is structurally like cinematic representation (as described by Williams), we can imagine a case where the subject loses this form of self-knowledge but not her ability to self-refer.

The second way in which the anonymity theory might attempt to explain our ability to self-refer in self-conscious thinking is by way of general rules of reference. The anonymity theorist could attempt to account for the structure of first-personal thinking and the reference of the "I" not by some special relation between self-reference and self-knowledge but by a general semantic rule. The reference of the "I" is not fixed by a special form of knowledge of the self; rather, it is fixed by a simple rule. The rule is the following token-reflexive rule: a token of the "I" refers to the creature that produces it. The token-reflexive rule says that the meaning of the "I" is that it refers to the creature that produced a token of the term and that a grasp of the meaning of the "I" is a grasp of this rule (cf. Barwise and Perry 1981; O'Brien 2007, ch. 4).

The problem for this account is that it has no good story to tell about why first-person thinking entails that the thinker knows and understands that she is thinking about herself in the first-person way. Recall that a person thinking a self-conscious thought necessarily refers to herself and understands that she is thinking about herself in such a way that she could not be thinking about someone else. The suggestion we are considering now is that this form of first-person understanding can be explained by a grasp of the token-reflexive rule that governs the use of the "I"-concept. The suggestion is confronted with a dilemma: either it over-intellectualizes first-person understanding and self-conscious thinking or it focuses exclusively on the causal role of first-person representations and it will be unable to explain self-*conscious* thinking.

On the first horn of this dilemma, the anonymity theory tries to explain the thinker's understanding of first-person self-reference by her conscious grasp of the token-reflexive rule. The thinker understands that when thinking an "I"-thought she is necessarily thinking something about herself. The thinker has this understanding in virtue of consciously grasping the rule that a token of the "I" (in thought and talk) is referring to the producer of it, i.e., to herself. This proposal immediately runs into the problem that the understanding that is supposed to ground the ability for first-person self-reference itself contains indexical elements and therefore presupposes exactly this kind of understanding. Furthermore, claiming that the ability to self-refer in thinking requires an ability to consciously grasp the token-reflexive rule is a non-starter. At least if conscious grasp is understood along the lines of an ability to state the rule explicitly. Most people can think self-conscious thoughts but only a few of them can state the token-reflexive rule that governs the use of the "I"-concept.

On the second horn, the anonymity theory understands the token-reflexive rule not as a rule that is explicitly represented by the thinker but as a law-like generalization that describes the workings of the system. The anonymity theory could claim that there is nothing more to first-person self-reference than the application of the token-reflexive rule in a particular context of thinking (the rule-governed production of mental symbols). The rule need not be explicitly represented or grasped by the thinker. The rule is applied in the sense that it seems to govern the way in which the cognitive system functions. This view can provide a nice account of the cognitive difference between first-person and third-person self-reference. It could, for example, be claimed that the token-reflexive rule describes a situation where the cognitive system sets up a processing rule that either relates information directly to the cognitive system or does not do so. Application of the rule in a particular context describes a situation where certain information is put into an information file with direct pragmatic relevance to the system (Perry 1986). We would thus have a functional story to tell about the motivational difference between the two forms of self-reference. This view also provides us with a story about guaranteed reference. It seems plausible that if a cognitive system produces a symbol to which token-reflexive rule finds application, then the symbol is guaranteed reference—after all, there must have been a producer of the symbol.

It might be true that our "I"-thinking is governed by the token reflexive rule; this, however, is not sufficient to explain some of the crucial properties of self-conscious thinking that we have discussed. If we are interested in the special form of understanding that is manifested in self-conscious thinking, then the functionalist proposal seems insufficient. Thinking an "I"-thought entails thinking a thought where the thinker understands that she is necessarily thinking something about herself. It is this understanding which is missing from or left unexplained in the functionalist story. An equivalent of Searle's Chinese Room argument might persuade us that this is so. Imagine a person inside the room sorting all incoming information into two files: information in one file is either immediately or later sent to the production system, whereas information in the other file simply stays there. Operating in a way that fits the rule does not entail that there is any understanding. Or think of zombies. A zombie is functionally equivalent to a conscious human being and might, consequently, be operating in accordance with the token-reflexive rule. We might want to say the same of a computer or mindless robot. But we should refrain from saying that any of these creatures think self-conscious thoughts and understand that they are referring to themselves.

The argument presented here is of course not conclusive. It only sketches the kind of pressure one may lay on the anonymity theory for not being able to explain or make sense of the most central features of self-conscious thinking. Our diagnosis of these problems (to be sure not the only possible diagnosis) is that the problems are caused by the fact that the theory is an anonymity theory: it denies any phenomenal presence of minimal self-awareness.

Concluding Remarks

Let us in conclusion again turn to the question of whether this theoretical discussion of consciousness and self-consciousness has implications for our understanding of psychopathological phenomena. We might return to the earlier discussion concerning thought insertion and the two different forms of ownership. The result of that discussion was that according to one form of ownership the schizophrenic cannot sensibly be said to lose the ability to self-refer in thinking. Insofar as he can report his delusional states and altered experiences he is making first-person reference, he is thinking about himself. According to a second form of ownership, however, he might feel that he cannot control his thoughts or that he is not their causal origin, and in this sense he might feel fundamentally alienated vis-à-vis his own experiential life. These distinctions can be understood on the background of a theory of minimal self-consciousness. If this theory is true, then there is a phenomenal feature present in experience, be it when a subject is consciously thinking, perceiving, or feeling. No matter how alien your own experience seems to you, it is still felt as occurring in your stream of consciousness. In short, since "one remains the subject of the alien thought, the foreignness of the experience cannot be due to a lack of ownership in the formal sense, but might rather be due to a lack of authorship" (Zahavi 1999, p. 154).

What is the argument? When a subject who experiences thought insertions or delusions of control reports that certain thoughts are not his thoughts, that someone else is generating these thoughts, he is also indicating that these thoughts are present, not "over there" in someone else's head, but within *his own* stream of consciousness, a stream of consciousness for which he claims ownership. Even if the inserted thoughts or alien movements are felt as intrusive and strange, they cannot lack minimal ownership altogether, since the afflicted subject is aware that it is he himself rather than somebody else who is experiencing these alien thoughts and movements. In short, some sense of ownership is still retained, and that is the basis for his complaint. This is also the view of Graham, who recently argued that subjects of thought insertion recognize that certain thoughts occur to them and that "the *subjectivity* sense" of ownership is consequently retained, but that their sense of self as agent, or the agency sense of ownership, is disrupted (Graham 2010, pp. 247–248).

Claiming that a patient suffering from thought insertion is not completely bereft of a sense of ownership and that such phenomena do not involve a complete effacement of the sense of mineness is not, however, to deny that the clinician should recognize that schizophrenia does in fact involve a fragile and unstable first-person perspective. But there is an important difference between claiming that thought insertion exemplifies a state of mind with no mineness, and saying that the mineness that is retained is frail (cf. Parnas and Sass 2011,

p. 532): frail in the sense that, for the patient, mineness can no longer simply be taken for granted, it has lost some of its normal obviousness and unquestionability. Some patients are able to articulate these subtle experiential disturbances better than others. One of Parnas's patients reported that the feeling that his experiences were his own always came with a split-second delay; another that it was as if his self was somehow displaced a few centimeters backwards. A third explained that he felt an indescribable inner change that prevented him from leading a normal life. He was troubled by a very distressing feeling of not being really present or even fully alive (Parnas 2003, p. 223).

One might mention that this experience of distance or detachment is often accompanied by a compulsive self-monitoring. This is what Blankenburg called a convulsive reflection or a reflective spasm (*Reflexionskrampf*) and is an aspect of what Sass has more recently dubbed *hyperreflexivity*. According to Sass, this hyperreflexivity manifests itself in a variety of different ways, depending on whether it occurs (1) as a facet of the basic defect itself, (2) as a consequence of, or (3) defensive compensation for the more basic disturbance (Sass 2000, p. 153). At first, hyperreflexivity is not a volitional kind of self-consciousness; it occurs in a more or less automatic manner and has the effect of disrupting experiences and actions that would normally remain in the background of awareness. Thus, the normal stream of consciousness is interrupted by sensations, feelings or thoughts that suddenly become the focus of attention with an object-like quality (*basal hyperreflexivity*). These primary disruptions and disturbances then attract further attention and thereby elicit a process of self-scrutiny and self-objectification, or reflective turning-inwards of the mind (*consequential hyperreflexivity*). Finally, such patients might voluntarily engage in reflective self-monitoring in an attempt to compensate for their diminished self-presence (*compensatory hyperreflexivity*). Needless to say, rather than restoring what has been lost, such excessive self-monitoring may only exacerbate the problem by further objectifying, alienating, and dividing the experiential life (Sass 1994, pp. 12, 38, 91, 95).

Having now pointed to the presence of a widespread consensus about how to describe cases of thought insertion, we can return a final time to the anonymity theory. Recall that one appealing way to make sense of the schizophrenic patient's statement that he is thinking a thought which is not really his own is to dissolve the apparent contradiction by saying that a thought is his in one sense of ownership (minimal ownership) and not his in another sense of ownership (ownership as authorship). In short, individuals suffering from thought insertion have not lost their ability to make first-person self-reference. One way to rephrase our argument against the anonymity theory would then be to say that insofar as it denies a minimal self-awareness (as part of the experience) it leaves out an important dimension of conscious life necessary for understanding the minimal form of ownership. The anonymity theory can account for the second form of ownership as authorship but would have problems of making sense of the minimal form. But if that is the case, the theory would have difficulties in explaining how the person with schizophrenia can succeed in making first-person self-reference even in those cases where the thought is disowned.

Acknowledgment

We are indebted to an anonymous reviewer for a number of helpful comments.

REFERENCES

Anscombe, G. E. M. (1975). The first person. In S. Guttenplan (Ed.), *Mind and Language: Wolfson College Lectures 1974*, pp. 45–64. Oxford: Clarendon Press.

Baker, L. R. (2000). *Persons and Bodies: A Constitution View*. Cambridge: Cambridge University Press.

Baron-Cohen, S. (1989). Are autistic children 'behaviorists'? An examination of their mental–physical and appearance–reality distinctions. *Journal of Autism and Developmental Disorders*, 19, 579–600.

Barwise, J. and Perry, J. (1981). Situations and attitudes. *Journal of Philosophy*, 78(11), 668–91.

Bermúdez, J. L. (1998). *The Paradox of Self-Consciousness*. Cambridge, MA: MIT Press.

Block, N. (2007). Consciousness, accessibility, and the mesh between psychology and neuroscience. *Behavioral and Brain Sciences*, 30, 481–548.

Burge, T. (1998). Reason and the first-person. In C. Wright, B. C. Smith, C. MacDonald (Eds), *Knowing One's Own Mind*, pp. 243–70. Oxford: Blackwell.

Burge, T. (2006). Reflections on two kinds of consciousness. In T. Burge (Ed.), *Philosophical Essays, Volume II: Foundations of Mind*. New York, NY: Oxford University Press, pp. 392–419.

Byrne, A. (2005). Introspection. *Philosophical Topics*, 33, 79–104.

Byrne, A. (2010). Recollection, perception, imagination. *Philosophical Studies*, 148, 15–26.

Campbell, J. (1994). *Past, Space and Self*. Cambridge, MA: MIT Press.

Campbell, J. (1999). Schizophrenia, the space of reasons, and thinking as a motor process. *The Monist*, 82(4), 609–25.

Cassam, Q. (1997). *Self and World*. Oxford: Clarendon Press.

Castañeda, H.-N. (1967). On the logic of self-knowledge. *Noûs*, 1(1), 9–21.

Castañeda, H.-N. (1968). On the phenomeno-logic of the I. *Proceedings of the XIVth International Congress of Philosophy III*, 260–6.

Caston, V. (2006). Comment on A. Thomasson, 'Self-awareness and self-knowledge'. *Psyche*, 12/2, 1–15.

Coliva, A. (2002). Thought insertion and immunity to error through misidentification. *Philosophy, Psychiatry, & Psychology*, 9(1), 27–34.

Coliva, A. (2006). Error through misidentification: Some varieties. *Journal of Philosophy*, 103(8), 407–25.

Crane, T. (2003). The intentional structure of consciousness. In Q. Smith and A. Jokic (Eds), *Consciousness: New Philosophical Perspectives*, pp. 33–56. Oxford: Oxford University Press.

Crane, T. (2009). Intentionalism. In A. Beckermann, B. P. McLaughlin, and S. Walter (Eds), *The Oxford Handbook of Philosophy of Mind*, pp. 474–93. Oxford: Clarendon Press.

Dainton, B. (2004). The self and the phenomenal. *Ratio*, XVII(4), 365–89.

Dainton, B. (2008). *The Phenomenal Self*. Oxford: Oxford University Press.

Dretske, F. (1995). *Naturalizing the mind*. Cambridge, MA: MIT Press.

Dretske, F. (1999). The mind's awareness of itself. *Philosophical Studies*, 95(1–2), 103–24.

Dretske, F. (2003a). Experience as representation. *Philosophical Issues*, 13(1), 67–82.

Dretske, F. (2003b). How do you know you are not a zombie? In B. Gertler (Ed.), *Privileged access*, pp. 1–14. Aldershot: Ashgate.

Evans, G. (1982). *The Varieties of Reference* (J. McDowell, Ed.). Oxford: Oxford University Press.

Finkelstein, D. (2003). *Expression and the Inner*. Cambridge, MA: Harvard University Press.

Flanagan, O. (1992). *Consciousness Reconsidered*. Cambridge, MA: MIT Press.

Frith, C. D. (1992). *The Cognitive Neuropsychology of Schizophrenia*. Hove: Lawrence Erlbaum.

Frith, U. and Happé, F. (1999). Theory of mind and self-consciousness: What is it like to be autistic? *Mind & Language, 14*, 1–22.

Gallagher, S. (2000). Self-reference and schizophrenia: A cognitive model of immunity to error through misidentification. In D. Zahavi (Ed.), *Exploring the Self*, pp. 203–39. Amsterdam: John Benjamins.

Gallagher, S. (2004). Neurocognitive models of schizophrenia: A neurophenomenological critique. *Psychopathology, 37*, 8–19.

Goldman, A. I. (1970). *A Theory of Human Action*. Princeton, NJ: Princeton University Press.

Graham, G. (2010). *The Disordered Mind: An Introduction to Philosophy of Mind and Mental Illness*. Abingdon: Routledge.

Hoerl, C. (2001). On thought insertion. *Philosophy, Psychiatry, & Psychology, 8*, 189–200.

Kriegel, U. (2003). Consciousness as intransitive self-consciousness: Two views and an argument. *Canadian Journal of Philosophy, 33*, 103–32.

Kriegel, U. (2009). *Subjective Consciousness: A Self-Representational Theory*. Oxford: Oxford University Press.

Levine, J. (2001). *Purple Haze: The Puzzle of Consciousness*. New York, NY: Oxford University Press.

Lewis, M. (2003). The development of self-consciousness. In J. Roessler and N. Eilan (Eds), *Agency and Self-Awareness*, pp. 275–95. Oxford: Oxford University Press.

McGinn, C. (1983). *The Subjective View: Secondary Qualities and Indexical Thoughts*. Oxford: Oxford University Press.

McGinn, C. (1991). *The Problem of Consciousness*. Oxford: Blackwell.

Mead, G. H. (1962). *Mind, Self, and Society. From the Standpoint of a Social Behaviorist*. Chicago, IL: University of Chicago Press.

Nagel, T. (1974). What is it like to be a bat? *The Philosophical Review, 83*, 435–50.

O'Brien, L. (2007). *Self-Knowing Agents*. Oxford: Oxford University Press.

Parnas, J. (2003). Self and schizophrenia: A phenomenological perspective. In T. Kircher and A. David (Eds), *The Self in Neuroscience and Psychiatry*, pp. 217–41. Cambridge: Cambridge University Press.

Parnas, J. and Sass, L. A. (2011). The structure of self-consciousness in schizophrenia. In S. Gallagher (Ed.), *The Oxford Handbook of the Self*, pp. 521–46. Oxford: Oxford University Press.

Perry, J. (1977). Frege on demonstratives. *The Philosophical Review, 86*(4), 474–97.

Perry, J. (1979). The problem of the essential indexical. *Nous, 13*, 3–21.

Perry, J. (1986). Perception, action, and the structure of believing. In R. E. Grandy and R. Warner (Eds), *Philosophical Grounds of Rationality. Intentions, Categories, Ends*, pp. 333–61. Oxford: Clarendon Press.

Proust, J. (2006). Agency in schizophrenics from a control theory viewpoint. In W. Prinz and N. Sebanz (Eds), *Disorders of volition*, pp. 87–118. Cambridge, MA: MIT Press.

Proust, J. (2010). Metacognition. *Philosophy Compass, 5*(11), 989–98.

Pryor, J. (1999). Immunity to error through misidentification. *Philosophical Topics, 26*, 271–304.

Sass, L. A. (1994). *The Paradoxes of Delusion*. London: Cornell University Press.

Sass, L. (2000). Schizophrenia, self-experience, and the so-called 'negative symptoms'. In D. Zahavi (Ed.), *Exploring the Self*, pp. 149–182. Amsterdam: John Benjamins.

Schear, J. (2009). Experience and self-consciousness. *Philosophical Studies, 144*/1, 95–105.

Searle, J. R. (1992). *The Rediscovery of the Mind*. Cambridge, MA: MIT Press.

Searle, J. R. (2005). The self as a problem in philosophy and neurobiology. In T. E Feinberg and J. P. Keenan (Eds), *The Lost Self: Pathologies of Brain and Identity*, pp. 7–19. Oxford: Oxford University Press.

Shoemaker, S. (1968). Self-reference and self-awareness. *Journal of Philosophy*, 65, 556–79.

Stephens, G. L., and Graham, G. (1994). Self-consciousness, mental agency, and the clinical psychopathology of thought insertion. *Philosophy, Psychiatry, & Psychology*, 1, 1–10.

Strawson, P. F. (1959). *Individuals: An Essay in Descriptive Metaphysics*. London: Methuen.

Strawson, P. F. (1966). *The Bounds of Sense: An Essay on Kant's Critique of Pure Reason*. London: Methuen.

Thomasson, A. (2006). Self-awareness and self-knowledge. *Psyche*, 12/2, 1–15.

Tye, M. (1995). *Ten Problems of Consciousness*. Cambridge, MA: MIT Press.

Tye, M. (2003). *Consciousness and Persons*. Cambridge, MA: MIT Press.

Tye, M. (2009). *Consciousness Revisited: Materialism without Phenomenal Concepts*. Cambridge, MA: MIT Press.

Vosgerau, G. and Newen, A. (2007). Thoughts, motor actions, and the self. *Mind & Language*, 22, 22–43.

Williams, B. (1973). Imagination and the self. In *Problems of the Self*, pp. 26–45. Cambridge: Cambridge University Press. (Original work published 1966.)

Young, G. (2006). Kant and the phenomenon of inserted thoughts. *Philosophical Psychology*, 19(6), 823–37.

Zahavi, D. (1999). *Self-Awareness and Alterity: A Phenomenological Investigation*. Evanston, IL: Northwestern University Press.

Zahavi, D. (2005). *Subjectivity and Selfhood: Investigating the First-Person Perspective*. Cambridge, MA: MIT Press.

CHAPTER 18

INTERPERSONAL RELATING

DANIEL D. HUTTO

Getting clear about the nature and basis of interpersonal relating is a central concern of many recent debates in the philosophy of mind. These debates should be of interest to psychiatrists for several reasons. First, the development of successful clinical practice may depend, at least partly, on having an accurate understanding of the basic character of unimpaired interpersonal relating because such understanding can shed light on the nature and source of its disturbed forms. Second, philosophical discussions may be of direct practical importance to psychiatry given that different theories suggest different potential ways of devising therapies. Finally, it is important that psychiatrists are aware of the implications of various philosophical frameworks and proposals because of the influence they exert on executive decisions about which interventions are most appropriate when dealing with psychopathological dysfunctions and disorders.

This chapter is divided into five parts. The first highlights some basic facts about the complexity and multifaceted character of interpersonal relating and briefly overviews some of its most prominent dysfunctions. The second part introduces popular mind minding hypotheses which claim that the dysfunctions in question are rooted in impaired capacities for attending to and attributing mental states to others. The third part summarizes recent evidence from cognitive psychology and neuroscience with which these mind minding hypotheses must be made compatible. The fourth part highlights the important differences between two main philosophical frameworks—frameworks that offer opposing ways of understanding the nature of mind minding capacities. Focusing on these differences, the final part highlights how adoption of these philosophical frameworks matters to thinking about the prognosis and strategies for the treatment of certain mental disorders.

COMPLEXITIES AND DYSFUNCTIONS OF
INTERPERSONAL RELATING

We relate to others in various ways and on many levels. This is always an enormously complicated affair, which requires us to bring an array of cognitive, emotional, and behavioral resources to bear flexibly and in concert.

Sometimes interpersonal exchanges call on high-level conceptual capacities, such as those needed for interpreting and attributing sophisticated psychological attitudes. In such cases a number of heuristics might be brought into to play to ensure more or less reliable attributions. These range from focusing on what another explicitly says and what this implies to making judgments based on what can be discerned by attending to more purely bodily based expressions. Thus, for example, I might conclude from your tight smile that you are really not as pleased about the proposed merger as you claim to be.

At other times our face-to-face encounters might be pitched entirely at a more basic and low level, such as those cases in which one picks up on and responds to another's psychological situation but without ascribing any mental states. Such responding involves being aware of another's expressed attitudes, emotions, and moods at some level and in making timely, affectively appropriate, and well-managed responses to them. Doing this, successfully, is partly a matter of picking up on subtle cues as well as controlling and regulating one's own emotions and expressions, keeping them within an acceptable range and register. More often than not, any given episode of interacting with others will require us to operate at both of these levels.

Due to its complex and multifaceted nature there are many ways that relating to others can go awry. Even those comfortably within the normal range of social competence differ widely in their abilities in this regard. Those diagnosed with specific types of mental disorder have systemic and selective problems in this domain. Their inabilities are often severe, profoundly disturbing, and difficult, if not impossible, to treat. Dysfunctional or unstable interpersonal relating is a prominent clinical feature of several major psychiatric disorders. The *Diagnostic and Statistical Manual of Mental Disorders, Fourth Edition* lists it as a criterion for the diagnosis of autism spectrum disorder (ASD) and borderline personality disorder (BPD), and as a characteristic symptom of schizophrenia.

The precise profile of impairment varies, however, not only across, but also within, these clinical populations. For example, there is no single pattern associated with the difficulties that individuals with ASD experience when relating to others (Wing 1996). Some are socially awkward, imposing their concerns and interests on others in a one-sided and insensitive manner. This leads to difficulties in relating to others that involves a mixture of poorly timed, badly coordinated, and inappropriate styles of engagement. These include problems in the way that attention is given and contact is made with others. Often this takes the form of a failure to understand what is permissible with respect to personal boundaries. Nonetheless, people with this style of ASD are strongly motivated to engage with others. In contrast, others on the spectrum are socially indifferent or unreachable by normal means; they can appear emotionally empty because of their unresponsiveness. But this is contradicted by the fact that these individuals are also given to outpourings of extreme emotion, indicating that their problem lies with an inability to connect emotionally with others and not with a lack of emotion. It has been observed, for example, that children with ASD sometimes exhibit quite sophisticated emotions, including shyness, pride, and jealousy but that they fail to display other-focused emotions, such as empathic concern or shame (see Hobson 2010). Others are not isolated in this extreme way. They can and do respond to others, to some extent, but they do not initiate social contact and are unable to play an active and competent role in sustaining such interactions. High-functioning individuals with ASD, those who are the most competent at interacting with others, often rely on strict, explicit rules as a means of navigating social situations. But as such rules are insensitive to the delicate requirements of specific situations; the style of interaction of such people is awkward and stilted.

People diagnosed with BPD exhibit a different array of problems in relating to others (Fonagy and Luyten 2010). They are prone to intense emotional arousal, often driven by the disappointment of excessive and alternating expectations that they place on significant others, including their therapists. This tendency is thought to be the consequence of childhood traumas—e.g. abuse or parental neglect or loss. When in an aroused state, those with BPD become incapable of providing reasonable interpretations of their own beliefs, attitudes, and motives and those of others to greater or lesser extents. Yet, at the same time, they display a heightened sensitivity to the emotions of others.

Those diagnosed with schizophrenia also have pronounced difficulties in their normal relations with others—difficulties that typically lead to social isolation and withdrawal—but the clinical picture is different again. Their problems in this domain make it difficult for them to form significant long-term relations, a fact that can exacerbate their condition (Hooley 2010). Like ASD, schizophrenia is a heterogeneous disorder; its symptoms vary greatly in presentation and course and they can co-occur, making it difficult to isolate well-defined subgroups (McCabe 2004). The presence of positive, or added, symptoms or unusual experiences—such as paranoid delusions and hallucinations—distort normal functioning. For example, formal thought disorder interferes with the performance of any task requiring well-ordered thought processes. Difficulties in relating to others, certainly where this requires complex social problem solving, might be expected when people with schizophrenia are thus disturbed in their thinking, in general, is disorganized and unclear. Thus, "in conversation, patients with schizophrenia show weaker verbal (e.g., clarity, negotiation, and persistence) and nonverbal skills (e.g., interest, fluency, and affect) than do nonpatient controls" (Hooley 2010, p. 239). The presence of negative or subtracted symptoms, by contrast, diminishes their normal functioning. When exhibiting negative symptoms, schizophrenics lack emotional expressiveness, are apathetic, have impoverished speech, and show little interest in, and take little pleasure from, social engagement.

There is no single pattern to the dysfunctional interpersonal relating associated with the clinical subgroupings of individuals diagnosed with any one of these disorders. There are different degrees and types of impairment. Although there is similarity in the way that interpersonal relating is disturbed in clinical subgroups within different disorders, for example, the profile of those with severe autism resembles that of those presenting negative symptoms in schizophrenia, there is no simple, common, pattern of dysfunction apparent in all of these disorders nor across all subpopulations (see Corcoran 2000 for a review).

IMPAIRED MIND MINDING HYPOTHESES

An extremely popular conjecture is that the core deficiency responsible for the diverse forms of impaired interpersonal relating found in all of the aforementioned disorders is that the individuals in question are impaired—in some way or other—in their capacities to respond to and understand the mental states of others. Such individuals are often described as having impaired theory of mind (ToM), mentalizing, mindreading, or folk psychological abilities.

This terminology has unfortunate connotations insofar as it suggests that the incapacities always and everywhere concern problems in the representation and attribution of the sophisticated mental states and their contents—including beliefs and desires—in complex, conceptually-based, and articulate ways.

As these considerations reveal, this cannot be the whole story. Humans, and many other non-human animals, can attend and respond appropriately to the mental states of others—such as another's anger or fear—without making any mental state attributions. Indeed, it seems wholly possible to respond fearfully to another's anger without invoking or even having a concept of fear. All that this requires is the exercise of low-level capacities for non-conceptual responding and attending to mental states of different kinds.

For this reason it is useful to adopt a more neutral terminology and to speak inclusively of mind minding abilities. This term can be used to denote, in a maximally liberal fashion, any and all capacities that require specialized abilities for recognizing, responding to and/or attributing mental states of all kinds. So conceived, anyone who believes that dysfunctional social relating is the result of incapacities in this domain can be thought of as endorsing an impaired mind minding hypothesis (or IMMH) of some kind or other. An IMMH claims that dysfunctional interpersonal relating that is symptomatic of these disorders is—in some way—rooted in problems with the awareness of, sensitivity to, and/or insight into the mentality of others.

Analyses of performances on standardized ToM tests attest to selective and dissociable deficits in high-level mind minding abilities for those with ASD and schizophrenia. ToM tests include first- and second-order false belief tasks (which, respectively, test the ability to ascribe beliefs contrary to one's own, and to ascribe beliefs about someone else's beliefs to another); intention inferencing tasks (which test the ability to infer a character's intention from information in a story); and tasks which examine understanding of indirect speech. It is acknowledged that our current understanding of the psychometric properties of these tasks is seriously impoverished, leading to questions about construct and criterion validity (Badgaiyan 2009; Bosco et al. 2009; Sprong et al. 2007). Even so, performance patterns on these tests provide at least a partial insight into the abilities of different clinical populations and subpopulations for making third-person mental state ascriptions, albeit an insight that is restricted to performances in restricted and artificial laboratory conditions.

Although it has been robustly shown that those individuals with ASD who have problems with joint attention tasks perform poorly on false belief tests, not all of those with ASD fail the latter tests—somewhere in the range between 15% and 60% pass (Happé 1995). A recent meta-analysis reveals that individuals with schizophrenia perform more poorly on ToM tests than those with other disorders and healthy controls (Sprong et al. 2007; see also Brüne 2005). However, the performance of individuals in different symptom subgroups varies;

those with negative and more severe symptoms—resembling the more extreme forms of ASD—perform comparatively worse than those in other schizophrenic subpopulations who display other active symptoms.

This data underlines the fact that it would be a mistake to characterize the impaired mind minding associated with these disorders as a total absence or loss of capacity—i.e. as a blanket mindblindness. This is further emphasized, in the case of schizophrenia, by studies conducted by McCabe et al. (2004). Using the ecologically sensitive techniques of conversational analysis, they examined routine encounters between people diagnosed with schizophrenia and their psychiatrists and therapists. The subjects were inpatients with active symptoms, but were not acutely ill. It was found that they are able enough in attributing mental states to themselves and others, and do so spontaneously when the need arises. They manage to navigate conversational twists and turns, showing awareness of communicative intentions. Their problems in interpersonal relating rest, rather, with the incredible nature of their attributions, their unconvincing justifications for making them, and their unwillingness to revise such attributions in the face of challenge and disagreement.

The situation is different with BPD patients. Although they too are unable to make coherent and credible mental attributions while emotionally aroused in certain contexts, they are able to pass standard ToM tests under experimental conditions (Fonagy and Luyten 2010; see also Arntz et al. 2009). Indeed, recent studies show that BPD patients are superior to healthy controls in the attribution of mental states to interaction partners when emotional cues are present (Franzen et al. 2011).

Summarizing, the performance data—from controlled experiments and ecological studies—suggests that individuals on the extreme end of the autistic spectrum and schizophrenics presenting with negative symptoms come closest to displaying a near total incapacity for understanding or complete indifference to the mental life of others. High-functioning individuals with autism who lack the normal means of relating and understanding mental states, sometimes develop alternate compensatory methods, such as employing basic rules of thumb, that enable them to get by in their dealings with others, even if awkwardly. Comparatively, although those in some subgroups of schizophrenia may perform more poorly in ToM tests compared with controls, they never fully lose their ability to attribute mental states. Rather their capacity for dealing with others is diminished by the fact that the content of their attributions are aberrant or unrealistic. The latter also seems to be the case with BPD patients.

It seems that while individuals with ASD might never acquire the capacity to recognize or attribute mental states in the normal way at all, those with other disorders are capable of making mental attributions but their ability to do so falls apart when other symptoms or complications take hold. When in such states these individuals are unable to bring at least some of their mind minding capacities to bear properly.

The existing data from ToM test performance in these populations line up with the fact that the profile of dysfunctional interpersonal relating varies across and within disorders. It also suggests that capacities for relating to and understanding mental states operates on multiple levels and comes in degrees.

There are several IMMHs now on the market that seek to explain specific patterns of dysfunction in ASD, BPD, and schizophrenia. In 1985, Baron-Cohen, and colleagues suggested that the fundamental problem autistic individuals have in relating to others is that they are to varying degrees, in effect, blind to other minds. Although not offered as an explanation of the full set of clinical features associated with ASD, proponents of this view claim that mindblindness may be the "core and possibly universal abnormality of autistic individuals" (Baron-Cohen 2000, p. 3). The mind minding deficits in question are thought to be essentially problems with the capacity to "imagine or represent states of mind that we or others might hold" (Baron-Cohen 1995, p. 2). But this version of IMMH thinks the problem lies with an inability to understand mental states of a quite sophisticated sort—such as beliefs and desires. Baron-Cohen (1995) admits, "my model of the mindreading systems says very little about the role of emotion" (p. 136). Rather, on his account, those with ASD are thought to completely lack or have only a shaky understanding of the basic axioms about how such mental states inter-relate. This is a wholly cognitivist kind of IMMH in that it assumes all the relevant work is done by forming mental representations about mental states.

In a similar vein, Frith (1992) suggested, more ambitiously, that the underlying deficit which explains the full range of positive and negative symptoms in schizophrenia might also boil down to problems in representing representational mental states, or metarepresentational capacities. According to Frith's model, metarepresentational failures result in an inability to recognize and keep track of one's own intentions. This, in turn, results in misattributions of self-produced states in the form of delusions of control, thought insertion, thought withdrawal, and auditory hallucinations. Equally, problems in attributing mental states to others allegedly give rise to paranoid delusions and delusions of reference. The negative symptoms of schizophrenia, he conjectured, stem from a more fundamental loss of the ability to represent mental states—a sort of mindblindness. This would explain the similar pattern of withdrawal and disinterest in socializing which is seen in schizophrenics presenting with negative symptoms and in certain autistic individuals.

Not all IMMHs are cognitivist in flavor. Opposing the intellectualist focus of the high-end cognitivist explanations, Hobson (1991, 1993, 2002, 2007, 2010) has consistently championed the idea that the central difficulties of autism stem from problems in more basic, emotionally charged ways, of engaging with others. He holds that "what is central to autism is an impairment in emotional aspects of interpersonal relatedness" (Hobson 2002, p. 14). These have to do primarily with inabilities to connect with others on an emotional level—inabilities that prevent those with ASD from engaging in shared practices that are critical for the development of more sophisticated ways of understanding others.

Other IMMHs focus on the way high and low mind minding activities interact. Fonagy and Luyten (2009, 2010) advocate a multidimensional theory, maintaining that the pattern of dysfunctions specific to BPD, for example, arise because of disturbed interplay between different modes of mind minding. Low-level mind minding capacities, those used for attending and responding to others' emotions, become heightened when BPD individuals are in aroused states. This, Fonagy and Luyten claim, interferes with and diminishes their, quite distinct, high-level capacities for successfully attributing mental states, like beliefs and desires.

It is beyond the scope of this chapter to comment on the plausibility of these different IMMHs. It is, however, worth observing that several branches of empirical work strongly support the hypothesis that adult humans do in fact have more than one way of minding minds. There is compelling evidence that there are at least two, functionally isolated and anatomically quite separate, networks for dealing with and making sense of other minds (Fonagy and Luyten 2010; Gallese 2007, 2010; Saxe 2009a, 2009b). These distinct modes of mind minding are called into service for different kinds of interpersonal relating.

Evidence From Cognitive Psychology and Neuroscience

Preliminary findings from cognitive psychology suggest that normally developing adults have a sophisticated competence for making mental state attributions but one that exists alongside more basic capacities for attending to and engaging with other minds.

Low-level capacities for responding to other minds are apparently enlisted during fast and fluid non-verbal intersubjective engagements. Such capacities appear to be preserved throughout development. Adults continue to call upon them in a default manner even after more sophisticated capacities for mental attribution and understanding others are fully in place (for a review see Apperly and Butterfill 2009). The existence of two parallel but distinct systems is apparently confirmed by interference patterns demonstrated in experiments that tax subjects' capacities for making mental state attributions while they are simultaneously engaged in tasks that require the low-level monitoring of others' perspectives. It seems that the price of speed is inflexibility—this way of attending and responding to other minds has signature limitations. Consistent with these findings, low-level mind minding is assumed to be automatic whereas reaction time data suggests that adults only actively and explicitly monitor and attribute contentful mental states, such as false beliefs selectively—i.e. when doing so is demanded by, and specifically relevant to, the interpretative task in hand (Saxe 2009b).

Capacities for low-level mind minding are thought to be part of a phylogenetically ancient system for dealing with others. Fonagy and Luyten (2010) identify the brain regions associated with it as including the amygdala, basal ganglia, ventromedial prefrontal cortex, lateral temporal cortex, and the dorsal anterior cingulated cortex.

An exciting possibility is that at least some low-level mind minding in humans might involve mirroring mechanisms. In such systems sets of cortical neurons tied to specific types of goal-related actions fire when actions of that type are perceived (visually or audibly) and also when observers execute actions of that type. Such systems are akin in functionality to those discovered in the premotor cortices of macaque monkeys (Gallese and Goldman 1998; Gallese et al. 1996). It seems that humans have several different neural systems that function in this way. Some, located in the premotor and posterior partial cortices, are implicated in the imitation of simple movements, imitative learning, and the detection of action intentions. Others involve the activation of brain regions associated with specific emotions, such as disgust, and sensations such as pain, which are set off by observing expressions of these emotions and sensations in others (see Gallese (2010) for discussion).

In line with the two-systems hypothesis, mirroring activity in humans is regarded as "immediate, automatic, and almost reflexlike" (Gallese 2005, p. 101). Some hold that mirroring activity is sufficient to enable a special variety of non-conceptual and pre-linguistic form of understanding of actions and intentions (Rizzolatti and Sinigaglia 2006, 2010; Sinigaglia 2009). Although the claim that mirror systems yield anything that might be properly called an understanding of minds is disputed, it is agreed that whatever precise role they play in interpersonal relating, mirror systems come before and below, and remain quite distinct from high-level folk psychological abilities of the sort that involve the ascription and interpretation of contentful mental states—such as beliefs that say or represent how things stand with the world—in systematic ways.

Not only are the two ways of minding minds separate, they do not appear to directly communicate. Saxe (2009a) observes:

> there is substantial evidence for co-opted mechanisms, leading from one individual's mental state to a matching state in an observer, but there is no evidence that the output of these co-opted mechanisms serve as the basis for mental state attributions. There is also substantial evidence for attribution mechanisms that serve as the basis for mental state attributions, but there is no evidence that these mechanisms receive their input from co-opted mechanisms. (p. 447)

This raises important questions about the extent to which and precisely how the different mind minding systems interact, but it further highlights the fact that a different set of brain regions is implicated in the reflective, controlled, and cognitively demanding tasks of explicit mental state attribution. For example, successfully attributing beliefs that diverge from one's own requires simultaneously inhibiting one's own current view of how things stand with the world. This entails keeping track of the inferential connections that hold between the attributed attitudes, professed and/or inferred, and checking these for coherence. For this reason, sophisticated attribution and interpretation is slower than low-level forms of engaging with another's attitudes and emotions. Apart from calling on specialized capacities for representing and understanding mental states it also involves deploying domain general, cognitively costly resources for inhibitory control, working memory, and language.

The high-level network for making sense of others in ways that involve the attribution of contentful mental states is thought to be formed by an alliance of dissociable brain regions including the right and left temporo-parietal junction, medial parietal cortex (including posterior cingulate and precuneus), and medial prefrontal cortex. These areas exhibit significantly greater hemodynamic activation, for example, when subjects read about beliefs as opposed to other purely, non-mentalistic topics (Saxe 2009b).

Functional magnetic resonance imaging (fMRI) experiments reveal that the right temporo-parietal junction (RTPJ), in particular, is selectively enlisted for tasks requiring the interpretatively complex attribution of mental states. Saxe and Wexler (2005) discovered that RTPJ activity is enhanced when the professed beliefs or desires of story protagonists conflicted with subjects' expectations about what such characters ought to believe or desire, based on background knowledge about them. Moreover, this region is not similarly recruited for other tasks that involve assessing other, more general, socially relevant facts about persons. Saxe and Wexler also reported that none of the other brain regions in the wider network for controlled mental state attribution—i.e. the left temporo-parietal junction (LTPJ), posterior cingulate (PC) and medial prefrontal cortex (MPFC)—exhibited equally selective activity. Summarizing Saxe (2009b) reports that the "fMRI literature suggests a division in the neural system involved in making social judgments about others, with one component (the RTPJ) specifically recruited for the attribution of mental states, while a second component (the MPFC) is involved more generally in the consideration of the other person" (p. 405).

In line with the Gogtay (2004) neurodevelopmental data about the stages of cortical maturation of gray matter, Saxe et al. (2009) found "that selectivity for thinking about people's thoughts emerges in the RTPJ between ages 6 and 11 years" (p. 1206). In attempting to understand what might drive this process they consider the "intriguing recent hint that middle childhood is a critical time for interactions between language and theory of mind" (p. 1207). The authors recognize that these new findings present a challenge "for theories of cognitive development that emphasize an innate and early-maturing domain-specific module for theory of mind" (p. 1207).

PHILOSOPHICAL PROPOSALS AND FRAMEWORKS

It is one thing to suggest that certain dysfunctions in interpersonal relating are in fact problems with various mind minding capacities; it is quite another to isolate and understand the true causes of such disturbances. A popular assumption is that dysfunctional mind minding, whether of the high or low variety, stems from the faulty performance of a cognitive mechanism, or set of mechanisms, that are imagined to literally house the rules and representations that are the basis of our mind minding competencies. Although the disturbances manifest at the cognitive level, it is assumed that such faults are ultimately rooted in damaged or disturbed bits of neural circuitry that implement the relevant mind minding competencies. If so, this gives us special reason to attend to the brain regions that instantiate these competencies when seeking to understand the underlying causes of such dysfunctions.

Influential versions of theory theory (TT) and simulation theory (ST), offered from within the fold of cognitive science, promote this general explanatory strategy. They suppose that our mind minding competencies strongly supervene, entirely, on representational activity in areas of the brain that can be specified in principle.

Proponents of pure TT approaches conjecture that mind minding depends on the use of internally represented rules that describe the behavior of mental states—rules that are required for making inference-based attributions of mental states. These rules enable inferences to be drawn from evidence (of perceived behaviors, testimony, and the like) in order to reach conclusions about which mental states might cause or might have caused a particular action. It is assumed that the network of principles—a theory of mind—that makes this possible is similar in all crucial respects to the theories scientists operate with, only the content of this theory is couched in mental representations and rules at the subpersonal, subdoxastic level.

Many versions of TT aim to explain the apparently unique human competence for making sophisticated mental state attributions; those that require an understanding of the full range of mental states and how they inter-relate (Fodor 1987, 1995; Leslie et al. 2004). However, in an attempt to explain the limited capacities of younger children and non-human animals, a number of theorists have posited the existence of naïve, weak, or minimal ToM as well. ToMs of this kind are thought to contain rules and representations detailing the interaction of primitive mental states, such as goals and simple intentions, not more sophisticated mental states such as beliefs and desires (Bogdan 2009; Tomasello et al. 2003). Having a theory about primitive states of mind, so the proposal goes, suffices to enable young infants, adults (sometimes) and other non-human animals (possibly) to conduct their social dealings.

Pure TTists subscribe to the strongest form of cognitivism about what explains mind minding abilities. As Goldman (2006) stresses, "According to all forms of TT ... mindreading is a thoroughly metarepresentational activity. It exploits data structures and computational procedures about first-order mental states" (p. 114). Advocates of TT assume that mind minding requires the possession and use of a core set of mentalistic laws or rules. If so, even the most rudimentary forms of social cognition depend on subpersonal processes involving mental representations—representations of mental states and their rules of inter- action. It is by having the relevant theory that such mental states can be recognized "as such," and thus can be targeted and tracked. Similarly, it is having the relevant theory that enables actions to be predicted and explained.

Modularist versions of TT take these ideas a step further. They propose that the rules and representations that form the basis of mind minding competencies reside in dedicated, informationally encapsulated and cognitively impenetrable, cognitive mechanisms— or modules—of a special kind; ToM mechanisms (or ToMMs). These devices contain the domain specific principles or theories that enable their owners to deal with and make sense of minds (Fodor 1983). ToMMs are mental modules that are hypothesized to contain infor- mationally encapsulated and cognitively impenetrable mental representations of these core folk psychological principles housed in a fixed and dedicated neural architecture.

Adherents of pure simulation theory (ST), in contrast, hold that our capacities for engag- ing with and understanding minds are not grounded in a set of represented rules. They propose, instead, that the insights into minds that underwrite our social dealings depend on using features of our own mental equipment in order to model the way in which some other may be thinking or experiencing. Specifically, this involves co-opting our own mental machinery, normally used for other tasks, for this alternative purpose. Because both our minds and those of others are assumed to operate in structurally similar ways it is at least possible to deal effectively with and make sense of other minds without invoking any theo- retical rules at all. For example, a prominent version of ST theory supposes that high-level mind minding is made possible by operations involving the practical reasoning mechanism. That mechanism, it is conjectured, is taken off-line from its usual task of manipulating men- tal states in order to produce actions to become the engine of the simulative process. This is achieved by feeding it with pretend beliefs and desires so that it produces predictions and explanations of another's behavior rather than generating one's own actions.

Importantly, because of this, ST yields different predictions from TT about where the relevant neural activity that underpins mind minding might occur. Like pure TT, pure ST comes in both high- and low-level varieties (see Goldman 2006). As such, defenders of ST believe that many different parts of the brain might be involved in different kinds of mod- eling or simulation processes.

It is possible to mix and match pure versions of these accounts—combining, for example, low-level ST with high-level TT or vice versa. Hybrid theories of TT and ST are also possi- ble at all levels. Indeed, it is widely held that theory or simulation might come into play and perform different sorts of roles in enabling mind minding. It is, however, incumbent on pro- ponents of hybrid theories to specify exactly which roles theory and simulation procedures are meant to play.

Despite important differences, combining TT and ST in these ways is possible because both proposals subscribe to a common framework. Theories of both types assume that the primary function of mind minding is to predict and explain actions and that the attribu- tion of causally efficacious inner mental states to others is required for this. Attribution is achieved by means of inference or analogy. As such, TT and ST approaches assume a certain characterization of what any kind of intelligent encounter with minds necessarily requires, despite local disagreements about how best to explain what enables such encounters to take place. In endorsing the idea that there is always an essential gap between people—even in our most basic encounters—defenders of TT and ST assume that mental phenomena cannot be directly perceived.

Both theories are motivated by the idea that we can only know of mental states indirectly. When engaging with others we are only ever acquainted with outward behavior, where such behaviors amount to nothing more than the causal product of behind-the-scenes mental activity. Such behavior counts as mindful if and only if it is generated by inner, mental states—which lie somewhere between perceptual inputs and behavioral outputs. Accordingly, in intersubjective encounters, there is always a gap to bridge if we are to make sense of behavior in terms of mental states. The explanations of TT and ST offer competing proposals about how we bridge this gap—how we solve the practical problem of getting at other minds—when encountering others.

Because they characterize what dealing with other minds essentially involves in this way, proponents of TT and ST also assume that our mind minding competencies, high and low, reside entirely within individuals. This commitment to individualism strongly encourages the idea that mind minding competencies must be located, wholly and solely, somewhere in the brain. It is only in finer details of their accounts that TT and ST disagree about what the engines of social cognition are, how they work and where they might be found in the brain.

Inspired by the phenomenological tradition and Wittgensteinian approaches to mind, a number of philosophers have questioned the legitimacy of the assumed framework within which TT and ST operate as well as criticizing details of particular TT and ST proposals (see Gallagher and Zahavi 2007; Hutto 2008; Ratcliffe 2007). It is argued that the idea that we are essentially cut off from other minds at a basic level mischaracterizes how we first encounter others. Primary intersubjective engagements, so these critics hold, are based not on inference or analogy, but on a direct responsiveness to the psychology of others. The psychological situation of others is perceived in and through their expressions. This is possible if mentality is conceived of as strongly embodied and thus integrally bound up with world-relating activities, including those in which we reciprocally engage and interact with others. Accordingly, mentality is constituted by nothing short of, and nothing beyond, concrete episodes and patterns of interactive engaging. On this account, to the extent that it is intelligible to ask where such experiences are located, the best answer is that they are extensive; they are to be found in interactions that spread across time and space—across brains, bodies, and environments.

From this vantage, at least in basic cases, there is no problem of other minds for individuals to solve. Barring impairments, we come ready made to attend to, and be moved by, others expressions and actions and vice versa. The expressions and actions of others are of immediate significance to us. Thus perceiving another's attitudes and emotions can transform and shape our psychological situation in direct and meaningful ways. To accept this is to assume that, rather than trying to solve a naturally occurring version of the problem of other minds in order to make social dealings possible, evolution equipped us with specialized capacities for engaging with one another in order that we might regulate our activities with respect to others. We are built to shape and share, but not read, minds (McGeer 2007; Zawidzki 2008).

Despite appearances, to conceive of mentality as constituted by embodied activity is not to endorse behaviorism, although it is often mistaken as having this implication. This is because to reject the idea that minds are hidden in a wholesale way is to reject idea that embodied activity is rightly identified with bodily movements that are not already mindful, experiential or purposeful.

The enactivist framework, first articulated by Varela and colleagues (1991) and now hailed as a new wave of thinking in cognitive science, offers powerful support to this alternative way of thinking about the nature of minds. It stresses the embodied, embedded and extensive nature of mentality. In its more radical variants, enactivism is a way of conceiving of the basic nature of minds and how we encounter them is completely antithetical to the intellectualism promoted by cognitivists. The most revolutionary varieties of enactivism deny that mentality must be, always and everywhere, mediated by mental representations (Chemero 2009; Hutto and Myin, 2013; Thompson 2007). Enactivist approaches that insist on a strong embodiment thesis regard mentality as concretely constituted by and consisting in the ways in which organisms interact with their environments, where these ways of interacting involve, but are not exclusively restricted to, what goes on in brains.

Consequently, enactivists of a radical stripe hold that mentality is, at root, extensive and not merely, as Clark and Chalmers (1998) famously argued, occasionally extended. The difference between these claims is that the extended mind hypothesis starts from the assumption that biologically basic mentality is, by default, brainbound. It then argues that in exceptional cases minds can extend, as when non-bodily add-ons are required in order to make the achievement of certain cognitive tasks possible. By contrast, those who endorse a strong version of the embodiment thesis assume that minds, in their basic nature, cross boundaries—they are wide-ranging and extensive.

Such approaches provide new tools for understanding the basis of primary interpersonal interaction while abandoning the idea that social interaction depends upon the capacity to represent mental states of any sort at all—even those of an immature or weak variety.

They offer a de-intellectualized characterization of what human interpersonal relations involve. Engaging with others takes the form of unprincipled embodied, interactions where the capacity for such engagement is not thought to be best explained by positing internal devices that manipulate subpersonal rules and representations or their equivalents (Gallagher 2005; Hutto 2006). Defenders of this view allow that it is possible to stand back and describe the rules of these engagements but they deny that in so doing one is describing or making explicit the set of rules that govern and causally explain how individuals manage to conduct their social exchanges.

Familiarity with traditions, institutions, roles, and local norms play a large part in molding our everyday expectations, hence, appeal to capacities for basic embodied engagements cannot be the whole story about what grounds human interpersonal relating (Gallagher and Hutto 2008). In the human case, it is conjectured that the mastery of more sophisticated social practices, involving pretense, conversation, and narratives, make different kinds of interpersonal relating and ways of understanding others possible. Highlighting this, Bruner (1990) argues convincingly that folk psychology is an instrument of culture.

The narrative practice hypothesis (NPH) is an advance on Bruner's idea. It shows why that proposal deserves a place at the table in current debates about the basis of our folk psychological abilities (Hutto 2008). The NPH says that our high-level capacity for making sense of others is normally acquired through engagement in narrative practices. It is by engaging in narrative practices (in which the participants jointly attend to stories about people who act for reasons) that children gradually come to see the connections between mental states and thereby acquire their full-fledged folk psychological competence. This occurs over the course of later childhood, especially from age five years onward. Through participating in narrative practices children gradually come by an articulate understanding of intentional attitudes such as beliefs, desires, hopes, and their possible relations.

The NPH recognizes that folk psychology is a highly structured, conceptually based, competence. But it assumes that it is an environmentally scaffolded competence and, hence, implies that it does not have a wholly internal, neural basis. Rather, in line with Sterelny's (2010) scaffolded mind hypothesis the NPH assumes that "human cognitive capacities both depend on and have been transformed by environmental resources" (p. 472).

IMPLICATIONS FOR PSYCHIATRY

These philosophical debates matter to psychiatry. One reason for this is that how we think about the basis of mind minding competencies influences how we think about the prognosis and possible treatment of dysfunctional interpersonal relating. Another reason is that philosophical frameworks influence the way we think about and evaluate possible psychiatric strategies. To illustrate these effects, it is instructive to compare and contrast two opposing classes of proposal about the basis of our high-level folk psychological competence: those that posit biologically inherited, hardwired mindreading devices and those that regard folk psychological capacities to be dependent upon special sorts of environmentally based activities and practices.

If it is true that folk psychological competence is wholly and solely based in neurally instantiated mindreading devices then it is theoretically possible that dysfunctions in this domain might be curable one day. This idea holds out the promise that it may be possible to completely eliminate the mental dysfunctions by intervening on the wiring of the brain. In principle, it should be possible to fit new parts into the existing cognitive structure and restore performance, in much the way that malfunctioning components in one's car can be fixed or new ones fitted. If it is assumed that such theories are true then the only way to fully deal with mind minding dysfunctions would be to intervene on the neural circuitry causing the disturbances.

Therefore, practically speaking, to assume that inherited mindreading devices are the source of the dysfunctions sets a certain agenda for psychopathological intervention. This assumption provides both a specific target and a rough idea of where to look for it: the task is to find the neural troublemaker that is the source of the dysfunctions. To approach this psychiatric task in this way would be to adopt the ambitions of the medical model, at least when dealing with mind minding dysfunctions. That model insists that all genuine mental disorders are to be understood as biological, brain-based pathologies (see Murphy 2010).

Conversely, theories that assume that malfunctioning biological devices are ultimately responsible for mind minding dysfunctions predict that it is impossible for such dysfunctions to be treated through education or training. For example, this is clearly true of modular TT since it assumes that the core rules of ToM are hardwired and cognitively impenetrable. Equally, there is no way to repair a faulty practical reasoning mechanism, assumed by prominent versions of ST to be the engine of high-level simulations, by means of exercise or education.

These predictions are consistent with evidence from various studies. It has been demonstrated that after explicit instruction individuals with autism can master basic ToM rules and can be taught to pass false belief tasks. Nevertheless, they are unable to bring this understanding to bear in non-experimental contexts (Begeer et al. 2011). Thus, even after successful training these individuals show no improvement in their ability to navigate everyday social interactions. Conversely, "several studies showed transfer from 'real life' scenarios to artificial tasks" (Sweetenham 2000, p. 453).

If mind minding dysfunctions are best explained by faults in biologically inherited devices then it is to be expected that explicit ToM training will not yield the requisite improvements in interpersonal relating. At best, such training might provide a different and limited means of getting by in the social arena. ToM training might, at best, compensate, imperfectly, for the lack of subpersonally grasped rules or simulative capacities but having true competence in this domain requires having a properly functioning and fitted mindreading device.

The neuroscientific evidence cited earlier suggests that there are devoted brain regions that can be pinpointed as being, uniquely and exclusively, implicated in sophisticated tasks involving the attribution of mental states. However, all of the neuroscientific data gathered by imaging and lesion studies relating to the exercise of folk psychological abilities is compatible with the non-existence of biologically inherited mindreading devices. In the neuroscience literature the ToM descriptor is widely used to describe these brain regions. It is generally assumed that there must be some place in the brain that manipulates mental representations and that house or enable our folk psychological competence. This is in line with the view that "the brain is the seat of most, if not all, mental events" (Goldman and de Vignemont 2009, p. 154). But, crucially, the evidence from neuroscience, taken on its own, does not necessitate this conclusion. The description of what the brain is doing, preferred by those who adopt a ToM framework, is not something that can be read off from the models of neural activity produced on the basis of fMRI scans. There is no logical connection between the existence of ToMMs and the robust findings of modern neuroscience about which brain regions are involved in specific mind minding tasks.

If there are no biologically inherited mindreading devices then we have to interpret the data in a new way. Reconfiguring our thinking along enactivist lines does exactly that—it asks us to rethink our understanding of the status and nature of the neuroscientific findings. To accept that minds are enactive and extensive in the ways described in the previous section is not to deny that the exercise of our mental capacities always and everywhere involves the brain. But if our mind minding competencies are extensive then brain activity alone cannot solely be responsible for them. For that reason attending exclusively to what goes on in brains, at best, can only ever give us a partial take on what is, in fact, a much more complicated and wide-reaching phenomenon. If our folk psychological competence does not in fact reside in a set of internally represented rules or modeling capacities located in the brain then dealing with any faults to neurology, even when necessary, is insufficient for curing dysfunctions of interpersonal relating.

More than this, not only do we lack any special justification for focusing our curative attention exclusively on individuals and their brains, we have positive reason to cast our gaze wider and seek to understand the nature and role of the environmental and interpersonal factors, such as our shared practices, as well. A number of promising therapies for addressing mind minding dysfunctions—including the use of relational development interventions and social stories—have been and are still being actively developed. These are designed to make focused adjustments to the style, timing, content, and rhythm of intersubjective interactions along specific parameters (Belmonte 2009; De Jeagher and Di Paolo 2007; Shanker 2004; Sparaci 2008).

Believers in biologically inherited mindreading devices can acknowledge the value of these therapies, pointing out that there is no conflict in supposing that they can be effective even if they do not get at the root cause of the dysfunctions. From a different philosophical vantage, however, the status of these therapies looks quite different. It may be that they primarily target what lies behind mind minding dysfunctions, as opposed to providing direct relief by dealing with collateral features. This shift of perspective raises the possibility that practice-based therapies can directly assist or educate individuals by helping them to acquire or recover the relevant mind minding capacities without having to intervene directly and invasively in the brain.

If so, this underlines the importance of identifying and better understanding the wider features that matter. Focusing on the high-end abilities, for example, one well-known version of TT rejects the idea that our mindreading capacities are wholly biologically inherited, arguing instead that our theory of mind is forged through active, scientific theorizing (Gopnik and Meltzoff 1997). If this version of TT is true, then it could provide insight into the sort of activities that would be required for engendering or restoring theory of mind abilities. If it is not, then we must look elsewhere. By the same token, if it is assumed that folk psychological competence is instead acquired by engaging in shared, social practices that make use of narratives with special properties then a better understanding of those practices, and the capacities required for engaging in them, may be of critical importance in developing effective treatments.

REFERENCES

American Psychiatric Association (2000). *Diagnostic and Statistical Manual of Mental Disorders, Fourth Edition, Text Revision*. Washington, DC: American Psychiatric Association.

Apperly, I. and Butterfill, S. A. (2009). Do humans have two systems to track beliefs and belief-like states? *Psychological Review*, 116(4), 953–70.

Arntz, A., Bernstein, D., Oorschot, M., and Schobre, P. (2009). Theory of mind in borderline and cluster-c personality disorder. *Journal of Nervous and Mental Disease*, 197(11), 801–7.

Badgaiyan, R. (2009). Theory of mind and schizophrenia. *Consciousness and Cognition*, 18, 320–2.

Baron-Cohen, S. (1995). *Mindblindness: An Essay on Autism and Theory of Mind*. Cambridge, MA: MIT Press.

Baron-Cohen, S. (2000). Theory of mind and autism: A fifteen-year review. In S. Baron-Cohen, H. Tager-Flusberg, and D. Cohen (Eds), *Understanding Other Minds: Perspectives from Developmental Cognitive Neuroscience*, pp. 3–20. Oxford: Oxford University Press.

Baron-Cohen, S., Leslie, A., and Frith, U. (1985). Does the autistic child have a 'theory of mind'? *Cognition*, 21, 37–46.

Begeer, S., Gevers, C., Clifford, P., Verhoeve, M., Kat, K., Hoddenbach, E., *et al.* (2011). Theory of mind training in children with autism: A randomized controlled trial. *Journal of Autism Developmental Disorder*, 41(8), 997–1006.

Belmonte, M. (2009). What's the story behind 'theory of mind' and autism. *Journal of Consciousness Studies*, 16(6–8), 118–39.

Bogdan, R. (2009). *Predicative Minds: The Social Ontogeny of Propositional Thinking.* Cambridge, MA: MIT Press.

Bosco, F. M., Colle, L., De Fazio, S., Bono, A., Ruberti, S., and Tirassa, M. (2009). Th.o.m.a.s.: An exploratory assessment of theory of mind in schizophrenic subjects. *Consciousness and Cognition, 18,* 306–19.

Brüne, M. (2005). 'Theory of mind' in schizophrenia: A review of the literature. *Schizophrenia Bulletin, 31*(1), 21–42.

Bruner, J. (1990). *Acts of Meaning.* Cambridge, MA: Harvard University Press.

Chemero, A. 2009. *Radical Embodied Cognitive Science.* Cambridge, MA: MIT Press.

Clark, A. and Chalmers, C. (1998). The extended mind. *Analysis, 58*(1), 7–19.

Corcoran, R. (2000). Theory of mind in other clinical conditions: Is a selective 'theory of mind' deficit exclusive to autism. In S. Baron-Cohen, H. Tager-Flusberg, and D. Cohen (Eds), *Understanding Other Minds: Perspectives from Developmental Cognitive Neuroscience,* pp. 391–421. Oxford: Oxford University Press.

De Jeagher, H. and Di Paolo, E. (2007). Participatory sense-making: An enactive approach to social cognition. *Phenomenology and the Cognitive Sciences, 6*(4), 485–507.

Frith, C. (1992). *The Cognitive Neuropsychology of Schizophrenia.* London: Erlbaum.

Fodor, J. A. (1983). *The Modularity of Mind.* Cambridge, MA: MIT Press.

Fodor, J. A. (1987). *Psychosemantics.* Cambridge, MA: MIT Press.

Fodor, J. A. (1995). A theory of the child's theory of mind. In M. Davies and T. Stone. (Eds), *Mental Simulation,* pp. 109–122. Oxford: Blackwell.

Fonagy, P. and Luyten, P. (2009). A developmental, mentalization-based approach to the understanding and treatment of borderline personality disorder. *Development and Psychopathology, 21,* 1355–81.

Fonagy, P. and Luyten, P. (2010). Mentalization: Understanding borderline personality disorder. In T. Fuchs, H. C. Sattel, and P. Henningsen (Eds), *The Embodied Self: Dimensions, Coherence and Disorders,* pp. 260–77. Stuttgart: Schattauer.

Franzen, N., Hagenhoff, M., Baer, N., Schmidt, A., Mier, D., Sammer, G., *et al.* (2011). Superior 'theory of mind' in borderline personality disorder: An analysis of interaction behavior in a virtual trust game. *Psychiatry Research, 187*(1–2), 224–33.

Gallagher, S. (2001). The practice of mind: Theory, simulation or primary interaction? *Journal of Consciousness Studies, 8*(5–7), 83–108.

Gallagher, S. (2004). Understanding interpersonal problems in autism: Interaction theory as an alternative to theory of mind. *Philosophy, Psychiatry, & Psychology, 11*(3), 199–217.

Gallagher, S. (2005). *How the Body Shapes the Mind.* Oxford: Oxford University Press.

Gallagher, S. and Hutto, D. D. (2008). Understanding others through primary interaction and narrative practice. In J. Zlatev, T. Racine, C. Sinha, and E. Itkonen (Eds), *The Shared Mind: Perspectives on Intersubjectivity,* pp. 17–38. Amsterdam: John Benjamins.

Gallagher, S. and Zahavi, D. (2007). *The Phenomenological Mind: An Introduction to Philosophy of Mind and Cognitive Science.* London: Routledge.

Gallese, V. (2006). Intentional attunement: A neurophysiological perspective on social cognition and its disruption in autism. *Cognitive Brain Research, 1079,* 15–24.

Gallese, V. (2007). Before and below 'theory of mind': Embodied simulation and the neural correlates of social cognition. *Philosophical Transactions of the Royal Society B: Biological Sciences, 362,* 659–69.

Gallese, V. (2010). Embodied simulation and its role in intersubjectivity. In T. Fuchs, H. C. Sattel, and P. Henningsen (Eds), *The Embodied Self: Dimensions, Coherence and Disorders,* pp. 77–91. Stuttgart: Schattauer.

Gallese, V., Fadiga, L., Fogassi, L., and Rizzolatti, G. (1996). Action recognition in the premotor cortex. *Brain*, *119*, 593–609.

Gallese, V. and Goldman, A. (1998). Mirror neurons and the simulation theory of mind-reading. *Trends in Cognitive Sciences*, *2*(12), 493–501.

Goldman, A. I. (2006). *Simulating Minds: The Philosophy, Psychology and Neuroscience of Mindreading*. New York, NY: Oxford University Press.

Goldman, A. I. and de Vignemont, F. (2009). Is social cognition embodied? *Trends in Cognitive Sciences*, *13*(4), 154–9.

Gopnik, A. and Meltzoff, A. N. (1997). *Words, Thoughts, and Theories*. Cambridge, MA: MIT Press.

Happé, F. (1995). The role of age and verbal ability in the theory of mind task performance of subjects with autism. *Child Development*, *66*, 843–55.

Hobson, P. (1991). Against the theory of theory of mind. *British Journal of Developmental Psychology*, *9*, 33–51.

Hobson, P. (1993). The emotional origins of social understanding. *Philosophical Psychology*, *6*(3), 227–49.

Hobson, P. (2002). *The Cradle of Thought*. Basingstoke: Palgrave Macmillan.

Hobson, P. (2007). We share, therefore we think. In D. D. Hutto and M. Ratcliffe (Eds), *Folk Psychology Re-Assessed*, pp. 41–61. Dordrecht: Springer.

Hobson, P. (2010). Autism: A disorder in the development of self. In T. Fuchs, H. C. Sattel, and P. Henningsen (Eds), *The Embodied Self: Dimension, Coherence and Disorders*, pp. 183–202. Stuttgart: Schattauer.

Hooley, J. M. (2010). Social factors in schizophrenia. *Current Directions in Psychological Science*, *19*(4), 238–42.

Hutto, D. D. (2006). Unprincipled engagements: Emotional experience, expression and response. In R. Menary (Ed.), *Radical Enactivism: Focus on the Philosophy of Daniel D. Hutto*, pp. 13–38. Amsterdam: John Benjamins.

Hutto, D. D. (2008). *Folk Psychological Narratives: The Socio-Cultural Basis of Understanding Reasons*. Cambridge, MA: MIT Press

Hutto, D. D. and Myin, E. (2013). *Radicalizing Enactivism*. Cambridge, MA: MIT Press.

Leslie, A., Friedman, O., and German, T. P. (2004). Core mechanisms in 'theory of mind'. *Trends in Cognitive Sciences*, *8*(12), 528–33.

McCabe, R. (2004). Do people with schizophrenia display theory of mind deficits in clinical interactions? *Psychological Medicine*, *34*, 401–12.

McGeer, V. (2007). The regulative dimension of folk psychology. In D. D. Hutto and M. Ratcliffe (Eds), *Folk Psychology Re-Assessed*, pp. 137–56. Dordrecht: Springer.

Murphy, D. (2010). Philosophy of psychiatry. In E. N. Zalta (Ed.), *Stanford Encyclopedia of Philosophy*. [Online.] Available at: <http://plato.stanford.edu/entries/psychiatry/>.

Ramsey, W. M. (2007). *Representation Reconsidered*. Cambridge: Cambridge University Press.

Ratcliffe, M. (2007). From folk psychology to commonsense. In D. D. Hutto and M. Ratcliffe (Eds), *Folk Psychology Reassessed*, pp. 233–44. Dordrecht: Springer.

Rizzolatti, G. and Sinigaglia, C. (2006). *Mirrors in the Brain: How Our Minds Share Actions and Emotions*. Oxford: Oxford University Press.

Rizzolatti, G. and Sinigaglia, C. (2010). The functional role of the parieto-frontal mirror circuit: Interpretations and misinterpretations. *Nature Reviews Neuroscience*, *11*(16), 264–74.

Saxe, R. (2009a). The neural evidence for simulation is weaker than I think you think it is. *Philosophical Studies*, *144*(3), 447–56.

Saxe, R. (2009b). Theory of mind (neural basis). In W. P. Banks (Ed.), *Encyclopedia of Consciousness*, pp. 401–9. Amsterdam: Elsevier and Academic Press.

Saxe, R. and Wexler, A. (2005). Making sense of another mind: The role of the right temporo-parietal junction. *Neuropsychologia*, 43(10), 1391–9.

Saxe, R., Whitfield-Gabrieli, S., Scholz, J., and Pelphrey, K. A. (2009). Brain regions for perceiving and reasoning about other people in school-aged children. *Child Development*, 80(4), 1197–209.

Shanker, S. (2004). The roots of mindblindness. *Theory and Psychology*, 14(5), 685–703.

Shapiro, L. (2011). *Embodied Cognition*. London: Routledge

Sinigaglia, C. (2009). Mirror in action. *Journal of Consciousness Studies*, 16(6–8), 309–34.

Sinigaglia, C. (2010). Mirroring and making sense of others. *Nature Reviews Neuroscience*, 11(6), 449.

Sinigaglia, C. and Sparaci, L. (2008). The mirror roots of social cognition. *Acta Philosophica*, 2(17), 307–30.

Sparaci, L. (2008). Embodying gestures: The social orienting model and the study of early gestures in autism. *Phenomenology and the Cognitive Sciences*, 7(2), 203–23.

Sprong, M., Schothorst, P., Vos, E., Hox, J., and van Engeland, H. (2007). Theory of mind in schizophrenia: Meta-analysis. *British Journal of Psychiatry*, 191, 5–13.

Sterelny, K. (2010). Minds: Extended or scaffolded? *Phenomenology and the Cognitive Sciences*, 9(4), 465–81.

Sweetenham, J. (2000). Teaching theory of mind to individuals with autism. In S. Baron-Cohen, H. Tager-Flusberg, and D. Cohen (Eds), *Understanding Other Minds: Perspectives from Developmental Cognitive Neuroscience*, pp. 442–58. Oxford: Oxford University Press.

Thompson, E. (2007). *Mind in Life: Biology, Phenomenology, and the Sciences of Mind*. Cambridge, MA: Harvard University Press.

Tomasello, M., Call, J., and Hare, B. (2003). Chimpanzees understand psychological states—the question is which ones and to what extent. *Trends in Cognitive Sciences*, 7(4), 153–6.

Wing, L. (1996). *The Autistic Spectrum: New Updated Edition*. London, Robinson.

Varela, F. J., Thompson, E., and Rosch, E. (1991). *The Embodied Mind: Cognitive Science and Human Experience*. Cambridge, MA: MIT Press.

Zawidzki, T. (2008). The function of folk psychology: Mind reading or mind shaping? *Philosophical Explorations*, 11(3), 193–210.

CHAPTER 19

INTERSUBJECTIVITY AND PSYCHOPATHOLOGY

SHAUN GALLAGHER

THEORIES

Psychiatrists and psychopathologists sometimes look to psychology, neuroscience, and/ or philosophy of mind for concepts useful in understanding the specific pathologies with which they deal. In regard to intersubjectivity or social cognition, what they find when they look to current discussions in these fields, is, for the most part, an emphasis on theory of mind (ToM). ToM characterizes intersubjective relations in terms of the cognitive practice of mindreading (sometimes called mentalizing).

There are two dominant models for ToM. The first, "theory theory" (TT), claims that one's understanding of the other person is a matter of theoretical inference to that person's mental states. That is, if one wants to understand another's behavior, one needs to infer the mental states (beliefs, desires, intentions, etc.) that may be motivating that behavior. Such inferences are based upon an appeal to a general and common sense theory of behavior and motivation—folk psychology. The second model, simulation theory (ST), claims that rather than appealing to folk psychological theory to understand others, we make use of our own mind by running a simulation routine. That is, we put ourselves in the other person's shoes and ask what we would do in their circumstances. We simulate a set of beliefs and desires, specifically pretend or "as if" beliefs and desires that would explain the observed behavior, and then project these into the mind of the other person.

One of the assumptions shared by both TT and ST, and the very motivation for the idea of mindreading, is that the mind of the other is not directly accessible. We are not able to directly perceive the other person's mental states, and therefore we need some extra-perceptual cognitive operation—either inference or simulation—to work out what those mental states must be. Working out their mental states is precisely what it means to understand other people. Another assumption shared by TT and ST is that mindreading (i.e., understanding behavior in terms of the desires and beliefs that motivate and rational-ize it) is the primary and pervasive way in which we understand others. It characterizes our everyday encounters with others. On such views, when mindreading is construed in explicit conscious terms involving metarepresentation or introspection, our ordinary and everyday understanding of others involves a high-level cognitive process (for TT, see e.g., Carruthers 2009; for ST, see Goldman 2006). If something goes wrong with regard to intersubjective understanding, it means that something goes wrong with this cognitive process.

In terms of neuroscience, it is thought that high-order mindreading abilities depend on the medial prefrontal cortex and posterior superior temporal sulcus (e.g., Frith and Frith 1999). Recently, however, neuroscience has provided evidence that our intersubjective social cognitive processes may not all be high-level cognitive operations, but may involve a lower-level sensory-motor process. Simulationists suggest that the discovery of mirror neurons in pre-motor and parietal areas supports the idea that our primary way of understanding others starts as an automatic, low-level simulation carried out in the mirror system (Gallese 2001). Some simulation theorists consider this to be a form of (or a basis for) mindreading.

Neuroscience tells us, then, that we have two candidate systems for social cognition. One system, involving medial prefrontal cortex and posterior superior temporal sulcus, subtends high-order, explicit mindreading; the other system, pre-motor and parietal areas, or more generally sensory-motor areas, subtend low-level automatic mindreading. Insofar as social cognition involves the latter sensory-motor processes, it is said to be embodied, although this is often cashed out in terms of somatic representations in the brain (see Goldman and de Vignemont 2009). To conceive of mirror neuron processes as simulations in this sense is to think of social cognition as, at best, minimally embodied—that is, as a set of processes or mechanisms occurring only "in the head" and reducible to specific kinds of neuronal activity (Gallagher 2011).

In contrast to these ToM approaches, a recently developed phenomenological approach to social cognition has shifted the focus away from mindreading to more fully embodied interaction processes that involve enactive perception of the other person's contextualized meaning (De Jaegher et al. 2010; Gallagher 2005). This is sometimes referred to as interaction theory (IT). IT involves a shift away from defining the problem of social cognition in terms of mental states hidden away in the mind of the other, and a correlative shift away from defining the solution in terms of neuronal states in the brain of an individual engaged in mindreading. Rather, the emphasis is put on perceived social affordances and the engaged interactions taking place in our shared, intersubjective world. This phenomenological approach borrows heavily from developmental studies of primary and secondary intersubjectivity. It is also part of a larger account that includes a theory of communicative and narrative competences to explain our more subtle and sophisticated folk psychological abilities (Gallagher and Hutto 2006; Hutto 2007).

In the remainder of this section I'll focus on some of the evidence that supports IT; then, in the sections that follow, I'll discuss IT accounts of autism and schizophrenia.

Briefly, "primary intersubjectivity" (Trevarthen 1979) refers to perceptual and motor processes that allow newborn and young infants to engage with others from birth. The newborn infant can pick out a human face from the crowd of objects in its environment, with sufficient detail that will enable it to imitate the gesture it sees on that face (Meltzoff and Moore 1977, 1994). Infants automatically attune to smiles (and other facial gestures) with an enactive, and sometimes mimetic, response (Schilbach et al. 2008). Infants are visually attracted to biological movement, and auditorily attracted to certain kinds of sounds, such as familiar voices. They "vocalize and gesture in a way that seems [affectively and temporally] 'tuned' to the vocalizations and gestures of the other person" (Gopnik and Meltzoff 1997, p. 131), and they demonstrate a wide range of facial expressions, complex emotional, gestural, prosodic, and tactile face-to-face interaction patterns that are absent or rare in non-human primates (Falk 2004; Herrmann et al. 2007). They are also able to see bodily movement as expressive of emotion, and as goal-directed intentional movement. For example, at nine months infants follow the other person's eyes (Senju et al. 2006), and they start to perceive various movements of the head, the mouth, the hands, and more general body movements as meaningful, goal-directed movements. At ten to 11 months they are able to parse some kinds of continuous action according to intentional boundaries (Baird and Baldwin 2001; Baldwin and Baird 2001).

Expressions, intonations, gestures, and movements, along with the bodies that manifest them, do not float freely in the air; we find them in the world, tied to specific contexts, and infants soon start to notice how others engage with the world. Thus, primary intersubjectivity is supplemented and enhanced by processes of *secondary intersubjectivity* (Trevarthen and Hubley 1978), starting in the first year of life with the advent of joint attention. Infants begin to tie actions to pragmatic and social contexts; they enter into *contexts* of shared attention—shared situations—in which they learn what things mean and what they are for. In joint attention and joint actions the child looks to the body and the expressive movement of the other to discern the intention of the person or to find the meaning of some object. Children begin to see that another's movements and expressions often depend on meaningful and pragmatic contexts and are mediated by the surrounding world. Others are not given primarily as minds that we encounter cognitively. We perceive them as agents whose actions are framed in pragmatic and socially defined contexts.

It follows that there is not one uniform way in which we relate to others, but that our relations are mediated through the various pragmatic (and ultimately, institutional) circumstances of our encounters. Indeed, we are caught up in such pragmatic circumstances, already existing in reference to others from the very beginning. We do not simply observe others; we are not passive spectators. Rather we interact with others and in doing so we develop further capabilities in the contexts of those interactions.

According to IT we understand the actions of others on the highest, most appropriate pragmatic level possible, and in an enactive way. In other words, we understand actions at an intentional, goal-oriented level, primarily in terms of social affordances—in terms of our real or potential interactions with those agents. Rather than *making an inference* to, or *simulating* what the other person is intending by starting with bodily movements and moving thence to the level of mental events, we see the other's action as meaningful and as something to which we can respond, in the context of the physical and social environment. Applying Gibson's (1979) theory of affordances to the social context, we see others in relation to their possible actions and our possible interactions with them. Our enactive perception of the other person is never of an entity existing outside of a situation, but rather of an agent in a pragmatic context, which is often a situation that includes ourselves, as participants and not just as observers.

From the ToM perspective, all such processes might be considered precursors to the later development of mindreading capability, traditionally thought to emerge around four years of age (Baron-Cohen 1995; Bradshaw 2001). On the IT account, however, primary intersubjective processes give the infant, by the end of the first year of life, a non-mentalizing, perception- and interaction-based embodied understanding of the intentions and dispositions of other persons. These capabilities do not disappear in adulthood, or get replaced by ToM capabilities; they mature and become more sophisticated. This can be clearly shown in a micro-analysis of the postures, movements, gestures, gazes and facial expressions of people as they engage in a novel task and where communication among them comes in their very actions (see Lindblom 2007; Niedenthal et al. 2005). Behavioral experiments support this analysis. For example, Manera et al. (2011) showed that adults are able to perceptually discern another's intention (reflecting cooperation, completion, or individual action) in grasping an object, approximately 76% of the time. They can even do it in the dark (72% of the time) when point-light displays of grasping movements are presented (also see Becchio et al. 2010, 2012; Dittrich et al. 1996). According to IT, in many and perhaps most everyday interactions we understand the intentions, emotions, and actions of others in their movements, gestures, facial expressions, vocalizations, and in the particular pragmatic and social contexts in which they act, without having to infer or simulate what is going on inside their heads.

In regard to understanding what goes wrong with intersubjective processes in psychopathology, then, we should expect three different stories from the three different accounts of social cognition, TT, ST, and IT. Let's start by looking at what is perhaps the test case in this context: autism.

Autism

ToM approaches have developed the "mindblindness" account of autism (Baron-Cohen 1995). We can think of this in either TT or ST terms. Autistic children have well-documented difficulties with social interaction. From the TT perspective such difficulties are best characterized as a lack of ToM, as demonstrated in the autistic child's inability to pass false belief tasks. "Even with a mental age of 7 years, these children mostly fail in tasks which are normally passed around ages 3 and 4" (Leslie and Frith 1988, p. 315).

The standard false belief test is conducted with children of three and four years of age. There are different versions of the test, but perhaps the most famous is the Sally–Anne version. This is often presented in terms of a narrative, sometimes using drawings or puppets. Sally places a toy in a basket and then leaves the room. Anne moves the toy to a box. Sally returns. The three-year-old who has been observing this and listening to the story is then asked by the experimenter, "Where will Sally look for the toy?" On average the three-year-old will answer that she will look in the box. That, of course, is the wrong answer, and the supposition is that the three-year-old is developmentally unable to mindread the false belief that Sally would have in this case, since Sally would clearly want to look in the basket where she thinks the toy is still located. In contrast, the four-year-old will, on average, give the correct answer that Sally will look in the basket. So the TT view is that children acquire ToM around the age of four years.[1]

---

[1] The timing of this development has been recently challenged by false-belief experiments that show children as young as 15 months seemingly able to recognize false beliefs (Baillargeon et al. 2010). This is troublesome for TT proponents since the experiments push them to suggest that the metarepresentational abilities that they regard as necessary for ToM ability are already operative in the pre-linguistic 15 month old (see e.g., Carruthers 2009). This, however, is a controversial claim, and a

Autistic children typically fail to pass the false belief test, as Leslie and Frith (1988) indicated, even if they demonstrate a strong level of general intelligence at seven or nine years of age. The conclusion is thus that autistic children fail to develop the ability to mindread. They lack "the relevant normally developing mechanism ... for creating and handling *meta-representations*" (Leslie and Frith 1988, p. 315). They are thus "mindblind," and this is claimed to be the "core and possibly universal abnormality of autistic individuals" (Baron-Cohen 2000, p. 491). The explanation is that some domain-specific mechanism (a ToM mechanism) is damaged, cashed out in terms of a malfunction of prefrontal cortex areas, and that this explains the problem of social cognition, but not, of course, all problems associated with autism.

The sense that this explanation is not wholly satisfactory, however, is motivated by the fact that not every autistic individual fails false belief tasks. Roughly, between 15% and 60% actually pass these tests (Happé 1995; Reed and Patterson 1990). Thus, "although most autistic children fail tests which assess their mentalizing ability, there is a substantial minority of such children who regularly succeed" (Coltheart and Langdon 1998, p. 143). In addition, there is good reason to think that, in contrast to what ToM theorists suggest, high-functioning autistic individuals may actually employ inferential mindreading. Zahavi and Parnas (2003) cite accounts of strategies used by high-functioning autistic individuals. Temple Grandin, a well-known academic with Asperger's syndrome, for example, reports that she reads about people and observes them in order to arrive at the various principles that would explain and predict their actions in what she describes as "a strictly logical process." As Zahavi and Parnas suggest, "Grandin's compensatory way of understanding others perfectly resembles how *normal* intersubjective understanding is portrayed by the proponents of the theory-theory" (2003, pp. 67–68). For example, she has to decode emotional behavior since, as Oliver Sacks explains, she lacks an "implicit knowledge of social conventions and codes" (Sacks 1995, p. 258). Working with high-functioning autistics and those with Asperger's syndrome, Ozonoff and colleagues conclude that the ToM deficit "may not be primary to all of the autistic continuum, but may be a correlated deficit, present in more severely affected autistic individuals" (Ozonoff et al. 1991, p. 1118).

Turning to ST, the high-level simulation view cites evidence that autistic individuals have problems with simulation (see, e.g., Gordon and Barker 1994). Goldman (2006) cites Baron-Cohen:

> Autism is an empathy disorder: those with autism have major difficulties in "mindreading" or putting themselves into someone else's shoes, imagining the world through someone else's eyes and responding appropriately to someone else's feelings. (Baron-Cohen 2003, p. 137)

Goldman (2006, p. 203) notes that the kind of empathy that depends on what he terms "E-imagination," which is the basis for high-level simulation, is lacking in autistic individuals. One could easily ask, however, whether this is the cause of their social interaction problems (i.e., since they cannot simulate, they have deficits in social cognition), or the result of their social interaction problems (i.e., since they have serious deficits in social interaction, they also have trouble imagining what another person is thinking or feeling). Goldman

---

number of alternative interpretations that do not involve claims about metarepresentation or the concept of false belief have been put forward (see Froese and Gallagher, 2012; Gallagher and Povinelli 2012; Ruffman and Perner 2005).

doesn't consider the second possibility; he quickly concludes that Baron-Cohen's diagnosis supports ST. He also goes on to suggest that other theories of autism (like executive dysfunction or weak central coherence) are equally consistent with high-level simulation. Being consistent with ST, however, doesn't justify the claim that the failure of explicit simulation processes can account for the social interaction problems found in autism.

A number of researchers have suggested a connection between autism and dysfunction of mirror neurons (I've done so myself in Gallagher 2001; also see Iacoboni 2005; Williams et al. 2001). A deficit in mirror neuron activation in autism (for which there is some indirect evidence; see Oberman et al. 2005), would suggest, on the ST interpretation of mirror neuron resonance, that autistic subjects are not capable of low-level, automatic simulation. The ST interpretation of mirror neuron activation, however, is controversial. There is some empirical evidence that weighs against the view that mirror neurons should be construed as *simulating*, understood as a *matching* of observed action with one's own motor possibilities (a definition advanced by Goldman 2006). A variety of studies suggest that mirror neuron activation does not involve matching in this sense (Catmur et al. 2007; Csibra 2005; Dinstein et al. 2008; also see Gallagher 2008). The more traditional conception of simulation that involves pretense doesn't seem to apply to mirror neuron activation (Gallagher 2007a); nor does the interpretation of neural simulation as an action-model "reuse" of motor control mechanisms (e.g., Gallese 2004, 2010; Hurley 2006). On the latter view, we use motor control mechanisms, which usually allow us to correct our actions as they are in process (a so-called forward model), to simulate the actions we see others do. It's not clear, however, why reuse of such mechanisms, which remain on the level of effector-related basic movement (reach, grasp, to move one's hand to a target, etc.) to model/simulate the other's action can deliver an unambiguous understanding of the other's intention or goal. That is, a motor control model based on reuse of efferent signals is too low level (too closely tied to effectors) to give us an understanding of anything close to the goal-related meaning of even a simple intentional action (see Gazzola et al. (2007) for a discussion of the difference between goal- and effector-matching in the mirror system). The claim here is not that mirror neurons are not activated in normal everyday intersubjective interactions, or that they are not dysfunctional in autistic subjects. Rather the claim is that even if this is the case, the best way to interpret such neuroscientific data is not in terms of intersubjective simulation, whether that is conceived as involving pretense, matching, or reuse of motor control mechanisms.

Let's turn to the account proposed by IT. Long before we see problems in ToM-mentalizing in autism, we see problems that affect the more basic intersubjective interaction characterized by primary and secondary intersubjectivity (see Gallagher 2004). On the IT account, the problem of specialized cognitive functions related to mindreading appears at the end of a long line of effects that are more primary. Specifically, sensory-motor problems may interfere with the development of social interaction and understanding at the level of primary intersubjectivity.

A variety of basic sensory-motor problems have been shown to exist in autistic children between ages three and ten years (see Damasio and Maurer 1978; Vilensky et al. 1981), and even before that in infants who are later diagnosed as autistic. Teitelbaum et al. (1998) studied videos of infants in their first year who were later diagnosed as autistic. Movement disturbances were observed in all of the infants as early as age four to six months, and in some from birth. These include problems in lying, righting, sitting, crawling, and walking, as well as abnormal mouth shapes. They involve delayed development, as well as abnormal motor patterns, for example, asymmetries or unusual sequencing in crawling and walking.

Developmental studies show that these kinds of sensory-motor processes may be important in explaining some basic aspects of social cognition. When I observe someone else performing a certain action, or imagine myself doing that action, neuronal patterns are activated in my premotor cortex, supplemental motor area, and other brain areas that may be preparatory for my enactive response to the other's action. Accordingly, problems with our own motor or body-schematic system could significantly interfere with our capacities for understanding others. Just such developmental problems involving sensory-motor processes may have an effect on the capabilities that make up primary intersubjectivity, and therefore the autistic child's ability to understand the actions and intentions of others. The use of ToM strategies in high-functioning autistic subjects, then, would be compensatory for the loss of the more primary processes.

In addition to problems with primary intersubjectivity, problems with "central coherence" (Frith 1989; Happé 1995) may also have an effect on secondary intersubjective processes. Frith (1989) suggested that autism involves an imbalance in the integration of information, and specifically in integrating parts and wholes. She refers to this as a problem with "central coherence." Perception and understanding are normally shaped by coherence or Gestalt principles. In autism these Gestalt principles seem to break down. Autistic subjects tend to focus on parts and miss the broader contexts that provide meaning for the parts. Thus, autistic subjects have difficulty seeing things (including other people) as they are in their contexts.

Not only problems with primary intersubjectivity, but also these central coherence problems in the perception of context can interfere with the capabilities that make up secondary intersubjectivity. Seeing another person move in a certain way could mean many different things if it is done outside of any particular context. If you see my right arm, with open hand, drop through the air, but nothing else that would provide the context for what it means, then it could mean many different things: a gesture of "hello" or "goodbye" or "get out of here" or "this point is important." Without context, my intention is simply not clear to anyone watching or trying to interact with me.

At the neurological level, research on apoptosis (the natural pruning of the excess of neuronal cells with which we are born) suggests that the normal timing of this process is disrupted in the autistic brain (see, for example, Courchesne et al. 2003; Fatemi and Halt 2001; Fatemi et al. 2001; Margolis et al. 1994). This is a more general problem than simply a dysfunction of mirror neurons. If this is the case, it is likely that many and diverse neurological problems affecting many different parts of the brain, and different kinds of dynamic processing in the brain, could result. It would not be surprising then to find abnormalities in the neuronal processes that underlie face recognition (the fusiform gyrus; Pierce et al. 2001), emotional perception (amygdala and limbic system; Bachevalier 2000; Bauman and Kemper 1994), and many other sensory, motor, and cognitive problems that can result from a variety of brain abnormalities.

This also suggests that we should acknowledge the limitations of any theory that focuses exclusively on the social problems in autism since there is an array of other symptoms that go beyond such problems—restricted range of interest, obsessive concern for sameness, preoccupation with objects or parts of objects, high cognitive ability for rote memory, non-semantic form perception, echolalia, and a variety of sensory and motor behaviors such as oversensitivity to stimuli, and repetitive and odd movements. Problems with central coherence may contribute to the explanation of these non-social problems as well. The ToM approach might suggest a connection between central coherence and metarepresentation, so that a deficit that affects the former may affect the capacity for metarepresentation, important for mindreading, but also for imaginative play. Happé notes, however, that weakness in central coherence is found even in autistic subjects who pass ToM tasks, and this has to qualify any proposed tie between central coherence and ToM (Happé, 1995; also see Frith and Happé, 1994).

Schizophrenia

In a recent review of the ToM literature with respect to schizophrenia, Martin Brüne makes the following claim: "functional or structural disruption of the neural mechanisms underlying ToM may give rise to various types of psychopathology, including schizophrenia" (2005, p. 21). Brüne attributes this position to Frith (1992) and suggests that impairment in ToM capacity to correctly attribute intentions to others and to oneself may account for a number of symptoms, including disorders of willed action, self-monitoring (which may give rise to delusions of alien control and auditory hallucinations) and problems involved in keeping track of other persons' thoughts and intentions (giving rise to delusions of reference and persecution). According to some theory theorists, we use ToM not only to understand others, but also to attribute mental states to ourselves (e.g., Carruthers 2009). The idea that we make theoretical inferences concerning our own mental states leads Graham and Stephens to an explanation of the loss of a sense of agency in schizophrenic thought insertion in terms of a problem with metarepresentation. That is, our ToM capacity allows us to develop explanations of our own thinking that "amount to a sort of theory of [... our own] agency or intentional psychology" (1994, p. 101).

> [Normally] the subject's sense of agency regarding her thoughts ... depends on her belief that these mental episodes are expressions of her intentional states. That is, whether the subject regards an episode of thinking occurring in her psychological history as something she does, as her mental action, depends on whether she finds its occurrence explicable in terms of her theory or story of her own underlying intentional states. (Graham and Stephens 1994, p.102)

In the case of schizophrenic delusions of control or thought insertion, the patient may do or think something which she cannot attribute to herself because it doesn't fit her self-theory. She can find no beliefs or desires to explain or rationalize the action or the thought; accordingly, the movement or thought appears to be something she does or thinks *without intention*. To make sense of it introspectively the subject *infers* that she is not the agent; she constructs an explanation that involves misattribution to others.

A view more consistent with ST is proposed by Hardy-Baylé (1994; Hardy-Baylé et al. 2003). Patients with executive or planning deficits and highly disorganized thought may be unable to monitor their own thought processes and therefore be unable to use their own mental states as a model for understanding others (Brüne 2005).

Studies that employ ToM tasks do show some differentiation among patient groups. Patients with negative or disorganized symptoms are most ToM impaired (similar to autistic individuals), and may have difficulty representing mental states at all. Those with paranoid symptoms overly monitor the intentions of others, and do so inaccurately (Abu-Akel 1999; Abu-Akel and Bailey 2000; Walston et al. 2000). Patients with passivity symptoms perform closer to normal on ToM tasks (Brüne 2005; Frith 2004; Pickup and Frith 2001).

Across these different ToM studies one should distinguish between: (1) the strong causal claim that problems with ToM may be causal factors in schizophrenia (Brüne 2005) or at least for some symptoms of schizophrenia (Graham and Stephens 1994); (2) a more moderate correlational view (e.g., Frith 1992, 2004; Frith and Gallagher 2002; Pickup and Frith 2001); and (3) a weak causal claim that suggests certain aspects of schizophrenic symptoms (such as executive and planning deficits) may cause problems in ToM (e.g., Hardy-Baylé 1994). In the latter case ToM deficits would not be domain specific. There is some evidence, however, that ToM deficits in schizophrenia are domain specific rather than the result of general cognitive impairments (Brüne 2005; Langdon et al. 2001; Pickup and Frith 2001).

Empirical studies of ToM performance in schizophrenia are complicated by a number of factors, not the least by the complexity of the schizophrenia syndrome (or spectrum). For example, it has been shown that brain areas involved in ToM are frequently abnormal in schizophrenia, although not always, and not exclusively. These include prefrontal cortex, paracingulate cortex, amygdala, and temporal cortex. Cortical connectivity is also an issue (e.g., Gallagher and Frith 2003; Lee et al. 2004; Narr et al. 2001). Also, the use of false-belief tests may be complicated by the more general loss of contact with reality that characterizes some schizophrenic processes. Thus, patients with schizophrenia not only fail to attribute the correct mental states to others but also often fail to correctly respond to the reality questions used as a control—e.g., in the Sally–Anne test, "Where is the toy *really* located?" (Drury et al. 1998; Frith and Corcoran 1996).

A study by McCabe et al. (2004) suggests some important limitations involved in the ToM approaches for understanding social cognition in schizophrenia. They showed that, in contrast to the difficulties shown by schizophrenics with ToM tasks in the various experimental studies, schizophrenics seem to show no such problems in clinical conversations and interviews. Patients respond to the clinician on the basis of what the clinician needs to know. Patients know that the clinician may have different beliefs from their own, and they take account of such differences in their replies. The difference between a ToM experiment and a clinical conversation is, of course, obvious. In the case of the clinical encounter, the patient is *interacting* with the clinician, whereas in the case of the typical experiment, the patient is asked to observe and make third-person judgments about another person's beliefs. Frith (2004, p. 387), reflecting on this difference, puts it this way:

> There is a fundamental difference between the use of mentalizing in discourse and the use of mentalizing in theory of mind tasks. In other domains this difference has been characterized as "on-line" versus "off-line" processing (e.g., Tyler, 1992). During discourse mentalizing is used implicitly and automatically in the service of communicating. In this sense it is used on-line. In most theory of mind tasks mentalizing is carried out off-line. The patient is not taking part in the interaction, but must make explicit use of mentalizing to answer questions about an

interaction that has been described. This requirement puts more weight on working memory and on meta-cognitive processes (i.e., reflecting on mentalizing).

In the typical false-belief test performed with children, the child is not asked to explain an interaction, but rather to explain what a third person with whom the child has not interacted, believes. That is, the test is designed to test mindreading from an observational rather than interactional perspective. Notably, however, even in such testing situations, the three-year-old child who fails the false-belief test shows no problem in understanding the experimenter, or what the experimenter wants. That's because the child is in a second-person, interactive relation with the experimenter. Generally speaking, from the IT perspective, the important and primary thing in everyday social encounters is interaction; ToM and the kind of mindreading it entails is derivative from this. In this regard, if schizophrenics do better in some cases of second-person interaction than in third-person ToM experiments, this suggests that at the very least the ToM explanations are not giving us the best accounts of the schizophrenic's problems.

There is, so far, no developed IT account of the intersubjective problems found in schizophrenia. Thomas Fuchs (2010), however, in a clinical context, suggests two guidelines that would define such an account. First, a realization that the patient as a person should be understood in the medium of interpersonal relationships, which includes the encounter of patient and psychiatrist; second, that the features relevant for diagnosis may only be grasped during and through the interaction. These clinical guidelines can also be considered principles that can inform scientific explanation (see Fuchs and De Jaegher 2009). Following these principles, one can hypothesize, based on the various problems that people with schizophrenia have with contextual cues, that there are important disruptions in abilities associated with secondary intersubjectivity, and that such deficits come to be reflected in problems with communicative pragmatics and narrative competency.

Secondary intersubjectivity involves joining in contextualized activities with others and recognizing the importance of contextual differences in the meaning of the other's actions. Patients with schizophrenia show impairments in using contextual information in intersubjective situations (Frith 1992; Langdon et al. 2001), reflected in problems with language (Andreasen 1986; Hardy-Baylé et al. 2003). Patients with schizophrenia also have a tendency to interpret metaphorical speech literally (Brüne 2005; Gorham 1956), show impaired pragmatics (Frith and Allen 1988), and impaired use of context-dependent information when presented with ambiguous verbal material (Bazin et al. 2000). All of this is further reflected in problems involving narrative competence (Gallagher 2003; 2007b; Gallagher and Cole 2011; Phillips 2003), problems that likely interfere with narrative-based false-belief tests (as in Frith and Corcoran 1996; see, e.g., Guajardo and Watson 2002). Patients with schizophrenia also have problems with autobiographical memory (Corcoran and Frith 2003). The contribution of autobiographical memory to self-narrative content is significant, as is apparent from cases in which such content is lost, as in amnesia or Alzheimer's disease. Bruner (2002, pp. 86, 119) points out that dysnarrativia (encountered for example in Korsakoff's syndrome or Alzheimer's disease) is destructive not only for self-understanding generated in narrative (also see Young and Saver 2001), but also for the ability to understand others' behavior and their emotional experiences.

TOM OR INTERACTION IN PSYCHOPATHOLOGY?

A variety of ToM studies suggest that deficits in social cognition are widespread in many psychopathologies, including depression (Wang et al. 2008), bipolar disorder (Kerr 2003; Wolf et al. 2010), Alzheimer's disease (Cuerva et al. 2001), and frontotemporal dementia (Adenzato et al. 2010). Studies of mindreading in non-pathological subjects, as well as in people with autism and schizophrenia, however, raise a number of methodological and substantial issues that researchers need to keep in mind when asking about intersubjectivity in these and other pathological cases.

In a study of ToM in cases of Alzheimer's disease involving mild dementia, for example, Cuerva et al. (2001) employed a series of short stories to assess false-belief understanding. Sixty-five percent of the patients failed the test. The same group who failed the false-belief test had more severe deficits on tests of verbal anterograde memory, verbal comprehension, abstract thinking, and naming, than the patients who passed the test. It's not clear that these other deficits, which may also suggest problems with narrative competency, were not the reason for the failures. It's also not clear how these same patients conducted themselves in ordinary "online" interactions with others.

Similar considerations are relevant to studies of ToM in bipolar disorder (Kerr 2003; Wolf et al. 2010), which involve frontal and temporal cortex areas, and the various studies reviewed by Adenzato et al. (2010) where traditional ToM/false-belief tests were used to test patients with the behavioral variant of frontotemporal dementia. The neurological picture complicates the interpretation of the results. Areas of the brain involved in studies of frontotemporal dementia—the areas of the medial prefrontal cortex especially, but also temporoparietal junction, and temporal poles, for example—are the same areas of the brain that have been associated with ToM functioning. These areas, however, are not specific for intersubjective understanding—since they also serve future planning, abstract representations, reflecting on values, and are involved in resting or default mode functions that may include self-monitoring, self-referential process, and self-generated thoughts. Indeed, in a recent review, Legrand and Ruby (2009) suggest that these areas, including the medial frontal cortex, are not specific for self (despite self-related processes), and by extension, are not specific for mindreading, future planning, or any of the other functions associated with them. Rather, their review indicates that these areas serve a general (reflective) evaluative performance over a wide scope of functions. In regard to mindreading, then, these brain areas may be called upon only because the tasks used in these experiments are all "offline" and call for reflective evaluation rather than online social interaction.

Studies of ToM in antisocial personality disorders (ASPD), where one might expect to find problems with intersubjective relations, showed that subjects with ASPD did no worse than controls on most of the standard ToM tests (Dolan and Fullam 2004; Richell et al. 2003). This suggests, as Frith (2004) has noted, that ToM should not be equated with social cognition in general. Indeed, rather than being the primary and pervasive way in which we understand and interact with others, mindreading (whether of the inferential or simulationist variety) should be considered a relatively rare and specialized ability that we may use when our normal everyday interactions break down, or when we are confronted by a puzzling case of behavior (Gallagher 2004, 2005).

Studies of intersubjectivity in psychopathologies, then, to the extent that they have focused on ToM functions, at best can explain only one small part of the puzzle, and they fail to address deeper problems with online, second-person, social interactions. Some of these problems are apparent in clinical settings but are difficult to study using current brain scanning technologies and the experimental techniques they require (see Schilbach et al. in press). Clearly, to gain a fuller account of both online and offline intersubjective impairments in various psychopathologies, one needs to employ and integrate a variety of approaches, including phenomenological, developmental, behavioral, clinical and narrative studies.

ACKNOWLEDGMENTS

My work on this chapter was supported in part by the focused research project on *Enactive and extended cognition in social institutional contexts* at the University of Hertfordshire, UK, funded by the Marie Curie Actions project, *Towards an embodied science of intersubjectivity* (TESIS), and by a 2012 Humboldt Foundation Anneliese Maier Research Award.

REFERENCES

Abu-Akel, A. (1999). Impaired theory of mind in schizophrenia. *Pragmatics and Cognition, 7*, 247–82.

Abu-Akel, A. and Bailey, A. L. (2000). The possibility of different forms of theory of mind. *Psychological Medicine, 30*, 735–8.

Adenzato, M. Cavallo, M., and Enrici, I. (2010). Theory of mind ability in the behavioural variant of frontotemporal dementia: An analysis of the neural, cognitive, and social levels. *Neuropsychologia, 48*, 2–12.

Andreasen, N. (1986). Scale for the assessment of thought, language, and communication (TLC). *Schizophrenia Bulletin, 12*(3), 473–82.

Bachevalier, J. (2000). The amygdala, social cognition, and autism. In J. P. Aggleton (Ed.), *The Amygdala: A Functional Analysis*, pp. 509–43. Oxford: Oxford University Press.

Baillargeon, R., Scott, R. M., and He, Z. (2010). False-belief understanding in infants. *Trends in Cognitive Sciences, 14*(3), 110–18.

Baird, J. A. and Baldwin, D. A. (2001). Making sense of human behavior: Action parsing and intentional inference. In B. F. Malle, L. J. Moses, and D. A. Baldwin (Eds), *Intentions and Intentionality: Foundations of Social Cognition*, pp. 193–206. Cambridge, MA: MIT Press.

Baldwin, D. A. and Baird, J. A. (2001). Discerning intentions in dynamic human action. *Trends in Cognitive Science, 5*(4), 171–8.

Baron-Cohen, S. (1995). *Mindblindness: An Essay on Autism and Theory of Mind*. Cambridge, MA: Bradford/MIT Press.

Baron-Cohen, S. (2000). Is autism necessarily a disability? *Development and Psychopathology, 12*, 489–500.

Baron-Cohen, S. (2003). *The Essential Difference: Men, Women and the Extreme Male Brain*. New York, NY: Penguin/Basic Books.

Bauman, M. L. and Kemper T. L. (1994). *The Neurobiology of Autism.* Baltimore, MD: Johns Hopkins University Press.

Bazin, N., Perruchet, P., Hardy-Baylé, M. C., and Feline, A. (2000). Context-dependent information processing in patients with schizophrenia. *Schizophrenia Research, 45,* 93–101.

Becchio, C., Manera, V., Sartori, L., Cavallo, A., and Castiello U. (2012). Grasping intentions: from thought experiments to empirical evidence. *Frontiers in Human Neuroscience, 6,* 117.

Becchio, C., Sartori, L., and Castiello, U. (2010). Towards you: The social side of actions. *Current Directions in Psychological Science, 19,* 183–8.

Bradshaw, J. L. (2001). *Developmental Disorders of the Frontostriatal Systems.* East Sussex: Psychology Press.

Brüne, M. (2005). 'Theory of mind' in schizophrenia: A review of the literature. *Schizophrenia Bulletin, 31*(1), 21–42.

Bruner, J. (2002). *Making Stories: Law, Literature, Life.* New York, NY: Farrar, Straus and Giroux.

Carruthers, P. (2009). How we know our own minds: the relationship between mindreading and metacognition. *Behavioral and Brain Sciences, 32*(2), 121–82.

Catmur, C., Walsh, V., and Heyes, C. (2007). Sensorimotor learning configures the human mirror system. *Current Biology, 17*(17), 1527–31.

Coltheart, M. and Langdon, R. (1998). Autism, modularity and levels of explanation in cognitive science. *Mind & Language, 13*(1), 138–52.

Corcoran, R., and Frith, C. D. (2003). Autobiographical memory and theory of mind: Evidence of a relationship in schizophrenia. *Psychological Medicine, 33,* 897–905.

Courchesne, E., Carper, R., and Akshoomoff, N. (2003). Evidence of brain overgrowth in the first year of life in autism. *Journal of the American Medical Association, 290,* 337–44.

Csibra, G. (2005). Mirror neurons and action observation. Is simulation involved? *ESF Interdisciplines.* Available at: <http://www.interdisciplines.org>.

Cuerva, A. G., Sabe, L., Kuzis, G., Tiberti, C., Dorrego, F., and Starkstein, S. E. (2001). Theory of mind and pragmatic abilities in dementia. *Neuropsychiatry, Neuropsychology, and Behavioral Neurology, 14,* 153–8.

Damasio, A. R., and Maurer, R. G. (1978). A neurological model for childhood autism. *Archives of Neurology, 35*(12), 777–86.

De Jaegher, H., Di Paolo, E., and Gallagher, S. (2010). Does social interaction constitute social cognition? *Trends in Cognitive Sciences, 14*(10), 441–7.

Dinstein, I., Thomas, C., Behrmann, M., and Heeger, D. J. (2008). A mirror up to nature. *Current Biology, 18*(1), R13–R18.

Dittrich, W. H., Troscianko, T., Lea, S. E. G, and Morgan, D. (1996). Perception of emotion from dynamic point-light displays represented in dance. *Perception, 25,* 727–38.

Dolan, M. and Fullam, R. (2004). Theory of mind and mentalizing ability in antisocial personality disorders with and without psychopathy. *Psychological Medicine, 34,* 1093–102.

Drury, V. M., Robinson, E. J., and Birchwood, M. (1998). 'Theory of mind' skills during an acute episode of psychosis and following recovery. *Psychological Medicine, 28,* 1101–12.

Falk, D. (2004). Prelinguistic evolution in early hominids: Whence motherese? *Behavioral and Brain Sciences, 27*(4), 491–503.

Fatemi, S. H., and Halt, A. R. (2001). Altered levels of Bcl2 and p53 proteins in parietal cortex reflect deranged apoptotic regulation in autism. *Synapse, 42*(4), 281–4.

Fatemi, S. H., Halt, A. R., Stary, J. M., Realmuto, G. M., and Jalali-Mousavi, M. (2001). Reduction in anti-apoptotic protein Bcl-2 in autistic cerebellum. *Neuroreport, 12*(5), 929–33.

Frith, C. D. (1992). *The Cognitive Neuropsychology of Schizophrenia*. Hillsdale, NJ: Lawrence Erlbaum Associates.

Frith, C. D. (2004). Schizophrenia and theory of mind. *Psychological Medicine, 34*, 385–9.

Frith, C. D. and Allen, H. A. (1988). Language disorders in schizophrenia and their implications for neuropsychology. In P. Bebbington and P. McGuffin (Eds), *Schizophrenia: The Major Issues*, pp. 172–86. Oxford: Heinemann.

Frith, C. D. and Corcoran, R. (1996). Exploring 'theory of mind' in people with schizophrenia. *Psychological Medicine, 26*, 521–30.

Frith, C. and Gallagher, S. (2002). Models of the pathological mind. *Journal of Consciousness Studies, 9*(4), 57–80.

Frith, C. D. and Frith, U. (1999). Interacting minds—a biological basis. *Science, 286*, 1692–5.

Frith, U. (1989). *Autism: Explaining the Enigma*. Oxford: Basil Blackwell.

Frith, U. and Happé, F. (1994). Autism: Beyond 'theory of mind'. *Cognition, 50*, 115–32.

Froese, T. and Gallagher, S. (2012). Getting IT together: Integrating developmental, phenomenological, enactive, and dynamical approaches to social interaction. *Interaction Studies, 13*(3), 434–66.

Fuchs, T. (2010). Subjectivity and intersubjectivity in psychiatric diagnosis. *Psychopathology, 43*, 268–74.

Fuchs, T. and De Jaegher, H. (2009). Enactive intersubjectivity: Participatory sensemaking and mutual incorporation. *Phenomenology and the Cognitive Sciences, 8*, 465–86.

Gallagher, H. L. and Frith, C. D. (2003). Functional imaging of 'theory of mind'. *Trends in Cognitive Sciences, 7*, 77–83.

Gallagher, S. (2001). Emotion and intersubjective perception: A speculative account. In *Emotions, Qualia and Consciousness*, pp. 95–100. London: World Scientific Publishers, and Naples: Instituto Italiano per gli Studi Filosofici.

Gallagher, S. (2003). Self-narrative in schizophrenia. In A. S. David and T. Kircher (Eds), *The Self in Neuroscience and Psychiatry*, pp. 336–57. Cambridge: Cambridge University Press.

Gallagher, S. (2004). Understanding interpersonal problems in autism: Interaction theory as an alternative to theory of mind. *Philosophy, Psychiatry, & Psychology, 11*(3), 199–217.

Gallagher, S. (2005). *How the Body Shapes the Mind*. Oxford: Oxford University Press.

Gallagher, S. (2007a). Simulation trouble. *Social Neuroscience, 2*(3–4), 353–65.

Gallagher, S. (2007b). Pathologies in narrative structure. *Philosophy* (Royal Institute of Philosophy) Supplement, *60*, 65–86.

Gallagher, S. (2008). Neural simulation and social cognition. In J. A. Pineda (Ed.), *Mirror Neuron Systems: The Role of Mirroring Processes in Social Cognition*, pp. 355–71. Totowa, NJ: Humana Press.

Gallagher, S. (2011). Interpretations of embodied cognition. In W. Tschacher and C. Bergomi (Eds), *The Implications of Embodiment: Cognition and Communication*, pp. 59–71. Exeter: Imprint Academic.

Gallagher, S. and Cole, J. (2011). Dissociation in self-narrative. *Consciousness and Cognition, 20*, 149–55.

Gallagher, S. and Hutto, D. (2008). Understanding others through primary interaction and narrative practice. In J. Zlatev, T. Racine, C. Sinha, and E. Itkonen (Eds), *The Shared Mind: Perspectives on Intersubjectivity*, pp. 17–38. Amsterdam: John Benjamins.

Gallagher, S. and Povinelli, D. (2012). Enactive and behavioral abstraction accounts of social understanding in chimpanzees, infants, and adults. *Review of Philosophy and Psychology, 3*(1), 145–69.

Gallese, V. (2001). The 'shared manifold' hypothesis: from mirror neurons to empathy', *Journal of Consciousness Studies*, *8*, 33–50.

Gallese, V. (2004). Intentional attunement. The mirror neuron system and its role in interpersonal relations. *ESF Interdisciplines*. Available at: <http://www.interdisciplines.org>.

Gallese, V. (2010). Embodied simulation and its role in intersubjectivity. In T. Fuchs, H. C. Sattel, and P. Henningsen (Eds), *The Embodied Self. Dimensions, Coherence and Disorders*, pp. 77–92. Stuttgart: Schattauer.

Gazzola, V., van der Worp, H., Mulder, T., Wicker, B., Rizzolatti, G., and Keysers, C. (2007). Aplasics born without hands mirror the goal of hand actions with their feet. *Current Biology*, *17*, 1235–40.

Gibson, J. J. (1979). *The Ecological Approach to Visual Perception*. Boston, MA: Houghton-Mifflin.

Goldman, A. (2006). *Simulating Minds: The Philosophy, Psychology and Neuroscience of Mindreading*. Oxford: Oxford University Press.

Goldman, A. and De Vignemont, F. (2009). Is social cognition embodied? *Trends in Cognitive Sciences*, *13*(4), 154–9.

Gopnik, A. and Meltzoff, A. N. (1997). *Words, Thoughts, and Theories*. Cambridge, MA: MIT Press.

Gordon, R. M. and Barker, J. A. (1994). Autism and the 'theory of mind' debate. In G. Graham and G. L. Stephens (Eds), *Philosophical Psychopathology*, pp. 162–81. Cambridge, MA: MIT Press.

Gorham, D. R. (1956). Use of the proverb test for differentiating schizophrenics from normals. *Journal of Consulting Psychology*, *20*, 435–40.

Graham, G. and Stephens, G. L. (1994). Mind and mine. In G. Graham and G. L. Stephens (Eds), *Philosophical Psychopathology*, pp. 91–109. Cambridge, MA: MIT Press.

Guajardo, N. R. and Watson, A. (2002). Narrative discourse and theory of mind development. *The Journal of Genetic Psychology*, *163*, 305–25.

Happé, F. (1995). *Autism: An Introduction to Psychological Theory*. Cambridge, MA: Harvard University Press.

Hardy-Baylé, M. C. (1994). Organisation de l'action, phénomènes de conscience et représentation mentale de l'action chez des schizophrènes. *Actualités Psychiatriques*, *20*, 393–400.

Hardy-Baylé, M. C., Sarfati, Y., and Passerieux, C. (2003). The cognitive basis of disorganization symptomatology in schizophrenia and its clinical correlates: Toward a pathogenetic approach to disorganization. *Schizophrenia Bulletin*, *29*(3), 459–71.

Herrmann, E., Call, J., Hare, B., and Tomasello, M. (2007). Humans evolved specialized skills of social cognition: the cultural intelligence hypothesis. *Science*, *317*(5843), 1360–6.

Hurley, S. L. (2006). Active perception and perceiving action: The shared circuits model. In T. Gendler and J. Hawthorne (Eds), *Perceptual Experience*, pp. 205–59. New York, NY: Oxford University Press.

Hutto, D. (2007). *Folk Psychological Narratives*. Cambridge, MA: MIT Press.

Iacoboni, M. (2005). Understanding others: Imitation, language, and empathy. In S. Hurley and N. Chater (Eds), *Perspectives on Imitation: From Neuroscience to Social Science* (Vol. 1), pp. 76–100. Cambridge, MA: MIT Press.

Kerr, N., Dunbar, R. I. M., and Bentall, R. (2003). Theory of mind deficits in bipolar affective disorder. *Journal of Affective Disorders*, *73*, 253–9.

Langdon, R., Coltheart, M., Ward, P. B., and Catts, S. V. (2001). Mentalising, executive planning and disengagement in schizophrenia. *Cognitive Neuropsychiatry*, *6*, 81–108.

Lee, K-. H., Farrow, T. F. D., Spence, S. A. and Woodruff, P. W. R. (2004). Social cognition, brain networks and schizophrenia. *Psychological Medicine*, *34*, 391–400.

Legrand, D. and Ruby, P. (2009). What is self-specific? Theoretical investigation and critical review of neuroimaging results. *Psychological Review*, *116*(1), 252–82.

Leslie, A. and Frith, U. (1988). Autistic children's understanding of seeing, knowing and believing. *British Journal of Developmental Psychology*, *6*, 315–24.

Lindblom, J. (2007). *Minding the Body: Interacting Socially through Embodied Action*. Linköping: Linköping Studies in Science and Technology, Dissertation No. 1112.

Manera, V., Becchio, C., Cavallo, A., Sartori, L., and Castiello, U. (2011). Cooperation or competition? Discriminating between social intentions by observing prehensile movements. *Experimental Brain Research*, *211*, 547–56.

Margolis, R. L., Chuang, D. M., and Post, R. M. (1994). Programmed cell death: implications for neuropsychiatric disorders. *Biological Psychiatry*, *35*(12), 946–56.

McCabe, R., Leudar, I., and Antaki, C. (2004). Do people with schizophrenia display theory of mind deficits in clinical interactions? *Psychological Medicine*, *34*, 401–12.

Meltzoff, A. and Moore, M. K. (1994). Imitation, memory, and the representation of persons. *Infant Behavior and Development*, *17*, 83–99.

Meltzoff, A. and Moore, M. K. (1977). Imitation of facial and manual gestures by human neonates. *Science*, *198*, 75–8.

Narr, K. L., Thompson, P. M., Sharma, T., Moussai, J., Zoumalan, C., Rayman, J., and Toga, A. (2001). Three-dimensional mapping of gyral shape and cortical surface asymmetries in schizophrenia. Gender effects. *American Journal of Psychiatry*, *158*, 244–55.

Niedenthal, P. M., Barsalou, L. M., Winkielman, P., Krauth-Gruber, S., and Ric, F. (2005). Embodiment in attitudes, social perception, and emotion. *Personality and Social Psychology Review*, *9*(3), 184–211.

Oberman, L. M., Hubbard, E. M., McCleery, J. P., Altschuler, E. L., Ramachandran, V. S., and Pineda, J. A. (2005). EEG evidence for mirror neuron dysfunction in autism spectrum disorders. *Cognitive Brain Research*, *24*, 190–8.

Ozonoff, S., Pennington, B. F., and Rogers, S. J. (1991). Executive function deficits in high-functioning autistic children: Relationship to theory of mind. *Journal of Child Psychology and Psychiatry*, *32*, 1081–105.

Phillips, J. (2003). Schizophrenia and the narrative self. In T. Kircher and A. David (Eds), *The Self in Neuroscience and Psychiatry*, pp. 319–35. Cambridge: Cambridge University Press.

Pickup, G. J. and Frith, C. D. (2001). Theory of mind impairments in schizophrenia: Symptomatology, severity and specificity. *Psychological Medicine*, *31*, 207–20.

Pierce, K., Muller, R. A., Ambrose, J., Allen, G., and Courchesne, E. (2001). Face processing occurs outside the fusiform 'face area' in autism: evidence from functional MRI. *Brain*, *124*(Pt 10), 2059–73.

Reed, T. and Paterson, C. (1990). A comparative study of autistic subjects' performance at two levels of visual and cognitive perspective taking. *Journal of Autism and Developmental Disorders*, *29*, 555–68.

Richell, R. A., Mitchell, D. G. V., Newman, C., Leonard, A., Baron-Cohen, S., and Blair, R. J. R. (2003). Theory of mind and psychopathy: Can psychopathic individuals read the 'language of the eyes'? *Neuropsychologia*, *41*, 523–6.

Sacks, O. (1995). *An anthropologist on Mars*. New York, NY: Vintage Books.

Schilbach, L., Eickhoff, S. B., Mojzisch, A., and Vogeley, K. (2008). What's in a smile? Neural correlates of facial embodiment during social interaction. *Social Neuroscience*, *3*(1), 37–50.

Schilbach, L., Timmermans, B., Reddy, V., Costall, A., Bente, G., Schlicht, T., *et al.* (in press). Toward a second-person neuroscience. *Behavioral and Brain Sciences.*

Senju, A., Johnson, M. H., and Csibra, G. (2006). The development and neural basis of referential gaze perception. *Social Neuroscience*, *1*(3–4), 220–34.

Teitelbaum, P., Teitelbaum, O., Nye, J., Fryman, J., and Maurer, R. G. (1998). Movement analysis in infancy may be useful for early diagnosis of autism. *Proceedings of the National Academy of Science of the United State of America*, *9*(23), 13982–7.

Trevarthen, C. and Hubley, P. (1978). Secondary intersubjectivity: Confidence, confiding and acts of meaning in the first year. In A. Lock (Ed.), *Action, Gesture and Symbol: The Emergence of Language*, pp. 183–229. London: Academic Press.

Trevarthen, C. B. (1979). Communication and cooperation in early infancy: A description of primary intersubjectivity. In M. Bullowa (Ed.), *Before Speech*, pp. 321–48. Cambridge: Cambridge University Press.

Tyler, L. K. (1992). The distinction between implicit and explicit language function: Evidence from aphasia. In A. D. Milner and M. D. Rugg (Eds), *The Neuropsychology of Consciousness*, pp. 159–178. San Diego, CA: Academic Press.

Vilensky, J. A., Damasio, A. R., and Maurer, R. G. (1981). Gait disturbances in patients with autistic behavior: A preliminary study. *Archives of Neurology*, *38*(10), 646–9.

Walston, F., Blennerhassett, R. C., and Charlton, B. G. (2000). 'Theory of mind', persecutory delusions and the somatic marker mechanism. *Cognitive Neuropsychiatry*, *5*, 161–74.

Wang Y. G., Wang Y. Q., Chen S. L., Zhu C. Y., and Wang, K. (2008). Theory of mind disability in major depression with or without psychotic symptoms: a componential view. *Psychiatry Research*, *161*(2), 153–61.

Williams, J. H. G., Whiten, A., Suddendorf, T., and Perrett, D. I. (2001). Imitation, mirror neurons and autism. *Neuroscience and Biobehavioral Reviews*, *25*, 287–95.

Wolf, F., Brüne, M., and Assion, H.-J. (2010). Theory of mind and neurocognitive functioning in patients with bipolar disorder. *Bipolar Disorders*, *12*, 657–66.

Young, K. and Saver, J. L. (2001). The neurology of narrative. *SubStance*, *30*(1&2), 72–84.

Zahavi, D. and Parnas, J. (2003). Conceptual problems in infantile autism research: Why cognitive science needs phenomenology. *Journal of Consciousness Studies*, *10*(9–10), 53–71.

....

CHAPTER 20

OTHER MINDS, AUTISM, AND DEPTH IN HUMAN INTERACTION

....

ANITA AVRAMIDES

INTRODUCTION

....

The philosophy of psychiatry is a relatively new discipline. Philosophy is accustomed to links with other disciplines; there is nothing new in that. The birth of modern science has philosophy attending as midwife, but as scientific disciplines have matured they have tended to move away from philosophy; the philosopher, however, can often be found still lurking in the conceptual shadows. The subject matter of psychiatry is disorders of the mind, and the mere mention of mind is enough to interest the philosopher. Although psychiatry has firm roots in medicine, the fact that its subject matter is characterized as *mental* disorders is enough to ensure that discussions concerning these disorders will include considerations that range from the purely biological to the less tractable social.

One disorder that has come to be of increasing concern and interest not only to psychiatrists and psychologists but also to philosophers is that of infantile autism. The characterization of autism in the *Diagnostic and Statistical Manual of Mental Disorders* (DSM-IV; American Psychiatric Association 2000) classifies it according to several of its symptoms, some of which involve abnormalities with regard to what I will call "involvement with others." Although the focus of much of the discussion of autism has been on this aspect of it, there have also been discussions that highlight symptoms that we might characterize as disorders with regard to the self.[1]

Philosophers have a long-standing interest in issues to do with the mind in relation to the body. They also have a fairly long-standing interest in the question of the self, as well as of

---

[1] Other characteristics have also been noted in connection with the behaviour of autistic individuals such as a restrictive range of interest, an obsessive concern with sameness, a preoccupation with objects or their parts, oversensitivity to stimuli, and ability for rote memory.

the self in relation to others. One of the problems that may be identified here is sometimes referred to as "the problem of other minds." It is interesting to note that, while the philosopher is often preoccupied by the central case or the normal, what drives the psychiatrist in his or her quest to understand is what is accepted to be an abnormal phenomenon. In his book *Psychological Explanation*, Jerry Fodor (1968, pp. 3–4) considers an idea that he claims to find in philosophy (or the philosophy of a certain time) to the effect that the impetus to explanation comes from the observation that something is "somehow untoward, abnormal, and unusual";[2] by extension, explanation of the normal or the usual is somehow misplaced (1968, p. 4). In opposition to this idea, Fodor cites the work of H. P. Grice which differentiates between that which is logically and that which is pragmatically implicated. Once this distinction is in place, we can say that the connection between the abnormal and the quest for explanation is merely pragmatic. Fodor then goes on to also point out that an explanation in the "abnormal case" commits us to a corresponding explanation in the "normal" case.[3]

Fodor claims to find this philosophical hostility to explanation of the usual in the work of Ludwig Wittgenstein and some of those who claim to follow in his philosophical footsteps. If Fodor is right in his interpretation of these texts, one would not expect to find rich sources for interdisciplinary work here. I am less sure than Fodor that this work is hostile to a certain sort of explanation. Indeed, I want to suggest that Wittgenstein's texts do offer us a rich source of thought concerning the self in relation to others, and that this thought might help guide the more empirically minded in their quest to understand certain abnormalities that can arise in these relations.[4] However, the concern of this chapter will not be to defend Wittgenstein's work here against Fodor's interpretation of it. I want simply to show how attention to this work—and to a certain age-old problem in philosophy—may be used to yield some interesting results when it comes to thinking about the problem of autism.[5]

One age-old problem in philosophy that I think might be used to shed some light on problems more recently of concern in both philosophy and psychiatry is that of skepticism.[6] Skepticism about the external world has a particularly long history, while skepticism concerning the minds of others has a somewhat shorter one.[7] In more recent times, some epistemologists have become impatient with skepticism, insisting that concern with it has only served to hold up work in epistemology. This "new" epistemology has introduced a divide between itself and the traditional "internalist" epistemology. This new

---

[2] The idea is one he claims to find in Hamlyn (1957).

[3] That is, "It wants explaining, hence its abnormal" expresses a pragmatic—not a logical—implication.

[4] One philosophically informed psychologist, Peter Hobson, has already understood this. See later.

[5] Comments concerning the relationship between explanations of the normal and the abnormal abound in the literature concerned with autism. I take one example, from Gallagher (2004, p. 7), who writes: "Defects in theory of mind [one prominent view] cannot explain autism because the theory of mind itself is not a good explanation of non-autistic intersubjective experience."

[6] This may seem an odd choice of issue to concentrate on. In recent times this traditional philosophical problem has been supplemented by what is called sometimes called the descriptive problem of other minds. It is arguably on this problem that theory theorists and simulation theorists concentrate. The question they ask is not, How do I know that another has a mind?, but, How do I go about attributing minds to others? And it is the work of these theorists that has been to the fore in much interdisciplinary, and empirically orientated, work. I want to try to show that there is interdisciplinary mileage in the older, more traditional, problem of other minds.

[7] See Avramides (2001, ch. 1).

"externalist" epistemology might be thought to have more in common with what was once referred to as "naturalized epistemology." One thing the externalist and the naturalist have in common is impatience with the skeptic. Just as the skeptic concerning the external world might be thought to be preoccupied with questions concerning the possibility that all the world is but a dream or the machinations of an evil demon or perverse scientist, the skeptic concerning the minds of others ponders the possibility that all those with whom s/he communes are no more than person-imitating automata or mindless zombies. Externalist epistemologists want an answer to the question, How do we know things about the world around us?, or the question, How do I know that my daughter is in pain or that the professor is angry? One could say that the externalist wants to place to one side the possibility of dream worlds and imitation people and to concentrate on how things go for *us*—for those of us in what we take to be the actual world surrounded by ordinary objects and others like us.[8]

Philosophers who take their lead from Descartes in his *Meditations* (and who are for the most part internalists) are caught up with the skeptic to the following extent: they believe that it is not possible to say how it is that we know ordinary things about ordinary people and the world around us unless and until we can say how it is that we know that we are not in the grip of an evil demon or perverse scientist. The skeptic's challenge is allowed to block all attempts to know. The externalist, as I have explained, is determined to find a way of explaining how it is that we know all sorts of thing—and if this means ignoring the skeptic, so be it.

If I am to say anything interesting or meaningful about the externalist epistemologist, it is time that I stop referring en masse to a large and diverse literature. For the rest of this chapter I want to take one such epistemologist, Fred Dretske, as my point of reference. Dretske's work in this connection is particularly of interest if one is largely concerned—as I shall be in the rest of this chapter—with the epistemological problem of other minds. This is because Dretske devotes more space in his writings than most epistemologists to addressing this problem, and what he has to say is both important and interestingly revealing.[9]

The problem of other minds has traditionally been thought of as the flip side of the problem of solipsism.[10] The problem is conceived of as what I shall refer to as a "thick problem," and the question raised can be taken to be a correspondingly "thick question." Thus, the question raised concerning other minds is to be understood as another way of asking the question, How do I know that I am not the only mind? More recently philosophers have tended to concern themselves with what I shall call the "thin problem" of other minds, and the question raised can be taken to be the "thin question," How do I know what another is thinking or feeling? (I explain the ideas of thick vs. thin later. For the moment I am simply labeling problems and questions.)

---

[8] Smith (2010, p. 3) distinguishes between skeptical questions and epistemological ones. Using Smith's distinction one could say that externalists aim to answer only epistemological questions while internalists run together epistemological and skeptical questions. Of course, from the point of view of traditional, internalist, epistemology there can be no separating out these two questions.

[9] As I explain later, Dretske would be considered by many epistemologists to be a controversial choice. But it is precisely the issue that raises the most controversy that I believe raises a most interesting issue—and one that may be revealing in connection with empirical research.

[10] The traditional way of asking the question is the way that fits in with Cartesian, internalist, epistemology.

If one looks at the history of philosophy one finds various attempts to respond to these questions. One response that dominated for centuries is the argument from analogy.[11] It was closely followed by the argument from induction (see, e.g., Ayer 1956). Both analogy and induction have, in more recent times, been challenged by the argument from best explanation (see, e.g., Pargetter 1984). These three approaches exemplify what has come to be referred to as "the inferentialist model." Much of the discussion has been dominated by this model, and I don't propose to consider it in this chapter. One response that is *not* to be found in the history of philosophy is the following: I know that another has a mind because I can perceive it. Alvin Plantinga (1966, p. 441) quotes Thomas Reid who writes: "The thoughts and passions of the mind are invisible, intangible, odorless and inaudible." For good measure, Plantinga adds: "And they can't be tasted either." Plantinga's attitude to the suggestion that we perceive other minds was the dominant one in philosophy until quite recently. This isn't to say that the idea didn't receive any support until now. Actually, around the time that Plantinga made his remarks, Dretske proposed a perceptual model in opposition to the dominant inferentialist one. That idea, however, received no attention that I am aware of.[12] About a decade later the idea was put forward by John McDowell (1978/1998a, 1982/1998b). One must not confuse this model in the hands of these two philosophers; they are very different. Nevertheless, the suggestion that we can use perception to counter the inferentialists' proposals is a powerful idea, and it is the one I want to explore in this chapter. I shall place McDowell's perceptual model to one side and concentrate on Dretske's model.[13] My reason for doing this is not that I think Dretske's model is the correct one, but that I think it poses the problem in a particularly fruitful way—especially when it comes to thinking about individuals suffering from the spectrum of disorders associated with autism.

Understanding How Knowledge of Other Minds Can be A Visual Achievement

Before we can assess Dretske's perceptual model we need to understand it. What follows is a very brief account. Dretske begins by distinguishing between simple seeing and epistemic seeing. Simple seeing involves a simple relation to a thing. As he writes (Dretske 1969, p. 6) in one place, "Seeing a bug is like stepping on a bug." Epistemic seeing, on the other hand, has what Dretske calls "positive belief content"; it involves recognition

---

[11] For a classic statement of this response see Mill (1872, pp. 242–244). For a more recent defence of this argument see Hyslop and Jackson (1972), and Hyslop (1995).

[12] I hazard the explanation that Dretske's proposal about seeing and knowing was itself so controversial that its extension to the case of other minds was simply ignored.

[13] The philosophically informed will appreciate that McDowell's perceptual model offers yet another way to think about things here. There is not time to explore both options in this chapter. My hope is that the way in which I pose the issues may stimulate further thought about how other models may be brought to bear on the issues raised.

or identification of what is seen; it is seeing *that*. Dretske explains that simple seeing and epistemic seeing can come apart in interesting ways. Here is one way: there can be simple seeing without epistemic seeing. This is relatively easy to grasp, and we can find examples of simple seeing alone in some non-human animals. There is another way in which these two kinds of seeing can come apart which is somewhat harder to grasp: there can be epistemic seeing without simple seeing. This is what Dretske thinks is going on when we perceive the mind of another. As this is going to be important to my discussion, let me explain how this can be.

Let's begin with Dretske's account of epistemic seeing:

A subject S *epistemically sees that p if*

(i) b is P
(ii) S sees (simple) b
(iii) The condition under which S sees b are such that b would not look the way it looks now to S unless it was P
And (iv) S, believing the conditions are as described in (iii), takes b to be P.

Thus one can come to see that the cake is in the shape of a heart or that the metal rod is bent. Furthermore, one not only sees that these things are the case, one knows that they are. Seeing for Dretske is a way of knowing.

Having introduced the idea, Dretske then explains that there can be two kinds of epistemic seeing: primary and secondary. The difference here relates to condition (ii). If S sees b in a direct, first-hand, or eye-witness way, then this counts as a case of primary epistemic seeing. If S sees b in an indirect way, then this counts as a case of secondary epistemic seeing. Say I want to know if the cake is cooked or if the metal rod is hot. Let's say I insert a toothpick and look to see if it comes out clean as a way of coming to know the former, and that I read the thermometer attached to the rod as a way of coming to know the later. If this is the way I come to know these things, then Dretske would say that I come to know these things in a *secondary* epistemic manner. Now consider again coming to know that the metal rod is hot. Say that, instead of reading the thermometer attached, I simply look at the rod and see it *glow in the manner characteristic of hot metal*. In this case I can come to know that the metal rod is hot in a *primary* epistemic manner.

Now let us return to the topic which is of central concern to this chapter: our knowledge of other minds. In so far as Dretske thinks we see other minds, what kind of seeing is involved? Dretske takes this to be an instance of primary epistemic seeing. Actually, there is a choice here. Whether one takes this to be a case of primary or secondary epistemic seeing will depend upon how one understands the relationship between mental states and behavior. If one thinks of this relationship on the model of the heat of the metal rod and the thermometer, then one will take this to be a case of secondary epistemic seeing. But Dretske rejects this model, or at least he rejects the idea that the mind is some private entity (see Dretske 1969, p. 185). According to Dretske I see that my daughter is in pain, for example, by seeing her behave in the manner characteristic of someone in pain. Behavior is crucial to what I know, but not on the model of the metal rod and the thermometer. Seeing that another is in pain is, for Dretske, a case of primary epistemic seeing. And now we have arrived at an understanding of how it is that Dretske thinks that our perception of other minds can provide us with an example of epistemic seeing without simple seeing. In order to see that, e.g., my daughter is in pain I need not see her pain or her mind.[14] It is this that Dretske thinks the inferentialist misses (see Dretske 1964, p. 32).

At this point it is important to pause to consider just what question we want answered with this perceptual model of other minds. Traditionally, the question philosophers asked has simply been,

Q I. How do I know that another has a mind?

I want to propose that this question admits of two readings, and can be taken as corresponding to the two ways I introduced earlier of understanding the problem of other mind: there is a thick and a thin reading of the question, and this corresponds to a thick and a thin understanding of the problem. The question in I. masks two questions that can be teased apart, thus:

q (i) How do I know *what* another thinks and feels? and
q (ii) How do I know *that* others think and feel?

These two questions are, on the whole, not differentiated in traditional discussions of other minds. Any attempt to understand how I can know that my daughter is, say, in pain is taken as, *in effect*, an attempt to understand how I can know that she is not a zombie (more on this later). For the traditional epistemologist the problem of other minds concerns both questions (with an emphasis on q(ii)) and is understood to be a *thick* problem.

Now, in so far as Dretske claims to have shown that we can use a perceptual model to achieve knowledge of other minds; can we take it that he thinks we can use the perceptual model to achieve knowledge that solipsism is false? The simple answer to this question is "no." Dretske insists that the perceptual model can only yield a reply to a question understood *thinly*. By this I mean that he takes it that we can separate q(i) from q(ii) and give an answer to q(i) but not q(ii). Indeed, that we cannot give an answer to q(ii) is Dretske's reason for believing that I cannot know that solipsism is false (more on this later). For epistemologists like Dretske, the only response that we can give to the problem of other minds is a response to a *thin* question.[15,16]

---

[14] Although Dretske writes of seeing that another is in pain, we need to be very careful. He does not intend that we see that another is not a zombie, but only that the other is in pain as opposed, to say, feeling a tickle. Seeing that someone is in pain is equivalent to knowing what that person is feeling—not knowing that they feel.

[15] As I explain later, it is not that Dretske does not think that the problem of other minds is not to be understood as a thick problem. However, the question he thinks the perceptual model gives an answer to is the thin question; it cannot give a response to the thick question.

[16] In footnote 17, I put forward a reason for why the perceptual model proposed in Dretske's work failed to receive much attention when it was first published. I now hazard a further explanation: as the traditional problem of other minds is taken to be a thick problem, Dretske's thin reply may have been thought to be missing the real point.

FROM DRETSKE TO WITTGENSTEIN

I introduced the problem of other minds earlier by explaining that it is frequently—and traditionally—taken to raise a skeptical worry. The skeptic challenges any claim that one is not alone in the world. Consider an excerpt from the writings of John Stuart Mill, one traditional source of material on this topic. Mill writes, just before he proposes his argument from analogy: "By what evidence do I know, or by what considerations am I led to believe, that there exist other sentient creatures; that the walking and speaking figures which I see and hear, have sensations and thoughts, or in other words, possess Minds?" (Mill 1889, p. 243). It seems clear that talk of "possessing a mind" is just another way of talking about having (we might say) *real* thoughts and feelings. The *dominant* question for the skeptic, then, is the question, How do I know that solipsism is false? The skeptic takes it that this question is the *first* question, and that without an answer to it I cannot know that others *really* have thoughts and feelings instead of presenting mere behavioral imitations of such. The question, What do others think and feel?, is necessarily secondary.

Now epistemologists who concern themselves with skeptical issues would insist that these two questions must be answered in a particular order: we must answer the first question *first*. Furthermore, we must answer the first question *in independence* of any questions concerning what others think and feel. The reason seems clear: there is little point is asking what another thinks and feels if I cannot rule out the possibility that the other is a zombie or automaton.

It is at this point that Dretske may be thought to disengage his epistemology from the traditional one. He holds that we can perceive that another is, say, in pain, but that we cannot see that the other is not a zombie or a cleverly constructed automaton. It follows that Dretske believes that I can know that my daughter is in pain but not know that she is not an automaton.

This result has seemed pretty counterintuitive to most philosophers, but Dretske is unrepentant. First let's be clear why Dretske believes he must reject the idea that we can see and thereby know that others are not zombies. The reason lies in condition (iii) in his account of epistemic seeing. According to condition (iii) the conditions under which I see that my daughter is in pain, say, are such that my daughter would not look the way she looks unless she was in pain. According to Dretske this condition is fulfilled in normal cases of seeing one's daughter crying, sucking her finger, and generally shaking. My daughter has cut her finger and is in pain. But if we consider whether condition (iii) is fulfilled for the case of seeing that my daughter is not a zombie, we get a very different result. Even if my daughter were a zombie the conditions under which I see that she is in pain are such that my daughter *would* look the way she looks now to me even if she were a zombie. That is because a zombie, as recent philosophical tradition conceives it, is designed to be a perfect imitation. I cannot tell the difference between a zombie and the real thing. Nevertheless, I can engage in all sorts of practices that require that I differentiate between my daughter being in pain and being angry, or being in pain and experiencing a tickle, and the like. One might say, I know what it is to be in pain, as opposed to being angry or experiencing tickles, and none of this requires that I first rule out that my daughter is not a zombie.

Thus, Dretske's account of epistemic seeing militates against getting any reply to the question about solipsism; and Dretske thinks this is as it should be (in other words, he thinks we shouldn't ditch the theory just because it throws up this result). After all, how could one *see* that others have minds, or are not zombies or cleverly constructed automata; you cannot *see* that solipsism is false. There is no way of knowing that solipsism is false, and therefore no way of answering the skeptic.

But has Dretske overlooked something? Perhaps it is possible to reply to the skeptic and the only thing we need to do in order to do so is reject the order of knowledge. While the skeptic insists that one needs to know that solipsism is false before one can know that, say, one's daughter is in pain, it might be possible to know that one's daughter is in pain and thereby know that solipsism is false. The line of thought would go like this: I know that my daughter is in pain. I know that, if my daughter is in pain, then she is not a zombie. So, I can conclude that my daughter is not a zombie. This line of thought employs what is known as the principle of epistemic closure to come by the knowledge needed to reply to the skeptic.[17] But Dretske won't have any truck with this principle. If there is no way of knowing that solipsism is false, then one should not be able to know this simply by employing the principle of epistemic closure. As far as Dretske is concerned there is no way, directly or indirectly, of answering the skeptic.

Philosophers have, over the centuries, adopted various strategies vis-à-vis the skeptic. Dretske's strategy is to place the skeptic off to one side. He does not argue that the skeptic makes any mistake in his argument, or that his approach involves some sort of incoherence. Nor does he assert that there is knowledge dogmatically and without regard to the skeptic. Rather, Dretske admits that the skeptic makes a good point, and agrees that there are certain things that we cannot know.[18] Nevertheless, despite not being able to know that solipsism is false we can, he suggests, have ordinary knowledge of other people's thoughts and feelings. This is what his analysis of epistemic seeing is designed to show.

Dretske's work drives a firm wedge between what we can see and thereby know—that, say, another is in pain, and what we cannot see and cannot know—that others are not zombies. There are those philosophers who try to argue, contra Dretske, that it *is* possible to perceive that others are not zombies (see, e.g., Cassam 2007, ch.5). There are yet others who insist on retaining the principle of epistemic closure, and so reject Dretske's account of knowledge in the form I presented it earlier.[19] One might say that those who distance themselves from Dretske's work in one or another of these ways want to maintain a connection between knowing another's thoughts and feelings and knowing the other isn't a zombie.

I think there is something interesting—indeed, correct—about Dretske's insistence that I cannot know that others are not zombies. How *can* one know this? This is something that was appreciated by Wittgenstein. In *On Certainty* (1969) Wittgenstein takes issue with the work of G. E. Moore. Moore famously claimed to have replied to skepticism by simply

---

[17] Employing the principle of epistemic closure might not be the only way of answering the skeptic by rejecting the order of knowledge here. See, for example, Cassam (2007, ch. 5).

[18] This is why I say in footnote 24, that Dretske does not deny that there is a thick understanding of the problem of other minds. What he denies is that we can give an answer to the question concerning others, considered as a thick question.

[19] See, for example, Stine (1976).

holding up one hand, and then another, and saying "I know here is a hand." He thought it followed from this knowledge that there is an external world. Transferring this to the case of another mind we might get: I know here is a person in pain, and here is another feeling ticklish, therefore solipsism is false.[20] What Wittgenstein objected to in Moore's work is the way Moore used knowledge of ordinary things to answer the skeptic. Now Wittgenstein's work is complex and there is not room here to do more than gesture at how I read the text. As I understand him, it is not that Wittgenstein objected to *Moore's* response to the skeptic. Rather, what he objected to was the fact that Moore thought he needed to respond to the skeptic at all, and furthermore that claiming to know such ordinary things is a way to do this.

In *On Certainty* §1 Wittgenstein writes: "If you do know *here is one hand*, we'll grant you all the rest." I take it that "all the rest" is what Moore wanted to prove. Wittgenstein rejected the idea that I could claim to know things as a way of responding to the skeptic. This isn't to say that Wittgenstein did not accept that there may not be situations where it would be perfectly in order to talk of knowing that one has a hand (perhaps there is some reason for believing it was amputated while one was under anesthetic). But this is not Moore's situation. Moore is claiming to know something about the world of bodies in order to show that the external world really does exist, and, by extension, to know about another's pain in order to prove that other minds really do exist.

It is at this point that Wittgenstein suggests that, unless there is something unusual or untoward, we do not correctly use the operator "I know that" in connection with ordinary things in life. When all is going along normally and the context involves no reason for pretense or subterfuge, I do not say "I know my daughter is in pain." I wipe my daughter's brow or call a doctor. When all is going normally I do not say "I know I have a hand." I pick up the post or wave to my friend.[21] One can see here hints of what Fodor seized upon in his discussion of the normal and the abnormal. It is true that Wittgenstein insists that in normal circumstances one does not say things like "I know I have a hand" or "I know my friend is in pain." In response to this, philosophers—including Fodor—cite the work of H. P. Grice and argue that, although such a locution would certainly be odd or unusual, we should not conclude that it is not strictly speaking true. But to make such a point in reply to Wittgenstein is, I believe, to miss the point. The point is that we must be careful not to fall into the trap of thinking that we can use our knowledge claims to show the skeptic the error of his ways. That would be the verbal equivalent of Dr. Johnson who kicked a stone and claimed to have refuted Berkeley's idealism in favor of realism.

One might think that Dretske and Wittgenstein are in basic agreement here. Both think that one cannot respond to the skeptic. And both allow for certain ordinary knowledge claims. But there is an important difference between the two. To appreciate the difference we must return for a moment to Dretske. I said that it is the sensitivity condition (condition (iii)) in Dretske's analysis of primary epistemic seeing that opens up a gap between what I can and cannot know. What the analysis shows us is that I can be sensitive to the fact that that my daughter is in pain despite not being sensitive to the fact that she is not a zombie.

---

[20] Although Moore insists the proof works for the case of other minds, he nowhere explains precisely how the proof would proceed in this case.

[21] In this connection consider *On Certainty* §10.

This is because my experience operates like an indicator that carries information about people in pain and children enjoying tickles, but not information about (what Dretske calls) the "heavyweight implications of these facts" (2005, p. 22). As I cannot know what I do not have information about, I cannot know these heavyweight implications. For this reason, Dretske says that my experience needs to be supplemented with what he in one place calls "proto-knowledge." Dretske explains that he used this term "to describe things that have to be true for what you perceive to be true but which (even if you knew that they had to be true) you couldn't perceive to be true" (2005, p. 14). In some places Dretske writes of "presupposition—something one simply takes for granted."[22] In the case of others what one takes for granted is that solipsism is false. One could say that Dretske holds that in the foreground one can see that another is in, say, pain, while in the background there operates a certain proto-knowledge or presupposition concerning what must be the case for one to be in a position to see what one sees.

This split between the foreground and the background is an interesting one. And, once again, it is tempting to read Wittgenstein as agreeing with this talk of a background. Time and time again we find Wittgenstein writing about what must be in place before we can talk of knowledge. So he, too, appears to want to differentiate between the background that cannot be known and what can be known in the foreground. But when we come to understand just what Wittgenstein means when he talks about the background to our knowledge, we find an important *difference* from Dretske. Consider what Wittgenstein writes in *On Certainty* §534:

> But is it wrong to say: "A child that has mastered a language-game must know certain things?"
>   If instead of that one said "must be able to do certain things," that would be a pleonasm, yet this is what I want to counter the first sentence with.

Wittgenstein is here showing us the way in which our knowledge is founded in our activities. These activities lay at the foundation of our language-game, and only once this is in place can we proceed to *know*. To insist that knowledge has anything to do with this foundational business is to miss the point. And it is precisely this point that Wittgenstein thinks the skeptic misses. Where Wittgenstein thinks there is a foundational practice, the skeptic thinks there is something to know.

Wittgenstein shows the skeptic the error of his ways.[23] The skeptic misunderstands how things operate at this foundational level. We might say, all of this activity and practice is what we need to understand as in operation "in the background." It is not a matter of knowing anything; it is a matter of having a certain nature which is such that I respond to the world and to others in a certain manner. Out of this response we build our practice, and with this practice in place I proceed to learn about my world and those around me. I take it that the reference here to our nature is important to what Wittgenstein is saying. The practice we build up is *our* practice; it is a practice constructed by individuals who share a—human—nature.

---

[22] Dretske (2005, p. 21). See also Dretske (1970/1999, p. 137). When Dretske writes of proto-knowledge his point looks to be a logical one; there is, however, a hint of the psychological about this presupposition.

[23] Which is not to say that that I take Wittgenstein as responding to skepticism. On this very interesting question of Wittgenstein's attitude to the skeptic I find I am in agreement with McGinn (2008).

Dretske, on the other hand, appears to be in agreement with the skeptic who holds that there is something to be known, but that we—humans—cannot know this. The only difference between Dretske and the skeptic is that he, Dretske, does not take the absence of knowledge here to stand in the way of ordinary knowledge. Dretske does not think, as Wittgenstein does, that for knowledge to proceed we need to have in place—in the background, if you like—a practice built up from activities in the world and with others.

From Philosophy to Psychiatry

The point to which I now want to draw attention is this: once we acknowledge the difference between a thick and a thin reading of the question concerning the minds of others, we can, perhaps, exploit different understandings of the background in such a way as to help us to understand aspects of psychological development and psychopathology.

Let us return to Dretske and Wittgenstein. We could say that Dretske holds that, while our knowledge is limited, we can nonetheless understand the thick reading of the question of classical philosophy. The thick question makes sense and we are making no mistake when we ask it. Wittgenstein, on the other hand, does not think the thick question makes sense, and he believes that the skeptic is making a mistake when s/he asks it. Consider what he writes in *On Certainty* §32:

> It's not a matter of Moore's knowing that there's a hand there, but rather we should not understand him if he were to say, "Of course I may be wrong about this." We should ask, "What is it like to make such a mistake as that?" E.g. what's it like to discover that it was a mistake?

Of course we should understand if a person were to make a mistake about having a hand if he were an injured soldier coming out of anesthetic after being caught in a mortar attack (consider what Wittgenstein writes in *On Certainty* §23). Similarly, we could understand someone whose daughter works in an automobile factory, where lifelike robots work on the assembly line along with bored teenagers, admitting that they may be mistaken when they aim to point out a teenager to a friend from a distance. What we should *not* understand is someone who thought something along these lines: of course I may be wrong and all those who I associate with on a day to day basis are mere automata or zombies.

In another passage Wittgenstein compares the person who employs the language of doubt regarding such things with a person whose mind is disturbed (cf. for example, *On Certainty* §71). The person who doubts is disturbed, while the person who is not disturbed is, as he puts it, "certain."[24] This certainty is not that of believing something that is guaranteed in some way. Such a guarantee might be the result of our perception/knowledge of the fact that the world is not a dream and that others are not zombies. But there is no such guarantee; and yet we are certain. Wittgenstein takes this certainty to be expressed in a surefootedness vis-à-vis the world and others. My daughter is chopping vegetables with a sharp knife when the knife slips and cuts her finger. She cries out in pain and I rush to help her. There is no

---

[24] The question of knowledge and certainty is a vexed one. Stanley (2008) distinguishes between what he calls epistemological certainty and subjective certainty. Wittgenstein introduces yet *another* idea of certainty.

doubt. I do not act on the knowledge that she is not a zombie merely feigning pain. She is my daughter and in pain.

Consider when Wittgenstein writes (*The Blue Book*, p. 48):

> Certainly we shouldn't pity him if we didn't believe that he had pains; but is this a philosophical, a metaphysical belief? Does a realist pity more that an idealist or a solipsist?

This talk of "a philosophical, a metaphysical belief" is the belief involved in q(ii). It is the belief that others are not zombies. Wittgenstein's point here is that our reaction to the other—in this case our pity—in no way depends upon what we believe or know. My nature is such that I respond to the other in a certain way. That response does not wait upon, or in any way require, belief. It just is. And in so far as it is, belief has no place. What Wittgenstein thinks we should learn from this is that we already have the certainty we hanker after when we look for knowledge *that* others think and feel.[25]

What if we pursue the idea that Wittgenstein introduces in various places, of the person who is disturbed? It is notable that Wittgenstein never considers *real* disturbances—the sort one might find in the textbooks of the psychiatrist. But he does explain what occurs in the *normal* case of the child learning a language. Wittgenstein refers to the child learning to "master a language game" (*On Certainty* §534), of the child who "learns to react in such-and-such a way" (*On Certainty* §538), and the like. The child learns from *someone*, and for this to occur the child and its teacher need to be able to respond to the world in a similar manner. When Wittgenstein writes about our practice he is, at the same time, writing about our natures. It is because we share a certain nature that the learning process can take place in the way that it does. Given the place that our shared natures play in building our practice, we might consider the impact on this practice if a particular child's nature is disturbed in some way. This would no doubt have an impact on the child's capacity to learn from her teacher, and on her capacity to be integrated into our shared practice.

Wittgenstein claims that in the course of a normal, healthy development, the child interacts with the world and the people around her in a particular way that we would all recognize. He gives, as an example, someone sitting by the bed of a very sick friend (*On Certainty* §10). He contrasts knowing the friend is sick with the actions of sitting by his bedside and looking attentively into his face. In *On Certainty* §281 Wittgenstein writes:

> I, L.W., believe, am sure, that my friend hasn't saw-dust in his body or in his head, even though I have no direct evidence of my senses to the contrary. I am sure, by reason of what has been said to me, of what I have read, and of my experience. To have doubts about it would seem to me madness—of course, this is also in agreement with other people; but *I* agree with them.

Think of how a child responds when a playmate falls over and badly injures herself. The child looks anxious; often a very young child will cry despite not being injured herself. It is this reaction that the teacher will build on when teaching the child about another's pains. But what if the child shows no interest, keeps bouncing her ball and showing no reaction whatever to this badly injured playmate? How do we teach this child?

---

[25] Cf. *On Certainty* §112: "And isn't that what Moore wants to say, when he says he *knows* all these things?—But is his knowing it really what is in question, and not rather that some of those propositions must be solid for us?"

Depending on just *how* different the child is, we may be able to teach such a child *some* of our practice or we may not be able to teach it *any*. A child may have a limited sympathy for others, or may show no interest whatsoever.[26]

Notice that, when an individual's nature is disturbed, two things (at least) are the result. Firstly, the child does not react to the world and to others in the same way as those around him/her. As a result of this different reaction the child, secondly, is not able to learn as those around him/her learn. This isn't to say that the child might not be able, as it were, to come up with deviant strategies (deviant from the point of view of the norm), and thereby learn to talk about the pain of others. Perhaps she simply learns that "pain" is what we say when a person cries out, bleeds, and attends the wounded body part. She might learn to attend to the playmate in much the same way we might respond to a "tiny tears doll." But the healthy child brings more to the learning situation. The healthy child responds to the injury and there is, as a result, what one might call an "added dimension" to her use of the word "pain." This added dimension can be thought of by comparison with the child who understands about adult sexuality from watching films and reading magazines, and then comes to the age when they experience sexual feelings themselves. In both cases we have individuals whose behavior is altered by an alteration in their natures. The child may understand about sexuality from films and magazines, but this understanding acquires another, call it a deeper, dimension after a certain age. Similarly, a child who experiences no concern or pity may nonetheless learn to help others who cry out and say they are in pain, but there is an undoubted difference in the quality of the response from someone who not only "reads the signs" but who also spontaneously responds with concern and pity.[27]

THE THICK PROBLEM VERSUS DEPTH OF PRACTICE

Stanley Cavell has written that skepticism pictures the field of everyday knowledge as "intellectually confined." The skeptic "presses the aim of reason itself, to know objectively, without stint; to penetrate reality itself" (1979, pp. 430–431). This is the skeptic who presses q(ii). This skeptic challenges us to solve the *thick* problem of other minds. As I have already explained, Dretske has some sympathy with this skeptic. He understands the problem of other minds to be a thick problem, despite the fact that he thinks we can only use the perceptual model to reply to the thin question here: I can perceive another's thoughts and feelings, and in order to do this I do not have to perceive that they are not zombies. Dretske also holds that a certain "proto-knowledge" must be in place, and we might think of this proto-knowledge as a surrogate for the knowledge that we cannot have.

---

[26] In connection with autism, Hobson (2009, p. 250) has noted: "I stress that in most cases of autism, the children's limitations in each [of the observed] respects are partial rather than absolute."

[27] I take the comparison from Kripke (1982, pp. 140–141). As Kripke is careful to point out, the comparison will only work if we leave aside Freudian theories of infantile sexuality and the latency period. Kripke draws this comparison in order to explain his understanding of how Wittgenstein sees the role of one's own feelings of pain when attributing feelings of pain to others. I am using the comparison to highlight the way in which a certain absence of attitude (such as pity) towards another can affect one's development.

Dretske quite rightly presses the question, How *could* we perceive that another is not a zombie? But in the light of this question, we might raise another: How are we to think of the proto-knowledge that Dretske insists must be in place whenever we perceive what another thinks or feels? Dretske says altogether too little about an idea which plays such an important role in his philosophy. When he writes about proto-knowledge it would seem that Dretske is largely concerned with what has to be the case *in the world*. The picture Dretske offers is one where we have limited knowledge of the other.[28]

What if we were to drop this idea that our knowledge here is limited? In opposition to this picture of our limited knowledge of others, Cavell (1979, p. 432) suggests that we turn the skeptic's picture on its head: instead of taking our everyday knowledge of others to be confined, we should think of it as "exposed." Cavell explains this idea of exposure as, in part, the idea of an exposure to my concept of the other. He writes (1979, p. 433):

> Being exposed to my concept of the other is being exposed to my assurance in applying it, I mean to the fact that this assurance is *mine*, comes only from me. The other can present me with no mark or feature on the basis of which I can *settle* my attitude. I have to acknowledge humanity in the other, and the basis of it seems to lie in me.

Following Wittgenstein, Cavell turns us away from looking to the other to settle questions here. It is *my* assurance that settles things; I must acknowledge the humanity in the other. It is this acknowledgment, evidenced in my assured behavior towards the other, which gives what I have been calling a "depth" to my talk about the thoughts and feelings of others.

This idea that, in the normal run of things, our practice in relation to each other possesses a certain depth is to be distinguished from the idea of a thick problem of other minds. Depth is a quality of the relationship between individuals; it is evidenced in the behavior of one individual towards another. Rather than holding (as Dretske does) that there is a limitation in our knowledge, we should understand why it is important to eschew knowledge here (as Wittgenstein does). It is not that our knowledge is limited, but that what knowledge we do have is grounded in our activities in the world and vis-à-vis others. Instead of agreeing with Dretske and the skeptic that there is a thick question that we cannot answer, we can look toward the work of Wittgenstein and say that our attitudes toward others provides a certain depth to our thought and talk about another's thoughts and feelings.

If we do favor our attitudes toward others as providing the depth we seek when we pose the thick question concerning other minds, we can then consider what disturbance might result from a defect in that attitude. A child might learn when to say that another is in pain or is happy, but that child's behavior towards others may still "lack a certain dimension." Peter Hobson (1993, pp. 229, 243) cites the case of a young man with Asperger's syndrome "who could not grasp the concept of friend."[29] The example is particularly apt, but the idea can be extended to other concepts. It should be clear that I am not suggesting that some

[28] Dretske (2005, p. 15) writes: "We can see (hear, feel, smell) that P, but some of the Q's that (we know) P implies are just too remote, too distant, to inherit the positive warrant the sensory evidence confers upon P."

[29] This young man was a high achiever academically, but claimed to be unable to grasp the concept of a friend. Hobson concludes that "it was my patient's lack of intersubjective sharing that led to his incomprehension of what it means to have to be a 'friend,' a conceptual deficit that stood in contrast to his understanding of sophisticated concepts that were beyond the grasp of many non-autistic teenagers."

people actively question whether those around them are zombies. Dretske holds that our perception of other minds is supplemented by proto-knowledge—something one "simply takes for granted."[30] One may question what the result might be of the absence of such proto-knowledge, but Dretske does not write in such a way as to leave room for such a possibility. If, however, we turn to the work of Wittgenstein, it is possible to raise the question what would happen if activities between individuals at a crucial developmental stage were affected by a disturbance in the nature of the developing individual. Furthermore, and importantly, we can see that the nature of the disturbance can lie on a spectrum from the very severely disturbed (where the development of language and attendant activities are hindered) to the mildly disturbed (which allows for the use of language and other sorts of engagement with others but where the quality of that use and that engagement is at odds with the norm). We could say that there is a certain *thinness* or lack of depth to the engagement with others in such situations and hence, a certain thinness or lack of depth to the understanding of what it is to speak of another's pain or anger.[31]

This idea that our interaction with others, in the normal case, exhibits a certain depth is an idea that is in sympathy with the work of Peter Hobson. Hobson is also drawn to the work of Wittgenstein from which he develops his own idea that an "infant's capacity for personal relatedness, the psychological bedrock for their understanding of persons, is partly constituted by innately determined perceptual-affective sensibilities towards the bodily appearances and behavior of others" (1991, p. 33). Hobson takes his work here to be a development of a proposal due to Kanner (1943) who observed that certain children "come into the world with innate inability [*sic*] to form the usual, biologically provided affective contact with people" (Hobson 1989, p. 22). What Hobson has tried to work out is the impact a disturbance in the way an infant relates to others can have upon that infant's social relations in later life. He believes that that impact is evidenced in much of the behavior which is cited as characteristic of the autistic individual: the inability to form certain social relations; the lack of a certain pragmatic dimension in their communication and use of language; and an impairment of imagination that manifests itself in an absence of creative play.[32] What marks Hobson's work, in contradistinction to other approaches that dominate the literature on this topic, is its emphasis on the *inter*personal. He rightly sees the dominant explanatory approach as predominantly individualistic.[33] As well as emphasizing the intersubjective, Hobson's work also emphasizes the importance of the quality of that intersubjectivity in early development. The quality of the intersubjective experience in infancy and early childhood should be seen, he argues, as playing a "foundational role," as providing "a kind of bedrock for subsequent relations with other people and attitudes towards oneself" (Hobson 2003). And he explains the way in which impairment of this intersubjective experience may be thought to explain the characteristics associated with autism. Hobson (1989, p. 42) concludes that "to arrive at a theory of autism, we need to reach beyond cognition." This is a lesson Hobson claims to have learned, inter alia, from Wittgenstein.

---

[30] Cf. footnote 35.

[31] This is not to say that such individuals could not characterize the difference between persons and puppets, or between real pain and sham pain.

[32] See footnote 1 for mention of other characteristics that also need explanation.

[33] See Hobson (2003). The dominant approach that Hobson has in mind here is the theory theory approach to be found in work influenced by Premack and Woodruff (1978).

Conclusion

I began this chapter by introducing one way—that due to the work of Fred Dretske—of answering the traditional problem of other minds. In the place of the various inferential-ist models, Dretske has proposed a perceptual model of our knowledge of other minds. However, when one looks closely at the model it soon becomes clear that Dretske does not think that that model answers quite the same question as the inferentialist model was designed to answer. While the problem of other minds is traditionally put forward as one undifferentiated question, Dretske proposes that we can separate out two questions. Once these questions have been separated out, Dretske's proposal is that we can use the perceptual model to provide an answer to q(i) but not to q(ii). Or, in the terminology I have introduced, he thinks the perceptual model provides an answer to the thin but not the thick question of other minds.

By way of contrast with Dretske's work here I also introduced some ideas from Wittgenstein's later work. It should be clear that in such a short chapter I have had to skim over various issues that would greatly complicate the picture I am trying to outline. Nonetheless, I believe there is some illumination to be gained by approaching Wittgenstein's work in the light of Dretske's. I have explained that where Dretske acknowledges a thick problem of other minds, Wittgenstein does not.[34] I also suggested that where Dretske intro-duces the idea of proto-knowledge, Wittgenstein explains the way in which our knowledge of others is grounded in our practices in relation to others. Furthermore, I explained the way in which these practices are conditioned by the natures of those who engage in them. The nature of those who engage in the practice not only determines how that practice devel-ops, but can also be taken to provide that practice with what I called a "depth."[35] Should this nature either be different or become, for some reason, disturbed, there will be repercussions for the practice that develops. It may be that the practice which develops will be noticeably at odds with the norm, or it may be that the difference will be found in some more subtle quality of the interaction between persons. What is important here is that the stage is set for asking the thin question concerning others at a very early stage in development.

Wittgenstein's last work in *On Certainty* provides an important conceptual framework which may help us to understand the psychopathology of autism.[36] By placing Wittgenstein's work in relation to Dretske's, we can also begin to appreciate how an age old problem in philosophy—that of skepticism and other minds—might shed light on this most perplexing of disorders.

---

[34] The issue of whether Wittgenstein would allow talk of *any* problem of other minds is one of those I have had to skim over here. Of course we *do* attribute thoughts and feelings to others, and this alone can be said to raise q(i)—whether or not one thinks of this as *problematic*.

[35] The importance of our nature is something also appreciated the eighteenth-century philosopher Thomas Reid (1764/1983, pp. 633–634) who observes: even before a child reaches its first birthday, it "clings to its nurse in danger, enters into her grief and joy, is happy in her soothings and caresses, and unhappy in her displeasure."

[36] Others have appealed to Wittgenstein's work in an attempt to understand another psychopathology, the certainty with which delusional belief is often held. See, for example, Campbell (2001) and Rhodes and Gipps (2008).

References

American Psychiatric Association (2000). *Diagnostic and Statistical Manual of Mental Disorders, Fourth Edition, Text Revision*. Washington, DC: American Psychiatric Association.

Avramides, A. (2001). *Other Minds*. London: Routledge.

Ayer, A. J. (1956). *The Problem of Knowledge*. Great Britain: Penguin Books Ltd.

Campbell, J. (2001). Rationality, meaning, and the analysis of delusion. *Philosophy, Psychology, & Psychiatry, 8*(2/3), 89–100.

Cassam, Q. (2007). *The Possibility of Knowledge*. Oxford: Oxford University Press.

Cavell, S. (1979). *The Claim of Reason*. Oxford: Oxford University Press.

Dretske, F. (1964). Observational terms. *Philosophical Review, 73*, 25–42.

Dretske, F. (1969). *Seeing and Knowing*. Chicago, IL: University of Chicago Press.

Dretske, F. (1999). Epistemic operators. In K. DeRose and T. A. Warfield (Eds), *Skepticism: A Contemporary Reader*, pp. 131–145. New York & Oxford: Oxford University Press. (Original work published 1970.)

Dretske, F. (2005). The case against closure. In M. Steup and E. Sosa (Eds), *Contemporary Debates in Epistemology*, pp. 13–26. Oxford: Blackwell's Publishing Ltd.

Fodor, J. (1968). *Psychological Explanation*. New York, NY: Random House.

Gallagher, S. (2004). Understanding interpersonal problems in autism: Interaction theory as an alternative to theory of mind. *Philosophy, Psychiatry & Psychology, 11*(3), 199–217.

Hamlyn, D. (1957). *The Psychology of Perception*. London: Routledge & Kegan Paul.

Hobson, P. (1989). Beyond cognition: A theory of autism. In G. Dawson (Ed.), *Autism*, pp. 22–48. New York, NY: The Guilford Press.

Hobson, P. (1991). Against the theory of 'theory of mind'. *British Journal of Developmental Psychology, 9*, 33–51.

Hobson, P. (1993). Emotional origins of social understanding. *Philosophical Psychology, 6*(3), 227–49.

Hobson, P. (2003). Between ourselves: psychodynamics and the interpersonal domain. *British Journal of Psychiatry, 182*, 193–5.

Hobson, P. (2009). Wittgenstein and the developmental psychopathology of autism. In *New Ideas in Psychology, 27*, 243–57.

Hyslop, A. (1995). *Other Minds*. Dordrecht: Kluwer Academic Publishers.

Hyslop, A. and Jackson, F. (1972). The analogical inference to other minds. *American Philosophical Quarterly, 9*, 168–76.

Kanner, L. (1943). Autistic disturbances of affective contact. *Nervous Child, 2*, 217–50.

Kripke, S. (1982). Postscript: "Wittgenstein on Other Minds." In *Wittgenstein on Rules and Private Language*, pp. 114–46. Oxford: Basil Blackwell.

McDowell, J. (1998a). On 'the reality of the past'. In *Meaning, Knowledge, and Reality*, pp. 295–314. Cambridge, MA: Harvard University Press. (Original work published 1978.)

McDowell, J. (1998b). Criteria, defeasibility, and knowledge. In *Meaning, Knowledge, and Reality*, pp. 369–95. Cambridge, MA: Harvard University Press. (Original work published 1982.)

McGinn, M. (2008). Wittgenstein on certainty. In J. Greco (Ed.), *The Oxford Handbook on Skepticism*, pp. 372–91. Oxford: Oxford University Press.

Mill, J. S. (1872). *An Examination of Sir William Hamilton's Philosophy* (4th edn). London: Longman, Green, Reader and Dyer.

Pargetter, R. (1984). Scientific inference to other minds. *Australasian Journal of Philosophy, 62*, 158–63.

Plantinga, A. (1966). Induction and other minds. *Review of Metaphysics*, *19*(3), 441–61.

Premack, D. and Woodruff, G. (1978). Does the chimpanzee have a theory of mind? *Behaviour and Brain Sciences*, *4*, 515–26.

Reid, T. (1983). *An Inquiry into the Mind on the Principles of Common Sense*. In R. E. Beanblossom and K. Lehrer (Eds), *Thomas Reid: Inquiry and Essays*. Indianapolis: Hackett Publishing Company, Inc. (Original work published 1764.)

Rhodes, J. and Gipps, R. G. T. (2008). Delusions, certainty and the background. *Philosophy, Psychiatry, and Psychology*, *15*(4), 295–310.

Smith, J. (2010). Seeing other people. *Philosophy and Phenomeological Research*, *81*(3), 731–48.

Stanley, J. (2008). Knowledge and certainty. *Philosophical Issues*, *18*, 33–55.

Stine, G. C. (1976). Skepticism, relevant alternatives, and deductive closure. *Philosophical Studies*, *29*, 249–61.

Wittgenstein, L. (1969). *On Certainty* (G. E. M. Anscombe and G. H. von Wright, Eds). New York, NY: Harper & Row.

CHAPTER 21

···

EMPATHIC FOUNDATIONS
OF CLINICAL KNOWLEDGE

···

NANCY NYQUIST POTTER

This chapter sets out several views of empathy that draw not only on psychology's literature but on philosophical and psychiatric writings. I consider empathy to be a complex
concept involving perception, emotion, attitudinal orientation, and other cognitive processes as well as an activity that expresses character traits and, hence, one of the virtues. In
other words, an examination of the philosophical and clinical literature reveals empathy to
be not one unified concept but instead a set of related characteristics and qualities needed
to be an ethical and therapeutically effective clinician. To this end, I offer reasons as to why
empathy is important to clinical work. I then distinguish empathy from a related concept
called "world"-traveling and situate its relevance to therapeutic relations. At the end, I bring
these ideas together by highlighting Iris Murdoch's (1970) idea of "just vision" and "loving
attention."

EMPATHY AND MORAL LIFE

···

Part of being a moral person is the recognition both that our actions, choices, and ways
of being in the world affect others, and that this connection to others matters to us. That
is to say, humans are relational, and our emotional, cognitive, and material connections
are constituents of moral life. Still, the fact that morality is relational can be difficult,
practically speaking. For one thing, it means that we have to get outside ourselves (what
Iris Murdoch (1970) calls "the fat relentless ego") and at times we feel conflicts between
what we want for ourselves and what we want for others. For another thing, the fact that
morality is relational presents difficulties because it sometimes requires us to imagine
and understand others' perspectives, needs, and values in ways that are epistemically and
imaginatively challenging. As William Ickes (1997, p. 1) writes in the introduction to
Empathic Accuracy:

the indeterminate, ever-elusive nature of the Other's subjective experience when the Other is immanently present is a central problem not just for phenomenologists and existential philosophers. It is a central problem for all of us. When the strange figure abruptly looms on Ortega [y Gasset's] horizon, or slips past the park benches to disorder [Jean-Paul] Sartre's private world, he reminds us all how difficult—and yet how important—it is to accurately infer the thoughts, feelings, motives, and intentions of other people.

While I do not think that epistemic (or empathic) incommensurability exists between self and other, I agree with Ickes that the inner world—and the material, lived experiences—of others can be puzzling, elusive, or very difficult to grasp. This may be the case especially for clinicians, whose therapeutic effectiveness relies on being able to understand what it is like for their patient, from the patient's perspective, to live with their illness (more on this in the section entitled "Strange landscapes"). To accurately understand the patient enough to empathize with him or her in ways that facilitate the patient feeling understood and empathized with is a learning process. That is, empathizing accurately (to frame empathy as Ickes does) requires both a general skill that is developed over time, and also an ongoing process of being able to apply these skills with a particular patient and as the relationship with each particular patient develops. And sometimes, feeling and expressing empathy for a patient is a daunting task as, for example, with patients diagnosed with borderline personality disorder (BPD) who many clinicians report feeling extreme frustration, dislike, and even hatred toward (cf. Potter 2009). Because the emotional and epistemic demands of empathy call upon us to develop qualities and skills within ourselves that make it more likely that we will become good at being appropriately empathic, even with incomprehensible or unlikeable patients, these demands suggest that one useful way to conceive of empathy is as a virtue. I discuss this idea in the later section "Empathy as something we can choose." But first we need to begin to clarify the concept.

As I intimated earlier, empathy is a vitally important character trait not only for individual flourishing but also for social harmony and morally good relationships. Empathy is oriented toward the concrete and subjective person, not an abstract and generalized other. As Arne Vetlesen (1994) says, "In moral performance a great deal turns on whether the other is perceived as an abstract, faceless, and 'formal' other or as a concrete other to which I can relate emotionally as well as intellectually" (p. 287). An empathetic cognitive and emotional orientation toward the particular person is key to recognizing the subjectivity and humanity of him or her. By this, I mean that central to being a good and accurate empathizer is that we conceptualize the other person as a subject in his or her own right. This idea is grounded in philosophical and feminist analysis of social relations that, historically, have been hierarchical and oppressive to some groups of people. In standard analyses of oppressive social systems, people who have more power and authority fail to perceive and treat those less powerful as fully human and as more than mere tools for the benefit of the oppressor class. The effect is that those in oppressed groups are seen and treated as objects, not as subjects who have projects, life goals, desires, hopes, and fears of their own. (The explanation and justification for these claims is beyond the scope of this article. But see, for example, Fanon (2008) for one analysis of the effects of oppressive systems on the subjectivity of those in subordinate groups.) While it might seem that a discussion of social systems is a digression here, it is relevant to the history of scientific research where the "subjects" of research are, in fact, *objects* of study. And it is pertinent to psychiatry in the sense that clinicians have sometimes viewed their patients in terms of their symptoms and their diagnoses instead of as a full subject who is living with a mental disorder. This is seen most starkly with respect to patients with BPD who are often referred to just as "that borderline." (The service user movement in Europe speaks to this problem of reducing a person to his or her diagnosis.) To sum up the points I have made so far: I have said that understanding *this situated* person—and *this* patient within *such-and-such* a context and history—is a process of recognizing the subjectivity of that patient while feeling and expressing empathy toward him or her.

> Vetlesen asks, what essential cognitive and emotional resources in the subject are required for him or her to recognize the other as a moral addressee? Emotions as well as cognitions anchor us to the particular moral circumstance, to the aspect of a situation that addresses us immediately, to the here and now. To "see" the circumstance and to see oneself as addressed by it, and thus to be susceptible to the way a situation affects the weal and woe of others—in short, to identify a situation as carrying moral significance in the first place--all of this is required in order to enter the domain of the moral, and none of it would come about without the basic faculty of empathy. (Vetlesen 1994, p. 4)

One way to understand empathy, then, is as a kind of moral perception that involves attentiveness and that requires both that we see and that we listen. But, as I indicated earlier, it is also a quality in us that takes time, energy, and practice to do well. Iris Murdoch (1970) emphasizes the moral effort required to be attentive, pointing out that being good is not merely a matter of discrete right actions but of the moral vision we cultivate in between the moments of choosing: "I can only choose within the world I can see, in the moral sense of 'see' which implies that clear vision is a result of moral imagination and moral effort" (1994, p. 37). That is, the choices we make over time create habits in us; they set in place (not necessarily rigidly, though) the sorts of things that we then tend to notice, to desire, to aim at, and to deem choiceworthy again. In other words, the development of moral vision is grounded in background conditions of past feelings and actions, choices and consequences. The moral choices we make, including the degree and accuracy of empathy we can offer to another are, ideally, grounded in reason and not just accident, gut reaction, or whim. Like other moral and epistemic endeavors, empathy draws upon practical reasoning.

Sara Hodges and Daniel Wegner capture the depth of the task we face in being empathetic for even one specific encounter:

> To empathize with a person in a situation involves more than simply changing one's spatial viewpoint; it also involves changing one's judgment of the situation, one's memory for events and one's emotional responsiveness to them, one's conception of the person's traits and goals, and even one's conception of oneself .... The occurrence of empathy involves such a generalized structural transformation in thought and emotion that it must be conceptualized more broadly than many less sweeping changes in mental content. (1997, p. 312)

In other words, empathy is epistemologically significant in that it allows us to understand and anticipate the behavior of others, and it is morally significant to our ability to apply reciprocity principles and the principle of universalizability. As Robert Gordon says, "That is a heavy load for one mental procedure to bear" (1995, p. 740). Gordon is right.

EMPATHY AS SOMETHING WE CAN CHOOSE

Elsewhere (Potter 2009) I have argued that empathy is not just an understanding attitude toward, or a way of perceiving, others but a virtue. Empathy contributes to flourishing, expresses an enduring state of character, and has an intermediate condition and extremes. I stated earlier that being empathetic requires a kind of reasoning and not just an intuition and this is because, on an Aristotelian account of virtue, displaying a virtue requires that we deliberately decide how to feel and what to do and that we make a choice based on it being the right way to feel and to act (Aristotle 1984). Practical reasoning directs us in finding the mean between the two extremes of being excessively empathetic (for example, by carrying the emotional burden for others or losing oneself in others) or being deficient in empathy (for example, by failing to be moved by the troubles of others or being unable emotionally and cognitively to imagine others' suffering). Although the mean is contextual and relative to the persons involved, it is also objective in that we can get it wrong about how much empathy to feel and to express. Practical reasoning picks up the nuances of the situation while assisting us in finding the objectively right way to express the virtue of empathy. A person who feels empathy can see how (and whether) a heuristic applies. The reasoning necessary for virtue is not abstract and detached; instead, it requires that we think about context, feelings, and social relations in a psychologically rich way—a way that attends to the full subjectivity of others—so as to determine the rightness or wrongness of particular actions. Without empathy, the moral agent is unable fully to grasp the moral features of certain situations, because part of what makes those situations the kind they are is the other particular person. Empathy plays a central role in coming to understand the context and potential implications for others of our contemplated actions so that we can reason well.

Treating empathy as a moral and epistemic virtue commits us to the view that empathetic responses are, at least to some degree, under our control. To what extent is the view warranted that empathy can be modulated and controlled? To address this question, let us look more closely at the way empathy is discussed in literature from clinical research.

Some researchers suggest that empathy is best thought of as a set of constructs that draws together a number of phenomena. In particular, that set includes (1) physiological responses of awareness and arousal; (2) a wandering imagination: a tendency to fantasize and daydream about fictional situations in an undirected manner; (3) fictional involvement: the ability to transpose oneself by imagination into the feelings and actions of fictitious characters in books, movies, and plays; (4) a humanistic orientation: a sensitivity to and appreciation for the emotional welfare of others; and (5) emotional contagion: a susceptibility to the emotions of those around one (Tamborini et al. 1990).

According to these researchers, empathetic processes are understood to involve the somewhat deliberate and conscious place-taking of another and thus are or can be under our control even though awareness and arousal are immediate responses to external stimuli. Reactions are considered empathetic when they are concordant with the observed or likely experience of another and exclude reactions that are discordant. When viewing a horror film, for example, subjects would experience distress and arousal while simultaneously appraising their reactions in terms of concordance or discordance with the victim. When viewers assess their actions as appropriate to the situation that the victim is in, they generate the appropriate emotion by imagining similar situations in their own lives that have produced intense emotional reactions. While this research suggests that there is a cognitive component to empathetic responses, it also shows that "individual differences on various dimensions of empathy have been shown to influence emotional reactions in several distressing contexts" (Tamborini et al. 1990, p. 616). Place-taking of another, for example, can occur without an emotional component, as when a con artist is calculating what it would take for the victim to act on her vulnerability. That is, place-taking in itself is not necessarily empathic.

Other research suggests that some empathetic responses (especially in infants) are purely non-cognitive in that they do not require recognition of someone else's mental state or a mechanism for converting cognitions into what they are cognitions of. The most basic levels of empathetic mapping occur in facial mimicry, in mimicry of direction of gaze, and in social referencing. In mimicry of the gaze, one tracks the gaze of another from her facial expression to the "cause" or "object" of the emotion, whereas in social referencing the process is reversed. Facial mimicry, together with these other levels of empathetic learning, are powerful socializing mechanisms (Gordon 1995, p. 730). What we learn to do, in effect, is to simulate the emotions of others. As Gordon explains, "simulation permits us to extend to others the modes of attribution, explanation, and prediction that otherwise would be applicable only in our own case" (1995, p. 730). This approach, Gordon explains, involves a kind of transformation by which one draws an inference from one's own emotion, state of mind, or situational experience (perhaps under a hypothetical situation) to that of another. "The imaginative shift in the reference of indexicals [from 'I' to 'you' or from 'here' to 'there' or from 'now' to 'then'] reflects a much deeper, more important shift. Many of our tendencies to action or emotion appear to be specially keyed to an egocentric map" (Gordon 1995, p. 734). So what we can do, through simulation, is to recenter our egocentric map.

Of course, we have to learn how to make adjustments for errors when simulating the emotions of others and this is part of the skill-building that clinicians must acquire in order to be accurate empathizers.

> Although we imaginatively project ourselves into the person's problem situation, it is always important, in giving advice, to hold back in certain ways from identification with the other person—that is, from making the further adjustments required to imagine being not just in that person's situation but *that person* in that person's situation. (Gordon 1995, p. 740)

Thus, Gordon draws an important distinction between two kinds of simulation: "between just imagining being in X's situation, and making the further adjustments required to imaging being X in X's situation" (p. 741). For the sake of empathic accuracy we would aim for the latter kind of simulation. Such an adjustment is crucial but, indeed, difficult for clinicians to accomplish with patients who are mentally ill (more on this later).

Recent research offers mirror neurons as a kind of embodied simulation theory to understand empathetic responses to others. Vittorio Gallese's work develops an expanded idea of empathy that explains how humans can understand others by forming mental representations, in the prefrontal cortex, of others. Gallese calls this way of understanding embodied empathy "the shared manifold of intersubjectivity" (2001, p. 34; cf. also Gallese 2003; Gallese et al. 2007). "Far from being *exclusively* dependent upon mentalistic/linguistic abilities," Gallese writes, "the capacity for understanding others as intentional agents is deeply grounded in the *relational* nature of action. Action is relational" (Gallese 2001, p. 34;

emphasis in original). This idea harks back to the earlier section "Empathy and moral life" where I discussed the relational aspect of morality. The deeper point that Gallese is making, I take it, is that our basic actions themselves are grounded in a hard-wired ability to learn how to coordinate hand–eye movement and other fundamental movements through the action of mirror neurons as we observe and imitate others. The import of actions being relational is that it highlights the deep effects that we can have on each other, even without our realizing it. But this just makes the question of whether or not such empathetic responses are really under our control even more complex. If we are relationally but neuronally mirroring others, thereby developing empathy, in what sense are we able to develop virtuous, as opposed to accidental, empathy? To address this question, I call upon Aristotle's theory of moral responsibility.

On an Aristotelian account, virtue and vice are voluntary:

> Now the virtues, as we say, are voluntary, since in fact we are ourselves in a way jointly responsible for our states of character, and by having the sort of character we have we lay down the sort of end we do. Hence the vices will also be voluntary; since the same is true of them. (*Nicomachean Ethics* (*NE*) 1114b22–25)

As I discussed earlier, when responding to situations with feelings and actions, the background conditions that we have cultivated over time will come into play in our current response. And those background conditions—our character—are developed, in part, through choices we have made and through what has appeared to us, in the past, as good to aim at, or good to do. On an Aristotelian account, our feelings and actions are up to us, because our characters are, at least in part, up to us. Aristotle argues against the notion that the virtuous person has an "inborn sense of sight" by which he can judge rightly. Furthermore, he suggests that one is in error who thinks that such a sense cannot be acquired or learned (*NE* 1114b3–10). In fact, virtue must be acquired: "Thus the virtues arise in us neither by nature nor against nature, but we are by nature able to acquire them, and reach our complete perfection through habit" (*NE* 1103a24). Nature, therefore, does not determine the outcome of our character. But, even though we do not have an inborn sense of right and wrong, or a natural feeling of empathy for others, we do have the ability to learn to perceive right and wrong. Because of our nature as human beings, we are able to acquire virtues if we receive the proper training and upbringing. This is compatible with the passage in which Aristotle makes a distinction between natural and full virtue:

> For each of us seems to possess his type of character to some extent by nature, since we are just, brave, prone to temperance, or have another feature, immediately from birth. However, we still search for some other condition as full goodness, and expect to possess these features in another way. For these natural states belong to children and to beasts as well [as to adults] but without understanding they are evidently harmful … But if someone acquires understanding, he improves in his actions; and the state he now has, though still similar [to the natural one], will be virtue to the full extent. (*NE* 1144b5–15)

Aristotle is making two points here. First, that although we have the capacity by nature to become virtuous, we need to deliberately and consistently work at it. As he says, we become just by doing just actions over and over again, not by getting it right on the occasional situation; over time, we develop habits of character that help us to more readily see and desire what is good to feel and act in a given situation. The second point is that different people's natural temperament will make it more or less easy to develop various character traits such as being appropriately and accurately empathetic. Some people are born with impatient temperaments, for example, and they may struggle to learn patience that comes more easily to others. Aristotle says that we must know ourselves and which character vulnerabilities we have so that we can correct for them, and this advice addresses the individual differences in natural virtue that makes developing full virtue particular to each person.

Aristotle admits that it is "hard work to be excellent" (*NE* 1144b5–15). Since becoming virtuous is not always "natural" or easy, it is a good thing that empathy is a state of mind that we can reflect upon (Hodges and Wegner 1997, p. 313). Sometimes, Hodges and Wegner say, we can take another's viewpoint and experience that person's world with no effort at all; we are drawn without thinking into another's perspective. This kind of empathy they call "automatic empathy." This clinical characterization is probably the equivalent to "natural virtue" in Aristotle's sense. But people can also consciously and intentionally produce empathy. This they call "controlled empathy." And controlled empathy seems to match up with the full virtue in the Aristotelian sense.

The clinical conception of empathy is consistent with the idea from virtue theory that empathy is an attitudinal orientation that can be learned and that is voluntary. I would add to the clinical picture, though, that although empathy has both cognitive and emotional components and can be automatic or controlled, past theories have tended to equate the emotional component of empathy with automatic empathy and the cognitive component with controlled empathy. In fact, both components are necessary for either kind. And exhibiting the full virtue of empathy, both from a clinical and from a philosophical point of view, engages both emotional and cognitive aspects of us.

Why Clinicians Need a Rich Understanding of Empathy

Clinicians need a rich understanding of empathy, not merely literature's evocation of empathy as good for clinician/patient relations. The first reason is that it is so important to have accurate knowledge of the other person in order to engage in diagnostic and therapeutic work. This analysis of empathy suggests that it is *epistemologically* significant in that it allows clinicians more accurately to understand, explain, and predict the behavior of their patients. For example, knower trustworthiness requires epistemic responsibility (Code 1991; Fricker 2007), and empathy is central to that process. In fact, empathic (and thus epistemic) accuracy is, I would suggest, connected to a thick description of evidence-based psychiatry (EBP). In order for EBP reliably and validly to yield results, clinicians must be able to do more than reason well scientifically; they must have knowledge of other persons. (I return to this point shortly.) It follows that empathy is necessary for *practical reasoning*. Because empathy is particular-directed, a clinician who feels empathy can see how (and whether) various therapies might apply in a given case. He or she can see how (and whether) confrontation, or boundary setting, or expressions of hopefulness are appropriate. In order to facilitate healing, the clinician must not only be therapeutically adept and morally attuned but also be able to assess beliefs and credibility claims (including his or her own.)

The second reason clinicians need a rich sense of empathy is due to the moral contributions that empathy makes to relationships. Empathy is necessary for collaboration which, in turn, is necessary to healing. Empathy makes it possible for the patient to feel understood in her distress, anger, fear, or confusion, and when she begins to feel understood, she is more likely to work with the carer rather than against him or her. Thus, empathy as an activity and attitude expresses the qualities a good clinician would bring to a therapeutic relationship.

Nevertheless, empathy is not the only virtue that one should bring in order to practice good EBP. Here I will develop the idea of a related characteristic that clinicians need to have in order to have knowledge of other persons. This contribution to the discussion moves beyond empathy per se and toward other ways to connect with patients with their own perspectives taken into account. Clinicians regularly face the task of constructing bridges between seemingly disparate worlds and the people who inhabit them. A bridge allows us to cross a difficult landscape to reach territory that is removed from us. Yet it matters *how* such bridges are built and how they are crossed. This section appraises and advocates a methodological stance toward other persons called "world"-traveling. Drawing on the work of María Lugones (1990), who argues that people who are at ease in a world need to experience other worlds in which they are outsiders, I discuss ways that clinicians can experience more immersion in a patient's experience and thereby provide better treatment for that patient. I argue that "world"-traveling is distinct from empathy and that each concept contributes to knowledge and treatment of patients.

Strange Landscapes

Eric Cassell says that suffering is experienced by *persons*, and it is in that capacity that clinicians must approach and treat them. This is why knowledge, including the epistemic grounds of EBP, is insufficient without knowledge of other persons. Let me briefly, albeit incompletely, fill in the prevailing view of knowledge that pervades epistemology in the philosophical tradition. Western mainstream accounts of knowledge privilege "simples"—statements that are easily verifiable or falsifiable such as "the cat is on the mat." These simples contain everyday objects that are considered to form the paradigm of knowledge (cf. Code (1991) for a full treatment on this.) But, as Lorraine Code argues, knowledge of other persons is at least as worthy a contender for basic knowledge as are objects (1991, p. 37). Code writes, "even if one could know all the facts about someone, one would not know her as the person she is. No more can knowing all the facts about oneself, past and present, guarantee self-knowledge" (1991, p. 40). This is because knowledge of other persons involves subjectivities, not just objective ordinary facts, which the mainstream view of epistemology holds as sharply dichotomous. Code is thus criticizing both the prevailing account of knowledge and the way that subjective knowledge gets discounted. (In her book, she provides a sustained argument about a more complex and less dichotomous way to conceptualize objectivity but a discussion of this argument would take us too far afield.) This is the point that Cassell presses: physicians deal with human suffering, and understanding and treating suffering requires knowledge of other persons. Code's addition is that, although knowledge of other persons has historically not been counted as genuine knowledge because of the long-assumed distinction between (objective) facts and (subjective) values, it should—and must—be counted as knowledge because it is a fundamental source of social and moral relating.

Suffering occurs when a person experiences himself or herself as having lost connection to the world of objects, events, and the web of relationships, including the person's work and habits (Cassell 1991, pp. 40, 162–164). Such loss can be profound in that it includes a sense of loss of oneself, one's values, one's hopes, and, indeed, one's identity. A central role of psychiatrists and psychologists is to help relieve the suffering that comes from mental illness. As indicated earlier, the task is, in part, one of reasoning: a clinician must apply general knowledge to specific individuals. The way to do this is to particularize the general. Many clinicians come to an encounter with a patient with a combination of theory, experience, general principles, and overall aims involved in being a good psychiatrist. When particularizing the general, the reasoning process may be a movement from those general standing beliefs and values, to the immediacy and practical idea of the sick patient, to discrimination, differentiation, and analysis producing separate ideas of the disease and the person, then again to a particular unity—*this sick person*. Aiming toward therapeutic healing is a matter, in part, of working to see that these ideas are systematically integrated (Cassell 1991, p. 179; emphasis in original).

Cassell discusses kinds of information that clinicians can gather about persons: empirical facts (medical history, current symptoms, blood pressure), moral judgments about qualities of the person (ambitious, trustworthy, shy), and aesthetic judgments (how the different aspects of the self relate to one another and hang together as a whole—relating to harmony and order). The knowledge acquired will be relevant to this particular patient because the actual experiences and perspective of this patient form part of the knowledge base upon which the clinician draws. In other words, theoretical knowledge and general frameworks about nosology and symptomatology are necessary but not sufficient in order to care appropriately for a patient, Cassell says (1991, p. 216). To gain the kind of knowledge needed to relieve patient suffering adequately, clinicians must understand not only a particular mental illness or a particular person who is ill, but how that specific person experiences his or her world. Illness is never a mere loss or excess, because patients always also react, trying to restore, replace, or otherwise compensate for the affliction (Sacks 1986, p. 4). Treating a person's illness or relieving suffering, therefore, requires that the clinician understand how that person attempts to restore him- or herself in relation to the world or to compensate for the illness. But reasoning from generals to particulars can be distorted when clinicians' world views dominate the clinical process. If clinicians have an inadequate understanding of the power of their cognitive, theoretical, and ideological schemas to frame their perceptions, interpretations, diagnoses, and treatment plans, they run the risk that their responses to patients will have more to do with the clinician than with the patient's problems and needs (Connolly 2003, p. 106). "Pasts are culturally saturated, and it is easy to lose one's way when navigating the cultural landscape of another. Indeed, one's own cultural landscape is often so complexly embedded that its impact on our beliefs and understandings can sometimes be underestimated" (Connolly 2003, p. 103).

Clinicians face a difficult task. Yet, as I noted earlier, I think it is a mistake to assume incommensurability. As Louis Sass argues, when we encounter those we do not readily understand, we appeal to a theory, and that theory typically works by analogy. We employ a model that builds on something we think we do understand to help us comprehend something initially less intelligible (Sass 1992, p. 10). To assume there are no such models that would serve as a bridge between the mentally ill and those better off is damaging in two ways: it does a disservice to the patient, who is then "banished from the community of human understanding," and it does a disservice to the rest of us, who are thereby "deprived of all access to what may be an important limit-case of the human condition" (Sass 1992, p. 7). Perhaps Thomas Nagel is right that we cannot know what it is like to be a bat (Nagel 1974), but it is offensive to classify the human mentally ill in the category of alien or animal. An alternative is to "take the uncanny and alien qualities of this condition as challenge rather than prohibition, as signs not of the impossibility but of the difficulty" of understanding others' experiences of madness (Sass 1992, p. 7).

The impulse behind my suggestions comes from Aristotle's *Rhetoric*, where he uses the concept of *suggnômê* (judging with) to characterize the stance required to make a proper assessment. Aristotle's idea seems to be that, to perceive particulars and make judgments accurately, we must see things from the other's point of view, for only then will we begin to comprehend what obstacles that person faces (Nussbaum 1995, p. 156). Empathy is one way to accomplish *suggnômê*; I now flesh out another idea, drawing on the work of Marìa Lugones (1990).

Lugones advocates the willful exercise of flexibility in shifting back and forth from one construction of life where a person is more or less "at home" to other constructions of life. This willful exercise she calls *world-traveling*. To understand this concept, we first have to understand what Lugones means by a *world*. A world is a kind of *experience*—where who we take ourselves to be is constructed through the concepts and norms, the language, history, and interpersonal relations of the inhabitants of that world (present living ones, ancestral ones, and even imaginary ones). For example, I may be constructed among black southern activists as a fairly conventional, white, middle-class philosopher, even though I may not understand or accept myself that way. "I may be animating such a construction," Lugones writes, "even though I may not intend my moves, gestures, acts in that way" (1990, p. 395). To world-travel, then, is to shift from one world to another, or to live in more than one world at the same time. Traveling involves a kind of shift in constructions of the self.

Lugones points out, however, that some people—for example, women of color—necessarily, as a matter of survival, become adept at world-traveling, whereas others—for example, white Western philosophers—have less experience, less facility, less need, and less interest in traveling to the worlds of others whose constructions of us might be ones we do not recognize (or do not want to recognize.) Genuine world-traveling is not a matter of merely acknowledging differences and honoring an abstract idea of plurality while implementing plans designed to improve others' lives as *I* understand them. To world-travel is to leave the familiarity of home. Being at ease involves being a fluent speaker in that world (in Wittgensteinian terms, knowing the language games); agreeing and being content with all the norms; being bonded to others through love; and having a shared history. World-traveling involves seeing myself as I am constructed in the world of that person and that I witness her own sense of herself in her world. To do this requires that I learn to perceive differently. And this, in turn, requires that I abandon the comfort of the worlds in which I am most at home. World-traveling is a way to have actual and material experiences of others' worlds, and Lugones emphasizes the normative aspects of what she calls "non-imperialist" world-traveling. By "non-imperialist" she means that the sort of traveling we do to other worlds is not based on an impulse to dominate or an unconscious attitude of superiority, or an assumption of our various roles, identities, values, and belief systems.

For Lugones, non-imperialist world-traveling is fluid, non-dominating, not competitive, and open to surprises. To better understand the normative force of these ideas, I suggest a connection between travel as metaphor, travel as literal experience, and genuine travel in Lugones' sense of *world*-traveling.

Travel as a metaphor of the mind suggests the idea of being open to new ways of looking at things. "That mind is a critical one to the extent that its moving beyond a given set of pre-conditions or values also undermines those assumptions" (Van den Abbeele 1992, p. xiii). In fact, the activity of traveling is paradoxical: it is always restrained by a sense of home yet liberated or liberating in its possibility of movement from home. The very notion of travel presupposes a home, or *oikos,* from which one departs and to which one might return. Yet if one circumscribes the travel by keeping home or *oikos* in sight, one does not really take the voyage. Suggestive of a link with world-traveling in Lugones' sense, Van den Abbeele says that the activity of traveling is both the menace of loss and the possibility of gain (Van den Abbeele 1992). His way of characterizing travel is resonant with that of Lugones: travel in which we remain oriented yet are willing to risk loss (including loss of orientation) changes us; it is a kind of travel in which we are open to being changed. "By traveling to their 'world,'" Lugones explains, "we can understand what it is to be them and what it is to be ourselves in their eyes." The degree to which we can see and witness depends on how much at ease we learn to be in the other's world, where the other's language, norms, historical landscape, and belongingness are centered.

WORLD-TRAVELING AND EMPATHY

World-traveling is distinct from empathy, although its ways of responding to another's suffering are *related* to world-traveling. *World-traveling* is a methodology, whereas *empathy* is a cognitive and moral experience and response. World-traveling answers the question of how I can *have* that experience and that response.

Much weight is given to the role of emotional contagion and imagination in learning how to empathize accurately (cf. Gordon 1995; Hodges and Wegner 1997; Ickes 1995). Yet even those considerations presuppose background conditions that may not exist: namely, the decentering of the ego (as Murdoch (1970) says is required in order to be ethical) along with the norms, historicity, and linguistic practices that animate the center of that ego. Empathy, then, is an important moral response to suffering, but it is apolitical in a way that world-traveling is not. World-traveling has the potential to provide clinicians with even more understanding of their patients' experiences. A world-traveler sees epistemic and political shifts in oneself as crucial to being a good clinician and the openness and commitment to change that a world-traveler brings to the therapeutic relation is a central way that a clinician can learn to help her patient relieve her suffering and distress. Lugones' conception of world-traveling thus helps create the space in which empathy toward the other may develop and flourish.

A richly sensitive understanding of another cannot be separated from the politics of difference. World-traveling may not give rise to empathy because, for example, one may never become enough at ease in that other world to be anything other than displaced and frightened. But world-traveling, because it is a methodology and not only an experience or moral and epistemic response, deepens and enriches the level of empathetic understanding of the other. Empathy is accurate to the extent that the empathetic person has engaged in genuine world-travel. "Only when we have traveled to each others' 'worlds' are we fully subjects to each other" (Lugones 1990, p. 401). The failure to recognize the other's subjectivity is partly because we fail to see ourselves in others who are quite different from us (p. 393).

Western conceptions of the self amplify the difficulty clinicians may encounter when trying to decenter themselves. That conception includes ideas of a unified, stable, bounded self. Experiences of living with mental illness may belie that self-conception. Consider these remarks by a person who suffers from schizophrenia, for example: "All that was my former self has crumbled and fallen together and a creature has emerged of whom I know nothing. She is a stranger to me … She is not real—she is not I … She is I—and because I still have myself on my hands, even if I am a maniac, I must deal with me somehow" (Sass, 1992, p. 215). Sass comments that, if one's cultural assumptions include the idea that a healthy person is one who is bounded, unified, and integrated, it is not surprising that one's encounter with a person who expresses such profound ontological insecurity would leave one finding that person incomprehensible (1992, pp. 215–216). My point is not to advance an alternative metaphysics of selfhood but, instead, to highlight an effect of maintaining one's home ideology and values in trying to understand others who seem strikingly different: sometimes another person seems different in part because we carry with us a paradigm-centered trope that should not be superimposed on that other world.

This problem of difference does not leave us with an unbridgeable gap. We need to, and can, travel. But the *way* we need to travel is lovingly, animatedly, and playfully—not imperialistically. As Murdoch puts it, "As moral agents we have to try to see justly, to overcome prejudice, to avoid temptation, to control and curb imagination, to direct reflection" (1970, p. 40). Responsibly done, world-traveling is a method by which clinicians can come to understand the full subjectivity of their patients. World-traveling can assist clinicians in avoiding exploitation and objectification of their patients because it requires clinicians to shift their perspective from that of a center of power and knowledge to one of being a relative outsider who is ill at ease in the patient's world. If the goal is to assist the patient in healing or in relieving suffering, a clinician needs a rich body of knowledge, understanding, and empathy, and world-traveling is a full-bodied way to bring about the appropriate cognitive states that will enable healing to unfold.

Conclusion

Some patients may not want their world(s) to be traveled to and may find it intrusive for clinicians to approach them this way. In these cases, a degree of empathy may be all the patient can accept. For still other patients, there may be no world in which they are at ease, and so no world in which the clinician can practice the decentering methodology in the way that Lugones' work, as I have applied it, suggests.

In-patient treatment may be one setting in which clinicians could practice world-traveling. But even that community may not be one where the patient feels most at ease and, so, cannot give a complete sense of how the patient experiences herself and her illness in a chosen or home community. Still, the clinician who can even partially understand what it is like never to be at ease in any world and never to feel at home will grasp to some degree the profound alienation those patients feel.

As I stated at the outset of this article, Murdoch says that "In the moral life the enemy is the fat relentless ego" (1970, p. 52). Egocentrism can prevent us from accurate empathy and from accurate epistemic experiences. Clinicians, in particular, need the background moral and epistemic skills in order to work effectively with patients. The background conditions are important to deliver because, as Murdoch suggests, they create the quality of attention that clinicians need to draw on in the moment (p. 67). "The background condition of such habit and such action, in human beings, is a just mode of vision and a good quality of consciousness" (p. 91). That, Murdoch says, is a *task* to achieve.

REFERENCES

Aristotle. (1984). *Nicomachean Ethics*. Indianapolis, IN: Hackett.

Cassell, E. (1991). *The Nature of Suffering and the Goals of Medicine*. Oxford: Oxford University Press.

Code, L. (1991). *What Can She Know? Feminist Theory and the Construction of Knowledge*. Ithaca, NY: Cornell University Press.

Connolly, M. (2003). Cultural components of practice: Reflexive responses to diversity and difference. In T. Ward, D. R. Laws, and S. M. Hudson (Eds), *Sexual Deviance: Issues and Controversies*, pp. 103–18. London: Sage.

Fanon, F. (2008). *Black Skin, White Masks* (R. Philcox, Trans.) (Revised edn). New York, NY: Grove Press.

Fricker, M. (2007). *Epistemic Injustice: Power and the Ethics of Knowing*. Oxford: Oxford University Press.

Gallese, V. (2001). The 'shared manifold' hypothesis. From mirror neurons to empathy. *Journal of Consciousness Studies*, 8, 33–50.

Gallese V. (2003). The roots of empathy: The shared manifold hypothesis and the neural basis of intersubjectivity. *Psychopathology*, 36(4), 171–80.

Gallese, V., Eagle, M. N., and Migone, P. (2007). Intentional attunement: Mirror neurons and the neural underpinnings of interpersonal relations. *Journal of the American Psychoanalytic Association*, 55(1), 131–76.

Gordon, R. (1995). Sympathy, simulation, and the impartial spectator. *Ethics*, 105, 727–42.

Hodges, S. and Wegner, D. (1997). Automatic and controlled empathy. In W. Ickes (Ed.), *Empathic Accuracy*, pp. 311–39. New York, NY: Guilford.

Ickes, W. (Ed.) (1997). *Empathic Accuracy*. New York, NY: Guilford.

Lugones, M. (1990). Playfulness, 'world'-traveling, and loving perception. In G. Anzaldua (Ed.), *Making Face, Making Soul/Haciendo Caras: Creative and Critical Perspectives by Women of Color*, pp. 390–402. San Francisco, CA: Aunt Lute Foundation.

Murdoch, I. (1970). *The Sovereignty of Good*. London: Routledge and Kegan Paul.

Nagel, T. (1974). What is it like to be a bat? *Philosophical Review*, 83, 435–50.

Potter, N. (2009). *Mapping the Edges and the In-Between: A Critical Analysis of Borderline Personality Disorder*. Oxford: Oxford University Press.

Sass, L. (1992). *Madness and Modernism: Insanity in the Light of Modern Art, Literature, and Thought*. New York, NY: Harper Collins.

Tamborini, R., Stiff, J., and Heidel, C. (1990). Reacting to graphic horror: A model of empathy and emotional behavior. *Communication Research*, *17*, 616–39.

Van den Abbeele, G. (1992). *Travel as Metaphor: From Montaigne to Rousseau*. Minneapolis, MN: University of Minnesota Press.

Vetlesen, A. J. (1994). *Perception, Empathy, and Judgment: An Inquiry into the Preconditions of Moral Performance*. University Park, PA: Pennsylvania State University Press.

CHAPTER 22

....

DISCOURSE AND
DISEASES OF THE PSYCHE

....

GRANT GILLETT AND ROM HARRÉ

Discursive psychology is interested in the way that human beings enact identities and agency through their engagement in discourses (Harré and Gillett 1994). It is a form of ethology—the study of natural creatures within a world to which they are adapted. Its ontology is laid out in Table 22.1, which defines the parameters of discursive theory.

The human mind or psyche is created and shaped by discourse to do things with words and we relate to those words in two ways—as *tools* and as *signs*, *symbols*, or *icons*. We position ourselves and create stories in which we take certain parts so as to negotiate a dual world which we both create and are created, in part, by our discursive tools. Images and icons, crafted by our discursive tools, make human beings complex by shaping our adaptation and the skills we use in the human life-world.

We could say that we live in "two worlds": a world of biology and physical causes and one subject to various influences reflecting the history, position, and current commitments of the person concerned (Harré and Gillett 1994, p. 99). They result in a dynamic and changing mode of being in which various facets of our engagement with others are relevant to various "mental disorders," best understood as dissolutions of our adaptation (Jackson 1887) to the discursively structured context of human function that is being-in-the-world-with-others (Gillett 2009).

The discursive approach to psychiatry, taking as it does an ethological approach to the human organism, directs us to rules and story-lines that structure our ways of dealing with the challenges thrown up by particular situated positions in our discursive world. By examining breakdowns in the relationship between a human organism, the psyche, and the world of speech in which the psyche is formed, the real dimensions of psychological dysfunction can be appreciated, only some aspects of which are open to physical or causal analysis of the type found in the core natural sciences. Therefore psychiatry impoverishes itself by focusing on biology to the exclusion of human discourse and the (partly symbolic) structure of our life-world (Husserl 1970).

The two components of the human life-world: (i) actual things and our interactions with them as beings of flesh and blood, and (ii) the meanings that inform our understanding of them and our many dealings with them, are completely entwined. For instance, I am given

Table 22.1 Two ontologies (Harré and Gillett, 1994, p. 29)

Ontologies	Locative systems	Entities	Relations
Newtonian	Space and time	Things and events	Causality
Discursive	Arrays of people	Speech acts	Rules and stories

a strange object and helplessly turn it this way and then that and look blankly at it. Then someone tells me that it is for screwing into a cork to remove it from a bottle and I can make sense of it: i.e., I know what to do with it. Similarly, if I am lost in a forest, depending on my bushcraft, I can look for telltale signs that will help me find my way out. But imagine that I am lost in a forest of bureaucracy, and disempowered by my clinical role—as a patient—and my uncertainty as to what is wrong with me. In that case, I lack the discursive skills I need to find my way about. Those skills, whatever the setting, straddle the worlds of symbol and physical causal interaction enabling us to construct stories and take up positions within them. These positions then impose constraints on all the characters involved as can be seen in the lived stories of hysteria (conversion reaction—DSM300.11) and dementia (multiple cognitive impairment—DSM290.0; American Psychiatric Association 1994).

The Discursive Psyche

Our understanding of the relation between the two aspects of the human life-world that form the psyche emerges from pursuing the conversation between Frege and Husserl, in two directions: into both Anglo-American (post-Russellian) philosophy and (post-structuralist) European thought.

Frege famously noted that in order to understand a thought we need to see how the thinker has constructed a representation of the world so as to frame well-grounded assertions, practicable imperatives, informative questions, and so on. To do this cognitive work, a thinker must develop skills that engage meanings with the world as it is lived in around here but that can happen in more than one way. Frege therefore identified the sense (*Sinn*) associated with a thought as something different from the actual thing or things being referred to. The planet *Venus* (which could also be thought of as *the morning star* or *the evening star*) and Dr. Gustav Lauben who remarks to a friend "I have been wounded" gave him examples where different senses provoked different thoughts (one person could think of Gustav Lauben as a friend, another impersonally, and yet a third as a historian.) The thoughts related to the same object (Gustav Lauben) even though they had different values or meanings according to the rules emerging within and regulating conversations and contexts where thinkers use the term. One thinker might think "Oh, my poor friend Gustav, I hope he isn't too bad" and another, "Oh, that poor chap from Number 16, I wonder how he is." Frege used the term "cognitive significance" and conceptualized that in terms of "inner" or psychological states (a Cartesian conception). For Frege, these states were primarily concerned with depicting states of affairs in the world as they related to objective conceptions of truth and falsity.

Discursive psychiatry rejects the Fregean foundations of language and thought and sees the human being as a situated individual in relation to others and the discourses that create meaning. In such a context, the rules that govern what can be said, by whom, and what positions are recognized in relation to what is actually said, are of primary importance and thoughts or sentences lose their direct and transparent relation to states of affairs objectively defined.

Frege had a problem accounting for the apparent objectivity (or intersubjectivity) of human knowledge. The sense of any term (Gustav Lauben as my friend, … as a man who lives in No.16, … as the figure who did this or that deed) might vary from one occasion of utterance to another, but this variation was not merely subjective and it reflected different "objective" (or intersubjectively shared) meanings. However, he could not reconcile his conception of the psyche as an inner realm of meaning and images with the public or "objective" norms required for unambiguous discourse. If the criterion of truth or accurate description with which a thinker is working is the "fit" between an inner picture of reality and the world, then we seem condemned to a systematic indeterminacy of meaning.

The idea of shared or common participation in meaningful situations where power and position are mutually understood did not enter the Fregean picture but Ludwig Wittgenstein (whom Frege hugely influenced) was not so hampered. He realized that sense (or *Sinn*) was central to understanding human beings as thinkers and pointed to contexts of use—language games, discursive contexts, and the positions of speakers in them—as the basis of the shared world of meaning or symbols that we all inhabit (1953). In that context we can do things with words and agree, not just in opinions but also in the ways we recognize each other and position ourselves so as to understand our varied subjective orientations. We can adopt positions so that what we say is inflected or colored by the position in which we find ourselves: thus "I see that you are a troubled soul" means something different from a friend to what it means in the mouth of a psychiatrist.

Our journey from Frege therefore leads fairly directly to the work of Wittgenstein and to the analysis of *Sinn*/sense in terms of discursive contexts, where language games and the rules operating in them enable us to think of things in a variety of ways because of the linguistic markers we use to locate them in our discourse. This path, developed by Winch (1958) and others, implicates sociocultural contexts where we find ways to mark patterns of significance in our world and converge in the ways we speak and think about them. For instance, the moral transition from youth and dependence to adulthood and responsibility is a pattern of great significance in one's dealings with others. The Anglo-American analytic route to a conception of the discursive psyche and positioned subjectivity therefore goes through Wittgenstein and his followers such as Winch and Austin (Harré 2002).

A different path, via Husserl and phenomenology, also focuses on *Sinn* and the norms (*noemata*) or rules governing the terms that we use to structure our thinking and the ways we communicate about and understand ourselves within a shared world. These norms, intersubjective and socioculturally generated, are inscribed within us and form our conceptions of who we are, what is happening to us, and the disorders to which we are prone (Hacking 1995).

Following the phenomenological path to Heidegger and beyond, we find the human being as a situated being who questions the world and his or her own place in it and organizes his or her dealings with it in the light of those questions (1953/1996). This continental or existential-phenomenological route to the discursive psyche is then extended to furnish concepts such as *ipseity* (a sense of oneself as a living presence in the life-world) and subjectivity (explored by feminist thinkers and thinkers like Zahavi or Stanghellini). The psyche is seen as a reification of our mode of relating to the world through discourses. In a lived and situated trajectory and an associated world of meaning and rules within which "I" can speak or think of myself, I learn the significance of things including myself as a being-in-the-world-with-others understood and evaluated by those others (Gillett and McMillan 2001). The ipseity of the subject is a joint product of the biological actuality that is embodiment and the ways we articulate that actuality in human discourses. I inhabit my own way of being and map it onto the rules and stories that tell me what to make of it (in both senses of that phrase). Biology and story are combined in a self, a being who is *you* or *he* or *me* and is therefore located in the human life-world (Harré and Gillett 1994) through conversations, discourses and modes of "speaking the self." The value of any human being originates in this discursive reality, where judgments are implicit and mutual recognition is perfused by power and the attitudes we take up toward each other.

How one makes sense of the world is grounded, therefore, in the fact that each of us is always already located in a historicocultural situation—a context of subjective being. The discursive analysis of my actions and self-conceptions examines the production of my subjective body and identifies ways in which biology, culture, interpersonal relationships, and political power have affected and currently affect that process. A human existence is articulated and lived among others as a focus of concern (*sorge*), concern for and care of the self, and concerned encounters with others whose attitudes toward me are inherently related to our dealings with each other.

Discursive analysis therefore reveals the human subject as a biopsychosocial being, dynamic and unfolding in self-articulating ways, who is to be understood within an ontology of others and the rules that govern their interactions. A phenomenological analysis reveals a subjective indwelling of a situation; and when we deconstruct the discursive context we see what it is to be the person at the center of a certain story and we understand why that person says certain things and acts in certain ways. Within that framework a way of being that is unsustainable creates strains that we can all understand and may come to the attention of psychiatrists and/or those who study "abnormal psychology." When the strains reach a breaking point the measures that a person is reduced to can become inaccessible to others as, for instance, when a conversion reaction makes a person unable to move her legs, or when anxiety and cognitive impairment may lead to incessant crying out for help. These however are best understood as relational and not as merely internal disorders (Gillett 2009).

These lines of analysis come together in figures like MacIntyre (1999), Taylor (1989), and Hacking (1995), who explore the activity of situated human beings in the human life-world while fully alert to the discursive context provided by history and biopolitics and to the human need to find a sociocultural niche to inhabit and a good-enough individual story to live by. They approach "the stories of the mad" alert to the clues which allow us to "join the dots" of otherwise fragmented subjectivities and thereby situate the inaccessible experience in a subjectively real world.

The dual nature of the human life-world (both physico-causal and rule-governed or meaningful), mandates a nuanced account of the social and interpersonal realities that contribute to fractures in the complex adaptation that is a livable human story. Discursive psychiatry uses an inclusive view of human ethology to understand the situations in which people find themselves and the rules and conventions that govern what they do and say. For instance, if one edits out the hesitancies and gaps in conversation in a recorded interview with

Alzheimer's disease patients, those conversations become far more intelligible and "normal" than they previously appeared. And if care-givers are warned about these time gaps then the infantilizing tendency to say what the patient might have been going to say is offset and conversations go much more easily and normally, albeit more slowly (Sabat and Harré 1992). In relation to the psychogenic disability of hysteria, it is almost unthinkable, if one has been disabled for a certain length of time, that any intervention might lead to the complete recovery of normal function, absent a "miracle" or something similar (Gillett 2009).

Human well-being arises within a life-world constructed in part from conversations, the layers of meaning they generate, the positions they make available, and the forces (both positive and negative) that form the discursive reality in which we live. Teasing apart the relative contributions of biology and the distinctly human sphere of meaning to the lived reality of any human life is the challenge that confronts the philosophy of psychiatry. Hysteria (and factitious illness) and dementia, the new epidemic of developed society, both center on what is intelligible or available as an enacted way of *being somebody* in the contemporary world.

Each of us uses ways of being that emerge in discursive contexts to create an agreed self to present (and have presented) to others (Harré and Gillett 1994, p. 103). Disorders like dissociation (the heart of conversion reactions) and dementia are distinctive ways of framing the situated interaction between subjective embodiment and the demands we make on each other but neither is adequately illuminated by the deficit model (and its focus on internal dysfunctions). In each case, we can lose sight of the living voice that has to construct a lived narrative subject to the disciplines which constrain the way that we give an account of ourselves and our trajectories through the discursive world (with its ontology of people, rules and stories, and speech acts).

Discursive psychiatry lies within an Aristotelian tradition, and examines the ways that the neurocognitive aspects of mental illness, situated human voices, and lived stories are co-constructed within our life-world. These connections are clarified by clarifying what discursive psychiatry adds to the broadly Aristotelian position on the soul, or psyche.

(i) The brain records significant regularities of excitation and information use captured by and central to language-related activity (Luria 1973).
(ii) The vehicle of the human soul is structured activity laid down in the brain and the patterns forming that structure are configured to realize disciplines and skills created in human discourse.
(iii) The symbolically mediated skills realized in human neurocognitive structure underpin perception, action, and cognitive connection.
(iv) Human discourse and the relationships that shape a segment of the human life-world write and re-write our souls (Hacking 1995).

Some conclusions follow that are closely relevant to discursive psychiatry:

(v) Our being-in-relation-to-others, told and lived out in stories of the self, rests on fragile patterns of brain function.
(vi) That function mediates our interactions with the world and we constantly remold ourselves (and our neurocognitive structures) as we subjectively participate in discourse.

It follows that we must be alert to the interaction between brain physiology and pathology and the need to learn skills through our dealings with others when we are faced by a human being who is not coping in terms of neurocognitive function. We can illustrate these claims by thinking about dementia and the cognitive decline of aging. Any person is adapted to the world and others through memories, learned routines of doing things in certain contexts, and the knowledge of what is called for in terms of emotional displays and problem-solving skills (Jackson's "reason, memory, emotion, and will," Jackson 1887). When the quasi-stable human neural network starts to internally disconnect (due to neuronal loss) then the discursive performance of the individual begins to disintegrate. A person therefore loses certain discursive skills such as certainty about context based on cumulative or indexical tracking on the basis of conversational cues, links between faces and words, secure expectations about what is coming next, and the imaginative reconstruction at will of where one has been and how one has got to the current situation. These performances are based on inscribed techniques of adaptation enabling one to get by in the human life-world by coping with information arriving at its normal rate. This process of adaptation, involving discursive techniques of mapping an implicit symbolic milieu ordered by schemata (this is a "meet and greet old friends" situation) onto actual happenings here and now (voices, actions, bodies moving toward me) is normally smooth and unproblematic and the discourse surrounding it is cursory so that a breakdown of recognition, self-placement, and framing may go undetected until some question calling for a substantive answer does not get the expected response and a judgment is passed ("If she does not recognize her own daughter she must have really lost her marbles"). These judgments are part of the currency of enacted worth and they condition the way one is presented to others as someone in whom there is a mental disorder of a certain shape and severity. The importance of the human and interpersonal context of brain development and activity is underscored when we realize that self and consciousness are modes of integration and coordination designed to function interactively (Clark 2008; Jackson 1887). Schemata for information use are set up in our neuronal networks that are designed to complete loops of action and reaction with life-enhancing results in the context to which they are fitted. The brain, through processes such as long-term potentiation (Bliss and Collingridge 1993) and dendritic pruning (McGowan 2006), becomes fitted for the demands of discourses, positions, and relations of power. The actual connections are formed during human development as a result of social experience (Eisenberg 1995, p. 1563) mediated by speech (Luria 1973), techniques of perception and action used around here (Dennett 1991), and other culturally mediated ways of being (Zhu et al. 2008). The brain is therefore both subject to disruption through its organic vulnerability and its activity is translated into a discursive performance according to cues and clues that frame our interactions with others (such as timing, conversational implicatures, and positional expectations). These are our ethological points of "fitness of function" and the world creating them is criss-crossed by the games people play (including language games). We normally meet the dual demands of dealing with contingencies thrown up by life and giving accounts of ourselves (according to accepted norms of discourse around here). Mental explanations chart the way that we deal with these demands of the human life-world and our ways of doing that may be quite idiosyncratic.

Imagine an elderly woman confronted with a Mini-mental Status Examination (MMSE):

> She refused to answer the question about where the interview was happening because she wanted to indicate the doctor's rudeness and make him alert to the political overtones of the situation in terms of the treatment of the elderly; that is why she said "It is taking place in The Castle" without any expectation that he would recognize the allusion to Kafka.

This comment explains her answer in a way that "Her failing brain was unable to recognize where she was because she is not oriented" does not (even if the latter description sounds more objective and scientific and may be partly true). But what is the human story connecting the elderly woman undergoing the assessment, the doctor, the MMSE as a test, the lived human interaction in which the conversation occurs, and *The Castle* and what is the "real" significance of such "incorrect" answers and given by other aged patients under similar discursive demands?

Imagine a young middle-aged man who cannot move his left side when conscious but can when partly disinhibited by a short-acting anesthetic. We can explain what is going on in terms of changed patterns of inhibition and excitation in his subcortical motor pathways. But why is that happening? Why has he developed a conversion reaction and what is sustaining it? When we subsequently find out that he had his "left-sided stroke" when trying to account for his being in a car at a well-known trysting spot with a woman who was not his wife, and that his wife was overbearing (to say the least), we might be getting closer to understanding him and to a therapeutic response to his quasi-neurological disorder (the "dissociation" in his psyche). Does he know that he has a mental disorder and not a neurological one? We should perhaps ask, "Under what strains is he trying to translate his bodily state into a self-report and what positions are open to him in this complex moral-emotive-interpersonal and culturally loaded discourse?"

Discursive explanation explores the reality of souls as beings-in-relation who do things to each other with words and demand certain accountings of each other. In this they read what is happening from the events going on in their brain and in the normal course of events they do not stumble very much in that task, exercising the skills they have learnt and translating in a way that obeys shared rules so that we can all position the person within the frame of reference of "the common behavior of mankind" (Wittgenstein 1953 §205). Allowances are made for disability and the exigencies of illness and, in the discourses structuring medical life, we articulate our subject matter in terms of biomedical discourse. The discourses of the soul lay bare the connections between events in terms of their significance to the individuals concerned in particular interpersonal and sociocultural settings. They try and discern meaning and translate the results of an interaction between a human being and the world into terms out of which one can make a story according to the rules we use to interpret our behavior. These two different types of story, necessarily related because of the embodiment of the central character and the series of events in which s/he has participated, are differently framed and obey different norms. The discursive story tells us about a person's self-positioning, how certain expectations are being perceived and responded to, and whether we are witnessing a self-presentation that is comprehensible in terms of the language games we use with patterns of events such as those we are witnessing. For that reason discursive accounts (that concern the psyche) "distinguish among events … differentiate the networks and levels to which they belong, and … reconstitute the lines along which they are connected and engender one another" (Foucault 1984, p. 56) according to their meaning or discursive profile.

We can take each of these in turn: the events are distinguished as moments of enactment of a story; they belong with our understanding of how people interact with each other and use words to position and influence each other. When we see the elderly woman as locating herself in a version of *The Castle*, we begin to understand the bewilderment and sense of hopelessness she feels. We realize that a guide is needed who gets to know her story and to limn the contours of her currently lived experiences replete with threats and points of impenetrability. Only so can we begin to know how the events and statements she wants to make could be connected with what happens around her. Reconstituting the ways events engender or connect to one another at a given level reveals the narrative production of a person's behavior. Why has this man got a "left-sided stroke" and what has to be done to relieve the (non-arterial) "blockage" causing it? The range of useful interventions and investigations now takes on a profile that is quite distinctive. That profile may focus on life skills and relationships that articulate his doings within an intense discursive context. We can choose which descriptions and connections are the most revealing in relation to a distressed human being who comes to us and, in doing so, we enter what Bolton and Hill (1996) call the domain of decision, where we give reasons for our choices and actions and take responsibility for the kind of knowledge we adduce. The moral or value-based dimension to the kinds of explanation we need in psychiatry is never far away despite the fact that the fit between a person and a complex discursive milieu may be profoundly affected by a physiological or cognitive "shift" (Bolton 2008).

The wayward husband and others like him are impaired in ways that are "lost in translation" so that their "neurological conditions" have a discursive significance. Such patients cannot be as others are (or expect them to be) and this inability or mismatch is presented according to the rules (including moral rules) we follow in treating and assessing neurological disorders. They suffer disabling breakdowns unable to be dealt with by insight or self-examination and the underlying causes and realities of their disorders are "lost in translation." Try, if that sounds unconvincing, holding your arm flexed and fist clenched until it goes numb and then see how good you are at moving and sensing it when you "unbend" and have to cope with the painful pins and needles that afflict you. This auto-experiment may help the reader imaginatively bridge the yawning gap between clarity of thought about and empathy for a patient with a conversion reaction (Gillett 2009). Your inability to move without "pins and needles" (or, for a certain kind of person, "searing pain") is based on neural function and can be linked to your story—you have voluntarily entered into an experiment this text has suggested to you and you know the pain or discomfort is self-induced and you are normal. But imagine it is otherwise, imagine you feel rotten and helpless, and doubt that bringing yourself to reoccupy your normal embodiment is a merely a matter of resolution and confidence. Imagine that you feel so sorry for yourself that your pain or inability is taken as self-vindication and that you are not convinced that your impaired state is as escapable as others seem to think it should be. We could say that you are crushed under a weight of (discursive) facticity that is inherently enervating[1] or alienates you from your ipseity (your familiar lived bodily experience as *me here*).

Alternatively, as in Alzheimer's disease (where depression may also go unrecognized), a person may, despite being cognitively impaired, assert their independence because s/he may

---

[1] Jean-Paul Sartre's "facticity" is the inertia of flesh and nature—a resistance to existence or emerging from oblivion or nothingness, and standing out as oneself—a being who can affirm him or herself.

realize that to request help when you are "stretched" in terms of your life skills and coping may be to confirm the infantilization that is increasingly defining your position in your own family and your everyday life. The institutionalization and marginalization that often follow infantilization (as an almost inevitable part of the story in developed urban society), for an older person with a fragile adaptation to a familiar life setting and a combination of cognitive impairment and anxiety, may be a daunting and hazardous prospect. In both cases, the discursive situation, and the rules that informally govern it, frame what is happening to the person and make certain subjective positions available that condition who one is and how one sees oneself. In such an impasse what is happening in the brain and how that is translated into experience and behavior must be viewed through a discursively informed lens.

In psychiatry, as elsewhere, decisions as to how we approach what is going on render the contours of the human situation in a certain way by picking out events and what is part of them (e.g., she was trying to answer a question about her current orientation), differentiate the networks in which they make sense (e.g., she was disoriented in time and place *versus* she experienced the hospital as the architectural expression of a bureaucracy that marginalized and disempowered her), and reconstitute connections between events that show how they engender one another (e.g., he had painted himself into a corner and only a drastic change of focus would save him, he felt smitten and like fainting and his left side suddenly felt queer, or did it really—he could not tell?). How we paint the picture of a disorder shapes our understanding of it, but there are levels that help and levels that only enmesh us in a series of incomprehensible complexities (of, for instance, dopaminergic and serotoninergic pathways and centers in the brain). None of these framings is more ultimate or realistic than the others. We tend to equate ultimacy or realism with a material or categorical basis (brain function and pathophysiology), but neurocognitive structure is shaped by its immersion in a human context of meaning and the models we make of it only help us answer a limited range of "why" questions. A discursive analysis of the subjective body as it is framed in discourse is likely to help us make sense of a wide range of human phenomena as they cause distress and present to a clinic. By contrast, to conceive of anorexia or hysteria in terms of neural changes susceptible to psychopharmacological intervention is to set out on an explanatory path with poor scientific validation (Giordano 2005; Pike et al. 2003). No regimen centered on drug treatments or neurophysiological interventions has proven efficacy in either condition, but to investigate how the young anorexic woman is positioned in relation to a livable life story and the demands she conceives herself as trying to meet may be very revealing. Both anorexia and hysteria can be seen as quasi-moral and interpersonal responses to life events creating insecurity about identity and the possibility of a life lived on your own terms. We can and do address them in terms of developing life skills that equip a person to face challenges that they currently find overwhelming and unable to be met.

Discursive realities like marginalization and political resentment may also need to be addressed to begin to understand aggression and violent crime (and here culturally informed responses cut straight through neuropsychobiological constructions based on models grounded in the scientific imaginary). For that reason, cognitive neuroscience can obscure actual patterns of adaptation between a human being and a particular ecological niche that become dysfunctional in another context. The human brain uses language-related activity to organize itself (Franz and Gillett 2011; Luria 1973). And the inscribed brain activation patterns that emerge realize (or physiologically inscribe) discursive relations enabling a life that is worth living in the human life-world. Brain malfunctions of various kinds (as in acute psychosis, where we see hyperactive associations, or antisocial personality disorder where we see under-developed integration of behavior causing impulsivity and regressive violence) cause the person to fail in our life-world. That failure will not be reversed without the person concerned developing more integrated and adaptive ways of responding to life events. Brain-world malfunctions throw a person "out of synch" with the rhythm of human activity and the give and take that is a pervasive feature of our life-world. They can occur in many different ways because, in part, the person does not adequately connect situations, his or her position within them, and the emotional and interpersonal responses required to meet the challenges presented. In antisocial personality disorder, for instance, the engagement between an individual and fellow members of "the kingdom of ends" is impaired because the aspects of one's story in which one attends to the value of others are lacking (Gillett 2010). A quite different failure of interpersonal resonance is seen in autistic spectrum disorder (Gillett 2009). Each of these discontents of the mind has echoes discernible in terms of cognitive neuroscience, but the dissolution of function (Jackson 1887) is in terms of our distinctly human adaptation to the world. This adaptation is configured in the context of a life history producing a singular outcome revealed through "thick" or narrative constructions rather than focused neuroscientific descriptions (Geertz 1973).

The complex nature and life of a discursive creature implies that a malady of the soul is not just a "natural kind" (as in natural science) with a causal/biological profile whose connections and production can be understood in terms of brain dysfunction. Each malady of the soul is unique or particular to a situated person (Kristeva 1995) such that the suffering patient, like every other human being, is an enigma (Levinas 1996). As enigma, every psychiatric patient is the product of a unique history in which are embodied the many and diverse traces of our dealings with him or her and a flesh and blood answer to the question "Who am I?" That answer is presented in a discourse that makes a particular moral demand on the rest of us, perhaps in the clinic. The woman with Alzheimer's disease says, however confusedly, "Let me address you!" or "Let me tell you about my life!" As a soul, she cries out to other souls, some of whom are paid to care, asking for recognition, witness, and a hand of compassion (or even healing) in a situation on which she may have an increasingly tenuous hold. The confluence of discourse, history, and a (di-)stressed human psyche creates a dis-ease (or malady) of the soul co-created in two worlds. The soul and its maladies are, therefore, cross-categorial (Armstrong 2004) bridging our ways of telling truth and the biological or physical world in which we are enmeshed as creatures who self-construct and can self-destruct in their task of soul-making. The messy realism (Cooper 2007) of discursive naturalism spans the "two worlds in one" that is human reality; "psychiatric disease" then is best understood as a metaphor (Pickering 2006). As metaphor, it assimilates a complex breakdown in the relation between a human being and the sociosymbolic world to a pathophysiological process, but it helps us to understand certain varieties of human suffering. Conversion reactions dissociate the story of the self and its states from what is happening between the brain and the world so that something is lost in translation. In dementia, a self-construction, previously held together in intricate and skillful ways, unravels because brain connectivity can no longer support it (Gillett 2002). The disease metaphor focuses on the neurocognitive functions used in human adaptation to a sociocultural milieu, and, in so doing reminds us that we are fragile cultural artifacts produced in an image (of the human and its variations) under the imperative of the word (Lacan 1977, p. 106). We live and die in discourse and construct ourselves accordingly, a realization that carries with it emancipation, angst, and responsibility (and even sickness unto death).

Attunement to the world, especially the world of the clinic and its workings, requires scaffolding (or cognitive support) by those with the relevant skills. Therefore the health care professional, or any other companion in the recovery journey, has a role in the illness story that is often understated. S/he is not only an arbiter of a regimen of treatment but also a judge, an educator, and a counselor, the one who compiles a dossier but also who cares for the person and helps to equip them for the discursive world. The discourse of the clinic cannot be separated from the discourse of life but often, through focusing on the brain and health deficits, disempowers. A psychiatric patient may find refuge in a diagnosis and the rules that mitigate all kinds of demands that would otherwise confront them, but also might find, in the midst of a being-in-the-world-with-others strained beyond its limits of tolerance, a further set of challenges to be overcome in establishing the self as a locus of life skills that enable one to enact an identity as part of a sustainable subjective being (Clark 1997). These challenges and their complexities are illustrated by the two conditions we have discussed.

Hysteria presents us with "dissociation," an apparent impairment in the neurological underpinnings of the psyche that is, in fact, not as it seems. The clinician, the patient, and the patient's significant others can find themselves caught in a discourse of neurological understanding which locates the signs and symptoms at a certain level of connections and causes that increasingly frustrate any progress in treating "the condition." Both often subscribe to a "Cartesian dualism" whereby "the condition" is either real (= neurological) or imaginary (= "all in the head," pretense and morally degenerate) so that the discursive or contextual skills that enable a person to cope with the world are "not in the frame." The dualistic construction shuts off any way forward but a realistic understanding of the dynamism of neurological states and the difficulty in translation from the brain-world interaction to the discursive presentation of the self, gives the problem a more tractable shape.

In hysteria, subjectivity is "lost in translation" as a thicket of troubles of the soul block effective enactment of a self with any worth so that skills must be developed that have a hope of overcoming that impasse. Both psychological and moral work has to be done and that work is so demanding and fraught with peril to lives and relationships that it can defy comprehension or acknowledgment (so that it is literally a sickness unto death, perhaps by suicide).

Dementia, as we have hinted, is quite otherwise. The psyche is willing and often resolved but the brain is weak. The psyche is often also beset with well-meaning but very real social hazards to a worthwhile continuation of a meaningful life. The effective discursive presence of the person has to be maintained when his/her normal methods of participation are failing (as is evidenced in the timing of conversations and the gaps that appear in them). Self-nourishment through meaningful activity and a full-blooded adaptation to the human life-world are often "frayed around the edges" and the person can no longer see themselves as the being of worth s/he used to be so that their "pathology" is intensified (Sabat 2001):

> Things began to happen that I just couldn't understand. There were times I addressed friends by the wrong name. Comprehending conversations seemed quite impossible. My attention span became quite short. Notes were needed to remind me of things to be done and how to do them. I would slur my speech, use inappropriate words, or simply eliminate one from a

sentence. This caused me not only frustration but embarrassment. Then came the times I honestly could not remember how to plan a meal or shop for groceries. (Post 2000, p. 83)

Cognition can be enhanced by improving biological functions underpinning memory and cognition, but we should also attend to the structures of personhood so as to allow a person to remain *somebody* around here and not be marginalized through the discourse of "decline-and-loss" (Holstein 2000). Human beings contribute to each other's lives and, in contemporary society, where planned obsolescence and executive efficiency rule the roost, our living repositories of memory and continuity may be marginalized so that we lose touch with our roots, our traditions, and the threads of value that bind us together. Unfortunately bedside (objective) assessments, like the MMSE, and unnatural modes of curation (or custodial care; "They just sit there, in their chairs") drain the worth from a person suffering dementia just as harmfully as any failure of neuronal metabolism. The preservation of voice and functioning identity is vital to respect for such a person (and much more so than artificial nutrition and hydration), given that the essence of human life, health and well-being is discursive and not merely biological.

The co-creation between the patient on the one hand and mental health professionals on the other, means that helping the patient through the illness journey of Alzheimer's disease must engage with the context of meaningful discourse in which self and mind are formed and given ways to function. Individuals need discursive skills apt to a given context in order to be recognized as the subjective beings they really are. That recognition is essentially other-involving and reflects the discursive context in which we position ourselves as beings of worth or value (however modest). Discursive interactions create and inform agency and shape the stories that we live and maladies of the soul are disruptions of the stories that engender, for each of us, a good-enough sense of well-being.

To become whole again is to re-integrate and coordinate a lived story through the very skills of self-expression impaired, in quite different but equally disabling ways, by hysteria and dementia. A patient with hysteria is wounded but dissociates from his or her real wounds because they lie in the liminal space between meaning and the body and are so "lost in translation" that they cannot be located in the networks and levels to which they belong. The affected individual deceives and is self-deceived. Therefore to heal such wounds requires a set of skills based on a secure mode of being in (moral and) discursive reality, and to reconstitute events according to the lines along which they are connected and engender one another. It is seductive to remain "lost" and resort to "surd" disease or bodily defect as the explanation of one's impairment.

The patient with dementia is wounded in the neural networks that enable them to integrate the levels of being to which they belong. Such a person may be helped by biological enhancements but needs support in discursive self-positioning so as to foster inclusion and respect and the preservation of ties that bind one together and relationships that constitute one's being somebody with individuality and worth.

Philosophy of psychiatry engages in reasoned discourse about the failures that disrupt personal being as it straddles the imaginary (or symbolic) and the actual (or existent). The discourses of mental disorder partly determine what happens to mental health patients or clients. We create or produce and address their suffering through our ways of dealing with them and our attempts to help must equip them for discourse—engaging mindfully, interpersonally, morally, socially, and politically with others who occupy certain subjective positions and do things with words.

Discursive approaches to psychiatry take the "two worlds"—mental symbols and mortal contingencies—of psychiatric thought and practice as equally important. Neuroscience tells us about the processes that form the vehicle of human being-in-the-world-with-others and discourse tells us what those processes are for. The skills we use in everyday life may be undermined by failures in brain function and impair a person's ability to see who s/he is and how to enact a self in a good-enough way. Being somebody, discursive identity, the basis of any person's participation in the human life-world, is the product of a triadic relation— between a human being, the discursive world of constructed meanings, and the actual contexts of life. Discursive skills link these three aspects of our being-in-the-world-with-others integrating and coordinating brain function so as to present "a self" at the heart of a human story. Being engaged and empowered as a discursive subject enables one to bring meaning to life (in both senses). When we are suitably supported in that complex activity, we can enjoy relative mental health, whatever maladies of the soul we struggle with.

References

American Psychiatric Association (1994). *Diagnostic and Statistical Manual of Mental Disorders, Fourth Edition*. Washington, DC: American Psychiatric Association.

Armstrong, D. (2004). *Truth and Truthmakers*. Cambridge: Cambridge University Press.

Bliss, T. V. and Collingridge, G. L. (1993). A synaptic model of memory: long-term potentiation in the hippocampus. *Nature*, 361(6407), 31–9.

Bolton, D. (2008). *What is Mental Disorder? An Essay in Philosophy, Science and Values*. Oxford: Oxford University Press.

Clark, A. (1997). *Being There: Putting Brain Body and World Together Again*. Cambridge, MA: MIT Press.

Clark, A. (2008). *Supersizing the Mind: Embodiment, Action and Cognitive Extension*. Oxford: Oxford University Press.

Cooper, R. (2007). *Psychiatry and Philosophy of Science*. Stocksfield: Acumen.

Dennett, D. C. (1991). *Consciousness Explained*. London: Penguin Press.

Eisenberg, L. (1995). The social construction of the human brain. *American Journal of Psychiatry*, 152, 1563–75.

Franz, E. and Gillett, G. (2011). John Hughlings Jackson's evolutionary neurology: a unifying framework for cognitive neuroscience. *Brain*, 134, 3114–20.

Geertz, C. (1973). *The Interpretation of Cultures: Selected Essays*. New York, NY: Basic Books.

Gillett, G. (2002). You always were a bastard. *Hastings Center Report*, 32(6), 23–8.

Gillett, G. (2009). *The Mind and its Discontents* (2nd edn). Oxford: Oxford University Press.

Gillett, G. (2010). Intentional action, moral responsibility and psychopaths. In L. Malatesti and J. McMillan (Eds), *Responsibility and Psychopathy: Interfacing Law, Psychiatry and Philosophy*, pp. 282–98. Oxford: Oxford University Press.

Gillett, G. and McMillan, J. (2001). *Consciousness and Intentionality*. Amsterdam: John Benjamins.

Giordano, S. (2005). *Understanding Eating Disorders*. Oxford: Oxford University Press.

Hacking, I. (1995). *Rewriting the Soul*. Princeton, NJ: Princeton University Press.

Harré, R. (2002) *Cognitive Science—a philosophical introduction.* Thousand Oaks, CA: Sage.

Harré, R. and Gillett, G. (1994). *The Discursive Mind.* London; Sage.

Heidegger, M. (1996). *Being and Time* (J. Stambaugh, Trans.). New York, NY: SUNY Press. (Original work published 1953.)

Holstein, M. (2000) Ageing, culture, and the framing of Alzheimer disease. In P. J. Whitehouse, K. Maurer, and J. F. Ballenger (Eds), *Concepts of Alzheimer Disease: Biological, Clinical and Cultural Perspectives*, pp. 158–80. Baltimore, MD: Johns Hopkins University Press.

Husserl, E. G. (1970). *The Crisis of European Sciences and Transcendental Phenomenology* (D. Carr, Trans.). Evanston, IL: Northwestern University Press.

Jackson, J. H. (1887). Remarks on the evolution and dissolution of the nervous system. *British Journal of Psychiatry, 33,* 25–48.

Kristeva, J. (1995). *The New Maladies of the Soul.* New York, NY: Columbia University Press.

Lacan, J. (1977). *Ecrits.* New York, NY: Norton & Co.

Levinas, E. (1996). *Basic Philosophical Writings.* Bloomington, IN: Indiana University Press.

Luria, A. R. (1973). *The Working Brain.* Harmondsworth; Penguin.

McGowan, D. (2006). Cell biology of the neuron: Pruning processes. *Nature Reviews Neuroscience, 7,* 685.

Pickering, N. (2006). *The Metaphor of Mental Illness.* Oxford: Oxford University Press.

Pike, K. M., Walsh, B. T., Vitousek, K., Wilson, G. T., and Bauer, J. (2003). Cognitive behavior therapy in the posthospitalization treatment of anorexia nervosa. *American Journal of Psychiatry, 160,* 2046–9.

Post, S. (2000). *The Moral Challenge of Alzheimer Disease.* Baltimore, MD: Johns Hopkins University Press.

Sabat, S. (2001). *The Experience of Alzheimer's Disease.* Oxford: Blackwell.

Sabat, S. and Harré, R. (1992). The construction and deconstruction of self in Alzheimer's disease *Ageing and Society, 12,* 443–61.

Stanghellini, G. (2004). *Disembodied Spirits and Deanimated Bodies.* Oxford: Oxford University Press.

Taylor, C. (1989). *Sources of the Self.* Cambridge, MA: Harvard University Press.

Winch, P. (1958). *The Idea of a Social Science and its Relation to Philosophy.* London: Routledge.

Wittgenstein, L. (1953). *Philosophical Investigations.* Oxford: Blackwell.

Zahavi, D. (2005). *Subjectivity and Selfhood.* Cambridge, MA: MIT Press.

Zhu, Y., Zhang, L., Fan, J., and Han, S. (2007). Neural basis of cultural influence on self-representation. *NeuroImage, 34*(3), 1310–16.

CHAPTER 23

PHILOSOPHICAL RESOURCES FOR THE PSYCHIATRIC INTERVIEW

GIOVANNI STANGHELLINI

THE PSYCHIATRIC INTERVIEW: A PHILOSOPHICAL PROBLEM?

The psychiatric interview is obviously a crucial step in the overall clinical process. Notwithstanding this truism, a cursory review of the literature reveals that a majority of authors and researchers are more interested in "what" should be assessed than "how" the assessment should be conducted. One reason for this neglect may be that the skill in asking questions and listening to answers is taken for granted as a commonplace habit of everyday life (Lazarsfeld 1935). Another cause may be the assumption that interviewing is an art that cannot be taught but only acquired (MacKinnon and Michels 1971). A third, and perhaps more profound, possibility could be that a critical reappraisal of interview principles and skills may become a rather puzzling enterprise requiring us to re-think some of the basic tenets of psychiatry as a science.

Studies concerned with the methodological problems of the psychiatric interview mirror a vexed question within the community of mental health professionals (Othmer and Othmer 2002; Shea and Mezzich 1988): Is the psychiatric interview a technique designed to objectively and reliably elicit signs and symptoms that allow nosographical diagnosis, or is it a special instance of interpersonal rapport exploring personal problems, including the problems that arise in this rapport and especially those connected to affective involvement? Attempts to answer this question have cemented a dichotomy between structured and symptom-oriented approaches, on the one hand, and free format and insight-oriented interview styles, on the other (e.g., Shea 1988).

What is lacking most in studies of both approaches is an analysis of the philosophical—namely epistemological and ethical—problems related to the psychiatric interview. A lot of work has been done to conceptually clarify psychiatric nosography and classification (e.g., Sadler et al. 1994), but very little effort has been made to bring to the fore the problems that arise in examining and assessing the psychiatric patient's behaviors, experiences, and expressions.

In this chapter, I will first review the basic tenets of mainstream psychiatric interviewing techniques—the so-called technical approach—highlighting their main drawbacks and limitations. Since the psychiatric interview is, first and foremost, a search for symptoms, I will then spend considerable time analyzing the different ways of conceptualizing symptoms in the biomedical, psychodynamic, and phenomenological-hermeneutical paradigms. The following step will be describing the *family of dispositives* in use during the interview, that is the first- (subjective), second- (dialogical), and third-person (objective) mode of interviewing. A short history of the discipline of psychopathology, the basic science for psychiatric assessment, will introduce three levels of the psychopathological inquiry: descriptive psychopathology, whose main purpose is to systematically study conscious experiences, order and classify them, and create valid and reliable terminology; clinical psychopathology, which is a pragmatic tool for bridging relevant symptoms to diagnostic categories; and structural psychopathology, which assumes that the manifold of phenomena of a given mental disorder are a meaningful whole and searches for meaningful units. I will conclude the chapter with a phenomenologically- and hermeneutically-informed flowchart for the psychiatric interview.

The Technical Approach to
Psychiatric Interviewing

In 1963, an article appeared in the *New York Post* in which the reporter wrote: "a young doctor at Columbia University's New York State Psychiatric Institute has developed a tool that may become the psychiatrist's thermometer and microscope and X-ray machine rolled into one" (Spitzer 1983, p. 400). The young doctor was obviously Robert Spitzer and the tool was a structured interview for the assessment of psychiatric symptoms.

Since the early 1970s, mental health professionals endorsing the biomedical paradigm have increasingly emphasized the need for standardization in psychiatric interviews (Endicott and Spitzer 1978). The magnitude of the variability between observers in research and clinical settings (Saghir 1971) was viewed as the main obstacle to the advancement of psychiatry as a scientific discipline. The variability of psychiatric diagnoses had become symbolic of the professionals' self-doubts and of the vulnerability of psychiatry to scientific and public criticism (Kirk and Kutchins 1992). A consensus emerged among psychiatric professionals that standardized procedures would eliminate the disarray that characterized the practice of psychiatric diagnosis (Bayer and Spitzer 1985). Improvement of the validity of the diagnostic schema and the reliability of the diagnostic method became a valued goal in itself (Spitzer 2001). Since that time, the importance of reliable assessment of psychiatric diagnosis has been taken for granted and been undisputed (Ventura et al. 1998).

In the technical approach, the effectiveness of the diagnostic process relies on two domains: diagnostic criteria and the interview method. Operational criteria are instrumental in achieving high reliability in the domain of the diagnostic schema, primarily because of their reduction of criterion variance. Structured interview methods help to improve the reliability of diagnostic assignment by reducing information variance (Spitzer 1983). These two domains are coupled in such a way that structured interviews are designed to explore only those symptoms that are relevant to establish a diagnosis according to the diagnostic criteria themselves. The interviewer's main goal is discovering whether a patient with a given set of signs and symptoms "meets criteria."

Accordingly, interviewing is seen as a technique that should conform to the technical-rational paradigm of natural sciences, namely laboratory techniques in biological sciences, in which psychiatry as a branch of biomedicine is positioned. Interviewing is thus conceived as a stimulus-response pattern of questions formulated in such a way as to reduce information variance (Kirk and Kutchins 1992) and to elicit only "relevant" answers (Mishler 1986).

To achieve the aim of reliable nosographical diagnosis, structured interviews are symptom-oriented, rather than insight-oriented (their aim, or at least their main aim, is not in-depth understanding of personal experiences). They rely on a descriptive method, and point to classification of the patient's complaints and dysfunctions according to defined diagnostic categories. The main epistemological tenet is that psychiatric disorders manifest themselves in characteristic sets of signs, symptoms, and behaviors that are in principle accessible to question-and-answer techniques (Othmer and Othmer 2002).

Early empirical studies comparing structured and unstructured psychiatric interviews seemed to support the belief that structured interviews are more comprehensive in covering symptomatology and in eliciting factual information and feelings (e.g., Hopkins et al. 1981; Saghir 1971). After more than 30 years, at least a part (if not the majority) of mental health professionals hold the view that structured interviews not only allow better statistical inter-rater agreement, but also, as reported by Ventura et al. (1998), improve non-specialists' assessment in clinical and research settings, permit standardization of formal training programs, and, finally, facilitate the development of ultra-rapid diagnosis (Zimmerman 1993), tele-video psychiatric assessment procedures (Stevens et al. 1999; Yoshino et al. 2001), and computer-assisted or self-administered interview (Peters and Andrews 1995).

MAin Criticisms of the Technical Approach

This approach to the psychiatric interview, and more generally its advocacy of the assimilation of psychiatry into general medicine as a branch of one the natural sciences, has of course raised many criticisms (e.g., Kirk and Kutchins 1992; Richardson 1996; Sadler et al. 1994; Stanghellini 2004).

Procrustean errors and tunnel vision

The technical-rational paradigm conceives interviewing as a stimulus–response pattern of questions designed to elicit only *relevant* answers. It follows a rigid pattern of questions oriented by operationalized criteria for nosographic diagnosis. This may entail so-called "procrustean errors," i.e., "to stretch and trim" the patient's symptomatology to fit criteria (McGuffin and Farmer 2001), and "tunnel vision" (van Praag et al. 1997), i.e., to avoid the assessment of those phenomena which are not included in standardized interview instruments since they do not reflect operational diagnostic criteria. Both are serious problems; but the second involves particularly important theoretical implications, including the perpetuation of systematic inattention to all those features that are not included in mainstream diagnostic schemas, potentially impeding the evolution of psychiatric knowledge. Tunnel vision and procrustean errors reduce validity—as argued, for instance, by Smolik (1999) who stigmatizes the low validity of operationalized diagnostic procedures of schizophrenia compared with expert clinician ratings.

Obviously, the relevance of some phenomena (and the irrelevance of all the others) is decided a priori—i.e., before the interview with that singular person takes place. The consequence is that a great deal of abnormal phenomena may pass unobserved. The criterion of a priori diagnostic relevance of a given set of symptoms may promote quite perplexing proposals in the clinical setting. Encouraged by the tenet that inquiring about specific symptoms is a more effective method of conducting a psychiatric interview since it eliminates the vagueness of general questions (Zimmerman 1993), clinicians may be encouraged to endorse a style that transforms the psychiatric interview into a *tele-ocular-dromic* performance: a distancing ("tele"), first-sight ("ocular"), quick ("dromic") scanning of the patient's mental status. But in fact psychiatric patients seem to report a very low number of symptoms in a structured interview that lasts only a few minutes, and the information gathered during this period does not allow accurate diagnosis (Herran et al. 2001).

The ineffectiveness of research interviews for clinical practice

The structured interview is a methodology imported into clinical practice from research paradigms, and as such is not responsive to the requirements of clinical settings and the clinician's need. For instance, it deliberately seeks to uncouple assessment procedures (getting information) from therapy, an untenable principle in practicing clinical psychiatry (Finn and Tonsanger 1997). Moreover, since it mainly relies on nosographic diagnostic categorization, it may be ineffective in guiding therapeutic (pharmacotherapeutic, and even more psychotherapeutic) decision-making which requires more subtle subgrouping and sometimes trans-nosographical categorization (van Praag et al. 1997).

The insufficiency of pure theoretical knowledge

To conceive of the psychiatric interview as a technique entails the presupposition that actual interviewing skills are subservient to the cognitive knowledge and application of diagnostic schemata. This idea has been challenged by several studies: there is a negative correlation between the understanding of interviewing principles (Ware et al. 1971), and a negative correlation between academic (theoretical) knowledge and skill in communicating with patients (practical knowledge) (Pollock et al. 1985). The possibility that cognitive understanding "gets in the way" of clinical performance may indicate that the clinical effectiveness of the interviewing process may entail something more than mere diligence in "learning about" a diagnostic algorithm that guides the interview.

The narrow dependence on the standard view of science

A more global criticism often raised against the technical approach to psychiatric interviews is its narrow dependence on the "'received,' 'standard' or 'traditional' view of science" (Pidgeon and Henwood 1996), which values detachment, objectivity, and rationality as guiding principles of Western science. This is the image of *true* science conveyed to medical students (and psychologists): objects in the natural world enjoy existence independent of human beings (human agency is basically incidental to the objective character of the world out there); scientific knowledge is determined by the actual character of the physical world; science comprises a unitary set of methods and procedures, concerning which there is, by and large, a consensus; and science is an activity which is individualistic and mentalistic (the latter is sometimes expressed as "cognitive") (Woolgar 1996). This image may reflect an inaccurate and misleading description of how science actually gets done.

The misunderstanding of empathy

Another problem with the technical approach is its idiosyncratic understanding of the notion of "empathy." For instance, to Ventura et al. (1998) empathy is the capacity to make emotionally congruent remarks, and Othmer and Othmer (2002) report sentences like "You must feel awful" or "I can see how that shook you up" as instances of empathic responses. Empathy is seen as a special technique to elicit trust in order to achieve rapport and relevant information (Turner and Hersen 1985/2003), rather than as itself the medium for understanding. In the standard interviewing process, empathy is conceptualized as a way of "putting the patient and yourself at ease" (Othmer and Othmer 2002) before proceeding to a purely objective assessment. Empathy, that is, is too often conceived as a mere precursor to the genuine article of psychopathological understanding, rather than as a core form that understanding may take. From a different perspective (Jaspers 1997), empathy is the basic method of psychopathological assessment that implies the ability to feel oneself into the situation of the other person (Oyebode 2008).

The avoidance of subjectivity and the praise of objectivity

In the past few decades, an objectifying trend has taken place not only in psychiatry but also in the philosophy of mind. This ongoing focus on objectively observable behaviors in contrast to subjective experiences as more reliable indicators of (normal or abnormal) psychic life has been criticized by many authors (e.g., Lieberman 1989). This celebration of sight as the noblest of senses was uncritically imported into psychiatry from scientistic philosophy as well as from "visually imbued cultural and social practices" (Jay 1994, p. 2). Ocularcentrism in psychiatry values a kind of practice that lets the observer avoid direct engagement, helps establishing a sharp subject–object distinction, and allows neutrality. The major criticism of this approach is that observable behaviors are mere "shells" whose content (i.e., motivations) is radically underappreciated from a purely "objective," third-person perspective. Behaviors are final common pathways, e.g., anorectic behavior may be motivated by very different mental states like the dread to appear deformed in one's bodily shape, the delusional fear of being poisoned (sitophobia), the hypochondriacal idea that fat will cause a disease, the value of asceticism, etc. Thus, the category that includes all persons displaying anorectic behavior is highly non-specific and has very low clinical utility, whereas in order to establish homogenous categories we must take into account the mental states that subtend (abnormal) behaviors.

The objectification of subjectivity

Another substantial criticism of the objectifying trend is evident in its avoidance of complex problems entailed by the exploration of subjectivity. It is questionable whether we do, in the ordinary sense, have empirical knowledge of the mental states of others and also of our own mental states. Mental states are subjective, i.e., I have *direct* access to my own and only to my own inner ("private") experience. But for me to access to the complex features (e.g., emotional nuances, motivations, etc.) of my own experiences can be highly problematic. For instance, it may necessitate my taking a third-person perspective on my own mental states and, so to say, to explore myself from without. The objectification of subjectivity may occur in the process of reflection, since reflection implies a third-person approach to oneself. Also, it may occur in the phenomenon of remembering—how does someone remember her past experiences as his or her own? Does remembering also imply a third-person perspective on oneself? A second shift from first-person to third-person perspective is obviously entailed when someone asks me to explicate my mental states, and this step can be even more problematic. As Zahavi (1999) puts is: Can subjectivity be made accessible for direct theoretical examination, or does such examination necessarily imply an objectivization and consequently a falsification? This is the fundamental issue addressed by phenomenology, namely how to approach consciousness. This shift is nonetheless necessary if we want to assess (e.g., measure) subjective phenomena underlying objective behaviors. The facts that a subjective mental states may be opaque to its owner, and that *errors in translations* may occur in the process of assessing someone else's mental states, do not seem to represent sufficient arguments for excluding subjectivity from the "objects" of psychology and psychopathology and for confining psychological and psychopathological sciences to the realm of the objectively observable.

Also, mental states are meaningful, and the meaning of a person's action is not visible, as is clear in the case of anorectic behavior. Mental states are subjective, and their complete content often cannot be captured simply by observing the behaviors in which they are expressed at any one time. Avoiding the exploration of human subjectivity is certainly not the best solution to these difficulties. The purpose of the psychiatric interview (to quote Paul Klee's famous formula) is not simply *to render the visible, but to render visible*.

The place of language

The exploration of subjectivity takes place in language. Words are one of the means through which currently opaque meanings are rendered more sensible. Here is raised a further problem: Can words always aptly express a mental state and its proper meaning? For some mental states (especially psychotic and, even more, pre-psychotic ones) are almost ineffable. The "assessment" of a mental state involves two kinds of reductions. The first is performed by the speaker who tries to find the propositional correlate of a given mental state, or the "right words" to communicate it. The other reduction is performed by the listener who must sometimes interpret the speaker's meaning by asking the speaker and himself "what does he mean by that?" This problem, which plagues psychopathological research and clinical practice, becomes even more acute in using standardized assessment, since when interviewees respond to questionnaires, they might have very different understandings of the questions, and this may lead to the inaccurate conclusion that different individuals or groups have similar experiences or beliefs.

An interview is a linguistic event. It is not a behavioral-verbal interchange simply *mediated by* language. Rather, it happens *in* language. Language is not a set of formal classes or boxes that we apply to reality (be it inner or outer reality) from without, but rather "a medium where I and world meet" (Gadamer 2004, p. 469). Language is the house of being—as Heidegger would put it. This has several implications in the psychiatric interview. First, language is not given as the "reflection" of something, be it external or internal reality. Although we do very often use language to represent, this does not mean that language can be understood as a representation of a world whose structure it reflects or mirrors (Rorty 1981). Rather than reflecting, language instead often "unconceals" (Heidegger 1962). A special instance of this problem emerges in a consideration of bodily sensations. What is the relationship between metaphors (i.e., the expressions we use to describe our bodily experiences) and bodily experiences themselves? Do metaphors directly arise from bodily sensations? Or are they similes (imperfectly) reflecting bodily experiences? Or, rather, do they partly constitute bodily experiences? Second, when reality comes into language a kind of interpretation is at work; and the words through which reality comes to be understood also necessitate an interpretation. Third, a patient's use of language is not simply descriptive of her inner experience, but is rather of a piece with it. The way that she lives in language is of a piece with her inner life, her subjectivity. It constitutes what the psychoanalyst Bollas (2003) calls the "personal idiom" of the patient—her unique set of resonances, affordances, and metaphors which strike her and which both express and construct her interiority.

Language does not always and everywhere constitute a universally agreed descriptive (non-expressive, non-metaphorical) medium of exchange, but rather is dwelled in idiosyncratically by its speakers. It is not possible, therefore, to treat a patient's language use as a straightforward reflection of her inner experience. This implies, in practice, that the coding of each item of an interview always requires an (often laborious) process of interpretation—rather than a pseudo-objective simple "ticking."

The avoidance of personal meanings and narratives

The technical approach to the psychiatric interview is dominated by *de-narratization*, i.e., by the neglect of intelligible relations between persons—the interviewer and the interviewee—and between the person's feelings, ideas, perceptions, sensations, etc. Narratives are the ordinary forms through which we attempt to order the sense and meaning of our actions, experiences, and beliefs. Narrative reasoning is the ability to use structure above the level of the sentence, hence above the level of single experiences. Narratives establish a form of organization in autobiographical memory providing temporal and goal structure, combining personal experiences into a coherent story related to the self. Structured interviews are usually not concerned with personal narratives since their aim is usually the assessment of bits of behavior and expression; they thereby avoid the problem of constructing interpersonally shared meanings (Mishler 1986).

In suppressing the natural occurrence of conversation and substituting for it the stimulus-response process in structured interviews, crucial epistemological and ethical problems arise: (i) The stimulus-response process disrupts the specific rhythm of natural conversation. A fragmentation of personal experience occurs. The intimacy of the relationship, based on the quality of the concentration of one individual on another and on the capacity to alter previously stated positions, is affected (Zinberg 1987). (ii) Shared meanings between interviewer and interviewees are assumed, and not investigated in the process of the interview itself. Serious questions should instead be raised about the validity of the assumption of real mutual understanding. Take the following example: one patient says, "I feel depressed." What exactly does she mean by that? Some patients may use the word "depressed" to describe themselves as feeling sad and downhearted, but others may use it to mean that they feel unable to feel, or also to convey their sense of inner void, lack of inner nucleus and/or of identity, feelings of being anonymous or non-existent. This is especially relevant in multicultural societies since mental disorders are often displayed in idiosyncratic culturally-bound phenomena. (iii) Answers to questions often display the features of narratives. But in the stimulus–response paradigm the interviewee's narratives are suppressed in that his responses are limited to "relevant" answers to narrowly specified questions. By doing so, storytelling, i.e., the primary way human beings make sense of their experiences by casting them in a narrative form, is discouraged. Thus, the search for understanding, i.e., meaningfulness and coherence, is discouraged; this process may even be iatrogenic. (iv) The idea of a neutral stimulus is chimerical. Every researcher and clinician knows very well that even in the stimulus–response approach interviewers often depart from standard questions. These departures from prescribed questions are not exceptions, but rather representative of a process that is inherent to interviewing, i.e., the matching of perspectives.

The overwriting of personal meanings and narratives

The technical approach to psychiatric interviewing may inappropriately assume a priori systems of meanings that can obscure (overwrite) personally structured meanings and narratives (Mishler 1986; Pidgeon and Henwood 1996). These a priori systems of meanings are diagnostic categories. The nosographical approach based on operational criteria for discrete disorders (as we have seen) may force researchers and clinicians to commit procrustean errors. Diagnostic categories are conceptualized as boxes ("category" originally means "box," "container") in which similar objects should find their place. The pattern of interviewer dominance and respondent acquiescence is emphasized and enhanced. This entails a shift from initial extended self-reports to simple a priori "relevant" yes-or-no answers. The relevance and appropriateness of questions and responses in an interview should instead emerge through the discourse itself, i.e., from the shared attempt to arrive at meanings that both interviewer and interviewee can understand. A symptom is reduced to the properties that correspond to one category or box.

There is little space for personal meanings and personal narratives, as well as for meanings and narratives negotiated during the psychiatric interview. Also significant is the fact that each psychopathological experience is accompanied by a personal meaning or value that the patient attributes to it; that is, each patient may take a certain position with respect to his abnormal experiences. For instance, the very same raw "depressive" experience of a sense of inner void may be rated by different persons either as the effect of a change in one's body and thus explained as the effect of a somatic disease; or passively suffered, thus leading to apathetic and disorganized behavior; or it may kindle a "fight" reaction, leading to dysphoric mood and auto/hetero-aggressive comportments. Or else it may be accompanied by an "exalted" reaction so that the person will say that this experience revealed to him his true nature as a disembodied automaton. The *position-taking* (meaning and value attribution) of each patient toward his experiences is obviously a relevant clinical feature since it shapes distinct clinical pictures and prognoses (Stanghellini 1997). Knowing a patient's interpretation of his condition also contributes to the design of his individual treatment plan.

The categorial versus the typological approach

A final set of critiques can be posed from a semantic stance. The standard interview is said to rely on categorization, i.e., the recognition of a special particular (e.g., a symptom) as the member of a class of other particulars that share common properties or criteria. Categorization in this sense can be described as the reconstruction of the "identity" of a certain object via the analytical or algorithmic apprehension of its multiple features in a bottom-up inferential process: "this object shows features 'x,' 'y,' and 'z,' therefore it must be my daughter Virginia." This is the way symptomatological-criteriological diagnosis is supposed to work—but in fact it does not work like this.

As a matter of fact, mental health professionals (as all other humans), in their diagnostic efforts, are instead engaged in a typification process (Rosch 1973; Schwartz and Wiggins 1987). Typification implies "seeing as," i.e., perceiving objects, automatically and pre-reflectively, as certain types of objects. The notion of typicality or prototype is crucial here: prototypes are central exemplars. The recognition of an object is founded upon a family resemblance (Wittgenstein 1953), a network of criss-crossing analogies between the individual members of a category. The typological approach to anomalous experience is concerned with bringing forth the ideally necessary feature(s) of such experience (see, e.g., Kraus 2003). The concept of typification also provides a way to rephrase notions like "intuition" and "holistic approach." The former advocates the primacy of pre-reflective and implicit over the reflective and explicit cognitive process; the latter emphasizes the importance of the global grasp of a phenomenon as an organizing and meaningful Gestalt over a particularistic focus of attention.

The Truth about Symptoms

A further set of criticisms of the technical approach stems from its understanding of the concept of "symptom." The psychiatric interview prescribes, first and foremost, a search for symptoms. Handbooks of psychiatry and clinical psychology usually present a list of phenomena that should be assessed and by doing so they establish a system of relevance concerning *what* should attract the clinician's attention. These *relevant* phenomena are called "symptoms." Of course, there are different psychopathological paradigms (among which the biomedical, the psychodynamic, the phenomenological, etc.) and each paradigm has its own hierarchy of priorities (what should be the clinician's focus of attention) as well as its own concept of symptom.

The concept of symptom covers a vast array of indexicalities. In biological medicine, a symptom is the epiphenomenon of an underlying pathology. Red, itchy and watery eyes, congestion, runny nose and sneezing, sometimes accompanied by itchy ears and buzzing sound, itchy and sore throat, cough and post-nasal dripping are known to be the manifestation of an inflammation of the respiratory apparatus. But long before we found out what was the cause of these disturbing phenomena (namely rhinovirus infection), we all knew that they were the symptoms of a mild, although distressing and untreatable, disorder called "cold." Within the biomedical paradigm, a symptom is first of all an index for diagnosis, i.e., it is used by clinicians to establish that the person who shows that symptom is sick (rather that healthy), and that he or she is affected by a particular illness or disease. The principal utility of any system of medical taxonomy relies on "its capacity to identify specific entities to allow prediction of natural history and response to therapeutic intervention" (Bell 2010, p. 1).

The biomedical paradigm

The biomedical understanding of "symptom" is clearly coherent with the technical approach described in the previous paragraph. Biomedical research aims to sharpen its tools to establish increasingly more reliable and valid diagnostic criteria. Its real ambition is not simply to establish a diagnosis through the assessment of clinical manifestations (i.e., symptoms), but to discover the causes of these symptoms (etiology) and the pathway that leads from etiology to symptoms (pathogenesis). "Ultimately, disease specification should be related to events related to causality rather than simply clinical phenotype" (Bell 2010, p. 1). It is assumed that progress in medicine is dependent on defining pathological entities as disease based on etiology and pathogenetic mechanism—rather than as clinical syndromes based on symptom recognition. So to say, in the biomedical paradigm the *truth* about a symptom is its *cause*. The main, more or less explicit, assumptions in the biomedical paradigm are the following: (i) each symptom must have at least one cause, (ii) this cause lies in some (endogenous or exogenous) *noxa* affecting the living organism, (iii) the presence of a symptom causes some kind of dysfunction (cause → symptom → dysfunction). Also, (iv) if we want to eliminate a symptom, we should eliminate its cause or interrupt the pathogenetic chain that connects its putative etiology with the symptom itself. Thus, the biomedical paradigm is a knowledge device based on the concept of "causality." In general, causality (in the biomedical paradigm) goes from etiology (in our example, the presence of a virus), to symptom(s) (breathing difficulties), to dysfunction (poor physical performance due to blood hypo-oxygenation, thus reduced adaptation of the person to his or her environment). An important, implicit, assumption is also that symptoms are considered accidental, i.e., non-essential (*synbebekos*, as in the sense stipulated in Aristotle's (1991) *Metaphysics*) to the living organism, whereas the absence of symptoms is considered essential—i.e., normal to living organisms. In other terms, health is considered normal, whereas disease is considered abnormal.

Many of these assumptions—if we apply this paradigm to the field of psychic pathology—are at least controversial, or even counterfactual. We will examine some of these controversies later in this chapter. What is of utmost interest here is the fact that in the biomedical paradigm, symptoms have causes, not meanings. This assumption has been challenged by the psychodynamic paradigm. But before we analyze the shift from the biomedical to the psychodynamic concept of "symptom," let's focus for a while on the relationship between symptom and dysfunction with the help of the criticism of the biomedical paradigm that arises from the evolutionary (Darwinian) medicine. Diagnosis, in the biomedical paradigm, puts emphasis on symptom profiles as symptoms are considered the most proximal indicators of a disorder. From an evolutionary viewpoint, a clinical assessment that focuses exclusively on signs and symptoms limits itself to explaining only partial features of disorders. According to Darwinian psychiatry, clinical assessment should focus primarily on *functional capacities* and *person–environment interactions* (Troisi and McGuire 1998). It is argued that the capacity to achieve biological goals is a better measure of health than the absence of symptoms because it is an indication that the individual possesses those optimal functional capacities that promote biological adaptation. From an evolutionary perspective, not only do symptoms cause dysfunction, but also dysfunction or maladaptation may generate symptoms. When classified from an evolutionary perspective, symptoms can be divided into two broad categories: symptoms as defects in the body's mechanisms and symptoms as useful defenses. For example, seizures, jaundice, coma, and paralysis have apparently no adaptive function and arise from defects in the organism. But many other manifestations of disease are defenses. Vomiting eliminates toxins from the stomach. The low iron levels associated with chronic infection limit the growth of pathogens. Coughing clears foreign matter from the respiratory tract (Troisi 2011). In the field of mental pathology, it is argued by evolutionary psychiatrists that some depressive symptoms may have adaptive functions serving in the regulation of behavior and psychological processes. For instance, crying elicits comforting behaviors and strengthens social bonds, whilst pessimism withdraws the individual from current and potential goals. Also, absence of positive emotions discourages approach behavior and risk-taking. More generally we could explain depressive behavior by saying that someone withdraws depressively in order to protect himself socially. Thus, the Darwinian concept of disorder—including mental disorder—encourages clinicians to consider re-prioritizing their selection of diagnostic criteria to ensure that the focus shifts away from mere symptom profiles and more toward a comprehensive data collection that includes functional capacities.

Symptoms in the psychodynamic paradigm

Early psychodynamic conceptualizations of "symptom" address both the cause of a symptom and its meaning. Before Freud, no one asked about the *meaning* of a symptom. Or better: no one posed this question systematically and rigorously. However, since the main aim of early psychoanalytic thinking is to answer the question "What is the origin or *cause* of this psychical symptom?," it still resents of a rather mechanistic view in touch with the biomedical model. But at the same time early psychoanalysis paved the way for the quest for the meaning of the symptom: "What does that symptom *mean*?"

Psychodynamic thinking develops its genealogy of symptoms around two main pathogenetic devices: trauma and conflict. The psychodynamic question of trauma was first posed by a French neurologist—Jean-Martin Charcot. We are in the year 1885. Charcot examines a group of patients who underwent a physical shock and developed a series of motor or sensory symptoms—typically some sort of paralysis or anesthesia. Charcot's careful medical assessment established that: (i) the physical shock was very mild and left no traces in the patient's organism, whereas symptoms still persist—these symptoms are (so to say) *sine materia*; (ii) the motor and/or sensory symptoms, their localization, the way they are correlated with each other, do not correspond to an organic lesion of the nervous system; that is these symptoms do not correspond to the symptoms one could expect as a consequence of any given lesion of an area of the nervous system. The localization of these symptoms—namely hysterical symptoms—in the patient's body does not reflect the rules of anatomy; rather, these symptoms mirror a kind of *imaginary anatomy* that imitates *true* anatomy. From these observations Charcot concludes that these symptoms are the outcome not of a physical, but of a psychic, trauma. Hysterical symptoms are not the epiphenomena of a neurological lesion, but rather the manifestation of a psychopathological syndrome. Hysterical symptoms force Charcot (and later Freud) to see behind the neurological body another kind of body—the "sexual body" (Foucault 2003). Medicine in general, and psychopathology in particular, from Charcot and Freud onward, must consider the existence of another kind of body, next to the neurological one: this new body is the psychological representation of the body or "representational body" (Leoni 2008, p. 18), whose imaginary anatomy does not correspond to the anatomy prescribed by the cortical homunculus discovered by neurology. The representational body, according to Charcot (as explained by Foucault), enters into the mind of a person during a traumatic event and will be inscribed in his cortex "as a kind of permanent injunction" (Foucault 2003, p. 274).

Some neurotic symptoms are the outcome of a conflict—usually a conflict between an unconscious drive (typically: a sexual desire) and a proscription or prohibition by the Ego. According to classic psychodynamic theory (Freud 1905), this conflict generates anxiety, and anxiety "alerts" the Ego that a defense is necessary. Defenses lead to a compromise between the Ego and the Id. This compromise is the symptom: a symptom is therefore a compromise that at the same time defends the patient from the desire that emerges from the Id, and satisfies this desire in a masked form. Freud (1926, p. 91) wrote:

> The main characteristic of the formation of symptoms have long since been studied and, I hope, established beyond dispute. A symptom is a sign of, and substitute for, an instinctual satisfaction which has remained in abeyance; it is a consequence of the process of repression. Repression proceeds from the ego when the latter—it may be at the behest

of the super-ego—refuses to associate itself with an instinctual cathexis which has been aroused in the id. The ego is able by means of repression to keep the idea which is the vehicle of the reprehensible impulse from becoming conscious. Analysis shows that the idea often persists as an unconscious formation.

It is clear that psychodynamically-oriented interviews cannot avoid delving into this profound dimension of abnormal behaviors entailing the reconstruction of traumatic events and the unearthing of conflicts. Suppose a young woman develops a paraplegia a few days before she is going to get married. Careful medical assessment excludes any sort of neurological deficit. Imagine that through careful interviewing we can ascertain that she suffers from the unconscious desire not to marry her promised husband (or not to get married at all, or to marry another person); and that she cannot manifest this desire, not even to herself. Her symptom, which impedes her walking to the altar, satisfies her desire in a masked form, and at the same time it *speaks* on behalf of her desire. In this example (if viewed from the psychodynamic angle) the symptom has a psychological cause (the conflict) which kindles a pathogenetic cascade (involving a disturbing affect like anxiety alerting defense mechanisms like repression and conversion).

Psychodynamic thinking has a number of basic assumptions or postulates. These underlying assumptions are nicely summed up by Brackel (2009). First, all psychological events have, at least as one of their causes, a psychological cause, and can thereby be at least in part explained on a psychological basis. Second, all psychological events can be understood as psychologically meaningful to the person who displays them. Third, there exists a dynamic unconscious that must be posited because without such a postulate many psychological events are neither psychologically explicable nor psychologically meaningful. In our example, the psychological cause of the young lady's paralysis is the conflict; the meaning of the symptom is her unconscious desire not to get married; and the psychodynamic unconscious must be postulated for the symptom to become psychologically explainable and meaningful.

As a consequence of these postulates the psychodynamically oriented interview will not merely focus on conscious phenomena like overt symptoms, but will try to elicit unconscious or pre-conscious mental phenomena (e.g., repressed thoughts, representations, fantasies, desires, etc.) by means of free associations (as well as by asking open questions, leaving certain kinds of pauses, not always trying to reduce the patient's anxiety, etc.); also, it will focus on unconscious defense mechanisms (e.g., displacement, idealization, projective identification, etc.), or other subpersonal devices (e.g., attachment styles, self- and other-representations, etc.), as well as on the patient's personal life-history (not merely the medical anamnesis) and interpersonal patterns that will complete the psycho(patho)logical picture. The *Psychodynamic Diagnostic Manual* (PDM Task Force 2006) clearly states that symptom patterns can only be understood in the context of the personality of the patient and of his mental functioning, since symptom patterns are the explicit expressions of the ways patients face and cope with their life experiences. The reason for this extended assessment beyond mere symptoms or isolated behaviors is exquisitely practical: treatments that focus only on symptoms are deemed ineffective in producing changes and recovery (Westen et al. 2004).

In a symptom, as we saw earlier, an unconscious desire seeks to make itself manifest. What is at stake within a symptom is a repressed desire repugnant to the consciously accepted self-conception and values of the person. This desire, if it is to gain satisfaction, needs to be expressed indirectly. Whilst some symptoms function to express repressed desire (or are a product of defense mechanism other than repression like projection, projective identification, splitting, etc.), others seem to be "unmentalized" (Fonagy and Target 1997) fragments of emotions or of self-experience (McDougall 1996). For instance, one way of understanding a patient who "somatizes" is conceiving of her symptom as a product of anxiety which cannot be understood by the patient and instead is experienced merely bodily. As if the meaningful affective component is not simply repressed, but has never really got the chance to develop—because of an inadequate early environment for example.

In contrast to the biomedical paradigm, in the psychodynamic-hermeneutic approach the symptom asks to be heard and deciphered (rather than to be explained and removed). Lacan's conceptualization of "symptom" is a good example of the turn from searching for the causes of a symptom to searching for its meaning in psychoanalytic thinking. According to Lacan (2005), a symptom (that he spells *sinthome*) is a special kind of speech act through which the unconscious is made manifest. The unconscious itself is structured as a language, and a symptom is a meaningful event. A symptom is a *signifier* that takes the place of a *signified* that has been repressed. It is a kind of embodied metaphor (Miller 1990). The Lacanian understanding of "symptom" completely reverses the biomedical concept. A person's symptom is not accidental (*synbebekos*) to that person; rather it is the manifestation of his or her true identity. Lacan even held that someone's symptom could be the most authentic thing he possesses. A symptom has the same structure of Heidegger's *aletheia* (literally: un-hiddenness). It is the place where truth about oneself manifests while hiding itself. The symptom is not an accident to that person; rather it displays his or her true essence. As such, it is the contingent opportunity of a possible encounter between the person and the repressed truth of his own desire.

Symptoms in the phenomenological-hermeneutic paradigm

The phenomenological-hermeneutic paradigm is essentially concerned with laying bare the structure of the *life-world* inhabited by a person. A symptom is a feature of a person's life-world whose meaning will be enlightened by grasping the deep architecture of the life-world itself and the person's invisible transcendental structure that projects it. The phenomenological-hermeneutic interview places the interviewer and the interviewee en route toward the unfolding of the phenomenal world by producing a *text* and, through that, establishing personal narratives. I will explicate here how this process is deployed during the interview. But before doing that, I need to clear the ground of a possible misunderstanding. To consider phenomenology as a purely descriptive science of the way the world appears to the experiencing subject is a serious mistake, although it is true that phenomenology sponsors a kind of seeing that relates to something already there, rather than to what stands before, beyond or behind what is existent. "Making the invisible visible" can instead be taken as the motto of phenomenology, as it was the passion that possessed many of the artists of the twentieth century and the intellectual motor of the major scientists of the "invisible century," including Einstein and Freud, and of their search for hidden universes (Panek 2005). Phenomenology shares with Modernism, and with the *Zeitgeist* of the twentieth century, a passion for the invisible, and a skeptical stance toward the way things are seen in the natural attitude, that is, in straightforward cognition.

Phenomenology sponsors a *sui generis* kind of seeing—enlightening the enigmatic poetry of familiar things. But, especially in its hermeneutic *coté*, it is also resolutely tied to hearing and the spoken word since—as Gadamer (2004, p. 458) has acknowledged—"the primacy of hearing is the basis for the hermeneutical phenomenon." The symptom, in the phenomenological-hermeneutic paradigm, is conceived as a part of a discourse, to be deployed and analyzed as a *text*. Patients are encouraged to report their experiences, including their symptoms, and position them in a meaningful context, that is, in a narrative format. These are not immediately given as a narrative. Before that they are given as a text—that is a discourse that contains a structure—but this is *prima facie* an *invisible* as well as *unintended* structure. The issue, then, is how to rescue this invisible and unintended structure, and through this the meaning of the symptom(s) (Stanghellini 2010).

All human deeds can be produced or reproduced as a text. The text—be it oral or written—is a work of discourse that is produced by an act of intentional exteriorization. One of the main characteristics of a text is that once it is produced, it is no more a private *affaire*, but is of the public domain. It still belongs to the author, but it also stays there "independent with respect to the intention of the author" (Ricoeur 1981, p. 165). An example of this is the following: A patient is overcome by a feeling of estrangement from himself when he recounts an event of his life during a therapy session: "Doctor, I have repeated to myself this story so many times, but now that I tell it to you it sounds to me completely different. I see it from a completely different angle!" Another, even more explicit, example is the *parapraxis*, that is the emergence of an unintended meaning while putting a fact into words. Consider a solitary and rather ascetic persons who, coming back from a trip during which he had the chance to meet a lot of people including several girls, tells the therapist: "You know, one evening I even made a photo with the *sex* of them" (of course, what he meant to say was "with the *six* of them"). The externalization of one's actions, experiences, and beliefs via the production of a text implies their objectification; this objectification entails a distantiation from the person herself and an automatization of the significance of the text from the intentions of the author. Once produced, the text becomes a matter for public interpretation. Now, the author's meanings and intentions do not exist simply for-himself, but also for-another.

This process of objectification and of automatization is nicely described in Hegel's theory of action (Hegel 1998). Indeed, there is a parallel between a text and an action because—as explained by Ricoeur (1981, p. 206)—"in the same way as a text is detached from its author, an action is detached from its agent and develops consequences of its own." Just as every action involves a *recoil* of unintended implications back upon the actor, every text implies a recoil of unintended meanings back to its author. "All action"—Berthold-Bond (1995, p. 123) explains, commenting on Hegel—"is a circle wherein our conscious purposes are projected outward, in a deed whose consequences inevitably express something beyond what was intended; the deed therefore recoils back upon the purpose, throwing it into question, exposing the disparity between its intended meaning and its actual outcome." This happens because the deed immediately establishes a train of circumstances not directly connected to and contained in the design of the person who committed it. All conscious intentions—Berthold-Bond concludes—are "incomplete, unable to anticipate and encompass the full train of consequences, unable through any sheer exertion of will to force the world to become a simple mirror of our purposes" (Berthold-Bond 1995, p. 123). The upshot of this is that whenever we act, via the externalization of our intentions, we experience a kind of alienation and estrangement from ourselves. We discover *alterity* within ourselves.

The symptom deployed as a text exposes its author to this very destiny (see Ricoeur 2004; Stanghellini 2011). A text is the product of an action—a linguistic action. Like all actions, once produced the text shows the disparity between the author's conscious intentions and unintended consequences. The symptom exposed like a text recoils back upon its author, displaying the discrepancy between the private intended sense and its public tangible result. As a text, in the symptom alterity becomes manifested. The text, as the tangible result of a linguistic act, with its unintended consequences, reflects—*makes visible*—the "mind" of the author much more faithfully than a simple act of self-reflection. To paraphrase Hegel, the "mind" cannot see itself until it produces a text objectifying itself in a social act. Because all conscious intentions are incomplete, self-reflection is just an incomplete form of self-knowledge. A person cannot discern alterity within himself until he has made of himself an external reality by producing a text, and after reflecting upon it. This is the effect searched for and produced by the phenomenological-hermeneutic interview.

Personal narratives are the result of the integration of alterity, revealed by the distantiation and autonomization of the text, in the discourse of the self (Ricoeur 1990). To note, the essential question is not to recover, *behind* the text, the lost intention of the author (as it is often the case with the psychodynamic paradigm); rather, to unfold "in front of the text, the *world* which it opens up and discloses" (Ricoeur 1981, p. 111). Alterity comes into sight, materializing in the pleats of the text I have produced. By unfolding the pleats of the text in front of me, I get a panoramic view of how the parts of the text are articulated. To paraphrase Merleau-Ponty (1964), the mystery is exposed in the exteriority of things perceived in their reciprocal intertwining. Consider a patient in his fifties who is going through a rather difficult period in his life. He says that he feels "anxious, unstable, precarious, and I don't know why." His mood is almost inscrutable and unintelligible to him, and this makes him more and more insecure, tense and nervous. During a session he tells the following story: "You know, this may sound irrelevant to you; none the less I will tell you what happened to me this week. I have been travelling a lot, and every morning I woke up in a different place. One day very early in the morning I took the elevator to the breakfast room, my eyes still half shut. All of a sudden I see a shade in the elevator and I think: 'What's my father doing here?' Of course, it was my image in the mirror of the elevator." During the following sessions he remembers that when he was about ten, and his father about 50, his parents had a horrible conjugal crisis apparently caused by their infidelities. His father, who was a businessman, was often away from home and—he says—"he could not take care of his marriage in a proper way." His bad mood was an allusion to the resemblance between his situation and that of his father when he was about his age, and a warning to take care of his family better than his father did. What could disclose the enigma of his bad mood was grasping the relation between his bad mood, being often away from home, and the analogies between his present situation and his father's when he was about his age, through the resemblance between his own and his father's image in the elevator. He could get a panoramic view over all these phenomena, see their connections—the bonds that tie each element of the story with the others. This patient could now see himself, his own present situation, from the vantage point of his father's story. He could also discover in himself his father as the alterity that was haunting him—his father as a destiny to be avoided. "Only after making these connections"—he once said—"I realized that my bad mood was the way through which all this was revealed.

My feeling shaky, wobbly, unsteady was indeed an admonition: 'Give yourself a form, a form different from that of your father!'"

This is a kind of understanding that "seeks to find the logos of the phenomena in themselves, not in underlying subpersonal mechanisms" (Fuchs 2008, p. 280). What can reveal the mystery of things is their mutual dependence—"the articulation of our field" (Merleau-Ponty 1964, p. 231), the architectural plan of the world over there? This is not simply a spatial arrangement; rather, it is a semantic ordering of things whose center is the *flesh* of the person who is seeing them—i.e., his being an embodied and situated agent, in the case reported earlier, the image of his body in a mirror. Things acquire their semantic order through the relations they have with each other and with my own lived body. We need to make visible the otherwise invisible texture of the world we inhabit. But this is just the first step of this process of unfolding, whose final aim is rescuing that which *makes the appearance of things possible*—the invisible (unconscious) existential pivot of our experiences, the *punctum caecum* of the self, what the self does not see in itself, and makes it possible for it to see, the backbone, the scaffolding, the spatiotemporal framework of the self, that derives from the sedimentation of all (voluntary and involuntary) experiences.

The key-question then is the following: How can this invisible (transcendental) structure become visible *for me*? Merleau-Ponty's answer is that it *cannot* become visible via an act of reflection of the self on itself; rather, it becomes perspicuous as the organization of the world *in front of me*. If I want to see the transcendental framework of my experience, I must turn my gaze away from my "mind," and also from the "world" as it appears in straightforward cognition, and look for the world's spatiotemporal architecture that lies in between the phenomena. Phenomenological understanding is a kind of knowledge "informed by an *explication* of the implicit constitutive structures of conscious experience" (Fuchs 2008, p. 280). The texture of the world bears the traces of this invisible transcendental structure. This means that if we want to rescue the implicit (unconscious) generating "vortex" that makes things appear as they appear to us, it must not be looked for in one's own depth, *behind* our own awareness, but *in front of us* (Merleau-Ponty 1964).

The symptom, then, in the phenomenological-hermeneutic paradigm is an *anomaly*, but not an abnormal, aberrant or *insane* phenomenon in strict sense. Rather, it is a salience, a knot in the texture of a person's life-world, like a *tear in the matrix*. It is a place that attracts someone's attention, which catches one's eyes, and awakens one's care for oneself in a double sense: since it reflects and reveals alterity in oneself—in it alterity becomes conspicuous; and since from the vantage it offers one can see oneself from another, often radically different and new, perspective.

THe Grammar of the Psychiatric Interview

Another key question (closely tied to the previous one) concerns the *family of instruments* in use during the interview. This question deserves an articulated analysis since different, and sometimes conflicting, paradigms are at play. There are three kinds of approaches, usually described as first-, second-, and third-person mode of interviewing (Stanghellini 2007).

Third-person approach

We have seen the third-person approach at work when describing the technical paradigm of psychiatric interviewing. This is often taken as a standard of scientific discourse for its emphasis on objectivity, detachment and quantification. The aim of the third-person approach is not to understand human subjectivity but to *explain* symptoms, and especially abnormal behaviors, i.e., reducing them to (or seeing them as mere epiphenomena of) a-priori-fixed subpersonal causes. "Explanation" (*Erklaerung*) means connecting a phenomenon with its cause(s) (*scire per causas*) and this is customarily the kind of knowledge in circulation in the natural sciences. Explanation orients knowledge in an outer space, outside the person's experience. Its focus is mainly on properties that do not belong to the patient's experiential field and is sometimes called "subpersonal," since these properties reside outside the field of personal conscious experience, and belong to our internal machinery—to goings on in our bodies, limbs, brains. They dwell in the pre-phenomenal (e.g., cognitive unconscious mechanisms) or the trans-phenomenal (e.g., neurological substrate), or else in the trans-personal (e.g., social dynamics and constraints) sphere. Explanation must be clearly distinguished from "explication" (*Auslegung*) that means displaying or unfolding the manifold of phenomena and their interrelation through language; and from "interpretation" (*Deutung*) which is the appropriation of a text by a reader.

The point of anchorage of the third-person approach in human subjectivity is narrow, often confined to the assessment of behaviors and expressions, since these are considered more reliably assessable features than personal experiences (see, e.g., Andreasen 1989). Its main limitations have been reviewed in the paragraph on the criticisms to the technical interview. It is worth adding here that the third-person approach tends to support the hegemony of vision over hearing. Indeed, it is tightly linked to the visual language of neuroimaging and its epistemology that privileges spatialization. It also promotes the spectatorial distance between viewing subject and viewed object, non-reciprocity since it denies that the "observer" and the "observed" belong to the same life-world, and de-narratization since it overshadows the relevance of personal history.

First-person (subjectivist) approach

The first-person approach is mainly centered on the *empathic understanding* of the other's experience. Empathy is a special kind of intentional experience in which my perception of the other leads me to grasp (or to feel that I grasp) his personal experience, e.g., his emotions, and to feel that and how he is an embodied person like me, animated by his own feelings and sensations and capable of voluntary movements and of expressing his experience. The intentional movement entailed in the experience of empathy is twofold: either I may (temporarily) feel that I incorporate the other's way of experiencing, or I may feel that I am transposed to the place or into the body of the other. In both cases, empathy implies a special kind of immediate resonance between my self (and especially my embodied self) and the one of the other person, and through this I feel that I understand him.

Usually, empathy does not require any voluntary and explicit effort. We may call this type of empathy, which is at play since the first seconds of our life, *non-conative*—a kind of spontaneous and pre-reflexive attunement between embodied selves through which we implicitly make sense of the other's behavior (Stern 2000). But in some cases the other's behavior becomes elusive. In these situations, while we deliberately put forward all our efforts to thematically understand the other (which may be called *conative* empathy), we also experience the limitations of this mode of understanding, In some cases—maybe the most relevant in clinical practice—we do not feel immediately in touch with the other, we do not immediately grasp the reasons and meaning of his actions, and thus purposively and knowingly attempt to put ourselves in his place. While performing this act of imaginative self-transposal we experience the radical otherness of the other. In this vein, early clinical phenomenologists (like Jaspers) and early psychoanalysts (like Freud) disclaimed empathy as a legitimate tool for understanding psychotic people's subjectivity.

This frustrating experience of the limitations of conative empathy is not the only motive for questioning the validity of empathy as a sound method to access the other's subjectivity. Whereas non-conative empathy mainly implies the resonance between my and the other's lived body as a means of understanding, conative empathy requires something more than a resonating body: it puts into play my personal past experiences and my personal knowledge of commonly shared experiences (common sense). Conative empathy is then a more cognitive and reflective task than immediate non-conative empathy, in which I actively look inside myself for stored experiences to make them resonate with those of the other. It implies a kind of understanding *by analogy.* An important epistemological concern arises here: How do I know that I am not projecting my own experiences onto the other?

In particular, understanding psychotic experiences like schizophrenic ones requires a kind of training that goes beyond non-conative, spontaneous and naïf empathic skills, and at the same time avoids the pitfalls of conative empathy based on the clinician's personal experiences and common-sense categories. The clinician's empathic capacities need some kind of education. In the clinical setting we cannot simply rely on standard empathic capacities. I suggest naming *second-order empathy* the method required to grasp those experiences that are not understandable via simply transposing oneself into another person and by doing so directly experience the "contagion" of belief and feeling (Golde 1970). To achieve second-order empathy is a complex process. First, I need to acknowledge that the life-world inhabited by the other person is not like my own. The supposition that the other lives in a world like my own—that is, that he lives time, space, his own body, others, the materiality of objects etc. just like I do—is often the source of serious misunderstanding. Take the example of lived time: existential time—as Erwin Straus (1967) wrote—cannot be detached from the life and history of the individual. One day for a young man can be lived as growth and fulfillment, whereas an old man may live it as consumption and decline. An anxious person may be afflicted by the feeling that time vanishes, inexorably passes away, that the time that separates her from death is intolerably shortened. Another patient in an early stage of schizophrenia may experience time as the dawn of a new reality, an eternally pregnant "now" in which what is most important is not present, what is really relevant is not already there, but is forever about to happen.

In order to empathize with these persons I must acknowledge the ontological difference which separates me from the way of being in the world that characterizes each of them. Any forgetting of this ontological difference, for instance between my own world and that of an anxious or a schizophrenic patient (but I would say, also, *mutatis mutandis* between my own and an adolescent's or an old man's world), will be an obstacle to empathic understanding, since these people live in a life-world whose structure is (at least in part) different from my own. Achieving second-order empathy thus requires bracketing my own pre-reflexive, natural attitude (in which my first-order empathic capacities are rooted), and approaching the other's world as I would do while exploring an unknown and alien country.

Second-person (intersubjectivist) approach

How can we improve the validity of first-person understanding, avoiding the risk that our first-person methodology "become[s] purely private or even solipsistic" (Varela and Shear 1999)? One possibility is that we turn to the second-person, intersubjective mode of understanding. The radical move that distinguishes the intersubjectivist approach from the subjectivist one is the presupposing of differences rather than merely analogies between my world and that of the other. More precisely, its prerequisites are both the awareness of a reciprocal extraneousness, and the awareness of belonging to a shared horizon of a common humanity. I am asked to bracket (which does not mean suspending but rather neutralizing by becoming aware of) my personal experiences and commonsense knowledge while approaching the other's world; and to explore it as if it were a world in which different categories are at work.

The guidelines for this exploration are the so-called *existentialia* (Heidegger 1962), its aim being the reconstruction of the other's lived world by grasping the form in which his experience is set in time and space, the mode in which he experiences his own body and others, and the way the physiognomy of material things appears to his senses. This reconstruction is obviously the outcome of a dialogue between interviewer and interviewee. The intersubjectivist approach envisions understanding not as the effect of the internal actualization in the interviewer of the interviewee's experience, but rather as the outcome of an exchange which posits knowledge of the other in an intersubjective, non-dogmatic, contextually sensitive and ongoing milieu. Thus understanding in this context is the point of intersection of two subjectivities that takes place in language. Its final aim is a shared narrative.

Of course, a kind of falsification is also at risk in co-constructing personal narratives, and in particular in attempting to realize the "fusion of horizons" between interviewer and interviewee and in the presupposition of sharing a common language. However, contrary to the third- and first-person mode of interviewing, here the differences between interviewer and interviewee can be a strength rather than a weakness—provided that difference and not only analogy is presupposed—since "in a true dialogue, the mirroring effect of question and answer, or give and take, produces a richer and more developed truth than was there before" (Jay 1989, p. 69) Also significant is that within the framework of the inter-subjectivist mode of understanding one seeks truth *in* words, in the way they are used to *approximate* internal or external reality. Rather than presuming that words *mirror* an observed object, they are seen as an index of the way the person appropriates an experience. Thus the object of the intersubjectivist approach is not experience per se (e.g., a perceived object or a felt emotion), but rather the way it is grasped and conveyed in language. In more radical terms, "*[a]ll that can be understood is language*" (Gadamer 2004, p. 474).

Much work in this area has been done in cultural anthropology and ethnography. This is the way ethnographer Rabinow (1977, p. 155) puts it: "Fieldwork […] is a process of intersubjective construction of liminal modes of communication. Intersubjective means literally more than one subject […]. [T]he subjects involved do not share a common set of assumptions, experiences or traditions. Their reconstruction is a public process." Rabinow depicts here the meeting of two alien worlds, using the language of separatedness and distance. The rapport between interviewer and interviewee is one of co-presence: a relevant consequence of this is the reduction of the power of the interviewer because of the transformation of his relationship with the other from a subject–object relation to a subject–subject partnership. In this context, interviewing means negotiating a cross-cultural construct, and looking for meaningfulness is connecting two distant horizons of meanings. Italian philosopher and ethnographer De Martino (1962/2002) asserts that in the encounter with a different culture pretending to be neutral is unfair and hypocritical; understanding implies a double thematization of myself and of the other; and questioning my own categories is not an abdication to relativism but a critical re-appropriation of them. He called this approach *critical ethnocentrism*.

Anthropological studies can provide an alternative and helpful way of thinking about the psychiatrist–patient encounter, emphasizing that each encounter with a patient is also the meeting with a separate culture, with an alter or alien way of being in the world. Cultural-anthropologic and ethnographic studies are a fitting metaphor for the clinical interview: as is the case with the ethnologist, (i) the cultural orientation of the clinician, even before influencing the formulation of the diagnosis and the attribution of meaning to certain signs and symptoms, has already come into play in the selection of the elements that are clinically relevant; (ii) the clinician cannot refrain from applying labels, first of all because in so doing he would be abdicating his role as specialist; secondly, because he needs a language to synthetically transmit and to translate into practice the knowledge that he has accumulated; (iii) the clinician can "improve—*by measuring*—the very units of measurement and the very tools for measuring" (De Martino 1977, p. 273) that he has at his disposal, and by re-establishing his own categories of evaluation through a systematic comparison of that which he knows and lives and the knowledge and lived experience of the other; (iv) the awareness that it is the clinician's own point of view that is assumed in the therapeutic setting allows him to displace his gaze, thereby making it possible to validate another vision, and to avoid leveling the other while he goes on along his own logical-emotional path; (v) finally, establishing an analogy between the ethnographic and the clinical encounter prevents us from uncritically accepting the view that the clinician and the other have of reality and in which they may feel entrapped.

This practice of negotiation and critical integration between "myself and the other" improves both narrative validity and clinical utility: it validates clinical narratives, avoiding that any kind of understanding becomes private or solipsistic, and it improves their clinical utility, kindling the patient's double thematization of his own narrative's background assumptions and his recognition of the therapist's and of common-sense or scientific knowledge about his (the patient's) behaviors and experiences. The upshot of this is an empowerment of the patient's intentionality, i.e., his capacity to adopt a *reflexive stance* over the feel and the meaning(s) of his experiences, thus reinforcing his subjective and inter-subjective sense of being a self.

THE MEANINGS OF PSYCHOPATHOLOGY

In this section I discuss the relevance of the discipline of psychopathology for the psychiatric interview. In 1913 Karl Jaspers published his psychiatric *opus magnum—General*

Psychopathology (Jaspers 1997). Jaspers was working at a time of rapid expansion in depth psychologies and (like our own) of the neurosciences and responded to the philosophical challenges that this raised. The idea inspiring his book was very simple: to bring order into the chaos of abnormal psychic phenomena by rigorous description and classification, and to empower psychiatry with a valid and reliable method for exploration of abnormal human subjectivity.

Now, as in Jaspers' times, the importance of psychopathology for psychiatry is threefold: psychopathology is the common language that allows psychiatrists to understand each other while talking about patients; it is the ground for classification and diagnosis; and it makes an indispensable contribution to understanding patients' personal experiences. For each of these aims we can distinguish a corresponding specialty or subarea of psychopathology (Stanghellini 2009a). *Descriptive psychopathology*, the *koiné* of psychiatry that allows specialists belonging to different school to understand each other, whose main purpose is to systematically study conscious experiences, order and classify them, and create valid and reliable terminology. *Clinical psychopathology*, a pragmatic tool for connecting relevant symptoms to diagnostic categories, thus restricts the scope of the clinical investigation to those symptoms that are useful for establishing a reliable diagnosis. *Structural psychopathology*, which looks for a global level of intelligibility, which assumes that the manifold of phenomena of a given mental disorder constitutes a meaningful whole, and which searches for meaningful units rather than subpersonal dysfunctions.

Descriptive psychopathology

Descriptive psychopathology is the common language that allows specialists each speaking their own dialect or jargon to understand each other. It consists of "the precise description and categorization of abnormal experiences as recounted by the patient and observed in his behavior" (Oyebode 2008, p. 4). Its "breeding ground" is the work of Karl Jaspers and the Heidelberg School (Janzarik 1976/1987). Descriptive psychopathology gives a concrete description of the psychic states which patients actually experience; it delineates and differentiates them as sharply as possible; and it creates a suitable terminology. The main objects of descriptive psychopathology are the patients' experiences. The form in which these experiences is presented is considered more significant than their contents. Perceptions, ideas, judgments, feelings, drives, and self-awareness are all forms of psychic phenomena, denoting the particular mode of existence in which a content is presented to us.

Interviewing a patient following the spirit of descriptive psychopathology involves relying on two main methodological assumptions: avoiding theoretical explanations and interpretations, and the centrality of empathic or first-person understanding (Jaspers 1997). Avoiding all theoretical prejudices is the quintessential methodological as well as ethical (i.e., maximum respect for the person as a subject of experience) prerequisite of descriptive psychopathology. Descriptive psychopathology is not concerned with any subsidiary speculations, psychological constructions, interpretations or evaluations, but solely with the phenomena that are present to the patient's consciousness. Everything that is not a conscious datum is considered non-essential. Descriptive psychopathology attempts to use empathy as a special kind of intentional experience through which the clinician tries to recreate in himself the subjective experience of a patient to obtain a valid and reliable description of it. In Jaspers' sense, descriptive psychopathology is methodologically based on the intuitive presentation of the other person's mental life through first-person understanding of his experiences. Since we cannot directly perceive the experiences of the other person, descriptive psychopathology attempts to make a representation of them based on the patients' own self-descriptions.

Clinical psychopathology

Clinical psychopathology is the doctrine bridging symptoms and diagnosis, essentially aimed at identifying those symptoms which are significant in view of nosographical distinctions (Schneider 1959). It is the ground for diagnosis and classification in a field like psychiatry where all major conditions are not etiologically defined disease entities, but exclusively clinically defined syndromes. Restricting the task of the interview to the search for pathognomonic, or clinically relevant, symptoms is the hallmark of clinical psychopathology (Lanteri-Laura 1985; Rossi Monti and Stanghellini 1996). The dominant focus on classifications and diagnosis (Broome 2008; Oulis 2008) of present-day psychiatry encourages an emphasis on the approach of clinical rather than descriptive psychopathology. This is probably a misunderstanding of Schneider's (the father of clinical psychopathology) legacy, since to Schneider psychopathological symptoms are conceived as "floating buoys" useful for clinical navigation, rather than as the exclusive focus for the clinician. Also, to Schneider psychopathological "symptoms" are not symptoms in the same sense of biomedicine (epiphenomena of a given etiology)—rather they are "characteristics" that may become criteria when it is established which of them are necessary and sufficient to justify a certain diagnosis (Kraus 1994). The approach of descriptive psychopathology tends to expand, rather than restrict, the area of relevant phenomena, suggesting that the psychiatric interview should "account for every psychic phenomenon" rather than resting "satisfied with a general impression or a set of details collected ad hoc" (Jaspers 1997, p. 56). By contrast, clinical psychopathology, as it was received and incorporated in current criteriological diagnostic manuals, goes in the opposite direction. As a consequence, clinical utility is confined to ad hoc bits of information useful for clinical decision-making. This excludes the scrutiny of the manifold manifestations of what is really there in the patients' experience—the essential methodological and ethical prerequisite to understand the worlds they live in.

Structural psychopathology

Structural thinking belongs to the mature phase of the evolution of psychiatry as a science (Lanteri-Laura 1998). Structural psychopathology goes beyond the description of isolated symptoms and the use of some of those symptoms to establish a diagnosis. It aims to understand the meaning of a given world of experiences and actions, grasping the underlying characteristic modification that keeps the symptoms meaningfully interconnected. Structural psychopathology assumes that the manifold of phenomena of a given mental disorder is a meaningful whole. The symptoms of a syndrome are supposed to have a meaningful coherence. One can find, and should look for, internal links between the various aspects of a person's experience and actions. Displaying this structure reveals how the parts that are present at a given moment stand in a relationship to each other of reciprocal expression. The most impressive example of a structure is a melody, which is made of the reciprocal rapport between its notes, and not of isolated notes. To change one note is to alter the whole melody. If one wants to keep the melody intact and transposes one note to the higher octave, one also needs to transpose all the other notes, since what counts here is the rapport between each note and all the others (Lanteri-Laura 1998).

Thinking of a syndrome as a structure is a clear invitation to look for meaningfulness within the elements of the syndrome itself, avoiding an assumption of external elements. Thus, the concept of structure bears close analogies with the hermeneutic concept of "text" described earlier. Danish linguist Hjelmslev succinctly defines a structure as "an autonomous entity of internal dependences" (Hjelmslev 1971, p. 28). This reflects the idea that a structure, as with the text, has an internal, immanent *sense*. "Autonomous entity" refers to the assumption that meaningfulness can be found in the structure itself, without involving elements that do not belong to the structure that can overwrite personally structured meanings. For instance, antecedent events should not be used to explain some bits of the structure as is the case with traumatic or genetic explanation (e.g., when dissociation of consciousness is understood as a consequence of an early experience of abandonment). "Internal dependences" refers to the assumption that meaningfulness emerges from the internal links between the elements of the structure. For instance, one should avoid symbolic or paradigmatic interpretation (e.g., when enjoying burning a tree is to be understood as enjoying burning a phallus).

All this may have serious implications for the recording of relevant facts and for making sense of them, perhaps the most important being the danger of eliminating time and history from the horizon of the psychiatric interview and encouraging a purely synchronic, a-temporal approach. Is there a space for the diachronic dimension of narratives in structural thinking? In the following section I will try to answer this question and to integrate the legacy of structural psychopathology into the overall process of the psychiatric interview as it results from the ideas gathered throughout this chapter.

FIVE LEVELS OF MEANINGFULNESS

A tentative, philosophically-rich, and phenomenologically-hermeneutically oriented framework for the assessment of mental abnormal phenomena includes five steps corresponding to five levels of meaningfulness.

Unfolding the phenomena of the life-world and rescuing its implicit structure

The first step considered here is *unfolding* the details of a given psychopathological world as a text—the explication of the case material. Unfolding means to exposit, open up, lay bare the pleats, creases, or corrugations of a text. The opposite of this is to garble, pervert, distort, twist/stretch/strain the text itself. What comes into sight is the *texture* that is immanent in the text itself, although it may remain invisible to or unnoticed by the author. Explication enriches understanding by providing further resources in addition to those which are immediately visible. The product of unfolding is a *text* that reflects the phenomenal world, the world as it appears to the subject of experience (Stanghellini 2007), including all those details that resist standard semiological classification. In a given psychopathological text, there is much more than what can be mapped using the catalogue of psychopathological symptoms (like phobias, formal thought disorders, or delusions).

The aim of this process is to rescue the *logos* of the phenomena in themselves, by "bringing unnoticed material into consciousness"—as Jaspers (1997, p. 307) would put it. The *logos* that is immanent in the intertwining of phenomena is called *sense*, i.e., the internal coherence between the clinical (as well as subclinical and existential) phenomena found in a given condition of suffering. Phenomenological psychopathology advocates the idea that the phenomena embedded in a given (normal or abnormal) form of existence are a meaningful whole. This has an important clinical implication. Whereas the standard understanding of the concept of "syndrome" in psychiatry is one which views it as a cluster of symptoms which happen to hang together not by any mutual phenomenological implication, but by their being otherwise unrelated effects of a common neurobiological cause, this alternative perspective has it that the manifold of (abnormal) phenomena in a syndrome are meaningfully interconnected, that is, they form a *structure*. A psychopathological syndrome is not simply a casual association of (abnormal) phenomena. To have a phenomenological grasp on these phenomena is to grasp the structural nexus that lend coherence and continuity to them, because each phenomenon in a psychopathological structure carries the traces of the underlying formal alterations of subjectivity.

Although this discourse is imbued with visual metaphors, it is important to note that this process of unfolding is profoundly rooted in hearing—or even better: *listening and dialoguing*—and in the power of the spoken word. The kind of seeing implied in this practice is—to adopt Levin's (1988) distinction—"aletheic" rather than "assertoric" since it is "multiple, aware of its context, inclusionary, horizontal and caring" (Jay 1993, p. 275). Hearing contributes to an ethics based on reciprocity and belonging, as well as to establishing a kind of knowledge focused on subjective experiences and personal narratives.

Rescuing the implicit structures of the self

The second stratum made visible by this process consists of the invisible conditions of possibility of the world disclosed in the first level. By rescuing the map of the world that is depicted in the text, we can approximate the architecture of the mind which projected it. This is an exploration of the implicit structures of experience, or into the *structures of the self* as the tacit and pre-reflexive conditions for the emergence of mental contents. It looks for the way the self must be structured to make phenomena appear as they appear to the *experiencing self*. Looking for structural relationships consists in the unfolding of the basic structure(s) of subjectivity, that is, the way the self appropriates phenomena. The guidelines for reconstructing the life-world a person lives in are the so called *existentialia*, namely, lived time, space, body, otherness, materiality, and so on (Heidegger 1962). In this way we can trace back this transformation of the life-world to a specific configuration of the embodied self as the origin of a given mode of inhabiting the world, perceiving, manipulating, and making sense of it. In order to grasp the transcendental framework of one's experience, one must turn one's gaze away from one's "mind," and also from the "world" as it appears in straight-forward cognition, and look for the world's spatiotemporal architecture which reflects it.

The reconstruction of the patient's life-world, and of the transcendental structures of his self, allows for the patient's behavior, expression and experience to become understanda-ble. An example of this could be taken from Conrad's (1966) analysis of the beginning of schizophrenia—*das Trema*, in Conrad's words—where behaviors look markedly inappro-priate and incomprehensible if seen from the angle of commonsense. To make the patient's comportments understandable, one must first unfold the phenomena of his life world and then rescue its implicit structure. To the patient everything feels strange, ominous, uncan-nily transformed. Reality has undergone some inexplicable, ineffable, ungraspable change. The world is suspended between meaninglessness and the imminent revelation of a new meaningfulness; it is pervaded by a kind of latent meaningfulness, having lost its habitual familiarity, and not yet acquired a new kind of significance. The patient's mood is a paradoxi-cal mixture of anguish, hope, despair, and suspicion. What kind of deep metamorphosis has the structure of the lived world undergone? Which changes in the structure of the self make possible this deep metamorphosis of the life world? It has been suggested that what is essen-tial to the beginning schizophrenia is a dissolution of one's familiar way to experience *space*. In normal conditions, the things present in the surrounding space are distributed according to a hierarchical order: only a few of them are in the foreground, while all the others remain unperceived in the background. This hierarchical order of things in space makes things in the background neutral and those in the foreground significant. Space is experienced as a structure of salience or relevance organized around the vital necessities of the embodied self.

In the trema stage, "the neutrality of the background gets lost." Lived space grows flat. Nothing is salient and evident anymore. The particularity of this experience is that the patient is not struck by what is actually happening but by what is not happening, e.g., not by what people do or say, but by what they don't do or say (Berner 1991). "The intermedi-ate spaces between the visible and what remains behind, all what is impalpable is no longer uncanny (...) What makes us tremble are not the trees and the bushes that we see, nei-ther is it the whisper in the treetops nor the ululate of the owl that we hear, rather all what constitutes the background, all the surrounding space from which trees and bushes, whis-per and ululate arise: they are precisely *the very obscurity and background*" (Conrad 1966, p. 41). The patient—it has been noted (Berner 1991)—behaves like an anxious child walking through a wood. His behavior (otherwise inappropriate and incomprehensible) becomes understandable in the light of this deep metamorphosis of lived space. This metamorphosis of the life-world discloses a profound change in the structures of the self. First and foremost the self organizes space according to the vital needs of the lived body in which it is rooted. This anchoring of the self in the lived body is lost in the early stages of schizophrenia (Sass and Parnas 2003; Stanghellini 2008), and the capacity to organize space as a structure of sali-ence and relevance is therefore also lost.

Narrating the transcendental origin of the life-world

This kind of practice connecting a given experience (abnormal or not) with its transcen-dental condition of possibility may have etiological or pathogenetic implications, thus link-ing the research on *meanings* to that on *causes* of mental symptoms. The path to genetic understanding in psychopathology was opened by Karl Jaspers, who described it as the "[i]nner, subjective, direct grasp of psychic connectedness" (Jaspers 1997, p. 307). Genetic understanding, according to Jaspers, is a kind of knowledge that establishes meaningful connections between psychic phenomena. Jaspers argued that psychic events emerge out of each other in a way which we can immediately understand. For instance, we immediately understand that attacked people become angry and spring to defense, or cheated person grow suspicious. The philosophical paragon inspiring Jaspers is Nietzsche's understanding of morality as connected to weakness: the awareness of one's weakness, wretchedness and suffering gives rise to moral demands and religion because in this roundabout way the psyche can gratify its will to power. Jaspers offers several examples of genetic understanding in psychopathology, among them psychic reactions and the development of passions. Jaspers insists on the character of immediateness and self-evidence in the grasping meaningful connections in someone's life. To him, genetic understanding in psychopathology "is a precondition of the psychology of meaningful phenomena (. . .) just as the reality of perception and of causality is the precondition of the natural sciences" (Jaspers 1997, p. 303).

Husserl also developed, beyond static or descriptive phenomenology, another kind of genetic or constructive phenomenology that he called "explanatory" (for recent discussion see Sass 2010). This is a kind of *developmental* or diachronic understanding studying the way complex modes of experience are constituted via the synthesis of more basic modes or lived experiences. The key dispositive of Husserl's explanatory phenomenology is motivation or motivational causality. It has been argued that "analyzing the basic constitution and explicating the implicit structure of experience, phenomenology offers another way of developmental understanding: it allows for a comprehension of the prereflective dimension of experience [. . .] from which manifest symptoms arise" (Parnas and Sass 2008, p. 280). In this way, the phenomenologically-informed psychiatric interview moves beyond pure description and static understanding toward "an understanding of both the overall unity of that person's subjectivity and its development over time" (Parnas and Sass 2008, p. 264). This kind of narrative, based on the understanding of the basic architecture of the life-world, and on the structures of subjectivity which allegedly generate them, may allow us to both make sense (rescue the personal *meaning*) and explain (rescue the *motivation*) of a given symptom, be it an action or a belief. An example of genetic phenomenology comes from the studies of symptom progression in schizophrenia (Klosterkoetter 1988). For instance, it has been demonstrated that patients who experience abnormal bodily sensations may later develop a delusion of alien control over their own body. Feelings of extraneousness, or numbness, or non-existence of parts of one's own body, sensations of paralysis, heaviness, abnormal lightness, of shrinking or enlargement, of movement or traction, etc.—occurring abruptly in early stages of schizophrenia, often migrating from one organ or bodily zone to another—may lead to typically schizophrenic symptoms like delusions of alien control. Delusions of being controlled, i.e., the most "bizarre" symptom of schizophrenia, become understandable as motivated by the patients' need to explain their disturbing changes in bodily experiences.

Appropriation (by the clinician) of the patient's life-world

The fourth level of meaningfulness made manifest by this exploration is the world that the text opens up in the patient when it is *appropriated* by the interviewer. The clinician "appropriates" the sense of the patient's experience and suggests his view of it. To appropriate a text means to acknowledge the way the text belongs to the reader, the way the reader *could inhabit it*. It is an attempt at reducing the distance between the text and its reader. If the *interpretandum* were completely extraneous, the understanding enterprise would be condemned to a checkmate, and if it were completely familiar, there would be no sense in making an effort at interpretation. The interviewer makes explicit his understanding *as his own*, that is, the vantage point from which he sees the interviewee's situation. This implies, in fact, a tension between extraneousness and familiarity. In this way, and only in this way, the interviewer may become a "You" for his interviewee. The interviewer appropriates the interviewee's world by means of his own imagination when he tries to reply to the question: "To make sense of the patient's otherwise absurd and otherwise meaningless behavior, I must imagine myself as if I were living in a world that has the following characteristics." This approximation to the patient's life-world is carried out by the clinician via as-if experiments which are *metaphorically* expressed.

One example of this is constructing the schizophrenic condition as a *disembodied* type of existence. A schizophrenic person describes a special kind of depersonalization experience: he perceives his body not as a living body, rather as a functioning body, a thing-like mechanism in which feelings, perceptions, and actions take place as if they happened in an outer space. It can be argued that the essential feature of schizophrenic existence is its being disembodied. This is the feature that unifies the varied dimensions of that existence. The disembodiment of the self, of the self-object relation and of interpersonal relationships all lead to a kind of world in which the schizophrenic person lives and behaves like a soulless body or a disembodied spirit (Stanghellini 2009b). The clinician may try to approximate the patient's experience and establish a dialogue with this by saying: "What you are telling me is what I would feel if I were a 'deanimated body' feeling distant from myself and lifeless." Or: "If I try to understand your experience and put myself in your shoes I feel as a 'disembodied spirit,' that is painfully aware of myself as if I were displaced from myself, observing me from without, from another place."

Grasping the *importance* of the patient's life-world

We have seen that the meanings that we find in a text may exceed the intention of the author. This is the case with the parapraxis, and more generally for any kind of symptom. By unfolding the structures of a text, we can understand an author better than the author himself. Also, during this process of unfolding, the text lays in front of its author who can adopt a third-person stance over the text itself—and in the case of the symptom the patient can take a reflexive stance over the feel and the meaning of his experience, thus reinforcing his subjective and intersubjective sense of being a self. The *importance* of a text reaches beyond this level of understanding and discloses the mode of being in the world of that individual patient as a universal problem. It reveals the way his existence belongs to human existence as a whole, to the *condicio humana*. The text may display meanings that transcend the situation in which the text was produced. To grasp the importance of a text is to unfold "the revelatory power implicit in his discourse, beyond the limited horizon of his own existential situation" (Ricoeur 1981, p. 191). The importance of a text is what "goes 'beyond' its relevance to the initial situation" (Ricoeur 1981, p. 207). In virtue of its importance, a text acquires a universal (not merely contingent) meaning, and its author embodies a universal problem (he stops being a merely contingent sufferer).

As an example of this we once again take the case of a person with schizophrenia. Schizophrenia reveals the human condition of eccentricity, that is of chronic decentralization and depersonalization. Schizophrenic persons feel *à coté* with respect to their own body, their mental processes and the social world. In particular, the position of a person with schizophrenia in the social world can be seen as reflecting his fragile anchoredness in common sense, the bracketing of ready-made social roles and rules and the tendency to be placed out of the boundaries of the social game. The schizophrenic is an existentially-vulnerable person since he is weakly anchored to common sense, and as a result he finds it difficult to adjust to social norms. The formation of an individual as a member of a Community requires a dialectical training, an oscillation between oneself and the Other, between one's own individuality and the alienation in the *corpus* of social rules. Our identity develops within this assimilation-differentiation dialectic, which is often stormy. The condition of *eccentricity* is the root of liberty, as well as of madness. The pre-requisite for liberty is the capacity to bracket the pre-established representations of the world (our common-sense knowledge), without losing our historical articulation with the common world. In the context of this eccentricity drama, we need both the capacity for distantiation and for assimilation—dialectically inter-related. But the pass between assimilation and differentiation is quite narrow. The importance of the schizophrenic condition is that it shows us what we have to lose if this dialectic gets polarized into one of the two extremes. As Binswanger (1957) had foreseen, psychosis is the failure to lead oneself between these two extremes, resulting in the subsequent pulling back of the antinomic tensions of living. Schizophrenic persons find intolerable the attrition by these tensions: they split up existence into rigid alternatives, and end up with withdrawing into a private world. The schizophrenic condition brings to its extreme the human condition, that is, of a cast off, both in terms of the aspirations and projects lying in wait in each of our private worlds, as well as in terms of the expectations and norms that regulate the societal life and the common world.

CONCLUSIONS

The psychiatric interview is not merely a clinical problem; rather, it may be considered a philosophical problem. By this I mean that there is a need for a philosophically-rich approach to the psychiatric interview, especially for the task of exploring the patient's subjectivity. There are many reasons for this. The most basic of them is that not every aspect of the science of the psyche can share the same kind of objectivity of the natural sciences. The objectivity we require from psychiatry depends on the nature of the phenomena under investigation in this discipline (Gabbani and Stanghellini 2008). A pathology of the psyche may have clear objective causes, i.e., biological bases, but such natural causes do not make of it simply a natural entity. This is not to deny the causal relevance of functional subagencies of our brain, but to insist that the assessment and the comprehension of a pathological psychic state requires a kind of analysis which exceeds the range of a naturalistic approach. Furthermore, a pathology is not simply an anomaly in the statistical sense at a functional or organic level: a strange deviation from normality would not represent in itself a pathology if this caused an experience felt by the person and recognized by others as a condition of well-being and judged as not being problematic in our shared form of life. A pathology of the psyche constitutes an experienced condition and a family of behaviors, emotions and beliefs, the peculiar significance of which first and foremost emerges within a personal history and a sociocultural context. Such a kind of pathology is, therefore, completely on view only because of what has been called the *personal level* of analysis. Only at this level, indeed, the real correlates of a psychopathological condition can be understood in their *peculiar feel, meaning and value* for the subjects affected by them (Stanghellini 2007).

In this chapter, I acknowledged the primacy of subjective experience over objective behavior. There are many reasons for this. First, subjective experiences are more specific phenomena to establish diagnosis. Second, a careful analysis of subjective experience is probably the only way at our disposal to make sense of otherwise odd and incomprehensible behavior. Last but not least, focusing on subjective experience may be more effective in guiding clinical work, including diagnostic procedures and therapeutic (pharmacotherapeutic, and even more so, psychotherapeutic) decision-making.

In endorsing the legacy of phenomenological psychopathology and its emphasis on the analysis of subjectivity by means of the first-person and second-person mode of understanding, I have sketched a framework for the psychiatric interview aimed to a wide-range, fine-grained assessment of the patient's morbid subjectivity, not constrained in a priori fixed schemata such as specific rating scales, that can be useful not only in the clinical, but also in the research setting. In the clinic this approach can provide the background for unfolding the phenomena of the life-world inhabited by the patient, including all those details that resist standard semiological classification; and it can rescue the architectural nexus that lends coherence and continuity to them. Phenomenological psychopathology assumes that the manifold of phenomena of a given mental disorder is supposed to have a meaningful coherence. Rather than being a mere aggregate of symptoms, they form a structure, i.e., a meaningful whole. Also, the method of phenomenological psychopathology is a prerequisite for moving beyond pure static description of the life-world toward the illumination of the structures of subjectivity that allegedly *generate and structure* the phenomenal world.

In research, it may prove helpful to rescue fringe abnormal phenomena that are not covered by those standard assessment procedures focused on symptoms relevant for nosographic diagnosis rather than on the reconstruction of the complexities of the patients' subjectivity and life-worlds. Thus it provides the basis for exploratory studies, for the assessment of real-world, first-personal experiences of subpersonal impairments since this approach is concerned with bringing forth the typical feature(s) of personal experiences in a given individual to establish objective, trans-personal constructs helpful for empirical research (Stanghellini and Ballerini 2008).

Also, reflection on the philosophical resources for the psychiatric interview may help to combat the hegemony of *de-narratization* in the mainstream biomedical model with its emphasis on matters of fact rather than on intelligible relations. Narrative reasoning is the ability to order the significance of our actions, experiences and beliefs above the level of the sentence, hence above the level of single experiences. Narratives are also the principal means to integrate the alterity of the symptoms into autobiographical memory, providing temporal and goal structure, combining personal experiences into a coherent story related to the self. Obviously, hermeneutics is a necessary complement to pure phenomenology in this context.

Hermeneutics is also important for re-thinking the relation between experience and language—a crucial issue for a discipline like psychiatry in which language is not simply a means of expression, but the *medium* in which the psychiatric interview takes place. The objectifying procedures of natural science, and their concept of objectivity, prove to be misleading when viewed the angle that all understanding is verbal. The idea of experience-in-itself is an abstraction. From the angle of hermeneutics, all personal experience is given in the linguistic medium, and from the angle of the second-person mode of understanding all that can be understood of another person's experience is a linguistic event—be it the other person's way of talking about his experience, or the way I re-enact through empathy his experiences in myself, since also my relation with my own "feel" is given in language.

Hermeneutic thinking is also helpful as an antidote to the *de-humanization* of psychiatry and of psychiatric patients. I have argued that the preliminary step is the unfolding of the phenomenal world the patient lives in, and the reconstruction of its invisible semantic ordering. The following step consists in the rescuing of the structures of subjectivity which project the world the patient lives in. A further step in the psychiatric interview is the *appropriation* by the clinician of the patient's life-world: to appropriate the patient's world means to acknowledge that it belongs to the clinician's ownmost possibilities as a vulnerable human being. Appropriation is not assimilation, since it preserves the tension between extraneousness and familiarity. Finally, the concept of *importance* stretches the meaning of a given mental symptom to its extremes. The way of being in the world of that individual patient transcends the concrete situation of the patient himself and can thus be envisioned as a universal problem since it belongs to human existence as such. The psychopathological condition of the patient unfolds its revelatory power, and acquires a universal meaning that sheds light on the *condicio humana*.

REFERENCES

Andreasen, N. A. (1989). Scale for the assessment of negative symptoms. *British Journal of Psychiatry*, 155 (7), 53–8.

Aristotle (1991). *The Metaphysics* (J. H. McMahon, Trans.). New York, NY: Prometheus Books.

Bayer, R. and Spitzer, R. S. (1985). Neurosis, psychodynamics, and DSM-III: History of the controversy. *Archives of General Psychiatry*, 42, 187–96.

Bell, J. (2010). *Redefining Disease: The Harveian Oration*. London: Royal College of Physicians.

Berner, P. (1991). Delusional atmosphere. *British Journal of Psychiatry*, 159(14), 88–93.

Berthold-Bond, D. (1995). *Hegel's Theory of Madness*. New York, NY: State of New York Press.

Binswanger, L. (1957). *Schizophrenie*. Pfullingen: Neske

Bollas, C. (2003). *Being a Character: Psychoanalysis and Self-Experience*. London: Routledge.

Brackel, L. A. W. (2009). *Philosophy, Psychoanalysis, and the A-Rational Mind*. Oxford: Oxford University Press.

Broome, M. (2008). Philosophy as the science of value: Neo-Kantianism as a guide to psychiatric interviewing. *Philosophy, Psychiatry, & Psychology*, 15, 107–16.

Conrad, J. (1966). *Die beginnende Schizophrenie*. Stuttgart: Thieme.

De Martino, E. (1977). *La Fine del Mondo*. Torino: Einaudi.

De Martino, E. (2002). Promesse e minacce dell'etnologia. In E. De Martino (Ed.), *Furore Simbolo Valore*, pp. 84–118. Milano: Feltrinelli. (Original work published 1962.)

Endicott, J. and Spitzer, R. (1978). A diagnostic interview schedule for affective disorders and schizophrenia. *Archives of General Psychiatry*, 35, 837–44.

Finn, S. E. and Tonsanger, M. E. (1997). Information gathering and therapeutic models of assessment: Complementary paradigms. *Psychological Assessment*, 9, 374–85.

Fonagy, P. and Target, M. (1997). Attachment and reflective function: their role in self-organization. *Development and Psychopathology*, 9, 679–700.

Foucault, M. (2003). *Le pouvoir psychiatrique*. Seuil: Gallimard.

Freud, S. (1905). *Three Essays on the Theory of Sexuality* (Standard edn, vol. 7). London: The Hogarth Press.

Freud, S. (1926). *Inhibition, Symptoms and Anxiety* (Standard edn, vol. 20). London: The Hogarth Press.

Fuchs, T. (2008). Comment: beyond descriptive phenomenology. In K. S. Kendler and J. Parnas (Eds), *Philosophical Issues in Psychiatry; Explanation, Phenomenology, and Nosology*, pp. 278–85. Baltimore, MD: Johns Hopkins University Press.

Gabbani, C. and Stanghellini, G. (2008). What kind of objectivity do we need for psychiatry? A commentary to Oulis' ontological commitments in psychiatric taxonomy. *Psychopathology*, 41, 203–4.

Gadamer, H. G. (2004). *Truth and Method* (2nd rev. edn) (J. Weinsheimer and D.G. Marshall, Trans.). New York, NY: The Continuum Publishing Company.

Golde, P. (1970). *Women in the Field*. Chicago, IL: Aldine.

Hegel, G. W. F. (1998). *Phenomenology of Spirit* (A. V. Miller, Trans.). Delhi: Motilal Banarsidass.

Heidegger, M. (1962). *Being and Time*. Oxford: Blackwell/Harper and Row.

Herran, A., Sierra-Biddle, D., de Santiago, A., Artal, J., Diez-Manrique, J. F., and Vazquez-Barquero, J. L. (2001). Diagnostic accuracy in the first five minutes of a psychiatric interview. *Psychotherapy psychosomatics*, 70, 141–4.

Hjelmslev, L. (1971). *Linguistic Essays*. Paris: Minuit.

Janzarik, W. (1987). Die Krise der Psychopathologie. In J. Cutting and M. Shepherd (Eds), *The Clinical Roots of Schizophrenia Concept*, pp. 134–43. Cambridge: Cambridge University Press. (Original work published 1976 in *Nervenarzt*, 47, 73–80).

Jaspers, K. (1997). *General Psychopathology* (J. Hoenig and M. W. Hamilton, Trans.). Baltimore, MD: The Johns Hopkins University Press.

Jay, M. (1989). The rise of hermeneutics and the crisis of ocularcentrism. In P. Hernadi (Ed.), *The Rhetoric of Interpretation and the Interpretation of Rhetoric*, pp. 55–74. Durham, NC: Duke University Press.

Jay, M. (1994). *Downcast Eyes. The Denigration of Vision in French Twentith Century Thought*. Berkeley and Los Angeles, CA: University of California Press.

Kirk, S. A. and Kutchins, H. (1992). *The Selling of the DSM: The Rhetoric of Science in Psychiatry*. New York, NY: Aldine de Gruyter.

Klosterkoetter, J. (1988). *Basissymptome und Endphaenomene der Schizophrenie*. Berlin: Springer.

Kraus, A. (1994). Phenomenological and criteriological diagnosis: different or complementary? In J. Z. Sadler, O. P. Wiggins, and M. A. Schwartz (Eds), *Philosophical perspectives in psychiatric diagnostic classification*, pp. 148–60. Baltimore, MD: John Hopkins University Press.

Kraus, A. (2003). How can the phenomenological-anthropological approach contribute to diagnosis and classification in psychiatry? In K. W. M Fulford, K. Morris, J. Z. Sadler, and G. Stanghellini (Eds), *Nature and narrative: An Introduction to the New Philosophy of Psychiatry*, pp. 199–216. Oxford: Oxford University Press.

Lacan, J. (2005). *Le Seminaire Livre XXIII. Le Synthome (1975–76)*. Paris: Seuil.

Lanteri-Laura, G. (1985). Psychopathologie et processus. *L'Evolution Psychiatrique, 50*, 589–610.

Lanteri-Laura, G. (1998). *Essay sur les Paradigms de la Psychiatrie Moderne*. Paris: Editions du Temps.

Lazarsfeld, P. (1935). The art of asking why: three principles underlying the formulation of questionnaires. *National Marketing Review, 1*, 26–38

Leoni, F. (2008). *Habeas Corpus. Sei Genealogie del Corpo Occidentale*. Milano: Bruno Mondadori.

Levin, D. M. (1988). *The Opening of Vision: Nihilism and the Postmodern Situation*. London: Routledge.

Lieberman, P. B. (1989). Objective methods and subjective experiences. *Schizophrenia Bulletin, 15*(2), 267–75.

Mackinnon, R. A., and Michels, R. (1971). *The Psychiatric Interview in Clinical Practice*. Philadelphia, PA: Saunders.

McDougall, J. (1996). *Theatres of the Body*. London: Free Association Books.

McGuffin, P. and Farmer, A. (2001). Polydiagnostic approaches to measuring and classifying psychopathology. *American Journal of Medical Genetics, 105*, 39–41.

Merleau-Ponty, M. (1945). *Phenomenology and Perception*. Paris: Gallimard.

Merleau-Ponty, M. (1964). *Le Visible et L'invisible*. Paris: Gallimard.

Miller, J.- A. (1998). *Le Symptôme-Charlatan, Textes Réunis par la Fondation du Champ Freudiaen*. Paris: Seuil.

Mishler, E. G. (1986). *Research Interviewing: Context and Narrative*. Cambridge. MA: Harvard University Press.

Othmer, E. and Othmer, S. C. (2002). *The Clinical Interview Using the DSM-IV, Vol.1: Fundamentals*. Washington, DC: American Psychiatric Publishing.

Oyebode, F. (2008). *Sim's Symptoms in the Mind. An Introduction to Descriptive Psychopathology*. Edinburgh: Saunders-Elsevier.

Oulis, P. (2008). Ontological assumptions of psychiatric taxonomy: main rival positions and their critical assessment. *Psychopathology, 41*, 135–40.

Panek, R. (2005). *The Invisible Century. Einstein, Freud, and the Search for Hidden Universes*. London: Penguin Books.

Parnas, J. and Sass, L. A. (2008). Varieties of 'phenomenology'. On description, understanding, and explanation in psychiatry. In K. S. Kendler and J. Parnas (Eds), *Philosophical Issues in Psychiatry; Explanation, Phenomenology, and Nosology*, pp. 239–78. Baltimore, MD: Johns Hopkins University Press.

Parnas, J. and Zahavi, D. (2002). The role of phenomenology in psychiatric diagnosis and classification. In M. Maj, W. Gaebel, J. J. Lopez-Ibor, and N. Sartorius (Eds), *Psychiatric Diagnosis and Classification*, pp. 137–62. Chichester: Wiley.

PDM Task Force (2006). *Psychodynamic Diagnostic Manual*. Silver Spring, MD: Alliance of Psychoanalytic Organizations.

Peters, L. and Andrews, G. (1995). The procedural validity of the computerized version of the Composite International Diagnostic Interview. *Psychological Medicine, 25*, 1269–80.

Pidgeon, N. (1996). Grounded theory: theoretical background. In J. Richardson (Ed.), *Handbook of Qualitative Research. Methods for Psychology and Social Science*, pp. 75–85. London: British Psychological Society.

Pidgeon, N. and Henwood, K. (1996). Grounded theory: Practical implementation. In J. T. Richardson (Ed.), *Handbook of Qualitative Research Methods for Psychology and the Social Sciences*, pp. 86–101. Leicester: British Psychological Society.

Pollock, D. C., Shanley, D. F., and Byrne, P. N. (1985). Psychiatric interviewing and clinical skills. *Canadian Journal of Psychiatry*, *30*(1), 64–8.

Rabinow, P. (1977). *Reflections on Fieldwork in Morocco*. Berkeley, CA: University of California Press.

Richardson, J. T. (Ed.) (1996). *Handbook of Qualitative Research Methods for Psychology and the Social Sciences*. Leicester: British Psychological Society.

Ricoeur, P. (1981). *Hermeneutics and the Human Sciences* (J. B. Thompson, Trans. and Ed.). Cambridge: Cambridge University Press.

Ricoeur, P. (1990). *Oneself as Another*. Chicago, IL: University of Chicago Press.

Ricoeur, P. (2004). *Parcours de la Reconnaissance*. Paris: Stock.

Rorty, R. (1981). *Philosophy and the Mirror of Nature*. Princeton, NJ: Princeton University Press.

Rosch, E. (1975). Cognitive reference point. *Cognitive Psychology*, *7*, 532–47.

Rossi Monti, M. and Stanghellini, G. (1996). Psychopathology: An edgeless razor? *Comprehensive Psychiatry*, *37*(3), 196–204.

Sadler, J. Z., Hulgus, Y. F., and Agich, G. J. (1994). On values in recent American psychiatric classification. *Journal of Medical Philosophy*, *19*, 261–77.

Sadler, J. Z., Wiggins, O. P., and Schwartz, M. A. (1994). *Philosophical Perspectives on Psychiatric Diagnostic Classification*. Baltimore, MD: Johns Hopkins University Press.

Sass, L. (2010). Phenomenology as descriptions and as explanation: The case of schizophrenia. In S. Gallagher and D. Schmicking (Eds), *Handbook of Phenomenology and the Cognitive Sciences*, pp. 635–54. Berlin: Springer.

Sass, L. and Parnas, J. (2003). Schizophrenia, consciousness, and the self. *Schizophrenia Bulletin*, *29*, 427–44

Schneider, K. (1959). *Clinical psychopathology* (5th edn). New York, NY: Grune & Stratton.

Schwartz, M. A. and Wiggins, O. P. (1987). Typifications: The first step for clinical diagnosis in psychiatry. *Journal of Nervous and Mental Disease*, *175*(2), 65–77.

Shea, C. S. (1988). *Psychiatric Interviewing: The Art of Understanding*. Philadelphia, PA: Saunders.

Shea, C. S. and Mezzich, E. J. (1988). Contemporary psychiatric interviewing: New directions for training. *Psychiatry*, *51*, 385–97.

Smolik, P. (1999) Validity of nosological classification. *Dialogues in Clinical Neuroscience. Special Issue Nosology and Nosography*, *1*(3) 185–90.

Spitzer, R. L. (1983). Psychiatric diagnosis: Are clinicians still necessary? *Comprehensive Psychiatry*, *24*(5), 399–411.

Spitzer, R. L. (2001). Values and assumptions in the development of DSM-III-R: an insider's perspective and a bleated response to Sadler, Hulgus, and Agich's "On values in recent American psychiatric classification." *Journal of Nervous & Mental Disease*, *189*(6), 351–9.

Stanghellini, G. (1997). *Antropologia della vulnerabilità*. Milano: Feltrinelli.

Stanghellini, G. (2004). The puzzle of the psychiatric interview. *Journal of Phenomenological Psychology*, *35*(2), 173–95.

Stanghellini, G. (2007). The grammar of psychiatric interview: a plea for the second person mode of understanding. *Psychopathology*, *40*, 69–74.

Stanghellini, G. (2008). *Psicopatologia del senso comune*. Milano: Raffaello Cortina Editore.

Stanghellini, G. (2009a). The meanings of psychopathology. *Current Opinion in Psychiatry*, *22*, 559–64.

Stanghellini, G. (2009b). Embodiment and schizophrenia. *World Psychiatry*, *8*, 56–9.

Stanghellini, G. (2010). A hermeneutic framework for psychopathology. *Psychopathology, 43*, 319–26.

Stanghellini, G. (2011). Phenomenology: A method for care? *Philosophy, Psychiatry, & Psychology, 18*(1) 25–9.

Stanghellini, G. and Ballerini, M. (2007). Values in persons with schizophrenia. *Schizophrenia Bulletin, 33*, 131–41.

Stanghellini, G. and Ballerini, M. (2008). Qualitative analysis. Its use in psychopathological research *Acta Psychiatrica Scandinavica, 117*, 161–3.

Stanghellini, G. and Lysaker P. H. (2007). The psychotherapy of schizophrenia through the lens of phenomenology: intersubjectivity and the search for the recovery of first- and second-person awareness. *American Journal of Psychotherapy, 61*, 163–79.

Stern, D. N. (2000). *The Interpersonal World of the Infant*. New York, NY: Basic Books.

Stevens, A., Doidge, N., Goldbloom, D., Voore, P., and Farewell, J. (1999). Pilot study of televideo psychiatric assessment in an underserviced community. *American Journal of Psychiatry, 156*, 783–85.

Straus, E. (1967). An existential approach to time. *Annals of the New York Academy of Sciences, 138*(2), 759–66.

Troisi, A. (2011). Mental health and wellbeing: Clinical applications of Darwinian psychiatry. In S. C. Roberts (Ed.), *Applied Evolutionary Psychology*, pp. 276–89. Oxford: Oxford University Press.

Troisi, A. and McGuire, M. (1998). *Darwinian Psychiatry*. Oxford: Oxford University Press.

Turner, S. M. and Hersen, M. (2003). The interviewing process. In M. Hersen and S. M. Turner (Eds), *Diagnostic Interviewing* (3rd edn), pp. 3–11. New York, NY: Spring Street. (First edition published 1985.)

van Dijk, T. A. (1980). *Macrostructures: An Interdisciplinary Study of Global Structures in Discourse, Interaction, and Cognition*. London: Erlbaum.

van Praag, H. M. (1993). *Make-Believes in Psychiatry*. New York, NY: Brunner/Mazel.

van Praag, H. M., Asnis, G. M., Kahn, R. S., Brown, S. L., Korn, M., Harvaky Frieman, J. M., et al. (1997). Nosological tunnel vision in biological psychiatry: A plea for functional psychopathology. *Annals of the New York Academy of Sciences, 600*, 501–10.

Varela, F. and Shear, J. (1999). First-person methodologies: what, why, how? In F. Varela and J. Shear (Eds), *The View from Within. First-Person Approaches to the Study of Consciousness*, pp. 1–13. Thorverton: Imprint Academic.

Ventura, J., Liberman, R. P., Green, M. F., Shaner, A., and Mintz, J. (1998). Training and quality assurance with the Structured Clinical Interview for DSM-IV (SCID-I/P). *Psychiatric Research, 79*, 163–73.

Ware, J., Straussman, H. D., and Naftulin, D. H. (1971). A negative relationship between understanding interviewing principles and interview performance. *Journal of Medical Education, 46*, 620–2.

Westen, D., Novotny, C. M., and Thompson-Brenner, H. (2004). The empirical status of empirically supported psychotherapies: Assumptions, findings, and reporting in controlled trials. *Psychological Bulletin, 130*, 631–63.

Wittgenstein, L. (1953). *Philosophical Investigations*. New York, NY: Macmillan.

Woolgar, S. (1996). Psychology, qualitative methods and the ideas of science. In J. T. Richardson (Ed.), *Handbook of Qualitative Research Methods for Psychology and the Social Sciences*, pp. 11–24. Leicester: The British Psychological Society.

Yoshino, A., Shighemura, J., Kobayashi, Y., Nomura, S., Shishikura, K., Den, R., et al. (2001).

Telepsychiatry: Assessment of televideo psychiatric interview reliability with present and next generation internet infrastructures. *Acta Psychiatrica Scandinavica, 104*, 223–6.

Zahavi, D. (1999). *Self-Awareness and Alterity: A Phenomenological Investigation*. Evanston, IL: Northwestern University Press.

Zimmerman, M. (1993). A five-minute psychiatric screening interview. *Journal of the Family Practitioner, 37*, 479–82.

Zinberg, N. E. (1987). Elements of the private therapeutic interview. *American Journal of Psychiatry, 144*, 1527–33.

SECTION IV

SUMMONING CONCEPTS

CHAPTER 24

INTRODUCTION: SUMMONING CONCEPTS

Earthworms don't need concepts. They spend most of their time burrowing in the ground. They possess neither separate sensory organs (unless one classifies their entire epidermis as a sensory organ) nor cognitive capacities. When they plug their holes with leaves, petioles, and twigs, they do not think, or presumably they do not think, of these things as classified into categories. Nor do they do what they do in order to intentionally keep their skins warm and moist. While they may profit from the result, they do not, or presumably they do not, conceive of the result as a result. They don't think "This twig here fits into that hole there." Or "Thank goodness, I am nice and warm now."

Human beings need concepts. Our powers of discrimination, selection, purpose, and deliberative reasoning depend upon them. Our thoughts have concepts as their constituent parts or elements. Science, literature, and, indeed, all of human culture exhibit our astounding conceptual powers and the multitudinous theoretical and practical roles that concepts perform.

There are few more stunning examples of human conceptual proclivity than the concepts exhibited by psychiatrists and the mental health profession. The field of psychiatry has a prodigious capacity for constructing concepts and categories for understanding and treating mental illness or disorder.

Dozens of concepts in psychiatry could be cited as examples. Some specific to particular theories of disorder (like the concepts of "Id" and "Superego" for Freud), and others parts of general psychiatric parlance (like "delusion" and "dissociation"). Given the basic roles of concepts in the understanding and treatment of mental illness or disorder, it is not feasible to summon forth or design apposite concepts for the discipline without taking sides in a number of issues in the philosophy of psychiatry. In fact, discussions of appropriate concepts for the discipline have become focal points for debating different orientations to the topics of mental health and illness. For instance, the theory of concepts for psychiatry is essentially bound up with issues such as whether there are real, observer independent mental disorders or whether concepts for disorder are descriptive, evaluative, or some mixture of the two. Or again: perhaps the most disturbing worry about the *Diagnostic and Statistical Manual of Mental Disorders* (DSM) as well as the *International Classification of Diseases* is their super-abundance of taxonomic concepts or classificatory categories for mental disorder. In the case of DSM, by the end of the 1980s it had become obvious to the mental health profession that the spiral notebook that was DSM-II in 1968, 150 pages in length, and available in the United States for three dollars and change was in danger in later versions or editions of becoming an unmanageable and expensive brick. Conceptual subtraction and excision was needed, urgently. As successive versions have revealed, such activity has yet to occur.

It's time to re-think and re-examine the concepts of the discipline, not just those used in diagnosis and classification, but in the whole theory and practice of the mental health profession. Chronic conceptual fatigue syndrome is settling in.

The aim of the fourth section of the book is to explore just which concepts and categories, which ways thinking about mental disorder, are worth summoning forth, and for which purposes. Naturalistic concepts? Normative or evaluative ones? Concepts derived from neurology and brain science, character assessment, or definitional considerations? Concepts apposite for assessments of rationality? Tackling the mind/brain problem?

Chapter 25 by Elselijn Kingma is the first in the section. It is aimed at clarifying just what makes a mental disorder a mental disorder. What is it *in nature* that makes for a mental disorder or illness? One possibility is that if this or that aspect of mind has its source of psychiatrically relevant functions in natural selection and contribution to genetic fitness, then appeal to failures in those adaptational functions should be used to describe the disorder of a mental disorder. According to such a failure-of-biological-adaptivity view, there is nothing in the distinctive elements of a mental disorder that concerns what we persons ourselves may value in mind and behavior. Human values and personal or social interests or preferences are irrelevant to the warranted attribution of a disorder. Kingma describes such an adaptationalist approach to characterizing mental disorder as resolutely naturalistic, and although he offers criticisms of the global utility or range of applicability of the approach, he believes that it may yet make a contribution to our understanding of a mental disorder.

Fulford and van Staden, in Chapter 26, share Kingma's worry about the makings of a mental disorder, in some very general way, but approach or interpret the topic from a different angle. They ask about the purposes that the worry or debate over definition serves. Who or what benefits by focusing on the very idea of a mental disorder? Concern with what makes a mental disorder a mental disorder serves, they claim, at least four purposes. Two are mentioned here. One: it signals a concern about the nature of bodily disorders, first and foremost, and not primarily, except by segregation from the domain of bodily disorder, mental disorder. Two: it helps to identify the value-laden concepts of disorder as a whole. Whatever makes a person disordered, sick, ill, diseased, or defective can only be understood, they claim, against background appreciation for the diverse values of human beings and of our evaluative practices and activities. These lessons, and others that they discuss in their chapter, derive, they say, from an appreciation of the tradition of ordinary language philosophy. The tradition urges that the analysis of any concept stems from the necessary philosophical field work and from discovery of the scope and roles of a concept—its full logical geography.

A variety of scientific disciplines have set as their task understanding and explaining mental disorder or illness, recognizing that in some way or another mental disorder or illness depends upon the brain, for the brain is the bearer of mind and meaning. Mind is what brain does. Thinking of the brain as the bearer of mind and meaning often is taken to require thinking of it as a mechanism that processes information. What is crucial to understanding the information that is processed requires not just studying the hardware implementation of that information (its physical vehicles) or embodiment (e.g., changes in sodium and potassium concentrations), but how an organism appropriately or inappropriately relates to or interacts with the surrounding environment—how it plans actions, remembers events, perceives changes in its surroundings, and so on.

Kelso Cratsley and Richard Samuels (Chapter 27) offer their chapter as a description and assessment of the roles of cognitive neuropsychology and cognitive neuroscience in the study of mental disorder. These two disciplines, primary members of the larger field of cognitive science, devote themselves to thinking of the brain as an information processing mechanism, and to thinking of a mental disorder as grounded in damaged, injured, defective, dysfunctional, or flawed information processing in the brain. Their chapter examines the most important explanatory strategies of cognitive science for understanding a mental disorder or illness, aiming in applied particulars at the examples of autism spectrum disorder and major depressive disorder. Various concepts associated with the cognitive science of mental disorder are introduced and discussed (subpersonal mechanisms and double dissociations, among them) as well as misgivings that some theorists have expressed about the purport and utility of mechanistic subpersonal information processing models of disorder.

Keith Bolton, in Chapter 28, takes us back to the question asked by Kingma. What makes a mental disorder or illness a mental disorder or illness? He asks his readers to imagine a patient awaiting diagnosis in a clinic, and wonders how a diagnosis of mental illness may be warranted as over and against thinking that the person is suffering from normal or ordinary troubles or heartaches. Sadness or loneliness is one thing; major depressive disorder another. Anxiety about meeting strangers is one condition; agoraphobia another. Bolton argues that DSM puts its diagnostic finger on two features of a disorder: serious distress and pronounced impairment. While these two features help to characterize disorders, they do not, Bolton claims, cleanly or clearly divide the domain of mental disorder from that of ordinary problems of living. So can (or even should?) science help to distinguish between the two domains more precisely or determinately? The chapter considers how far a science of disorder may assist in drawing boundaries about mental illness.

Next, in Chapter 29, John Sadler examines several of the philosophical issues that surround mental illness concepts and the various roles that those concepts play, not just in the mental health professions but in the criminal justice system and in intellectual disability services and systems. He argues that there is a tight connection, both historically and in contemporary terms, between attributions of wrongful conduct, socially and morally speaking, and of mental disorder or illness. This is not to say that being "bad" is being "mad," but the boundaries between the two are both vague and porous and cannot be distinguished without addressing a welter of metaphysical commitments and philosophical issues about the nature of moral and criminal responsibility, the character of forensic psychiatry, and much else besides.

In Chapter 30 Lisa Bartolotti examines a topic introduced at the start of the book. Sanity. Or more exactly, irrationality. While forms of irrationality are often cited as criteria for mental illness or disorder, Bartolotti argues that many psychiatric disorders are not best understand as violations of reason's norms. In part, she says, this is because many non-ill people are just as irrational in their attitudes or behavior as individuals properly classified as mentally ill. So, irrationality is not generally sufficient for disorder. In part, it is also because serious deficits or malfunctions in one or more cognitive and emotional capacities may also be constitutive of a mental disorder—rather than persistent irrationality. So, irrationality often fails to be necessary. Much for Bartolotti depends on just what it means to be irrational as opposed to rational, and how far the rationality (or irrationality) of a state of mind or behavior can be differentiated from non-rational components.

Jennifer Church, in Chapter 31, refrains from general claims about the nature or identity of mental disorder. She focuses quite specifically on disturbances and disorders that reflect various and heart-breaking failures to negotiate and establish effective personal boundaries between one person and another, boundaries, in particular, of personal responsibility and of gain and loss. One person's identity or sense of self, she says, should not always compete with another person's. Just because you are responsible should not mean that I am not responsible. Just because you have gained (or lost) should not mean that I have lost (or gained). But human suffering, she says, often results from unhealthy misjudgments about gains or losses to one's person or threats to one's personal responsibility posed by the actions or inactions of other people. Such misjudgments occur in cases of depression as well as in instances of borderline personality disorder and threaten the integrity and sense of self of persons who are characterized by such disorders. Mistakes about personal boundaries deflect emotional energy away from more productive goals or ends.

Suppose mind is brain based. Does this mean that mental disorders are a subtype of brain disorder? George Graham, in Chapter 32, is skeptical of the temptation to conceive of mental disorders as a subtype of brain disorder. For him, disorders of mind, although based in the brain, are not disorders of the brain. Brain science, he says, is useful for understanding certain aspects of a mental disorder, to be sure, but not for various other aspects for which psychological understanding is needed. The need for psychology is not a matter of idle metaphysics, but is directly relevant to appreciating the significance of therapies and treatments for one sort of condition (a brain disorder) as opposed to another (a mental disorder). Grouping or ordering disorders into mental and brain disorders may depend, in part, he says, on which therapies or treatments succeed or fail. If a successful therapy works through reason or appeal to a person's reason responsive psychology, the corresponding disorder may be a mental disorder. If sound and sensible treatment may occur only when a person's rational capacities as such are bypassed, as happens under the knife of neurosurgery, the corresponding disorder may be best classified as a brain disorder. Truth of a diagnosis is a matter of fit—fit with a body of background theory and fit of theory with (among other things) past facts about successful and failed interventions.

In the last chapter in the section, Chapter 33, Eric Matthews offers an approach to the topic of mental disorder inspired by the French phenomenologist, Maurice Merleau-Ponty (1908–1961). In the spirit of Merleau-Ponty, Matthews claims that psychiatry should conceive of a mental illness or disorder as above all meaningful to the subject of the disorder and as rooted in the conceptual world of the individual. Mental health medicine requires, he says, both a humanistic understanding of a mental disorder and one that appeals to the neurosciences. Some aspects of a disorder may be explicable in brain science terms, but others require an understanding of the concepts that a subject of mental disorder uses or fails to use. To neglect or bypass the conceptual world of a patient with a mental disorder is to neglect what makes a mental disorder a disorder of mind and mentality.

CHAPTER 25

NATURALIST ACCOUNTS OF MENTAL DISORDER

ELSELIJN KINGMA

Whether one is believed to have a mental disorder or not has consequences: it can give access to special and/or medical treatment as well as other social, economic, and emotional benefits, but it can also result in significant harms or risks of harm such as stigma, social exclusion, and infringement of rights. Less often mentioned, but perhaps more importantly, whether a person is thought to have a mental disorder affects how she and others view, interpret, respond to—and thereby partially form—who she is and what she does (Hacking 1995, 1998).

It seems crucial, then, to get our judgment on whether someone has a mental disorder right. This chapter shall examine part of that judgment: it shall ask what mental disorder *is*. There are at least three possible versions of that question. First, what makes a disorder a *mental* rather than a *physical* or *somatic* disorder?; second, what makes a *particular* mental disorder different from *another*?; third, what makes a condition an instance of *disorder*?[1] This essay focuses on the third question.[2]

THE DEMARCATION PROBLEM

IN PSYCHIATRY

The question of what distinguishes disorder from health, the *demarcation problem*, sparks considerable controversy and is most hotly debated in the context of psychiatry. But it does

---

[1] Because the contrast is between *disorder* and *health*, I take the former to denote all departures from health. That is not entirely consistent with either medical or ordinary language use, but in keeping with an established tradition in the literature (e.g., Boorse 1975; Cooper 2002). Boorse and Cooper use the term "disease," Clouser et al. (1981, 1997) speak of "malady," Wakefield (1992b) of "disorder," and Boorse in his later work (1997, 2011) prefers "pathological condition." All intend the same inclusive denotation.

[2] See Murphy (2006) for a recent treatment that touches on all three questions.

not belong there exclusively: obesity, deafness, and high blood pressure have all posed demarcation problems in somatic medicine. Still, there are good reasons for worrying especially about mental health. First, mental disorders seem more controversial and elusive than somatic ones; most of us, including doctors and scientists, have a clearer idea of broken legs than broken personalities, and a better grasp on high blood pressure than low moods. Second, psychiatry seems more easily "polluted" by values and social considerations than somatic medicine—indeed the idea that psychiatry is a mere "tool for social and political control," as opposed to a scientifically or biomedically founded enterprise that has the interest of its patients at heart, is an enduring critique of psychiatry (see e.g., Foucault 1961; Laing 1959; Szasz 1960, 1972).

The history of psychiatry provides a wealth of examples that support this latter view. Masturbation, hysteria, and nymphomania were widely considered to be disorders in the nineteenth century, for example, as was homosexuality.[3] A more outlandish example is "drapetomania," the disorder supposedly exhibited by slaves who ran away from their master (Cartwright 1851; Engelhardt 1974). Viewed from our present perspective, these misdiagnoses result not just from an inferior scientific understanding of the natural world, but seem to indicate a conception or understanding of mental disorder that embodies contemporary—and morally dubious—social and evaluative standards rather than scientific ones: gender norms, sexual morality, and racism.

The worry that mental disorder constitutes social rather than biomedical deviance is not confined to the distant past either; our present-day expansions and increases in the prevalence of certain psychiatric diagnoses, such as depression and attention-deficit/hyperactivity disorder (ADHD), are still being challenged as *merely* reflecting social norms (about how long children should sit still, for example, or about how happy we should be) rather than scientific facts about *actual* disorder (see, e.g., Hawthorne 2007; Horwitz and Wakefield 2007). Indeed the definition of mental disorder was a heavily contested topic in the construction of the third edition of the *Diagnostic and Statistical Manual of Mental Disorders* (DSM-III), when precisely such worries played a role in the process that ultimately resulted in the exclusion of homosexuality from the DSM (Bayer 1987). The literature on the demarcation problem very much exists against the background of these particular worries, which also explain and motivate its two main and opposing positions: naturalism and normativism.[4]

NATURALISM AND NORMATIVISM

According to naturalism, the concepts of health and disorder are predominantly driven by objective natural categories, that is, categories that exist independent from our values and interests: *biological function* and *dysfunction*.[5] Whilst these categories may interact with

---

[3] Boorse (2011, pp. 13–14) lists many examples and sources.

[4] The terms "naturalism" and "normativism" are most widely used, but Murphy (2009), following Kitcher (1996), contrasts "objectivism" and "constructivism."

[5] See Boorse (1975, 1976b, 1977, 1987, 1997, 2011), Kass (1975), Kendell (1975), Scadding (1988, 1990), Schramme (2007), Szasz (1960) and most recently Ananth (2008). The disease-as-dysfunction approach is defended in most detail by Boorse (1977, 1997) and Wakefield (1992b).

values, social considerations, and/or social norms to generate more complex judgments about what conditions qualify for particular social and medical treatment,[6] and whilst values may also play a role in our identification of these categories (Murphy 2009), naturalists maintain that these values or social norms do not determine what disorder/dysfunction is; nature does. On the naturalist view, then, the history of psychiatry is purely one of mistaken science and illegitimate social influence. Indeed, to criticize past or present boundary shifts in our application of mental disorder as (merely) reflecting values or social norms is to assume already that a category of "real disorder" exists that is independent from those values and social norms.

Normativism, by contrast, must give an alternative account of the history of psychiatry; according to normativism, the demarcation between health and disorder is not a matter of nature alone.[7] Normativists therefore tend to present past and present psychiatry not as illegitimately influenced by values, but as illustrative of the way in which shifting values and social norms have driven changes in mental disorder.[8] Indeed, if normativism is correct, there is no non-evaluative notion of "real" disorder that a shifting diagnostic pattern of ADHD is a deviation from.

In the rest of this chapter I focus on naturalist accounts of mental disorder and examine its three most influential positions: Szasz's rejection of mental disorder, Boorse's biostatistical account of disease, and Wakefield's evolutionary account of disorder. I conclude that the statistical concept of dysfunction offered by Boorse tracks medical usage more closely than the evolutionary account offered by Wakefield. But neither succeeds in offering a completely value-free account of disorder.

Szasz and Mental Functional Architecture

The modern debate on mental disorder has been deeply influenced by Thomas Szasz (1960), whose "The Myth of Mental Illness" put pressure on both the concept of mental disorder and psychiatry as a whole. Here is a version of Szasz's argument against mental disorder:

P1. (Naturalist premise): what constitutes disorder is a dysfunction or lesion at a structural, cellular, or molecular level.
P2. (Empirical premise): "mental disorders" present without such a physical lesion.[9]
C. (Conclusion): mental disorders do not exist.

---

[6] Boorse (1975, pp. 54–55, 60, 1977, p. 544, 1997, pp. 11, 12–13, 55, 95–99). See also Wakefield (1992a).

[7] See Agich (1983), Clouser et al. (1981, 1997), Cooper (2002), Engelhardt (1976, 1986), Goossens (1980), Margolis (1976), Nordenfelt (1987, 2001, 2007), Reznek (1987), and Whitbeck (1978). See Simons (2007) for an overview and comparison of different normativist positions, which are far more heterogeneous than is generally presented.

[8] This position is certainly found in, e.g., Foucault (1961), but it is also implicit in, e.g., Cooper's (2002) definition of disease.

[9] Some mental disorders, such as neuropsychiatric conditions, do present with physical lesions of course—and presumably these would have to be recognized as disorders by Szasz. It should be remembered that he wrote his essay in the 1960s, on the basis of contemporary knowledge.

Szasz argued, not that the things we call mental illnesses do not exist, but that they are not *disorders*—naturalistically conceived of by him as dysfunctions. Instead they are problems in living and/or departures from "psychosocial, ethical, and legal" norms. To apply the term "disorder" to these problems is to use the term metaphorically, which Szasz considered both illegitimate and obfuscating. Illegitimate because it is employed to excuse inexcusable behavior and justify unjustifiable measures, such as forced treatment and isolation. Obfuscating because "the concept functions as a disguise; for instead of calling attention to conflicting human needs, aspirations, and values, the notion of mental illness provides an amoral and impersonal 'thing' (an 'illness') as an explanation for problems in living" (Szasz 1960, p. 116).

Szasz's criticisms map neatly onto the naturalist/normativist divide: he defends a *naturalist* concept of dysfunction as the only legitimate concept of disorder, then criticizes psychiatry for illegitimately employing a *normativist* conception of disorder as deviation from social norms. Subsequent normativists have mostly argued that Szasz was right to think that mental disorder is a non-naturalist concept, but wrong to think this makes it illegitimate. Naturalists, by contrast, agree with Szasz's contention that dysfunction is the only legitimate construal of disorder, but tend to disagree with his views on mental disorder; where Szasz thought that naturalism undermined psychiatry, most naturalists attempt to *support* and *legitimize* (at least part of) psychiatry. For this latter project to succeed Szasz's argument that the mind does not instantiate dysfunction has to be answered—and such an answer is provided by David Papineau (1994).

Against Szasz: Minds over brains

One way to argue that Szasz is wrong about mental disorders is to question his second premise: "mental illnesses present without a structural, chemical or molecular-level lesion." It is conceivable that this premise is wrong, and that unbeknownst to us every instance of mental disorder is the result of some structural or physiochemical deviation in the brain/body. I believe, with Szasz, that this is unlikely, but settling that question is not relevant here: we can grant Szasz his second premise and *still* conclude, on the basis of his first premise, that his argument against the existence of mental disorders is unsound.

Szasz's first premise supposes that biological dysfunctions can only manifest in physical lesions. But contemporary philosophy of mind gives us good reason to think that there could be natural mental dysfunctions that are not reducible to abnormalities in the structural and physiochemical make-up of the body/brain. Papineau helpfully uses the software/hardware analogy to illustrate this: a bug in a computer program need not be a problem in the hardware of your computer, because the physical substrate of your computer can run a multitude of software programs, including dysfunctional ones. Similarly a structurally and functionally intact *brain*—that is to say all neurons working as they should, and no neuronal or structural lesions are present—can *run* (instantiate) a variety of mental patterns, including dysfunctional ones (Papineau 1994).

By driving a wedge between the functional integrity of the brain and the functional integrity of the mind, Szasz's challenge to the existence of mental disorders/dysfunctions can be answered. Subsequent naturalists have thus been freed to discuss the mind and its functions without reference to the brain, and can thus attempt to construct a naturalist account of mental disorder as mental dysfunction that could support psychiatry.

Mental dysfunction and functional architecture

Once we can posit the mind as a legitimate object of inquiry, we can proceed to uncover its functions. But that is only possible if the mind possesses a functional architecture. Now in somatic medicine, conceiving of the organism as having a functional architecture has been a successful approach. But when it comes to the mind, our understanding of mental functional architecture is far less developed, and the scientific project of carving the mind into traits that have functions falls far short of the success that its somatic counterparts enjoy. Compare, for example, physiological descriptions of the working of the ear with functional description of the *mental* component of auditory processing. Ear physiology includes detailed accounts of cells and processes that have particular functions, which have mostly achieved the status of scientific fact. In accounts of auditory processing, by contrast, multiple and mutually exclusive models remain in contention.

Still, in absence of agreement on the functional structure of the mind, we can ask what the truths about mental functional architecture would have to be if we are to end up with a suitable account of disorder as dysfunction. I contend there are at least two such truths. First, the mind must be modular, with different modules having distinct functions. Second, this modular structure must not exist merely at a broad level, but at a level of considerable detail. Both, I suggest, are problematic, and let me start with the second point.

Although we can easily agree upon certain broad-level functions of the mind, such as "tracking the environment" or "social interaction," a considerably more detailed account of mental functions is needed to support an account of mental illness as mental dysfunction. Take, for example, "tracking the environment." Most of us are pretty bad at that; we suffer not only from a range of well-described systematic biases such as self-serving bias and attribution error, but are also subject to optical illusions and attentional deficits. An accurate account of mental function and dysfunction needs to be sensitive to this: it should explain, or at least accommodate, that sometimes our inability to track the environment is not a dysfunction, even though in other circumstances, in the case of hallucinations, for example, it is.

This is particularly important for psychiatry, because conceiving of mental functions broadly, as "successful social interaction" or "tracking the environment" means that any lack of social functioning or false belief becomes a disorder. And that would violate both our ideas about mental disorder and the core expectation that motivated the search for a naturalist account of disorder in the first place. This is the expectation that such account of disorder should help distinguish between false beliefs per se—of which we have many—and false beliefs that are, or indicate, mental dysfunctions; between impaired interaction that results from different values and ideas—all too common—and impaired interaction that is mental disorder; between problems that beset a healthy mind, and those that indicate something wrong. A broad description of mental function does not allow for that distinction, therefore a very detailed account is necessary if an account of mental disorder as dysfunction is to succeed.

Levels of detail aside, we should also question whether the mind has a modular functional structure at all. This is not an unpopular proposition: the modular theory of mind supports a considerable research program in cognitive psychology. This presents the mind as consisting of distinct but cooperating, hierarchically and sequentially organized "specific modules" that have functions, and non-specific or general modules that support other modules.[10] Such a modular mind would be a good candidate for supporting an account of disorder as dysfunction. But it is not *obvious* that our minds should have such a structure. It may be the case that our minds operate in diffuse ways that do not lend themselves to easy carving into traits and functions, or that do not lend themselves to carving at all.[11] To use a well-trodden metaphor, minds may not have joints—and if they do, they may have so many that there are multiple possible yet mutually incompatible ways of carving them.

If such a pluralist stance to mental organization was justified, and multiple functional descriptions of the mind are true,[12] then that would pose problems for a naturalist account of mental disorder: multiple true functional descriptions of the mind means multiple true demarcations between function and dysfunction, which means multiple true accounts of mental disorder. And this (I argue in the next section) undermines naturalism about mental disorder.

Boorse and Requirements of Naturalism

The most widely known and well-discussed naturalist account of disorder is Christopher Boorse's "biostatistical theory" (BST):

1. The *reference class* is a natural class of organisms of uniform functional design; specifically, an age group of a sex of a species.
2. A *normal function* of a part or process within members of the reference class is a statistically typical contribution by it to their individual survival and reproduction.
3. A *disease* is a type of internal state that is either an impairment of normal functional ability, i.e., a reduction of one or more functional abilities below typical efficiency, or a limitation on functional ability caused by environmental agents.[13]
4. *Health* is the absence of disease.[14]

In other words, health is normal function, where normal function is the statistically typical contribution to survival and reproduction in a reference class. Disorder, on this account, is dysfunction, which is an adverse departure from normal function.

---

[10] See Cosmides and Tooby (1987), Murphy and Stich (2000), and Tooby and Cosmides (1990a, 1990b, 1992) for more detail.

[11] Such a conception of the mind may be supported by another research program in cognitive psychology: connectionism. See, e.g., Bechtel and Abrahamsen (1990) and Garson (2010).

[12] And pluralism already is a well-respected position in philosophy of biology when it comes to both species (Dupré 1993; Ereshefsky 2001; Kitcher 1984) and functions (e.g., Godfrey-Smith 1993; Griffiths 1993; Perlman, 2004).

[13] The clause on environmental agents is controversial. It appeared in Boorse's (1977, p. 567) original proposal, but in 2011 (p. 27) following discussion in 1997 he proposed to drop it. For an objection to Boorse that is based on environmental agents see Kingma (2010); Hausman (2011) responds.

[14] Boorse (1997, pp. 7–8). See also Boorse (1977, pp. 562, 567).

To illustrate, let us suppose that visual perception can be understood as the mind's interpreting of visual information to facilitate its tracking of environmental happenings. This is a statistically typical contribution the mind makes to survival and reproduction. The normal execution of this function is determined by what is statistically typical in my reference class. Therefore if I interpret visual information as accurately as most humans of my sex and age, I am healthy. Optical illusions cause me to interpret visual information in a manner that fails to track environmental happenings in the world correctly, but since that is statistically normal in my reference class, this is not a disorder. Hallucinations, by contrast, are interpretive failures to track the environment that are *not* statistically typical. They are thus an adverse departure from normal function, and a (form of) disorder on Boorse's account.

Boorse's account of disorder has attracted criticism proportional to its notoriety,[15] and his account of biological *function* is subject to a separate and additional set of objections in the literature on philosophy of biology.[16] In this chapter I want to focus on just one, so far unanswered, objection to Boorse, which does not question the accuracy of the BST, but contends that even *if* Boorse's account were to accurately depict disorder, it does not succeed in being completely interest-independent or value free.

Against naturalism: Reference classes

The BST performs statistical abstractions to determine what is normal, and therefore healthy, functional performance in humans. But normal functional performance varies tremendously within the human species. What counts as normal mental function in a two-year-old would not be normal in a twenty-year-old, for example, and normal hormone levels vary considerably amongst sexes, over a lifetime, and even during the day. The BST therefore employs *reference classes*, in which it calibrates statistics separately to determine what the normal function is. These reference classes divide the population by sex, age, and (for certain purposes only) ethnicity.

Reference classes are at the core of an objection against Boorse's account, that I defend in more detail elsewhere (Kingma 2007). Imagine different reference classes than the ones proposed by Boorse. If we allow such different reference classes, then different accounts of function, and of health and disorder, would emerge. For example, if people with depression or ADHD formed a separate reference class on the BST, then depression or ADHD would be statistically normal in these groups. These would then no longer be a disorder according to the BST. This move could be repeated for many conditions such that they become "healthy": all we need to do is create a BST-type account of function that admits a separate reference class for the condition in question. Note that these different accounts of functions would be just as value-free as the BST presented by Boorse, provided that the reference classes they admit are grounded in natural or value-free categories.

Presumably Boorse wants to maintain that the BST provides the correct analysis of function and health, and that alternative concepts generated by alternative reference classes do not. If so, he needs to provide a non-circular justification for why the reference classes he proposes are admissible, and alternative reference classes are ruled out.

[15] Boorse (1997) provides a near-complete treatment of objections to that date. He summarizes several more in 2011 (pp. 29–32). For subsequent objections see Kingma (2010) and Guerrero (2010).

[16] See Lewens (2004) for an overview, and Boorse (1976a, 2002) for a response to some objections.

In other words, Boorse needs to justify, without prior reference to health and disorder, why out of all possible ways of groupings humans, only age, sex, and perhaps race are the groupings that underpin an account of health and disorder. And since Boorse is committed to arguing that the BST is *value-free*—i.e., that a preference for the BST over alternatives represents a *value-free* choice or objective representation of reality and not a value-laden preference—this justification for admitting certain reference classes only should be value-free too.

Such a non-circular, value-free justification cannot be provided: restricting reference classes to healthy groups of humans would be circular, and other proposals either fail to generate the correct results or appeal to values (Kingma 2007). We therefore lack a reason to think the reference classes Boorse admits, and thereby the BST, are value-free or interest-independent. Instead they are likely to reflect prior, and possibly value-laden, assumptions about which groups are normal and healthy—assumptions that are deeply embedded in this account of disorder.

The example of the "XST" illustrates the problem that the BST is in. Suppose the XST is an account of disorder that closely resembles the BST, with one exception: sexual orientation is a reference class on the XST. According to the BST homosexuality is a disorder, because non-heterosexual attraction is a worse-than-typical contribution to reproduction.[17] On the XST, however, homosexuality is normal in the reference class of people with homosexual orientation, and therefore healthy. In the absence of an objective justification of the kind that Boorse should but cannot provide, i.e., an objective justification for favoring the BST over the XST (or vice versa), we lack a way to settle the demarcation problem regarding homosexuality. And since XST-type accounts can be generated for many if not all "disorders," the BST—even if it appears successful at delineating our concept of disorder—lacks the resources, let alone a value-free method, to withstand challenge posed by such accounts. The BST is therefore neither a value-free account, nor is it able to provide a value-free justification for our actions or a value-free method for settling controversy.

Naturalists' burden of justification

The earlier argument has wider implications for naturalist accounts of disorder: it increases their burden of justification. Naturalists' central claim is that disorder is not a reflection of social values or norms, but a feature of the natural world. Following Boorse, naturalists have attempted to defend this view by demonstrating that health and disorder can be defined in value-free terms, most notable in terms of *dysfunction*. But the earlier argument suggests that this is not enough; giving a definition or account of the concepts "health" and "disorder" in value-free terms does not suffice for proving that these concepts are completely value-free. As the example of the XST demonstrates, accounts stated in value-free terms can still embody deeply held social values. It follows that if naturalists are to defend their main claim, they have to meet an additional challenge: demonstrate that there is some value-free justification for employing the particular naturalistic concept they define, *rather than* another one.

---

[17] Although Boorse grants that homosexuality is a pathology on the BST, he maintains that it is not a bad thing and therefore should not be treated (1975, p. 63, 1997, p. 99). See also footnote 22.

One might object that that is too demanding. We cannot be expected to give a value-free justification for why we employ concepts in certain roles rather than other ones, and it is quite plausible that our ultimate reason for employing the concept "disorder" in its present role is a social or evaluative one: disordered conditions are worthy of attention as a group because they are painful, disabling, and so on.[18] The challenge for naturalists is therefore slightly narrower: *given* that we are interested in certain conditions that are disabling, painful, and so on, naturalists have to provide a value-free justification for favoring one possible naturalist extension of these conditions over another. In other words, *given* that pneumonia, cancer, and arthritis are disorders, naturalists have to justify why the category "disorder" that they belong to is described by—say—the BST rather than the XST. It is this justification that Boorse cannot provide. Without it, accounts of disorder in value-free terms cannot on their own deflect the worry that the concept "disorder" might reflect underlying evaluative categorical judgments. Naturalists have considerable extra work to do.

Naturalism and pluralism

At this point, it is worth recalling a suggestion made in the "Mental dysfunction and functional architecture" section, which is that the structure of the mind may be such that a pluralist stance toward mental functional architecture may be justified. In that case—*whatever* the right account of function turns out to be—we end up with a problem very much similar to the one the BST faces: any particular account of disorder as dysfunction, whilst describing disorder in value-free terms, has to choose and employ a particular way of carving up functional architecture, rather than another one, to determine what are disorders. Such an account will therefore reflect the values that drove this choice, and—just like the BST—be unable to withstand challenges that can be framed in terms of employing a different method of carving up the mind. Pluralism, in this case, would put the view that disorder is a value-free concept on shaky grounds.

At the same time we should also not overstate the force of this argument. If naturalism were to modify its commitments and restate its aims, much of the problems outlined would disappear. Naturalism could admit that disorder was a value-laden category in the limited sense I have outlined, and restrict its aims to identifying and defining this category in clear factual terms so that questions can be settled by first-order appeal to facts without having to *explicitly* agree or disagree about values. This much weaker and pragmatic version of naturalism may be defensible, and it could possible help us settle some disputes, conflicts, and boundary cases by allowing us to move straight from the facts about a condition to a judgment about its disordered status, without further appeal to values or norms. As the example of the XST illustrates, however, it would lack the resources to answer many challenges or resolve all problems.

---

[18] This latter observation is often employed as an argument by normativists in order to show that health and disease must be value-laden categories (see, e.g., Cooper 2002, p. 271, 2005, p. 22; Engelhardt 1975, pp. 127, 136, 1976, p. 226; Goosens 1980, p. 106; Margolis 1976, p. 242; Nordenfelt 2007a). I argue elsewhere that the normativist conclusion does not follow (Kingma 2012; see also Schramme 2007).

Wakefield and Evolutionary

Accounts of Disorder

The main naturalist alternative to Boorse's BST is Jerome Wakefield's "harmful dysfunction analysis" (HDA) of disorder. This account also defines disorder in terms of *dysfunction*, but gives an account of function that is explicitly grounded in evolutionary theory.[19] Such an evolutionary account of disorder has two prima facie advantages. First, it might provide a response to the challenge posited in the previous section. For where Boorse had to construct unjustified and arbitrary reference classes to extract a particular account of function out of several possible closely related ones, an evolutionary account of function is based in a more substantive metaphysical claim: given a contingent evolutionary history, there exists a specific way in which biological systems should function. Thus *if* disorder is indeed (harmful) dysfunction, evolutionary history provides a non-arbitrary and naturalistic extension of the concept "dysfunction."[20] Second, the other apparent advantage of an evolutionary account of function is that it enjoys considerable support in the literature of philosophy of biology.[21]

Cashing out evolutionary dysfunction

The core idea behind the evolutionary account of disorder is that evolution, as a design-like process, can create and explain biological norms of functioning that are non-evaluative. But that idea needs development, for not every effect or trait produced by evolution is useful or has a function. Congenital disorders, for example, are just as much the product of evolution as the absence of them; disease agents are products of evolution too; and detailed evolutionary explanations have been posited for a variety of acquired diseases and/or disease susceptibilities.[22] What the evolutionary disorder naturalist therefore needs is a distinction between those products of evolution that are functioning as designed, and other results of evolution that count as a dysfunctions and disorders.

One way to generate this distinction is to contrast evolution by *natural selection* with other forms of evolutionary processes, such as drift.[23] On this proposal, functions are effects

---

[19] There is another difference between Wakefield and Boorse: Wakefield defines disorder as *harmful* dysfunction, whereas Boorse defines disease as dysfunction per se. But since Boorse agrees with Wakefield that only harmful dysfunctions are the kind of conditions that we should treat, this difference is merely semantic, and has no practical or theoretical implications (Boorse 1975, p. 54–55, 60, 1977, p. 544, 1997, p. 11, 12–13, 55, 95–99).

[20] Though it may still lack the resources to define the boundary between normal function and dysfunction (Schwartz 2007). See also Lilienfeld and Mario (1999, p. 404) and, for a response, Wakefield (1999).

[21] See Godfrey-Smith (1993, 1994), Griffiths (1993), Millikan (1984, 1989), and Neander (1991a, 1991b, 1995) for a development and defense of evolutionary accounts of biological function, and Lewens (2004) and Ariew et al. (2002) for overviews.

[22] See, e.g., Williams and Nesse (1996), Gluckman et al. (2009), McKenna et al. (2008).

[23] Simply put, drift happens when the outcomes of selection are different from what one would expect based on the fitness of the traits involved. This can happen, amongst others, because of a founder effect

of traits that are a result of evolution *by natural selection*. But this fails to get at the desired distinction: first, *traits* that have spread in the population as the result of natural selection can include disorders. For example, sickle-cell anemia, a homozygous trait, has spread in the populations in which it exists as a consequence of natural selection for malaria-resistant heterozygous sickle-cell trait.[24] Second, *effects* that have spread in the population as a result of natural selection for underlying traits can also include diseases. Atherosclerosis, for example, is understood as an effect of the very good immune system that may have evolved by natural selection when humans lived in crowded cities in very unsanitary conditions.

A better interpretation of an evolutionary account of dysfunction/disorder does therefore not appeal to the traits or effects that are the *result* of evolution by natural selection but those that were the *drivers* of evolution by natural selection.[25] In the earlier examples, sickle-cell anemia may be the result of natural selection, but only malaria resistance drove natural selection by contributing to the inclusive fitness of ancestors. Therefore only malaria resistance is a function of heterozygous sickle-cell trait. Homozygous sickle-cell anemia, in contrast, has no function. Similarly atherosclerosis—although a result of natural selection—did not drive its selection because it did not contribute to the inclusive fitness of ancestors, and therefore has no function. Superior bacterial immunity, by contrast, does have a function, and is indeed what drove the natural selection of an aggressive immune system.

In keeping with this, Wakefield states: "The natural function [...] is not just any benefit or effect provided by a mechanism but a benefit or effect that explains, through evolutionary theory, why the mechanisms exists or has the form that it does."[26] This statement is too strict, however; in philosophy of biology a distinction is routinely drawn between exaptations and adaptations. A trait is an *adaptation* when it has an effect that enters into the explanation of the structure or form of that trait. Turtles' flippers, for example, have probably gotten their present shape because of their fitness-enhancing swimming effects—and are therefore adaptations for swimming. But turtles also use their flippers to bury eggs. This effect does not explain how flippers got their present form, although it may explain why flippers continue to exist. Flippers are therefore an *exaptation* for burying eggs (Gould 1991; Gould and Vrba 1982). Whether exaptations are legitimately called functions is "perhaps to be settled by one's taste for neologisms" (Allen 2009). But in the context of defining function for the purposes of defining disorder it is best to take a permissive account of selected effects that includes exaptations.[27] We might, then, replace Wakefield's original account with something like Neander's: "It is the/a proper function of an item (*X*) of an organism (*O*) to do that which items of *X*'s

---

in a small population; a freak accident that killed all fitter types; or the inherent variability involved in probabilistic sampling. See, e.g., Brandon (2005, 2006), Matthen and Ariew (2002), and Walsh et al. (2002).

[24] See also Wakefield (1999, p. 389).

[25] Sober (1980, 2004) calls the former "selection of" and the latter "selection for."

[26] Wakefield (1992a, p. 236). For similar definitions see Wakefield (1992b, pp. 382, 384, 1995).

[27] Wakefield (1999, pp. 380–381) in response to Lilienfeld and Marino (1995, p. 412) and McNally (1994). See also Murphy and Woolfolk (2000a). On the same pages Wakefield makes clear that "maintenance selection" should also subsumed under natural selection on his account. In maintenance selection a trait does not increase in frequency in the population, but is maintained at present frequencies by natural selection—for example because new mutations are being selected against. See, e.g., Godfrey-Smith (1994) and Griffiths (1993).

type did to contribute to the inclusive fitness of *O*'s ancestors, and which caused the genotype, of which *X* is the phenotypic expression, to be selected by natural selection."[28]

One problem for evolutionary accounts of functions and disorder is that they depend heavily on the details of our evolutionary history. And we rarely, if ever, have access to those details. This is a problem at two levels. First, it means that if the etiological account is the correct account of disorder, it might not be of much use to the naturalist or society more broadly. For though this means that what health and disorder are is a matter of fact, we will never be in a position to access all those facts; we are lucky to have access to any.[29] The second problem is directly relevant to our present task: if our lack of epistemic access to selective histories makes it difficult to determine whether a condition is a disorder *if* etiological accounts are correct, how do we judge that this is the right approach to disorder in the first place?[30] This problem will crop up repeatedly in the rest of this chapter, but I will attempt to proceed in a way that is least affected by this.

Against Wakefield: "Selected disorders"

Like Boorse's BST, Wakefield's evolutionary account of disorder has been widely discussed.[31] In this section I wish to focus on two main objections to his account, one of which Wakefield can absorb—at a price—and one that I believe he cannot.

The first possible problem for Wakefield is that of *"selected disorders."* These are selected effects or strategies that have very negative effects in our present society. Possible examples include forms of antisocial behavior: rape, a violent disposition, or dependent or attention-seeking behavior. All of these may have been beneficial in selective terms: serial rape can be a good strategy for increasing one's reproductive output, for example, and violence, dependence, or attention-seeking may all increase one's access to resources that in turn increase fitness.[32] But if it is true that these conditions have been selected, then they are not a disorder according to Wakefield—and this countervenes our current way of thinking about these conditions.

In response, Wakefield sticks to his guns: if "attention seeking" is an effect of a trait that drove the selection of that trait, then it cannot be a disorder—no matter how much we dislike it.[33] Indeed, he argues, there is historical precedent for this. When we discovered fever

---

[28] Neander (1991a, p. 174). See also Godfrey-Smith (1993, 1994), Griffiths (1993), Millikan (1984, 1989), and Neander (1991b, 1995).

[29] Bolton (2008) argues that if an evolutionary account of disorder were correct, it would put the DSM in an epistemic situation barely different from the one it is at present.

[30] This problem is very evident in discussions between Murphy and Woolfolk (2000a, 2000b) and Wakefield (2000) that very much revolve around competing "just-so" stories about evolutionary histories.

[31] See, e.g., Cosmides and Tooby (1999), Fulford (1999), Klein (1999), Kirmayer and Young (1999), Lilienfeld and Marino (1995, 1999), Richters and Hinshaw (1999), Sadler (1999), Sadler and Agich (1995).

[32] These examples and others can be found in Bolton (2008), Cooper (2002), Lilienfeld and Marino (1995), Murphy and Stich (2000), Murphy and Woolfolk (2000a), and Richters and Hinshaw (1999) all of whom discuss a version of the problem of "selected disorders."

[33] See, e.g., Wakefield (1999a, 1999b, pp. 466–467, 2000). See also Murphy and Stich (2000) who attempt a detailed classification of the different kind of problems that can beset an "evolve mind,"

was both functional and naturally selected we stopped seeing it as a disorder (Wakefield 2000, p. 259).

Whether Wakefield's response to these "selected disorders" is tenable depends, of course, on what conditions turn out to fall into the category outlined (which we cannot know without knowledge of the relevant evolutionary facts). But it also depends on our willingness to revise the DSM and our treatment attitudes in light of such facts. It seems possible that we would adjust our opinion of such conditions, as Wakefield predicts, but that is not inevitable; we could also continue to treat them as disorders, which would put pressure on the idea that defining a naturalistic concept of disorder has practical relevance (see also Bolton 2008).

Against Wakefield: "Non-selected effects"

The second and more damaging problem for Wakefield is that of *non-selected effects*. As we saw earlier, not all of our mental traits have been *selected* for effects that they themselves perform; in some cases the presence of a trait is explained by the effects of a different trait. For example, the presence of blue eyes is not explained by an effect of blue eyes, but by the increased ability of lighter skin to absorb ultraviolet B radiation (which helps with vitamin D production). This can happen because the trait "blue eyes" is *linked* to the trait "light skin." Such linkage can happen in various ways: traits can be genetically linked, when their genes appear close together on chromosomes; they can be pleiotropically linked, when they result from genes that give rise to or are involved in the development of multiple traits; or they can be developmentally linked, when physical and other constraints on human development are such that the development or evolution of one trait cannot happen without giving rise to or changing another.[34]

Such linked traits pose a serious problem for Wakefield's account of disorder. As discussed, the selected effect account of function to which he is committed is very strict: it *only* ascribes a function to effect e of trait t if e was causally responsible for the selection of t.[35] Accordingly, traits that are not selected for their own effect, but are selected because of their linkage to other successful traits, do not have a function on Wakefield's account.

An example will illustrate this problem, and how Wakefield proposes to deal with it. Take the human ability to learn how to read. If this ability were a function, the effects of reading would have to explain why we find this ability in humans. But that is not borne out by the data. Humans developed script very recently even in non-evolutionary terms—a couple of thousand years BCE—and only in a few human subgroups in the Middle East, Mesoamerica, and perhaps China. Even within those groups only a small proportion of the population has been exposed to script until quite recently. Thus if the effects of reading had driven the natural selection of our ability to learn how to read, we would expect to find that ability

---

including a further distinction between selected traits that are disliked and presently maladaptive, and selected traits that are disliked but not presently maladaptive.

[34] All of this is an oversimplification of course; the development of organisms, the relations between traits and genes, and indeed the very notion of a gene itself, are all highly complex (see, e.g., Kitcher 1982).

[35] Even on the permissible interpretation outlined here that includes exaptations and recent selection. See also footnote 27.

only in small proportions of the aforementioned populations. Since, however, the ability to learn how to read is found universally around the globe, some effect other than reading must explain its selection.[36] Reading, then, is not a function on Wakefield's account. And this means that a problem in our ability to read, such as dyslexia, would not be a disorder.[37]

Wakefield responds to this example by acknowledging that reading cannot be a function, but denying that this would stop dyslexia from being a disorder (Wakefield (1999a, pp. 382–383, 1999b, 2000). When our ability to learn to read is compromised, he argues, it is because a mechanism underlying this ability is not working as it should. And since that mechanism must have been selected for something, it has a function that is compromised. Strictly speaking, then, dyslexia is not a dysfunction of our ability to learn to read, but a dysfunction of whatever effect it was that *did* drive the selection of our ability to learn how to read.[38]

Problems for Wakefield's response

There are two problems with Wakefield's response.[39] First it depends heavily on the mistaken assumption that when the effect of a trait is selectively explained by an effect elsewhere, a failure to produce the former effect *must* indicate a dysfunction of the latter. But even though the selection of blue eyes is explained by the effects of fair skin, it is entirely possibly for something to happen to the blueness of my eyes without my skin being affected. We therefore have no reason to accept this assumption. In fact the multiple ways in which traits can be linked, the developmental complexity of human organisms, and the length of the human lifespan all give active reason to reject it. The combination of these factors means that it is not just possible, but in fact overwhelmingly likely, that all manner of things—either later in life or during development—could affect one out of a pair of genetically or developmentally linked traits without affecting the other.

Second Wakefield's response seems terribly ad hoc. Of course it *may* be the case that our ability to read is produced by a mechanism that was selected for a particular effect, and that dyslexia indicates a breakdown of that that mechanism. But it is just as plausible that that mechanism is itself a by-product of the selection of a different, linked trait, and therefore

---

[36] See also Gould (1991) and Gould and Lewontin (1979).

[37] Lilienfeld and Marino (1995) first raised this as an objection to Wakefield.

[38] Wakefield (1999b, p. 466, 2000, pp. 255–256). Wakefield does not think that all inabilities to read are dysfunctions; only those that are due to a hypothesized underlying dysfunction. Illiteracy due to lack of schooling, for example, is not a dysfunction on his account. To avoid potential confusion I have been talking about the *ability* to learn to read.

[39] Note that Wakefield in his responses talks about spandrels rather than non-selected effects. Spandrels are the decorated triangles between the skeletal support-structures in churches, which Gould and Lewontin (1979) famously claim are the necessary side effect of churches having roofs. I prefer to speak of non-selected effects for two reasons. First, because it is broader and more in line with the literature in philosophy of biology: not every non-selected effect is a spandrel, even if every spandrel is a non-selected effect. In fact it is the very spandrel analogy that leads Wakefield to suppose that a failure in the non-selected effect must indicate a failure in the selected mechanism producing it (Wakefield 2000, pp. 244–245). This may be true for actual spandrels, if they *have* to exist if a church has a roof, but I argue in the upcoming paragraph that this is not the case for every non-selected effect. Second, Gould and Lewontin were wrong about spandrels, even if they weren't wrong about adaptationism (e.g., Houston 2009).

lacking in function. Or that both the normal ability to learn to read and dyslexia are on a spectrum of normal variation in non-selected effects produced by a functioning underlying mechanism. And then there is a fourth option, which is that dyslexia itself is explained by its linkage to an adaptive trait, such as superior visual-spatial ability. In that case, dyslexia is indicative not of dysfunction, but of superior function. All four explanations are conjectures, of course, and I am not committed to any particular one of them. But Wakefield is: out of these four—on the face of it equally plausible and equally adaptive explanations for dyslexia—only one would make dyslexia a disorder. Wakefield, therefore, seems to be making a risky bet.[40]

This second problem is more damaging than might seem at first. Remember that the discussion here is not really about dyslexia—which is just an example—but about whether Wakefield can provide a successful account of *all* mental disorders. Wakefield can bet against the odds in one case, dyslexia, and either win or lose. But if very many of our mental capacities are like reading—that is, effects of traits that do not themselves explain why those traits were selected, and that are therefore not functions—Wakefield's position starts to look more precarious. Now he is betting in a series, and at least some of those bets he must lose. Whatever the truth on dyslexia, then, Wakefield's account of disorder will end with a substantial group of conditions that it cannot label as disorders, even though they are according to our folk concepts and the DSM.

Here is one reason to suppose that more rather than fewer of our mental capacities will be like reading. Recall a point made at the beginning of the chapter, which is that the mind, if it is to allow for an account of disorder as dysfunction, must consist of distinct modules with distinct functions. That—I argued—was contentious on the face of it. But if a selected effect account is to bear out that mental modules have functions, an even more demanding picture emerges: modules should not only be distinct and have distinct effects, but those effects should also—in every single case—have been the drivers of the selection of those very modules. In other words, every single mental module or capacity must have been "visible to natural selection" via its own effect rather than through any of the other possibilities discussed: pleiotropic, developmental or genetic linkage, or other effects of that module. Given the developmental complexity of our mind, that seems extremely unlikely. The moment that we allow, however, that mental modules are genetically, developmentally or pleiotropically linked, and that the selection of some traits and effects may be explained by effects elsewhere, Wakefield's account is already in a position where at least some apparent mental dysfunctions turn out not to be dysfunctions at all. Wakefield's account of disorder, it turns out, is very strongly revisionist.

Wakefield: More revisionist than he realizes

What should be done with the observation that Wakefield's account is so very revisionist? Bolton (2008) thinks it invalidates his account. Wakefield (1999a, 1999b, 2000) insists that it is not a large problem, and that where necessary we will adjust our ideas in the light of evolutionary facts. But Murphy and Woolfolk (2000b) point out—and I fully agree—that

---

[40] See also Murphy and Woolfolk (2000a).

Wakefield is not really owning up to the degree of revisionism that his account is committed to. Wakefield has yet to acknowledge explicitly that his dyslexia bet is a slim one, or that he is committed to maintaining that dyslexia, schizophrenia, and a host of other disorders would not be disorders if it turns out that they are not, in fact, failures of a selected effects—which is a distinct possibility.

Wakefield in his later work (2000, pp. 244–245) explicitly commits to the narrow selected effect account of function that I have outlined, which means he is subject to the problems that accompany it. But the bulk of his defense remains devoted to insisting that his account would not be terribly revisionist because the evolutionary facts will bear out our common-sense judgments—which is implausible. What Wakefield is not defending is that his account of disorder would be correct even if these facts go radically against the grain of common sense judgments. And that is the far more likely situation.[41]

We cannot settle this stalemate without access to the relevant evolutionary facts. But we can say with confidence that there is something deeply inconsistent about Wakefield's claim that his account won't be so terribly revisionist. In making this claim Wakefield assumes adaptive explanation for traits we like, such as reading, but not for ones we do not like, such as dyslexia. If one is favorably disposed toward adaptive explanations in general, however— as Wakefield appears to be—then one should be willing at least in principle to expect them equally in instances of health and in instances of disorder, unless one has good reason not to. And Wakefield has not given us such good reasons.

What we do have, of course, are bad reasons to assume adaptive explanations for traits we like, where we do not assume them for traits we dislike. One such bad reason is the prior judgment that the traits we do not like are disorders. This justification is occasion-ally offered by Wakefield (1999, 2000), but it is a bad one because it makes Wakefield's core claim circular; Wakefield believes that a condition's being a *dysfunction* should determine our judgment that it is a disorder. That point becomes rather hollow if our judgment that something is a disorder becomes our main, if not only, reason for thinking that condition is a dysfunction.[42]

A second bad reason is the usefulness or complexity of a trait, as the example of reading illustrates. It seems almost impossible that our ability to learn to read would not be designed: it is unique to humans, complicated, widespread, and incredibly useful, so how could it be a fluke? But it is a mistake to think that something is either selected, or a fluke. There is a good explanation for why we seem so well adapted to reading, but this explanation points not from script to our traits, but rather from our traits to script: the usefulness of reading does not explain why we developed the ability to read, but rather our ability to learn to read explains the discovery—or rather creation—of script and why it is useful to us. Therefore the fact that our traits seem beautifully adapted to what they do should not tempt us into think-ing that they were selected for what they do.[43] Rather, in some cases, a trait doing things well is what explains why it was and continues to be put to the use to which it is suited.

---

[41] See Murphy and Woolfolk (2000b) for a more detailed argument that Wakefield seems to hold evolutionary science hostage to folk concepts of mental disorder and psychiatric practice, and seems not truly committed to the idea that science may prove our folk concepts to be radically wrong—which science does regularly.

[42] See also Murphy and Woolfolk (2000b) and Bolton (2008).

[43] Famously illustrated by Gould and Lewontin (1979).

In summary, then, we have only bad reasons to accept Wakefield's claim about the lack of revisionism implied by his account, and good reasons to reject it on both theoretical and empirical grounds, even if we are not in possession of *all* the empirical facts. It is overwhelmingly likely that we have an abundance of traits that fulfill important roles for us and in our culture, particularly in the mental realm, but whose effects may not be what drove their selection. These traits therefore lack functions and, by consequence, the ability to dysfunction.

And this leads us to the final and most damaging aspect of the non-selected effects objection, which has not been raised so far. I take it that most if not all of our physical, and the vast majority of our mental traits, fall within the domain of health and disorder. That is to say, they are either disordered, and if not, they are healthy.[44] But an evolutionary account of disorder can never bear this out. As argued earlier, on such an account only those effects with the right evolutionary causal role can function and dysfunction. All other effects—that is, all effects of traits that did not drive the selection of those traits, and all effects produced by traits that were not selected for their own effects—neither have a function nor can they dysfunction. A consequence of this is that the revisionism of Wakefield's account lies not just in its labeling certain common-sense disorders as non-disorders. It also lies in the creation of an account of health and disorder that applies only to a subset of our traits. For whatever the precise evolutionary facts, Wakefield's account of disorder places a substantial portion of our physiological and mental traits out of the realm of health and disorder altogether. And that seems a clear violation of one core conceptual element of the health and disorder dichotomy, which is that all of our physical and mental traits seem to fall within them.

Naturalist Accounts of Disorder: Conclusions

Naturalism about disorder consists of two claims that should be kept separate. First, the claim that disorder can be defined at least in part in terms of biological dysfunction. Second, the claim that disorder and dysfunction are value-free concepts.

With respect to the former claim, I have examined two dominant accounts of dysfunction in philosophy of medicine and philosophy of biology: the causal role account defended by Boorse and the etiological account defended by Wakefield. A careful examination of the latter reveals it is highly revisionist in two ways. First, it relabels many conditions we now consider disorders as non-disorders. Second, and more problematically, it places many conditions—both normal and uncommon—out of the realm of disorder altogether. That latter revision is particularly hard to stomach as it seems to be a departure not merely from the extension of our current concepts of health and disorder, but from their very structure. In terms of tracking our actual concept of disorder, then, something like the forward-looking statistical causal role account offered by Boorse appears superior to Wakefield's.

---

[44] Indeed this is the very assumption that underlies most of the interest in and literature on division between health and disease. See also footnote 1.

One could decide to stick with Wakefield's account and accept its revisionism neverthe-less. But I strongly suggest that this is undesirable. Medicine and psychiatry are pragmatic disciplines; they are primarily interested in the effects of our bodies and minds that are use-ful to us in the here and now, not in how those effects were selected under different circum-stances in the past. Being able to learn how to read, for example, is an important function in modern life. But whether it is even included in the realm of functions, health and medicine, in Wakefield's account, depends entirely and crucially on the precise details of its causal role within a contingent evolutionary history. That does not do justice to how we want our con-cepts of health and disorder, and the disciplines that use them, to operate. If we are going to accept Wakefield's highly revisionist proposals we need a good defense of his revisionism first. Pretending that it does not exist or is marginal, as Wakefield does now, is not good enough.

With respect to the second claim I argued that it should be rejected; even if health and dis-order can be defined in terms of function and dysfunction, there is no reason to think that this makes these concepts value-free. The reason is that a concept definable in value-free terms can still embody the values that caused us to classify the natural world using this concept in the first place, rather than an alternative one. This argument only gains serious traction, however, if the natural world is such that alternatives are available. I have given sev-eral reasons to think that this is the case. First, the core role of reference classes in Boorse's account of health means that naturalist alternatives can readily be constructed. Second, any kind of pluralism about detailed descriptions of mental functional architecture would afford alternative classifications of mental disorder, and thereby undermine the second naturalist claim.

I conclude that our concepts of health and disorder are not value-free. Naturalism in that sense fails. But a weaker form of naturalism can survive. This weaker naturalism offers an account of disorder in value-free terms but does not claim that this makes the concept of disorder value-free. Such an account might be helpful in settling some controversy and in clarifying our thinking. But it will be based in the forward-looking model created by Boorse, not the backward-looking one by Wakefield.

References

Agich, G. J. (1983). Disease and value: a rejection of the value-neutrality thesis. *Theoretical Medicine*, 4, 27–41.

Allen, C. (2009). Teleological notions in biology. In E. N. Zalta (Ed.), *The Stanford Encyclopedia of Philosophy* (Winter 2009 Edition). [Online.] Available at: <http://plato.stanford.edu/archives/win2009/entries/teleology-biology/>.

Ananth, M. (2008). *In Defense of an Evolutionary Concept of Health: Nature, Norms and Human Biology*. Aldershot: Ashgate.

Ariew, A., Cummins, R., and Perlman, M. (2002). *Functions: New Essays in the Philosophy of Psychology and Biology*. Oxford: Oxford University Press.

Bayer, R. (1987). *Homosexuality and American Psychiatry: The Politics of Diagnosis*. Princeton, NJ: Princeton University Press.

Bechtel, W. and Abrahamsen, A. (1990). *Connectionism and the Mind: And Introduction to Parallel Processing in Networks*. Cambridge, MA: Blackwell Publishing.

Boorse, C. (1975). On the distinction between disease and illness. *Philosophy and Public Affairs*, 5, 49–68.

Boorse, C. (1976a). Wright on functions. *Philosophical Review*, 85, 70–86.

Boorse, C. (1976b). What a theory of mental health should be. *Journal for the Theory of Social Behaviour*, 6, 61–84.

Boorse, C. (1977). Health as a theoretical concept. *Philosophy of Science*, 44, 542–73.

Boorse, C. (1987). Concepts of health. In D. Van de Veer and T. Regan (Eds), *Health Care Ethics: An Introduction*, pp. 359–93. Philadelphia, PA: Temple University Press.

Boorse, C. (1997). A rebuttal on health. In J. M. Humber and R. F. Almeder (Eds), *What is Disease?*, pp. 1–134. Totowa, NJ: Humana Press.

Boorse, C. (2002). A rebuttal on functions. In A. Ariew, R. Cummins, and M. Perlman (Eds), *Functions: New Essays in the Philosophy of Psychology and Biology*, pp. 7–32. Oxford: Oxford University Press.

Boorse, C. (2011). Concepts of health. In F. Gifford (Ed.), *Philosophy of Medicine*, pp. 13–64. Oxford: Elsevier.

Bolton, D. (2008). *What is Mental Disorder? An Essay in Philosophy, Science and Values*. Oxford: Oxford University Press.

Brandon, R. N. (2005). The difference between selection and drift: a reply to Millstein. *Biology and Philosophy*, 20, 153–70.

Brandon, R. N. (2006). The principle of drift: biology's first law. *Journal of Philosophy*, 103, 319–35.

Cartwright, S. A. (1851). Report on the diseases and physical peculiarities of the negro race. *The New Orleans Medical and Surgical Journal*, 7, 707–9.

Clouser, K. D., Culver, C. M. and Gert, B. (1981). Malady: a new treatment of disease. *The Hastings Center Report*, 11, 29–37.

Clouser, K. D., Culver, C. M. and Gert, B. (1997). Malady. In J. M. Humber and R. F. Almeder (Eds), *What is Disease?*, pp. 175–219. Totowa, NJ: Humana Press.

Cooper, R. (2002). Disease. *Studies in History and Philosophy of Biological and Biomedical Sciences*, 33, 263–82.

Cooper, R. (2005). *Classifying Madness: A Philosophical Examination of the Diagnostic and Statistical Manual of Mental Disorders*. Dordrecht: Springer.

Cosmides, L. and Tooby, J. (1987). From evolution to behavior: evolutionary psychology as the missing link. In J. Dupre (Ed.), *The Latest on The Best: Essays on Evolution and Optimality*, pp. 277–306. Cambridge, MA: MIT Press.

Cosmides, L. and Tooby, J. (1999). Toward an evolutionary taxonomy of treatable disorders. *Journal of Abnormal Psychology*, 108, 453–64.

Dupré, J. (1993). *The Disorder of Things: Metaphysical Foundations of the Disunity of Science*. Cambridge, MA: Harvard University Press.

Engelhardt, H. T. (1974). The disease of masturbation: values and the concept of disease. *Bulletin of the History of Medicine*, 48, 234–48.

Engelhardt, H. T. (1975). The concepts of health and disease. In H. T. Engelhardt and S. F. Spicker (Eds), *Evaluation and Explanation in the Biomedical Sciences*, pp. 125–41. Dordrecht: Reidel.

Engelhardt, H. T. (1976). Ideology and etiology. *Journal of Medical Philosophy*, 1, 256–68.

Engelhardt, H. T. (1986). *The Foundations of Bioethics*. New York, NY: Oxford University Press.

Ereshefsky, M. (2001). *The Poverty of the Linnaean Hierarchy: A Philosophical Study of Biological Taxonomy*. Cambridge: Cambridge University Press.

Foucault, M. (1961). *Madness and Civilisation: A History of Insanity in the Age of Reason* (R. Howard, Trans.). London: Tavistock.

Fulford, K. W. M. (1999). Nine variations and a coda on the theme of an evolutionary definition of dysfunction. *Journal of Abnormal Psychology*, 108, 412–20.

Garson, J. (2010). Connectionism. In E. N. Zalta (Ed.), *The Stanford Encyclopedia of Philosophy* (Winter 2010 Edition). [Online.] Available at: <http://plato.stanford.edu/archives/win2010/entries/connectionism/>.

Gluckman, P., Beedle, A., and Hanson, M. (2009). *Prinicples of Evolutionary Medicine*. New York, NY: Oxford University Press.

Godfrey-Smith, P. (1993). Functions: Consensus without unity. *Pacific Philosophical Quarterly*, 74, 196–208.

Godfrey-Smith, P. (1994). A modern history theory of functions. *Noûs*, 28, 344–62.

Goosens, W. (1980). Values, health and medicine. *Philosophy of Science*, 47, 100–15.

Gould, S. J. (1991). Exaptation: a crucial tool for an evolutionary psychology. *Journal of Social Issues*, 47, 43–65.

Gould, S. J. and Lewontin, R. C. (1979). The spandrels of San Marco and the Panglossian paradigm: a critique of the adaptationist programme. *Proceedings of the Royal Society of London, Series B*, 205, 581–9.

Gould, S. J. and Vrba, E. S. (1982). Exaptation—a missing term in the science of form. *Paleobiology*, 8, 4–15.

Griffiths, P. E. (1993). Functional analysis and proper functions. *The British Journal for the Philosophy of Science*, 44, 409–22.

Guerrero, J. D. (2010). On a naturalist theory of health: a critique. *Studies in the History and Philosophy of Biological and Biomedical Sciences*, 41, 272–8.

Hacking, I. (1995). The looping effects of human kinds. In D. Sperber, D. Premack, and A. J. Premack (Eds), *Causal Cognition: A Multi Disciplinary Debate*, pp. 351–83. Oxford: Clarendon Press.

Hacking, I. (1998). *Mad Travelers: Reflections on the Reality of Transient Mental Illnesses*. Charlottesville, VA: University Press of Virginia.

Hausman, D. (2011). Is an overdose of paracetamol bad for one's health? *British Journal for the Philosophy of Science*, 62, 657–68.

Hawthorne, S. (2007). ADHD drugs: values that drive the debates and decisions. *Medicine, Health Care and Philosophy*, 10, 129–40.

Horwitz, A. V. and Wakefield, J. C. (2007). *The Loss of Sadness: How Psychiatry Transformed Normal Sorrow into Depressive Disorder*. Oxford: Oxford University Press.

Houston, A. I. (2009). San Marco and evolutionary biology. *Biology and Philosophy*, 24, 215–30.

Kass, L. R. (1975). Regarding the end of medicine and the pursuit of health. *The Public Interest*, 40, 11–42.

Kendell, R. (1975). The concept of disease and its implications for psychiatry. *British Journal of Psychiatry*, 127, 305–15.

Kingma, E. (2007). What is it to be healthy? *Analysis*, 67, 128–33.

Kingma, E. (2010). Paracetamol, poison and polio: why Boorse's account of function fails to distinguish health and disease. *British Journal for the Philosophy of Science*, 61, 241–64.

Kingma, E. (2012). Health and disease: Social constructivism as a combination of naturalism and normativism. In H. Carel and R. Cooper (Eds), *Health, Illness and Disease: Philosophical Essays*, pp. 37–56. Durham: Acumen Publishing.

Kirmayer, L. J. and Young, A. (1999). Culture and context in the evolutionary concept of mental disorder. *Journal of Abnormal Psychology*, 108, 446–52.

Kitcher, P. (1982). Genes. *British Journal for the Philosophy of Science*, 33, 337–59.

Kitcher, P. (1984). Species. *Philosophy of Science*, 51, 308–33.

Kitcher, P. (1996). *The Lives to Come: The Genetic Revolution and Human Possibilities*. New York, NY: Touchstone.

Klein, D. F. (1999). Harmful dysfunction, disorder, disease, illness, and evolution. *Journal of Abnormal Psychology*, 108, 421–9.

Laing, R. D. (1959). *The Divided Self*. London: Tavistock.

Lewens, T. (2004). *Organisms and artifacts*. Cambridge, MA: MIT Press.

Lilienfeld, S. O. and Marino, L. (1995). Mental disorder as a Roschian concept: a critique of Wakefield's "harmful dysfunction" analysis. *Journal of Abnormal Psychology*, 104, 411–20.

Lilienfeld, S. O. and Marino, L. (1999). Essentialism revisited: Evolutionary theory and the concept of mental disorder. *Journal of Abnormal Psychology*, 108, 400–11.

Margolis, J. (1976). The concept of disease. *The Journal of Medicine and Philosophy*, 1, 238–55.

Matthen, M. and Ariew, A. (2002). Two ways of thinking about natural selection. *Journal of Philosophy*, 49, 55–83.

McKenna, J., Trevathan, W., and Smith, E. O. (2008). *Evolutionary Medicine and Health: New Perspectives*. Oxford: Oxford University Press.

McNally, R. J. (1994). *Panic Disorder: A Conceptual Analysis*. New York, NY: Guilford.

Millikan, R. G. (1984). *Language, Truth and Other Biological Categories*. Cambridge, MA: MIT Press.

Millikan, R. G. (1989). In defense of proper functions. *Philosophy of Science*, 56, 288–302.

Murphy, D. (2006). *Psychiatry in the Scientific Imagine*. Cambridge, MA: MIT Press.

Murphy, D. (2009). Concepts of disease and health. In E. N. Zalta (Ed.), *The Stanford Encyclopedia of Philosophy* (Summer 2009 edition). [Online.] Available at: <http://plato.stanford.edu/archives/sum2009/entries/health-disease/>.

Murphy, D. and Stich, S. (2000). Darwin in the madhouse: evolutionary psychology and the classification of mental disorders. In P. Carruthers and A. Chamberlain (Eds), *Evolution and the Human Mind: Modularity, Language and Meta-Cognition*, pp. 62–92. Cambridge: Cambridge University Press.

Murphy, D. and Woolfolk, R. L (2000a). The harmful dysfunction analysis of mental disorder. *Philosophy, Psychiatry, & Psychology*, 7, 241–52.

Murphy, D. and Woolfolk, R. L (2000b). Conceptual analysis versus scientific understanding: an assessment of Wakefield's folk psychiatry. *Philosophy, Psychiatry, & Psychology*, 7, 271–93.

Neander, K. (1991a). Functions as selected effects: the conceptual analyst's defense. *Philosophy of Science*, 58, 168–84.

Neander, K. (1991b). The teleological notion of 'function'. *Australasian Journal of Philosophy*, 69, 454–68.

Neander, K. (1995). Misrepresenting and malfunctioning. *Philosophical Studies*, 79, 109–41.

Nordenfelt, L. (1987). *On the Nature of Health: An Action-Theoretic Approach*. Dordrecht: Reidel.

Nordenfelt, L. (2001). *Health, Science and Ordinary Language*. Amsterdam: Rodopi.

Nordenfelt, L. (2007). The concepts of health and illness revisited. *Medicine, Health Care, and Philosophy*, 10, 5–10.

Papineau, D. (1994). Mental disorder, illness and biological dysfunction. In A. Griffiths (Ed.), *Philosophy, Psychology and Psychiatry. Royal Institute of Philosophy Supplement 37*, pp. 73–84. Cambridge University Press.

Perlman, M. (2004). The modern philosophical resurrection of teleology. *The Monist*, 87, 3–51.

Reznek, L. (1987). *The Nature of Disease*. London: Routledge.

Richters, J. E. and Hinshaw, S. P. (1999). The abduction of disorder in psychiatry. *Journal of Abnormal Psychology*, *108*, 438–45.

Sadler, J. Z. (1999). Horsefeathers: a commentary on 'evolutionary versus prototype analyses of the concept of disorder. *Journal of Abnormal Psychology*, *108*, 433–7.

Sadler, J. Z. and Agich, G. J. (1995). Diseases, functions, values, and psychiatric classification. *Philosophy, Psychiatry, & Psychology*, *2*, 219–31.

Scadding, J. G. (1988). Health and disease: what can medicine do for philosophy? *Journal of Medical Ethics*, *14*, 118–24.

Scadding, J. G. (1990). The semantic problem of psychiatry. *Psychological Medicine*, *20*, 243–8.

Schramme, T. (2007). A qualified defence of a naturalist theory of health. *Medicine, Health Care, and Philosophy*, *10*, 11–17.

Simons, J. (2007). Beyond naturalism and normativism: reconceiving the 'disease' debate. *Philosophical Papers*, *36*, 343–70.

Sober, E. (1980). Evolution, population thinking and essentialism. *Philosophy of Science*, *47*, 350–83.

Sober, E. (2004). *The Nature of Selection: Evolutionary Theory in Philosophical Focus*. Cambridge, MA: MIT Press.

Szasz, T. S. (1960). The myth of mental illness. *American Psychologist*, *15*, 113–18.

Szasz, T. S. (1972). *The Myth of Mental Illness*. London: Paladin.

Tooby, J. and Cosmides, L. (1990a). On the universality of human nature and the uniqueness of the individual: the role of genetics and adaptation. *Journal of Personality*, *58*, 17–67.

Tooby, J. and Cosmides, L. (1990b). The past explain the present: emotional adaptations and the structure of ancestral environments. *Ethology and Sociobiology*, *11*, 375–424.

Tooby, J. and Cosmides, L. (1992). The psychological foundations of culture. In J. Barkow, L. Cosmides, and J. Tooby (Eds), *The Adapted Mind: Evolutionary Psychology and the Generation of Culture*, pp. 19–136. Oxford: Oxford University Press.

Wakefield, J. C. (1992a). Disorder as harmful dysfunction: a conceptual critique of DSM-III-R's definition of mental disorder. *Psychological Review*, *99*, 232–47.

Wakefield, J. C. (1992b). The concept of medical disorder: on the boundary between biological facts and social values. *American Psychologist*, *47*, 373–88.

Wakefield, J. C. (1995). Dysfunction as a value-free concept: a reply to Sadler and Agich. *Philosophy, Psychiatry, & Psychology*, *2*, 233–46.

Wakefield, J. C. (1999a). Evolutionary versus prototype analyses of the concept of disorder. *Journal of Abnormal Psychology*, *108*, 374–99.

Wakefield, J. C. (1999b). Mental disorder as a black box essentialist concept. *Journal of Abnormal Psychology*, *108*, 465–72.

Wakefield, J. C. (2000). Spandrels, vestigial organs, and such: reply to Murphy & Woolfolk's "the harmful dysfunction analysis of mental disorder." *Philosophy, Psychiatry, & Psychology*, *7*, 253–69.

Walsh, D., Lewens, T., and Ariew, A. (2002). Trials of life, natural selection, and random drift. *Philosophy of Science*, *69*, 452–73.

Whitbeck, C. (1978). Four basic concepts of medical science. *PSA: Proceedings of the Biennial Meeting of the Philosophy of Science Association*, *1*, 210–22.

Williams, G. and Nesse, R. M. (1996). *Why We Get Sick: The New Science of Darwinian Medicine*. New York, NY: Vintage Books.

CHAPTER 26

VALUES-BASED PRACTICE: TOPSY-TURVY TAKE-HOME MESSAGES FROM ORDINARY LANGUAGE PHILOSOPHY (AND A FEW NEXT STEPS)

K. W. M. FULFORD AND C. W. VAN STADEN

Values-based practice is a new skills-based approach to working with complex and conflicting values in health care that is proving to be a fast growing force at the practical cutting edge of the philosophy of psychiatry. This chapter outlines the theoretical basis of values-based practice in ordinary language (or linguistic analytic) philosophy as exemplified mainly by the work of J. L. Austin, Gilbert Ryle, Philippa Foot, R. M. Hare, Geoffrey Warnock, and others of the mid-twentieth-century "Oxford School."[1] Ordinary language philosophy has been something of a philosophical back-water in recent decades: when Fulford's extended essay in ordinary language philosophy, *Moral Theory and Medical Practice*, was published (in 1989) it was described by an Oxford philosopher, no less, as a "philosophical coelacanth." It was aptly so named. Like the coelacanth, ordinary language philosophy has proved to be a survivor. In values-based practice, as we will show, ordinary language philosophy lives on and indeed thrives as one of the key bridges supporting the rich two-way trade between theory and practice that is the hallmark of the philosophy of psychiatry.

The chapter has three main sections. The first section shows how ordinary language philosophy suggests a novel angle on the long-running debate about the concept of mental disorder. This in turn leads in the second section to a review of the findings from ordinary language philosophy first for mental disorder and then for bodily disorder. It is these findings that in the third and final main section provide the philosophical starting point for values-based practice. We start with a brief resume of what ordinary language philosophy is and what it is not.

---

[1] The practice of values-based practice is described more fully in our chapter in the companion volume to this book (Fulford and van Staden forthcoming), the *Oxford Handbook of Psychiatric Ethics*.

Ordinary Language Philosophy: What It Is and What It Is Not

Like most philosophical "schools," ordinary language philosophy is not a well-defined discipline.[2] At its heart it is perhaps best understood as a method or way of tackling philosophical problems. Austin, it is true, resisted the idea that ordinary language philosophy amounted to anything as grand as a method (reported by Warnock 1989, chapter 1). Ordinary language philosophy nonetheless does have a number of distinctive features and it will be worth reviewing these briefly before turning to how the approach can be helpful in medicine.

The starting point for ordinary language philosophy is the observation that by and large we are better at using higher-level concepts than at defining them. This observation is not original to ordinary language philosophy. St Augustine, for example, in a widely cited passage from his fourth-century *Confessions* (book 11, chapter 14, no. 17) observed "What then is time? Provided that no one asks me, I know. If I want to explain it to an enquirer, I do not know" (Chadwick 1992). A moment's reflection shows exactly what Augustine meant. We *use* the concept of time all the time pretty much effortlessly; and yet if pressed we find we are unable to define what we mean by it. Lower-level concepts by contrast present no problem of definition at all. A "watch," for example, is readily defined along the lines of "a small instrument used for measuring time." Similarly, the definitions of subcategories of watch (wrist watch, fob watch, etc.) and of subparts of a watch (second hand, winder, etc.) all follow without undue difficulty. But these definitions only work *as* definitions (they only tell us what the lower-level concepts in question mean) to the extent that we are already able to *use* the (higher-level) concepts in terms of which they are expressed with understanding, including in this case the concept of time.

This cluster of ideas—that we are better at using than defining higher-level concepts; that definition nonetheless works fine with lower-level concepts; but only because we are already able to use the higher-level concepts in terms of which lower-level definitions are expressed—will be important later when we come to the language of medicine. There is though more to ordinary language philosophy. For ordinary language philosophy builds on the priority of use over definition to suggest a particular way of understanding conceptual problems (to the extent that these involve higher-level concepts), a particular method for tackling them, and a particular expectation of the outputs to be derived in terms of improved understanding if things go well. Again, each of these will be important to us later on:

- *Conceptual problems as grammatical illusions.* Ordinary language philosophy takes (at least some) conceptual problems to derive from partial or distorted views of the meanings of complex concepts, views which have become tacitly embedded in the ways that philosophical questions are posed. Wittgenstein (to borrow from the

---

[2] Even the term "ordinary language philosophy" is far from settled. Austin himself expressed dissatisfaction with it and with its (continuing) cognates such as "linguistic philosophy" and "linguistic analysis." One option he suggested in "A Plea for Excuses" (p. 25) might be "'linguistic phenomenology,' only that is rather a mouthful."

"Cambridge school") used psychopathological metaphors like "grammatical illusions" (Wittgenstein 1953, section 110) and "delusion" (Wittgenstein 1958, p. 158) to capture the way in which conceptual problems can arise from the "bewitchment of our intelligence by means of language" (Wittgenstein 1953, section 109).

- *The method of philosophical field work.* Ordinary language philosophy piggy-backs on our enhanced ability to use complex concepts, i.e., instead of passively reflecting on their meanings (as in definition), ordinary language philosophy involves actively observing how the concepts in question are used in the relevant range of ordinary (i.e., non-philosophical) everyday contexts. Austin called this quasi-empirical look-and-really-see approach philosophical "field work" (Austin 1956/1957, p. 25).[3]

- *The outputs as logical geographies.* Philosophical field work has the modest aim of helping to dispel grammatical illusions by producing a more complete picture of the full meaning of the complex concept(s) in question. Gilbert Ryle compared ordinary language philosophy in this respect with the way a geographer maps out the features of a complex terrain, describing it as producing a more complete view of the relevant "logical geography"" (Ryle 1949/1963, p. 10).

From the start, ordinary language philosophy was subject to a number of objections (Fann 1969): it was suggested, for example, that ordinary usage incorporates precisely those difficulties (about truth, justification, and so forth) that it is the task of philosophy to explicate; that many of the problems of philosophy, as in the philosophy of mathematics, have precious little to do with ordinary usage; and that philosophy is anyway a normative rather than (as any empirical approach must be) a descriptive venture. In a recent defense of the approach, on the other hand, the American philosopher Avner Baz (2012) has argued that a number of now widely accepted critiques of ordinary language philosophy (notably by Searle, Geach, and Soames) have attributed to it a theory of meaning that it was its precise aim to reject. These critiques, Baz concludes, were therefore misdirected.

Either way, it is important always to bear in mind the limitations of ordinary language philosophy as spelled out by no less an exemplar of the approach than Austin. Investigating ordinary language use, Austin said, is no more than "one way of getting started with some kinds of philosophical problem" (cited in Warnock 1989, p. 6); and again, it may sometimes be a useful "first word," but never the last (Austin 1956/1957, p. 27). These limitations, we believe, provide the basis for a balanced understanding of the place of ordinary language philosophy within analytic philosophy as a whole. Taken together with its look-and-really-see empirical orientation, furthermore, Austin's limitations show ordinary language philosophy to be well matched to the requirements of a practical discipline like psychiatry. Looking-and-really-seeing is after all very much what psychiatry like other areas of scientific medicine is all about. So a descriptive rather than normative approach works well at least as a "first word." Looking-and-really-seeing furthermore in a complex field like psychiatry requires more than one kind of methodological spectacles. Ordinary language philosophy, therefore, as only "one way of getting started," becomes a natural partner in combined-methods research protocols in which complex problems are distributed across a team of researchers with expertise in different fields (philosophical, empirical, and clinical). Austin, drawing on his experience as an intelligence officer in World War II, advocated

---

[3] Page references to Austin 1956/1957 are to the reprint of his article in White (1968).

just such a "team work" approach (Warnock 1989, chapter 1). While as to Austin's limitation to "some kinds of philosophical problem," it is precisely within the ordinary language of psychiatry (and related disciplines such as the neurosciences) that the problems with which the philosophy of psychiatry is concerned arise. We need indeed look no further again than Austin for a direct endorsement of the prima facie appropriateness of psychopathology as an area for philosophical field work (Austin 1956/1957, p. 42).[4]

So, how do things turn out? Austin died relatively young and before he could put his ideas for philosophical (team) field work into effect. In the next two sections we will look at some of the results from this approach as applied first to the long-running "debate about mental disorder" and then to successor debates about concepts of disorder generally.

The Debate about Mental Disorder

Current debates about concepts of disorder (as reflected in a number of chapters in this book; e.g., Bolton, Chapter 28; Kingma, Chapter 25) have their origins in the psychiatry versus anti-psychiatry debate that developed in the 1950s and ran through into the 1960s and 1970s. Psychiatry over this period came under attack from various disciplines including psychology (Eysenck 1960), sociology (Scheff 1974; Sedgewick 1973), and history (Foucault 1971); but also and importantly from the then nascent patient-power movement (Campbell 1996) supported by many from within psychiatry's own ranks (Laing 1960; Laing and Esterson 1964; Szasz 1960).

These attacks on psychiatry were motivated in one way or another by concerns about the then dominant medical model of mental disorder. Mental disorder, everyone acknowledged, was a real enough aspect of human experience and behavior: but it was a mistake, the anti-psychiatry movement argued, to assimilate mental disorders to the model of disorder that (it was true) worked so well in bodily medicine. Widely differing views were expressed about what mental disorders really were: maladaptive learned behaviors (Eysenck); a construct of social processes such as labeling (Scheff, Sedgewick); mechanisms of political control (Foucault); spiritual experiences (Campbell); attempts to make sense of conflicting family messages (Esterson, Laing); or, simply, life problems (Szasz). But one way or another, mental disorders, the anti-psychiatry movement all agreed, were not just another kind of bodily disorder. The pro-psychiatry movement on the other hand countered that, to the contrary, mental disorders, although certainly distinctive in some respects really were, when it came down to it, properly understood in essentially the same way as bodily disorders (Kendell 1975; Roth and Kroll 1986; Wing 1978).

The conceptual issues at the heart of the anti-psychiatry versus psychiatry debate are shown particularly clearly by an exchange over this period between two psychiatrists (both professors of psychiatry), Thomas Szasz (Syracuse University, New York) and R. E. Kendell (Edinburgh Medical School, Scotland). Szasz (1960) argued that "mental illness is a myth"; Kendell (1975), replying directly to Szasz, argued that it was not. Szasz and Kendell were

---

[4] In the concluding section of Austin's "A Plea for Excuses" (p. 42) he gives two examples from psychopathology ("displacement behaviour" and "'compulsive'" behaviour (as in) compulsive washing for example") to illustrate the way in which language use in the sciences can usefully supplement "ordinary speech."

Szasz (1961): The myth ...

Target problem is mental illness: My aim in this essay is "to raise the question 'Is there such a thing as mental illness?' and to argue that there is not." (p. 113)

Meaning of bodily disorder the paradigm: Bodily disorder is defined by deviation from the clearly defined norms of the "structural and functional integrity of the human body." (p. 114)

Does mental disorder measure up?: NO—by contrast with bodily disorders the norms deviation from which are regarded as mental illness "are psychosocial, ethical, and legal." (p. 114)

Conclusion: Mental disorder is essentially *different* from bodily disorder and thus "mental illness is a myth." (p. 118)

Kendell (1975): The concept ...

Target problem is mental illness: "The purpose of this essay is to examine (the) proposition ... that what psychiatrists regard as mental illnesses are not illnesses at all." (p. 305)

Meaning of bodily disorder the paradigm: Bodily illness is defined by "biological disadvantage" which ... "must embrace both increased mortality and reduced fertility." (p. 310)

Does mental disorder measure up?: YES—epidemiological evidence (pp. 310–314) shows that at least some mental illnesses "carry with them an intrinsic biological disadvantage" (p. 314) as defined by increased mortality and/or reduced fertility.

Conclusion: Mental disorder is essentially *similar* to bodily disorder and thus in answer to Szasz "At least part of the territory regarded by psychiatrists as mental illness fulfils the same criteria as those required for physical illness." (p. 314)

FIGURE 26.1 The parallel forms of argument adopted by Szasz and Kendell.

well-matched and able protagonists and the differences between them in these and subsequent publications have been extensively rehearsed elsewhere (Schaler 2004). Relatively neglected, however, have been three important similarities between them in the assumptions underlying their respective positions. We illustrate these three similarities with sample quotes from Szasz and Kendell in Fig. 26.1. Briefly, Szasz and Kendell both assumed that:

1. it is the meaning of mental disorder that is their target problem
2. the meaning of bodily disorder is (relatively speaking) not a problem, and hence,
3. the legitimacy or otherwise of the concept of mental disorder depends on the extent to which its meaning tracks that of the concept of bodily disorder.

Given their three shared assumptions, it is perhaps remarkable that the contrary conclusions to which Szasz and Kendell came about mental disorder (respectively that it is and is not a myth) turned on differences between them in the way they interpreted the meaning not of mental disorder (their shared target problem) but rather of the (so they supposed) relatively unproblematic *bodily disorder*. Thus, Szasz argued that bodily disorder is defined by anatomical and physiological norms of the "structural and functional integrity of the human body" (Szasz 1960, p. 114); but the norms of mental disorder, he suggested, are by contrast "psychosocial, ethical and legal" (Szasz 1960, p. 114); hence Szasz concluded that mental disorder is a myth because it is essentially *different from* bodily disorder. Kendell, on the other hand, defined bodily disorder in broadly evolutionary terms as involving "biological disadvantage" (Kendell 1975, p. 309) which (whatever else it means) "must embrace both increased mortality and reduced fertility" (Kendell 1975, p. 310); but many mental disorders, Kendell pointed out, drawing on epidemiological data of reduced fertility and increased mortality among people with conditions like schizophrenia, also involve biological disadvantage; hence he concluded *contra* Szasz that mental disorder is not a myth because it is essentially *the same as* bodily disorder.

Things might have gone differently between Szasz and Kendell. They might, for example, have agreed about the meaning of bodily disorder while disagreeing about whether mental disorder mapped onto it. Or they might have agreed about the meaning of bodily disorder but disagreed about whether the validity of mental disorder stood or fell by whether or not it mapped onto it. As it was, the pivotal point of disagreement between them was about the meaning of bodily disorder.

And that with some refinements is more or less where matters stand today. Some have argued recently that "anti-psychiatry is dead" (Fulford and Sadler 2000). But anti-psychiatric concerns from the 1960s and 1970s, about the dominant medical model of mental disorder, continue to surface, for example in the currently growing "critical psychiatry" movement (Bracken and Thomas, Chapter 11, this volume); and the challenge from that period to the hegemony of psychiatry has been translated into "boots on the ground" through the development of multidisciplinary models of service delivery (Department of Health 2007) and a growing influence of the "service user voice" (Department of Health 2005; Williamson 2004). These developments in turn have provoked ongoing debates within and beyond psychiatry about what has become known as the "boundary problem," i.e., the problem of where medical involvement with mental disorder properly begins and ends. A key aspect of the boundary problem, moreover, directly reflecting Szasz's concerns, has been the boundary between mental disorders (medically understood) and moral categories such as delinquency; and, directly reflecting Kendell's "biological disadvantage" definition of disorder, evolutionary theory has been the dominant theme in debates about where the boundary of mental disorder properly lies (we return to the boundary problem in the next section). These debates indeed, about the concept of mental disorder, far from being dead have been given a particular urgency in recent years with the launch of revision processes leading to new editions of the world's two major psychiatric classifications, the World Health Organization's *International Classification of Diseases* (the ICD; World Health Organization 1992) and the American Psychiatric Association's *Diagnostic and Statistical Manual of Mental Disorders* (the DSM; American Psychiatric Association 2000) (Poland and Von Eckardt, Chapter 44, this volume). The key conceptual issues were indeed highlighted in a major publication from the American Psychiatric Association in 2002 setting out the research agenda for the new DSM (Kupfer et al. 2002; see also Chapter 1, this volume).

Subsequent refinements to the debate between Szasz and Kendell are important. The American philosopher, Christopher Boorse, for example, was among the first to explore the distinction between illness and disease (Boorse 1975, 1997); and the American academic social worker, Jerome Wakefield, has written extensively on how concepts of "harm" and "dysfunction" come together in the concept of disorder (see, e.g., Wakefield 1995, 1999a, 2000). (We return to Boorse and Wakefield's work in the next section.) There have been other approaches too: the Swedish philosopher Lennart Nordenfelt's "action theoretic" model (Nordenfelt 1987, 1992); Derek Bolton's concept of "intentional causality" (Bolton and Hill 1996; see also Bolton, Chapter 28, this volume); Chris Megone's derivation of Aristotelian norms of flourishing (Megone 1998; see also Irwin, Chapter 4, and Harcourt,

Chapter 5, this volume); and Tim Thornton's innovative use of the concept of "salience" to cut across the evaluation/description divide (Thornton 2000). But the dominant themes remain essentially as first set out in the debate between Szasz and Kendell: the concept of mental disorder remains the target problem (albeit cast now as a problem of boundary setting rather than about whether or not mental disorder as such is a myth); the concept of bodily disorder remains the resource to which most turn (albeit with many refinements in how bodily disorder itself is understood); and the boundary between mental disorder (medically understood) and moral categories (of one kind or another) is taken by a large majority to be defined (in one way or another) by norms derived from an evolutionary understanding (of one kind or another) of the concept of bodily disorder.

This no-further-forward bottom line comes as no surprise from the perspective of ordinary language philosophy. To the extent that the whole debate about mental disorder has been an extended exercise in definition it is no surprise that it has been ultimately unproductive. For definition, so ordinary language philosophy suggests, is simply the wrong tool for the job (i.e., the job of exploring the meanings of a higher-level concept like disorder). True, the exercise in definition shows no sign of running out of steam but, to the contrary, continues to be pursued with ever greater subtlety and determination: "Just one more definition and we'll get it right!" those involved seem to be saying. But by extension from Wittgenstein's metaphor of the linguistic "delusion," this is fully understandable as an example of what in descriptive psychopathology would be called "delusional elaboration" (perhaps combined with a large dose of "folie à deux").[5] There was certainly no a priori reason why in the 1960s and 1970s definition should not have been adopted as the tool for the job. After all, who is to say, a priori, where in any given area of discourse definitions of lower-level concepts give way to the need for other ways of exploring the meanings of higher-level concepts (the move as in our earlier example from the lower level "watch" up to the higher level "time"). Indeed, the many successes over this period with the use of definition for lower-level psychopathological concepts (as in the Present State Examination; Wing et al. 1974) is sufficient justification for the initial adoption of a similar approach to exploring the meanings of higher-level concepts of disorder. And the expectation at the time was that with advances in the sciences underpinning psychiatry, the concept of mental disorder would come increasingly to look like that of bodily disorder (see, e.g., Boorse 1976). But now with the benefit of a no-further-forward bottom-line reality check, it is surely time to try a different approach.

This is what we will be doing in the next two sections: first, recasting the debate along ordinary language philosophy lines as a debate about concepts of disorder in general, and then, in the final main section, seeing where in the spirit of Austin's "getting started" this takes us.

THE DEBATE ABOUT DISORDER

In this section we will first outline how, recast in the terms of ordinary language philosophy, mental disorder instead of being the target problem becomes a resource for philosophical field work on concepts of disorder in general. We will then summarize some of the

---

[5] Where people close to someone with delusions get drawn into their delusional thinking.

early findings from philosophical field work in this area. In the next section we will offer an interpretation of these findings that draws on work in ordinary language philosophy on value terms (sometimes called philosophical value theory) and indicate how this "ordinary values-language interpretation" underpins values-based practice.

Mental disorder as a resource for philosophical field work

Ordinary language philosophy turns the traditional debate about mental disorder upside down in the sense that the concept of mental disorder, instead of being the target problem, becomes a key resource for philosophical field work on concepts of disorder as a whole. This is essentially because in ordinary language philosophy the most fruitful areas for philosophical field work are often where the concepts in question cause trouble. It is where concepts run into trouble that, as Austin put it, we are able to break through the "blinding veil of ease and obviousness" by which the full complexity of their meanings is normally hidden from us (Austin 1956/1957, p. 23). There is a natural parallel here with medicine in that it is often where things go wrong with our bodies that we gain new insights into normal functioning (diabetes leading to the discovery of insulin, for example).

Mental disorder, we should add hastily, is still part of the problem as well as being a resource. But in the terms of ordinary language philosophy it is a problem specifically *in use*. More precisely, there are problems about the boundaries of (medical models of) mental disorder that there are not, or not to the same degree, with the corresponding boundaries of (medical models of) bodily disorder. The qualification "not to the same degree" is important: there *are* boundary problems also with bodily disorder; indeed the concept of "biological disadvantage" and its interpretation in evolutionary terms on which Kendell and so many of his successors draw in interpreting mental disorder, was derived from the work of E. J. M. Campbell, R. E. Scadding, and R. S. Roberts (1979) who as general medical physicians were trying to establish the boundary of disease conditions such as chronic bronchitis and asthma.[6] But the boundary problems are certainly wider and deeper in psychiatry. So much so that in the DSM classification (see earlier) the American Psychiatric Association felt it necessary to introduce what they called "criteria of clinical significance" in an attempt to demarcate the proper boundary of psychiatric interventions in the diverse range of human experiences and behaviors with which psychiatry might in principle be concerned. We return to the DSM's criteria of clinical significance later. But the point for now is that no such criteria of clinical significance have been felt to be necessary in the diagnostic manuals of areas of bodily medicine such as cardiology and gastroenterology.

If, however, part of the problem in the debate as now recast is the (relative) difficulty in use of the concept of mental disorder, another and no less important (conceptually speaking) part of the problem is the (relative) *ease of use* of the concept of bodily disorder. The problem for analysis, that is to say, is two-sided: one side of the problem is to explain why the concept of disorder is relatively *difficult to use* in connection with *mental* conditions;

---

[6] Published in a medical journal, and widely debated at the time among clinicians, this paper is of particular interest philosophically in that although drawing on Scadding's earlier work (in the 1960s) defining disease in terms of "biological disadvantage," it adopts what is in effect an empirical philosophical field work approach looking at the "... common usage [of] 'disease.'" (p. 757, column 2).

the other (and no less significant) side of the problem for analysis is to explain why the concept of disorder is relatively *easy to use* in connection with *bodily* conditions. The point is one of logical geography: the more complete view of the logical geography of the concept of disorder that it is the aim of philosophical field work to provide, must explain *both* sides (both difficult and easy sides) of the use of the concept of disorder in the contexts respectively of mental and of bodily conditions. There is no requirement here to validate or indeed invalidate this or that use of the concept of disorder (mental or bodily). Such validations or invalidations may or may not follow from a more complete understanding of the relevant logical geography. But the requirement of understanding as such extends even-handedly as much to the (relatively unproblematic in use) concept of bodily disorder as to the (relatively problematic in use) concept of mental disorder. Bodily disorder and mental disorder are in this respect equal and opposite sides of the logical geography of disorder.

With these considerations in mind, then, philosophical field work in this area might reasonably start with the (relatively problematic in use) concept of mental disorder. This is not, however, because mental disorder is (in any particular still less exclusive sense) the target problem, but because, as the more problematic concept in use, it is the more likely to prove productive as an area for philosophical field work aimed at producing a more complete understanding of the logical geography of concepts of disorder as a whole. There are many different ways in which starting with mental disorder might be done. There are many different ranges of the use of the concept of disorder in connection with mental conditions. There are many different disciplines (philosophical and empirical) that might be used, together and/or separately, to explore this or that range of uses of the concept of disorder in connection with mental conditions. We will describe here just one example of each: a combined-methods philosophical-empirical study of the use of the concept of mental disorder; and then a single-method philosophical study of the use of the concept of bodily disorder.

Philosophical field work: Some findings for mental disorder

We owe the combined-methods study to the British social scientist Anthony Colombo and colleagues (Colombo et al. 2003). Colombo had become interested in concepts of disorder in mental health when he was working as a doctoral student with the criminologist Nigel Walker in Cambridge in the 1990s (Colombo 1997). Colombo's DPhil was about the boundary problem. A key issue in criminology as in psychiatry is the boundary between, as it is often put, "mad and bad" and Colombo's DPhil explored how perceptions of where the boundary lay are influenced by different models of disorder. In pursuit of this he reviewed the by then already very extensive literature on concepts of mental disorder and showed that all of the widely diverse models currently on offer could be reduced to five main categories (medical, social, psychological, psychoanalytic, and political) each of which could be analyzed in terms of just twelve elements (covering key aspects of how the various models suggest mental disorders should be understood and managed). The resulting five-by-twelve "models grid" combined with a semistructured questionnaire and a standardized scoring scheme, thus allowed Colombo to locate a given individual or group of individuals within what amounted to a logical geography of mental disorder (Fulford and Colombo 2004).

We show two of Colombo's models grids together in Fig. 26.2. These are based on the results of a study that Colombo subsequently carried out with others at Warwick University

	Medical (biological)	Social (stress)	Cognitive behavioral	Psycho-therapeutic	Family (interaction)	Political
1 Diagnosis/ description	P			S		
2 Interpretation of behavior	P			S		
3 Labels	P			S		
4 Etiology	P			S		
5 Treatment	P	S			S	
6 Function of the hospital	P S	P S				P
7 Hospital and community	P	S		S		
8 Prognosis	P			S		
9 Rights of the patient	P S	S				S
10 Rights of society	P S					
11 Duties of the patient	P		P S			
12 Duties of society	P	S				

FIGURE 26.2 Models grids comparing two groups of practitioners, psychiatrists (P) and social workers (S).

combining his empirical work on models with Fulford's work in ordinary language philosophy (Fulford 1989). This particular study used responses to a standardized case vignette (of an imaginary person called "Tom") to explore the implicit models of disorder in play in the community care of people with a diagnosis of schizophrenia. The model of mental disorder adopted explicitly by clinicians then (as now) is called the "biopsychosocial model," i.e., a model in which biological, psychological, and social factors all play equal roles in how a given person's condition is understood and managed. The implicit models of those concerned, however, turned out to be very different. Figure 26.2 illustrates the differences between psychiatrists (expressing a predominantly biological (or medical) implicit model) and social workers (expressing predominantly psychological and social implicit models); and there were further differences for each of the other groups studied (psychiatric nurses, service users, and carers).

On first inspection Colombo's study might be thought to be nothing more than a (clever) piece of social science research. Its place of first publication after all was a (leading) social science journal (*Social Science & Medicine*); and the methodology too is derived from the empirical social science methodology he developed for his DPhil (although Colombo's initial literature review of concepts of disorder in itself amounts to an exercise in philosophical field work). But in this case at least, the empirical social science methodology was combined with an ordinary language philosophy theoretical approach that provided both a framework for interpreting the results of the study and a basis for converting those results subsequently into a series of practical initiatives in policy, training, and service development.

We return to the practical roll-out of the study in our chapter in the sister volume to this book (Fulford and van Staden, forthcoming). But the theory in outline runs like this. The differences found in implicit models reflect differences in *values*, i.e., differences in what this or that group perceived to be important about the test case vignette, "Tom." Thus, psychiatrists were concerned about diagnosis, medication, and so forth; while by contrast the priorities for social workers were to identify stress factors and to support self-management through psychological interventions. So far, so good, as it were. But now the question raised is how these differences in values should be understood and hence what we should do about (or with) them. One reaction—a natural enough reaction perhaps, faced with such apparently contradictory values—is to call for a top value: one of the referees for the paper subsequently published in *Social Science & Medicine* complained that we had made "not the slightest effort" to say whose sense of priorities was best. Yet understood as an exercise in logical geography, the Colombo study is (for better or worse, dare we say) a descriptive not a prescriptive exercise. Ordinary language philosophy as we will show in our chapter on the practical roll-out of values-based practice (Fulford and van Staden, forthcoming) does have something perfectly definite to say about "Whose values?" But an adjudication of the kind for which this referee was calling is not it.

A second reaction, an extension of the first really, is that further studies should be carried out to determine the clinical impact of the different models expressed and the values they embody. "Clinical trials" after all, as they are called, of just this kind are what would be expected of a new medication. But this begs the question of the outcome criteria by which the impact of this or that model of disorder and its embedded values should be judged. With a clinical trial of a new medication outcomes are at least centrally set by the condition for which the medication is intended. That is to say, the relevant values determining the criteria of "good and bad" outcomes are pre-set by the research history leading up to the clinical trial (though the relevant values are in general mainly implicit). But in a clinical trial of values there are no such pre-set values on which to draw. Indeed, the call for a clinical trial of values instead of resolving actually begs in a particularly acute form the question of "Whose values?" Here ordinary language philosophy as a descriptive exercise has no prior right of determination.

But surely, we can imagine our original critical referee now saying, the needs of patients provide a natural candidate outcome value criterion. And this is clearly true. But in this case at least, in the case that it is by reference to the needs of patients that outcome criteria should be set, a further aspect of the logical geography of disorder revealed by the study itself suggests that *both* kinds of model (both biological and psychosocial models) are needed. For as Fig. 26.3 shows, as judged by their reactions to "Tom,"[7] patients expressed essentially the same two kinds of implicit model (biological and psychosocial) as psychiatrists and social workers: the way some patients reacted to Tom reflected an essentially biological model like that expressed by psychiatrists: the way other patients reacted to Tom reflected psychological and social models essentially similar to those expressed by social workers. Translating these reactions therefore (as earlier) into values, it would seem that for some patients a broadly biological model would meet their needs, while for others a psychosocial model would be more appropriate.

---

[7] The study was based on a "level playing field" design in which patients and carers were involved throughout in the same way as practitioners, including playing an equal role in the study design (see Fulford and Colombo 2004).

	Medical (biological)	Social (stress)	Cognitive behavioral	Psycho-therapeutic	Family (interaction)	Political
1 Diagnosis/ description	PP			SP		
2 Interpretation of behavior			PP	PP SP		
3 Labels	PP		SP	SP		
4 Etiology	PP			SP		
5 Treatment	PP	SP		SP		
6 Function of the hospital	PP SP	PP				PP SP
7 Hospital and community		PP SP		PP SP		
8 Prognosis	PP			SP		
9 Rights of the patient	PP SP	SP				PP SP
10 Rights of society		PP SP				
11 Duties of the patient		PP SP	PP SP			
12 Duties of society	PP		PP SP			PP SP

FIGURE 26.3 Models grids comparing two groups of patients, one like psychiatrists (PP), the other like social workers (SP).

That both kinds of model (biological and psychosocial) are needed is the answer also to a third natural reaction to the results of the study. This third reaction can be put thus: If there is to be no top model, if even after further clinical trials it is clear that both biological and psychosocial models will be needed, perhaps there should be some form of "super model" in which the distinct elements of different models are in one way or another merged.

The call for a super model of this kind was the most common reaction among practitioners (psychiatrists, social workers, and others) involved in the study when presented with the findings in feedback sessions. It amounts after all to a call for an implicit biopsychosocial model corresponding with the explicit biopsychosocial model with which those involved in the study were already familiar. There were also clear clinical concerns driving their reaction. The practitioners involved in the study were all working in the then recently much expanded multidisciplinary mental health teams; and multidisciplinary team work depends critically on shared decision-making based on effective communication between team members; but at the time of the study there was growing evidence of poor communication and failures of shared decision-making within the multidisciplinary teams of the day. Practitioners themselves were correspondingly quick to realize that such failures were readily explained by the fact that despite their shared explicit commitment to a biopsychosocial model, they were all working unawares with widely different, and in some respects conflicting, implicit models. Surely, then, it was natural for these same practitioners to suggest, some form of consensus was needed; and given their already shared explicit biopsychosocial super model, why not merge their different implicit models into a shared implicit biopsychosocial super model?

Fig. 26.3, however, shows that although this is again a natural enough reaction, an implicit super model of the kind suggested (even if it proved to be psychologically possible to achieve) would actually be in conflict with the differentiated models (and correspondingly different needs) of patients. Hence while a consensual super model among practitioners might well increase the level of shared decision-making between them, it would by the same token reduce the extent to which the actual decisions they reached mapped onto the diverse needs of individual patients. In the "outcome language" of a clinical trial then, a consensual implicit super model would have better outcomes for practitioners but worse outcomes for patients.

Consensus, as we will show in our chapter in the sister volume to this book, does indeed have a part to play in the practice of values-based practice (as the basis of shared frameworks of values). But the central finding from the Colombo study as an exercise in philosophical field work is that *diversity* of values is as important as diversity of skills to the clinical effectiveness of multidisciplinary teams in meeting the diversity of needs (values) of individual patients and carers. This conclusion is consistent with much other field work evidence. We noted earlier, for example, the criteria of clinical significance at the heart of the DSM. These criteria, although of course assessable against descriptive criteria, are explicitly values-laden; and John Sadler's work on the DSM classification illustrates the extent to which values of many different kinds permeate concepts of mental disorder of more or less every stripe (Sadler 2005; see also Sadler, Chapter 45, this volume). It was indeed the value-laden-ness of mental disorder compared with bodily disorder that as we saw earlier, led Szasz to argue that the concept of mental disorder is a myth. And Kendell's introduction of evolutionary criteria and the many refinements thereon by subsequent apologists, have been motivated throughout by attempts to show mental disorder to be, really, just like bodily disorder by eliminating (or at any rate delimiting) the evaluative element in its meaning. Ordinary language philosophy reverses this, suggesting that values are an irreducible and clinically important feature of the logical geography of the concept of mental disorder.

But now comes the ordinary language philosophy "killer app" as they say. For in ordinary language philosophy, remember, it is where concepts run into trouble that we are more likely to break through what Austin (1956/1957, p. 23) called the "blinding veil of ease and obviousness" to their full meanings. That values are important in the logical geography of (the relatively more problematic in use) mental disorder thus suggests that despite appearances values might be important across the logical geography of concepts of disorder as a whole, including therefore and *contra* both Szasz and Kendell and indeed a majority of their "medical model" successors, the (relatively less problematic in use) concept of bodily disorder. This brings us to our example of single- (as opposed to combined-) method philosophical field work, in this case on the concept of bodily disorder.

Philosophical field work: Some findings for bodily disorder

One perhaps surprising place where philosophical field-work evidence is to be found of the importance of values across concepts of disorder as a whole, is in the language use of the very authors who have sought to define disorder (in part at least) value-free. We mentioned two such authors earlier as having added important refinements to the debate about mental disorder, Christopher Boorse and Jerome Wakefield. Both are concerned with the boundary problem presented by mental disorder; both respond to the boundary problem by seeking to define (by reference in one way or another to evolutionary theory) parts of the concept of disorder that are value-free, "disease" in Boorse's definition, "dysfunction" in Wakefield's. Yet both continue (in different ways) to use evaluative language in relation to their respective value-free (as they believe) concepts (disease for Boorse, dysfunction for Wakefield). We will not have space here to do justice to the contributions of either author to our understanding of evolutionary concepts of disorder (this is covered in more detail elsewhere in this book; see Kingma, Chapter 25, and Bolton, Chapter 28, this volume). Our aim here will instead be restricted to the philosophical field-work aim of describing the continued use of evaluative language by these two authors and what this suggests about the meaning of disorder.

The philosophical field work in Boorse's case is the observation that having defined disease value-free he slips more or less immediately into using evaluative language in relation to it. This slip from value-free definition to value-laden use is clear in his first paper on this subject, "On the distinction between disease and illness" (Boorse 1975).[8] He opens this paper with the boundary problem as represented by the expanding range of moral and social issues that at the time he was writing were being increasingly subsumed to the concept of mental disorder. The proper boundary of mental disorder, he argued, should be set by "a value-free science of health" (p. 49) that, turning now like others to examples of bodily disorder, was the province of (value-free) disease as distinct from (value-laden) illness. For disease, he continued, could be defined as "a deviation from the natural [= statistically typical] functional organization of the species" (p. 59, parenthesis added). There is much clear and persuasive argument behind Boorse's value-free definition of disease as set out like this at this point in his paper. But the philosophical field-work point to take is that despite his careful development of a value-free definition of disease, Boorse goes straight on only four lines later to write of disease in terms that are to all appearances value-laden. "In general" he says, "diseases are *deficiencies* in the functional efficiency of the body" (p. 59, emphasis added). We find a similar shift from value-free definition to value-laden use a little later in the same passage when (extending his definition to include endemic diseases) Boorse adds a causal criterion: in this instance the value-free "mainly due to environmental causes" shifts just three lines later to become the value-laden "action of a *hostile* environment" (both p. 59, emphasis added). A wide variety of further value terms make their appearance in both this and a later paper in which Boorse applies his definition of disease to mental conditions (Boorse 1976; see Fulford 1989, p. 38).

Boorse has had a good deal more to say about concepts of illness and disease in subsequent publications (e.g., 1997, 2004). We return in a moment to his later work and to the significance, notwithstanding, of the persistence of his use of evaluative language in writing of disease as just described. First, though, we will turn to the corresponding persistence of evaluative language in the more recent work of Jerome Wakefield on the concept of dysfunction.

Wakefield has published widely in recent years on what he calls the "harmful dysfunction" definition of disorder (see earlier). Like Boorse, Wakefield's target is the boundary problem presented by mental disorder; and like Boorse he draws on evolutionary theory as a resource for carving out a value-free element in the meaning of disorder that he intends should be used to set proper medical boundaries to the use of mental disorder. Where Boorse (in the papers noted earlier) focuses on disease, however, Wakefield focuses on dysfunction; and

---

[8] These shifts from value-free definition to value-laden use are described in more detail in Fulford 1989, chapter 3.

where Boorse draws on evolutionary criteria such as survival and reproduction as a source of (putative) value-free criteria, Wakefield draws (as others have drawn, e.g., Millikan 1998) on natural selection. Again, we do not have space here to do justice to Wakefield's substantive position. The key point though, the key philosophical field-work point, is that just as Boorse continues to use evaluative language in relation to disease notwithstanding his value-free definition of the term, so Wakefield continues to use evaluative language in relation to dysfunction notwithstanding his claim to having defined dysfunction value-free. In Wakefield, moreover, the persistence of evaluative language is even closer to (his definitional) home. In Boorse's account of disease his use of evaluative language comes a few lines after his value-free definitions (four lines and three lines respectively, noted earlier). In Wakefield's work evaluative language persists actually within what he nonetheless claims to be a value-free definition of dysfunction.

The philosophical field work required to show the persistence of evaluative language in Wakefield's definition of dysfunction is rather more involved than with Boorse's work on disease. This has been set out in detail by one of us in an invited commentary on an article by Wakefield (1999a) in a special issue of *The Journal of Abnormal Psychology* on concepts of disorder (Fulford 1999).[9] The concept of disorder, Wakefield suggested here as elsewhere, is a hybrid fact–value concept: it means "harmful (value) plus dysfunction (fact)"; and drawing (again like Millikan) on the idea of natural selection as a particular kind of cause–effect story he concluded that "dysfunctions are failures of internal mechanisms to perform the functions for which they were naturally selected."[10]

On first inspection, "failure" as used here in Wakefield's definition of dysfunction looks straightforwardly to be an evaluative word. But as Fulford (1999) noted, "failure" is ambiguous as to fact and value: it is often used with evaluative force (as in "he failed the exam") but it also has non-evaluative uses (Fulford's example was brown dwarf stars being described in the popular science magazine, *The New Scientist,* as "failed stars"). So Wakefield could claim that it is just the non-evaluative side of the meaning of "failure" that is essential to his definition. But then the question is, why did he not find an unambiguously value-free form of words? There is nothing to prevent this: one such form of words would be "a dysfunctional *condition of an* internal mechanism is *one in which it is not* performing the functions for which it was naturally selected" (Fulford 1999; emphases in the original and show changes from Wakefield's definition). True, this is a little more long-winded but at least it avoids the fact–value ambiguities of "failure." And in his commentary Fulford went on to show that with a series of further such substitutions, Wakefield's definition of dysfunction could indeed be purged of evaluative language (ambiguous or otherwise) altogether. *But* (and it is a *big* "but") in stripping Wakefield's definition of evaluative language, Fulford showed: first, that we strip it also of its ability to distinguish what Millikan has called the proper function of a functional object from its other properties; second, that this in turn means it no longer serves as a sufficient definition of dysfunction; and third that, in consequence, it was after all the *evaluative* side of the meaning of "failure" (and other similar fact–value terms) that was operative in Wakefield's original definition.

---

[9] This article can be read together with a subsequent article (Fulford 2000) responding to Wakefield's (2000) Aristotelian defence of his position.

[10] This summary definition combines two statements of Wakefield's definition of dysfunction, in the abstract to his paper and on p. 375, respectively: but the words are his—see Fulford (1999, 2000).

Wakefield then, like Boorse, despite arguing for a value-free definition of (part of) the concept of disorder continues to use evaluative language in relation to (that part of) the concept. In neither case, of course, does this as an observational point from philosophical field work provide anything in the way of a knockdown argument against these authors' respective claims to having defined a value-free part of the concept of disorder. Boorse indeed has suggested that his use of evaluative language is "harmless...rhetoric" (Boorse 1997, p.105, note 14); Wakefield in his response to Fulford's commentary focused on other issues (Wakefield 1999b). And the point after all, as an observational point, is, simply, evidential. The continued use of evaluative language in the ways described is, simply, evidence (philosophical field-work evidence) that there may be an evaluative element of meaning in concepts of disorder as a whole including bodily disorder. It is, though, evidence that at the very least is worth taking seriously: for the continued use of evaluative language in these instances is not just by any hoi polloi but by two authors from very different backgrounds (being, respectively, a philosopher and a practitioner) both of whom are persuaded of (and in the process of seeking to persuade others of) the value-free nature of (some part of) the concept of disorder. In the final main section of this chapter we will look at where taking the philosophical field-work evidence seriously leads.

VALUES-BASED PRACTICE

One place to which taking the evidence seriously leads is the practical spin-off of values-based practice. We do not have space here to set out in detail the full pathway from theory to practical spin-off but a key step along the way is provided by the work of R. M. Hare, Geoffrey Warnock, and others of the Oxford School on the language of values. Sometimes called "philosophical value theory" this work adds an ordinary language philosophical angle to the long-running "is–ought" debate. Concerned as philosophical value theory is with the relationship between descriptive and evaluative meaning, it offers a potentially rich (though thus far largely untapped) resource of ideas for understanding the relationship between descriptive and evaluative meaning in debates about concepts of disorder (Fulford 1989).[11] One such idea is Hare's (1952, 1963) observation (made also in a different way by Warnock (1971)) that can be summed up in the equation "visible values = diverse values." This observation, as we will see, explains at a stroke both sides (both easy and difficult sides) of the use of the concept of disorder (respectively of bodily and of mental conditions) thus satisfying the key constraint on theory outlined earlier, and, as we will see, leading directly to values-based practice.

This is how the argument runs. The Hare/Warnock observation is that values are like the air we breathe, around us all the time and vital to everything we do but largely unnoticed

---

[11] Thus, not covered in this chapter is the idea that concepts of disorder might be understood in terms of the "descriptivist" account of value terms developed by Warnock (1971) and Foot (1958–1959): descriptivism allows in principle for concepts of disorder to be defined value-free while at the same time carrying in relevant contexts evaluative meaning (Fulford 1989, chapter 3): descriptivism though fails as an under-pinning theory for values-based practice (as a resource for working with complex and conflicting values) because the dual-aspect (fact-plus-value) use it allows is available only where the values concerned are largely shared.

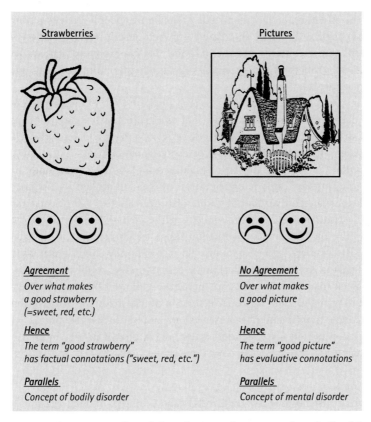

FIGURE 26.4 "Good strawberry" and "good picture" compared with "bodily disorder" and "mental disorder."

until in one way or another they cause trouble. In the case of the air we breathe trouble might come with the air being in short supply (on a high mountain, say) or difficult to access (as in an asthma attack): in circumstances like these the normally taken for granted and unnoticed air suddenly becomes all too visible. Correspondingly with values then, although like the air we breathe vital to everything we do, they go largely unnoticed until they cause trouble: and trouble with values tends to come when the values in question are diverse and hence likely to come into conflict. One of Hare's examples of "visible values = diverse values" is shown diagrammatically in Fig. 26.4. People have largely shared values for "good strawberry" (left-hand side of the figure); these shared values are reflected in shared descriptive criteria for "good strawberry" (that it is red, sweet, grub free, etc.); hence the use of the value term "good" in "good strawberry" carries predominantly factual associations reflecting these shared descriptive criteria (say "good strawberry" and most people think "red, sweet, grub free, etc. strawberry"[12]). When it comes to

[12] This is borne out by experience of using this as the basis of a training exercise in values-based practice (Fulford 2009, table 1.5.2.1).

pictures on the other hand (right-hand side of the figure) people's values are highly diverse (vide the Turner prize[13]): hence there are no shared descriptive associations of the term "good picture"; to the contrary, the use of "good" in "good picture" carries overtly evaluative connotations reflecting disagreements about which pictures are good pictures (vide the Turner prize again).

All this may seem blindingly obvious to a philosopher. Yet it puts a completely different spin on the debate about mental disorder. For as Fig. 26.4 also shows, the Hare/Warnock observation about the use of "good" maps directly onto the use of "disorder": "disorder" in "bodily disorder" (factual connotations) corresponds directly with "good" in "good strawberry"; "disorder" in "mental disorder" (value connotations) corresponds directly with "good" in "good picture." This is not because (as Kendell argued) the science of mental disorder is less advanced than that of bodily disorder; still less is it because (as Szasz suggested) bodily disorders are scientific concepts while mental disorders are moral concepts. It is because (the Hare/Warnock observation suggests) the criteria for the value judgment expressed by disorder are largely shared in the case of bodily conditions but highly diverse (and hence likely to come into conflict) in the case of mental conditions. Again, this merits more setting out than we have space for here (see Fulford 1989, part II). But we can see broadly that the parallel holds: disorder is used in bodily medicine of conditions like heart attacks and cancer that (in and of themselves) are bad by anyone's standards (= shared values); in psychiatry by contrast "disorder" is used of conditions defined by emotions, beliefs, desires, sexuality, and other areas in which our values (what we take to be good or bad) are highly diverse.

In the terms of our two-sided challenge for analysis, then, "bodily disorder" is relatively unproblematic in use because it is (relatively) values-simple: "mental disorder" by contrast is relatively problematic in use because it is (relatively) values-complex. Again, this may seem blindingly obvious to a philosopher. But it leads to a completely different practical strategy for tackling the problems in use presented by mental disorders. Szasz's strategy of exclusion won't do: mental disorders are disorders albeit values-complex rather than values-simple; and even if it were possible to exclude them from medicine they would take their (values-complex) problems with them. But neither will Kendell's call for more science (and corresponding calls by Boorse, Wakefield, and others) do. More science as such is fine of course. But more science as a way of converting psychiatry from a values-complex to a values-simple area of medicine could if successful prove positively counter-productive. For the only way that scientific advances could reduce the (values-complex) problems presented by mental disorder is by reducing the diversity of human values that these problems reflect. Yet much of our very individuality as human beings consists in this same diversity of values. The Kendell/Boorse/Wakefield "less-values-by-way-of-more science" agenda therefore, although motivated by the need to improve practice, risks abusively dehumanizing consequences. Importantly, it was just such abusive consequences (arising from an overuse of a supposedly value-free medical model) that motivated the anti-psychiatry movement (see earlier) and continues to motivate current concerns (see Bracken and Thomas, Chapter 11, this volume). And that such concerns are well founded is clear from the extent to which some of the worst abuses of psychiatry have been underpinned by

---

[13] An annual prize for modern art in the UK that regularly evokes heated debate by its highly contentious choice of winners.

a value-free scientific medical model (as in the former Soviet Union; see Fulford et al. 1993).[14]

Enter then values-based practice. For values-based practice as we indicated at the start of this chapter is a new skills-based tool for working with complex and conflicting values in health care. As such it is a direct response to and meets head-on the (values-complex) problems presented by mental disorders. Again, we describe the practical operation of values-based practice in our chapter in the sister volume to this book (Fulford and van Staden, forthcoming). But a couple of points are worth emphasizing here, one about the relationship between values-based practice and science, the other about the relationship between values-based practice and philosophy.

Values-based practice and science

A common misunderstanding about values-based practice is that it is inimical to (or at any rate somehow a balancing factor against) science. But there is nothing in either the theory or practice of values-based practice that is anti-science. As to theory, the criteria for the value judgments with which values-based practice is concerned are (as earlier) *descriptive* criteria: as such they define the proper scope of descriptive science in medicine; and to the extent that the value judgments concerned are complex nothing less than the best of (both clinical and laboratory) science is required for effective values-based practice. As to practice, the need for values-based practice (or some equivalent) as a partner to evidence-based practice was explicitly foreshadowed by the early pioneers of evidence-based practice (Sackett et al. 2000); the two come most fully together at the cutting edge of the clinical encounter in the exercise of clinical judgment (Fulford et al. 2012, chapter 2); and far from being made redundant by scientific advances in medicine (as Boorse and others have suggested, see earlier), such advances will inevitably increase rather than decrease the need no less for values-based as for evidence-based practice in all areas of health care.[15]

That last point is important. Scientific advances increase the need for evidence-based practice because such advances increase the complexity of the evidence bearing on clinical decision-making. But scientific advances also increase the need for values-based practice essentially because scientific advances open up new choices and with choices go complexity of values. Reproductive medicine is a case in point. Infertility, you will recall, was one of the evolutionary criteria for biological disadvantage on which Kendell, Boorse, and others drew in attempting to mark out a value-free concept of disorder. Translating this into the terms of philosophical value theory, then, this suggests that infertility is a condition that being (in and of itself) negatively evaluated by most people most of the time is values-simple and thus (consistently with the Hare/Warnock observation) appears to be value-free. And before Steptoe and Edwards' announcement of the first test-tube baby,

---

[14] We look at abuses of psychiatry and how they arise from a supposedly value-free medical model in our chapter in the sister volume to this book (Fulford and van Staden, forthcoming).

[15] Science itself is of course not value free: epistemic values aside, a wide variety of values come into every stage of the research process. Again, there is nothing anti-science in this. As we describe in our chapter in the sister volume to this book (Sadler et al., forthcoming), it is a matter rather of coming to a more realistic view of science as a step to developing the tools (including values-based tools) needed for better (clinically better) science.

Louise Brown, infertility might just as well have been value-free since there was little, if anything, that could be done about it in most cases. After Louise Brown, however, as a whole range of new "assisted reproduction" choices began to be opened up, the diversity of individual human values has come to count. Indeed, the key clinical variables in infertility treatment now include emotion, desires, needs, sexuality, and so forth, in other words precisely those aspects of human experience and behavior in which (as in psychiatry) human values are inherently diverse (Fulford et al. 2012, chapter 12). Scientific advances in reproductive medicine have thus shifted infertility treatment from its former status as a values-simple to a currently values-complex area; and with values-complexity goes the need for values-based practice.

The idea that science increases rather than decreases the role of values in medicine explodes a number of twentieth-century myths. It shows, first, that the problems in use of concepts of mental disorder arise not from psychiatry being (as Szasz argued) outwith science or (as Kendell and others supposed) a primitive science but rather from it engaging with people as unique individuals in areas in which their values are highly diverse. Psychiatry is thus not science-simple but values-complex. It shows, second, that the problems in use of concepts of disorder in psychiatry today will increasingly become the problems in use also of bodily disorder tomorrow. In other words, with advances in medical science, far from psychiatry coming to look increasingly like bodily medicine, bodily medicine will increasingly come to look (in this respect) like psychiatry. And it shows, finally, that psychiatry in developing the philosophically-based tools of values-based practice for working with complex and conflicting values is leading the way for the rest of health care.

Psychiatry in the twentieth century was stereotyped as lagging behind bodily medicine. This stereotype is reflected in the three assumptions guiding the traditional debate about mental disorder (as described earlier). Ordinary language philosophy shows instead that psychiatry is leading the way in developing a health care for the twenty-first century that is not only fully science-based but also fully person-centered.

Values-based practice and philosophy

A further common misunderstanding about values-based practice is that it depends on (perhaps even embodies) fact–value dualism. It does not. Certainly, it uses the language of fact and value (or, if you will, description and evaluation). And central to its training objectives is the aim of increasing awareness of values especially where the values concerned are masked by or presented as facts. But all that is required for values-based practice is what the American philosopher Hilary Putnam has called a *distinction* between fact and value (Putnam 2002). In other words, for values-based practice, all that is required is that fact and value (description and evaluation) should be distinguishable, not that, as with a dualism, the distinction can be driven all the way back.

There is indeed direct (philosophical field-work) evidence from values-based practice itself that the distinction between fact and value cannot be driven all the way back. This evidence comes from the clinical phenomenology of delusion. Fact–value dualists tend to emphasize the (linguistic) fact that any value is logically (though of course not always psychologically) possible: this was Hare's point, for example, in developing his prescriptivist account of evaluative meaning (Hare 1952, 1963). Descriptivists like Warnock and

Foot would put forward examples of situations that "anyone" would have to say were good (or bad). Hare would counter that psychologically compelling as such situations might be, the compulsion was always only psychological (reflecting what our values actually are) rather than logical (reflecting the very meaning of good or bad).[16] Well, delusion presents a counterexample to any value being logically possible at least to the extent that any fact is logically possible. This is because delusions may take the logical forms not only of the well-recognized false factual beliefs but also of true factual beliefs, and, crucially, of value judgments (Fulford 1989, chapter 10, 1991). Reflecting their many challenges to philosophy, delusions have, of course, been widely discussed in the philosophy of psychiatry (see a number of chapters in this book[17]). But the key (philosophical field work) point to set against Hare's "any value is logically possible" is that each of these logical forms of delusion carries *the same implications for practice*. In other words, by the test of (ordinary language) implication, in whatever sense a factual delusion (true or false) is wrong, in the same sense an evaluative delusion is wrong.

Evaluative delusions are important conceptually in providing one of the sharpest tests of theories of the meaning of mental disorder (and hence of disorder as a whole). To pursue their importance in this respect further would take us into a number of issues that are beyond the scope of this chapter. One such issue is that of the particular kind of negative value judgment that is expressed by disorder (how does disorder differ from, say, ugliness or foolishness, madness from badness). One of us has set out in detail elsewhere the beginnings of a response to this issue building on an agentic account of psychopathology (Fulford 1989, part III); and delusion emerges naturally from this account as a failure of practical reasoning rather than of cognitive functioning (Fulford 1989, chapter 10). There are still deeper epistemological issues (Gipps and Fulford 2004) and indeed ethical issues (Fulford and Radoilska 2012) that are raised by evaluative delusions. In each of these further philosophical areas, moreover, as in the philosophy of values, not only is theory a resource for understanding delusion but delusion is a resource for advancing theory. Once again, then, in philosophy as in science, the negative concept (to adapt another of Austin's aphorisms) "wears the trousers" (Austin 1956/1957, p.32).

TOPSY-TURVY TAKE HOME MESSAGES ...

Wittgenstein famously claimed that philosophy "leaves everything [to do with ordinary language use] as it is" (Wittgenstein 1953, section 124, parenthesis added). Ordinary language philosophy, consistently with Wittgenstein's aphorism, is as we have emphasized essentially descriptive. It leaves our ordinary use of the language of disorder (bodily and mental) as it is. Yet in focusing our attention carefully on that same ordinary usage, ordinary language philosophy turns our understanding of it in a number of key respects upside down. Ordinary language philosophy allows us to see: (1) that, if the language use of those concerned is any guide, the debate about mental disorder is, really, a debate about bodily disorder; (2) that mental disorder, rather than being "the problem" is, really, a resource for work on concepts

---

[16] See Fulford (1989, chapter 3) for exchanges of this kind.
[17] For example, Chapters 39, 41, and 42 in Section V, this volume.

of disorder as a whole; (3) that the value-laden nature of mental disorder, instead of being an embarrassment to the scientific status of psychiatry and hence in need either of limitation or of elimination, is, really, a linguistic signal of the essentially evaluative nature of concepts of disorder as a whole; and hence (4) that the need for values-based practice (or some equivalent) to stand alongside evidence-based practice, is a mark, not of a primitive medical science, but rather of an advanced medical science that in opening up new choices carries with it a requirement to engage with the diverse values of the unique individuals concerned in a given clinical decision. Merely to see all this is, certainly, to leave things as they are. But in dispelling the grammatical illusions by which, as Wittgenstein might have put it, recent debates about concepts of disorder have been bewitched, ordinary language philosophy at the very least helps us to see things as they *really* are. This indeed was the point of Ryle's metaphor of ordinary language philosophy giving us a more complete view of the logical geography of a given area of discourse.

And note, again, that phrase—a *more* complete view. This is vital. It is vital to appreciate that what is delivered by ordinary language philosophy is only a more complete view and not a different or substitute or competitor or even a once-for-all complete view. There is in particular (and this bears repetition) nothing in this more complete view that is anti-science. Philosophical value theory itself, as we have seen, demands (through the central logical role of descriptive criteria for the value judgments expressed by disorder) the best of science. The point is rather that there is more to the logical geography of medicine than (irreducibly important as it is) science. The terrain (the logical geography) includes science. The more complete view derived from ordinary language philosophy shows that the terrain includes values as well. It includes no doubt much else besides science and values. But the science is irreducibly important if medicine is to do its job. Ordinary language philosophy reinforces the irreducible importance of science in medicine while at the same time showing the irreducible importance also of values. Science is irreducible as the research base of medicine. Values are irreducible in linking up the sciences of medicine effectively with the unique individuals who (as patients, carers, clinicians, and others) are at the heart of the clinical encounter. This is why values-based practice is about "linking science with people" (Fulford et al. 2012). Which is where, finally, with the development of values-based practice, ordinary language philosophy has started to go beyond merely showing us how things really are, to actually changing them.

... And A Few Next Steps

These then are the topsy-turvy take-home messages of our title. Ordinary language philosophy, far from leaving everything the same, turns everything upside down and in the process provides a basis for changing them. Lest though we be accused of hubris, it is important to recall Austin's caution that ordinary language philosophy is only ever a first step. As to practice, there are, as we will describe in our chapter in the sister volume to this book, a number of important (and indeed exciting) next steps, some already under way, others yet to be taken.[18] But there are many other and no less important (and indeed exciting) next steps for theory.

[18] For recent developments in values-based practice see <http:go.warwick.ac.uk/values-basedpractice>.

Some of these we have signaled already in this chapter, notably the potential kickbacks from practice to philosophy: we gave by way of example the significance of the clinical phenomenology of delusion for epistemology, ethics, the philosophy of action, and philosophical value theory. That there is potential for a wider two-way dynamic between philosophy and psychiatry is evident in the extent of overlap between on the one hand the deepest problems of philosophy and on the other the sharpest challenges of psychiatric practice: both disciplines (philosophy and psychiatry) are concerned centrally with consciousness, causality, mind and brain, meaning, experience, rationality, cognition, thoughts, perceptions, determinism, intentionality, reasons, the nature of persons, not to mention the (logical) relationships between fact and value.

Philosophy and psychiatry thus occupy (extending Ryle's metaphor) a shared logical geography. And there is another twist to Ryle's metaphor. For ordinary language philosophy, rich as its returns have been, has thus far been limited to ordinary *English* language philosophy. Think therefore what results might flow from extending the Rylean territory to other language groups reflecting very different traditions of thought and practice. Philosophers working in the tradition of the Oxford School, such as Rom Harré (1983),[19] have recognized the potential here. The future though for philosophical field work beyond the territory of English is surely not with lone researchers but in what we called earlier Austin's philosophical *team* field work with people from different language groups working together in collaborative partnerships.

One of us (WvS), being based in Pretoria at the heart of the "rainbow nation" of South Africa, is well placed to take such collaborative, philosophical team field work forward through the development of an African version of values-based practice called "Batho Pele." Batho Pele is a term of the Sesotho language for which, consistently with the priority of use over definition, there is no direct translation into English that would account adequately for its embedded concepts. A mere translation as "people first" would miss, for example, the embedded African concepts of interpersonal and social connectedness and interdependence as expressed in the "African cogito," reading along the lines of "I am because you are, you are because we are."[20] Batho Pele, then, as an African version of values-based practice might do much to dispel the excessive individualism that, as yet another grammatical illusion, has come to dominate so much of the English language logical geography in recent years. Individualism, too, is important of course. But as a grammatical illusion unbalanced by community, individualism has become one of the key drivers for what the British philosopher Onora O'Neill has characterized as the loss of trust by which "Western" societies have been increasingly plagued in recent decades (O'Neill 2002). Behind excessive individualism, the Wittgensteinian diagnosis may reach even deeper in so far as these African concepts may serve to expose the grammatical illusion that pitches individualism against communitarianism (van Staden 2011). Breaking free from grammatical illusions and restoring trust then, through a collaborative partnership between one or more of the ordinary African language philosophies and ordinary English language philosophy: now that really would be a next step worth taking.

---

[19] Harré (1983, pp. 85–92) explores Inuit and Maori languages in his study of our conceptions of ourselves as "selves."

[20] The concept "Batho Pele" is related to the concepts "ubuntu" and 'unmuntu ngumuntu ngabantu." It is the latter concept that may be partially translated as "I am because you are, and you are because we are." The theoretical enrichment in ethics afforded by these concepts is explored in the sister volume together with an exploration of the African *practices*, concordantly with values-based *practice*, as entrenched in the relevant concepts.

References

American Psychiatric Association (2000). *Diagnostic and Statistical Manual of Mental Disorders, Fourth Edition, Text Revision*. Washington, DC: American Psychiatric Association.

Austin, J. L. (1956/1957). A plea for excuses. *Proceedings of the Aristotelian Society*, 57, 1–30. (Reprinted in White, A. R. (Ed.) (1968). *The Philosophy of Action*, pp. 19–42. Oxford: Oxford University Press.)

Baz, A. (2012). *When Words are Called For: A Defense of Ordinary Language Philosophy*. Cambridge, MA: Harvard University Press.

Bolton, D. and Hill, J. (1996). *Mind, Meaning and Mental Disorder: The Nature of Causal Explanation in Psychology and Psychiatry* (2nd edn 2004). Oxford: Oxford University Press.

Boorse, C. (1975). On the distinction between disease and illness. *Philosophy and Public Affairs*, 5, 49–68.

Boorse, C. (1976). What a theory of mental health should be. *Journal for The Theory of Social Behaviour*, 6, 61–84.

Boorse, C. (1997). A rebuttal on health. In J. M. Humber and R. F. Almeder (Eds), *What is Disease?*, pp. 1–134. Totowa, NJ: Humana Press.

Boorse, C. (2004). *Four Recent Accounts of Health*. Delaware, DE: University of Delaware Press.

Campbell, E. J. M., Scadding, J. G., and Roberts, R. S. (1979). The concept of disease. *British Medical Journal*, 2, 757–62.

Campbell, P. (1996). What we want from crisis services. In J. Read and J. Reynolds (Eds), *Speaking Our Minds: An Anthology*, pp. 180–3. Basingstoke: Macmillan/Open University.

Chadwick, H. (Trans.) (1992). *St Augustine: Confessions*. Oxford: Oxford University Press.

Colombo, A. (1997). *Understanding Mentally Disordered Offenders: A Multi-Agency Perspective*. Aldershot: Ashgate.

Colombo, A., Bendelow, G., Fulford, K. W. M., and Williams, S. (2003). Evaluating the influence of implicit models of mental disorder on processes of shared decision making within community-based multi-disciplinary teams. *Social Science & Medicine*, 56, 1557–70.

Department of Health (2005). *Creating a Patient-led NHS: Delivering the NHS Improvement Plan*. London: Department of Health.

Department of Health (2007). *Mental Health: New Ways of Working for Everyone: Developing and sustaining a capable and flexible workforce*. London: Department of Health.

Eysenck, H. J. (1960). Classification and the problems of diagnosis. In H. J. Eysenck (Ed.), *Handbook of Abnormal Psychology*. London: Pitman Medical Publishing Company Ltd.

Fann, K. T. (Ed.) (1969). *Symposium on J. L. Austin*. London: Routledge and Kegan Paul.

Foot, P. (1958–1959). Moral Beliefs. *Proceedings of the Aristotelian Society*, 59, 83–104. Reprinted in P. Foot (Ed.) (1967, chapter 6) *Theories of ethics*. Oxford: Oxford University Press.

Foucault, M. (1971). *Madness and Civilization: A History of Insanity in the Age of Reason* (R. Savage, Trans.). London: Tavistock.

Fulford, K. W. M. (1989). *Moral Theory and Medical Practice* (reprinted 1995, 1999, 2nd edn 2000). Cambridge: Cambridge University Press.

Fulford, K. W. M. (1991). Evaluative delusions: Their significance for philosophy and psychiatry. *British Journal of Psychiatry*, 159, 108–12.

Fulford, K. W. M. (1999). Nine variations and a coda on the theme of an evolutionary definition of dysfunction. *Journal of Abnormal Psychology*, 108(3), 412–20.

Fulford, K. W. M. (2000). Teleology without tears: Naturalism, neo-naturalism and evaluationism in the analysis of function statements in biology (and a bet on the twenty-first century). *Philosophy, Psychiatry, & Psychology, 7*(1), 77–94.

Fulford, K. W. M. (2009). Values and values-based practice in clinical psychiatry. In M. G. Gelder, N. Andreasen, and J. Geddes (Eds), *New Oxford Textbook of Psychiatry* (2nd edn), Oxford: Oxford University Press.

Fulford, K. W. M. and Colombo, A. (2004). Six models of mental disorder: A study combining linguistic-analytic and empirical methods. *Philosophy, Psychiatry, & Psychology, 11*(2), 129–44.

Fulford, K. W. M., Peile, E. P., and Carroll, H. (2012). *Essential Values-based Practice: Clinical Stories Linking Science with People.* Cambridge: Cambridge University Press.

Fulford, K. W. M. and Radoilska, L. (2012). Three challenges from delusion for theories of autonomy. In Radoilska, L. (Ed.), *Autonomy and Mental Disorder*, pp. 44–74. Oxford: Oxford University Press.

Fulford, K. W. M. and Sadler, J. Z. (2000). Editorial overview: History and philosophy. *Current Opinion in Psychiatry, 13*, 679–81.

Fulford, K. W. M. and Van Staden, C. W. (forthcoming). In J. Z. Sadler, K. W. M. Fulford, and C. W. Van Staden (Eds), *The Oxford Handbook of Psychiatric Ethics.* Oxford: Oxford University Press.

Gipps, R. G. T. and Fulford, K. W. M. (2004). Understanding the clinical concept of delusion: from an estranged to an engaged epistemology. *International Review of Psychiatry, 16*(3), 225–35.

Hare, R. M. (1952). *The Language of Morals.* Oxford: Oxford University Press.

Hare, R. M. (1963). Descriptivism. *Proceedings of the British Academy, 49*, 115–34.

Hare, R. M. (1972). *Essays on the Moral Concepts.* London: The Macmillan Press Ltd.

Harré, R. (1983). *Personal Being.* Oxford: Basil Blackwell.

Harré, R. (1997). Pathological autobiographies. *Philosophy, Psychiatry, & Psychology, 4*(2), 99–110.

Kendell, R. E. (1975). The concept of disease and its implications for psychiatry. *British Journal of Psychiatry, 127*, 305–15.

Kupfer, D. J., First, M. B., and Regier, D. E. (Eds) (2002). *A Research Agenda for DSM-V.* Washington, DC: American Psychiatric Association.

Laing, R. D. (1960). *The Divided Self.* London: Tavistock.

Laing, R. D. and Esterson, A. (1964). *Sanity, Madness and the Family.* London: Tavistock.

Megone, C. (1998). Aristotle's function argument and the concept of mental illness. *Philosophy, Psychiatry, & Psychology, 5*(3), 187–202.

Millikan, R. G. (1998). In defence of proper functions. In C. Allen and G. Lauder (Eds), *Nature's Purposes: Analyses of Function and Design in Biology*, pp. 295–312. Cambridge, MA: MIT Press.

Nordenfelt, L. (1987). *On the Nature of Health: An Action-Theoretic Approach.* Dordrecht: D. Reidel Publishing Company.

Nordenfelt, L. (1992). *On Crime, Punishment and Psychiatric Care.* Stockholm: Almquist and Wiksell International.

O'Neill, O. (2002). *A Question of Trust: The BBC Reith Lectures 2002.* Cambridge: Cambridge University Press.

Putnam, H. (2002). *The Collapse of the Fact/Value Dichotomy and other Essays.* Cambridge, MA: Harvard University Press.

Roth, M. and Kroll, J. (1986). *The Reality of Mental Illness*. Cambridge: Cambridge University Press.

Ryle, G. (1963). *The Concept of Mind*. London: Penguin Books Ltd. (Original work published 1949.)

Sackett, D. L. Straus, S. E., Scott Richardson, W., Rosenberg, W., and Haynes, R. B. (2000). *Evidence-Based Medicine: How to Practice and Teach EBM* (2nd edn). Edinburgh: Churchill Livingstone.

Sadler, J. Z. (2005). *Values and Psychiatric Diagnosis*. Oxford: Oxford University Press.

Sadler, J. Z., van Staden, C. W., and Fulford, K. W. M. (Eds) (forthcoming). *Oxford Handbook of Psychiatric Ethics*. Oxford : Oxford University Press.

Schaler, J. A. (Ed.) (2004). *Szasz Under Fire: The Psychiatric Abolitionist Faces His Critics*. Chicago, IL: Open Court Publishers.

Scheff, T. J. (1974). The labelling theory of mental illness. *American Sociological Review*, 39, 444–52.

Sedgwick, P. (1973). Illness—mental and otherwise. *The Hastings Centre Studies*, 1(3), 19–40.

Szasz, T. S. (1960). The myth of mental illness. *American Psychologist*, 15, 113–18.

Thornton, T. (2000). Mental illness and reductionism: Can functions be naturalized? *Philosophy, Psychiatry, & Psychology*, 7(1), 67–76.

Van Staden, C. W. (2011). African approaches to an enriched ethics of person-centred health practice. *International Journal of Person-Centred Medicine*, 1, 11–17.

Wakefield, J. C. (1995). Dysfunction as a value-free concept: A reply to Sadler and Agich. *Philosophy, Psychiatry, & Psychology*, 2(3), 233–46.

Wakefield, J. C. (1999a). Evolutionary versus prototype analyses of the concept of disorder. *Journal of Abnormal Psychology*, 108, 374–99.

Wakefield, J. C. (1999b). Mental disorder as a black box essentialist concept. *Journal of Abnormal Psychology*, 108, 465–72.

Wakefield, J. C. (2000). Aristotle as sociobiologist: The "function of a human being" argument, black box essentialism, and the concept of mental disorder. *Philosophy, Psychiatry, & Psychology*, 7(1), 17–44.

Warnock, G. J. (1971). *The Object of Morality*. London: Methuen & Co Ltd.

Warnock, G. J. (1989). *J. L. Austin*, London: Routledge.

Wing, J. K. (1978). *Reasoning about Madness*. Oxford: Oxford University Press.

Wing, J. K., Cooper, J. E., and Sartorius, N. (1974). *Measurement and Classification of Psychiatric Symptoms*. Cambridge: Cambridge University Press.

Williamson, T. (2004). User involvement—a contemporary overview. *The Mental Health Review*, 9(1), 6–12.

Wittgenstein, L. (1953). *Philosophical Investigations*. Oxford: Blackwell.

Wittgenstein, L. (1972). *The Blue and Brown Books: Preliminary Studies for the 'Philosophical Investigations'*. Oxford: Basil Blackwell. (Original work published 1958.)

World Health Organization (1992). *The ICD-10 Classification of Mental and Behavioural Disorders: Clinical Descriptions and Diagnostic Guidelines*. Geneva: World Health Organization.

COMMENTARY: VALUE-BASED PRACTICE BY

A DIFFERENT ROUTE

ROGER CRISP

One set of questions raised by Fulford and van Staden concerns what ordinary language philosophy amounts to and how its resources might underpin value-based practice. I want to address a different question: whether it is possible to arrive at value-based practice (or some reasonable conception of value-based practice) without commitment to ordinary language philosophy. I shall suggest that it is.

Our first move must be to deny the philosophical pessimism of Fulford and van Staden, who believe that because we find it hard to define "higher-level" concepts, and because we have failed to find consensus on the nature of mental disorder over the last few decades, we should give up on trying to provide a definition and move to the study of how the concept is actually used by practitioners and patients. Such pessimism would be catastrophic if carried over into other areas of philosophy. For millennia, philosophers have failed to agree on the nature of reality and knowledge, truth and meaning, personhood, the mind, God, beauty, and many other fundamental concepts. And yet they continue to try, through careful argument and analysis, to provide accounts of these basic concepts. It would certainly be worrying if philosophers could not come up with accounts which even they, as individuals, could accept. But since that is not the case, I suggest that we continue the project, in philosophy of psychiatry and in other areas, at least for the present.

Move two consists in asking which values *should* underpin the practice of psychiatry. One way to answer that question, as Fulford and van Staden explain, is to ask relevant parties what they *value*. But it is not clear why we should allow practice in any area to be led, without question, by what people *say* they value. What matters is *what is valuable* (and if this commits me to denying Fulford and van Staden's version of the fact–value distinction, so be it). In the medical context, the obvious answer must be the value of *well-being*—that is, what makes people's lives go well *for them* (where "for them" is not to be understood as "from their point of view" or "in their opinion"). Here there seem to be some cases involving facts, at least in some fairly unfreighted sense. Imagine that I suffer ten years of appalling agony and then die. Almost any sane person who understands the concept of well-being will agree that this outcome is bad for me.

Of course, there is no consensus on what well-being is among philosophers. Some accept hedonism, others some desire- or preference-fulfillment account, and yet others some more objective conception. But those who wish to take my alternative route to value-based practice at this point may be encouraged to develop their own account. This will be to take my third move, which will also involve mapping that conception of well-being onto alleged forms of mental disorder. The implications for treatment of those suffering from such disorders should not be thought to be obvious. On any plausible conception of well-being, it will probably turn out that a disorder comes to be classified as such primarily because, *in general*, it tends to make sufferers' lives worse than they would otherwise have been. But in the case of certain disorders—bipolar disorder being often mentioned in this connection—it is not obvious that it is always harmful. Here one's conception of well-being may be relevant. If my bipolar disorder leads to my life being, overall, quite unhappy, though hugely creative, a hedonist will advocate treatment, while an objective theorist who values creativity might not.

At this point, it may be objected that this conception of value-based practice, in ignoring the views of experts and patients, is excessively authoritarian, and in practice would result in the widespread violation of patient autonomy. This need not be so, however, for at least two reasons. The first is that, on any plausible conception of well-being, the benefits of many medical and other therapeutic interventions will depend on what the patient values, believes, and wants. So, if, for example, I am considering providing some drug to deal with your bipolar disorder, it would be highly irresponsible of me not to make serious enquiries of you in advance concerning your attitude to your condition and the possible effects of treatment. If I don't do that, then I'm not unlikely to make you worse off even by my own lights.

The second reason—or set of reasons—is more fundamental. Imagine that I, as practitioner, come to some substantive view of well-being (hedonism, let's say) then seek to guide my practice entirely in the light of that theory. I am ignoring the deep disagreement among practitioners, and of course philosophers, about the nature of well-being, disagreement which is, in effect, in many cases between *epistemic peers*. At this point, let me quote the last of the three great "classical utilitarians," Henry Sidgwick:

> Since it is implied in the very notion of Truth that it is essentially the same for all minds, the denial by another of a proposition that I have affirmed has a tendency to impair my confidence in its validity … And it will easily be seen that the absence of … disagreement must remain an indispensable negative condition of the certainty of our beliefs. For if I find any of my judgments … in direct conflict with a judgment of some other mind, there must be error somewhere: and if I have no more reason to suspect error in the other mind than in my own, reflective comparison between the two judgments necessarily reduces me temporarily to a state of neutrality.[21]

If we take Sidgwick seriously, as I think we should, will this not paralyze both thought and practice, since we will be forced to suspend judgment on almost every fundamental issue? I think not. We can hold on to our considered judgments, but rather than insist in discussion that others have got it wrong, we can say: "This is how things look to me." And we can ask: "How do things look to you?" When we disagree, whether in theory or in practice, we should seek to find as much agreement as possible. Where there is disagreement, philosophical debate can continue, and so can medical practice. But such practice should proceed not by practitioners' imposing their own judgments of well-being on their patients (unless these patients appear not only not to be epistemic peers, but to be making what nearly all would agree to be terrible mistakes about their own interests), but by their informing themselves carefully about their patients' views. And this is not because there is no right answer to the question of the values that should underpin psychiatric practice. It is because we do not know what that answer is, and assuming that we have got that answer and others haven't would, if it resulted in coercive psychiatric practice, lead to the usual very bad consequences of tyranny, arrogance, and overbearingness.

Roger Crisp
St Anne's College, Oxford
Oxford Uehiro Centre for Practical Ethics, Oxford, UK

[21] Henry Sidgwick, *The Methods of Ethics* (London: Macmillan, 1907), p. 342.

CHAPTER 27

COGNITIVE SCIENCE AND EXPLANATIONS OF PSYCHOPATHOLOGY

KELSO CRATSLEY AND RICHARD SAMUELS

INTRODUCTION

The past two decades have witnessed a striking convergence in the interests and methods of cognitive science and psychiatry. On the one hand, cognitive psychologists and cognitive neuroscientists have increasingly sought to model various forms of psychopathology; in part because they promise to illuminate our understanding of normal cognition, but also because such phenomena are now viewed as intriguing in their own right. At the same time, researchers within psychiatry have increasingly come to adopt the methods and assumptions of the cognitive sciences—especially cognitive neuropsychology and cognitive neuroscience—with an attendant commitment to a particular pattern of explanation which depends upon the construction of mechanistic models (Broome and Bortolotti 2009; Kendler 2008, Kendler et al. 2011). The study of psychopathology has thus become an important facet of the cognitive sciences, and the cognitive sciences have, in turn, exerted an important influence on many regions of psychiatry.

While these developments have led to significant research findings, the application of a cognitive scientific approach to psychopathology is still very much in its infancy, and the scope and limits of the research strategy remain to be determined. The aim of this chapter, then, is to explore the prospects for a developed cognitive science of psychopathology. In "Core explanatory assumptions" we outline the core theoretical assumptions of much cognitive science with a specific focus on the sorts of explanatory strategies that cognitive scientists typically seek to produce. In "Explaining psychopathology" we consider the extension of these explanatory strategies to the study of psychopathology. Then, in "Some cognitive accounts of psychopathology" we briefly illustrate how these strategies have been applied to two specific pathological phenomena: Autism Spectrum Disorder and Major Depressive Disorder. Finally, in "Two challenges to the cognitive science of psychopathology," we discuss a pair of challenges to standard cognitive scientific approaches to psychopathology, one that focuses on the pervasive role of dissociative data in theory construction, and another, more "philosophical" challenge which purports to establish in-principle limits on the sorts of explanations of psychopathology that cognitive scientists have sought to provide.

CORE EXPLANATORY ASSUMPTIONS: INFORMATION PROCESSING AND MECHANISM

Though cognitive scientists do not share a single vision of how explanation ought to proceed, large regions of the field cleave to a set of familiar assumptions about the sorts of models that ought to be developed. For heuristic purposes, we divide up these assumptions into two related families of commitments. The first concern the idea that cognitive processes and capacities depend on *information processing*. The second concern the idea that cognitive explanations are in some appropriately broad sense *mechanistic*. Neither family of assumptions has gone unchallenged in cognitive science. So, for example, advocates of situated or dynamical approaches sometimes reject them (Chemero 2009). For present purposes, however, we are concerned with research that adheres to these assumptions. And in what follows, we sketch them in a bit more detail and identify a range of explanatory strategies to which they give rise. In practice these different strategies are seldom pursued in isolation from each other, but are instead combined in different admixtures within individual research programs. Nevertheless, it will be useful to separate them out since in doing so we will be better placed to appreciate the range of strategies available in understanding psychopathology.

Information processing

Amongst the core assumptions of much cognitive science is that cognitive capacities –vision, reasoning, language production, memory, and so on—depend upon *information processing* of some sort. This general assumption has been articulated in a range of different ways, invoking different notions of information and different conceptions of the sorts of processing that is involved (see, e.g., Piccinini and Scarantino 2011). But in practice cognitive scientists typically assume that the relevant processes involve *representations*: roughly, physical states and structures have *semantic contents* in that they mean something or denote aspects of the world (Clark 2000; Thagard 2012; Von Eckardt 1993). Further, it is widely assumed that the relevant sort of processing is in some sense *computational* (Cummins and Cummins 2000; McDonald and McDonald 1995). This much is true of the sorts of "classical" computational models that dominated much early cognitive science (Fodor and Pylyshyn 1988), but it is also true of mainstream connectionist research as well (Smolensky 1988). Further, even amongst researchers who are less explicit in their computational assumptions, there is a pervasive tendency to characterize cognition in terms of representations and operations thereon. Such assumptions are, for example, widespread in developmental psychology (Carey

2009), linguistics (Pinker 1994), and cognitive neuroscience (Gazzaniga 2009), even though much of this research does not provide any very perspicuous computational characterization of the phenomena under discussion.

Suppose, as most cognitive scientists do, that psychological capacities and processes involve the sort of information processing we sketched earlier. Then it will be possible to explain cognitive capacities and processes in a range of different ways, or, roughly equivalently, to characterize them at a number of different *levels of description*. First, it will be possible to describe cognition at what has variously been called the *intentional*, *semantic* or *knowledge* level (Newell 1990; Pylyshyn 1984). Roughly put, we can explain what people do with reference to the semantic contents of their representational states—for example, what they believe and what their goals are—and the meaningful connections that hold between such states. Thus we might describe the cognitive development of infants in terms of their learning new concepts or beliefs on the basis of perceptual experience, and we might explain the decision-making behavior of an adult in terms of their preferences and their beliefs about the world. Such explanations abstract away from the computational (and neurobiological) details of psychological processes, but can nonetheless be exceedingly useful for making sense of human behavior and cognition.

Second, if an information processing account of cognition is correct, then it will be possible to describe psychological processes in more computationally perspicuous terms—at what is sometimes called the *representational/algorithmic level* (Marr 1982). Commitment to such a level of description in exceedingly natural in light of the following broadly held assumptions:

- The semantic contents of mental states are somehow encoded by information carrying states and structures of the brain, what are sometimes called *representational vehicles*.
- Such representational vehicles are created, utilized, and transformed by the computational processes in which they figure.

Under these assumptions, it is plausible to suppose that psychological capacities and processes can be explained by characterizing the computations they involve and the properties of representational vehicles that allow for them to figure in such computations.

To take one well-known example, it is common to characterize aspects of visual perception—such as binocular vision—by providing some account of the representational vehicles involved, and a computational characterization of the systems that allow for the exercise of the capacity—for example, the extraction of depth information from binocular disparity (Marr 1982). As with intentional level description, this strategy is exceedingly commonplace in cognitive science.

Mechanistic commitments

So far we have sketched some widespread assumptions about cognition, and highlighted the way in which they give rise to two commonplace explanatory strategies. We now turn to another commitment, also widespread amongst cognitive scientists, which concerns the *mechanistic* character of cognition. To a first approximation, it is widely supposed that cognitive capacities—such as, language production, memory and visual perception—depend upon the operation of cognitive *mechanisms*: roughly, physically realized information processing systems that are hierarchically decomposable into functionally specifiable components, whose individual activities and mutual interactions are responsible for the production of cognitive phenomena (Bechtel 2008). So characterized, this mechanistic assumption constitutes a rough-and-ready piece of metaphysics—a claim about the sorts of entities that cognitive systems are.[1] But it is a piece of metaphysics that has important methodological ramifications, and in what follows we spell these out in more detail.

A first ramification of the mechanistic assumption is that any comprehensive account of cognition must ultimately explain how representations and computational operations are dependent on—or *implemented* by—physical structures, states and processes. For if cognition depends on the activity of *physical* systems, then presumably there should be some explanation of how these physical systems—paradigmatically parts of the brain[2]—are able to perform the relevant computational operations. Such descriptions are sometimes said to comprise a distinctive *implementation* or *physical* level of description (Marr 1982; Pylyshyn 1984). Crudely put, theories couched at this level are analogous to descriptions of computational hardware in that they characterize those physical states and structures in virtue of which a system is able to perform information processing tasks of the relevant sort.

A second ramification of the mechanistic assumption is that cognitive phenomena can be explained by affecting a *decomposition* of the system into subparts (Bechtel and Richardson 1993; Cummins 1975). Roughly put, the idea is that if cognitive capacities depend on hierarchically decomposable physical systems, then it should be possible to explain the cognitive capacity of an organism by decomposing the relevant system into its parts and describing how their individual activities and mutual interactions give rise to the capacity in question. Indeed, the typical goal of such decompositions is to "break up" the system into parts so simple that they manifestly involve no intelligence at all (Fodor 1968).

It is important to be clear, however, that there are two quite different sorts of decompositional analyses to be found in cognitive science. These two approaches, though not always clearly distinguished, differ in the sorts of *parts* that they specify. The first approach, sometimes called *functional analysis* (Cummins 1975), involves a decomposition of a process—a system performing a task—into its various component *subprocesses*.[3] So, for example, one might decompose the process of visual perception into a range of subprocesses, such as those involved in extracting light intensity gradients from the retinal image, those involved

---

[1] For example, the mechanistic assumption appears to rule out various metaphysical theses about the mind, such as substance dualism. But it is largely neutral with respect to such issues as whether some form of functionalism is true, and whether some version of the type-identity theory is correct.

[2] Though see Clark (2008) for a defense of the view that much cognition depends on extra-neural physical structures.

[3] Functional analysis is sometimes characterized not in terms of the decomposition of processes into subprocesses, but in terms of the decomposition of the system's dispositions into subdispositions, or capacities into subcapacities. But in the present context such differences are not important. This is because any exercise of a psychological disposition or capacity that involves the exercise of subcapacities/disposition will be a process, and any psychological process of this sort will be an exercise of a capacity/disposition. Thus any given functional analysis can equally well be construed as an analysis of a process *or* as an analysis of a capacity/disposition.

in determining depth discontinuities, and those involved in determining the spatial orientation of objects (Marr 1982). Further, these various subprocesses will themselves typically be decomposed, in iterative fashion, so that the final analysis represents the overall process as a *hierarchically* organized informational process of the sort that is naturally represented as a flowchart or a program (Cummins 2000). For this reason functional analysis is exceedingly closely related to what we earlier called the algorithmic level. Specifically, such analyses are often a prelude to—and indeed ultimately represented as—an algorithmic level description of the system.

The second sort of decomposition does not merely seek to decompose a system performing a task into subprocesses, but aims to characterize the *structures* from which the system is composed. More specifically, such *mechanistic decompositions* aim to explain a phenomenon (or capacity) by decomposing the system into its functionally salient components, and describing the individual components, the activities in which they engage, and how they interact with each other in order to produce the phenomena in question. Moreover, such structural components are themselves typically decomposed further, in iterative fashion, so that the final analysis describes the system as a *hierarchically* organized set of causally interacting structural components—i.e., a *mechanism*. Thus the present explanatory strategy advocates that in understanding the mind, cognitive scientists in effect pursue the same approach that might be adopted in explaining the operation of a complex artifact, such as an internal combustion engine or a digital computer.

In our view, both functional analysis and mechanistic decomposition are legitimate explanatory enterprises. Indeed, we think that functional analysis is an important step toward developing mechanistic accounts of cognition. Nonetheless, the discovery of mental mechanisms is, as we see it, *the* central task of contemporary cognitive science. And many of the developments that have occurred over the past few decades—especially those associated with the emergence of cognitive neuroscience—are motivated largely by this explanatory goal. Though the identification of mental mechanisms gives rise to many kinds of issues, one that will figure prominently in later sections of this chapter concerns the extent to which the study of psychopathology can help illuminate the structure and organization of the human mind. In view of this, we propose to conclude our overview of cognitive science with a brief discussion of the methods most commonly deployed in drawing inferences about normal cognition from the study of pathology.

Evidence for mechanistic hypotheses: The importance of pathology

There are many different sorts of evidence that are relevant to the assessment of hypotheses about the structure and organization of the human mind, including chronometric data, developmental evidence, neuroimaging data, and computational simulations. But arguably *the* major source of evidence, and one central to the topic of this chapter, comes from the study of *pathology*. For just as experimental interventions can help tell us about the structure of the mind, "natural" interventions, such as disease, nonstandard development, or accidental damage, can provide opportunities to discover properties of the mechanisms normally responsible for our mental capacities (Bechtel 2008; Bechtel and Richardson 1993). A focus on accidental damage is traditionally the business of *cognitive neuropsychology*, which has been primarily interested in building models of normal cognition by studying the deficits incurred by patients with acquired brain injuries (Caramazza 1986; Coltheart 1985; Ellis and Young 1988; Shallice 1988). And a relatively recent variation on this approach, *cognitive neuropsychiatry*, pursues a similar agenda by focusing on pathological conditions traditionally classified as psychiatric disorders (David 1993; Frith 2008; Halligan and David 2001).

One central idea common to both cognitive neuropsychology and cognitive neuropsychiatry is that the functional organization of the human mind can be discerned by charting associations between pathologies and performance on different cognitive tasks. In particular, it is commonplace to study *double dissociations* in order to discern the component mechanisms responsible for cognitive capacities. In brief, double dissociations are instances of paired *single* dissociations, where a pathological condition (or experimental intervention) affects one particular capacity but not another. More specifically, suppose that we test at least two different patients (or groups) on at least two different tasks. In a double dissociation, a patient (or group) X is impaired on Task A but performs normally on Task B, whereas a patient (or group) Y shows the opposite pattern. In such situations, it is plausible to infer that the patients (or groups) differed in some cognitive variable that was differentially tapped by the two tasks. Moreover, the fact that the dissociation goes in *both* directions allows us to rule out task difficulty as an explanation of the data.[4] As a consequence, it is often plausible to conclude that the best explanation of the pattern is that different cognitive mechanisms are involved in the performance of tasks A and B; and that these mechanisms are differentially impaired (and spared) in the patients (or groups). Archetypical cases of this kind of inference include the comparison of patients with damage to Broca's area to patients with damage to Wernicke's area, or patients with deficits in long-term memory to those with deficits to short-term memory. (For classic results see Shallice 1988.)

The virtues of using dissociative data have been debated extensively elsewhere (Coltheart and Davies 2003; Dunn and Kirsner 2003; Davies 2010; Shallice 1988), and we defer any critical discussion to the section entitled "Two challenges to the cognitive science of psychopathology." For the moment, however, two comments are in order. First, notice that double dissociations appear to provide prima facie evidence for the existence of cognitive mechanisms that are distinct, at least to the extent that they are susceptible to selective impairment (and sparing). Thus the study of dissociations appears to provide some basis for claims about the mechanisms responsible for our normal cognitive capacities.[5] Second, and by the same token, double dissociations also appear relevant to understanding the cognitive *incapacities* characteristic of different psychopathologies. For it is by establishing conclusions about deficit cases that one is able to infer conclusions about the normal case. It is to the issue of explaining psychopathology that we now turn.

---

[4] Single dissociations may simply be the products of a single neural region, with two cognitive tasks sharing the same physical location, or the products of "resource artifacts" (Shallice 1988), where one task is impaired simply due to it being more difficult to carry out than the other.

[5] These issues are often couched in terms of modularity (e.g., Davies 2005), though in the present instance the relevant notion of modularity is that of separate modifiability. This notion of modularity is significantly different from those deployed by Fodor (1983) and others (e.g., Barrett and Kurzban 2006).

Explaining Psychopathology

So far we have outlined a range of commonplace explanatory strategies in cognitive science that are routinely combined in various admixtures within different research programs. Specifically, we noted that cognitive capacities and systems can be characterized in the following related ways:

- Intentional (semantic or knowledge) level descriptions
- Algorithmic level descriptions
- Implementation (physical) level descriptions
- Functional analyses
- Mechanistic descriptions.

In this section we set out a range of different ways in which these various strategies might be extended to the case of psychopathology. Specifically, in "Three approaches to the explanation of psychopathology" we highlight three importantly different approaches to the explanation of psychopathology, and in "A menu of explanatory strategies" we show how these approaches cross-classify with the strategies outlined in "Core explanatory assumptions" in order to yield a menu of different approaches to psychopathology. As with much research in cognitive science, different explanatory strategies are deployed in different combinations. In "Some cognitive accounts of psychopathology: Autism and depression" we illustrate this point by considering a couple of well-known attempts to understand psychopathology in cognitive scientific terms.

Three approaches to the explanation of psychopathology

There are a number of importantly different ways in which one might apply the resources of cognitive science to the study of psychopathology, which differ in the assumptions they make about the relationship between explanations of normal cognition and those invoked in the case of pathology. In our view, three such approaches are especially important, what we call deficit-based models, input-based models and direct pathology models.

Deficit-based models

On a deficit-based approach to psychopathology, one starts with a proposal about how the relevant regions of cognition operate in the normal, non-pathological case and then seek to explain the phenomena associated with a psychopathological condition by citing respects in which the normal cognitive system is (selectively) impaired, paradigmatically as a consequence of environmental insult or genetic disorder. In the most extreme cases, deficits are explained by hypothesizing the complete breakdown of a given cognitive mechanism. To take a relatively uncontentious case, extreme forms of cortical blindness can be explained in terms of widespread damage to the visual regions of occipital cortex. Or to take another, more contentious example, one might explain prosopagnosia—the inability to recognize faces—in term of the total breakdown of face recognition mechanisms realized in the fusi-form gyrus (see recent articles in Young et al. 2008).

But deficits need not be an all-or-nothing affair. It need not be the case that the system either works exactly as it should or is entirely inoperative. Instead, a mechanism can be damaged in particular respects and to varying degrees; and as a consequence, it may be that the explanatorily relevant deficit is more fine-grained and partial than complete breakdown. For example, it may be the case that in specific language impairment (SLI) only a highly dis-crete component of the language system is damaged, and perhaps only partially so (van der Lely and Marshall 2010). Indeed, the idea that various core pathological phenomena are a result of partial impairment has recently become quite common, for example, in research on delusions (Coltheart et al. 2011; Davies and Coltheart 2000).

Input-based models

A second approach to the explanation of psychopathology is what we call the input-based approach. Though less commonplace than deficit models, such an approach is still quite familiar from the literature. On this approach, the pathology is not entirely explained in terms of a deficit or breakdown of the normal system, but is instead explained, at least in part, with reference to the character of the inputs to *normally* functioning cognitive systems, inputs that are in some sense problematic or at least relatively unusual.[6]

What is the relationship between input-based and deficit models? Both approaches are parasitic on some prior conception of how relevant regions of normal cognition operate. But in contrast to deficit models, input-based models focus on the sorts of inputs that normally functioning systems receive. In some cases, which we might call *pure* input-based models, the divergence between normal and pathological cases is wholly explained in terms of the character of inputs that normally functioning systems receive. So, for example, in the lit-erature on depressive disorders, both early formulations of the learned helplessness account (Seligman 1975), as well as the social competition hypothesis (Price et al. 1994), maintain that some kinds of depression result from normally functioning cognitive systems receiving inputs that are in some way nonstandard (e.g., inputs that induce in the subject the percep-tion that they lack any control over their circumstances). Similarly, in research on addiction it is routine to explain drug dependencies in terms of the normally functioning reward sys-tem being "hijacked" by chemical stimulants (see, e.g., papers in Poland and Graham 2011).

But it is important to note that input-based and deficit-based strategies can be combined in various ways so that the overall explanation of the pathology is a *hybrid* that recruits both input-based and deficit-based components. For instance, one sort of hybrid model proposes that abnormal inputs to normally functioning developmental mechanisms are responsible for producing *malfunctioning* cognitive mechanisms. So, for example, in some cases of language impairment, such as "feral" children growing up in highly impoverished linguistic environments, the deficits observed in adulthood are plausibly attributed to the character of the input that the child received in the course of development, as opposed to any malfunction of the learning mechanisms themselves. Nevertheless, the *products* of this

---

[6] This approach supposes that some pathologies are strongly analogous to what computer scientists sometimes call garbage-in-garbage-out (or GIGO) phenomena.

developmental process, the mechanisms for language production and comprehension, are also plausibly viewed as pathological. Thus the overall account of such profound linguistic deficits plausibly recruits both an input-based component and a deficit-based component.

A second sort of hybrid model proposes that a normally functioning mechanism might be responsible for producing pathological symptoms because the inputs it receives are generated by some other mechanism that is malfunctioning. Such proposals are well known from the literature on delusions. For example, according to Maher's influential theory of delusion, although delusional beliefs are the output of systems for reasoning, these systems are in no way damaged or malfunctioning (Maher 1988). Instead, normally functioning reasoning systems produce delusional beliefs as a consequence of endeavoring to make sense of the bizarre sensory inputs that they receive from malfunctioning sensory systems. On this view, then, delusion is to be explained by combining a deficit-based account of sensory processing with an input-based account of reasoning processes.

Direct pathology models

The third and final kind of approach to understanding psychopathology is what we call a *direct pathology model*. In contrast to deficit and input-based models, direct pathology models do not seek to explain pathology in terms of some deviation from normal conditions. Rather, researchers instead seek to model directly the pathological condition or process. Although direct pathology models are rather less common than the alternatives, it is still the case that a number of cognitive accounts of pathology conform to this explanatory pattern. This is especially so of accounts which hold that a given psychiatric condition does not result from some manipulation to normally functioning cognitive systems, but instead maintain that the condition results from the existence of a stable polymorph—a distinct form of neurocognitive organization—within the relevant human subpopulation. So, for example, Annette Karmillof-Smith and her collaborators (D'Souza and Karmiloff-Smith 2011; Karmiloff-Smith 1992) have argued that for people with developmental disorders, such as Williams syndrome, the mature brain may be so different that their cognitive systems will need to be modeled in their own right, as opposed merely to characterized in contrast to neurotypicals. Such a view is also suggested by some of Baron-Cohen's more recent work on autism (Baron-Cohen 2005).

A menu of explanatory strategies

In the "Core explanatory assumptions" section we identified a range of related explanatory strategies, commonplace in cognitive science. Then in "Three approaches to the explanation of psychopathology" we drew an orthogonal three-way distinction between approaches to psychopathology, approaches that differ in the assumptions that they make about the relationship between the target pathology and normal cognitive processes. When combined, these distinctions yield a remarkably rich array of explanatory strategies. Indeed, even ignoring the hybrid approaches discussed, there are at least fifteen distinct strategies, each of which has been applied within research on psychopathology.

Moreover, these various strategies are routinely combined in various ways by those interested in psychopathology. For example, amongst those who adopt a deficit approach to a given pathology, it will be natural to seek: (a) an intentional characterization of both the normal process and the deficit, (b) to provide algorithmic and functional characterizations of the normal and pathological processes involved, and (c) to specify the cognitive mechanisms on which such processes depend (and the brain organization that allows for the realization of such mechanisms). Indeed we suspect that there is a widespread consensus amongst cognitive scientists that all of these various explanatory tasks should ideally be performed in the course of comprehensively characterizing a disorder. As a matter of fact, however, much extant research only roughly approximates this ideal, and it is quite uncommon for all of these strategies to receive equal weighting. In the next section we briefly review two examples that help illustrate the mixed—and often incomplete—nature of many cognitive models of psychopathology.

Cognitive Accounts of Psychopathology: Autism and Depression

In the previous section we provided a taxonomy of different cognitive scientific strategies for explaining and describing psychopathology. We noted that in general these strategies are not incompatible and that they are often combined within a single research program. These strategies have been applied to a broad range of psychopathologies, and we encourage readers to see other sources for further illustration (e.g., discussion of delusions in Davies and Egan, Chapter 42, this volume; Murphy 2006). In this section we very briefly sketch some well-known accounts of two forms of psychopathology that have long been the focus of cognitive scientific research: autism spectrum disorder (ASD) and major depressive disorder (MDD). In doing so, we make no attempt at being comprehensive; nor do we aim to adjudicate between competing proposals. Rather our aim is to illustrate the explanatory strategies outlined earlier.

Autism spectrum disorder

Although cognitive approaches to ASD have produced a range of competing hypotheses, the most common approach is one in which the social and communicative problems associated with the disorder are caused by impairment to a "theory of mind" mechanism or module: a system normally dedicated to processing information about beliefs, desires and other mental states (Baron-Cohen 1995; Frith 1989; Leslie 1994).[7]

Notice that the sort of model on offer here is *deficit-based*. As one might expect, then, much of the evidence comes from studies showing that people with ASD are significantly impaired on a range of social cognition tasks, including joint attention (following another's gaze), the use of pretense, and the understanding of deception (Baron-Cohen 1995). But perhaps the most frequently cited evidence comes from studies of the so-called "false belief"

---

[7] For a recent commentary on research in this area see Frith (2012).

task, where Leslie, Baron-Cohen, and others have argued that there is dissociative evidence for the selective impairment of a theory of mind mechanism (or ToMM). In particular, ToMM theorists argue that high functioning children with ASD perform poorly on this task compared to children with Down's syndrome, even though this latter group have far more profound general cognitive deficits (Baron-Cohen et al. 1985).

In elaborating their account of ASD, ToMM theorists operate at a number of descriptive levels. So, for example, they provide intentional descriptions of the relevant phenomena (e.g., detailing the supposed inability of patients to form accurate representations of mental states), and they also sketch the processing stages involved in, say, determining the content of another's belief. But perhaps the central focus of this approach is on the mechanistic decomposition of the systems responsible for "mindreading," and in what follows we focus on this issue.

Although ToMM theorists agree that there is a neurocognitive mechanism whose impairment is responsible for central aspects of ASD,[8] there is considerable disagreement on a range of related issues. One such issue concerns how best to characterize the functional and neuroanatomical organization of ToMM. So, for example, it remains a topic of ongoing research how best to decompose ToMM into its component parts, and what neural regions are primarily responsible for our capacity to attribute mental states to ourselves and to others (Baron-Cohen 2005; Carruthers 2009; Saxe and Kanwisher 2003).

Another issue concerns what mechanisms in addition to ToMM are implicated in "mindreading". So, for instance, according to Baron-Cohen's (1995) influential proposal, in addition to ToMM, the mindreading system contains highly specialized mechanisms for processing various sorts of perceptual information, including: an intentionality detector (ID) that interprets the movement of agent-like stimuli in terms of goals and desires; an eye-direction detector (EDD) that detects eye-like visual stimuli and tracks direction of gaze; and a shared attention mechanism (SAM), which takes inputs from ID and EDD and thereby enables the infant to work out whether they are attending to the same thing as another person (Baron-Cohen 1995).[9] In contrast, Leslie et al. (2004) have argued that, in addition to whatever specialized modules there are, we must posit a relatively unspecialized "selection processor"—an executive system that is, amongst other things, responsible for inhibiting a default bias in normal adults toward attributing true beliefs to others.

A third issue concerns the extent to which the phenomena associated with ASD are fully explained as a deficit to ToMM. While it has long been recognized that social deficits are central symptoms of this disorder (Wing and Gould 1979), more recent studies indicate that there are a range of other anomalies—for example, in executive function and memory (Happe and Frith 2006; Hill 2004). But the precise nature of the relationship between these anomalies and deficits to ToMM remains unclear. In particular, it remains a matter of active debate whether these anomalies are a downstream, developmental effect of ToMM impairment, or whether they are the products of other relatively independent deficits.

---

[8] For example, there is neuroimaging evidence that areas normally activated during social cognition are underactive in individuals with ASD (Frith and Frith 2003).

[9] For further additions and modifications see Baron-Cohen (2005).

A final issue regarding the ToMM hypothesis concerns its reception amongst ASD researchers more broadly. In particular, its adequacy has been challenged on a number of grounds. Some have, for example, recruited evidence about the degree of functional, neuroanatomical and developmental overlap between theory of mind capacities and executive function more broadly in order to argue that ToMM may not be a specialized, independent system (Carlson and Moses 2001; Perner and Lang 1999). Similarly, Gerrans and Stone (2008) have argued that normal theory of mind capacities are not supported by a dedicated ToMM but rather are the product of the developmental interaction between relatively domain-general, high-level systems, such as those underwriting executive function, and domain specific modules for low-level perceptual processing (though see Adams 2011 for critical discussion).

Major depressive disorder

Though a wide array of factors have been implicated in the etiology of MDD, most current cognitive models generally adhere to a "vulnerability-stress" conceptualization, according to which depression results from the activation of cognitive biases by stressful life events. Perhaps the most influential version of this approach was originally proposed by Beck (1967, 1976, 1987), with a model based on the idea that an interplay of dysfunctional "schemas" (or belief frameworks) and negative life events can lead to a pattern of negatively biased appraisals and thoughts. On this view, the characteristic signs and symptoms of MDD—including feelings of hopelessness and despair, suicidal ideation, and anhedonia—are downstream effects of these negatively valenced cognitive states.

Notice that the sort of explanation on offer here differs in a range of respects from the models of ASD considered in the "Autism spectrum disorder" section. First, on the most natural interpretation, Beck's model of MDD is substantially input-based in that the impact of negative life experiences is central to the explanation of depressive episodes. That is, the input-based approach takes depression to be the result of standard-issue cognition having fallen prey to the influence of stress and trauma over time. That said, whether the relevant cognitive "vulnerabilities" constitute a set of underlying deficits remains a point of active enquiry.[10] In which case, it may be that a fully articulated version of the proposal will ultimately constitute a hybrid model.

Second, Beck's model does not appear to provide any mechanistic decomposition. Instead, the model seems primarily concerned with recruiting familiar concepts from cognitive science, such as the notion of a schema, in order to provide an intentional level description of the processes implicated in MDD. What results is a kind of functional analysis—a decomposition of the process into intentionally characterized subparts—though one largely lacking in precise computational analyses. It should be noted, however, that in recent work Beck and his collaborators (Beck 2008; Clark and Beck 2010) have sought

---

[10] There is a large literature on the cognitive profiles of individuals with MDD, detailing their divergence from the non-depressed on a range of cognitive tasks, most significantly in the domains of attention, memory, and aspects of executive functioning (Gotlib and Joorman 2010; Kircanski et al. 2012). This profile of behavioral variation may then signal underlying deficits of some sort.

to develop an implementation level account of the neural structures involved in these processes.

Two Challenges to the Cognitive Science of Psychopathology

In the previous sections we outlined some of the main explanatory strategies to have emerged from cognitive science, and illustrated their application to the study of psychopathology. In this section we conclude by briefly considering two challenges to the prospects of a developed cognitive science of psychopathology. The first is methodological in character, and concerns the pervasive role of dissociative data in theory construction. The second challenge is rather more philosophical in spirit, and concerns whether cognitive scientific approaches to psychopathology will turn out to be subject to serious *in-principle* limitations.

Challenge 1: The role of dissociative data

As noted in the "Core explanatory assumptions" section, it is exceedingly common, especially within cognitive neuropsychology, to use *double dissociations* in order to provide evidence for the existence of distinct neurocognitive mechanisms, and to identify the underlying deficits responsible for neurological and psychiatric disorders. Indeed this method of dissociation (or MD) is arguably *the* main source of evidence for such hypotheses. In recent decades, however, this method has been a focus of much criticism, especially in its application of psychiatric disorders. In what follows, we outline three such criticisms (for a more comprehensive review see Davies 2010).

Objection 1: The instability of symptoms

A first worry with applying the MD to psychiatric disorders concerns the relative instability of psychiatric symptoms. While these considerations have not been extensively elaborated, the worry appears to concern the fact that many psychiatric symptoms—for example, suicidal and delusional ideation—tend to wax and wane in their occurrence, form, and severity (e.g., see Young 2000 on delusions). In view of this, it may be that the MD cannot be used to support conclusions about the underlying deficits responsible for such symptoms. Specifically, the idea seems to be that if, on the one hand, symptoms are unstable whilst, on the other, neurocognitive mechanisms are stable, enduring structures, then dissociative data will not license inferences regarding which specific underlying deficit is responsible for the symptoms—i.e., which neurocognitive mechanism is damaged. Thus it may be necessary to revise, supplement, or even replace the MD in cognitive neuropsychiatry.

Though symptom instability no doubt raises interesting methodological issues, we doubt that it poses a serious challenge to the use of dissociative data in the study of psychopathology. One obvious, and in our view convincing, response is that when studying psychopathology it may often be appropriate to characterize deficits in terms of *partial* impairment, as opposed to construing symptoms as products of completely impaired systems (again, see work on delusions by Coltheart et al. 2011; Davies and Coltheart 2000). In this way, the fact that some psychiatric symptoms appear to wax and wane is explained by supposing that the dysfunctional informational products of cognitive deficits are occasionally over-ridden—or compensated for—by other processes.[11]

Objection 2: "Impure" cases

A second challenge to the MD centers on the notion of *impure* cases, and the epistemic problems that such cases generate (Van Orden et al. 2001). In brief, a *single* dissociation is pure when it involves damage to exactly one neurocognitive mechanism; otherwise it is impure. A *double* dissociation is pure, when it combines two pure single dissociations; otherwise it is impure. In order to appreciate the significance of the distinction, it is important see that pure and impure double dissociations have quite different inferential properties. If a double dissociation is pure, then it *deductively* follows that there are two distinct mechanisms, each of which is impaired with respect to a task. In which case, if one has strong evidence that a case is pure, then one *also* has good reason to conclude that there are two, distinct cognitive mechanisms, and that the observed pattern of performance is explained by their selective impairment (and sparing).

The logical implications of impure dissociations are quite different. If a dissociation is impure, it does *not* deductively follow that there are two distinct mechanisms whose selective impairment and sparing is responsible for the pattern of performance. Instead there is a range of alternatives that are compatible with the impure case. So, for example:

1. It is possible that the dissociable tasks depend at least partially on some shared resource.
2. It may be that different components within a *single* mechanism are differentially affected and that this is responsible for producing different patterns of performance.
3. It is even possible that the dissociable tasks are the products of some kind of continuous processing space that wholly lacks separate and identifiable mechanisms (Shallice 1988).

But if this is so, if impure cases are consistent with all these possibilities, then having evidence of such a dissociation does *not* provide good reason to conclude that the pattern of performance is produced by the selective impairment of two distinct mechanisms. That is, impure cases neither provide strong evidence for distinct cognitive mechanisms nor for the underlying deficit responsible for a given pathology.

What are we to make of these observations? The appropriate response may seem obvious. If pure cases provide strong evidence and impure cases do not, then in using the MD we should restrict ourselves to pure cases. But this alone does not resolve the matter. First, we should expect the vast majority of dissociations to be impure since there is no reason to

---

[11] And this also leaves space open for the study of the role of factors external to the impaired mechanism, such as environmental stressors, that might explain the more-or-less acute presentation of certain symptoms.

suppose that the causes of neurocognitive insults—for example, blows to the head or chromosomal abnormalities—should respect the boundaries between cognitive mechanisms. In which case, if impure cases fail to provide a basis for dissociative inferences, then it would seem that the vast proportion of data that cognitive neuropsychologists have amassed is of little relevance to the task of discerning cognitive structure.

A second and apparently more serious worry is that in order to pursue a policy of restricting ourselves to pure cases, it would seem that we need some reasonably reliable method for determining *which* cases are pure and which impure. Yet (so the objection continues) there is no such reliable method; or at any rate, we have no good reason to suppose that there is. Indeed some go so far as to claim that there exists no noncircular way of determining whether a given case is pure or otherwise. For in order to know that a double dissociation is pure one must already have established what the dissociative evidence is supposed to show, viz., that there are two distinct mechanisms whose impairment is responsible for the pattern in performance (Van Orden et al. 2001). Thus critics conclude that the MD cannot support conclusions about the mechanistic structure of the mind or about the underlying causes of psychopathology.

In our view, the distinction between pure and impure cases does raise problems for the MD, if only because it suggests that such data typically provide rather less support for conclusions about neurocognitive structure than advocates have traditionally supposed. That said, we are inclined to think that the worries raised by impure cases are somewhat allayed by noting that the MD may well allow for respectable abductive inferences, even in the absence of any highly reliable means of discriminating pure from impure cases (Coltheart and Davies 2003; Davies 2010). This is because although *possible* alternative explanations will be routinely available, in many cases the *best* explanation—the simplest, most conservative, most powerful explanation—may well appeal to the existence of functionally distinct neurocognitive mechanisms. Of course, the strength of any particular inference will depend upon the details of the case. For example, it will depend on the degree of dissociation between the disorders being compared and between the neural regions that are associated with these disorders. But if used judiciously, we are inclined to think that, despite the existence of impure cases, the MD can still yield insight into the functional organization of the mind/brain and its pathologies.

Objection 3: The problem of developmental dissociations

Another potential challenge to the MD, especially as it extends to psychiatry, comes from the study of disorders that are thought to be the product of nonstandard development. Until quite recently, it was commonly assumed that dissociations arising from developmental psychopathology could provide good evidence for the existence of specialized cognitive systems. For example, as we saw in "Explaining psychopathology," many researchers were led to infer that the impairments in autism were the product of a dysfunctional mechanism normally responsible for theory of mind. Similarly, Williams syndrome, a developmental disorder marked by impairments to a child's spatial recognition capacities, has garnered considerable theoretical attention in large measure because there appear to be double dissociations between Williams and a range of other disorders, including: autism; prosopagnosia, which involves deficits in facial recognition; and SLI, which is characterized by syntactic impairments. Further, these dissociations have been taken to support conclusions regarding the existence of specific cognitive mechanisms whose selective impairment and sparing is responsible for the various disorders involved.

Though such inferences have been challenged on a number of grounds, perhaps the most theoretically interesting concerns the developmental presuppositions implicit in the application of the MD to developmental disorders. Annette Karmiloff-Smith and her collaborators (D'Souza and Karmiloff-Smith 2011; Karmiloff-Smith 1992) have argued, for instance, that the application of the MD to developmental disorders presupposes that developmental anomalies tend only to affect relatively autonomous neurocognitive systems, whilst leaving the rest of the brain "residually normal". In contrast, Karmiloff-Smith maintains that the brain is more plausibly construed as a massively interconnected system that develops in holistic fashion, so that early emerging pathological disruption will tend to be amplified in the course of develop, and ultimately produce *comprehensively* atypical neural organization. But if this is so, if developmental disorders, such as Williams, probably result in comprehensively atypical brains, then it is no longer safe to assume that the signs and symptoms associated with such disorders are produced by selective impairments to an otherwise intact or "residually normal" brain. In which case, it would seem that the MD, at least as typically applied, fails to license conclusions about the existence of specific cognitive mechanisms or about the underlying causes of psychopathology (for further discussion see Machery 2011).

Challenge 2: In-principle limitations?

Let us turn to the second, more principled, of our challenges. Though the cognitive sciences have made considerable progress in explaining aspects of the human mind and its various disorders, no one would be so sanguine as to suggest that the project is complete, or even nearly so. On the contrary, success to date has been fragmentary; and it remains a largely open question whether—and to what extent—efforts to explain mental disorder will prove successful. In view of this, we propose to conclude this chapter by discussing considerations that some (e.g., Murphy 2006) have recently taken to suggest that the cognitive science of psychopathology may well be subject to serious limitations.

The relevant considerations are familiar to cognitive scientists, and received their canonical expression almost three decades ago in the final sections of Fodor's *Modularity of Mind* (1983). In this work, Fodor famously advocates a conception of our mental architecture on which peripheral systems for motor control and low-level perception are *modular* in character. That is, they are highly specialized and informationally *encapsulated* in the sense that they only utilize a restricted range of the information available to the organism as a whole. In contrast, Fodor maintains that *central systems* responsible for such "higher" cognitive tasks as reasoning and decision-making are radically non-modular, or unencapsulated: that they can utilize virtually any sort of information in the course of their computations. According to Fodor, this is likely to have important implications for the scope and limits of cognitive science. In particular, he maintains that the sort of cognitive science we currently have, one wedded to an information processing model, is unlikely to make much headway in providing models of highly unencapsulated central processes. Indeed Fodor goes so far as to claim "the limits of modularity are also likely to be the limits of what we are going to be able to understand about the mind, given anything like the theoretical apparatus currently available" (Fodor 1983, p. 126). In what follows, we propose to explore the implications of this *Fodorian pessimism* for the cognitive science of psychopathology.

Reasons for Fodorian pessimism?

What reasons are there for supposing that non-modular systems will likely prove recalcitrant to the explanatory strategies of cognitive science? Fodor provides two main considerations, and though clearly neither are conclusive, many have found them prima facie compelling. The first focuses on the prospects of providing *implementational* (e.g., neurobiological or neuroanatomical) descriptions of central systems. If a cognitive system is modular and, hence, processes only a restricted range of inputs, and bears limited informational relations to other systems, then it is reasonable to suppose that it will have a reasonably well-defined neural architecture: that it will be localized and have well-defined connections to other systems. (This appears to be true in the case of early vision, for example.) In contrast, if central systems are, as Fodor claims, radically non-modular, bearing elaborate informational relations every which way, then they are also unlikely to exhibit a clearly articulated neural architecture. Further, the same will likely be true of the *components* of such mechanisms. As a consequence, according to Fodor, lesion studies, deficit studies, neuroimaging, and other strategies designed to aid in the identification of structurally characterizable units are unlikely to prove successful.

The second consideration focuses on the prospects of providing *algorithmic* specifications of central processes. On the assumption that cognitive systems are information processing devices, we should expect to be able to specify the sorts of information that a cognitive system deploys and the sorts of computations involved in the processing of such information. In the case of low-level perceptual processes, the task of doing so appears tractable. We are, for example, able to determine with reasonable clarity what sorts of information are deployed in early vision, and how it is being processed. According to Fodor, however, the problem we confront in understanding central processes is that there appear to be few discernible constraints on information processing. We are able to think about almost anything, the informational relations appear to go every which way, and they are highly sensitive to context. In which case, the task of specifying such processes in information processing terms will likely prove an extraordinarily difficult one.

Psychopathology in the shadow of Fodorian pessimism

Though the case for Fodorian pessimism is far from overwhelming, it is suggestive enough to merit consideration of its implications. Let us suppose for the sake of argument, then, that it is correct, and ask what its implications are for a cognitive science of psychopathology. In our view they are likely to be profound. In particular, Fodorian pessimism has bleak implications for the prospects of cognitive models of psychopathologies that involve central processes.

The point is perhaps clearest in the case of *deficit-based* models that seek to describe the pathology in algorithmic or mechanistic terms. Such models aim to explain how some pathological phenomenon is produced by citing some abnormality—or malfunction—in those mechanisms or computational processes responsible for normal cognition. But such models *presuppose* some prior account of normal cognition. In which case if Fodorian pessimism is correct, then such deficit-based models will be not be forthcoming for pathologies that involve central cognition. This will simply be because there will be no mechanistic or algorithmic account of normal function to work from in the first place.

Much the same is true of *input-based* models of psychopathologies that involve central processes. In such models one seeks to explain some pathological phenomena in terms of abnormal inputs to normally functioning mechanisms or processes. But again, such explanations *presuppose* a prior mechanistic account of normal function. In which case if Fodorian pessimism is correct about central processes, no such models of the psychopathologies will be forthcoming.

The issues are perhaps least clear in the case of *direct pathology models*. Rather than presupposing some account of normal cognition, such models instead proceed directly by constructing an account of the pathology itself or of the mechanism(s) that are responsible for the pathology in question. It is harder to assess the implications of Fodorian pessimism for such approaches, in large measure because it remains unclear, for any pathology, how much of central cognition needs to be characterized in order to provide such models. As a consequence, one cannot argue directly from Fodorian pessimism to conclusions about the prospects of such models. For all that, if Fodorian pessimism is correct, we should expect that direct models of pathologies that crucially depend upon central cognition—for example, thought disorders and delusional disorders—will be hard to produce in much the same way as indirect (deficit and input-based) models are.

Of course, none of this precludes the possibility of models of psychopathology that do not seek to provide mechanistic or algorithmic descriptions of the pathologies involved. But for present purposes, the point we wish to stress is that the search for such descriptions is very typically the ultimate goal of cognitive science. And what goes for cognitive science in general also goes for cognitive scientific explanations of psychopathology. In which case, if Fodorian pessimism is correct, this explanatory quest may turn out to be forlorn.

REFERENCES

Adams, M. (2011). Modularity, theory of mind, and autism spectrum disorder, *Philosophy of Science*, 78, 763–73.

Baron-Cohen, S. (1995). *Mindblindness*. Cambridge, MA: MIT Press.

Baron-Cohen, S. (2005). The empathizing system: A revision of the 1994 model of the mindreading system. In B. Ellis and D. Bjorklund (Eds), *Origins of the Social Mind*, pp. 468–92. New York, NY: Guilford Publications Inc.

Baron-Cohen, S., Leslie, A., and Frith, U. (1985). Does the autistic child have a 'theory of mind'? *Cognition*, 21, 37–46.

Barrett, H. C. and Kurzban, R. (2006). Modularity in cognition: framing the debate. *Psychological Review*, 113(3), 628–47.

Bechtel, W. (2008). *Mental Mechanisms: Philosophical Perspectives on Cognitive Neuroscience*. New York, NY: Routledge.

Bechtel, W. and Richardson, R. C. (1993). *Discovering Complexity: Decomposition and Localization as Strategies in Scientific Research*. Princeton, NJ: Princeton University Press.

Beck, A. T. (1967). *Depression: Causes and Treatment*. Philadelphia, PA: University of Pennsylvania Press.

Beck, A. T. (1976). *Cognitive Therapy and the Emotional Disorders*. New York, NY: International University Press.

Beck, A. T. (1987). Cognitive models of depression. *Journal of Cognitive Psychotherapy*, 1, 5–37.

Beck, A. T. (2008). The evolution of the cognitive model of depression and its neurobiological correlates. *American Journal of Psychiatry*, 165, 969–77.

Broome, M. and Bortolotti, L. (2009). *Psychiatry as Cognitive Neuroscience: Philosophical Perspectives*. Oxford: Oxford University Press.

Caramazza, A. (1986). On drawing inferences about the structure of normal cognitive systems from the analysis of patterns of impaired performance: the case for single patient studies. *Brain and Cognition*, 5, 41–66.

Carey, S. (2009). *The Origin of Concepts*. Oxford University Press: Oxford.

Carlson, S. M. and Moses, L. J. (2001). Individual differences in inhibitory control and children's theory of mind. *Child Development*, 72(4), 1032–53.

Carruthers, P. (2009). How we know our own minds: the relationship between mindreading and metacognition. *Behavioral and Brain Sciences*, 32, 121–82.

Chemero, A. (2009). *Radical Embodied Cognitive Science*. Cambridge, MA: MIT Press.

Clark, A. (2000). *Mindware: An Introduction to the Philosophy of Cognitive Science*. New York, NY: Oxford University Press.

Clark, A. (2008). *Supersizing the Mind: Embodiment, Action, Cognitive Extension*. New York, NY: Oxford University Press.

Clark, D. A. and Beck, A. T. (2010). Cognitive theory and therapy of anxiety and depression: Convergence with neurobiological findings. *Trends in Cognitive Sciences*, 14, 418–24.

Coltheart, M. (1985). Cognitive neuropsychology and the study of reading. In M. I. Posner and O. S. M. Marin (Eds), *Attention and Performance XI*, pp. 3–37. Hillsdale, NJ: Erlbaum.

Coltheart, M. and Davies, M. (2003). Inference and explanation in cognitive neuropsychology. *Cortex*, 39, 188–91.

Coltheart, M., Langdon, R., and McKay, R. (2011). Delusional belief. *Annual Review of Psychology*, 62, 271–98.

Cummins, D. D. and Cummins, R. (2000). *Minds, Brains and Computers*. Oxford: Blackwell.

Cummins, R. (1975). Functional analysis. *Journal of Philosophy*, 72, 741–64.

Cummins, R. (2000) "How does it work?" vs. "What are the laws?" Two conceptions of psychological explanation. In F. Keil and R. Wilson (Eds), *Explanation and Cognition*, pp. 117–45. Cambridge, MA: MIT Press.

David, A. S. (1993). Cognitive neuropsychiatry? *Psychological Medicine*, 23, 1–5.

Davies, M. (2005). Cognitive science. In F. Jackson and M. Smith (Eds), *The Oxford Handbook of Contemporary Analytic Philosophy*, pp. 358–94. Oxford: Oxford University Press.

Davies, M. (2010). Double dissociations. *Mind & Language*, 25(5), 500–40.

Davies, M. and Coltheart, M. (2000). Pathologies of belief. *Mind & Language*, 15(1), 1–46.

D'Souza, D. and Karmiloff-Smith, A. (2011). When modularization fails to occur: A developmental perspective. *Cognitive Neuropsychology*, 28(3&4), 276–87.

Dunn, J. C. and Kirsner, K. (2003). What can we infer from double dissociations? *Cortex*, 39, 1–7.

Ellis, A. W. and Young, A. W. (1988). *Human Cognitive Neuropsychology*. Hove: Erlbaum.

Fodor, J. (1968). *Psychological Explanation*. New York, NY: Random Rouse.

Fodor, J. (1983). *The Modularity of Mind: An Essay on Faculty Psychology*. Cambridge, MA: MIT Press.

Fodor, J. and Pylyshyn, Z. (1988). Connectionism and cognitive architecture: A critique. *Cognition*, 28, 3–71.

Frith, C. (2008). In praise of cognitive neuropsychiatry. *Cognitive Neuropsychiatry*, 13(1), 1–7.

Frith, U. (1989). *Autism: Explaining the Enigma* (2nd edn 2003). London: Blackwell.

Frith, U. (2012). Why we need cognitive explanations of autism. *The Quarterly Journal of Experimental Psychology*, 65(11), 2073–92.

Frith, U. and Frith, C. D. (2003). Development and neurophysiology of mentalizing. *Philosophical Transactions of the Royal Society B: Biological Sciences*, 358(1431), 459–73

Gazzaniga, M. S. (2009). *The Cognitive Neurosciences* (4th edn). Cambridge, MA: MIT Press.

Gerrans, P. and Stone, V. E. (2008). Generous or parsimonious cognitive architecture? Cognitive neuroscience and theory of mind. *British Journal of Philosophy of Science*, 59, 121–41.

Gotlib, I. H. and Joorman, J. (2010). Cognition and depression: Current status and future directions. *Annual Review of Clinical Psychology*, 6, 285–312.

Halligan, P. W. and David, A. S. (2001). Cognitive neuropsychiatry: towards a scientific psychotherapy. *Neuroscience: Nature Reviews*, 2, 209–15.

Happe, F. and Frith, U. (2006). The weak coherence account: detail-focused cognitive style in autism spectrum disorders. *Journal of Autism and Developmental Disorders*, 36(1), 5–25.

Hill, E. L. (2004). Executive dysfunction in autism. *Trends in Cognitive Sciences*, 8(10), 26–32.

Karmiloff-Smith, A. (1992). *Beyond Modularity: A Developmental Perspective on Cognitive Science*. Cambridge, MA: MIT Press.

Kendler, K. S. (2008). Explanatory models for psychiatric illness. *American Journal of Psychiatry*, 165, 695–702.

Kendler, K. S., Zachar, P., and Craver, C. (2011). What kinds of things are psychiatric disorders? *Psychological Medicine*, 41, 1143–50.

Kircanski, K., Joorman, J., and Gotlib, I. H. (2012). Cognitive aspects of depression. *WIREs Cognitive Science*, 3, 301–13.

Leslie, A. (1994). ToMM, ToBY, and agency: core architecture and domain specificity. In L. Hirschfeld and S. Gelman (Eds), *Mapping the Mind*, pp. 119–48. Cambridge: Cambridge University Press.

Leslie, A. M., Friedman, O., and German, T. P. (2004). Core mechanisms in 'theory of mind.' *Trends in Cognitive Sciences*, 8(12), 528–33.

Machery, E. (2011). Developmental disorders and cognitive architecture. In P. Adriaens and A. De Block (Eds), *Maladapting Minds: Philosophy, Psychiatry, and Evolutionary Theory*, pp. 91–116. Oxford: Oxford University Press.

Maher, B. (1988). Anomalous experience and delusional thinking: the logic of explanations. In T. F. Oltmanns and B. A. Maher (Eds), *Delusional Beliefs*, pp. 15–33. New York, NY: Plenum Press.

Marr, D. (1982). *Vision: A Computational Investigation into the Human Representation and Processing of Visual Information*. Cambridge, MA: MIT Press.

Murphy, D. (2006). *Psychiatry in the Scientific Image*. Cambridge, MA: MIT Press.

Newell, A. (1990). *Unified Theories of Cognition*. Cambridge, MA: Harvard University Press.

Perner, J. and Lang, B. (1999). Development of theory of mind and executive control. *Trends in Cognitive Sciences*, 3(9), 337–44.

Piccinini, G. and Scarantino, A. (2011). Information processing, computation, and cognition. *Journal of Biological Physics*, 37(1), 1–38.

Pinker, S. (1994). *The Language Instinct*. New York, NY: William Morrow.

Poland, J. and Graham, G. (2011). *Addiction and responsibility*. Cambridge, MA: MIT Press.

Price, J., Sloman, L., Gardner, R., Gilbert, P., and Rohde, P. (1994). The social competition hypothesis of depression. *British Journal of Psychiatry*, 164, 309–15.

Pylyshyn, Z. (1984). Computation and cognition. Cambridge, MA: MIT Press.

Saxe, R. and Kanwisher, N. (2003). People thinking about thinking people: the role of the temporo-parietal junction in 'theory of mind.' *NeuroImage, 19*, 1835–42.

Seligman, M. E. P. (1975). *Helplessness: On Depression, Development, and Death.* San Francisco, CA: W. H. Freeman.

Shallice, T. (1988). *From Neuropsychology to Mental Structure.* Cambridge: Cambridge University Press.

Smolensky, P. (1988). On the proper treatment of connectionism. *Behavioral and Brain Sciences, 11*, 1–23.

Thagard, P. (2012). Cognitive science. In E. N. Zalta (Ed.), *The Stanford Encyclopedia of Philosophy* (Fall 2012 Edition). [Online.] Available at: <http://plato.stanford.edu/archives/fall2012/entries/cognitive-science/>.

van der Lely, H. K. J and Marshall, C. (2010). Grammatical-specific language impairment: A window onto domain specificity. In J. Guendouzi, F. Loncke, and M. Williams (Eds), *Handbook of Psycholinguistics and Cognitive Processing Perspectives in Communication Disorders*, pp. 403–19. Hove: Psychology Press.

Van Orden, G. C., Pennington, B. F., and Stone, G. O. (2001). What do double dissociations prove? *Cognitive Science, 25*(1), 111–72.

Von Eckardt, B. (1993). *What is Cognitive Science?* Cambridge, MA: MIT Press.

Wing, L. and Gould, J. (1979). Severe impairments of social interaction and associated abnormalities in children: epidemiology and classification. *Journal of Autism and Developmental Disorders, 9*, 11–29.

Young, A. W. (2000). Wondrous strange: the neuropsychology of abnormal beliefs. *Mind & Language, 15*(1), 47–73.

Young, A. W., de Haan, E. H. F., and Bauer, R. M. (2008). Face perception: a very special issue. *Journal of Neuropsychology, 2*(1), 1–14.

CHAPTER 28

WHAT IS MENTAL ILLNESS?

DEREK BOLTON

How Do We Get to the Clinic?

In the 1970s the American Psychiatric Association was obliged to ask itself the question whether homosexuality, which it had included as a mental illness in the second edition of the Association's *Diagnostic and Statistical Manual of Mental Disorders* (DSM-II; American Psychiatric Association 1968), really was such, and in particular whether it should or should not be included in the third edition. This raised the general question what mental illness, or mental disorder, is. And among the many difficulties raised by this question was the fact that there was no definition in the DSM-II. On reflection it seemed to several contemporary commentators that no definition had seemed to be needed, that the "mental illnesses" were just the conditions that physicians regularly attended to in the clinic. Donald Klein, for example, commented (1978, p. 41):

> Strikingly there is no explicit statement within the *Diagnostic and Statistical Manual of Mental Disorders* [second edition] that defines the sort of condition categorizable within this document. Such a logical lapse is not restricted to psychiatry, however, since the *International Classification of Diseases* also lacks such a statement. It seems plain that these compendia are actually compilations of the sorts of things that physicians treat; a circular classificatory principle but a useful historical clue. Our definitions of illness are derived from medical practice.

While the great majority of psychiatry literature comprises mainly work on classification, causes, and treatments of conditions, there is a smaller but important literature on the definition of mental illness. Aspects of this will be covered in this chapter, particularly the conceptualization that came to be used in the DSM from its third edition onward, and influential subsequent approaches relying on concepts from evolutionary biology and psychology. There are also literatures on the social processes involved in diagnosis of illness and its consequences, related to medical power, prescribing, excuse from social role obligations, and sometimes from legal responsibility. Relatively less attention has been paid in the academic literatures to what goes on before the doctors and other health care professionals get involved, to what goes on at home, among family and friends, and in the individual's mind.

What conditions do people take to the clinic, and why? Here we could list the several hundred conditions in the current edition of the DSM, the DSM-IV (American Psychiatric Association 1994), though it should be said that many of these are subtypes, and many are relatively rare, so we could draw up with a much shorter list of the common mental health problems, anxiety and depressive disorders, severe mental illness such as schizophrenia, a variety of developmental or neurodevelopmental problems such as autism and attention-deficit/hyperactivity disorder (ADHD), and some others familiar in the culture such as obsessive-compulsive disorder and bipolar disorder, previously manic depression. All these conditions, so characterized, are of course as seen through the mental health care gaze; they are the phenomena as conceptualized following an assessment by the mental health care professional and a diagnosis. These diagnostic formulations are, on the other hand, increasingly what the person or family brings to the clinic, because they have looked up their symptoms on the Internet, following their own searches or suggestion from a friend.

Before the diagnostic formulations are the sets of symptoms, so a description of the conditions people take to the clinic could be a list of symptoms or patterns of symptoms, and these are very well laid out in the diagnostic manuals, the American Psychiatric Association's DSM-IV and the World Health Organization's *International Classification of Mental and Behavioural Disorders*, tenth revision (ICD-10; World Health Organization 1992). Here we find patterns of symptoms of *many, many kinds*, such as: long periods of uncontrollable, distressing worrying; paralyzing anxiety in social situations; suicidal thinking or intent; withdrawal to isolation; hearing persecuting voices when none are there; no friends as a child; and episodes of couldn't care less activities, instances of which would be, for example, temporarily forgetting about the children and spending large sums of money on credit cards which can't be paid back.

The compilations of symptoms and syndromes in the DSM and ICD are clear descriptions of the kinds of mental health problems people bring to the clinic, but they are descriptions from the outside, of an observer, and they are indeed *clinical descriptions*, based on what is ascertainable in the clinic from one or more informants. Descriptions from the inside, from the person who has the difficulties, or from the families who live with the person and the troubles, who have seen these troubles unfold in their loved ones, notwithstanding all efforts—are to be found elsewhere, in life-writing of people who have experienced mental health problems in themselves or in their family.[1]

There is also a strong, rich, and complex history of phenomenology in psychiatry that aims to elucidate the quality of inner experience involved in mental health problems. Psychiatrists early in the twentieth century gave clear descriptions, based on fine attention to the patient's experience, to the subjective quality of, for example, a "delusion" and how it differs from an "obsession" (these descriptors being those of the doctors of course). This so-called "descriptive phenomenology" may be distinguished from, and it has contested linkages with, philosophical phenomenology originating in the nineteenth and early twentieth centuries. Both aspects continue to play an important role in elucidating the experience

---

[1] The mental illness life-writing literature is extensive; see, e.g., Campbell (1999), Campion (2012), Mental Health Foundation (1999), and Read and Reynolds (1996).

of mental illness—its appearance from the inside—and as counterpoint to the objectivity and materiality of neuroscience.[2]

A person attends the clinic for themselves—or the family takes a person to the clinic—because they believe that something serious is, or may be, wrong with them, and that a doctor or other health care professional may be able to advise or help. In the case of mental health problems—as they will be called when the decision to attend the mental health clinic has been taken—coming to this belief can be, though is not always, complex, difficult, and protracted. There is, according to the person himself, or family, something wrong with the person, in a range between not quite right and very wrong, something not as it should be—some deviation in the wrong direction, it may be said, from the normal. What "the normal" is taken to be is a complex question, signaling large sets of issues involved in the conceptualization of mental illness. Standards immediately available to us, the clinic aside, in our everyday lives, include: the person is not themselves, they are not feeling or behaving as they usually do—there is a rupture in the personal narrative. And/or: the person is not feeling or behaving as is usual for comparable people—this often being the standard parents use, for example, when trying to assess their child and his development. And/or: the person is falling below commonly endorsed social standards, for example, in a child's showing some concern for other children, or paying attention and learning at school; or self-care. In all these cases there is the question: How much is too little, or too much? The standards are not clearly marked. How much variation within the person over time, or relative to others or to social standards, is within the normal range—so not to worry after all? *Normalizing* in this way is always an option, at least until things get very bad, or come to a crisis. A variation on this theme is finding an explanation which means the problem is self-limiting: it's just a temporary thing, he will grow out of it as he gets older; it's because he's upset because of such-and-such an event, he will get over it. Or consider another reaction in our repertoire: coping. There is a problem but we can help manage it; I can talk to the teacher and we can put in more support; I can try harder; I just to have put up with all this upset; it's just the way I am/he is. All these options interweave with just how serious the problem is thought to be, a matter likely to be revisited on a continuous basis. What does "seriously something wrong" amount to? There is much that can be said about this, but to cut the story short it probably means: gets in the way of activities which are essential to our way of life, to what people or myself in particular can and should be—highly valued things. So, for example, for children these might be: making use of educational opportunity, being able to get along with the peer group, make some friends or a friend, have some fun. For adolescents: begin to be able to get on with their increasingly independent activities (peers, sexual, work) without coming to harm, without causing too much harm. For adults: work, friendships, developing and consolidating a worthwhile life, if they have children, raising them well enough. In old age: respect, safety. This is just a list I have composed and we can all make one up and refine it, personalize it—but what we mean by "something seriously wrong" is disruption in these kinds of areas. But then, should we go for help to an expert? This problem interacts with many personal and social variables. Should we not be self-reliant? Can we trust doctors anyway? What about the shame; or the stigma? And there is, to complicate the position further, a whole other set of issues more or less raised to different extents in different cultures and subcultures: even if there is something seriously wrong, and we need expert help, why

---

[2] See, e.g., Berrios (1989), Kendler and Parnas (2008), Ratcliffe (2008), and Stanghellini (2004).

go to a doctor, why to the health care clinic? Why not, for example, to a priest? Or to a traditional healer for advice and remedies regarding spirits? The question of appropriate expertise will depend on how the problem is framed, on how the world and human beings in it are understood, and different cultures and subcultures have different options, inclinations, and decision-procedures.

It can be seen in this very brief review that coming to the decision to attend the clinic can be, though is not always, complex, difficult, contested, and protracted, within the person himself, and within the family, as different points of view are taken through time or across time. The brief review indicates the processes and constructions that lie beneath the conceptualization of something as a problem of the sort to be taken to the mental health clinic, being recognized as such by the health care professional, and either being or perhaps on its way to becoming a "mental disorder" in the DSM and ICD.

THE DSM CONCEPTUALIZATION

Following its deliberations as to the meaning of mental illness (or mental disorder) for the purposes of inclusion in its DSM, it was proposed that *distress and/or impairment* were fundamental. This idea was adopted, with elaborations and qualifications, in the DSM-III (American Psychiatric Association 1980), and it remains, with some modifications to the qualifications, in the current DSM-IV (American Psychiatric Association 1994):

> In DSM-IV, each of the mental disorders is conceptualized as a clinically significant behavioral or psychological syndrome or pattern that occurs in an individual and that is associated with present distress (e.g., a painful symptom) or disability (i.e., impairment in one or more important areas of functioning) or with a significantly increased risk of suffering death, pain, disability or an important loss of freedom. In addition, this syndrome or pattern must not be merely an expectable and culturally sanctioned response to a particular event, for example, the death of a loved one. Whatever its original cause, it must currently be considered a manifestation of a behavioral, psychological or biological dysfunction in the individual. Neither deviant behavior (e.g., political, religious, or sexual) nor conflicts that are primarily between the individual and society are mental disorders unless the deviance or conflict is a symptom of a dysfunction in the individual, as described above. (pp. xxi–xxii)

The fundamental idea then, is that mental disorders are associated with present distress or disability/impairment. This idea is also in the ICD-10, though with less conviction, elaboration, and qualification,[3] and a recent proposed amendment of the DSM-IV conceptualization for the DSM-5 does not attempt to change it (Stein et al. 2010). The lesson here, I suggest, is that for all its problems, the emphasis on distress/impairment is essentially correct. Distress and impairment constitute the fundamental personal and social phenomenology of the conditions people bring to the clinic, and so will appear at the very least as operationalized markers of whatever else we may suppose illness/disorder really is.

---

[3] The ICD-10 has: "'Disorder' is not an exact term, but it is used here to imply the existence of a clinically recognizable set of symptoms or behaviour associated in most cases with distress and with interference with personal functions. Social deviance or conflict alone, without personal dysfunction, should not be included in mental disorder as defined here" (World Health Organization 1992, p. 5).

Let us consider key points of the DSM-IV conceptualization, the key idea and the elaborations and qualifications, in turn:

Distress and impairment. This was the key idea of the conceptualization proposed for and incorporated into the DSM-III, and it served as a principled ground to exclude homosexuality from the third edition.[4] It captures a very sound and presumably very ancient healthcare principle: people attend to the clinic in states of distress and impairment—as noted in the first section.

Should not be an expectable response to an event. Much hangs on this qualification. It is meant to exclude "normal" responses to life's problems. Put another way: if we—for good reason—put distress and impairment center stage in our understanding of mental illness, how do we distinguish normal distress from "pathological" distress warranting health care attention? This is a good question to which there is no straightforward answer; in effect it re-asks the question: what is mental illness/disorder? Invoking "expectability" raises the question but does not answer it. Many physical and mental health problems are (somewhat) "expectable" in any readily available sense, such as broken limbs following a road traffic accident, or depression in the context of several major adverse life-events and chronic difficulties. What matters is that there is something seriously wrong that may be helped by healthcare attention, and what the "seriously wrong" means is open to the same options as "what is mental illness?" The DSM emphasizes distress and impairment as fundamental; other options will be reviewed in the next section.[5]

Another aspect of the problem of distinguishing what is normal from what is illness arises in connexion not with life-events but with traits, though this is not expressly addressed in the DSM conceptualization. Issues here include, for example, differentiation between

---

[4] The background to the construction of the definition adopted for the DSM-III is given in papers by Robert Spitzer and colleagues on the American Psychiatric Association's working party set up for this purpose, particularly Spitzer and Endicott (1978), Spitzer and Williams (1982, 1988), and Klein (1978). These papers are essential reading for understanding why the DSM conceptualizes mental disorder in the way that it does, and they remain, in the present author's opinion, among the very best theoretical papers on the definition of mental illness and illness generally.

[5] The vexed nature of the issue shows up in the fact that DSM apparently envisages a range of expectable responses to events that, while distressing/impairing, are not illness but rather expectable (normal), only bereavement is cited as an example; while in the diagnostic criteria for Major Depressive Disorder, only bereavement (not any other major loss) is permitted to exclude diagnosis. This has raised the question, vigorously discussed in the literature in the context of the DSM-5 revision: given that bereavement is an expectable (or understandable) reason for depressed mood, thinking and behaviour which isn't illness, and which therefore may exclude diagnosis of illness, why should other major losses also not mitigate against diagnosis; or, should the major losses not be added, and the bereavement exclusion deleted for consistency, in effect removing the non-expectability issue from the diagnosis of depression. Recent positions and reviews include Kendler (2010) and Maj (2012). Discussions of this issue revolve mainly around the course and outcomes of depression with and without bereavement and other major adverse life events and are not primarily theoretical. Theoretical issues are however in the background, particularly whether expectability/understandability of responses in relation to context excludes attribution of disorder, or whether it is distress/impairment, regardless of context, that are the crucial considerations for diagnosis (Bolton 2008; Horwitz and Wakefield 2007).

normal shyness and Social Anxiety Disorder (Lane 2007), and between the high end of normally distributed activity levels in children especially boys, and ADHD (Timimi and Taylor
2004). Again, the DSM emphasizes distress and impairment as key considerations in making such distinctions.

Not culturally sanctioned. This qualification acknowledges cultural differences, relativizing
the appraisal of patterns of mental life and behavior to cultural norms. That said, there
are very vigorous debates as to whether and to what extent Western psychiatry gives
due weight to cultural differences (e.g., Alarcón 2009; Kleinman 1987; Littlewood
1990).

Not social deviance. Spitzer and Williams (1982, p. 21) explain that the last statement
in the DSM definition of mental disorder "was added to express indignation at
the abuse of psychiatry, as when, in the Soviet Union, political dissidents without
signs of mental illness are labelled as having mental disorders and under that guise
incarcerated in mental hospitals." Related concerns have been expressed recently
regarding use of psychiatry in China (Birley 2002). Aside from political abuse of
psychiatry, the distinction between mental disorder and social deviance invoked
in the DSM-IV conceptualization of mental disorder is not straightforward.
Inside the book there are mental disorders defined apparently in such terms. For
example the primary criterion (A) in the DSM-IV diagnostic criteria for Antisocial
Personality Disorder, (American Psychiatric Association 1994, p.649–650), refers
to a "pervasive pattern of disregard for and violation of the rights of others,"
followed by examples including "failure to conform to social norms with respect
to lawful behaviors." Compulsory admission to hospital of people under the UK
Mental Health Act raises related issues, in authorizing detention under state
powers for public safety, without guilt of crime, in the context of mental disorder.
In an important paper on the political abuse of psychiatry, Richard Bonnie argues
that the key issue is not the definition of mental disorder as opposed to social
deviance, but the political and legal context in which psychiatry services operate
(Bolton 2008; Bonnie 2002).

In general, it is plain enough that the "definition" of mental disorder raises far more and
too complex issues than can be sorted out in the space of an introductory page of the DSM
or any other psychiatric textbook. The DSM cannot be expected to solve these problems,
and in any case its main purpose is something else, to specify reliable and as valid as possible diagnostic criteria for diagnosis. The DSM conceptualization is helpful, however, in my
opinion, as something more like a *position statement*. Key features of which are:

- "Mental disorder" is essentially linked to distress and impairment.
- It is to be distinguished from normal distress (and impairment) [somehow].
- It is not to be muddled up with other cultural/subcultural ways of doing things.
- Being in conflict with society, in the absence of something being wrong with the
  person (on which the first two points), is nothing to do with health care.

In this way the DSM definition is reasonable and very well constructed. As to what mental
illness really is, as to elaborations of the qualifications and conundrums to which the DSM

signals, this is left to others, in the surrounding literatures, in the sciences, professions, and cultures.

WHOSE NORMS ARE THESE?

The DSM conceptualization of mental disorder was constructed in the midst of and in response to much controversy. The background was the so-called anti-psychiatry critiques of the 1960s of Foucault, Laing, Szasz, Rosenhan, Goffman, and others.[6] The critiques of the 1960s laid major charges against mainstream psychiatry and its medical model: that it medicalized and pathologized what were essentially socially and morally defined problems.

Most of the explicit debate about the concept of mental disorder since the 1960s has revolved around the question of whether mental disorder attributions rest on some hard, medical fact or whether they are rather expression of social norms and values (see Sadler, Chapter 45, this volume). Here is the psychiatrist Robert Kendell reviewing the problem in the 1980s:

> The most fundamental issue, and also the most contentious one, is whether disease and illness are normative concepts based on value judgements, or whether they are value-free scientific terms; in other words, whether they are biomedical terms or socio-political ones. (Kendell 1986, p. 25)

Kendell was one of the first theoreticians to note that the current understanding of illness as physical lesion, well grounded in nineteenth-century biomedicine, was hardly plausible in psychiatry and was in fact losing traction, and was being joined by other paradigms, even in physical medicine (Kendell 1975). He was among the first to turn attention in this context to concepts of evolutionary theory (Kendell 1975; Klein 1978). The key idea is that evolutionary theory can deliver—is what is needed to deliver—objective norms of function and dysfunction which will underpin illness diagnosis. "Objective" here means: ascertainable by scientific method and biomedicine specifically. But in particular, it (also) means: *independent of social/sociopolitical norms and values*. The theoretical literature since has struggled with the issue of whether and how the evolutionary theoretic approach really works.

Kendell (1975) considered a simple and verifiable start to the evolutionary theoretic approach, understanding illness in terms of conferring "biological disadvantage," marked by lower life expectancy and fertility for example. He found, however, that the matter of biological disadvantage was less clear-cut than might have been hoped (social disadvantage appearing as a possible confound), and that it did not provide anything like a plausible demarcation criterion between mental health and illness. Since that simple or at least

---

[6] See Foucault (1965, 2006), Goffman (1961), Laing (1960), Rosenhan (1973), and Szasz (1961). Reactive defenses of psychiatry included Clare (1976); Spitzer (1976); Roth and Kroll (1986); and Resnek (1991). The critiques remain essential reading for the project of understanding how and why psychiatry and mental health services generally have been shaped and have shaped themselves over the past half-century—including in the microcosm, as it were, of the conceptualization of mental disorder in the DSM. Recent critiques of psychiatry from social science perspectives include Kutchins and Kirk (1997) and Horwitz (2002).

empirically testable hypothesis did not work well, the evolutionary theoretic approaches have been more *theoretical*. Christopher Boorse proposed defining "normal" functioning in (theoretical) statistical terms, as average for the human species, so that abnormal functioning is a matter of functioning below this species-typical level (e.g., Boorse 1975/1981; and for critical commentary, e.g., Fulford 2001; and Kingma, Chapter 25, this volume). Another approach to normal functioning—proposed in the early 1990s by Jerome Wakefield (1992)—is in terms of functioning "as designed" (as selected for). This has been the most influential version of the evolutionary theoretic approach to defining "mental illness" and will be considered briefly here.[7]

Wakefield's proposal has come to be called the "harmful dysfunction" analysis and it can be stated briefly along the following lines: "A 'mental disorder' is a harmful disruption of a natural function, where 'natural function' is to be understood in terms of functioning in the way 'designed' (selected for) in evolution." According to the first component in the analysis—"harmful"—negative evaluation, by the person with the condition, and/or because of deviance from social norms, is necessary for a condition to be a disorder. Its inclusion in the definition is consistent with the social science perspectives in the 1960s anti-psychiatry critiques. On the other hand, Wakefield emphasizes that his approach puts a definite limitation on what legitimately counts as a mental disorder, namely that it *also* has to involve, as a necessary condition, a failure of a natural function.

There have been many and diverse criticisms of Wakefield's analysis.[8] I will focus here on the question of the norms that are involved in illness attribution, specifically on the fundamental question whether it is valid to distinguish *natural/biological* norms from *social/evaluative* norms, given the context of the new genetic science paradigms of the past decade or so.

Wakefield's analysis is based on the plausible assumption that concepts of function and dysfunction refer to systemic "design": normal functioning is functioning as designed, abnormal functioning is otherwise. In relation to abnormal functioning invoked in illness attribution, Wakefield's plausible view is that we are not concerned with social norms of social functions, but rather—this making the required contrast—with natural norms of natural functions. He then supposes, again plausibly, that the current best science of the "design" of natural functions is evolutionary theory, with "design" in scare quotes since

---

[7] Before leaving evolutionary theoretic approaches in psychiatry generally it should be noted that they are not at all limited to serving as a possible basis for defining (the norms involved in) mental disorder. Also important to note in the context of the broad evolutionary theoretic approach to psychopathology is that it broadens out the range of possible pathways by which people may come to be in serious mental and behavioral trouble, to include not only lesions, or failing evolutionarily "designed" mechanisms, but also e.g., "design"/environment mismatch, and unhelpful learning. Key papers on these implications are Cosmides and Tooby (1999) and Richters and Hinshaw (1999). In addition there is the approach—often known as "evolutionary psychiatry"—which would stress the adaptive value of what we think of as psychopathology, in the present environment or at least in the environment of evolutionary adapativeness (see, e.g., Baron-Cohen 1997; Brune 2008).

[8] Criticisms include that it has a limited or oversimplified approach to evolutionary psychology (Cosmides and Tooby 1999; Richters and Hinshaw 1999), that it implies modularity in mental architecture that may not apply for some mental disorders (Murphy 2006), and that it makes diagnosis of mental disorder a speculative and unreliable hypothesis that is unsuited for both clinical and research purposes (Bolton 2007). Another problem is that the dichotomy between the natural (or "biological") and the social, which is basic both to Wakefield's analysis and to the problem it is designed to solve, is out of date in terms of the current science (Bolton 2008); this line of criticism is summarized in the text.

there is no designer. Putting all these plausible assumptions together—and adding the "harmful" proviso, delivers the "harmful (evolutionary theoretically defined) dysfunction" analysis.

However, recent developments and new paradigms in genetics question the crucial assumption that social functions can be identified as a separate class contrasted with natural functions, understood in this context as what are evolved and genetically transmitted. This dichotomy has broken down in two main ways:

1. Because human evolution has been in social groups, some evolved functions are social, in which case the contrast between the natural and the social breaks down. Examples include courtship, mating, child-rearing, and social collaboration.

2. In the case of psychological and behavioral phenotypes, genes may contribute a predisposition to particular outcomes, depending on subsequent social (and other) environmental factors, from infancy and beyond. The emphasis in current genetics on gene–environment interactions brings out that psychological/behavioral phenotypes are typically not simply evolved functions, on the one hand, or produced by environmental conditions alone, including by social processes, but are typically the product of interaction between the two.[9]

In this context, so far as concerns our mental life and behavior, who or what is responsible for design and function? These are the two familiar options:

1. Our natural constitution—how we are at birth—how we "naturally" are, prior to
2. Socialization processes (education, training, culturalization).

In the 1960s and 1970s these were the only two players on the pitch, conscripted then into the question of mental illness: in illness, what norms have broken down? Social, or natural? Given the forced choice, the answer has to be "natural," or both; and Wakefield is right about this—given the forced choice.

In the 1970s and 1980s evolutionary biopsychology and genetic theory were seen as giving specific content to the first proposition, so we have as influences on psychological and behavioral phenotypes:

1.* Evolutionary natural selection; genetic inheritance; prior to
2. Socialization processes (education, training, culturalization).

But while these two have plausibility as exclusive and exhaustive, and this is relied on in Wakefield's analysis, the plausibility derives only from what went before, prior to the new evolutionary biopsychology and genetics. The *dichotomy* between what is natural, meaning evolved and inherited, and what is social, did not survive, as already indicated. Rather, it has turned out on the one hand that socialization processes are profoundly influenced by genes, and on the other, that for mental and behavioral phenotypes, typically both sets of influence interact with each other to produce the outcome.

---

[9] The literature on gene–environment interactions is extensive and rapidly expanding; reviews include Belsky et al. (2009) and Rutter et al. (2005).

Further, in addition to the breakdown of the dichotomy between what is natural and what is social, to their entanglement, the new genetics has also highlighted a *third* kind of influence responsible for "design and function" of human behavior:

3. Individual choice—signaled by individual differences notwithstanding 1* and 2

In the new genetics, psychology, in this context in its role as study of individual differences, becomes a third factor alongside, or rather interwoven with, our natural makeup, the genes we inherit, and socialization processes. The origin and design of psychological functioning typically include a complex mixture of genetic, evolved factors, and social factors, with individual differences running through them both. Depending on which is dominant, or which is thought to be dominant, we can attribute the origin—the design—of the behavior to human nature, to society, to subculture, to family (to family genes or behavior or both), or to the individual's constitution, character, or personal values.

Given the linkage between functional norms and design, to each kind of the three kinds of design there corresponds a type of norm: evolutionary/genetic, social, and individual—but again with no clear divisions, and interplay between them. It follows then that a mental state or behavioral response can be said to be *dysfunctional*—to deviate from design norms—in one or more of three ways:

1. It fails to operate in the way selected for in evolution.
2. It fails to operate in the way taught and sanctioned by the culture.
3. It fails to work in the way the person intends, according to his needs and values as he sees them.

These three kinds of dysfunction are not clearly separated, and they interact. The first kind belongs to an evolutionary theoretic framework and is relative to conditions in the Environment of Evolutionary Adaptiveness. The second kind of dysfunction is the one accessible to social theory; it is immersed in the present, in more or less diverse social realities. There is however a third reading of dysfunctional psychic life, the one at the individual level involving deviation from personal norms and values, evident to the person involved. This meaning has been neglected, to do with the fact that "madness" was silenced—though it is apparent in discourse led by service users. These are not, however, three meanings of psychological function and dysfunction—the evolutionary, the social, and the individual—they are rather three interwoven themes which run through all kinds of cases.

So where does this leave Wakefield's approach to the analysis of mental disorder? It has survived notwithstanding the burdens of many shortcomings and this may be due not so much to its fitness but to having no distinguished competitors in this particular environment. On the other hand its insistence on the key idea that the concept of illness is distinct from the concept of social deviance is correct. We have a term—in fact many terms—for what we believe is (just) failure to keep to social norms: naughty, lazy, rude, bad, criminal, etc. (and terms with neutral or positive evaluations: free thinking, original, eccentric, innovative—etc.). However, if the argument proposed earlier is correct, we cannot make out this difference between mental/behavioral disorder and social deviance by positing, on the one hand, a class of mental/behavioral functions that are entirely "natural"/evolved, as opposed to, on the other hand, a class that is entirely "social"—with failure of one of the former class then being a "natural" dysfunction rather than a "social" dysfunction. According to current paradigms in genetics, the former class—of psychological functions that are entirely natural/evolved without social environmental influence—is probably empty; the main point being that the natural/social dichotomy is no longer valid.

So to preserve something of what is correct in Wakefield's analysis we might say something like: mental disorder typically involves either or both failure to comply with socially or personally identified norms (hence, by the way, there is no need then to add "harmful" except to emphasize severity)—but either or both of those is not enough: there also has to be a breakdown in a "natural function." "Natural function" would presumably have to be understood here as a psychological function which is common to human beings, the population variance in which is attributable to a high genetic component. However, making distinctions here is difficult since probably all psychological functions have some genetic heritability component, and how high is high? And on the other hand, probably all psychological functions are operational in personal and social activities. In brief all our activities involve the natural/genetic as well as the personal and social, so again there is no clear way here of distinguishing a subclass of psychological functions that do, as opposed to a class of functions that do not, involve the natural/genetic as well as the personal and the social. The latter class—psychological functions with no natural/genetic component—is again probably empty, and it is in any case unclear how anything like a demarcation criterion could be made out in these terms. Further, since psychological functions cannot be identified independent of the activities in which they operate, it is unclear what their "breakdown" would amount to other than breakdown in those personal and social activities, pointing again to the fundamental importance of personal and social phenomenology in the attribution of illness or disorder. Let us consider these implications further, with reference again to the core feature of the conceptualization of mental disorder in the DSM.

Unmanageable Distress and Impairment

We have terms for what we believe is (just) failure to keep to social norms: naughty, lazy, rude, bad, criminal, etc. (and with neutral or positive evaluations: eccentric, innovative—etc.). We also have terms for a person failing to keep up with his own standards, such as—and these are all negative—lazy, weak-willed, insincere and hypocritical. Crucially, all these negative terms circle around the discourse of illness; illness discourse, the discourse of the clinic, is the *alternative* we acknowledge. In brief, illness attribution protects from condemnation. At least, all being well; otherwise, in a less positive outcome, the person suffers double trouble: the condemnation plus the illness. This refers to the discrimination faced by people with a diagnosis of mental illness (Hinshaw and Cicchetti 2000; Thornicroft 2006).

All being well, illness attribution protects from condemnation. The idea is that the persons cannot do what they are supposed to be doing, according to social expectations or their own standards—not because they are naughty, lazy, rude, bad, weak-willed, or insincere—*but because they are ill*. And the underlying principle is: illness involves incapacity—the person just cannot help not doing what they are not doing, or help doing what they are doing.

This insight into the logic of illness attribution is explicit though not elaborated in the conceptualizations of mental disorder in the DSM and ICD, in the references to distress and disability or impairment. I considered earlier the question then arising about the difference between illness distress and normal distress. It is possible to make out this difference by adding the qualification "unmanageable" or "disabling." We are all often distressed, upset, and anxious, with variations according to life circumstances, with different frequencies and degrees—but to the extent that a person can manage, with their own resources or social supports, then that person does not typically seek professional help. Conversely, people are more likely to go to the clinic to the extent that they cannot manage. Unmanageability means that the distressing anxiety or mood state is too intense or too frequent to allow the person to get along satisfactorily with their lives as they usually do or want to lead them; in brief, it blurs into impairment. Emphasis is put here on unmanageable, disabling distress rather than what is expectable or not, or normal or not. So, it may be normal and expectable for a person to be unable to sleep much when they have high levels of worry and low mood levels while going through one or more life stresses or losses, at work or in personal relationships or both, but to the extent that the person is finding their mental state unmanageable and disabling, a visit to the clinic and healthcare may be warranted. Obviously many therapeutic approaches could be considered, including pharmacotherapy and brief psychotherapy, or simply rest, or a change of job; or, especially important to note explicitly, just keep a health care eye on things, "watchful waiting" as it is sometimes called, because the problem may well be self-limiting.

The possibility that illness in general and mental illness in particular may be explicated in terms of the person not being able to help doing or not doing as they are—in terms of "incapacity" in this sense—has been relatively neglected in the theoretical literature, perhaps due to the relatively high amounts of attention paid in the sociological literature to the social influences and power plays at work in diagnosis, on the one hand, and, on the other, to claims and counterclaims about the "natural dysfunction" that illness attributions allegedly track. It is possible, in some contrast with both these approaches, that illness attributions actually track our intuition that people sometimes cannot help what they are doing, or not doing, that they are sometimes not in control of their own actions. However, what this amounts to may be different for different conditions, as has recently begun to be explored in the literature.[10]

There is no objective hard and fast diagnostic threshold available here. What counts as intolerable distress, and what counts as serious impairment, what counts as disability (as being unable to do) all depend not only on individual psychological differences and individual life-circumstances but those in interaction with cultural expectations—all of these general headings themselves covering much diversity, and admitting opinions from many points of view.

BIOMARKERS: CAUSES AND BOUNDARIES

Can we expect science to deliver some clarity here? Are there objective factors which would tell us what are illnesses and what are not?

---

[10] For example, Bolton and Banner (2012), Kennett and Matthews (2003), and Pearce and Pickard (2011).

There is currently an extensive research effort in physical medicine to identify internal markers of disease processes reliably, to plan appropriate management, and early, to optimize prognosis under treatment, with progress in many areas. Similar benefits could accrue in psychological medicine, in psychiatry, if biomarkers could be identified. In addition, there would be the promise of clearer distinctions between mental illness and non-illness conditions, of tightening up the difference and distinction between, e.g., depressive illness and normal life distress, or normally distributed populations traits and ADHD, or Autistic Spectrum Disorder. There would be a proper laboratory test to bring clarity to what are otherwise vague and contested areas. So far, however, it would be fair to say that no well replicated, reasonably sensitive and specific biomarkers have been identified for any mental illnesses.[11] But is this just a matter of time? Can we look forward to having, one day, a clear scientific grasp of what mental illness is?

Important background here is the stunning success of biomedicine between approximately the mid-nineteenth and mid-twentieth centuries. For some conditions it constructed the notions of signs and symptoms, and of syndromes, taking into account course over time; then in key breakthroughs it identified processes at the cellular level that causally explained those complex, variable surface features. Further, with the development of penicillin, treatment was developed too. In addition, the understanding of causes and processes of transmitted diseases enabled prevention through public health interventions. Game, set and match to nineteenth/twentieth-century biomedicine and its disease theory. The nineteenth/twentieth-century biomedical disease paradigm was taken into the new psychiatry at the turn of the century—along with, it should be added for completeness, quite distinctive paradigms from neurology and psychology. As is well-known the biomedical paradigm had a stunning success early on with syphilis: it all worked in the new psychiatry too. Very diverse signs and symptoms at and over time were unified into a syndrome caused by a kind of bacterium, a spirochete, invading the central nervous system, and which was treatable by penicillin. This early achievement of the biomedical model applied to psychiatry has not been repeated since, and there are, as is well known, ample reasons from research in the past half-century—as alluded to earlier—to cast doubt on whether it will ever be repeated, and indeed reason to believe that it will not be. As Kendler put it in a recent paper on the philosophical framework for psychiatry: no more spirochete-like discoveries, but rather multiple causes at multiple levels (Kendler 2005).

Research in psychiatry in the past few decades has revealed much about causes of/risks for psychiatric conditions, including: genetic risks, typically involving multiple (perhaps hundreds) of genes adding relatively small risk; prenatal placental nutrient and hormonal environment affecting fetal programming; birth complications; early maternal and child rearing practices including neglect and abuse; life-stressors; maladaptive cognitive styles; social determinants such as social exclusion, poverty, and wealth inequality; and so on and on; and all interacting, and all, presumably, affecting brain development and functioning in some way.

---

[11] A publisher's announcement for a recent major edited volume on biomarkers in psychiatry states: "Biological markers, as physiological indicators of disease, hold immense promise for diagnostics and clinical drug trials. While for other complex disorders like diabetes and heart disease a limited number of markers are at hand, there are currently no biomarkers available for psychiatric disorders." (Springer 2009). The science is rapidly expanding and is to be found usually under specific conditions.

In this context the possibility arises that the complex array of biopsychosocial causes may reduce to a single final common biological pathway, underlying the thought referred to at the end of the previous paragraph, that all the distant (early) biopsychosocial causes and the current psychosocial causes must somehow be implemented in the brain. This line of thought is a complex combination of philosophy of mind, especially mind–brain identity theory, and the philosophy of explanation, especially the assumption that causes must be proximate to their effects, and an empirical theory of illness, especially the theory of illness as disease. The philosophy is plausible enough but the thinking that derives from the disease model in particular needs closer examination. One point is that it is an empirical matter, not an a priori one, whether or not there is a final common pathway leading from multiple pathways to a single clinical syndrome, especially when, as is often observed, the clinical spectrum, a biomarker may be just an (other) sign of the illness, *internal* (inside the skin) as opposed to external, but as yet hardly worth distinguishing from the *external* signs and symptoms of the illness, from the point of view of the etiological model, which, we may suppose, stays as highly complex and multifactorial as before. Or, at the other end of the spectrum, the biomarker may be something like a spirochete, in which case it has, let us suppose, a relatively simple mode of appearance in the body, in principle perhaps preventable, and a reliable response to treatment. But, as noted earlier, it looks implausible now to continue supposing that there are spirochete-like discoveries still on offer in psychiatry—and in this case biomarkers, even if we find them, won't much change the current paradigms of complexity of etiology and features of the conditions that interest us.

But if biomarkers were found in psychiatric conditions, would this solve the boundary problems? Well they probably would if they were as precise, as specific, as the linkage between the bacterium *Treponema pallidum* and syphilis: identification of the bacterium fixes the diagnosis. Otherwise, the biomarker will associated, correlated with the condition in some degree, and its presence or absence will not necessarily fix the boundaries of mental illness, but would rather be another factor to be taken into account in the context of the personal and social phenomenology of the conditions that we describe as mental health problems.

REFERENCES

Alarcón, R. D. (2009). Culture, cultural factors and psychiatric diagnosis: Review and projections. *World Psychiatry*, 8, 131–9.

American Psychiatric Association (1968). *Diagnostic and Statistical Manual of Mental Disorders, Second Edition*. Washington, DC: American Psychiatric Association.

American Psychiatric Association (1980). *Diagnostic and Statistical Manual of Mental Disorders, Third Edition*. Washington, DC: American Psychiatric Association.

American Psychiatric Association (1994). *Diagnostic and Statistical Manual of Mental Disorders, Fourth Edition*. Washington, DC: American Psychiatric Association.

Baron-Cohen, S. (Ed.) (1997). *The Maladapted Mind. Classic Readings in Evolutionary Psychopathology*. Hove: Psychology Press.

Belsky, J., Jonassaint, C., and Pluess, M., Stanton, M., Brummett, B., and Williams, R. (2009). Vulnerability genes or plasticity genes? *Molecular Psychiatry*, 14, 746–54.

Berrios, G. (1989). What is phenomenology? A review. *Journal of the Royal Society of Medicine*, 82, 425–8.

Birley, J. (2002). Political abuse of psychiatry in the Soviet Union and in China: A rough guide for bystanders. *The Journal of the American Academy of Psychiatry and the Law*, 30, 145–7.

Bolton, D. (2007). The usefulness of Wakefield's definition for the diagnostic manuals. *World Psychiatry*, 6, 164–5.

Bolton, D. (2008). *What is Mental Disorder? An Essay in Philosophy, Science and Values*. Oxford: Oxford University Press

Bolton, D. and Banner, N. (2012). Does mental disorder involve loss of personal autonomy? In L. Radoilska (Ed.), *Autonomy & Mental Health*, pp. 77–99. Oxford: Oxford University Press.

Bonnie, R. J. (2002). Political abuse of psychiatry in the Soviet Union and in China: Complexities and controversies. *The Journal of the American Academy of Psychiatry and the Law*, 30, 136–44.

Boorse, C. (1975). On the distinction between disease and illness. *Philosophy and Public Affairs*, 5, 49–68. (Reprinted in M. Cohen, T. Nagel, and T. Scanlon (Eds), *Medicine and Moral Philosophy*, pp. 3–22. Princeton, NJ: Princeton University Press.)

Brune, M. (2008). *Textbook of Evolutionary Psychiatry: The Origins of Psychopathology*. Oxford: Oxford University Press.

Campbell, P. (1999). The service user/survivor movement. In C. Newnes, G. Holmes, and C. Dunn (Eds), *This is Madness: A Critical Look at Psychiatry and the Future of Mental Health Services*, pp. 195–209. Ross on Wye: PCCS Books.

Campion, E. (2012). *Through the Unknowable: Family Life with Mental Illness, Alcohol, Loss, and Love*. New York, NY: Vantage Press.

Clare, A. (1976). *Psychiatry in Dissent. Controversial Issues in Thought and Practice*. Tavistock: London.

Cosmides, L. and Tooby, J. (1999). Toward an evolutionary taxonomy of treatable conditions. *Journal of Abnormal Psychology*, 108, 453–64.

Foucault, M. (1965). *Madness and Civilisation: A History of Insanity in the Age of Reason* (R. Howard, Trans.). London: Tavistock.

Foucault, M. (2006). *History of Madness* (J. Murphy and J. Khalfa, Trans.). London: Routledge.

Fulford, K. W. M. (2001). 'What is (mental) disease?' An open letter to Christopher Boorse. *Journal of Medical Ethics*, 27, 80–5.

Goffman, E. (1961). *Asylums. Essays on the Social Situation of Mental Patients and Other Inmates*. Harmondsworth: Penguin.

Hinshaw, S. and Cicchetti, D. (2000). Stigma and mental disorder: Conceptions of illness, public attitudes, personal disclosure, and social policy. *Development and Psychopathology*, 12, 555–98.

Horwitz, A. V. (2002). *Creating Mental Illness*. Chicago, IL: University of Chicago Press.

Horwitz, A. V. and Wakefield, J. C. (2007). *The Loss of Sadness: How Psychiatry Transformed Normal Sorrow into Depressive Disorder*. New York, NY: Oxford University Press.

Kendell, R. (1986). What are mental disorders? In A. M. Freedman, R. Brotman, and I. Silverman, and D. Hutson (Eds), *Issues in Psychiatric Classification: Science, Practice, and Social Policy*, pp. 23–45. New York, NY: Human Sciences Press.

Kendell, R. E. (1975). The concept of disease and its implications for psychiatry. *British Journal of Psychiatry*, 127, 305–15.

Kendler, K. (2005). Toward a philosophical structure for psychiatry. *American Journal of Psychiatry*, 162, 433–40.

Kendler, K. S. (2010). *A statement from Kenneth S. Kendler, M.D., on the proposal to eliminate the grief exclusion criterion from major depression, by Kenneth S. Kendler, M.D., Member, DSM-5 Mood Disorder Work Group.* Available at: <http://www.dsm5.org/Pages/Default.aspx> (accessed November 4, 2011).

Kendler, K. S. and Parnas, P. (Eds) (2008). *Philosophical Issues in Psychiatry: Explanation, Phenomenology, and Nosology.* Baltimore, MD: Johns Hopkins University Press.

Kennett, J. and Matthews, S. (2003). The unity and disunity of agency. *Philosophy, Psychiatry and Psychology, 10,* 305–12.

Klein, D. F. (1978). A proposed definition of mental illness. In R. L. Spitzer and D.F. Klein (Eds), *Critical Issues in Psychiatric Diagnosis,* pp. 41–71. New York, NY: Raven Press.

Kleinman, A. M. (1987). Anthropology and psychiatry: The role of culture in cross-cultural research on illness. *British Journal of Psychiatry, 151,* 447–54.

Kutchins, H. and Kirk, S. A. (1997). *Making Us Crazy. DSM—The Psychiatric Bible and the Creation of Mental Disorders.* New York, NY: Free Press.

Laing, R. D. (1960). *The Divided Self.* Harmondsworth: Penguin.

Lane, C. (2007). *Shyness: How Normal Behavior Became a Sickness.* Boston, MA: Yale University Press.

Littlewood, R. (1990). From categories to context: A decade of the new 'cross-cultural psychiatry'. *British Journal of Psychiatry, 156,* 308–27.

Maj, M. (2012). Editorial: Bereavement-related depression in the DSM-5 and ICD-11, *World Psychiatry, 11,* 1–2.

Mental Health Foundation (1999). *The Courage to Bare Our Souls.* London: Mental Health Foundation.

Murphy, D. (2006). *Psychiatry in the Scientific Image.* Cambridge, MA: MIT Press.

Pearce, S. and Pickard, H. (2010). Finding the will to recover: Philosophical perspectives on agency and the sick role, *Journal of Medical Ethics, 36,* 831–3

Ratcliffe, M. (2008). *Feelings of Being: Phenomenology, Psychiatry and the Sense of Reality.* Oxford: Oxford University Press.

Read, J. and Reynolds, J. (Eds) (1996). *Speaking Our Minds: An Anthology.* London: Macmillan, Open University Press.

Richters, J. E. and Hinshaw, S. P. (1999). The abduction of disorder in psychiatry. *Journal of Abnormal Psychology, 108,* 438–45.

Rosenhan, R. (1973). On being sane in insane places. *Science, 179,* 251–8.

Roth, M. and Kroll, J. (1986). *The Reality of Mental Illness.* Cambridge: Cambridge University Press.

Rutter, M., Moffit, T. E., and Caspi, A. (2005). Gene-environment interplay and psychopathology: multiple varieties but real effects. *Journal of Child Psychiatry and Psychology, 47,* 226–61.

Spitzer, R. L. (1976). On pseudoscience in science, logic in remission, and psychiatric diagnosis: A critique of Rosenhan's 'On being sane in insane places'. *Journal of Abnormal Psychology, 84,* 442–52.

Spitzer, R. L. and Endicott, I. (1978). Medical and mental disorder: Proposed definition and criteria. In R. L. Spitzer and D. F. Klein (Eds), *Critical Issues in Psychiatric Diagnosis,* pp. 15–40. New York, NY: Raven Press.

Spitzer, R. L. and Williams, J. B. (1982). The definition and diagnosis of mental disorder. In W. R. Grove (Ed.), *Deviance and Mental Illness,* pp. 15–31. Beverly Hills, CA: Sage.

Spitzer, R. L. and Williams, J. B. (1988). Basic principles in the development of DSM-III. In J. E. Mezzich and M. von Cranach (Eds), *International Classification in Psychiatry: Unity and Diversity,* pp. 81–6. Cambridge: Cambridge University Press.

Springer Publishing (2009). Publisher's announcement for *Biomarkers for Psychiatric Disorders* (C. Turck, Ed.). Available at: <http://www.springer.com/biomed/neuroscience/book/978-0-387-79250-7> (accessed August 10, 2012).

Stanghellini, G. (2004). *Disembodied Spirits and Deanimated Bodies*. Oxford: Oxford University Press.

Stein, D. J., Phillips, K. A., and Bolton, D., Fulford, K. W., Sadler, J. Z., and Kendler, K. S. (2010). What is a mental/psychiatric disorder? From DSM-IV to DSM-V. *Psychological Medicine*, *40*, 1–7.

Szasz, T. (1961). *The Myth of Mental Illness: Foundations of a Theory of Personal Conduct*. New York, NY: Harper & Row.

Thornicroft, G. (2006). *Shunned: Discrimination Against People with Mental Illness*. Oxford: Oxford University Press.

Timimi, S. and Taylor, E. (2004). In debate: ADHD is best understood as a cultural construct. *British Journal of Psychiatry*, *18*, 8–9.

Wakefield, J. C. (1992). The concept of mental disorder: on the boundary between biological facts and social values. *American Psychologist*, *47*, 373–88.

World Health Organization (1992). *The ICD-10 Classification of Mental and Behavioural Disorders: Clinical Descriptions and Diagnostic Guidelines*. Geneva: World Health Organization, Division of Mental Health.

CHAPTER 29

....

VICE AND MENTAL
DISORDERS

....

JOHN Z. SADLER

Like the philosophical consideration of values in psychiatric diagnosis (Sadler, Chapter 45, this volume) the philosophical consideration of "vice" and mental disorders opens up a vast realm of philosophical problems which converge upon compelling social problems involving crime, mental illness, and ordinary immorality and wrongdoing. These questions range from defining issues in legal and political philosophy, such as "What is crime?" and "Is criminal punishment justified?" to the puzzling twists and turns of concepts pertinent to the philosophy of psychiatry: from "Do humans have free will, and what significance does it have for mental disorders?" to "Should the concept of mental disorder include criminal and immoral thought and conduct?"

This chapter cannot discuss such a philosophical range. Instead, it presents a conceptual roadmap for a few of the philosophical questions posed by the interactions of vice and mental disorders. The first section considers a definition of "vice" suitable for the philosophy of psychiatry. The second section explores this vice concept in the context of the ongoing discussion of the concept of mental disorder (see also Bolton, Chapter 28, this volume). The third section presents a very attenuated summary of the historical relationships between vice and madness/mental disorder. This section serves as a historical background for the main section of the chapter, which addresses seven key issues in the vice–mental disorder relationship (VMDR). The seven key issues involve: (1) the confounding of vice and mental disorder, (2) questions about psychopathology of morality, (3) the meaning of "medical morality" for psychiatry, (4) regulating deviance and the role of the state, (5) forensic and correctional psychiatry, (6) moral and criminal responsibility, and (7) irrationality and evil. As will be shown through the discussions, these problem areas are richly interrelated, both from the perspective of philosophy as an intrinsically worthwhile intellectual activity and the perspective of philosophy as a tool in addressing clinical and social policy problems. As one of the most fascinating and neglected areas in the philosophy of psychiatry, a goal for this chapter is to stimulate scholars to work in this field.

A Concept of Vice for the Philosophy
of Psychiatry

In ordinary discourse today, "vice" typically describes immoral or self-damaging habits such as cigarette smoking, frequent inebriation, or womanizing, as well as specific categories of criminal offenses pursued by police "vice squads": prostitution, gambling, or the selling of illegal drugs. In the history of philosophy and literature, however, vice and vices typically reflected broader concerns: counterpoints or antonyms of culturally favored virtues of the time (Thomson 1993). For Homeric Greeks the lionizing of courage contrasted with the vice of cowardice. For Plato, vices included the failure of practicing classical virtues: courage, justice, moderation, and wisdom—as well as the failure of other virtues elaborated by Aristotle (MacIntyre 1998; Sidgwick 1888). Plato's influential account of wrongdoing—that only illness, ignorance, or compulsion by another could cause a person to choose wrongly—persists in philosophical discussions of *akrasia* or weakness of will today. Platonic notions of wrongdoing reflect a rationalistic psychology that befuddles and provokes contemporary psychiatrists, steeped as the latter are in Freudian dynamic conflicts, operant conditioning (behaviorism), as well as naturalistic neural networks and neuroanatomical hierarchies of function and neuroregulation. The differentiation of monotheistic Mediterranean religions (Judaism, Islam, Christianity) in the early Roman through the medieval era led to a parallel rethinking of vice (MacIntyre 1998; Sidgwick 1888). Vice was transformed into a spiritual failing of human nature—sin—which was universal and perennial; metaphysically etched into human nature by Augustine's elaboration of original sin. Through the conceptual transitions of the Reformation, Renaissance, and Enlightenment, vice made a pluralistic transition from its relationship to sin, expanding into naturalistic and social-science formulations as disease: vice as mental illness, vice as a consequence of social failures and social constructions, and vice as the consequence of bad policy and government.

So the philosophy-of-psychiatry challenge to contemporary concepts of vice is significant. A vice concept should reflect, with maximum metaphysical neutrality, an idea which practicing psychiatrists would recognize intuitively, which would fit into the intellectual history of vice, which would implicitly recognize and permit social and cultural variation of particular examples, and which could be analyzable as a conceptual component of other psychiatric ideas. So redefining vice in a technical sense—as simply criminal and/or immoral thought or conduct, seems a reasonable response to these demands (Sadler 2008). The concepts of "crime" and "immorality" are recognized by philosophers and psychiatrists as being (at least) primarily the products of culture (Duff 2008; Sadler 2005). The broad concept of vice as criminal and immoral thought/conduct fits easily into a semantic analysis of other psychiatric concepts and (specifically) categories of mental disorder (Sadler 2008). While this notion of "vice" is likely broader than Classical and Medieval ideas (permitting as it does broader cultural notions of moral wrong) while at the same time adding more contemporary dimensions through adding the concept of criminality, this technical notion of vice can perform for much of the intellectual work to follow.

VICE AND THE CONCEPT OF MENTAL DISORDER

The concept of mental disorder has posed perhaps the premier interest of contemporary philosophy of psychiatry, if such interest would be measured by the duration of ongoing scholarship in the area, the numbers of pertinent publications, and evidence for the joint interest of philosophers and psychiatrists in this area. For these reasons, as well as the fine contribution by Professor Bolton in Chapter 28 (this volume), I will not review this literature and instead highlight a few of the common themes pertinent to the consideration of vice and mental disorders.

The literature on concepts/definitions of mental disorders converges upon several themes, four of which are particularly pertinent here: (1) mental disorders involve a recognizable pattern of problematic experience and behavior (symptoms), (2) such a pattern represents a failure in normative functioning of the (3) individual, and (4) not just any normative failure, but only certain kinds of normative failure contribute to calling such failure a "mental disorder" (see, e.g., American Psychiatric Association (APA) 2000; Bolton 2008; Fulford 1989, 1999; <http://www.dsm5.org/proposedrevision/Pages/proposedrevision. aspx?rid=465#>; Wakefield 1992; Sadler and Agich 1995; Stein et al. 2010). Let us consider each of these in turn.

1. Mental disorders are a recognizable pattern of experience and behavior. The core ideas here are that a mental disorder is not an idiosyncrasy of the moment, but an ongoing feature of the affected person over time—a pattern of experience and/or conduct. In the case of the *Diagnostic and Statistical Manual of Mental Disorders* (DSM) and *International Classification of Diseases* (ICD) diagnostic criteria, the time frames are usually specified. These time frames may include a minimum time for symptoms to persist, or describe fluctuations in symptoms (e.g., "episodes" of illness) and specify how long the symptoms may persist.

2. Mental disorders involve a failure of normative functioning. I have selected this phrase to be agnostic about which account and key terminology to "endorse" for my purposes here. A large portion of the debate around the definition/concept of mental disorder involves disputes about the metaphysical kinds and locations of these failures of normative functioning. For example, Wakefield situates the failure of normative functioning in two core concepts: "harm" and "dysfunction." For Wakefield, mental disorders require harmful dysfunctions. The former (harm) is embedded in social contexts and involves social value judgments, while the latter (dysfunction) depicts failures of a person's evolved biological mechanisms as determined by evolutionary biology/psychology (Wakefield 1992). For Wakefield, the value-ladenness of psychiatric diagnosis resides in the "harm" component, while dysfunctions reflect value-free failures of natural functions. In contrast, Sadler and Agich (1995; Sadler 1999) contend that the metaphysical background assumptions within evolutionary biology/psychology's explanations of psychopathology have their own presuppositions about what is adaptive and desirable for human organisms. From this standpoint, even an

evolutionary science-defined concept of dysfunction has deeply assumed value preferences buried within concepts like "adaptation." (See also in this volume Sadler, Chapter 45, on "Values and Psychiatric Diagnosis and Classification," as well as Bolton, Chapter 28 on the concept of mental disorder.) In any case, these failures of normative functioning should possess some negative evaluation; mental disorder concepts are fundamentally value-laden and action-guiding: people generally don't want to have a mental disorder.

3. A third key feature of the concept of mental disorder is that the prevailing ontology of mental disorder concepts makes assumptions about the ontological "space" of the mind, which appears, for instance, in the recent DSM definitions of mental disorder as disorders occurring "in an individual" (APA 2000; see also Stein et al. 2010). Mental disorders under this rubric are causally driven from within persons, the disturbances and features are manifestations of structural or functional impairments of the brain/mind, and the social–environmental context contributes to the unique individual expression of a mental disorder in a particular person. Sadler calls these kinds of assumptions "disease naturalism" in that mental disorders are extrapolated or analogized to naturalistic physical diseases (see Sadler 2005, Chapter 45, this volume). Similarly, what mental disorders are *not*, in this account, are functional failures in reciprocal interpersonal functioning (as described by family systems approaches; Kaslow 1993, 1996) nor are they normative expressions of (or reactions to) social–political disturbances like poverty, slavery, or political mayhem (see Rothblum et al. 1986). The conventional individualistic ontological account of psychopathology becomes crucially important below when contemporary accounts of mental disorder stipulate certain kinds of failures of function.

4. Failures of function typically conform, rightly or wrongly, to our cultural intuitions and conventions about what a mental disorder is. If I am an inept cook, a bank robber, or illiterate because of no education, none of these conditions alone, regardless of any patterns of failures of normative function they imply, qualify me for a mental disorder. Since DSM-III, the DSMs have included a definition of mental disorder that stipulates that: (a) culturally sanctioned "abnormal" behavior does not qualify as a mental disorder (Stein et al. (2010) give tribal trance states as an example) and (b) mental disorders are not conditions due to "a conflict between the individual and society."

This latter stipulation generates a problem directly related to the vice–mental disorder relationship (VMDR): psychiatry already classifies a number of conditions that could be construed as primarily a conflict between the individual and society. These include disorders which are "vice-laden" (Sadler 2005, 2008, in press), DSM conditions such as Antisocial Personality Disorder, Conduct Disorder, Intermittent Explosive Disorder, Paraphilias that involve a victim (e.g., Pedophilia), to name a few examples (Sadler 2005, 2008). Chapter 45 describes some of the debate around Pedophilic Disorders and the normative judgments involved with this group of conditions.

Madness and Vice in Historical
Perspective

The tight relationship implied by this chapter about vice and mental illness has not been suitably explored by historians—few to no studies explore these relationships. Studies of "madness" (pre-Enlightenment mental illness) and vice as parallel historical developments provide valuable perspective in understanding the contemporary cultural tropes, idioms of distress, and iconography of social deviance that contribute to not just professional presuppositions and concepts, but also the diverse public/lay perspectives on the VMDR. Similarly, the study of the history of psychiatry along with the history of morality in the post-Enlightenment era sheds important light upon the ideological frameworks involving the VMDR as well as the interplay of sociopolitical structures that regulate social deviance. Unfortunately, no single resource exists that undertakes such an ambitious set of parallel histories, though one is in the works (Sadler, in press). For the purposes of this chapter, I will provide some very brief notes and references that sketch some of the most important historical contexts.

Referring to the social expression of the frailties of the human condition as "social deviance" provides a relatively neutral starting point for observing the differentiation of said deviance over history. (In this setting, "deviance" and "deviant" are used, however regrettably, to also signal the persistent theme of stigma for people so labeled.) Humankind has struggled over how to parse social deviance since prehistory, mingling religious and supernatural accounts, and later, early medical (e.g., Hippocratic) accounts (Porter 1988, 1998, 2002, 2004; Thomson 1993). Ancient views of madness described it as demon-possession, and from a moral perspective, often as a consequence of, or punishment for, wrongdoing (Porter 1988, 2002). In the early centuries of the monotheistic religions (Judaism, Christianity, Islam) madness was described both as a punishment for wrongdoing and possession by evil demonic entities (Mora 2008a; Scurlock and Anderson 2005). Not until the Enlightenment did rational-scientific viewpoints gain credence, but then and now, magico-religious accounts of mental disorder prevail in many cultures and even Western subcultures. In the early medieval Roman Catholic era, many of the vices identified by the Greek philosophers came to be formulated as sins. The cardinal ("seven deadly") sins included gluttony, lust, greed, wrath, sloth, pride, and envy. These iconic moral wrongs have persisted as Western cultural tropes for centuries into the present day (Newhauser 2007; Sadler in press). Indeed, the values reflected in these seven deadly sins are encoded into current DSM-IV and proposed DSM-5 mental disorder categories: Binge-Eating Disorder for gluttony; Hypersexual Disorder for lust; the "miserly spending style" of DSM-IV-TR Obsessive-Compulsive Personality Disorder for greed; various anger-related criteria in DSM Personality Disorders and Intermittent Explosive Disorder for wrath; Narcissistic Personality Disorder for pride and envy; to name a few (see Sadler, in press, for a detailed account).

In addition to these metaphysical frameworks for wrongdoing and madness, considerations of moral and criminal responsibility were equally early in history. The circa 1700 BCE Babylonian Code of Hammurabi explicitly addressed situations that invoke contemporary concerns about criminal intent and responsibility: "If during a quarrel one man strikes another and wounds him, then he shall swear 'I did not injure him wittingly', and pay the physicians" (Code of Hammurabi, <http://avalon.law.yale.edu/subject_menus/hammenu.asp>).

Regarding both morality and madness, Western history can be described as exhibiting a normative pluralism—prevailing attitudes, social mores, and tolerance for deviance have shifted around over the two millennia of recorded history. Bronze Age Egyptian artifacts indicate early versions of weapons and war, both of which have occupied humankind, with varying severity, ever since. Oliver Thomson's *The History of Sin* (1993) describes a wide cultural and temporal fluctuation of moral and religious accommodations for violence, slavery, sexual diversity, and respect for women, even among and within religious orthodoxies like Roman Catholicism and Islam. Indeed, these four areas of sociomoral substance appear to be among the most variable in the normative pluralism of the Western world, from both the moral and "madness" perspectives (Sadler, in press).

The Renaissance, Reformation, and Enlightenment served to differentiate the metaphysical frameworks of morality and madness, leading to parallel ontological universes: on the one hand, religious accounts of morality and madness; on the other, medical/scientific accounts of morality and mental illness. The secularization of the Western world, however, was initiated by wealthy intellectuals and aristocrats using the new printing-press technology. The secularist, naturalistic viewpoint of (particularly) mental illness was an elitist one in the late medieval and early modern periods (Mora 2008b). Ordinary people, by and large, varied in their viewpoints, and magico-religious accounts of morality and madness persisted into the discovery of the New World and beyond, into the present day (Sadler, in press).

The modern era, characterized by the fading of Church influence, industrialization, urbanization, educational and childrearing shifts from family to schools, stimulated both humanistic and stigmatizing responses to social deviance. Once a tolerated if begrudged part of every community, social deviants of various kinds began to be perceived as threats to safety, property, and morality (Rafter 1997, 2000; Rothman 2000). This shift from tolerance and familiarity to fear and loathing provoked new social responses, the differentiation of proto-professional and lay language for deviance conditions, and novel social institutions and professions. The poor became widows, orphans, and vagabonds, provoking the development of almshouses, workhouses, and jails. Sinners differentiated into criminals, drunkards, and ordinary sinners; the former subject to the stocks, the gallows, and the newly invented jails. Simpletons and fools became idiots, imbeciles, and wayward women, requiring new techniques of education and schooling, moral monitoring, and even confinement and sterilization (Rafter 1997). The mad became lunatics, hysterics, and maniacs, and the new asylum doctors became "alienists" and later "psychiatrists" to run the new institutions and social systems that cared for a new kind of patient (Grob 1983; Porter 1988, 2002; Rothman 2002a, 2002b).

The late modern era leading to the birth of psychiatry also led to the formulation of classical vice-laden diagnostic categories—the genealogies and conceptual histories for each of these, while important, are beyond the scope of this chapter. From "homicidal insanity" came psychopathy, Antisocial Personality Disorder, and Intermittent Explosive Disorder (Colaizzi 1985; Sadler, in press). From juvenile delinquency came Conduct Disorder,

Oppositional Defiant Disorder, and (to a lesser extent) Attention Deficit Hyperactivity Disorder (Costello and Angold 2001). From "abomination," "pederasty," and "perversion" came various Paraphilias, Gender Identity Disorder, and Homosexuality (the latter being first in, then out, as a twentieth-century mental disorder) (Garton 2004; Laqueur 1990; Sadler 2005, in press).

The development of differentiated institutions, care systems, schools, and professionals to deal with social deviance was typically, and regrettably, associated with the lack of a unitary social/political vision. The new institutions and systems developed in large part independent of each other, even as many deviants had cross-identities—widows could be mad or criminal; the intellectually impaired could be poor and orphaned. The asylum system grew into the mental health system, the criminal courts and jails grew into the criminal justice system, the juvenile justice system, prisons; and new "status" dispositions appeared, like probation and parole. Schools for idiocy grew into custodial and educational institutions for the mentally retarded. Juvenile courts developed juvenile detention and "reform schools" for youthful offenders. While Western countries and jurisdictions have made inroads in providing coordinated, efficient, and decent care, these collected services for "deviants" remain inchoate and inefficient into the present day, and especially in the USA (Grob 1983, 1992, 1994, 2005; Sadler in press).

For a variety of social, political, and professional reasons and interests that are characteristic of the twentieth century, psychiatry came to partner with many of these differentiated institutions addressing social deviance in its many forms, contributing to a "normalization" of society (Connolly 1987; Foucault 1980, 2006). Normalization, the tendency to homogenize rather than differentiate individuals within society, emerged from the conditioning of society by these deviance-regulating institutions, shifting the social balance toward collective interests and away from individual freedom. Forensic and correctional psychiatrists came to serve, for the former, the courts in determinations of guilt or excuse, while the latter came to care for the prisoner's mental health needs. Child and adolescent psychiatry, at least in the USA, emerged from the involvement of American physicians in the prevention and care of youth offenders, aka "juvenile delinquents" in the mid-twentieth century. Psychiatrists partnered with adult and juvenile courts, reform schools, and prisons, while developing their own asylums and treatment programs for the "criminally insane" and "sex offenders."

Through this whirlwind summary of the history of vice and mental disorders, what emerges is a powerful cultural nexus of muddled concepts, systems, values, and priorities, setting the stage for philosophical issues in the VMDR that encompass ethics, political theory, philosophy of mind, phenomenology, philosophy of law and criminology, and epistemology. The remainder of this chapter introduces some of these matters for philosophers of psychiatry.

PHILOSOPHICAL PROBLEMS POSED BY THE VICE–MENTAL DISORDER RELATIONSHIP

For the purposes of this handbook chapter the philosophical problems of the VMDR are organized into seven areas: (1) the confounding of wrongful conduct and mental disorder,

(2) questions about psychopathologies of morality, (3) the meaning of "medical morality" in psychiatry, (4) regulating deviance and the role of the state, (5) forensic psychiatry and relationships with the law/criminal justice system, (6) moral and criminal responsibility, and (7) irrationality and evil. As will be shown, all of these issues intertwine.

Mad and bad: The confounding of wrongful conduct and mental disorder

The other chapters in this "Summoning Concepts" section of the handbook explore in detail naturalistic and value-laden accounts of mental disorder. However, the "mad versus bad" trope in the philosophy of psychiatry requires its own comment in a chapter about vice and mental disorders (Prins 1980). As noted in the previous section, mental disorders have a long history of being alternately viewed as "bad" conditions involving moral wrongfulness, as well as "mad" conditions implying disease and illness frameworks, as well as frameworks of irrationality. What is less appreciated is the "mad *and* bad" problem, which describes the commingling of mental disorder and vice concepts.

This confound of vice and illness is prominently encoded into the descriptive terms of DSM categories of mental disorder, and enumerated in diagnostic criteria. Several brief examples can be given.

> DSM-IV-TR Antisocial Personality Disorder
>   Criterion A: There is a pervasive pattern of disregard for and violation of the rights of others. (APA 2000 p. 706)

For this category, the conceptual core is built around the idea that *rights*, a political and legal concept, are being violated by the disordered individual. Moreover, rights imply a *moral* demand by the state, leaving open the question what explicitly is *medical* about this condition (Charland 2006, 2010; Potter and Zachar 2010a, 2010b).

> DSM-IV-TR Intermittent Explosive Disorder
>   Criterion A: Several discrete episodes of failure to resist aggressive impulses that result in serious assaultive acts or destruction of property. (APA 2000 p. 667, other criteria omitted)

Here the language of rights is not invoked but rather ordinary criminal acts are described. What violent crimes do not involve the failure to resist aggressive impulses?

> DSM-IV-TR Pedophilia
>   Criteria A and B:
>   A. Over a period of at least 6 months, recurrent, intense sexually arousing fantasies, sexual urges, or behaviors involving sexual activity with a prepubescent child or children.
>   B. The person has acted on these sexual urges, or the sexual urges of fantasies cause marked distress or interpersonal difficulty. (APA 2000 p. 572, other criteria omitted)

For this category, personal experiences (fantasies, urges) as well as behaviors qualify as diagnostically relevant. Criterion B offers two directions for the criterion to be satisfied—either acting (molesting one or more children), or experiencing distress or interpersonal difficulty. Other than the age qualifiers (which were not reproduced above), ambiguities abound in deciding what constitutes recurrent sexually arousing fantasies (couldn't many, even most, sexual fantasies be intense and recurrent?). The Criterion B requirement for only a sexual offense against children ("acted on these urges") leaves "DSM-IV-TR Pedophilia" a concept whose meaning largely overlaps with the criminal concept of the child molester. The American Psychiatric Association views pedophilia as both a mental disorder and a criminal behavior (APA 2003). (See Sadler (Chapter 45, this volume) for a more extended discussion of the conceptual and normative difficulties of DSM Pedophilia.)

Sadler (2008, in press) has described disorders like these as "vice-laden," meaning the evaluational content of the concepts is substantively *moral* rather than *nonmoral* (Frankena 1973). Non-moral evaluations characterize other psychiatric disorders and general medical illnesses, with typical disease-related values involving incapacities, pain, suffering, injuries, or disabilities (Sadler 2005, 2008).

These vice-laden disorders pose puzzling historical questions. Why has one kind of vice become an official psychiatric condition while other forms of vice do not? Not just the presence of these official vice-laden disorders, but the *absence* of other potential vice-laden disorders, is puzzling: Why not classify other forms of vice (e.g., white-collar insider trading, sex work, drug dealing, serial murder), or for that matter, moral failings (e. g., racism (Bell 2004) or lying) as mental disorders? Vice-ladenness poses problems of both commission and omission vis-à-vis mental disorder concepts.

Vice-laden categories also suffer from other conceptual problems. The diagnostic criteria are often scant in their phenomenological detail, leading Sadler (2008) to describe some criteria sets as *impoverished*. Consider Intermittent Explosive Disorder and Pedophilia as examples, and compare the rich and differentiated detail of diagnostic criteria for conditions like Schizophrenia or Bipolar Disorder (APA 2000; Sadler 2008). Moreover, vice-laden disorders tend to depend upon "loud" symptoms—symptoms that are obvious to anyone, blatantly problematic, and unsubtle—which also appear to lead to comorbidities with other conditions, including those of ordinary experience (Sadler 2008, 2010). Vice-laden categories also lead to questions about the metaphysical assumptions and principles upon which mental disorders, moral conduct, and criminal conduct are built. One scientist working in the psychobiology of criminal behavior suggests that criminal conduct should be understood as a mental disorder (Raine 1993, 2001). Thomas Szasz, in contrast, exhorts us to rethink mental disorders as personal misconduct subject to regulation by the religious, educational, and criminal justice systems—and not the medical (Szasz 1961). For Szasz, if such (mis)conduct infringes on others, then criminal consequences should follow.

If these polarities of Raine and Szasz are stated in the extreme, the former might be characterized as the medicalization account of vice conditions, where potentially all criminal deviance is disordered, while the latter might be characterized as a "moralization" account of vice conditions, where all criminal and wrongful deviance is considered autonomous and morally responsible. Raine would be distrustful of ontologies that claim free will and autonomous choice for criminal conduct; Szasz is definitely distrustful of ontologies that would medicalize wrongful or criminal conduct. Within this polarity, where the DSMs and mainstream psychiatry land is in an inconsistent and incoherent middle ground, where some moral/criminal vice is medicalized, and other kinds of moral/criminal vice is not. As later subsections will demonstrate, the differing metaphysical assumptions between law and medicine drive these kinds of muddles, and alternative accounts are much needed.

Knowing and caring: Questions about psychopathologies of morality

So powerful have been the metaphysical commitments to Kantian and other faculty psychologies in psychiatry (Radden 1994) that until recently, the idea of an explicit and selective defect in moral capacity has not been explored consistently (Sadler, in press). Even classical concepts like "moral insanity" which invoke associations to right and wrong, actually referred to general psychological features than explicitly ethical ones (Hunter and MacAlpine 1963; Wallace 1994). Classical (nineteenth-century) psychopathology centered on three mental faculties: cognition, affection, and conation (Berrios 1996) each with an ambiguous relationship to moral being. (See Colaizzi 2002 for a genealogy of eighteenth- and nineteenth-century "homicidal insanity" as an example.) As a consequence, the field of psychopathology has been dominated by classical mental disorders which co-vary in reference to these faculties, separately or in complex combination: cognition (e.g., dementia), affection (e.g., mood disorders), and conation (e.g., impulse control disorders) (Berrios 1996; Radden 1994; Sadler, in press). Only in the latter half of the twentieth century has an expanded interest in psychopathology of specifically moral thought, capacity, and action been explored substantively.

However, over the past twenty-five years, activity in philosophy, social and clinical psychology, and neuroscience has greatly expanded research into moral psychology, contributing to a new and vast literature, and re-stimulating expanded clinical interest in the concept of psychopathy, and to a lesser extent, DSM-defined Antisocial Personality Disorder. Psychopathy is, according to a recent comprehensive review, a key issue for contemporary philosophical moral psychology (Sinnott-Armstrong 2008a, 2008b, 2008c).

Such a large literature on moral psychology, much less psychopathy, cannot be discussed here. However, one facet of the debate about psychopathologies of morality warrants mention in a chapter on vice and mental disorders. That facet addresses the variable exclusion of criminality and wrongful conduct as potential categories of psychopathology (see subsection A), and raises the question about whether human moral capacities can be disordered just as cognitive, affective, and motivational processes can be disordered. The neglect of moral psychopathology is likely rooted historically by the Enlightenment's rejection of moral-religious explanations of madness, substituting medical-scientific formulations of psychopathology and relegating criminal and ordinary moral wrongdoing to the religious metaphysical sphere. By the nineteenth century however, this Enlightenment dichotomy of misconduct and madness began to break down as European alienists contended with the disposition of mad criminal offenders, creating bridging institutions and bridging concepts for the criminally mentally ill, and leading to the confounding of vice and madness, and the legacy of vice-laden mental disorders described in subsection "Mad and bad" (Sadler in press).

Contemporary psychopathology, however, is still dominated by the Enlightenment idea that moral deviance is for religion and law, and madness is for medicine. The vice-laden mental disorders of subsection "Mad and bad" still represent a minority of classified disorders in the DSMs and ICDs. Vicious deviance in all its manifold depravities is still left to the largely retributive criminal justice system and not medicalized. Retributive models of justice are themselves based upon Judeo-Christian metaphysics of free will, individual

Table 29.1 Abbreviated PCL-R items sorted by factor groupings

Item	Factor group
1. Glibness/superficial charm	Interpersonal
2. Grandiose sense of self-worth	Interpersonal
3. Need for stimulation/boredom prone	Lifestyle
4. Pathological lying	Interpersonal
5. Conning/manipulative	Interpersonal
6. Lack of remorse or guilt	Affective
7. Shallow affect	Affective
8. Callous/lack of empathy	Affective
9. Parasitic lifestyle	Lifestyle
10. Poor behavioral controls	Antisocial
11. Promiscuous sexual behavior	–
12. Early behavior problems	Antisocial
13. Lack of realistic, long-term goals	Lifestyle
14. Impulsivity	Lifestyle
15. Irresponsibility	Lifestyle
16. Failure to accept responsibility	Affective
17. Short-term marital relationships	–
18. Juvenile delinquency	Antisocial
19. Revocation of conditional release	Antisocial
20. Criminal versatility	Antisocial

Adapted from Hare and Neumann (2006); not all clinical features empirically fit into the four factors.

choice, and personal responsibility (Braithwaite 1999; Timasheff 1937; Wenzel et al. 2008), and a moral culture of laws largely tied to Judeo-Christian norms of punishment and penance (Duff 2008; Dworkin 1977).

So contemporary philosophical moral psychology raises the question about whether psychopathy qualifies as explicitly, and primarily, a disorder of moral function. Sinnott-Armstrong's (2008a, 2008b, 2008c) series of comprehensive volumes exploring contemporary moral psychology present a majority view that indeed psychopathy represents a specific moral disorder. The debate is not about whether, but what is the significance of a disorder of moral capabilities. Table 29.1 summarizes the clinical features of psychopathy as described by Robert Hare's Psychopathy Check List- Revised (PCL-R) (Hare and Neumann 2006).

Hare's inspiration was Hervey Cleckley's mid-twentieth-century formulation of psychopathy (Cleckley 1988), and Hare's career has explored the empirical basis for Cleckley's clinical descriptions (Cleckley 1988; Hare and Neumann 2006). While virtually all of these clinical features of psychopathic individuals exhibit at least a potential for moral censure in Western industrialized cultures, what is evident and verified in the empirical studies is that a psychopath, in meeting clinical features excluding Hare's antisocial factors, could well avoid criminal prosecution or even criminal conduct yet still qualify as a "psychopath" (Hare 1998; Patrick 2006).

Hare's psychopathy construct has proven useful in a variety of neuroscience and psychology research programs, with one of the central debates centering on the criminal responsibility of the psychopathic offender. (In this regard, see also "Agents of misfortune" subsection.) Does a psychopathic offender have responsibility for his actions and should said offender be subject to punishment? Briefly, the debate revolves around research that indicates substantive biopsychological differences in psychopathic individuals and particularly the failure of psychopathic individuals to discriminate conventional rules from moral rules. Preschool children on up to adults can discriminate the difference between conventional rules invoked by authorities (e.g., sitting still in class in response to a teacher) and moral rules which regulate the welfare, human rights, or trust of others. The idea here is that conventional rules can be removed by the appropriate authority (e.g., you can move around in class if the teacher says so) while moral rules are not excused by authorities (e.g., you never stab your neighbor with a pencil even if the teacher says it's OK). Psychopathic individuals, however, treat both kinds of rules as the same, as authority-driven conventional rules. Moreover, they present conformist responses to both moral and conventional rules in experimental situations. Psychopathic individuals also differ in a number of morality related capabilities; for instance, they are less likely to learn from punishment situations, and generate feeble autonomic responses to stress and punishment situations (Aniskiewicz 1979; Blair 1999, 2001, 2007, 2010; Blair et al. 1997; House and Milligan 1976; Sutker 1970). As one group of scholars characterized psychopathic individuals, they know, but don't care, about moral rules (Jotterand et al., in press). The psychopathic individual can recognize that moral situations are supposed to invoke a normative cultural response, but their moral "response" carries little to no emotional weight in motivating conduct.

The extensive literature generated around the psychopathy concept (only a small portion of which is mentioned here) would seem to suggest that psychopathy would warrant inclusion as a particularly well-validated mental disorder, yet so far this has not been the case. Instead, the DSMs proffer a personality disorder category called Antisocial Personality Disorder which identifies a subgroup of psychopathic individuals who are more likely to be criminal offenders (Widiger 2006), leaving Hare's other varieties of psychopathic individuals with no place in the DSM.

Regarding the issue of criminal responsibility, the debate consolidates around two positions. One group is capably represented by Cordelia Fine and Jeanette Kennett (Fine and Kennett 2004; see also their contributions to Sinnott-Armstrong 2008a, 2008b), while the contrary view is represented by James Blair (2008) and Hare himself (1998) among others. Fine and Kennett's detailed arguments are recommended reading, but the gist of their position is that the psychopathic individual's impairment of moral understanding undermines criminal responsibility in similar ways to other forms of severe psychopathology, similar to the insanity defense for psychotic individuals. The retributive justice model (see subsection "Punishment versus restoration") is dependent upon the offender as capable of autonomous choice, and for Fine and Kennett, such choice is undermined by the well-established impairment of psychopathic moral understanding. The contrary viewpoint promulgates the argument that the psychopathic offender can be judged and punished because of the preservation of the psychopathic person's understanding of conventional rules. The psychopathic offender may not care that it's against the law, but knows that it is and is capable of conforming his conduct to the law. In this viewpoint, knowing that laws exist that say you shouldn't rob banks or commit rape is sufficient to satisfy the law's requirement for the capacity for choice (Blair 2008).

The paradigmatic example of psychopathy is crucial for the vice–mental disorder relationship in that it initiates a frame of discussion for the concept of specifically *moral* psychopathology. As neuroscience and psychology unravel additional frameworks for social cognition, social action, and motivational constraints on the individual's behavior, philosophical reflection on the interface of the law, criminal justice, and clinical concepts will only become more indispensable.

Good doctors: The meaning of "medical morality" in forensic psychiatry

Psychiatry's framing of vice-laden disorders in its nomenclature, and engagement with patients involved in vice, raises questions about the psychiatrist's professional role, ethical identity as physician, and social contribution to the general welfare. Should psychiatrists be involved in addressing vicious conduct and reforming offenders? Should psychiatrists—healers by professional identity—contribute to the criminal justice system whose prevailing goal in most jurisdictions is to punish (e.g., harm) offenders? Should public policy in democratic societies endorse a psychiatry whose aims are both to treat illness as well as diminish vicious conduct? (This latter question is taken up in this and the next section.)

Medicine, and psychiatry as a subspecialty, has always had an explicitly moral/ethical identity, going at least as far back as the Hippocratics:

> First I will define what I conceive medicine to be. In general terms, it is to do away with the sufferings of the sick, to lessen the violence of their diseases, and to refuse to treat those who are overmastered by their diseases realizing that in such cases medicine is powerless. (Hippocrates cited in Pellegrino 1999 p. 61. See also Hippocrates, *The Art*, Loeb Classical Library, Volume II, 1923)

The American philosopher of medicine, Edmund Pellegrino, argues that medicine's ends are the "need of sick persons for care, cure, help, and healing" (Pellegrino 1999, pp. 60–61). For Pellegrino, these ends of medicine are not negotiable, bound by a "covenant of trust" (p. 65) where patient needs prevail over personal, economic, or political needs. A moral community of physicians reinforces, supports, and protects these ends through training, ethical guidelines, and peer-regulation of conduct (Flexner 1915; Pellegrino 1999).

The Hastings Center, an American non-partisan ethics think tank, issued a consensus statement of the goals of medicine in 1999:

> (1) The prevention of disease and injury and the promotion of the maintenance of health. (2) The relief of pain and suffering caused by maladies. (3) The care and cure of those with a malady, and the care of those who cannot be cured. (4) The avoidance of premature death and the pursuit of a peaceful death. (Hanson and Callahan 1999, executive summary, p. 1)

These benchmark, and typical, statements of medical morality pose challenges when applied in the arena of forensic psychiatry's contributions as expert witnesses in the criminal court, as well as the general psychiatrist's role in addressing vice behavior in patients seen in ordinary clinical settings. I'll consider each of these two settings in turn.

As will be discussed in the "Agents of misfortune" section, outside the USA, for example, the UK, there are two functions within "forensic psychiatry"—one provides the clinical care of prisoners in criminal justice settings, and the other serves as expert witnesses in criminal and civil trial proceedings. These two identities tend to be separated in US forensic psychiatry, with the latter role, activity in criminal/civil trials, more characteristic, while the care of prisoners is labeled increasingly in the USA as "correctional" psychiatry.

The US forensic psychiatrist's identity as expert witness in trial settings has posed fundamental ethics challenges for the subspecialty. Former APA President Alan Stone posed these in a provocative article published in 1984, raising a number of issues with the American forensic psychiatry field:

> First, there is the basic boundary question. Does psychiatry have anything true to say that the courts should listen to?
>
> Second, there is the risk that one will go too far and twist the rules of justice and fairness to help the patient.
>
> Third, there is the opposite risk that one will deceive the patient in order to serve justice and fairness.
>
> Fourth, there is the danger that one will prostitute the profession, as one is alternately seduced by the power of the adversarial system and assaulted by it.
>
> Finally, as one struggles with these four issues—Does one have something true to say? Is one twisting justice? Is one deceiving the patient? Is one prostituting the profession?—there is the additional problem: forensic psychiatrists are without any clear guidelines as to what is proper and ethical, at least as far as I can see. (Stone 1984/2008, pp. 167–168)

Stone's comments amounted to a challenge to the profession to formulate its own ethics, which was answered shortly thereafter in several papers by Paul Appelbaum, who was to become an APA President and who had served as President of the American Academy of Psychiatry and the Law (AAPL). Appelbaum's viewpoint of forensic psychiatry's ethics was based on the idea that forensic psychiatrists do not perform clinical duties, and in that context, should be exempted from many aspects of traditional medical ethics:

> Forensic psychiatrists, however, work in an entirely different ethical framework, one built around the legitimate needs of the justice system. Their duties are to seek and reveal the truth, as best they can, whether or not that advances the interests of the evaluee. (Appelbaum 1997, p. 445)

This grounding, however, of forensic psychiatry ethics in the "legitimate needs of the justice system" was to prove controversial for some (Halpern et al. 1998). Halpern et al. were concerned that psychiatrists in service to the justice system permitted them to participate in evaluation the competency of prisoners for the death sentence, or to be involved in political use of psychiatry as in Soviet psychiatry's "treatment" of dissidents (Fulford et al. 1993).

Forensic psychiatrists, whose Appelbaumian first duties are to the justice system, are then contradicting Pellegrino's ends of medicine and the Hastings Center's goals of medicine. Such transfer of medical agency from patient to the justice system then sets the stage for the abuses of psychiatry that worried Halpern et al. Moreover, a related question is not explicitly raised, which concerns what the forensic psychiatrist is to do when the justice system is corrupt, evil, or misguided. The closest Appelbaum comes to addressing this question is "To determine which moral rules and ideals a group of professionals ought to observe with particular zealousness, we look to the values that society desires that profession to promote" (Appelbaum 1997 p. 238.)

From an ethics perspective, the grounding of forensic psychiatry in crime prevention and social justice for criminals is questionable on two fronts. Because a key function of Anglo-American criminal justice systems is to punish criminals, thus causing them harm, the status of the forensic psychiatrist as an ethically true physician is under question, if we are to take the Pellegrino and Hastings Center guidance on the moral ends of medicine seriously. Second, a grounding of forensic psychiatry ethics in the "legitimate needs of the justice system" raises questions about what to do when the needs of the justice system are illegitimate or corrupt—or even in serious dispute in the most democratic of polities. Situating the grounding of forensic psychiatry in "the values that society desires that profession to promote" seems an endorsement of a crudely relativistic concept of forensic ethics that both undermines traditional medical ethics duties and fails to address the problem of corrupt, evil, or misguided social values.

The meaning of medical morality in the forensic psychiatry setting remains ambiguous and is an open question of central professional and public policy importance.

Punishment versus restoration: Regulating deviance and the role of the state

A core function of government has been to regulate social deviance, and the regulation of deviance has been a core challenge for democratic theory and democratic governments since the Enlightenment (Hampsher-Monk 1992; Kelly 1999; Kymlicka 1990). The very brief historical background supplied in this chapter suggests that two primary standpoints regarding regulation of deviance have emerged in Western political culture: that of punishment and (sometimes) rehabilitation of deviant offenders on the one hand, and the provision of welfare and restoration to victims on the other. The varieties of punishments for (primarily) antisocial deviance are many, from fines to public whippings to imprisonments. Rehabilitation taken broadly, however, takes much more expansive forms. Medical care and the medical model of social deviance imply that deviance results from illness or disease, and rehabilitation requires therapy. Rehabilitation of the criminal deviant, however, has (particularly recently) included medical perspectives and medicalization, but more commonly has involved a concatenation of techniques including education, humanistic role modeling, peer support, and vocational training. Rehabilitation of the poor or unemployed involves providing job training and opportunities. All rehabilitation efforts are either supported or undermined by the relative adequacy of the public welfare for the general polity.

Disease/illness-related deviance, as opposed to criminal deviance, as considered earlier, involves profound ontological differences. People were sick, and recognized as such, long before there was anything resembling a polity or government; sickness is an ancient and perennial existential fact. Moreover, physicians tended to the ill in a dyadic relationship, while wrongdoing was addressed by rulers and, much later, the polity. Crime, however, implies more than the most primitive deviance from social cooperation. Crime requires a polity, authority, and declaration in a way that makes it distinctively social and political in a manner that sickness is not. Having slept with one's neighbor may not be a crime until the polity declares it so; but having a fever makes one sick regardless of what the polity says. The ancient Sumerian Code of Ur-Nammu, circa 2011 BCE, is the oldest code of moral instruction known and is thoroughly social in its orientation, addressing what today would be called civil disputes over property and personal injury as well as "crimes" like theft and murder (Roth and Hoffman 1995). While wrongdoing may be an existential fact of similar status to sickness, the concept of "crime" is much more dependent upon a polity than the concept of "illness" or "disease," and in this sense crime is more of a "social construct" than illness. Correspondingly, the criminal law is explicitly placed within the polity while medicine's relationship with the polity was indirect and much slower in evolving to its highly socially regulated practice today.

A third crucial difference between criminal law and medicine involves their moral structures discussed in the "Good doctors" subsection. Retributive criminal law that characterizes much of American and British policy intends to protect the collective at the moral expense of, at minimum, constraining the freedom of the offender, and at worst, causing frank harm to offenders through punishments. Medicine however, is all about "first doing no harm" and reducing the harm of illness and providing benefits to the patient.

These existential differences between crime and illness, and their associated social practices of criminal law and medicine, provide an ontological background for the kind of conflict and confusion that pervades the vice–mental disorder relationship.

A large portion of the philosophy of criminal law is occupied by a range of questions that emerge from the paradox of doing good for the majority polity through causing harm (e.g., punishing) for the relative few "offenders" (see Duff (2008) and Shiner (2009) for succinct reviews). These questions, for example, address the moral justifications for a criminal justice system, explore the proper relationship between crime and immorality, argue the respective benefits of punishment, rehabilitation, and containment of criminal deviance, address the tension between instrumental versus moral justifications for criminal law, and consider the sources of legal authority, to name a few (Tonry 2011). While many of these are relevant to the vice–mental disorder relationship, review of these cannot feasibly be done here. The "Good doctors" subsection describes in more detail one example of the moral conflict between criminal law and medical practice. The remainder of the discussion in this section considers the role of psychiatry in two approaches to criminal justice, that of "retributive" justice and "restorative" justice. My intent here is not to adjudicate the debate between the two forms of criminal justice, but rather briefly sketch some of their conceptual and ethical implications for mental health professional involvement in the criminal justice system.

Some definitional caveats are warranted. Both retributive and restorative justice are more family-resemblance concepts than crisply bounded, essential ones. Moreover, in application within particular countries and cultures, each is formulated, practiced, and regulated in different ways. Restorative justice in particular is experimental in many jurisdictions, is discussed under many names, and often represents innovative programs, applications, and structures of delivery. Finally, the rhetoric and advocacy from proponents for the two models tends to emphasize differences rather than shared elements (Daly and Proietti-Scifoni 2011). So the following descriptions of each should be taken with a grain of salt.

Retributive justice addresses criminal deviance through a moral model that emphasizes personal responsibility and accountable choosing between right and wrong. Its European roots belong in both Enlightenment social contract theory as well as Judeo-Christian mores (Braithwaite 1999). From a social psychological perspective, the function of retribution is not only protection of the community and the enforcement of shared/social values, but also motivationally linked to revenge (Wenzel et al. 2008). Legally, retributive justice emerges from the moral concept of desert and the ancient idea that people should get what they deserve (McLeod 2008; Timasheff 1937). In this latter regard, one may consider desert as the ancient expectation of punishment for the sinner, in this world or another. Desert applies to positives as well as negatives—people who work hard, hold the faith, and follow the law should be rewarded, and people who cheat and steal should be punished. Crime represents an unbalancing of desert, as worthy citizens are robbed (figuratively and literally) of their due. Justice is served through the imposition of punishment. In practice retributive justice marginalizes the role of the victim in the justice process, limiting victims' role to testimony and evidence-giving at trial; and largely excludes them during the conviction and sentencing phases. In the retributive justice model, the victim is relegated largely to a passive provider of information and observer role.

Restorative justice models address criminal deviance through a moral model that emphasizes the involvement of the victim and community in the justice process. The ethic of restorative justice is communitarian rather than individualistic (Braithwaite 1999). Metaphysically, crime is cast as a social problem where causality is distributed among the community and social system, rather than the individual-actor driven metaphysics of retributivism. Rather than focusing exclusively on punishment as a consequence for wrongdoing and as the instrument of justice, restorative justice focuses on making repairs to the harm done by the offender, eliciting discussion between victim(s), offender, and community about the reparative actions to be taken. While punishment may be a consequence of the discussions, the focus is on "restoring" the losses of the victim and community, through mechanisms such as apology, community service, financial reparations, as well as punishment—neatly summarized by Wenzel et al. as "restitution, compensation, and censure" (2007, p. 379).

In a recent international conference on restorative justice, a working definition of restorative justice declared:

> Restorative justice is a process whereby all the parties with a stake in the particular offense come together to resolve collectively how to deal with the aftermath of the offense and its implications for the future. (Tony Marshall quoted in Braithwaite 1997, p. 5)

As mentioned earlier, the labels for this orientation to justice are many: community justice, reconciliation, relational justice, and redress to name a few (Braithwaite 1999; Kurki 2000). Pioneering work in the area was inspired by tribal forms of justice, through communities as diverse as Native American ones in the USA to Maori communities in New Zealand (Braithwaite 1999; Kurki 2000). Another alternative to conventional retributive justice, therapeutic jurisprudence, is more a humanistic diversion technique in sentencing, often, perhaps usually, embedded in the retributive model of justice, and therefore not appropriate for discussion here (Allan 2003; James 2006; Wexler 2008; Winick 2003).

In the West, restorative justice is primarily distinctive in the sentencing phase, where the stakeholder discussion replaces the judge/jury appointment of punishment. From the social psychological perspective, restorative justice appeals more to the emotion of shame (of the offender)—while the community, face-to-face involvement of the offender in sentencing, and reparations add a motivational element of group conformity and belonging (Wenzel et al. 2007, 2012). The literature exploring the efficacy of these two criminal justice approaches is diverse, extensive, and difficult to interpret for the reasons suggested by the diversity of approaches, settings, and the fluidity of the concepts and practices sketched here.

As the reader can now recognize, in explicating the restorative alternative to retributive justice, most of this chapter has focused on *retributive* justice in reference to psychiatry and mental disorders. What remains to explore is the normative, conceptual, and practical relationships between psychiatrists and restorative justice. However, the literature on restorative justice and psychiatry is scant (Gatti and Verde 2012; Loeffler et al. 2010; Petrucci 2002) and is limited to specific applications (e.g., domestic violence) and historical studies. In closing this section I sketch some questions for the philosophy of psychiatry about the psychiatrist's role in restorative justice settings, questions that demand more scholarship.

Forensic psychiatry ethics in restorative justice settings

In the "medical morality" subsection, I considered the ethics of forensic psychiatry over against a traditional beneficence-centered ethics for doctors. The retributive justice setting, where the orientation of courts is punishment and harm, contradicts the conventional physician–ethics role of care/cure/healing/helping. What about the setting of restorative justice?

On the face of it, a restorative justice model based upon a psychology of shame and a reparative, conjoint process for key stakeholders may appear less objectionable to, and more compatible with, physician beneficence ethics than the revenge-and-punishment orientation of retributive justice. A focus on restoration promises a return to civil well-being for the community, including the offender if possible. Many restorative processes are explicitly intended as healing encounters (Kurki 2000), and from that standpoint are analogous, perhaps synergistic with, psychiatry's healing role while avoiding a medicalization of criminality. Moreover, the restorative justice model draws from a set of ontological assumptions that are more "friendly" to psychiatrists—that abnormal behavior is "biopsychosocial," causally emerging from complex interactions with a variety of causal vectors.

Alternatively, because restorative justice enters primarily in the sentencing phase of the criminal justice process, the role of a forensic psychiatrist (or, for that matter, a treating psychiatrist) in the trial phase is ambiguous when there is no guarantee of a particular, non-punitive restorative intervention after sentencing. Moreover, the explicitly medical contribution of psychiatry seems marginal in that restorative processes presuppose peer-competent relationships, and psychopathological concepts typically have not entered into the restorative discussion as yet. This concern prompts questions about what clinical role, if any, psychiatry offers restorative justice, and how the psychiatrist as agent to a patient/client fits into a restorative process.

What role? Whose agent? Even in the most "healing" restorative justice setting, the purpose of a psychiatrist is ambiguous. Should a treating clinician participate in the roundtable discussion? For the victim(s)? For the offender? The qualifications of a clinician to contribute to the restorative discussion are also unclear, whether the treating clinician is serving a victim or an offender as her client. The concept of the psychiatrist as agent-for-a-client is also questionable from the standpoint of the communitarian and egalitarian framework of restorative justice. The restorative discussion is of collective advocacy, not individual advocacy. On the other, more positive, hand, an offender's clinician may be able to assess, augment, or reinforce the behaviors of remorse and apology, and having first-hand knowledge of the proceedings may be of interest and benefit to a psychotherapist for either a victim or offender. But such participation raises a new set of questions about clinician duties, role responsibilities, and ethical constraints.

I noted that clinician participation in a restorative process raises the question of loyalty, agency, and related concepts like informed consent and confidentiality. To whom does the clinician owe alliances? The psychiatrist acts as the agent of whom? The patient's? The legal process? In this sense, the questions around agency in restorative settings are very similar to the questions posed in the retributive setting, e.g., is the psychiatrist in service to the state or in service to the "patient"? These questions of agency require clarification if an ethics for psychiatry in restorative justice is to be developed. Indeed, the question of psychiatrist participation altogether, in a restorative justice setting, is yet to be worked out.

Agents of misfortune: Forensic psychiatry and the law/criminal justice system

Up to this point, the moral and political framing of forensic psychiatry has privileged an American perspective on what defines this field. In several papers authored from the UK perspective, Gwen Adshead and Sameer Sarkar describe two "paradigms" within UK forensic psychiatry: the "welfare paradigm" and the "justice paradigm" (Adshead and Sarkar 2005; see also Adshead 2000). While not explicitly addressed by the authors, these two UK paradigms for a unitary "forensic psychiatry" relate closely to American conceptions of "forensic psychiatry" (for the justice paradigm) and American conceptions of "correctional psychiatry" (for the welfare paradigm) and are therefore of Anglo-American interest and perhaps wider international interest.

As noted in subsection "Good doctors," Adshead and Sarkar assign the traditional role of physician as beneficent and altruistic healer to the welfare paradigm. Linking this ethic of beneficence and altruism to a parental analogy, they argue that a role for paternalism in (particularly forensic) psychiatry is strong. The situation for which paternalism is most commonly demanded from forensic psychiatrists is the case where the patient lacks autonomy, which is formalized in legal language through such concepts as competency, capacity, duress, and responsibility. In dealing with mentally ill criminal offenders, the authors suggest that the broader social ethic of welfare is appropriate; incapacitated criminal offenders are a challenge not just for their own personal welfare but also the welfare of the community. The forensic psychiatrist then serves double-duty in provision of welfare: to the patient and to the community, whereupon the earlier discussed agency conflicts arise. However, these authors are most interested in the broader argument for morally justified priorities regarding patient welfare versus public welfare.

They contrast what I might call an encompassing-paternalism (EP) professional role for psychiatrists over against a restricted-paternalism (RP) role. Advocates of the EP role, which Adshead and Sarkar present as compatible with the official UK government stance, claim that public interests should trump patient interests in terms of their explicitly professional psychiatric responsibilities. This responsibility cashes out most commonly in decisions about involuntary (even preventive) detention and involuntary treatment. The justification for EP psychiatry is that public health interventions without consent are common outside of psychiatry, and indeed, the "basis for the duty of public welfare is actually an extension of the duty to the patient, because of the patient's interest to be prevented from causing harm to others" (Adshead and Sarkar 2005, p. 1013). This position is in turn supported by the impairment or lack of autonomy, or diminished responsibility, of psychiatric patients. In contrast, the RP role recognizes that the empirical evidence recognizes that mental illness usually does not impair the patient's ability to make decisions, including the decision to harm others. In response to the EP argument that public welfare extends to the patient welfare, they reply that promoting public welfare over patient welfare poses its own problem: "the individual duty of care to the patient is in danger of being abandoned: which itself may be a cause of harm to the patient" (p. 1014).

Adshead and Sarkar are worried that psychiatrists will be held responsible for patients' criminal behaviors, which will lead then to widespread abuse of involuntary detention, as psychiatrists will be unwilling to take any chances against even the most unlikely of patient-aggressors. They recommend splitting this role of psychiatry into two, one the traditional healer and the other as agent of the state whose role is to protect the public against dangerous mentally ill individuals. (By way of critique here, this solution does remove the clinician-therapist from the public welfarist role and therefore the ethical role conflict, but to my mind shifts the temptations to abuse involuntary detention to a now potentially wanton public-interest psychiatrist!)

In their consideration of the traditional American emphasis in forensic psychiatry with the expert-witness role in criminal trials and civil disputes, Adshead and Sarkar situate American forensic psychiatry within the justice paradigm. Here the forensic psychiatric role is to assure that the criminally accused are "fully responsible for their actions; if they 'own' their actions, as an individual choice" (Adshead and Sarkar 2005, p. 1014). They are cautious about psychiatric endorsements of judgments about the moral issue of guilt or punishments, but note that for principlist (deontological) medical ethics, supporting "justice" implies an obligation of forensic psychiatrists to participate in the justice process. They then explore the ethics of forensic experts addressing many of the features considered in the "Good doctors" subsection, as well as more that space here does not permit. They conclude by defending justice as the prevailing value for the forensic psychiatrist (in this setting under both the welfare and justice paradigms), making the argument (among others) that harm-doing in the trial phase of criminal procedures does not guarantee any particular harm/no-harm outcome for a particular defendant. Just as the forensic psychiatrist may contribute to harming a defendant by providing an incriminating evaluation, the psychiatrist may also protect a defendant by finding her incapable of participating in her own defense.

Taken together, the subsections discussed so far describe a metaphysical and moral minefield for practitioners as they attempt to navigate their professional roles in the face of manifold formulations of justice, social and professional duties, political pressures, and novel forensic case situations. As criminal justice systems work out their own priorities, moral frameworks, and practical applications, the need for philosophical reflection on psychiatrist participation will only increase.

Theaters of vice: Moral and criminal responsibility

Philosophical discussions of moral and criminal responsibility are among the most vigorous in relation to psychiatry, perhaps because of excusing illegal conduct in response to serious mental illness—e.g., the "insanity defense." This topic, along with the definition of mental disorder, may possess the biggest literatures under the umbrella of "philosophy of psychiatry." For this reason I'd like to limit my brief discussion to the views of Stephen Morse, a psychologist and attorney who has been among the most outspoken and articulate on the debate around criminal responsibility (Morse 1998; see also Morse 2002, 2008).

But first, a few words about what is meant by "criminal responsibility," and in contrast to "moral responsibility." Moral responsibility refers to a person being subject to praise or blame depending upon whether the person fulfills, or fails to fulfill, a particular moral obligation or duty (Klein 2005). Under this frame, moral responsibility may address, but not be limited to, criminal actions. Criminal responsibility, in Anglo-American law, refers in general to two contexts of meaning: (1) to fulfill legal requirements for liability for illegal acts or illegal omissions (or failures to act); and (2) the version of criminal responsibility most relevant to this discussion: the ability of the criminally accused to understand their actions and conform their behavior to the law (Garner 2004). A conventionally clear-cut case of impairment of criminal responsibility (in the latter sense) is the psychotic individual who, delusionally believing his employer means him harm, shoots his boss in self-defense in order to survive.

The idea for this kind of "excuse" for criminal conduct is ancient, and over the centuries the law has tinkered with how to make judgments about mad (mentally ill) offenders. Moreover, the use of "excuse" here is a general one, and may range from exemptions of guilt, as under the insanity defense (Perlin 1994; Robinson 1996), to the recognition of mitigating factors regarding both guilt and punishment phases: for the former, the downgrading to a less severe sentence, and for the latter, altering, deferring, or diminishing the sentence.

Morse provides a straightforward account of conditions where the criminal law might excuse an offender. First, he provides an account of "the law's concept of the person" which requires that persons act in response to reasons: "The reason-giving explanation accounts for human behavior as a product of intentions that arise from the desires and beliefs of the agent" (Morse 1998, p. 338). He contrasts this account with a mechanistic, deterministic account such as that provided by the sciences, which frame explanations of behavior in these terms, stepping outside the folk-psychological explanations of behavior depending upon reason-giving for actions. Morse notes that the social sciences, especially including psychology and psychiatry, are "uncomfortably wedged between the reason-giving and the mechanistic accounts of human behavior" (p. 338), sometimes offering explanations in terms of one or the other, depending on circumstances, predilections of the expert, and the kinds of explanatory evidence available. In my interpretation of Morse, it is the laissez-faire meandering in the courtroom between the reason-giving and mechanistic accounts of human behavior that generates the majority of confusion in criminal law in handling offenders who are mentally disordered or otherwise face psychologically powerful circumstances. Morse acknowledges the thesis that reason-giving folk-psychological accounts of behavior as causal is controversial in philosophy, and also dependent upon a solution to the mind-body problem. Recognizing that the law cannot wait for philosophers to solve definitively the problem of meanings-as-causal, he notes "the law presupposes that people use legal rules as premises in the practical syllogisms that guide human action" (p. 339).

For Morse, only two circumstances warrant excuse from criminal wrongdoing: (1) the offender was irrational and (2) the offender faced a "hard choice." The former means the offender's capability to formulate rational reasons for his behavior was compromised, at least at the time of the offense, and was therefore unable to choose with the normative competence (rationality) that is presupposed by the law's folk-psychological account of human action. The latter refers to circumstances of crime where the offender is coerced into wrongdoing; the example Morse gives is of an individual who is forced to kill two other people or else be killed by an additional malefactor.

Morse then systematically works through counterarguments, which can only be very briefly sketched here. He is especially vigorous in arguing against the relevance of scientific determinism, arguing that if universal determinism/causation is true, then it applies to all facets of human behavior, which leaves the reasons-giving account intact as a practical and salient approach to the problem of criminal offending, as everyone involved is subject to the same mechanistic causal forces at work regarding the criminal offense. Moreover, he appeals to everyday practices in situating the mechanistic account: If the mechanistic account is true, then infants and adults are equally determined, e.g., mechanistic causes don't lose their grip on the individual simply because s(he) is older. What in fact changes is that adults are more rational in their actions compared to children. Morse identifies problems with "free will" and "volitional impairments" as "placeholders" (Morse 1998, p. 353) in arguments that actually concern rationality of the offender, e.g., "the defendant lacks free will" versus "the defendant lacks rationality." Arguments attributed to the offender having "no choice" are more typically examples of hard choice, which are nonetheless excusing. Claims of lack of self-control are handled adequately by the circumstances of the offense. This may involve either falling under the rubric of irrationality or hard choice, or falling into provocations of ordinary life to which we all are expected to respond in a normatively respectable manner, e.g., I don't assault the police officer for giving me a speeding ticket. If I do assault the officer under such circumstances, that fails under normative social expectations and few juries will acquit me.

By way of commentary, I confine my comments to two broad ones: (1) the problem of rationality determinations in the criminal court setting; and (2) the role of criminal procedure in contributing to problematic excuse situations.

Morse's account of criminal excuse clarifies the muddy waters flowing from case law, as well provides some practical order in understanding both courtroom debate about excuse as well as mystifications surrounding criminal excuse. Moreover, Morse is right in situating discussions about excuse in the setting of social expectations of conduct, which at root are what define crime in the first place. He is forthright in not presenting a general account of rationality suitable for application in a courtroom. He acknowledges the tough cases for criminal excuse demand a theory of rationality—which we don't have. What he does provide is a framework to analyze criminal excuse and pinpoint the conceptual location of normative ambiguities. Moreover, his approach could account for jurisdictional variations in application of excuse defenses: jurisdictions that are less tolerant and more stigmatizing of mental illness may well constitute juries of a mindset that are intolerant of mental-illness mediated, irrationality excuses. What Morse's work demands from psychiatry and clinical psychology is a more precise means for determining "normative competence" as well as clinical tests for such. From this standpoint, the use of psychiatric diagnosis as a placeholder for the evaluation of normative competence misses the point; the diagnosis is much less important than the particular capabilities or incapabilities that a defendant exhibits or has exhibited. Such a clinical theory of rationality should account for not just more straightforward phenomena as delusional distortions in criminal offense settings, but more challenging assessments that are made with disorders that often fall outside the criminal excuse arena. Conditions such as

Intermittent Explosive Disorder (Coccaro 2000), Pedophilia, and drug addiction introduce new questions about the rationality (and perhaps, hard choices) posed by these conditions. What brand of irrationality, if any, is offered by an individual whose anger outbursts far exceed the provocation? To use Morse's language, what brand of irrationality marks anger outbursts which far exceed the normative expectations of the community for a given provocation? As another example, what kind of hard choice is faced by the pedophilic offender, whose desires may, or may not, be more severe than normative desires in heteronormative individuals? Moreover, does hard choice extend to expecting the pedophilic individual to forego all sexual expression of his pedophilic desires? To do so extends a normative expectation that is more demanding than that for a heteronormative individual—that is, heterosexuals are not required to be celibate if they are not married, and can have sex at will with a consenting adult. It appears that the normative requirement for pedophilic individuals to not molest children imposes a higher burden of sexual self-control than for heteronormative individuals, which implies some kind of hard(er) choice. Yet, pedophilic individuals are not typically excused, under either the rational or hard-choice framework, for their criminal offenses. Similar ambiguities appear in the case of drug addiction. The criminal status of the offender is dependent upon the illegality of the drug use—in jurisdictions where use of the drug is legal, then the burden of choice is lessened. What about the setting where drug use is illicit and illegal? Does not the addict face a hard(er) choice to use or not use? What is the normative competence standard in this situation? Today, at least in the USA, drug offenders of all kinds are not excused, regardless of their drug-dependent state.

The problem of criminal excuse is especially difficult in nations like the USA where enormous jurisdictional variability exists, from state to state and even within individual states' jurisdictions. Each jurisdiction has its own variations on criminal procedure, as well as its own interpretation of procedural law and local traditions of interpretation and practice. The adversarial approach to criminal procedure that is favored in the USA (Davis and Elliston 1986) produces a procedural setting where obfuscation around criminal excuse can be advantageous to prosecutors. Prosecutorial rhetoric in persuading juries in convicting the defendant may depend upon confusing, rather than clarifying, the issues around criminal excuse. Psychiatry and clinical psychology may be the only common thread in clarifying the excuse issue, and philosophical reflection on rationality and hard choice in criminal settings should assist them.

Bonfire of the ontologies: Human nature, irrationality, and evil

The foregoing discussions of the vice–mental disorder relationship betray fundamental metaphysical differences in the historical development as well as contemporary presuppositions of law and psychiatry. What has emerged in the foregoing discussions is two ontological worldviews on human conduct: one based in Judeo-Christian religious tradition and dependent upon the folk-psychological concepts of free will, individual choice, vengeance, desert, and punishment for wrongdoing, and another based upon Enlightenment rationalism, scientific fact-finding, and complex multifactorial causal reasoning. As noted by Morse, the center of this bonfire of the ontologies is forensic psychology and psychiatry, where moral objectives differ radically (punishment for criminal conduct, therapy for illness). The law-friendly Morse dualism of criminal responsibility (presence of rationality and absence of hard choice) is often challenged in application by the behavioral sciences which often, perhaps usually, view human conduct as a complexly determined organism-environment interaction where the very meaning of rationality and difficulty of choice is context-dependent and dimensional rather than essential and categorical (Erickson and Erickson 2008), as demanded by criminal law. Juries in contrast see the innocent, on the one hand, and "bad guys," on the other. The dichotomization of moral and non-moral psychological faculties, challenged by conditions like psychopathy, introduces further clashes between a moralistic criminal justice system and a secular rationalistic behavioral science and mental health system. These deeply metaphysical schisms between concepts of vice and concepts of mental disorder should keep philosophers of psychiatry busy for years to come.

References

Adshead, G. (2000). Care or custody? Ethical dilemmas in forensic psychiatry. *Journal of Medical Ethics, 26*(5), 302–4.

Adshead, G. and Sarkar, S. P. (2005). Justice and welfare: Two ethical paradigms in forensic psychiatry. *The Australian and New Zealand Journal of Psychiatry, 39*(11–12), 1011–17.

Allan, A. (2003). The past, present and future of mental health law: A therapeutic jurisprudence analysis. *Law in Context, 20*(2), 24–53.

American Psychiatric Association (2000). *Diagnostic and Statistical Manual of Mental Disorders, Fourth Edition, Text Revision*. Washington, DC: American Psychiatric Association.

American Psychiatric Association (2003). *American Psychiatric Association Statement Diagnostic Criteria for Pedophilia, June 17, 2003*. [Online.] Available at: <http://www.psych.org>.

Aniskiewicz, A. S. (1979). Autonomic components of vicarious conditioning and psychopathy. *Journal of Clinical Psychology, 35*, 60–7.

Appelbaum, P. S. (1997). A theory of ethics for forensic psychiatry. *Journal of the American Academy of Psychiatry and the Law, 25*(3), 233–47.

Bell, C. (2004). Racism: A mental illness? *Psychiatric Services, 55*(12), 1343.

Berrios, G. E. (1996). *The History of Mental Symptoms: Descriptive Psychopathology Since the Nineteenth Century*. Cambridge: Cambridge University Press.

Blair, R. J. (1999). Responsiveness to distress cues in the child with psychopathic tendencies. *Personality and Individual Differences, 27*(1), 135–45.

Blair, R. J. (2001). Neurocognitive models of aggression, the antisocial personality disorders, and psychopathy. *Journal of Neurology, Neurosurgery, and Psychiatry, 71*(6), 727–31.

Blair, R. J. (2007). The amygdala and ventromedial prefrontal cortex in morality and psychopathy. *Trends in Cognitive Sciences, 11*(9), 387–92.

Blair, R. J. (2008). Normative theory or theory of mind? A Response to Nichols. In W. Sinnott-Armstrong (Ed.), *Moral Psychology, The Cognitive Science of Morality: Intuition and Diversity*, pp. 275–8. Cambridge, MA: MIT Press.

Blair, R. J. R. (2010). Neuroimaging of psychopathy and antisocial behavior: A targeted review. *Current Psychiatry Reports, 12*(7), 6–82.

Blair, R. J. R., Jones, L., Clark, F., and Smith, M. (1997). The psychopath: A lack of responsiveness to distress cues? *Psychophysiology, 34*, 192–8.

Braithwaite, J. (1999). Restorative justice: Assessing optimistic and pessimistic accounts. *Crime and Justice, 25*, 1–127.

Charland, L. C. (2006). The moral nature of the cluster B personality disorders. *Journal of Personality Disorders*, 20(2), 119–28.

Charland, L. C. (2010). Medical or moral kinds? Moving beyond a false dichotomy. *Philosophy, Psychiatry, & Psychology*, 17(2), 119–25.

Cleckley, H. (1988). *The Mask of Sanity: An Attempt to Clarify Some Issues About the So-Called Psychopathic Personality* (5th edn., private printing for non-profit educational use). Augusta, GA: Emily S. Cleckley.

Coccaro, E. F. (2000). Intermittent explosive disorder. *Current Psychiatry Reports*, 2(1), 67–71.

Colaizzi, J. (2002). *Homicidal Insanity, 1800–1985*. Tuscaloosa, AL: University Of Alabama Press.

Connolly, W. E. (1987). *Politics and Ambiguity*. Madison, WI: University of Wisconsin Press.

Costello, J. E. and Angold, A. (2001). Bad behaviour: An historical perspective on disorders of conduct. In J. Hill and B. Maughan (Eds), *Conduct Disorders in Childhood and Adolescence*, pp. 1–10. Cambridge: Cambridge University Press.

Daly, K. and Proietti-Scifoni, G. (2011). Reparation and restoration. In M. Tonry (Ed.), *The Oxford Handbook of Crime and Criminal Justice*, pp. 207–53. Oxford: Oxford University Press.

Davis, M. and Elliston, F. A. (1986). *Ethics and the Legal Profession*. Buffalo, NY: Prometheus.

Dworkin, R. (Ed.) (1977). *The Philosophy of Law*. Oxford: Oxford University Press.

Duff, A. (2008). Theories of criminal law. In E. N. Zalta (Ed.), *The Stanford Encyclopedia of Philosophy* (Fall 2008 Edition). [Online.] Available at: <http://plato.stanford.edu/archives/fall2008/entries/criminal-law/>.

Erickson, P. E. and Erickson, S. K. (2008). *Crime, Punishment, and Mental Illness*. New Brunswick, NJ: Rutgers University Press.

Fine, C. and Kennett, J. (2004). Mental impairment, moral understanding, and criminal responsibility: Psychopathy and the purposes of punishment. *International Journal of Law and Psychiatry*, 27, 425–43.

Flexner, A. (1915). Is social work a profession? *Proceedings of the National Conference of Charities and Correction, Baltimore, MD*, Chicago, IL: National Conference of Charities and Correction.

Foucault, M. (2006). *Psychiatric Power: Lectures at the Collège de France, 1973–74*. Basingstoke/New York, NY: Palgrave Macmillan.

Foucault, M. and Gordon, C. (1980). *Power/Knowledge: Selected Interviews and Other Writings, 1972–1977*. New York, NY: Pantheon Books.

Frankena, W. K. (1973). *Ethics* (2nd edn). Englewood Cliffs, NJ: Prentice-Hall.

Fulford, K. W. M. (1989). *Moral Theory and Medical Practice*. Cambridge: Cambridge University Press.

Fulford, K. W. (1999). Nine variations and a coda on the theme of an evolutionary definition of dysfunction. *Journal of Abnormal Psychology*, 108(3), 412–20.

Fulford, K. W. M., Smirnov, A. Y., and Snow, E. (1993). Concepts of disease and the abuse of psychiatry in the USSR. *British Journal of Psychiatry*, 162, 801–10.

Garner, B. (2004). Responsibility. In B. Garner (Ed.), *Black's Law Dictionary* (8th edn). St. Paul, MN: Thomson West.

Garton, S. (2004). *Histories of Sexuality*. New York, NY: Routledge.

Grob, G. N. (1983). *Mental Illness and American Society, 1875–1940*. Princeton, NJ: Princeton University Press.

Grob, G. N. (1992). Mental health policy in America: Myths and realities. *Health Affairs*, 11, 7–22.

Grob, G. N. (1994). *The Mad Among Us: A History of the Care of America's Mentally Ill*. New York, NY: Free Press.

Grob, G. N. (2005). The transformation of mental health policy in twentieth-century America. In M. Gijswijt-Hofstra, H. Oosterheis, J. Vijselaar, and H. Freeman (Eds), *Psychiatric Cultures Compared: Psychiatry and Mental Health Care in the Twentieth Century: Comparisons and Approaches*, pp. 141–61. Amsterdam: Amsterdam University Press.

Halpern, A. L., Freedman, A. M., and Schoenholtz, J. C. (1998). Ethics in forensic psychiatry. Letter to the editor. *American Journal of Psychiatry*, 155, 575–6.

Hampsher-Monk, I. (1992). *A History of Modern Political Thought*. Oxford: Blackwell.

Hanson, M. J. and Callahan, D. (1999). *The Goals of Medicine: The Forgotten Issues in Health Care Reform*. Washington, DC: Georgetown University Press.

Hare, R. D. (1998). Psychopaths and their nature: Implications for the mental health and criminal justice systems. In T. Millon, E. Simonsen, M. Birket-Smith, and R. D. Davis (Eds), *Psychopathy: Antisocial, Criminal, and Violent Behavior*, pp. 188–213. New York, NY: Guilford.

Hare, R. D. and Neumann, C. N. (2006). The PCL-R assessment of psychopathy: development, structural properties, and new directions. In C. J. Patrick (Ed.), *Handbook of Psychopathy*, pp. 58–88. New York, NY: Guilford.

House, T. H. and Milligan, W. L. (1976). Autonomic responses to modeled distress in prison psychopaths. *Journal of Personality and Social Psychology*, 34, 556–60.

Hunter, R. and Macalpine, I. (1963). *Three Hundred Years of Psychiatry, 1535–1860: A History Presented in Selected English Texts*. London: Oxford University Press.

James, D. V. (2006). Court diversion in perspective. *Australian & New Zealand Journal of Psychiatry*, 40(6–7), 529–38.

Jotterand, F., Pascual, J., and Sadler, J. Z. (in press). Neuroimaging technologies, psychopaths and criminal responsibility. In J. Giordano (Ed.), *Toward a Neuroethics of Self and Other: Neurosciences, Neurotechnology, and the Enigma of Mind*. New York, NY: Cambridge University Press.

Kaslow, F. W. (1993). Relational diagnosis: An idea whose time has come? *Family Process*, 32, 255–9.

Kaslow, F. W. (Ed.) (1996). *Handbook of Relational Diagnosis and Dysfunctional Family Patterns*. New York, NY: John Wiley & Sons.

Kelly, J. M. (1999). *A Short History of Western Legal Theory*. Oxford: Oxford University Press.

Klein, M. (2005). Responsibility. In T. Honderich (Ed.), *The Oxford Companion to Philosophy* (2nd edn), pp. 815–16. Oxford: Oxford University Press,

Kurki, L. (2000). Restorative and community justice in the United States. *Crime and Justice*, 27, 235–303.

Kymlicka, W. (1990). *Contemporary Political Philosophy: An Introduction*. Oxford: Oxford University Press.

Laqueur, T. W. (1990). *Making Sex: Body and Gender from the Greeks to Freud*. Cambridge, MA: Harvard University Press.

Loeffler, C. H., Prelog, A. J., Unnithan, N. P., and Pogrebin, M. R. (2010). Evaluating shame transformation in group treatment of domestic violence offenders. *International Journal of Offender Therapy & Comparative Criminology*, 54(4), 517–36.

MacIntyre, A. (1998). *A Short History of Ethics*. South Bend, IN: University of Notre Dame Press.

McLeod, O. (2008). Desert. In E. N. Zalta (Ed.), *The Stanford Encyclopedia of Philosophy* (Winter 2008 Edition). [Online.] Available at: <http://plato.stanford.edu/archives/win2008/entries/desert/>.

Mora, G. (2008a). Mental disturbances, unusual mental states, and their interpretation during the Middle Ages. In E. R. Wallace IV and J. Gach (Eds), *History of Psychiatry and Medical Psychology*, pp. 199–226. New York, NY: Springer.

Mora, G. (2008b). Renaissance conceptions and treatments of madness. In E. R. Wallace IV and J. Gach (Eds), *History of Psychiatry and Medical Psychology*, pp. 227–54. New York, NY: Springer.

Morse, S. J. (1998). Excusing and the new excuse defenses: A legal and conceptual review. In M. Tonry (Ed.), *Crime and Justice: An Annual Review of Research*, pp. 329–406. Chicago, IL: University of Chicago Press.

Morse, S. J. (2002). Uncontrollable urges and irrational people. *Virginia Law Review*, 88(5), 1025–78.

Morse, S. J. (2008). Vice, disorder, conduct, and culpability. *Philosophy, Psychiatry, & Psychology*, 15(1), 47–9.

Newhauser, R. (Ed.) (2007). *The Seven Deadly Sins: From Communities to Individuals* (Studies in Medieval and Reformation Traditions, volume 123). Leiden: Brill.

Patrick, C. J. (Ed.) (2006). *Handbook of Psychopathy*. New York, NY: Guilford.

Pellegrino, E. (1999). The goals and ends of medicine: How are they to be defined? In M. J. Hanson, and D. Callahan (Eds), *The Goals of Medicine: The Forgotten Issues in Health Care Reform*, pp. 55–67. Washington, DC: Georgetown University Press.

Perlin, M. L. (1994). *The Jurisprudence of the Insanity Defense*. Durham, NC: Carolina Academic Press.

Petrucci, C. J. (2002). Apology in the criminal justice setting: Evidence for including apology as an additional component in the legal system. *Behavioral Sciences & the Law*, 20(4), 337–62.

Porter, R. (1988). *A Social History of Madness: The World Through the Eyes of the Insane*. New York, NY: Weidenfeld & Nicolson.

Porter, R. (1998). *The Greatest Benefit to Mankind: A Medical History of Humanity*. New York, NY: W.W. Norton.

Porter, R. (2002). *Madness: A Brief History*. Oxford: Oxford University Press.

Porter, R. (2004). *Flesh in the Age of Reason*. New York, NY: W.W. Norton & Co.

Prins, H. A. (1980). Mad or bad-thoughts on the equivocal relationship between mental disorder and criminality. *International Journal of Law and Psychiatry*, 3(4), 421–33.

Radden, J. (1994). Recent criticism of psychiatric nosology: A review. *Philosophy, Psychiatry, & Psychology*, 1(3), 193–200.

Rafter, N. H. (1997). *Creating Born Criminals*. Urbana, IL: University of Illinois Press.

Raine, A. (1993). *The Psychopathology of Crime: Criminal Behavior as a Clinical Disorder*. New York, NY: Academic Press.

Raine, A. (2001). A reply to Dolan's and Cordess' reviews of *The Psychopathology of Crime*. *Cognitive Neuropsychiatry*, 6(4), 304–7.

Robinson, D. N. (1996). *Wild Beasts & Idle Humours: The Insanity Defense from Antiquity to the Present*. Cambridge, MA: Harvard University Press.

Roth, M. T. and Hoffner, H. A. (1995). *Law Collections from Mesopotamia and Asia Minor*. Atlanta, GA: Scholars Press.

Rothblum, E. D., Solomon, L. J., and Albee, G. W. (1986). A sociopolitical perspective of DSM-III. In T. Millon and G. L. Klerman (Eds), *Contemporary Directions in Psychopathology: Toward the DSM-IV*, pp. 167–89. New York, NY: The Guilford Press.

Rothman, D. J. (2002a). *The Discovery of the Asylum: Social Order and Disorder in the New Republic*. Hawthorne, NY: Aldine de Gruyter.

Rothman, D. J. (2002b). *Conscience and Convenience: The Asylum and its Alternatives in Progressive America*. Hawthorne, NY: Aldine de Gruyter.

Sadler, J. Z. (1999). Horsefeathers: A commentary on "Evolutionary vs. Roschian analyses of the concept of disorder" by Jerome C. Wakefield. *Journal of Abnormal Psychology, 108*(3), 371–3.

Sadler, J. Z. (2005). *Values and Psychiatric Diagnosis*. Oxford: Oxford University Press.

Sadler, J. Z. (2008). Vice and the diagnostic classification of mental disorders: A philosophical case conference. *Philosophy, Psychiatry, & Psychology, 15*(1), 1–17.

Sadler, J. Z. (2010). Watch out for "loud" symptoms. *Psychiatric Times*, December 2. Available at: <http://www.psychiatrictimes.com/blog/DSM-5/content/article/10168/1745539>.

Sadler, J. Z. (in press). *Vice and Psychiatric Diagnosis*. Oxford: Oxford University Press.

Sadler, J. Z. and Agich, G. J. (1995). Diseases, functions, values, and psychiatric classification. *Philosophy, Psychiatry, & Psychology, 2*(3), 219–31.

Shiner, R. A. (2009). Theorizing criminal law reform. *Criminal Law and Philosophy, 3*, 167–86.

Sidgwick, H. (1888). *Outlines of the History of Ethics for English Readers*. London: MacMillan and Co. Ltd.

Sinnott-Armstrong, W. (Ed.) (2008a). *Moral Psychology. The Evolution of Morality: Adaptations and Innateness*. Cambridge, MA: MIT Press.

Sinnott-Armstrong, W. (Ed.) (2008b). *Moral Psychology. The Cognitive Science of Morality: Intuition and Diversity*. Cambridge, MA: MIT Press.

Sinnott-Armstrong, W. (Ed.) (2008c). *Moral Psychology. The Neuroscience of Morality: Emotion, Brain Disorders, and Development*. Cambridge, MA: MIT Press.

Stein, D. J., Phillips, K. A., Bolton, D., Fulford, K. W. M., Sadler, J. Z., and Kendler, K. S. (2010). What is a mental disorder? From DSM-IV to DSM-V. *Psychological Medicine, 40*(11), 1759–65.

Stone, A. A. (2008). The ethical boundaries of forensic psychiatry: A view from the ivory tower. *Journal of the American Academy of Psychiatry and the Law, 36*(2), 167–74. (Original work published 1984.)

Sutker, P. B. (1970). Vicarious conditioning and sociopathy. *Journal of Abnormal Psychology, 76*(3), 380–6.

Szasz, T. S. (1961). *The Myth of Mental Illness: Foundations of a Theory of Personal Conduct*. New York, NY: Hoeber-Harper.

Thomson, O. (1993). *A History of Sin*. Edinburgh: Canongate Press.

Timasheff, N. S. (1937). The retributive structure of punishment. *The Journal of Criminal Law and Criminology, 28*(3), 396–405.

Tonry, M. (2011). Crime and criminal justice. In M. Tonry (Ed.), *The Oxford Handbook of Crime and Criminal Justice*, pp. 3–25. Oxford: Oxford University Press.

Wakefield, J. C. (1992). The concept of mental disorder. On the boundary between biological facts and social values. *American Psychologist, 47*(3), 373–88.

Wallace, E. R. (1994). Psychiatric nosology: An historico-philosophical overview. In J. Z. Sadler, O. P. Wiggins, and M. A. Schwartz (Eds), *Philosophical Perspectives on Psychiatric Diagnostic Classification*, pp. 16–86. Baltimore, MD: Johns Hopkins University Press.

Wenzel, M., Okimoto, T. G., and Cameron, K. (2012). Do retributive and restorative justice processes address different symbolic concerns? *Critical Criminology Journal, 20*, 25–44.

Wenzel, M., Okimoto, T. G., Feather, N. T., and Platow, M. J. (2008). Retributive and restorative justice. *Law and Human Behavior, 32*(5), 375–89.

Wexler, D. (2008). *Rehabilitating Lawyers: Principles of Therapeutic Jurisprudence for Criminal Law Practice*. Durham, NC: Carolina Academic Press.

Widiger, T. A. (2006). Psychopathy and DSM-IV Psychopathology. In C. J. Patrick (Ed.), *Handbook of Psychopathy*, pp. 156–71. New York, NY: Guilford.

Winick, B. J. (2003). Outpatient commitment: A therapeutic jurisprudence analysis. *Psychology, Public Policy, & Law*, 9(1–2), 107–44.

Zachar, P. and Potter, N. N. (2010a). Personality disorders: moral or medical kinds—or both? *Philosophy, Psychiatry, & Psychology*, 17(2), 101–17.

Zachar, P. and Potter, N. N. (2010b). Valid moral appraisals and valid personality disorders. *Philosophy, Psychiatry, & Psychology*, 17(2), 131–42.

CHAPTER 30

RATIONALITY AND SANITY: THE ROLE OF RATIONALITY JUDGMENTS IN UNDERSTANDING PSYCHIATRIC DISORDERS

LISA BORTOLOTTI

The view that the insane person is irrational, and vice versa, is as old as the idea of mental illness itself.

Szasz *Insanity* (1997, p. 62)

INTRODUCTION

What is the relationship between rationality and sanity?

Thomas Szasz detects at least two distinct attitudes toward the mentally ill. First, he describes the perspective of the psychiatrist who believes that the insane are *diseased*. Szasz rejects the analogy between physical and mental illness. According to him, the differences between the two phenomena, in terms of causes, effects, and societal repercussions, are so great that talking about *illnesses of the mind* is misleading. One point he stresses on numerous occasions is that the people we regard as insane are not treated like the people who have physical diseases. Whereas the person diagnosed with a physical disease preserves all of her fundamental rights, the person diagnosed with mental illness may be confined, treated against her will, or lose custody of her children—depending on the nature of the diagnosed condition.

Second, Szasz considers the attitude of the lawyer who believes that the insane are *irrational*. Szasz is unhappy with this view, and denies the claim that irrationality is the mark of insanity. People are *regarded as* insane when they are *judged as* irrational, but he is not comfortable with the idea that one can be the judge of the rationality of another's behavior and he is very wary of the notion of rationality itself, as it can be used to comprise a variety of culturally relative norms, including social acceptability and conformity. In particular, he challenges the assumption that the insane are not to be held accountable for their actions because of their alleged irrationality and failures of autonomy.

What Szasz calls the psychiatrist's view, the view that insanity is essentially a disease, may lead us to doubt that there is anything distinctly mental in the phenomenon of mental illness. Some have recently argued that what we call "mental illness" consists of neurobiological malfunctioning (e.g., Taylor 1999) that happens to manifest in deviant behavior. In the context of what Szasz calls the psychiatrist's understanding of mental illness, irrationality plays no fundamental role in the diagnosis and classification of psychiatric disorders. A certain condition may still be diagnosed on the basis of the observation of deviant behavior, but the expectation is that neuroscience will soon provide more scientifically respectable diagnostic means. What Szasz calls the lawyer's view equally suggests a reinterpretation of mental illness, but in the opposite direction. According to the lawyer's view, psychiatric disorders are essentially mental and behavioral and irrationality plays a fundamental role in their detection. Mental illness is not strictly speaking an illness; it is a (radical) failure of rationality and autonomy (e.g., Edwards 1981). No amount of progress in the neurobiological sciences will bring to an end the way in which we currently detect the mentally ill, by judging their thought or behavior as irrational.

These opposing views of the phenomena commonly called "mental illness" are still defended in contemporary debates on the nature and status of psychiatry. My hope is that, from a careful consideration of the strengths and limitations of these rival positions, we can gain a better understanding of psychiatric disorders. It is important to recognize that the behavioral manifestations of psychiatric disorders include local failures of rationality and autonomy, and at the same time accept that such disorders have neurobiological and sometimes genetic bases as well as environmental and social triggers. For many psychiatric disorders, the explanation of their pathological nature makes explicit reference to behavioral manifestations. But this is perfectly compatible with conceiving of psychiatric disorders as diseases in a literal, not just metaphorical sense.

Here my main objective is to examine the role of judgments of rationality in the current understanding of psychiatric disorders. The relationship between rationality and sanity was an important theme in the anti-psychiatry literature but remains a timely question today, due to the need to update and revise the criteria for the classification and diagnosis of psychiatric disorders. To what extent are such criteria independent of judgments of rationality? The typical symptoms of many psychiatric disorders are described as instances of epistemic, procedural, or emotional irrationality, and references to such forms of irrationality are frequently made in the current classificatory and diagnostic criteria for schizophrenia, dementia, depression, and personality disorders. That said, I shall defend the view that irrationality is neither necessary nor sufficient for a behavior to be characterized as symptomatic of a psychiatric disorder.

In the first section, I shall review and assess a version of the lawyer's attitude toward mental illness. In the second, I shall turn my attention to instances of the psychiatrist's attitude. In the final section, on the basis of the partial conclusions reached in the previous sections, I shall develop an account of the relationship between rationality and sanity and suggest what a proper understanding of psychiatric disorders might require.

Is Mental Illness Really an Illness?

Mental illness as a persistent form of irrationality

Following some of the ideas put forward by the anti-psychiatry movement, it has been argued that the label of "mental illness" is applied to those who are judged to have lost rationality and moral responsibility for their actions, where the evidence for this loss is constituted by the breaking of social conventions and rules. The medical model which views insanity as a disease is often explicitly rejected, and so is the analogy between mental and physical illness. For instance, Ben Edwards (1981) argues that the application of the concepts "mental health" and "mental illness" is a moral issue, because these labels involve both a descriptive and a normative element. The descriptive element refers to statistical normality or abnormality, whereas the normative element refers to that subset of deviations from statistical normality that are the objects of approval or disapproval. According to Edwards, in our secular society human behavior is increasingly musicalized, and physicians and psychiatrists end up playing the same role that priests had in the religious society:

> Physicians and psychiatrists become the secular priests and final arbiters of what we should value and disvalue—in the name of "empirical" medicine. (Edwards 1981, p. 310)

The comparison between the role of psychiatrists and that of priests is a common theme in Szasz's writings too:

> The priest believed, and people agreed, that he was entitled to coerce individuals to live so that they maximized their chances of going to heaven and minimized their chances of going to hell. […] Today, doctors threaten and coerce people so as to make them healthy and live as long as possible. (Szasz 1997, p. 129)

For Edwards, psychiatrists are *arbiters of value* where the relevant values are rationality and autonomy. He observes that "mental illness" denotes those undesirable behaviors which are associated with the incapacity to act rationally and autonomously. The notion of rationality deployed in this context includes the capacity for means-ends reasoning, the possession of logically consistent and empirically supported beliefs, the capacity to give reasons for one's beliefs and behavior, clear thought, and fair mindedness. For Edwards, to have a mental illness is to deviate from such standards of rationality:

> Definition: "Mental illness" means only those undesirable mental/behavioral deviations which involve primarily an extreme and prolonged inability to know and deal in a rational and autonomous way with oneself and one's social and physical environment. In other words, madness is extreme and prolonged practical irrationality and irresponsibility. Correspondingly, "mental health" includes only those desirable mental/behavioral normalities and occasional abnormalities which enable us to know and deal in a rational and autonomous way with ourselves and our social and physical environment. In other words, mental health is practical rationality and responsibility. (Edwards 1981, p. 312)

The position defended by Edwards is implicit in many philosophical and lay conceptions of mental illness, but one problem with it is that some of the deviations from good reasoning and clear thinking considered to be paradigmatic of irrationality are so widespread in the non-clinical population as to count as the statistical norm. Rarely do human agents have logically consistent and empirically supported beliefs. Even more rarely do they engage in reason-giving that is not confabulatory, think clearly, and are fair-minded. Edwards anticipates this objection (although in my view he underestimates it) and characterizes mental illness not as any *temporary* violation of norms of rationality, but as irrationality that is *persistent* and *severe*.

Even with this qualification, Edwards' account is less than satisfactory. One might ask how persistent a form of irrationality needs to be in order to count as mental illness. Some symptoms of mental illness (e.g., a psychotic or depressive episode) are not persistent and several psychiatric disorders feature acute and less acute phases, thereby undermining the claim that persistent and severe irrationality is a distinctive feature of mental illness. Other two potential objections can be made to the identification of mental illness with irrationality. First, not all manifestations of irrationality, whether temporary or persistent, signal the presence of mental illness. For instance, a disposition toward basic reasoning mistakes or a tendency to form epistemically ungrounded beliefs can affect a person's behavior pervasively without necessarily leading to a diagnosis of mental illness. Second, it is conceivable that one may suffer from mental illness without exhibiting behavior that is persistently irrational—and is this part of the reason why diagnostic criteria that are based exclusively on the detection of irrational behavior often fail to demarcate mental illness successfully. Some forms of anxiety and depression may seem reasonable responses to life events and give rise to true beliefs and accurate predictions, as the literature on depressive realism has shown.

Another potential problem for Edwards' account lies in the relationship between the mental and the physical. How do persistent manifestations of irrationality relate to brain dysfunction or to other processes commonly regarded as the causes of mental illness? Is the claim that mental illness is primarily characterized by irrationality compatible with regarding insanity as a neurobiological dysfunction? Edwards argues that there are predictable *correlations* between mind and brain that can be experimentally tested and should inform treatment options. However, this concession may not be enough to capture the relationship between the mental and the physical in contemporary psychiatry. When information about the physical bases of at least some psychiatric disorders is getting increasingly detailed, it is at best an understatement to describe the relationship between mind and brain as a correlation. A good understanding of cognitive and affective disturbances in people who manifest statistically deviant behavior strongly supports the view that physical (biological, chemical) processes are causally linked with mental and behavioral deviations from the norm, although the direction of causation may be hard to establish in some contexts and a precise etiological story remains an aspiration for at least some disorders.

The disanalogies between mental and physical illness

Szasz offers a number of reasons to reject the notion of mental illness as analogous with that of bodily illness. First, he agrees with Edwards on the tenuous link between mental disturbance and biological dysfunction. Second, he argues that people diagnosed with a bodily illness are voluntary patients and preserve their rights, whereas people diagnosed with a mental illness are involuntary patients and lose their rights.

Szasz defines illness in general as "a structural or functional abnormality of cells, tissues, organs or bodies" (1997, p. 12). On the basis of such a definition, he argues that bodily illness is deviation from *biological* norms whereas psychological or insanity is intended as a deviation from *social* norms. Strictly speaking, then, there is no mental "illness." An indication of the difference between insanity and physical illness, according to Szasz, is that, in the case of latter, both the physician and the patient recognize the presence of an illness and cooperate in an attempt to eradicate it. In the case of insanity, however, the view of the physician might be very different from that of the person who receives treatment. Often the insane do not acknowledge the need for treatment. Szasz does not deny that some people see themselves as "mental patients," but makes a distinction between the way in which the notion of "patient" is used in psychiatry and in other medical contexts. Usually, a patient is someone who willingly assumes that role: you can be ill without being a patient if you have cancer but refuse treatment. In psychiatry, this is not the case: even those who refuse treatment are considered mental patients, if they are ascribed this role as a result of other people's concerns about their behavior or even as a result of a court proceeding.

It is true that on some occasions people diagnosed with a psychiatric disorder do not spontaneously seek the assistance of health care professionals, but this is not a generalized phenomenon, as it is suggested by the copious literature on *insight* (e.g., Amador and David 2005; Estroff et al. 1991; Roe and Davidson 2005). The overall picture we get from case studies and statistical information is a heterogeneous one, where some individuals affected by severe psychiatric disorders present themselves as normal, or as endowed with a special gift that makes them superior to the people around them, whereas others explicitly embrace their diagnoses and report that they thought there was something wrong with them well before they received medical attention. Thus, it is not clear whether voluntariness is really a core, essential feature of being patients, and it is not clear that there is a deep disanalogy between mental and physical patients to be made on the basis of voluntariness. There are non-psychiatric contexts in which it is considered acceptable to refuse treatment, as the debate on blood transfusions for children of Jehovah's witnesses testifies.

This issue is made more complicated by the difference between: (i) recognizing that something is amiss with oneself, and (ii) accepting a specific diagnosis. Many of the involuntary mental patients the psychiatric literature tells us about might recognize that they are different from those around them in a way that causes them distress, or they may even concede that they need help. However, they often reject a specific diagnosis of a psychiatric disorder or they are opposed to some specific treatment option. The fact that there is some insight in many of these cases renders the disanalogy with other medical patients much less radical. People who are diagnosed with mental or physical illness may equally refuse to accept their diagnosis or refuse treatment recommended to them on the basis of their beliefs and values.

Apart from voluntariness, one of the reasons why Szasz believes that the mental patient is different from other patients is that her rights are suspended. The fact that the mental patient may lose some of her personal rights as a result of being diagnosed with a psychiatric disorder is not sufficient reason to believe that mental illness is necessarily about loss of personal rights. *Some* of the rights of people diagnosed with *some* psychiatric disorders can occasionally be suspended, but this is not entirely due to their diagnosis as such, but to a judgment that they are incapacitated in relevant ways. Consider the case of parents with psychopathic tendencies who lose custody of their children after proven abuse:

> Often, [parents who inflict abuse] are described as psychopathic or sociopathic characters. Alcoholism, sexual promiscuity, unstable marriages, and minor criminal activities are reportedly common amongst them. They are immature, impulsive, self-centered, hypersensitive, and quick to react with poorly controlled aggression. Data in some cases indicate that such attacking parents had themselves been subject to some degree of attack from their parents in their own childhood. Beating of children, however, is not confined to people with a psychopathic personality or of borderline socioeconomic status. It also occurs among people with good education and stable financial and social background. (Kempe et al. 1985, p. 145)

Trivially, not all those who are diagnosed with a psychiatric disorder experience a suspension of their personal rights such as the revoking of child custody rights, and thus such a suspension is not a reliable way to distinguish people with psychiatric disorders from people without. As the earlier passage shows, the reason why people lose the right to have their children in custody is not they have been diagnosed with a certain disorder, but that they are found to abuse their children, whether they have a diagnosis of a psychiatric disorder or not. Child abuse is obviously not a phenomenon which is confined to parents with psychopathic tendencies and any parent found to beat her children would also be likely to have child custody rights suspended.

Mental illness is not exhausted by irrational behavior!

Some authors who believe that irrationality and lack of conformity are markers of mental illness nonetheless take distance from a simplistic identification of mental illness with irrationality or the breaking of social norms. Two examples of this more balanced attitude are found in the work by Len Bowers and Peter Sedgwick. Bowers (1998) re-describes mental illness as the "irrational or inexplicable breaking of social rules," that is, rule-breaking that happens with no apparent reason (p. 154). But on the same page, he also concedes that irrationality is not sufficient for mental illness. He openly acknowledges that suffering and lack of social functioning are the distinctive features of a psychiatric disorder, and that they are the most relevant when decisions about treatment need to be made. Bowers goes on to list other ideas that are central to mental illness, although they are not necessary conditions for it, and the list includes socially disruptive behavior, physiological deficits affecting brain functions, loss of control, lack of responsibility, and incapacitation.

Similarly, Sedgwick rejects the "elimination" of mental illness, but recognizes that the anti-psychiatry movement reacted to an excessively positivistic trend which aimed at purging all normative notions from the language of psychiatry. Sedgwick argues that we need to find a middle ground which avoids an unsophisticated contrast between the socially constructed nature of psychiatric classifications and the objective nature of other medical classifications (Sedgwick 1973, p. 21). In his view, the contribution of the anti-psychiatry movement is to show that diagnosis and treatment in psychiatry are grounded on moral and social norms that are often left implicit. Sedgwick rightly observes that this consideration should apply to the whole of medicine, and not to psychiatry alone, thereby rejecting the proposed disanalogy between physical and mental illness. Are tooth-loss and obesity *illnesses*? He argues that illness (whether physical or mental) is characterized by "deviancy" but this is a necessary, not a sufficient condition. There are deviancies that are not illnesses. To those that are illnesses further conditions apply: (i) the explanation of the deviance belongs to a set of causal factors that can be seen as "internal" to the individual, and (ii) therapy, or an investigation of possible treatment, is an appropriate response to the deviance. Sedgwick concludes that all forms of illness involve both a value judgment and an attempt at an objective causal explanation (Sedgwick 1973, p. 36).

Sedgwick's position is enlightening and well-balanced in an otherwise polarized debate, but his positive suggestion raises concerns. Is it always true that the explanation of deviance in psychiatry has to be found *in the individual*? There can be at least two interpretations of this question. One interpretation invites us to explore the metaphysics of psychiatric illness and draw an analogy between psychiatric disorders and lesions. Lesions seem to occur within an individual and to affect the individual's well-being independent of the existence of other individuals, or independent of the external environment. The alternative interpretation concerns either the etiology or the pathological nature of a psychiatric disorder. Can these be satisfactorily explained by exclusive reference to properties of the individual? It is not at all obvious that psychiatric disorders have no external (environmental or social) causes, and it may be difficult to account for the disabling nature of psychiatric disorders independently of the individual's environment or social context. To insist that the causes of psychiatric disorders or the reasons for their being pathological are necessarily or exclusively internal to the subject, would not be compatible with the fascinating results of epidemiological studies, suggesting higher occurrence of some psychiatric disorders in vulnerable populations immersed in stressful environments or subject to traumatic experiences (e.g., more frequent occurrence of psychosis in urban settings and late-onset schizophrenia in refugees or asylum seekers).

To sum up, in this section I have reviewed some attempts to characterize mental illness not as a disease, but as a failure of rationality. For Edwards, the mentally ill are people exhibiting severe and persistent irrationality. For Szasz, they are people judged by the rest of society as irrational and lacking in autonomy. Although there is a link between irrational behavior and the diagnosis of psychiatric disorders, this is not a necessary link and I offered some reason to think that we can have behavioral manifestations of persistent irrationality independent of a psychiatric disorder, and psychiatric disorders independent of behavioral manifestations of persistent irrationality. Now, it is time to assess the opposing view, and ask to what extent insanity can be medicalized.

IS THERE ANYTHING "MENTAL" IN
MENTAL ILLNESS?

Analogies between mental and bodily illness

Sedgwick is not alone in stressing the importance of values in the whole of medicine (see also Fulford 2004) and in believing that the search for a causal explanation for the purposes of finding effective treatment is a common feature of psychiatry and the rest of medicine. Here are some further examples:

> Diabetes mellitus is analogous to schizophrenia in many ways. Both are symptom clusters or syndromes, one described by somatic and biochemical abnormalities, the other by psychological. [...] There is also evidence that genetic and environmental influences operate in the development of both. The medical model seems to be quite appropriate for the one as for the other. (Kety 1974, p. 962)

> I argue that disorder lies on the boundary between the given natural world and the constructed social world; a disorder exists when the failure of a person's internal mechanisms to perform their functions as designed by nature impinges harmfully on the person's well-being as defined by social values and meanings. (Wakefield 1992, p. 373)

If it is true that psychiatric disorders are diseases, then is there anything distinctively mental about them? The opposed view to that defended by the anti-psychiatry movement tends to emphasize the extent to which psychiatric disorders are analogous to other medical disorders, and underplays the role of mental phenomena in psychiatric classification and diagnosis. In this section I shall review the recent attempts to reduce psychiatry to neurobiology and challenge some of the more radical conclusions in this area.

Whilst it is natural to suppose that psychiatric conditions share some feature with other disorders (e.g., they present obstacles to the satisfaction of an individual's interests and negatively affect the well-being of that individual), they also seem to have features that are adequately characterized only by using the vocabulary of the mental: they are pathological because of their manifestations, and such manifestations are disturbances of the mind.

The relationship between neurobiology and psychiatry has been revolutionized first by some important discoveries about the etiology of Alzheimer's disease and Tourette's syndrome, and more recently by the use of functional neuroimaging:

> Remarkable advances were made at the end of the 20th century in understanding the genetic basis of many diseases affecting the brain and the special senses. New drugs have been developed, and new theories have been espoused. It is increasingly difficult to distinguish scientifically between the disciplines of neurology and psychiatry. (Martin 2002, p. 695)

> In the past, mental disorders were defined by the absence of an "organic" lesion. Mental disorders became neurological disorders at the moment a lesion was found. With the advent of functional neuroimaging, we can now visualize patterns of regional brain activity associated with both normal and pathological mental experience. [...] If mental disorders are brain disorders, then it follows logically that the basic sciences of psychiatry must include neuroscience and genomics, and that the training of psychiatrists in the future needs to be profoundly different from what it has been in the past. (Insel and Quirion 2005, p. 2221)

> Now, [...] with the tools of modern neuroscience, a deeper understanding of causal pathways to major neuropsychiatric illness is evolving, thus rendering artificial the boundary between psychiatry and neurology. The artificiality of this boundary has profound implications for psychiatry's future. Our thesis is that the two disciplines, which were once united, should be, at least partially, reintegrated as clinical neuroscience. (Reynolds et al. 2009, p. 447)

It is increasingly difficult to preserve the distinction between organic and functional disorders—that is, disorders that have an organic cause and disorders that do not—and this has had a significant impact on the conception of psychiatry as a discipline and on the current understanding of psychiatric disorders. The dominant role of neurobiology in explaining the occurrence of behavioral symptoms contributes to strengthening the analogy between mental and physical illness that defenders of the anti-psychiatry movement wanted to challenge.

> By re-defining the foundation of psychiatry as clinical neuroscience, we also accelerate the integration of psychiatry with the rest of medicine. The separation of psychiatry from other medical specialties has contributed to the stigma of those who treat mental disorders as well as those who suffer from these illnesses. (Insel and Quirion 2005, p. 2225)

The question is, then, whether there is a role for the phenomena that are characterized as predominantly mental in psychiatry, either in classification, diagnosis, or treatment. Michael Taylor (1999, p. viii) states that "mental illness is not 'mental' at all, but the behavioral disturbance associated with brain dysfunction and disease." The assumption in much of the current psychiatric literature is that there is only one player in the game of validating psychiatric categories, and that is neurobiology. With very few exceptions, there is no debate about whether disorders can be validated psychoanalytically, cognitively, socially, or by clinical course, although there is some recognition of the appropriateness of non-pharmacological treatments in tackling some aspects of rehabilitation and recovery. Neurobiological psychiatry has become the paradigm in the field and thus it has led to a rejection of the potential contributions of alternative approaches in clinical practice and psychiatric research. Neurobiology has an important explanatory role, and can enlighten the connections between disorders and other aspects of normal or abnormal functioning. However, one of the tasks that cannot be performed by neurobiology alone is the characterization of a pattern of behavior as pathological. When we look for the standard classifications of common psychiatric disorders in diagnostic manuals, we find that disorders are distinguished from other disorders and from non-pathological behavior on the basis of their manifestations (Broome and Bortolotti 2009).

Behavioral criteria for the diagnosis of mental illness

Let's first consider the description of schizophrenia in the tenth revision of the *International Statistical Classification of Diseases and Related Health Problems* (ICD-10):

> The schizophrenic disorders are characterized in general by fundamental and characteristic distortions of thinking and perception, and affects that are inappropriate or blunted. Clear consciousness and intellectual capacity are usually maintained although certain cognitive deficits may evolve in the course of time. (ICD-10, F20)

This is not very different from criteria A in the account of schizophrenia proposed for the fifth edition of the *Diagnostic and Statistical Manual of Mental Disorders* (DSM-5):

> Characteristic symptoms: Two (or more) of the following, each present for a significant portion of time during a 1-month period (or less if successfully treated). At least one of these should include 1–3:
>
> 1. Delusions
> 2. Hallucinations
> 3. Disorganized speech
> 4. Catatonia
> 5. Negative symptoms, i.e., restricted affect or avolition/asociality. (DSM-5, May 2010)

There is a heavy usage of terms that refer to irrationality in thought and emotion, such as "distortions of thinking and perception" and "restricted" or "inappropriate" affect.

Similarly, the general description of personality disorders is characterized by references to irrationality and inappropriateness:

> They represent extreme or significant deviations from the way in which the average individual in a given culture perceives, thinks, feels and, particularly, relates to others. Such behaviour patterns tend to be stable and to encompass multiple domains of behaviour and psychological functioning. They are frequently, but not always, associated with various degrees of subjective distress and problems of social performance. (ICD-10, F60)

In the description of specific personality disorders, the language of moral failure is also abundantly used:

> Paranoid: Personality disorder characterized by excessive sensitivity to setbacks, unforgiveness of insults; suspiciousness and a tendency to distort experience by misconstruing the neutral or friendly actions of others as hostile or contemptuous [...]. (ICD-10, F60.0)

> Emotionally unstable: Personality disorder characterized by a definite tendency to act impulsively and without consideration of the consequences; the mood is unpredictable and capricious. (ICD-10, F60.3)

The paranoid are described as "unforgiving" and the emotionally unstable as "impulsive agents."

In the proposed revision of the DSM (DSM-5, May 2010), personality disorders are generally described as involving an "impaired sense of self-identity" and a "failure to develop effective interpersonal functioning," which suggests that they are framed as failures of self-knowledge, self-directedness, and socialization.

Dementia is also defined in terms of epistemic and emotional irrationality. In the ICD-10 (F00–F09), evidence of the condition includes decline in memory and in cognitive abilities, with deterioration of judgment and thinking, and decline in emotional control and motivation. In the proposed DSM-5 (May 2010), the term "dementia" is no longer used, and replaced with "major neurocognitive disorder." Name change aside, the characteristics of the phenomenon are those we found listed in ICD-10: cognitive decline in attention, executive ability, language, learning and memory, perception and social cognition.

Delusions

In my own research I spent some time thinking about the phenomena of delusions and confabulations, which are defined respectively as unjustified beliefs and inaccurate narratives (Bortolotti 2009, 2011). Both delusions and confabulations are defined on the basis of their surface features (e.g., how people with delusions and confabulations behave) and these features are described in epistemic terms, that is, they make explicit reference to the notions of truth, rationality, justification and belief. In particular, many of the epistemic features attributed to people with delusions and confabulations constitute infringements of norms of rationality for beliefs, such as resistance to counterevidence, inconsistency, lack of evidential support, failure of action guidance, or as failures of self-knowledge, such as distorted sense of one's personal boundaries, double bookkeeping, inaccurate autobiographical narratives, and fabricated memories (Bortolotti and Cox 2009).

Here are some examples of definitions where there is no *specific* reference to etiology or to the psychiatric disorders in which delusions and confabulations occur:

> A person is deluded when they have come to hold a particular belief with a degree of firmness that is both utterly unwarranted by the evidence at hand, and that jeopardises their day-to-day functioning. (McKay et al. 2005, p. 315)

> Confabulations are typically understood to represent instances of false beliefs: opinions about the world that are manifestly incorrect and yet are held by the patient to be true in spite of clearly presented evidence to the contrary. (Turnbull et al. 2004, p. 6)

It is easy to conceive of the psychiatric disorders considered earlier (schizophrenia, personality disorders, and dementia) and of the phenomena of delusions and confabulations as mental, given the way in which they are diagnosed and classified in manuals such as the ICD and the DSM, and given the way in which they are described by clinical psychologists working on their etiology and their treatment. Although psychological testing and neurobiological techniques can contribute to a better understanding of these disorders and of phenomena such as delusions and confabulations, behavioral evidence is key to diagnosis, and the criteria are phrased in mental terms with explicit reference to the deviation from epistemic and moral norms. As Lipowski reminds us in his lecture on the future of psychiatry, Szasz insists that we should choose between *mindless* or *brainless* psychiatry, but neither approach will work in isolation.

> I would argue that neither brainless nor mindless psychiatry could do justice to the complexity of mental illness and to the treatment of patients. A comprehensive biopsychosocial approach to our field is needed. (Lipowski 1989, p. 253)

To sum up, in this section I have assessed the psychiatrist's attitude to insanity as a neurobiological dysfunction. I argued by examples that principles of classification and diagnosis informing clinical practice and even neuropsychological research into psychiatric disorders are still parasitic on the behavioral manifestations of such disorders.

RATIONALITY, SANITY, AND RESPONSIBILITY

Familiar and radical irrationalities

In the previous section I have defended the central role of irrationality in the current classificatory and diagnostic practices in psychiatry. Here I shall offer some reasons to challenge the necessity and sufficiency of irrationality for insanity.

As we saw in the assessment of Edwards's account of mental illness as persistent manifestation of irrationality, irrationality does not seem to be sufficient for mental illness. As cognitive and social psychologists have insisted for fifty years now, widespread irrationality is a feature of normal cognition and is not reserved to those who have a diagnosis of mental illness. One obvious example comes from the domain of rationality for beliefs, according to which a belief is rational if well supported by, and responsive to the available evidence. There are copious instances of beliefs that do not meet these standards of epistemic rationality, even if they are not pathological (or at least, they don't contribute to the diagnosis of a psychiatric disorder). The racist belief that members of a certain ethnic group are violent or lazy is not obviously less irrational than the delusional belief that my neighbor is a spy paid by the government to follow my movements. Beliefs about alien abductions or about nights of full moon causing accidents share many of the epistemic features of delusions. They are false, they are badly supported by the available evidence, and they are often resistant to counter-evidence or counter-argument. The reason why racist and superstitious beliefs come across as less puzzling as delusions is that they are all but uncommon beliefs and that they do not seem to cause as much distress to the person reporting them—but they are likely to be just as unsupported by evidence as delusions are (Bortolotti 2009, chapter 3).

There is a possible objection to the claim that irrationality is widespread in the non-clinical population. What if the irrationality that characterizes mental illness were different in kind from the forms of familiar irrationality I have been talking about? Edwards suggested that the irrationality typical of mental illness is persistent and severe, but others make more specific suggestions. An influential thought (that we find in the work by Greg Currie, Richard Gipps, Shaun Gallagher, Luis Sass, and German Berrios with respect to delusions) is that the type of irrationality that characterizes mental illness has to do with a failure of reality testing, or a lack of contact with reality. The idea would be that someone with a delusion, say, conflates what she imagines to be the case with what she believes (Currie 2000) or lives in a parallel reality that at times she herself perceives as distinct from the actual reality (Gallagher 2009; Sass 2001). Although these accounts of delusions make perfect sense of some of the characteristics of psychotic behavior, they do not capture the sense in which people of delusions are often strongly committed to the content of their delusions, and change their whole lives to accommodate their "new" perception of reality.

More important to our purposes here, I want to challenge the assumption that familiar, everyday irrationality does not involve losing touch with reality. Thus, I reject the alleged disanalogy between the irrationality of the clinical and of the non-clinical populations. In my understanding, any form of epistemic irrationality does involve a departure from reality. The person with racist beliefs who refuses to acknowledge evidence against the view that black waiters provide as good a service as white waiters shuts herself off from the game of evidential support that all rational believers should play. The person who is driven to act by superstitious beliefs and refuses to drive in nights of full moon by fear of accidents is blind to the counterexamples that reality provides to the alleged regularities that she lives by. These failures to engage with reality may not be always as dramatic as the presence of hallucinations and bizarre delusional experiences and beliefs, but they are on a continuum with them, and it is not a surprise that some of the biases that are responsible for the maintenance of delusions are responsible for bad reasoning in everyday cognition.

Irrationality is not even necessary for mental illness. As I briefly mentioned earlier, it has been argued that, when people are depressed, they make more accurate predictions than people who are not. This is because the statistically normal way in which predictions are made seems to be characterized by excessive optimism. The literature on depressive realism is instructive in this respect (for a review, see Abramson et al. 2002). Even if critics suggest that the phenomenon of depressive realism turns out not to apply to the clinical population (for recent evidence against the phenomenon of depressive realism, see Baker et al. 2011), it is certainly possible to imagine situations in which the reasoning tendencies partially responsible for the formation of pathological beliefs or underlying pathological behavior can have epistemic benefits with respect to the reasoning tendencies found in the non-clinical population.

For instance, psychologists find that people tend to be very conservative and fail to update beliefs that have been long disconfirmed by the evidence. Rarely are we disposed to abandon a hypothesis that we have previously regarded as true, even if robust evidence against it becomes available at a later stage (*belief persistence*). This is partly due to *confirmation biases*, according to which we tend to focus our attention on information that seems to support our initial hypothesis, and we don't search for or tend to discount information that seems to conflict with it. On the background of this phenomenon, a tendency which leads people to come to a conclusion on the basis of limited evidence, such as the jumping-to-conclusions bias, can in some contexts balance-out excessive conservatism. But jumping to conclusion has been associated with the formation of delusions, as people with delusions are found to have this bias, and among the population at risk of psychosis the presence of the bias can predict which individuals will make the transition from at-risk to psychotic (Broome et al. 2007). Such examples suggest that, if we adopt a notion of rationality that includes norms of good reasoning as its criteria, the so-called insane can be as rational as the sane, or even more so.

Failures of autonomy and moral responsibility

As it would be wrong to believe that people diagnosed with a psychiatric disorder are distinctively irrational with respect to the rest of the population, so it would be wrong to uncritically assume that people diagnosed with a psychiatric disorder are by this very fact also lacking in autonomy and responsibility for their actions. People diagnosed with psychiatric disorders do not necessarily lose the capacity to develop self-narratives and, arguably, it is this capacity that underlies autonomy, as it provides a sense of self that can shape future decisions and behavior.

> The prevailing, clinical view of schizophrenia, as reflected in the psychiatric literature, suggests both that people with schizophrenia have lost their sense of self and that they have a diminished capacity to create coherent narratives about their own lives. Drawing on our empirical research in the growing area of recovery, we describe not only the disruptions and discontinuities introduced by the illness and its social and personal consequences, but also the person's efforts to overcome these, to reconstruct a sense of self, to regain agency and to create a coherent life narrative. (Roe and Davidson 2005, p. 89)

In a recent paper discussing the effects of certain forms of psychopathology on autonomy and moral responsibility, Kennett and Matthews (2009) argue that one condition that is necessary for a person to be autonomous is the capacity to make choices and decisions that commit one's future self to certain courses of action (p. 329). Kennett and Matthews make a case for the necessity of well-functioning episodic memory for forward planning:

> M.L. suffered a severe brain injury and was in the immediate post-injury period amnesic both for events and persons as well as suffering impairments in semantic knowledge. He made a good recovery from his semantic deficits and he re-learned significant facts about his own

past. However, his recall of events from his personal past remained fragmentary. Moreover and significantly, M.L. was unable to episodically re-experience post-injury events to the same extent as control subjects, although he could use familiarity or other non-episodic processes to distinguish events he had experienced from those he had not experienced. He continued to report a feeling of subjective distance from recall of events occurring after his recovery. He displayed errors of judgement and failures to understand his responsibilities as a parent that required supervision of his behaviour and structured routines. He was unable to secure paid employment [...]. Cases such as M.L. bring out the importance of the kind of access we have to past episodes for the purposes of planning and deliberation. An effective agent is the true author of the project, fully invested in its completion, and above all she has a knowledge of it that is part and parcel of her self-knowledge. (Kennett and Matthews 2009, p. 340)

In conditions similar to that of M.L., where access to previous thoughts, commitments and experiences is lost due to memory impairments, the agent can be thinking or doing things for reasons that are not accessible to her, because relevant biographical data are not available and thus cannot inform and constrain her self-narrative. As M.L. cannot have episodic memories of events that occurred after his accident, his capacity for deliberation and his moral responsibility for his actions are both compromised. There are good reasons to believe that seriously impaired access to autobiographical information of this type and lack of narrative integration result in the loss of the capacity for self-governance.

But in other conditions, where memory is not so dramatically impaired and biographical information is available to the agent, local failures of rationality and self-knowledge do not necessarily mean that the agent cannot be held accountable or morally responsible for her actions (Bortolotti et al. 2012; Broome et al. 2010). Failures of epistemic and emotional rationality and of self-knowledge do not necessarily compromise the capacity to construct self-narratives, and thus the capacity for self-governance, but can result in decisions and actions that are not conducive to the agent's well-being. Although (trivially) you don't need to be a successful self-ruler in order to be a self-ruler, self-knowledge and rationality help you become a successful self-ruler, while lack of self-knowledge and irrationality may interfere with the exercise of the capacity for self-governance.

It has been argued that psychological well-being ensues from self-narratives that are coherent and fairly accurate representations of autobiographical events (Wilson 2002). In psychiatric disorders (such as schizophrenia and dementia) accompanied by far-fetched delusions and confabulations which are integrated in the self-narrative, a gulf between the story and reality is created. This tension might compromise social functioning, as the way in which the agent sees herself is significantly different from the way in which others see the agent, and her account of key events might also diverge from the account provided by others.

Thus, a diagnosis of a psychiatric disorder does not necessarily signal a lack of capacity for autonomy as self-governance, but serious deficits in perception and cognition (memory in particular) can compromise the capacity agents have to shape their future decisions and actions, and might lead in some cases to reduced accountability.

Conclusions and Implications

I have revisited the relationship between rationality and sanity by assessing contributions to the anti-psychiatry debate and the debate on whether psychiatry can be reduced to neurobiology. The objective was to make progress toward an understanding of psychiatric disorders that captures both what psychiatry has in common with the rest of medicine, and what is distinctive about it.

Questions of value are inevitable components of medicine. But if the role of neurobiology in the explanation of psychiatric disorders is compatible with accounting for the pathological nature of psychiatric disorders in terms of deviations of behavior from accepted norms, then the alleged disanalogy between mental and physical illness is no longer a threat to an understanding of insanity as disease. Judgments of irrationality play an important role in psychiatric classification and diagnosis, but it would be a mistake to infer from this observation that irrationality is sufficient, or even necessary for mental illness. The forms of irrationality, lack of self-knowledge, and moral failure that are referred to in the ICD and DSM and are used in clinical practice and neuropsychological research in order to demarcate psychiatric disorders are not exclusive to the mentally ill, and there are many psychiatric disorders that do not involve any significant departure from epistemic or moral norms.

The acknowledgment that there is no necessary link between insanity and irrationality has some positive consequences. First, it is compatible with the view that there is continuity between insanity and sanity, and no categorical difference between the two in terms of conformity to norms of rationality. One view of mental illness as essentially a failure of rationality and moral responsibility that sharply divides clinical and non-clinical populations has led to a conception of the mentally ill as necessarily worse parents, friends, citizens, etc. than people without. In contrast, the view that mental illness is at bottom due to a different conception of reality that society interprets as deviant has promoted the idea that there is something romantic about mental illness—as if engaging in unconventional behavior were a special instance of courage or a manifestation of freedom which deserves admiration and not repression. My impression is that stigmatization and idealization of mental illness seem less justified if the behavior of people diagnosed with a psychiatric disorder is seen as continuous with the behavior of people without such a diagnosis. Both the mentally ill and the rest of the population engage in irrational behavior, and often lose touch with reality. For instance, when we form and retain beliefs that are not well-supported by the available evidence, and when we develop self-narratives that fail to integrate life events and past experiences coherently and accurately, psychological well-being and social functioning can be compromised. People with mental illness are distinguished from the rest of the population by the extent to which contact with reality is lost and the extent of the consequences that this has for their psychological well-being and social functioning.

Second, as we saw, the idea that irrationality is a distinguishing feature of mental illness contributes to a view of the mentally ill as people who cannot make autonomous decisions or be held accountable for their actions. This is due to rationality being considered as a prerequisite for autonomy and accountability in the most influential theoretical accounts of these notions. However, the necessity of the link between mental illness and failure of autonomy should be challenged. In psychiatric disorders where capacities that are necessary to self-directedness and self-governance (e.g., autobiographical memory) are severely compromised, then doubts about autonomy legitimately emerge. Similarly, where the capacity to read the emotions of others or the capacity to feel empathy for the suffering of others cannot be exercised, then behavior that results in other people's interests being frustrated or other people being harmed seems to be morally less blameworthy. But these considerations do not apply to psychiatric disorders in general, and thus they should not appear as defining features of mental illness. Thus, the equation of insanity with lack of autonomy, accountability, or moral responsibility is to be resisted.

ACKNOWLEDGMENTS

I acknowledge the support of the Wellcome Trust Research Expenses Grant entitled "Rationality and Sanity: Implications of a Diagnosis of Mental Illness for Autonomy as Self Governance" [WT092835MF]. I am also grateful to Matthew Broome for useful discussion on the themes of the chapter, and to Richard Gipps for extensive comments on an earlier version of it.

REFERENCES

Abramson, L. Y., Alloy, L. B., Hankin, B. L., Haeffel, G. J., MacCoon, D. G., and Gibb, B. E. (2002). Cognitive vulnerability-stress models of depression in a self-regulatory and psychobiological context. In I. H. Gotlib and C. L. Hammen (Eds), *Handbook of Depression*, pp. 268–94. New York, NY: The Guilford Press.

Amador, X. and David, A. (2005). *Insight and Psychosis: Awareness of Illness in Schizophrenia and Related Disorders*. New York, NY: Oxford University Press.

American Psychiatric Association (2010), *Diagnostic and Statistical Manual of Mental Disorders* (DSM-5), proposed revision May 2010. Accessed at www.dsm5.org in April 2011.

Baker, A. G. and Msetfi, R. M., Hanley, N., and Murphy, R. A. (2011). Depressive realism: sadder but not wiser. In M. Haselgrove and L. Hogarth (Eds), *Clinical Applications of Learning Theory*, pp. 153–78. Hove: Psychology Press.

Bortolotti, L. (2009). *Delusions and Other Irrational Beliefs*. Oxford: Oxford University Press.

Bortolotti, L. (2011). Psychiatric classification and diagnosis: Delusions and confabulations. *Paradigmi*, *XXXIX*(1), 99–112.

Bortolotti, L. and Cox, R. (2009). Faultless ignorance: strengths and limitations of epistemic definitions of confabulation. *Consciousness and Cognition*, *18*(4), 952–65.

Bortolotti, L., Cox, R., Broome, M., and Mameli, M. (2012). Rationality and self-knowledge in delusions and confabulations: implications for autonomy as self-governance. In L. Radoilska (Ed.), *Autonomy and Mental Disorder*, pp. 100–22. Oxford: Oxford University Press.

Bowers, L. (1998). *The Social Nature of Mental Illness*. New York, NY: Routledge.

Broome, M. R. and Bortolotti, L. (2009). Mental illness as mental. In defence of psychological realism. *Humana Mente*, *11*, 25–44.

Broome, M. R. and Bortolotti, L. (2010). What's wrong with 'mental' disorders? [Commentary on D. Stein et al.'s "What is a mental/psychiatric disorder? From DSM-IV to DSM-V"]. *Psychological Medicine*, *40*(11), 1783–5.

Broome, M. R., Johns, L. C., Valli, I., Woolley, J. B., Tabraham, P., Brett, C., *et al.* (2007). Delusion formation and reasoning biases in those at clinical high risk for psychosis. *British Journal of Psychiatry*, *191*, s38–42.

Broome, M. R., Mameli, M., and Bortolotti, L. (2010). Moral responsibility and mental illness: a case study. *Cambridge Quarterly of Healthcare Ethics*, *19*(2), 179–87.

Currie, G. (2000). Imagination, delusion and hallucinations. *Mind & Language*, *15*(1), 168–83.

Edwards, B. (1981). Mental health as rational autonomy. *Journal of Medicine and Philosophy*, 6(3), 309–22.

Estroff, S. E., Lachicotte, W. S., Illingworth, L. C., and Johnston, A. (1991). Everybody's got a little mental illness: Accounts of illness and self among people with severe, persistent mental illnesses. *Medical Anthropological Quarterly*, 4(5), 331–69

Fulford, K. W. M. (2004). Ten principles of values-based medicine. In J. Radden (Ed.), *The Philosophy of Psychiatry: A Companion*, pp. 205–34. New York, NY: Oxford University Press.

Gallagher, S. (2009). Delusional realities. In M. R. Broome and L. Bortolotti (Eds), *Psychiatry as Cognitive Neuroscience: Philosophical Perspectives*, pp. 245–68. Oxford: Oxford University Press.

Insel, T. and Quirion, R. (2005). Psychiatry as a clinical neuroscience discipline. *Journal of the American Medical Association*, 294(17), 2221–4.

Kempe, C. H., Silverman, F. N, Steele, B. F., Droegemueller, W., and Silver, H. K. (1985). The battered-child syndrome. *Child Abuse & Neglect*, 9, 143–54.

Kennett, J. and Matthews, S. (2009). Mental time travel, agency and responsibility. In M. R. Broome and L. Bortolotti (Eds), *Psychiatry as Cognitive Neuroscience: Philosophical Perspectives*, pp. 327–50. Oxford: Oxford University Press.

Kety, S. (1974). From rationalization to reason. *American Journal of Psychiatry*, 131, 957–63.

Lipowski, Z. (1989). Psychiatry: Mindless or brainless, both or neither? *Canadian Journal of Psychiatry*, 34(3), 249–54.

Martin, J. B. (2002). The integration of neurology, psychiatry, and neuroscience in the 21st century. *American Journal of Psychiatry*, 159, 695–704.

McKay, R., Langdon, R., and Coltheart, M. (2005). Sleights of mind: Delusions, defences, and self-deception. *Cognitive Neuropsychology*, 10, 305–26.

Reynolds, C., Lewis, D., Detre, T., Schatzberg, A., and Kupfer, D. (2009). The future of psychiatry as clinical neuroscience. *Academic Medicine*, 84(4), 446–50.

Roe, D. and Davidson, L. (2005). Self and narrative in schizophrenia: time to author a new story. *Medical Humanities*, 31, 89–94.

Sass, L. (2001). Self and world in schizophrenia: Three classic approaches. *Philosophy, Psychiatry, & Psychology*, 8(4), 251–70.

Sedgwick, P. (1973). Illness: Mental and otherwise. *Hastings Center Studies*, 1(3), 19–40.

Szasz, T. (1997). *Insanity*. Syracuse, NY: Syracuse University Press.

Taylor, M. A. (1999). *The Fundamentals of Clinical Neuropsychiatry*. Oxford: Oxford University Press.

Turnbull, O., Jenkins, S., and Rowley, M. (2004).The pleasantness of false beliefs: An emotion-based account of confabulation. *Neuro-Psychoanalysis*, 6(1), 5–45.

Wakefield, J. C. (1992). The concept of mental disorder. *American Psychologist*, 47(3), 373–88.

Wilson, T. D. (2002). *Strangers to ourselves*. Cambridge, MA: Belknap Press.

World Health Organization (2010). *International Statistical Classification of Diseases and Related Health Problems 10th Revision* (ICD-10), online version. Accessed at www.who.int/whosis/icd10 in April 2011.

CHAPTER 31

....

BOUNDARY PROBLEMS: NEGOTIATING THE CHALLENGES OF RESPONSIBILITY AND LOSS

....

JENNIFER CHURCH

Many psychiatric disorders involve problems with the recognition and preservation of personal boundaries. Dramatic cases of problematic boundaries include delusions of thought insertion (where the thoughts one is experiencing are attributed to someone else), disowned limbs (where the leg that extends from one's body is not recognized as one's own), and dissociation (where several different people seem to inhabit a single body). Less dramatic, and more common, are so-called personality disorders in which the boundaries between people, or the integration within a person, is problematic in some way. Narcissists attribute all good things to themselves and all bad things to others; dependent personalities subsume their own identities under the identities of others; borderlines experience themselves as fragmented and empty; and so on. Indeed, the upcoming fifth edition of the *Diagnostic and Statistical Manual of Mental Disorders* (DSM-5) defines personality disorders as adaptive failures involving an "impaired sense of self-identity" and a "failure to develop effective interpersonal functioning."[1]

An impaired sense of self-identity can certainly contribute to failures in interpersonal relationships—as a person who is confused about herself is bound to confuse others as well, and a person who fails to respect herself is less likely to receive the respect of others. But personality disorders can also complement each other in such a way as to support successful relationships—as when a megalomaniac and a dependent personality find reassurance through each other, and are each able to function more gracefully as a result, or when

---

[1] The planned DSM-5 no longer describes personality disorders as *structural* disorders, referring instead to *adaptive* and *functional* failures. It is interesting to recall Freud's (1915/1953–1974) discussion of structural versus functional characterizations of consciousness—a discussion in which he initially favors the functional approach but ultimately concludes that the two characterizations really amount to the same thing.

two antisocial personalities relax into the undemanding companionship of each other. Furthermore, a self that is fully-integrated and clearly distinguished from others can lack the humility and the flexibility that is necessary for successful relationships. The DSM characterizes a healthy or "unimpaired" sense of self in terms of experienced uniqueness, clarity of boundaries between self and others, coherence over time, and stability of self-appraisals. Successful or "unimpaired" interpersonal functioning is characterized in terms of one's capacity for empathy and intimacy. But these two measures of mental health are in tension with one another insofar as empathy requires one to relinquish boundaries and recognize similarities rather than uniqueness, and intimacy depends on accepting (indeed, welcoming) a certain amount of incoherence and instability over time. Indeed, the person with an obsessive-compulsive personality disorder might well be regarded as someone whose commitment to clear boundaries and coherence across time undermines the development of truly intimate relationships.

Just *where* the boundaries of self should be located, and *how rigidly* those boundaries should be upheld will depend, then, on *who* else is involved in *what social context*. In a world of like-minded people who are mutually supportive, a narrowly-circumscribed sense of self with firmly-enforced boundaries may lead to a "failure to develop effective interpersonal functioning"; on the other hand, in a world governed by competition, the failure to maintain a more narrowly-circumscribed sense of self will almost certainly lead to a failure to develop effective interpersonal functioning.[2] Potter (2009) rightly questions theorists such as Edwards and Varelius (2009) who propose autonomy as the criterion of mental health. She highlights the fact that autonomy is valued more highly in the West than in the East, and more highly in men than in women. But, of course, there are many factors other than cultural and gender identities that affect the ways we value autonomy. Family contexts are different than work contexts, some family contexts are different from other family contexts, some work contexts are different than other work contexts, and so on. None of us exists within a single culture, and none of us plays a single role in the cultures we do inhabit. And even when the social expectations are relatively straightforward, sometimes it is better to accept a mismatch between self-integration and societal fit;[3] and sometimes it is better to try to change contexts rather than fit in.

The question I want to pursue is not about what counts as appropriate boundaries in different social contexts but, rather, what it is that is being negotiated when we seek to establish personal boundaries. What is at stake, both socially and phenomenologically? What changes when boundaries change? It doesn't help to respond: "our own sense of self in distinction from others"; for my question, then, becomes: What is at stake in determining our own sense of self in distinction from others? The answer I will provide focuses on assignments of responsibility and loss. It is not a very surprising answer, and it is certainly not a complete answer, but it helps to expose the lived significance of boundaries and, I argue, it helps to explain why certain symptoms of mental disorder tend to occur together. In "Section I," I relate boundaries to responsibility and loss on broadly philosophical grounds—i.e., on

---

[2] Cooperation—even cooperation with one's rivals—can sometimes help one to reach one's own goals, but the situation should no longer be characterized as competitive in such cases.

[3] Indeed, one could argue that some degree of mismatch between one's own perspective and the perspectives of others is essential for a strong sense of self and for genuinely ethical relations with others. See Mishara (2009) and Church (unpublished) on the importance of ambivalence.

the basis of philosophical understandings of responsibility, resentment, and ownership. In "Section II," I focus on borderline personality disorders to show how the list of symptoms that the DSM uses to define this disorder revolve around problematic determinations of responsibility and loss. In "Section III," I explore some implications of these observations for the understanding of some other personality disorders, and for some ongoing controversies regarding the categorization of disorders.

Section I

I have certain rights and responsibilities over what is *mine*—over my body, my house, my family, my country, and so on. I may also have rights and responsibilities regarding things that are yours—your health care, for example, or your education—but these rights and responsibilities are usually derivative from the rights and responsibilities I have with regard to what is mine: because you are part of my family I have a responsibilities to care for you, or because your education is part of my job I have a responsibility to further it.[4] A strong claim would be that my having the relevant rights and responsibilities concerning x is *constitutive* of x being mine—that a house, or a child, say, only qualifies as mine insofar as I am granted certain rights and responsibilities regarding that house, or that child. A weaker claim would be that my having the relevant rights and responsibilities concerning x is an important part of what *matters* about x being mine—that having certain rights and responsibilities regarding my house, or my child, is part of why we care that they are mine—without that care being necessary to them being mine. The more we view our social practices as the source rather than the outcome of personal identity, the more we will incline toward the stronger claim.[5] Either way, however, the practical significance of where one draws the boundaries between mine and yours is largely a matter of what rights and responsibilities accrue to me versus you.

There are important differences between what is mine and what is *me* (my house is mine, it is not me; when I sell it, I am not selling a part of myself). But insofar as the boundary between me and you helps to determine what is mine versus yours, the practical significance of interpersonal boundaries will be closely tied to the allocation of rights and responsibilities. Indeed, according to many philosophers, it is precisely by holding someone responsible that we treat them as a person.[6] When we stop praising and blaming, we cease to regard others as persons at all. (Again, a strong version of this claim maintains that our personhood is constituted by the recognition afforded us by others' praise and blame, such that we cannot be said to even achieve the ontological status of persons if we do not receive such responses (or, at least, the recognition that such responses are appropriate). A weaker version claims that our willingness to extend praise or blame is crucial to our recognition of

---

[4] There are also many negative rights and responsibilities—the right not to be enslaved, or the responsibility to allow others to pursue their lives, for example—that derive from the positive rights of others.

[5] There are a number of different ways in which social practices can contribute to the formation of a particular identity—some more direct than others, and some more influential than others. See Church (2004) for a discussion of various possibilities.

[6] This view, that reaches back to Kant, became particularly influential after the publication of Strawson's essay "Freedom and Resentment" (1976). More recent books in its defense include those by Rovane (1997) and Scher (2006).

personhood but not to the existence of personhood. On either view, though, the experiential and sociological significance of what counts as a person is closely tied to our attribution of responsibility.) To the extent that we are not responsible for a particular bodily event (the twitching of a thumb, the aching of a foot) we consider the event to be something that happens *to* us, not an event that is part *of* us. When we suppose that a three-year-old is not fully responsible for her behavior (for hitting a sister, for flirting, or for having a temper tantrum), we are supposing that the behavior is not fully a part of herself.

Jennifer Radden (1996) describes ways in which different selves can exist within a single body and explores appropriate allocations of rights and responsibilities in light of such division (conditions under which a present self may be responsible for the actions of a past or coexisting self, conditions under which a present self may have rights over a future self's options). I am approaching the connection between selves and responsibilities from the opposite direction, exploring how our assignments of responsibility (apt or unapt as they may be) help to determine the way we draw boundaries between selves. Insofar as I am not held responsible for my rudeness when stressed, or for my regression to childhood given a history of sexual abuse, then that rudeness, or that childishness, can be attributed to another self or to no self at all; they are not part of my identity.

It is not easy to specify the criteria that determine our assignments of responsibility, nor the criteria that *should* determine our assignments of responsibility (or our willingness to withhold assignments of responsibility). Oft-cited criteria include responsiveness to reasons, capacity for control, and self-directedness or autonomy. But each of these criteria is elusive in its vagueness (Responsive in what way? How much capacity? Self-directed at what stage?), they are not always compatible (responsiveness to reasons can inhibit the single-mindedness needed for control and self-direction), and these criteria are not given the same weight in all cultures (many Asian cultures, for example, are said to put a high value on self-control but a low value on autonomy[7]). As a result, we are all likely to experience some confusion about what is and what is not our responsibility as we struggle to apply the criteria we have and as we shift between different criteria and cultures. On the one hand, vague and conflicting assignments of responsibility risk leading to the feeling that we are responsible for nothing *and* for everything; on the other hand, overly-rigid interpretations of relevant criteria tend to prompt escapist behavior for which one disowns responsibility. Either way, confusions about the boundaries of responsibility feed confusions about the boundaries of self. (In "Section II," I investigate the alignment of these boundary confusions in more detail as I consider so-called "borderline personality disorders"; and in "Section III," I suggest their relevance for other personality disorders as well.)

Assignments of responsibility are inextricable from praise and blame. Praise and blame, in turn, are closely tied to feelings of admiration and pride, in the case of praise, and anger and guilt, in the case of blame.[8] In some cases, an attribution of responsibility may lead to a surge of affect; in other cases, the attempt to explain a surge of affect may lead to an attribution of responsibility. Causal connections between judgments and affects run in both directions,

---

[7] The impact of these differences on psychiatric diagnoses and treatments is nicely illustrated in Browne (2001).

[8] It is, of course, possible to express praise or blame without feeling admiration or anger. But the social practice of praise and blame, and its effectiveness, is deeply dependent on their association with such feelings.

but directed feelings or emotions require the presence of both judgment and affect. What is important for our purposes is simply this: certain feelings or emotions will co-vary with certain attributions of responsibility. Thus, because the boundaries of persons are so intimately related to the boundaries of responsibility, we should expect those who experience abnormal personal boundaries to have abnormal experiences of emotions such as anger, resentment and guilt, on the one hand, and admiration and pride, on the other. Judgments about responsibility are already embedded in feelings of anger and guilt, admiration and pride; they are a necessary part of experiencing affect as anger, guilt, admiration, or pride.

So far we have been considering how judgments of responsibility and feelings of anger, etc. are indicative of where we locate the boundaries around selves and between selves. Confusion about the boundaries of selves is understandably correlated with confusion about the allocation of responsibility, and confusion about the meaning of a surge in affect. In addition to the challenges and confusions that accompany our attempts to *ascertain* the relevant boundaries, there are challenges and confusions that result from our need to *change* the relevant boundaries. The first is the challenge of finding boundaries that make sense of who one is in relation to others, the second is the challenge of altering one's boundaries in the face of changed circumstances. A mother may or may not draw clear boundaries between herself and her child, and she may draw the boundary differently in different circumstances. That is one challenge, inextricable from judgments about responsibility. As a child grows up and leaves home, though, the boundaries between parent and child will usually change—shifting more and more responsibility onto the child, extending the parent's identity in different directions. That is another challenge, inextricable from judgments about loss. A mother who remains deeply identified with her child will experience the child's independence as a loss to herself; if, on the other hand, she is able to revise the boundaries of her own identity as the child matures, the change will not be experienced as a loss so much as a transformation. Likewise, a person who moves from lover to lover, identifying with each in turn, redrawing his boundaries accordingly, will not experience a loss of self so much as a change of self.

Judgments of what counts as a loss, like judgments of who is responsible, are not just the result of how we experience personal boundaries; they help to establish those boundaries. (Again, I am putting aside the question of whether the boundaries that we establish are the correct ones, and whether there is any standard for correctness here apart from a culture's norms.) Insofar as a parent regards a child's independence as a loss to herself, her identification with that child will be reinforced; and insofar as a lover views a breakup as a change rather than a loss, his boundaries will shift more easily. Because peer groups and cultural contexts have a large role to play in determining judgments of responsibility and judgments of loss, they also have a large role in determining how we draw the boundaries around and between people. When the end of a marriage is considered a bigger loss for the woman than for the man (despite extensive data showing that unmarried women tend to be happier than unmarried men, and married women less happy than married men[9]), it reinforces differences in how we

---

[9] Numerous studies (summarized at numerous websites) have concluded that marriage tends to improve the happiness (and health) of men more than it improves the happiness (and health) of women. A more extreme contrast was defended in Bernard (1972/1982)—namely, that married men are happier than single women, that single women are happier than married women, and single men are the least happy of all. Bernard's conclusion continues to be cited despite having been effectively discredited. Gender contrasts become more complicated, of course, when socioeconomic conditions are factored

regard the boundaries of women versus men (with women's boundaries being more encompassing) and how willing we are to see those boundaries change (more acceptable in men than in women). There is a clear sense, then, in which the boundaries of selves are socially constructed by judgments about loss as well as judgments about responsibility.

The affect corresponding to loss is grief or depression (and the affect corresponding to gain is joy or euphoria). Indeed, the presence of grief or depression is a good indication of whether a loss—of a child, a lover, a job, or an ability—is experienced as the loss of a part of oneself. Women, for a variety of socioeconomic reasons, are more prone to loss, and are more likely to experience a change in relationships as a personal loss, and they are also more likely to become depressed (and they make up the majority of those diagnosed as bipolar). There is a logical as well as an empirical correlation between more encompassing boundaries, more experiences of loss, and more depressed affects; insofar as we seek a psychological explanation, as opposed to a merely physical explanation, of a person's suffering, this trio comes as a package.

Much has been written about the differences between ordinary grief or sadness and depression. Depression is variously described as more intense, more debilitating, longer-lasting, less clear about its object, and more focused on oneself. Theories of depression, of which there are many, try to explain these differences by appeal to past versus present losses, identification and internalization of the lost object, resentment of the lost object, low self-esteem, and much else.[10] What is important here, though, is simply the existence of, and the intelligibility—indeed, the inevitability—of, a correlation between how we draw the boundaries around selves, when we experience changes as losses to those selves, and when we become sad or depressed.

While it is tempting to view depressed affect as resulting from judgments of loss, and judgments of loss as resulting from the way personal boundaries have been drawn, it is important to recognize the causality that runs in the opposite direction as well. Judgments about what does and what doesn't constitute a loss (a child leaving home, for example) can play a role in determining the boundaries of one's self; and insofar as a depressed affect serves to cut one off from a range of stimuli, and a range of interactions, it can lead to a diminished sense of self.[11] (With euphoria, in contrast, there is a heightened sensitivity to stimuli and a broadened sense of self.)

Section II

"Borderline personality disorder" is a relatively recent but now prevalent diagnosis.[12] The DSM-IV estimates that 2% of the American population, 10% of the outpatients at American

in, when different sorts of companionship are considered, and when different sorts of health problems (including mental health problems) are sorted out.

[10] A thorough and thoughtful set of essays on contrasting definitions and contrasting theories of depression can be found in Radden (2009).

[11] In Church (2002), I discuss the way in which depression "flattens" perceptions as well as emotions. Kunzendorf (2011) reports on some empirical work that supports this hypothesis.

[12] Borderline personality disorder first appeared in DSM-III as a bona fide psychiatric diagnosis in 1980. The International Classification of Disease, tenth revision (ICD-10) diagnosis of "emotionally unstable personality disorder, borderline type" may also be used.

mental health clinics, and 20% of inpatients at American psychiatric hospitals suffer from this disorder. As we shall see, its distinctive features cluster around problems with personal boundaries, problems with responsibility and loss, and problems with anger and depression. When and whether these problems constitute a "disorder" will depend on how pervasive and how lasting they are, which is at least partly determined by what resources one has—both internal and external—to correct the problem or to limit the damage. What is striking for our purposes, though, is the way that certain types of problems regularly cluster together.

The DSM-IV introduces borderline personality disorder as "a pervasive pattern of instability of interpersonal relationships, self-image, and affects, and marked impulsivity." It goes on to elaborate on these characteristics, highlighting what is distinctive about the borderline's problems with interpersonal relation, with self-image, with affect, and with impulsivity. Unlike antisocial personalities, whose relationships suffer from widespread disregard of others, borderline personalities cling to their relationships with others, fear abandonment, and feel undermined and betrayed whenever others insist on greater independence or distance. "They experience intense abandonment fears and inappropriate anger even when faced with a realistic time-limited separation or when there are unavoidable changes in plans." "These individuals can empathize with and nurture other people, but only with the expectation that the other person will 'be there' in return to meet their own needs on demand. These individuals are prone to sudden and dramatic shifts in their view of others, who may alternately be seen as beneficent supports or as cruelly punitive."[13] Unlike narcissists, whose self-image is over-rated and inflated, borderlines suffer from a fragmented, fluctuating self-image, and from chronic feelings of emptiness or an absence of self. "There are sudden and dramatic shifts in self-image, characterized by shifting goals, values, and vocational aspirations." ... "Although they usually have a self-image that is based on being bad or evil, individuals with this disorder may at times have feelings that they do not exist at all."[14]

Unlike depressive or bipolar personalities, whose despondency persists (and then lifts) for weeks at a time, borderline's moods fluctuate hour by hour. "The basic dysphoric mood of those with Borderline Personality Disorder is often disrupted by periods of anger, panic, or despair and is rarely relieved by periods of well-being or satisfaction." "Individuals with Borderline Personality Disorder frequently express inappropriate, intense anger or have difficulty controlling their anger. They may display extreme sarcasm, enduring bitterness, or verbal outbursts.... Such expressions of anger are often followed by shame and guilt ... Symptoms tend to be transient, lasting minutes or hours." Finally, unlike the impulsivity of bipolar personalities, which is high-strung and ambitious, the impulsivity of borderlines tends to be self-destructive and rebellious. "Self-mutilative acts (e.g. cutting or burning) and suicide threats and attempts are very common.... These self-destructive acts are usually precipitated by threats of separation or rejection or by expectations that they assume increased responsibility." It is this particular combination of symptoms, then—as opposed

[13] See also Potter (2009, p. 25): "For the BPD patient, the other typically is either held rigidly at bay or is viewed as another to absorb, dominate, or become. Permeable boundaries are experienced as threatening but, at the same time, the desire for recognition from the other and to fill one's emptiness propels the BPD patient into boundary disruptions."

[14] In the words of Kernberg (1977): "Borderlines can describe themselves for five hours without your getting a realistic picture of what they're like."

to relationship problems or self-image problems more generally—that constitute what has come to be known as borderline personality disorder.

"Section I" emphasized the close connection between determining personal boundaries and determining responsibility, such that problems with determining where one's self begins and ends are bound to be accompanied by problems with assigning responsibility. It is well known that children who are abused have a tendency to dissociate from the self that was abused—erecting a boundary between the "other" who was helpless in the fact of an attack and the "self" that enjoys control over its life. Given the tight connection between one's sense of self and one's sense of responsibility, identifying with the abused self is sure to trigger feelings of inadequacy, guilt, and shame ("If I was punished, I was bad," "If I wasn't loved, I wasn't lovable") that are intolerable as well as ineffectual. Dissociation from that other self is a way to avoid the crippling effects of such feelings. It should not be surprising, then, to find that many borderlines were abused or neglected as children. But rather than protectively walling off parts of themselves (as do severely dissociative personalities), borderlines find it difficult to establish any stable boundaries at all. If parts of herself are disowned, the disowning is fleeting; and if taking responsibility is uncomfortable, it is uncomfortable because of the way that it assumes separation from others rather than the way it precludes dissociation. Indeed, many borderlines come from "too perfect" families, where avoiding a clear separation between self and other may protect one from taking responsibility for a self that could only seem less than perfect in comparison.[15]

A realistic self-image requires one to include both good and bad characteristics within the boundaries of self, and within the boundaries of ones' responsibilities. The borderline personality, however, has a tendency to either idealize or demonize herself and others. A borderline is easily enamored of a happy encounter, and easily enraged by an unhappy encounter; interpersonal problems lead to hatred of others and/or hatred of oneself rather than more nuanced attempts to work through the good and the bad; and responsibility for a damaged relationship is attributed to one or the other party rather than to both together.[16] The result is an inherent instability of personal identity; when expectations of the ideal or the demonic are threatened, and when relationships are continually dissolved, the borderline will oscillate between idealizations and demonization in a doomed attempt at circumventing the complexities and ambiguities of interpersonal responsibility and loss. Gilman (1985) notes that idealizing and demonizing stereotypes function to secure self-other boundaries when inner coherence is threatened. But it is equally true that idealizing and demonizing stereotypes themselves undermine inner coherence, giving rise to a vicious cycle in which the borderline turns to stereotypes (whether positive or negative) to provide a coherent self-image only to discover the unviability of those stereotypes, prompting a need for still more stereotypes to shore up a constantly disintegrating sense of self.[17]

---

[15] Potter (2009) makes this point.

[16] Psychoanalytic theories often understand these patterns as instances of projection or introjection. Here I have tried to avoid psychoanalytic terminology and, more importantly, psychoanalytic theories about the genesis of such patterns. Judith M. Hughes (2008) makes valuable observations, from within the psychoanalytic (Kleinian) tradition, about problematic experiences of guilt and responsibility.

[17] Clarkin et al. (2006) maintain that the borderline's simplistic good-bad dichotomy is used to distinguish relationships ("dyads") as well as individuals. "Splitting is not only the stark contrast between a good self-representation and a bad object representation within the same dyad, but it is even more fundamentally the unbridgeable gap between a dyad totally imbued with negative, hateful affect and

The borderline personality is notable in experiencing any withdrawal or withholding on the part of another (however normal it may be) not only as a personal betrayal (as does the narcissist) but as a devastating abandonment—a personal betrayal, a loss to one's very self. In the absence of another person's attention and care, the borderline personality feels empty, without a self. Again, this points to a characteristic inability to establish clear lines and maintain firm boundaries between self and other; without the other, there is no self. There is some truth in this perception, of course; meaningful lives depend on meaningful relationships, and the loss of a loved one is rightly experienced as the loss of some part of oneself. Borderline's experience of (and fear of) loss is extreme, however; they have trouble distinguishing genuine losses from temporary absences or lapses in attention; and they are unable to accept and move on from the losses that do occur.

The borderline's reaction to loss (whether actual or imagined) fluctuates between anger at others and anger at oneself. Anger toward others is easy to recognize, while anger toward oneself tends to be more disguised. Certain forms of depression, for example, are usefully understood as anger turned against oneself,[18] and self-destructive behavior is often an expression of self-hatred or self-punishment.[19] As noted earlier, the borderline personality has a tendency to either idealize or demonize people, including herself. Her affective responses are, accordingly, more focused and less qualified—purer in a way—with the result that anger directed at herself (absent external controls on that anger) is very powerful indeed. On the other hand, precisely because the over-simplified character of a borderline's self-conception is inherently unstable, periods of self-loathing (especially if relieved by self-punishment) will often be compensated for by periods of self-indulgent, impulsive behavior.

Cutting oneself is one of the most widespread kinds of self-destructive behavior among borderlines, and there is clearly an element of self-loathing or self-punishment in many cases of such self-mutilation. But there are other aspects of this phenomenon that seem especially relevant to the borderline personality: (1) Cutting identifies and inscribes a bodily boundary in a context where psychic boundaries are unstable and confusing. It enables one to see, vividly and unambiguously, where one's edges are. (2) Cutting causes pain that reassures one that there is a self, a mind, an inside—contrary to a persistent feeling that one lacks a self, or that one's insides are "empty." (3) Cutting is an assertion of power and agency, a rather violent reclaiming of one's right and one's ability to prevail over the domain that is one's body.[20]

---

one imbued with positive, loving affect.... This dissociation serves the defensive purpose of protecting each dyad from contamination or destruction by the other.... It may at first be less clear why the hateful dyad should be protected, but in borderline pathology a clear and unadulterated sense of hatred can provide a temporary respite from the confusion of identity diffusion and can protect against guilt feelings (attributions of responsibility) that could stem from the patient's own aggression towards what is at other times the good object" (pp. 56–57).

[18] Radden (2009), though, notes an absence of self-loathing in non-Western occurrences of depression.

[19] There is an important difference; however, between behavior that aims at self-destruction (suicidal behavior) and behavior that disregards the self-destructive implications of one's behavior (various kinds of substance abuse).

[20] Noted in McLane (1996). This function of cutting has interesting relations to Freudian theories of hysteria according to which social problems outside of one's control are displaced onto one's body.

In addition to showing something about the logic that unites the borderlines' symptoms, the analysis I have developed, described earlier, may help to explain why 75% of borderlines are female. For being a woman makes one a more likely recipient of conflicting, and therefore confusing, messages about responsibility and loss. Women are granted less control over their lives but are also blamed for more that is outside of their control. Women are alternately idealized and demonized—the perfect mother versus the despicable whore syndrome. A woman's anger at second-class status is inevitable but a woman's anger is not socially acceptable. A woman is supposed to extend her boundaries to include others and a woman is supposed to stay out of the way of others. Being a woman brings, in its wake, an interlocking set of problems concerning personal boundaries, the assignment of responsibility, and the negotiation of loss—precisely the problems that go into creating borderline personalities.[21]

Section III

In "Section I," we saw how problems with personal boundaries, problems with the assignment of responsibility, and problems dealing with loss are *logically* related to each other, and in "Section II" we saw how this set helps to make sense of an *empirical* list of symptoms that are attributed to borderline personalities. In general, it is helpful to discover the logic behind the way people act, and it is helpful to find the unity behind an otherwise disjointed set of symptoms. On the other hand, it is possible to regard people as acting more rationally than they do, and it is possible to view symptoms as more unified than they are. There are dangers of over-interpretation and over-unification, and there are dangers of under-interpretation and fragmentation.[22]

These dangers, easily recognizable on a theoretical level, can also be dangerous at a practical level. Over-interpretation can encourage one to justify rather than abandon harmful tendencies and, in more extreme cases, can contribute to psychosis or schizophrenia insofar as it requires one to fill in the gaps in one's narrative with various sorts of confabulations.[23] Under-interpretation, on the other hand, can feed one's despair at being out of control and, in more extreme cases, can contribute to dissociative and borderline disorders insofar as it fails to support a stable and integrated sense of self. (I do not mean to suggest that over-interpretation is a common cause of schizophrenia; only a potential contributor. Developing fuller interpretations can sometimes be very helpful to schizophrenics and psychotics.) How highly "medicalized" physiological explanations of mental problems fare with respect to these opposed dangers is an interesting and important question. On the one hand,

---

[21] Many of the cited contradictions are applicable to the poor and to other second-class citizens as well. Correlations between personality disorders and poverty are hard to measure, however, since the poor are less likely to have access to social services and, perhaps, because they have fewer options, their outsider status is more likely to lead to psychosis.

[22] Graham (2010) defends the attribution of "truncated rationality"—looking for what is rational about disordered minds while recognizing that their (and our) rationality is always incomplete and faulty.

[23] See Aviv (2010) for an interesting set of observations and reflections on this topic.

they offer explanations that are highly unified; on the other hand, they forego the attempt to discern a *rational* unity in one's experiences, thereby abandoning traditional means of establishing the unity of a *self*. Do those who suffer from a fragmented sense of self experience more or less unity when they accept physiological explanations of their condition?

Finding a way between these dangers—the danger of false fragmentation and the danger of false unification—is a challenge for any attempt at understanding people (oneself or another, the sane or the insane), and it is at the forefront of ongoing disputes over announced changes in the next DSM. The new DSM proposes to reduce the number of categories under which problematic symptoms are listed while lengthening the list of symptoms within each category. On the face of it, this encourages a more unified understanding of a wider range of patient symptoms. In reaching a diagnosis, however, practitioners are supposed to register applicable symptoms from a variety of lists and be more willing to assign cross-categorical identities to their patients. Using the new DSM, a patient that was formerly categorized as simply bipolar (despite less than perfect conformity to the current bipolar list), might now be categorized as having significant bipolar tendencies and significant antisocial tendencies and somewhat less significant obsessive-compulsive tendencies, for example. Diagnoses are more individually tailored on this approach, but they also encourage a more fragmented view of personalities and persons. The ongoing controversy over these proposed changes largely revolves around the question of whether dysfunctional personalities usually conform to recognizable types, or whether the problematic tendencies of dysfunctional personalities tend to be highly idiosyncratic and fragmented. This controversy is intertwined with a long-standing controversy over the Gestalt judgments of clinicians (i.e., those who spend most of their time talking with their patients) versus the statistical findings of researchers. Given the way that major funding is now largely dependent on statistical research, it is not surprising that the outlook of the researchers has prevailed over the outlook of the clinicians. More submerged but equally important, I think, is an ethical and practical controversy over whether categorizing people—in particular, people who are social misfits—in terms of personality types is helpful or harmful. Giving a name to an otherwise puzzling combination of problems can be a great relief; it can encourage one to seek appropriate treatment and to seek out fellow-sufferers. But naming can also function as a stigma, and it can encourage greater passivity in the face of life's problems.

One alternative to the DSM approach that has generated some excitement promises to locate otherwise disparate symptoms and otherwise disparate personality types along a single continuum. The so-called "autism spectrum," for example, which has been familiar for some time, understands various aspects of Asperger's syndrome (including seemingly anomalous "savant" aspects) as manifestations of a less extreme form of the same disabilities that constitute full-fledged autism. More recently, it has been hypothesized that the very same spectrum extends through normal to its opposite extreme in schizophrenia.[24] This hypothesis is underwritten, in part, by neurological findings that suggest a deficit of neural connections on the part of autistic people and a surfeit of neural connections on the part of schizophrenic people. (The same hypothesis gains support from psychological observations as well: autistic people become fixed on the details while schizophrenic people can't stay focused, autistic people lack imagination while schizophrenic people do too

[24] See, for example, Crespi and Badcock (2008).

much imagining.[25]) Likewise, the manic–depressive continuum has been familiar for some time, but a more recent hypothesis positions schizophrenia at an opposite pole from depression, arguing that the schizophrenic occupies a perspective that is almost purely subjective and in-the-body while the depressive occupies a perspective that is almost purely objective and outside-the-body (and where being normal requires one to occupy a position that combines both perspectives).[26] What is noteworthy about these spectrum hypotheses, in the context of our earlier discussion of DSM categorizations, is their ability to break out of the too-much-unity versus too-little-unity dilemma. Different symptom groups are unified as manifestations of a single position along a given continuum, but divisions and labels along that continuum are viewed as rather arbitrary ways of marking an infinitely divisible spectrum of possibilities. Problematic symptoms do fit together to form intelligible wholes, but those wholes do not coalesce around discrete personality types; rather symptoms are united by locating their source at a particular point along a physiological or existential continuum.

The approach that I have pursued in this chapter is somewhat different again. I have highlighted the importance of certain interconnections between the establishment of personal boundaries, the allocation of responsibility, and the experience of loss. These are, broadly speaking, rational or constitutive relations.[27] (It is rational to allocate responsibility for thoughts and actions that are part of oneself; one's self is at least partly constituted by what one experiences as a loss; and so on.) We are not always rational, of course, nor is our society, but because we all need to negotiate boundaries, responsibilities and losses across a wide range of circumstances, it is helpful to recognize how problems in any one of these areas are likely to generate problems in the others as well. In "Section II," I used the symptoms associated with borderline personality disorder to illustrate this point. Ultimately, though, I am not concerned with establishing the unity or the legitimacy of a "borderline personality" diagnosis[28] so much as I am concerned with showing how some seemingly unrelated symptoms are indicative of an interlocking set of difficulties. Furthermore, I suggest (but won't try to argue here) that many of the same difficulties underlie other disorders on the DSM list. Bipolar disorder, for example, might also be understood as a distinctive sort of solution to the problem of determining boundaries, responsibilities, and losses—namely, a "solution" in which one repeatedly alternates between overly-narrow and overly-wide construals of personal boundaries, responsibilities, and losses. And narcissism (a category that is about to be dropped from the DSM[29]) might be understood as a stance that solves these same challenges by refusing to acknowledge one's own boundaries, responsibilities, and

---

[25] See Fujii et al. (2009), Jansen (2005), and Sack et al. (2005).

[26] Kraus (1980) understands depressive as too stuck in social role/body-as-object while schizophrenic is too stuck in subjective/being body. Cutting (1999) proposes the opposite; Mishara (2009) notes the conflict between these two views, but agrees that mental health depends on incorporating both perspectives and tolerating the ambivalence—something that can be achieved to different degrees. See also Fuchs (2005) and Ratcliffe et al. (2009) for more recent discussions of how different ways of being in one's body might be indicative of different types of mental problems.

[27] I would prefer the term "reasonable" to "rational"; see Church (1987).

[28] Elsewhere (2004), I have suggested that it is probably a socially constructed category and open, therefore, to pragmatic arguments for or against its continuation.

[29] Critics of this change have wondered whether our society is now more accepting—more encouraging, even—of narcissistic personalities; also, whether we are more reluctant to pathologize personality types that are predominantly male.

losses.[30] If this is right, then, as the continuum hypotheses suggest, a variety of disorders can be seen as alternate responses to a single challenge. Unlike the continuum hypotheses mentioned earlier, however, the unifying thread is not a one-dimensional problem (the problem of balancing focus and free-association, or the problem of balancing subjective and objective perspectives) but rather a three-dimensional problem (the problem of setting stable but not overly-ridged boundaries, the problem of attributing enough but not too much responsibility, and the problem of recognizing some but not all change as loss).

I am not in a position to make any specific recommendations about the categorization of, or the treatment of mental disorders. I would, however, like to close with two broad reminders concerning the background within which we determine boundaries, responsibilities, and losses. First, it is important to realize how much happens that is not a part of any one person's identity, or any one person's responsibility, or any one person's losses. My identity does not always compete with yours, your responsibilities do not always alleviate me of mine, and your gains are not always my losses. There are many important contexts in which we share identities, responsibilities, and losses; and there are many important contexts in which no one's identity is at stake, no one is responsible, and no one sustains a loss. Given the very real challenges of negotiating identity, responsibility, and loss, and the very real suffering that results from failure to negotiate these things successfully, it is good to remember that much of life and much of what matters to us—simple pleasures, the riches of nature, the power of art—falls outside of this domain. Second, bad as it is to suffer from a mental disorder, it may sometimes be preferable to normal functioning (and, indeed, is often reported as preferable by those who suffer from mental disorders)—preferable to the individual on account of the pleasures and the insights that may be inextricably tied to the disorder, and preferable to the society at large insofar as that individual forces us to rethink our own boundaries, responsibilities, and losses.

ACKNOWLEDGMENTS

Relevant pleasures include the pleasure of relinquishing responsibilities, and relevant insights include the insights that accrue from remaining outside of mainstream society. I am grateful to Richard Gipps for raising good questions and making helpful suggestions about this and many other points in this essay.

REFERENCES

Aviv, R. (2010). Which way madness lies. *Harpers, December*, 35–46.

Bernard, J. (1972). *The Future of Marriage* (2nd edn 1982). New Haven, CT: Yale University Press.

Browne, K. (2001). Sakit Jiwa, Ng(amuk), and schizoaffective disorder in a Javanese Woman. *Culture, Medicine, and Psychiatry*, 25(4), 411–25.

---

[30] To fill out this suggestion, quite a lot would have to be said about what I mean by "acknowledge." Important and rich explications of the notion can be found in Cavell (1979), Fingarette (1969), and Moran (2001).

Cavell, S. (1979). *The Claim of Reason*. Oxford: Oxford University Press.

Church, J. (1987). Reasonable irrationality. *Mind*, 96(3), 354–66.

Church, J. (2002). Depression, depth, and the imagination. In J. Phillips and J. Morris (Eds), *Imagination and its Pathologies*, pp. 335–60. Cambridge, MA: MIT Press.

Church, J. (2004). Making order out of disorder: On the social construction of madness. In J. Radden (Ed.), *The Philosophy of Psychiatry: A Companion*, pp. 393–407. Oxford University Press.

Church, J. (unpublished manuscript). *On the Moral Significance of Emotional Ambivalence*. Presented at the CSMN Research Center, Oslo, Norway, 2008.

Clarkin, J. F., Yeoman, F. E., and Kernberg, O. F. (2006). *Psychotherapy for Borderline Personality: Focussing on Object Relations*. Washington, DC: American Psychiatric Publishing.

Crespi, B. and Badcock, C. (2008). Psychosis and autism as diametrical disorder of the social brain. *Behavioral and Brain Sciences*, 31(3), 241–61.

Cutting, J. (1999). Morbid objectification in psychopathology. *Acta Psychiatrica Scandinavica, Supplement*, 395, 30–3.

Edwards, C. (2009). Ethical decisions in the classification of mental conditions as mental illness. *Philosophy, Psychiatry, & Psychology*, 16(1), 73–90.

Fingarette, H. (1969). *Self-Deception*. Abingdon: Routledge Press.

Freud, S. (1953–1974). The unconscious. In *Standard Edition of The Collected Works of Sigmund Freud, Vol XIV* (J. Strachey, Ed.), pp. 166–215. London: The Hogarth Press. (Original work published 1915.)

Fuchs, T. (2005). Overcoming dualism. *Philosophy, Psychiatry, & Psychology*, 12(2), 115–17.

Fujii, D., Aleman, A., and Laroi, F. (2009). Just my imagination running away with me. *Journal of Clinical and Experimental Neuropsychology*, 31(7), 893–6.

Gilman, S. (1985). *Difference and Pathology: Stereotypes of Sexuality, Race and Madness*. Ithaca, NY: Cornell University Press.

Graham, G. (2010). *The Disordered Mind: An Introduction to Philosophy of Mind and Mental Illness*. Abingdon: Routledge.

Hughes, J. M. (2008). *Guilt and its Vicissitudes: Psychoanalytic Reflections on Morality*. New York, NY: Routledge.

Jansen, J. (2005). On the development of Husserl's transcendental phenomenology of imagination and its use for interdisciplinary research. *Phenomenology and the Cognitive Sciences*, 4(2), 121–32.

Kernberg, O. (1977). The structural diagnosis of borderline personality organization. In P. Hartocollis (Ed.), *Borderline Personality Disorders*, pp. 87–122. New York, NY: International Universities Press.

Kraus, A. (1980). Bedeutung und Rezeption der Rollentheorie in der Psychiatrie. In U. H. Peters (Ed.), *Die Psychologie des 20. Jahrhunderts, Vol X*, pp. 125–45. Zurich: Kindler.

Kunzendorf, R. G. (2011). Depression, unlike normal sadness, is associated with a "flatter" self-perception and a "flatter" phenomenal world. *Imagination, Cognition, and Personality*, 30(4), 447–61.

McLane, J. (1996). The voice on the skin: Self-mutilation and Merleau-Ponty's theory of language. *Hypatia*, 11(4), 107–18.

Mishara, A. L. (2005). Body self and its narrative representation in schizophrenia. In H. DePreester and V. Knowckaert (Eds), *Body Image and Body Schema*, pp. 127–52. Amsterdam: John Benjamins.

Mishara, A.L. (2009) Human Bodily Ambivalence: Precondition for Social Cognition and ITs Disruption in Neuropsychiatric Disorders. *Philosophy, Psychiatry, & Psychology* 16(2): 133–7.

Moran, R. (2001). *Authority and Estrangement: An Essay on Self-Knowledge.* Princeton, NJ: Princeton University Press.

Potter, N. N. (2009). *Mapping the Edges and the In-Between: A Critical Analysis of Borderline Personality Disorder.* Oxford: Oxford University Press.

Radden, J. (1996). *Divided Minds and Successive Selves: Ethical Issues in Disorders of Identity and Personality.* Cambridge, MA: MIT Press.

Radden, J. (2009). *Moody Minds Distempered: Essays on Melancholy and Depression.* Oxford: Oxford University Press.

Ratcliffe, M. and Varga, S. (2009). Feelings of being: Phenomenology, psychiatry, and the sense of reality. *Phenomenology and the Cognitive Sciences,* 8(4), 607–11.

Rovane, C. (1997). *The Bounds of Agency.* Princeton, NJ: Princeton University Press.

Sack, A. T, van de Ven, V., Etschenberg, S., Schatz, D., and Linden, D. E. (2005). Enhanced vividness of mental imagery as a trait marker of schizophrenia? *Schizophrenia Bulletin,* 31(1), 97–104.

Scher, G. (2006). *In Praise of Blame.* Oxford: Oxford University Press.

Strawson, P. F. (1976). *Freedom and Resentment and Other Essays.* Abingdon: Routledge.

Varelius, J. (2009). Defining mental disorder in terms of our goals for demarcating mental disorders. *Philosophy, Psychiatry, & Psychology,* 16(1), 35–52.

CHAPTER 32

ORDERING DISORDER: MENTAL DISORDER, BRAIN DISORDER, AND THERAPEUTIC INTERVENTION

GEORGE GRAHAM

There once was a man who aimed to compose a general theory of mental disorder or illness.[1] When given the opportunity, the man would appear at professional conferences and offer his theory.

In stating his theory he began by providing for his audience a list in PowerPoint of illnesses, disorders, or diseases. Some one hundred conditions appeared on the list. The list named such disorders as the following: addiction, agoraphobia, Alzheimer's disease, clinical depression/major depressive disorder, diabetes, epilepsy, ergotism (a type of poisoning that causes gangrene), Parkinson's disease, polycythemia vera, post-traumatic stress disorder, and ninety other afflictions. He said that some of the disorders on the list (such as major depressive disorder and post-traumatic stress disorder) were mental disorders or illnesses, others not. Some (like diabetes and ergotism) were bodily aliments or somatic disorders.

He then offered a theory about those cases that he said were cases of mental disorder or illness. He never offered the same theory at any two distinct conferences, however. In fact, he proposed conflicting theories at different conferences. At one conference, he said that a mental disorder is a disease with law-like patterns of progression and precise lines separating it from normal variations in human mental health. While at another he called mental disorder a culturally relative and intractably arbitrary social construct. At two other conferences, he called it, alternately, a type of brain or neurological disorder, and, then, at a fourth conference, a morally odious myth reference to which must be expunged from a properly scientific theory of mind and behavior. At still other conferences he made still other claims, offered still other theories. None were consistent with the others.

---

[1] I use "mental disorder" and "mental illness" interchangeably.

The man's utterly bizarre activity elicited the curiosity of an editor of a distinguished interdisciplinary journal, who was prone to attend conferences and liked to listen to talks on theories of mental disorder. When she inquired of the man, "To what final set of claims are you committed?," he replied that he was aiming for a perfectly *general* theory that would encompass all such claims. He said that the only way in which to achieve a truly general theory is to make many different and conflicting claims and then conjoin them by use of the word "and." He said he called his theory the Conjunction Theory of Mental Disorder. He promised to publically commit to all of the conjuncts at some future conference. The editor silently intended to avoid the occasion.

Gilbert Ryle once remarked that to say of a person that he enjoys digging "is to say that he [digs] with his whole heart in this task." "His digging [is] his pleasure" (Ryle 1949, p. 108). Well, no doubt, the man who aspired to construct a Conjunction Theory of Mental Disorder enjoyed his task, with his whole heart, but, of course, he was digging a conceptually bottomless pit. Into a category in which all theories are deposited, no matter how contrarian or incompatible with each other, none are saved or distinguished.

If we are to have a general theory of mental disorder or illness, if we are to possess an account of what a mental disorder is, we must be concertedly critical and diligently discriminatory. We must order disorder. We must dissent from unpromising theories and save and work only within promising ones. The catch, of course, is which is which and just how to tell the difference between them.

My intent in this essay is to defend dissent from one of the claims or theories about mental illness or disorder mentioned earlier. This is the claim that a mental disorder is a type of brain or neurological disorder. It is the thesis that any disturbance or condition that qualifies as a mental disorder or illness is, in its nature or foundation, a brain disorder—a kind of disorder of the brain and central nervous system. So, for example, if mental disorders are a type of brain disorder then disorders like major clinical depression and post-traumatic stress disorder (which presumably are mental disorders) are the same general type of disorder as, say, disorders like epilepsy, Parkinson's, and Alzheimer's (which presumably are brain disorders). They are a type of brain or neurological disorder.

The thesis is popular. Instances or versions of it often appear in the literature. One, in fact, appeared at the founding of the journal of the *Archives for Psychiatry and Nervous Disease* in 1867 by Wilhelm Griesinger. In an opening editorial Griesinger wrote that "so-called 'mental illnesses' are really ... illnesses of the nerves and brain" (quoted in Bentall 2004, p. 150).

In recent years, with neuroscience now a major influence in psychiatry, the claim that a mental disorder actually is a brain disorder has become increasingly frequent. The clinical neurologist Michael Allen Taylor writes: "[A] mental illness is not 'mental' at all, but the behavioral disturbance associated with brain dysfunction and disease" (Taylor 1999, p. viii). Taylor's claim possesses at least one ambiguity (what does he mean by "associated"?). But the thrust of his claim is clear: Mental disorder, thy name is brain disorder.

Though the argument of my essay is negative or critical, its lesson, I hope, is positive and constructive. What I want to suggest is that one important consequence of denying that mental disorders are brain disorders is that this helps to identify, construct, or make categorical elbow room for a distinctive domain or class of disorders or illnesses viz., conditions of mind and behavior that truly deserve to be called *mental* disorders or illnesses. By "distinctive" I do not mean a domain or class that necessarily precludes borderline or hybrid cases, viz., cases that are part mental disorder; part something else entirely.

I mean a type of disorder that can be reasonably demarcated from other phenomena—from non-disorders as well as from non-mental disorders—at least in prototypical or exemplary instances (see Graham 2010, 2013). I also do not mean a domain with empirical or epistemological credentials that are a priori guaranteed. I mean a domain that we *currently* have good reason to believe exists and is available for the application of the concept of a mental disorder and for theories of mental disorder that do not privilege brain science. In particular, a domain in which mental disorders or illnesses insofar as they are mental possess proximate or immediate causes or aspects of their causal explanatory foundations that in our current epistemic existential situation are best described (in robust part) in the language of psychology or mentality and without fear of displacement, elimination or evisceration by neuroscience (see Graham 2010, 2013; see also Graham in press; Graham and Stephens 2007).

Earnest and elaborate efforts to devise a characterization or concept of mental disorder are always being engaged. The most promising, in my judgment, share a common premise. This is that the most sound and sensible reason for having a concept or characterization of mental disorder is as follows: We need to explain, predict, understand and treat certain forms of human behavior in terms of it. We need to refer to mental disorders. Applicability of a characterization of mental disorder is a matter of overall evidential fit, however. So, if given a total assemblage of evidence for the application of a concept of mental disorder, alternative concepts to that of a mental disorder (for example, the alternative concept of a brain disorder or neurological illness) fit better than talk of mental disorder, there may be no alternative save giving up talking about mental disorders. Constructing epistemic elbow room for a domain of mental disorder that does not identify mental disorders with brain disorders is not enough to warrant application of the concept of a mental disorder; it is at most a necessary condition.

My course in the chapter is as follows. I shall proceed by first stating why some theorists believe or claim that mental disorders are brain disorders or disorders of the brain. Then, I shall criticize the hypothesis that just because the brain is the existential material base of a mental disorder, which I assume is true, means or implies that mental disorders are disorders of the brain. As the argument unfolds, I shall briefly describe the very idea of a brain disorder as this concept appears in the medical scientific field of neurology. I assume that the field of neurology encompasses all of the sciences of the brain that are germane to describing *being a brain disorder*. These include neuroanatomy (which studies the structural components of the brain), neurochemistry, neurobiology, and neurodynamics (which study, respectively, the molecular, biological, and electrical foundations of behavior), and neuropsychology (which attempts to localize mental activity in particular neural processes or systems). I shall conclude by describing how a distinction between mental and brain disorder may be supported, at least if only in part, by interpreting and distinguishing between the patterns of success and failure of different sorts of therapies or treatments for a behavioral disturbance or affliction.

Just what general type or class of disorder a disorder or illness is, whether, specifically, it is mental or neural, may be discoverable, in some measure, by learning how effectively or ineffectively to reconstruct or rebuild a person's mental health and psychological well-being. The successful applications of certain types of reconstruction may suggest that a disturbance in question is a mental disorder. Successful applications of other types may suggest that a disturbance is a brain disorder.

I

To begin with, suppose the following: You are a psychiatrist. A disturbed patient sits before you in your clinic, exhibiting signs of a possible mental disorder or illness. Do they really have a mental disorder or illness? Or do they suffer from some other sort of afflicted condition or illness entirely?

Consider the following diagnostic answer:

> (MD) This person sitting before you in the clinic is the subject of a mental disorder or illness.

A claim like (MD), a claim of mental disorder, is made true by the condition or state of mind and behavior of the person who is the subject of the diagnosis, viz., a condition in virtue of which the diagnosis is true—when it is true. Call the truth maker for any medical diagnosis a *diagnostic truth maker*.[2]

Are mental disorders a subset or species of brain disorder? Is being a brain disorder part of the diagnostic truth maker for being a mental disorder?

If mental disorders are a type of brain disorder, then part of the diagnostic truth maker for being a mental disorder is being a brain disorder. Nothing is a mental disorder unless it is a brain disorder.

I, for one, as indicated earlier, believe that being a brain disorder is not part of the diagnostic truth maker for being a mental disorder.[3] In saying that being a brain disorder is not part of the diagnostic truth maker for being a mental disorder, I do not mean that the brain or central nervous system is not the existential base of a mental disorder. Mental disorders are physically based, realized, or implemented in the brain and central nervous system. Or so I assume. But I do mean that if a condition is a mental disorder, properly so-called, then the subject's brain is not damaged, diseased, or disordered. It is not ill, sick, defective, injured, contaminated, or mechanically or chemically malfunctioning. So, mental illnesses or disorders are not brain disorders or diseases. They are based in the brain, or *in* the brain, as I like to put it, but not *of* the brain. They are not instances of a disordered brain.

So, why claim to the contrary that mental disorders are a subset or type of brain disorder? The attraction of some theorists to this subset thesis must be strong given the language in which certain individuals endorse it and their impatience with anything contrary.

The main source of attraction seems to be a fear of the scientific implications of metaphysical dualism, which, it is assumed, is not a theoretical option for an empirically informed and systematically integrated medical science (see Vogeley and Newen 2009). So understood, the fear is that unless mental disorders are classifiable as a type of brain disorder, then minds

---

[2] Diagnostic truth makers exist at different levels of specificity or determinacy. The determinable of being a mental disorder, for example, may be exemplified in any number of determinate or individual types of mental disorders.

[3] Various other theorists also deny that mental disorders are (or must be) brain disorders (Arpaly 2005; Poland, in press). I may be alone, however, in making the denial central to a large-scale theory of mental disorder (Graham 2010, 2013a, in press; Graham and Stephens 2007; Stephens and Graham 2009a). I make no effort in the present chapter to describe or even to outline the large-scale theory. Aside from reasons of space, this is because the denial that mental disorder is a type of brain disorder, I believe, is defensible independent of commitment to that theory.

and brains can, to use a crisp metaphor of Fred Dretske appropriated from another context, "march off in different directions" (Dretske 1988, p. ix). And that (it is assumed) is scientifically unacceptable.

But suppose we reject metaphysical dualism. Suppose we assume (as I do) that mental disorders are physically based or realized and not themselves something inherent in a non-physical substance. To assume that a mental disorder possesses a physical or neurophysical base does not to require that the disorder requires classification as a brain disorder. A mental disorder may have an existential physical platform *in* the brain without being a disorder *of* the brain. It is, I believe, only after we have a better understanding of what is to be explained in the explanation of disorders, and in particular whether the causal explanation of mental disorders, properly so-called, is to be conducted in the same terms as the causal explanation of brain disorders, that we will be able to appreciate that just because a disorder is in the brain does not mean it is a brain disorder or of the brain.

To appreciate this logical or conceptual point as well as to illustrate how an "in/of" distinction may be used when talking about disorder, consider five analogies. Neither is precisely like the in/of distinction that I make for brain and disorder, or like one another, for that matter, but the set of five expresses the spirit of the distinction. The distinction's conceptual relevance to the negative thesis of this chapter will be specified momentarily.

Suppose I am traveling through Paris, Texas. I am spending the night in a motel there. I have my travel alarm clock with me. The timing mechanism in the clock fails to show the correct time in Paris, Texas, however, for I had earlier set it for Atlanta, Georgia, my point of departure (which is in another time zone). I have not reset it for Texas. So, an incorrect time is registered *in* the clock, although this does not mean that there is a physical malfunction *of* the clock. It does not mean that the clock is damaged. Quite the contrary, my clock works well.

I am staying in a room that has an external entrance from the parking lot. Its door is equipped with a door bell. In normal circumstances, the ring of the doorbell carries the information that someone is at the door. But suppose a squirrel somehow pushes the doorbell button. The ring does not indicate that someone is at the door. The bell is failing to do what it is designed or supposed to do. There is no short circuit of the wiring, however. The wiring is in perfectly good working order. But the wrong information is contained in the ring.

I have brought my computer laptop with me. The motel has a WiFi hotspot. I am trying to use my laptop to make motel reservations for my final destination, which is San Diego, California. Alas, the computer's reservations-making software program possesses an annoying glitch or malfunction. Each time I type the word "Diego," it processes this as "Francisco." So, I am having trouble completing the reservation. The software program is running *in* the hardware or physical machine states of the computer, of course. However, just because the program is in the hardware does not mean that the computer has a disorder *of* the hardware. The hardware mechanism is not impaired. Rather, the reservations software is not functioning correctly.

In the lobby of the motel sits a newly pregnant woman, complaining of nausea. She is suffering from morning sickness. Morning sickness is a bodily condition, no doubt—a condition in the soma or body. But this does not necessarily mean that the woman's body is biologically unhealthy, has broken down, or is diseased. Not only is it quite normal to feel morning sickness, when pregnant, but, except in severe cases, as when, for example, serious dehydration occurs (say, because of protracted vomiting), it may express a proper or healthy bodily function in biological or adaptational terms. Morning sickness may be an evolutionary adaptation that protects first-trimester fetuses from food poisoning (Profet 1992). It may be a "healthy" defense mechanism, nothing inescapably pathological, and not a true somatic sickness per se, except in severe instances, such as when the defense mechanism itself, for whatever reason, overshoots its designed or adaptational function.[4]

The woman's husband currently is not in the motel with her. He is rowing a boat on a nearby lake. He has never been on a lake before or rowed a boat. To his surprise when he places a straight oar down in the water, it appears bent at the point at which it meets the surface of the water. Unbeknownst to him the human visual system fails to compensate for the optical effect of refraction. It furnishes him with misinformation, yet this does not mean that the system is functioning improperly or damaged. It means that the failure to furnish proper information about a perfectly straight oar takes place in the system. Not that there is disease or damage of the system.

The shared point behind mentioning the above five examples is this: "Disorders" or failures in an X (clock, doorbell, computer, soma, visual system, or then also, I argue, brain), should not be assumed to be disorders of an X (clock, etc.) without independent or additional argument. We must distinguish the question of where something occurs or is housed or inheres from the distinct question of whether the "house" itself is in good and proper working order. So, therein, a person may conceivably suffer from a mental disorder that is in the brain or is, in some sense, neurally (neurobiologically/neurochemically/neurodynamically) based or inherent, but this does not *necessarily* mean that the disorder is a brain deficit, illness, dysfunction, or disease. Physicalistic basal sentiment, depending upon its causal explanatory details, permits explanatory or categorical elbow room for disentangling the very idea of a mental disorder from that of a brain disorder.

Nancy Andreasen recognizes the temptation to believe that if a disorder of mind and behavior is brain based, then this must mean that something is wrong (broken, damaged, etc.) within the brain and she yields to it. Andreasen writes: When "cells in our brains go bad [this is] expressed at the level of systems such as attention and memory" and in such disorders as "schizophrenia and depression" (Andreasen 2001, p. 7). For Andreasen a mental disorder is a type of brain disorder, i.e. a condition that is a disorder or illness both in and of the brain, and possessed of psychological and conscious symptoms. (Brain disorders without psychological symptoms, if there are any, for Andreasen apparently fail to qualify as mental disorders period.) Just when a brain disorder or case of brain damage or malfunction has symptoms of a psychological or conscious sort, it makes good sense, Andreasen suggests, to maintain that the condition is a mental disorder.

Do the psychological symptoms or behavioral effects of neural damage alone constitute a mental disorder? One problem with Andreasen's suggestion is that the domain of mental disorder is inadequately specified by assuming, as she does, that the presence of psychological symptoms suffices as warrant or evidence for attribution of a mental illness (that is supposed also to be a brain disorder or reflection of brain damage). Closed head injuries may produce blurred vision, headaches, irritability, and depression (psychological symptoms), but they are not for this reason in the domain of mental disorder or illness. Numerous other

---

[4] The key assumption in assuming that morning sickness may be something healthy is that some plants are laced with toxins to prevent ingestions by predators and such toxins are, of course, a problem for a developing fetus. So it is "natural" or adaptational for a pregnant female to develop an aversion to toxins in various foods in order to protect the fetus.

counterexamples to Andreasen's suggestion may also be cited. Progressive visual blindness (a psychological symptom) due to causes such as macular degeneration, glaucoma, or diabetic retinopathy is another. For help with such conditions one consults an ophthalmologist, not a psychiatrist.

Suppose mental disorders are understood in the style or manner of the third edition of the *Diagnostic and Statistical Manual of Mental Disorders* (DSM-III; American Psychiatric Association (APA) 1980, 1987) and its successors (APA 2000; DSM-5). DSM-III insists that mental disorders can be individuated or classified by reference to "their clinical manifestations" (symptoms alone) and not in terms of "how the disturbances [symptoms] have come about" (because of, say, cells that have gone bad) (APA 1980, p. 7). The thesis that mental disorders are brain disorders certainly is incompatible with a DSM-style of disorder classification. This is because a consequence of the thesis that mental disorders are brain disorders is that a condition's categorization as a mental disorder has to be made (as I explain in a moment) in terms of the neural structures or neurobiological/neurochemical/neurodynamical systems assumed to be causally responsible for its symptoms, and these structures or substrates must be instances or areas of brain damage, disorder, or neuropathology. A mental disorder if it is a brain disorder must reflect a neuropathology, viz., a relevantly diseased, malfunctioning, damaged, or "ill" neuromechanical system, systems or connectivity (circuitry) between systems. Andreasen, in fact, entitles one of her books on mental disorder *The Broken Brain* (1984).

Why is that? Why does both the very idea of a brain disorder and a fortiori that of a mental disorder, if it is to count as a type of brain disorder, require reference to the neurological-causal foundations of a disorder? Why isn't reference to psychological symptoms alone enough? The obvious answer is that unless the causes or foundations of a disorder, if it is a brain disorder and not some other sort of disorder, such as a bone marrow disorder or cardiovascular illness, can be described in neural or brain science terms, then it should not be thought of as a brain disorder. The disorder of polycythemia vera (also known as Vaquez–Osler disease), for instance, has psychological effects. Patients with the illness normally become highly irritable, restless, demanding, and easily moved to anger. But its psychological effects are not what make it a disorder. It is a bone marrow disorder involving the overproduction of blood cells and increasing the risk of forming clots and of heart attack. The brain is not the problem. Bone marrow is.

Contrary to the taxonomic conventions of DSM, neurological medicine is anything but silent or neutral about the necessity or diagnostic desirability of a causal explanatory understanding of the foundations of a disorder. The known (or, depending on the current epistemology of the case, hoped to be known) immediate causes or foundations of a brain disorder must also be of a pathological or damaged neural sort. Indeed, even when no scientific consensus now exists about just which specific brain states, activities, or conditions are foundational for a disorder, as is the case with current brain science's incomplete understanding of, say, the proximate source of Alzheimer's and its symptomatic autobiographical memory loss, there is no tolerance in neurology and clinically attendant fields (such as neuroanatomy and neurobiology) for presupposing that a brain disorder is completely and ultimately classifiable just in syndromic or symptom cluster terms.

Neurologists want to develop nosologies or taxonomies for brain disorders, to predict the progression of their course and symptoms, and to treat symptoms and the underlying disorders or forms of damage or disease. In order to do that, it is presupposed, possessing at least some hypotheses about causally proximate and damaged or malfunctioning neural origins or foundations is required. In the words of two advocates of the taxonomic tradition in brain science, mental activities and cognitive functions "break down selectively following a brain disorder, whether due to a focal injury such as a stroke, or more diffuse degeneration" (Kosslyn and Dror 1992, p. 49). "Some parts of the brain [may be] more severely [affected] than others," therein producing different clinical manifestations or symptoms of disorder (Kosslyn and Dror 1992, p. 56).

Neurologists working on brain disorders are guided by something like the following causal explanatory principle or methodological assumption. Call it the principle or assumption of the *casual explanatory power of the damaged neural-physical foundations* of a disorder. If a condition is a brain disorder, it has a neural-physical cause or causes that admit of neural-physical description and the cause or causes are themselves states or conditions that merit classification as damaged or disordered. So, if the very idea of a brain disorder is applied to that of a mental disorder, if, that is, the domain of mental disorder constitutes a subdomain of brain disorder, then the category of mental disorder, too, must observe or follow the same methodological or explanatory principle. Mental disorders must be understood in terms of the brain states or conditions that are, as it were, disordered, pathological, damaged, or ill. This principle goes beyond requiring merely that the causal explanatory understanding of a mental disorder is loosely consistent with brain science or may or must use neuroscience to supplement non-neural types of explanation of a condition (such as types of psychological explanation or explanations that are couched in terms of mental causation; see Graham 2010, 2013). Rather, the principle insists that a brain science understanding is required of a mental disorder if it is to qualify as brain disorder. Indeed, no other type of explanation truly suffices or is apt enough to qualify a disorder as a brain disorder.

To be sure, the standards for satisfying the earlier mentioned principle, and for falling within the category of brain disorder, currently available in neurology are neither stably fixed nor the product of uniform consensus among medical brain scientists. In its use, interpretation, or application within neurology (neuroanatomy and so on), the application of the concept of a brain disorder often relies on presuppositions or assumptions, sometimes quite speculative and controversial, about the biological functions or adaptational purposes of various neural systems or components in the brain and of their causal explanatory role in controlling behavior. Clinical neurologists focus on tests, observations, and reports of current behaviors in current environments (in a clinic, for example), and the historical adaptiveness or evolutionary pedigree of a relevant neural capacity or system is not examined, of course, but only (when presumed relevant) presupposed.

Clinical neurological inquiry begins with the behavioral difficulties or incapacities that a patient confronts and then infers that the difficulties are maladaptive or dysfunctional and that a brain deficit or disorder is responsible for the difficulties. However, despite controversy over the very ideas of adaptivity and of standards or norms for a damaged or disordered brain, certain conditions of brain and behavior enjoy pride of place in the neurological literature as exemplary or prototypical brain disorders. What unites the otherwise rather loose collection of conditions and taxonomic categories of brain disorder that derive from such judgments and are presumed to be brain disorders, when consensus obtains, is the manner in which exemplars or consensus applications of the concept of a brain disorder are best understood. These include conditions such as Alzheimer's dementia, epilepsy, and

Parkinson's, for examples. Conditions that unquestionably count as brain disorders. One feature held in common by each of them (aside, of course, from their harmfulness) is that each and every condition receives or hopes to receive the best description of its proximate causal foundations and behavioral powers from within neuroscience/brain science alone or in a manner that conforms to the earlier mentioned methodological principle. No psychological non-neural vocabulary whatsoever is used in prototypical cases to identify the immediate causal springs or sources of a brain disorder's symptom manifestations or causal foundations.

People harbor Parkinson's, for example, not, it is assumed, because of job related emotional distress or imprudent beliefs or desires, but because they suffer from "a degenerative disorder of the brain," to quote one text, that "is responsible for [the condition's] motor and cognitive disturbance" (Litvan 1996, p. 559). Damage to dopaminergic, serotoninergic, and various other neurochemical pathways, in particular, may produce the condition's distinctive deficits.

To infer from neurological practice, a constraining assumption or norm, then, behind the very idea of a brain disorder as a disorder of the brain goes something like this: If a disorder's causal foundations and powers *cannot* be best described or sufficiently understood in brain science terms alone, if, that is, such terms are insufficient, and need to be complemented by, say, psychological terms, then the condition should not be thought of as a brain disorder. This constraint, which may be called the *brain science closure constraint*, holds firm in current neurology and closely attendant sciences in spite of repeated failure to find a precise or universally acceptable formula for just which sorts of brain states or conditions qualify as dysfunctional or pathological. In any case, with the closure constraint in explanatory place for a brain disorder, then if or when a disorder is a brain disorder, there is no epistemological or explanatory elbow room to step outside of brain science to describe or help to describe its foundational content or character. Such a description is closed off from causal explanatory reference to forces or events conceived in non-neuroscientific, say, psychological or mentalistic terms.

II

Of course, an investigator may ask, why describe the foundations or behavioral impact of *any* disorder in terms of causes or sources understood in brain science terms? Why *ever* encapsulate causal foundations in neural specifications? The neuroscientific literature contains or presupposes different arguments for or descriptions of the character of behavior or aspects of behavior that necessitate or warrant explanatory reference to the brain. I have no space to identify or explore the arguments here. But I shall briefly look at one argument for illustrative purposes and because it helps to identify an approach to the topic of causation that is relevant to understanding different types of disorder.

The argument may be called an argument from the *failure of neural agnosticism* about the proximate or immediate origins of behavior. Neural agnosticism? Failure? What do I mean by such terms?

As witness the daily practical success of ordinary belief-desire or commonsense folk psychology, it is possible to identify psychological states or conditions (such as beliefs, desires, emotions, decisions, whatever) as states or conditions that play causal or causal explanatory roles in behavior and are described in abstraction from the physical or compositional details of their brain base or realizing mechanisms. Ordinary psychological explanations of normal human behavior in terms of people's beliefs, desires, emotions, decisions, and so on, are topic neutral or agnostic about how the subpersonal neural activity that undergirds or implements such processes is best described (Dennett 2009). When, however, a pattern of behavior is taken by neurologists to be symptomatic of a brain disorder, neural damage, malfunction, or disease, the behavior is thought not to be plausibly interpretable other than in terms of the neural structures or biochemical processes or systems that (are assumed to) produce or account for it. Physical details behind behavior matter to understanding a brain disorder. When that happens, i.e., if neural damage or pathology is thought to occur and to produce behavior or symptoms, then reference to beliefs, desires, and continued allegiance to abstraction from neural details must ultimately be pushed aside for an understanding of behavior that is captured or described in neuroscientific terms. An investigator must seek out the internal neural processes or subpersonal mechanisms that constitute or underlie the breakdown in performance.

Here is one quick example of what I have in mind by talk of the attitude of neural agnosticism and its failure in a case of behavior that is symptomatic of a brain disorder. Suppose I ask Auntie Anne, at the family dinner table, to pass the pepper shaker to me. In order to explain why she passes the shaker to me, if she does, I need only to assume that she knows what I request, how to hand the shaker to me, and desires to do so. There is no need for me to nominate a brain area or neural network to explain how or why she passes it. If, however, I have good reason to believe that her hand is outside of her volitional control, and that she is the subject of a neural or brain disorder, malfunction or deficit, then I may need to learn something about callosal tumors or infarcts—my request for the pepper notwithstanding— to understand why she misbehaves as she does and instead tosses the shaker over my head and out of the (fortunately open!) dining room window.

Though scores of papers and stacks of books have been written on the differences between behavior that is best explained in psychological or mentalistic terms and behavior that can only be explained in neuroscientific terms, arguably one of the best papers ever written by a philosopher that is germane to the topic was written not on causality or causal explanation per se, but on the meaning or semantics of terms or linguistic expressions. It is David Lewis's "Scorekeeping in a Language Game" (1979). According to Lewis, so-called "rules of accommodation" operate in many spheres of discourse that contain context-sensitive terms or expressions. Rules of accommodation indicate when a statement is made using such a term or expression. As the context of use changes, rules of accommodation may indicate that the "conversational score" needs to change in order to make the statement true. For example, the term "flat," according to Lewis, is a term that is context sensitive. Just how flat a surface has to be in order for a sentence describing it as "flat" to be true is a variable and not invariant matter, which is determined by conversational context. A surface flat by standards for a game of soccer or field hockey is not flat by standards for a game of billiards, where the norms for flatness need to be changed. If I were to say "The surface is flat," what I say would be false if the "score" is kept by standards suitable for billiards. But by accommodating standards suitable for soccer or field hockey, the statement is true.

Lewis's basic semantically contextualist strategy may be applied to expressions like "causal explanation," "cause," and the like. Or so I assume. I assume "causal explanation" and "cause" are context sensitive expressions.[5] It is a variable matter as to what counts as a cause or causal explanation, a matter that is determined by the explanatory context—the context in which an explanation is sought—and the standards for explanation operative in that context. So, for example, supposing that the mind of my Uncle Max is in relevantly good working order, viz., nothing wrong with his ability to understand or follow a request, then a common sense psychological explanation for why he passes the shaker to me may be true. Max knows what I want, desires to help, and passes the shaker to me. Not so in the case of Auntie Anne's frustrated attempt. In her case the standards for scoring (explaining) must be changed so as to accommodate causal explanatory reference to neurophysiological particulars. In her behavior a different sort of game is being played. Not that of responding successfully to a request to pass. But a form of behavior reflective of a brain disorder—a stymied attempt to satisfy a nephew's request. The standards of folk psychology are not suitable for keeping score when involuntarily throwing tableware out of the window.[6]

If mental disorders are a type of brain disorder, medical scientists had better be spending their research time and dollars focusing on the possible proximate causes of and forces within a disorder described in neurophysical/neurological terms and the supposed damaged or impaired properties of the brain. The mere metaphysical embrace of physicalist sentiment about the mental is not enough to warrant saying that mental disorders are brain disorders. Causal explanatory success of a special sort is required. Basal physicalism about mind/brain, if true, insures that disorders are in or realized or harbored in the brain, but only the success of a disorder's brain science explanation empirically warrants saying that a disorder is of the brain. A brain disorder.

It is the epistemological or evidential fact or probability that brain science is *not* enough in cases of certain disorders or illnesses, viz. those disturbances or conditions of mind and behavior properly called *mental* disorders, and specifically that psychological explanation is needed to help to uncover the foundations and force or power of a mental disorder that, I claim, provides the categorical elbow room needed for the very idea of a mental disorder that is not itself a brain disorder (Graham 2010, 2013). One rough way of putting this

---

[5] Contextualism about causation has defenses in Hart and Honore's discussion of the topic of causation and the law, van Frassen's analysis of the context sensitivity of explanation, and contextualist accounts of mental causation. See, for examples, Hart and Honore (1985), Maslen et al. (2009), and Van Frassen (1980). It should be mentioned that contextualism about causation and causal explanation is not an uncontroversial position or assumption. I do not defend it here. I assume, as stated in the text, that some version of it is true.

[6] Causal claims about behavior are context sensitive because, in part, causal inquiry is context sensitive. Causal explanations are answers to "why"-questions. Differences in the background assumptions and explanatory contrast spaces of "why"-questions produce differences in the warrant or justification of the resulting causal claims. So, in particular, suppose we wish to identify some feature of Max that distinguishes him as an agent from Annie, then the following causal claim might well be acceptable: "Max's desire to honor my request caused him to pass the pepper shaker." Whereas if we are wondering why Annie failed to honor the request in contrast to Max, we may relegate her desire to satisfy the request to the status of a background condition, and embrace a more explanatorily salient or immediate alternative (a better "score keeper") than reference to her desire. So, the following causal claim might well be acceptable: "A physical incapacity in Annie's system of neuromuscular control caused her to throw the shaker out of the window." It is not as if Annie's desire to pass the shaker made no contribution to her failure. It set a background condition for the failure. But it did not itself cause her to throw the shaker out of the window.

particular explanatory or epistemic possibility is to say that if reference to an agent's beliefs, desires, and conscious states or experiences is required to understand certain critical or essential aspects of a condition of disorder—such as its immediate sources and influence on behavior—then it qualifies as a mental disorder even if or though the disorder is brain based and even if or although various other or related and interacting aspects of the condition may be best understood in brain science terms.[7]

Presumably, Mother Nature has not designed the brain so that each and every failure of the brain to support behavior that is healthy from a psychiatric point of view also is unhealthy from a brain centered, neurological or biologically adaptational point of view. If Mother Nature had endowed us with a brain that is exclusively and exquisitely dedicated to preserving mental health and psychiatric or personal well-being, wherein any serious psychological disruption or negative disturbance signals cells gone bad, then, yes, just to be, for example, clinically depressed or addicted to gambling at a race track or casino means being the subject of a brain disorder. However, nothing we know about the natural history of the brain and the parameters of genetic fitness is consistent with such an evolutionary hypothesis (Allman 1999). Whatever the true evolutionary story of the brain is, surely the historical facts are compatible with the brain's underwriting markedly unwelcome behavior in individuals without its being neurologically damaged or impaired. The historical facts are compatible with an enormous gap between what brains have been designed to do and what is best or psychiatrically or psychologically healthy for us as individual persons to do.

The brain, for one quick representative example, supports learning on a so-called variable ratio schedule of reinforcement. The evolutionary advantages or adaptational utilities of learning in such a manner—in a variable ratio schedule there is only occasional and unpredictable reinforcement—are quite clear. Counterintuitive as this may appear, a behavior that is only reinforced on some occasions becomes more deeply entrenched, and more impervious to change. This is an ideal form of learning in environments or settings in which food sources and other rewards are highly unpredictable and variable. Our neural reward mechanisms are designed not to abandon the hunt just because of a single failure or two. We persons may need to attempt numerous times to secure a prey in a bush or banana up a tree.

Biologically speaking, we often must be "driven to persist with [a behavior] as long as it works often enough to make it worthwhile" (West 2006, p. 93). But, alas, our variable ratio reinforcement-theoretic learning capacity is robustly compatible with individual persons tumbling into addictive behavior patterns at a race track or casino. The impulses to engage in such addictive patterns and that are generated by the brain's learning mechanisms can be so strong that they overwhelm a person's rational or reflective and considered preferences (see Stephens and Graham 2009). A mental disorder ensues, but not because the brain is disordered, damaged, or malfunctioning. Or, again, the nature of much human learning (not just on a variable ratio schedule) is compatible with embarking on a course of life that

---

[7] I think of myself as a type of "explanatory pluralist" about human behavior (see McCauley 2007). There are different types of apt explanations for different types of behaviors or aspects of behavior. Ascertaining the criteria for distinguishing between different types of explanations is an important project in the philosophy of science and of interdisciplinary cognitive science, and one that far outstrips the narrow confines of this chapter. Yet a fully systematic and detailed development of the notion of a mental disorder requires it. (See also footnote 10.)

is devoid of the consistent "sucrose" or psychological or personal nourishment needed to insulate a person against the depressive strains and despairing stresses of a life's learned helplessness setbacks (see Abramson et al. 1978). The complicated and general mechanism of the brain allows us to direct our lives along pathways that may be psychologically or prudentially unhealthy without violating the adaptive general utilities or design specifications of the mechanism itself.

The fact that we are not equipped with a psychiatrically fail-safe neurological system or brain means only that evolution is an imperfect, in certain respects, design process. It does not mean that mental disorders are best understood as breakdowns of the brain or that mental illnesses arise from disorders in or malfunctions of the mechanism.

III

To make good the thesis that mental disorders are not brain disorders, it helps, of course, to find empirical or clinical means, for a particular disorder, to determine or decide whether it is a mental or brain disorder. Because of several puzzling issues, among them issues about appropriate norms for disorder, vagueness in the boundary between disorder and non-disorder, and so on, this surely is a complicated topic. I discuss the topic of how to decide if a condition is a mental or brain disorder at length elsewhere (Graham 2010, 2013). Here I describe just one clinical-empirical way in which it may be done.

"A major purpose of diagnosis," as Jackson and McGorry note, "is to indicate the type of treatment that is required for the presenting patient" (Jackson and McGorry 2009, p. 178). A physician goes from diagnosis to treatment. However, it may also be worthwhile to travel in the reverse direction. By this I mean the following: If in cases of some disorders, it proves beneficial to psychotherapeutically guide a patient to reflect on their own condition and to undertake deliberate efforts to change how they feel, think and act, recognize situational vulnerabilities, their recent history of conscious experience, and so on, then part of the best explanation for the success of this course of therapy may be that the condition is a mental disorder and not a brain disorder. It is a disorder in which the brain itself is not broken or damaged. If, contrarily, such "mind-centered" therapies do not work, and the constituent symptoms of a disorder can only be effectively treated or managed by, say, drugs or electroconvulsive therapy, this may be because a patient's condition is a brain disorder, wherein a subject's understanding of their symptoms and ability to reason about their situation is beneficially irrelevant or relevantly causally ineffectual.

Quite clearly, different therapies, treatments, and clinical (including surgical) interventions are designed to build, rebuild, or restore a person's neural and/or mental health or at least to ensure that the harmfulness of a disorder is halted or reduced. A distinction may be made between two different general types of therapies or interventions (Graham 2010, 2013; Graham and Stephens 2007; Levy 2007). One type deploys or works through a person's reason responsiveness and overall rational sensitivity and reasoning capacities (of which more later). A second type does not. This second type consists of purely non-reason orientated, non-psychological mechanical forms of treatment that bypass a person's rational powers, broadly understood. It focuses directly on the brain or central nervous system and its subsystems. This second type of intervention, which may be referred to as *mechanical stance* or *bypass reason responsiveness* therapies, includes the following modes of intervention (among others):

- Psychosurgery
- Transcranial magnetic stimulation of superficial brain structures
- Deep brain stimulation
- Pharmacology (neuroleptics, antidepressant drugs, mood stabilizers, etc.).

The first type, which may be called *intentional stance* or *pass through reason responsiveness* therapies, includes the following (among others):

- Freudian psychotherapy (psychoanalysis)
- Rational emotive therapy (RET)
- Interpersonal therapy
- Reality therapy
- Cognitive behavioral therapy (CBT)
- Mindfulness therapy.

Pass through reason therapies that target a person's rational powers or agentive and deliberative capacities (including emotional sensitivities), aim for the following goal or result: to redirect and improve a person's self-knowledge and situational self-understanding. The assumption behind intentional stance therapies is that a relevant disorder distorts, truncates, irrationally regulates, or in some other manner is an incapacitating deficit and harmful liability in a person's self-knowledge and situational self-assessment. Different forms of pass through therapy or intervention differ in how the goal or aim is approximated or achieved. A Freudian psychoanalyst may include reflection on the continued and unwelcome force of a childhood trauma to act as a controlling variable of a person's current behavior. A RET or CBT therapist may put emphasis on dealing with a person's immediate circumstances, independent of childhood memories. They may try to help a patient to understand negative emotions or irrational thoughts that are harmful for them in current situations and to change their thinking or affective styles.

Intentional stance or pass through therapies typically seek to give persons good reasons, incentives, evidence, warrant, or sometimes just plain thoughtful or self-conscious means for changing, modulating, or regulating their thought and behavior. CBT, for instance, sometimes deploys performance-based and verbal-based interventions to help a patient change their thinking styles, which, in turn may bring about changes in their affect or behavior. A CBT patient in a case of learned helplessness depression, for example, may appreciate that they have failed in certain aspects of their life, but the global interpretation of themselves that they favor (in which they may existentially feel themselves to be a total failure) is presumed to be an unhealthy distortion. So, the patient may be shepherded by a therapist into re-describing their situation more accurately or with more situational grain and less affectively condemnatory detail.

Mechanical stance interventions or therapies deal explicitly with mechanisms as mechanisms—with the brain as brain. They leave direct or explicit appeal to a person's reasons for action or attitudes out of the interventional equation and focus on non-rational or non-psychological underpinnings of behavior change. Deep brain stimulation, for example, may be used to treat movement disorders arising from Parkinson's disease. Selective serotonin reuptake inhibitors may be used to help to lift a person's despondent mood. In a case of Alzheimer's drugs (like donepezil and memantine) may be deployed in hopes of preventing further neuronal loss and atrophy in those areas of the brain (like the hippocampus) implicated in episodic and semantic memory storage. A limbic leucotomy may be targeted at an area of the brain presumed to regulate emotion processing in the case of a severely depressed patient, who has failed to be responsive to pass through therapy.

Given the types of therapies or interventions (and those mentioned represent just examples of the two main types) deployed for disorders, we may ask what can be learned from their patterns of success and failure about a mental/brain disorder distinction? At least two tentative, empirically falsifiable lessons suggest themselves. One is that if the key phases or defining symptoms of a disorder are utterly unaffected and unrelieved by treatments that address a person's psychological responsiveness, then this lends prima facie credence to the proposition that the disorder in question is a brain rather than mental disorder. The bradykinesia (slowness of movement), and rigidity that are characteristic of Parkinson's disease, for example, are uncontrollable (incurable, etc.) by any form of therapy aimed at a patient's reasons for action or inaction, although some elements of the condition are improved, at least temporarily, with dopaminergic replacement therapy (although, alas, reaction to prolonged therapy of this sort may fluctuate and sometimes cause further deterioration of performance). What is reasonable to believe under such circumstances? The hypothesis that Parkinson's is a brain disorder (and not a mental disorder), made on the basis of the evidence of failed and successful therapy patterns, tends, other things being equal, to make sense, at least if we can assume that successful therapies target and help to control the types of causally degenerative processes or foundations responsible for the disorder. There is, we may assume, a disorder, damage or dysfunctionality of neural mechanisms. Parkinson's as a disease is not under the control of a subject's beliefs, thoughts, or attitudes. Rather the disorder is under the control of mechanisms whose causal powers can be described in brain science terms and that satisfy the closed under brain science constraint.[8]

The second lesson is: If a disorder favorably responds to intentional stance or pass through reason therapies, then, again, other things being equal, such evidence helps to warrant the claim that the condition is a mental rather than a brain disorder. Consider post-traumatic stress disorder (PTSD). We could, of course, reduce its frequency of occurrence in a population by focusing on its situational causes (wars, terrorist attacks, and violent assaults) and eliminating them. But assuming that such utopian events will not occur, and given that the power and intensity of reminders of past trauma are crippling to some people and produce PTSD, how are we to treat this vexing and deeply distressing condition?

There is a quasi-Darwinian school of thought that says that PTSD involves the improper activation of an otherwise biologically adaptational mechanism to never forget the location of danger or other risky situations that threaten survival. This school cautions that interfering with the relevant mechanism by neurochemical interventions (say, by taking a drug that takes the sting or vividness out of traumatic memories) could be, all costs and benefits considered, immensely imprudent or unwise. As Neil Levy remarks in a helpful discussion, a

---

[8] A word with more precision is in order here, as urged by Kenneth Kendler in helpful correspondence. Some symptoms (such as tremors) in some cases of Parkinson's disease can be reduced or partially controlled through mental effort and Intentional stance therapies.

drug capable of attenuating such memories "might [unhelpfully] prevent people from learning from [trauma] … or encourage risky behavior" (Levy 2007, p. 184).

Suppose some (if perhaps not all[9]) victims of PTSD respond favorably to various intentional stance therapies that help them to examine and moderate the emotional significance of certain traumatic memories—of military tours in Iraq, for example. It may be proposed that such cases of PTSD are mental and not brain disorders. Assume, for instance, that the guided opportunity to think through one's memories and to reassess them, and then to recognize oneself as not "mired" in a particular past trauma, may substantially reduce their vividness without interfering with the general capacity to learn from unpleasant memories or traumatic experiences. If a person with PTSD may be shepherded in therapy to deal with distressing memories, traumas, and recollections of negative events, this is not because PTSD fails to be implemented "in" the brain or to be a neurally based condition. It is not as if Descartes has risen from the grave to warn against prescribing a beta-blocker. Rather, the case may be one in which the brain itself is not in the wrong, not disordered or damaged. PTSD, or some cases of PTSD, may be mental disorders housed in a more or less sound brain—at least by Mother Nature's complex and gerrymandered standards.

Each of these inferences, whether about Parkinson's or PTSD, possesses complications and should be tempered with "other things being equal" clauses. Neither inference is unadulterated. Just why or how a therapy works often is an empirically complicated issue. So, for example, the hypothesis that a form of pass through or Intentional stance therapy succeeds because the relevant disorder is a mental disorder, must be methodologically humbled by the fact that sometimes therapies "work" just because a disorder is transient or circumstantial by nature. It disappears of its own and perhaps developmental accord. It does not evaporate because RET or CBT extirpates its forces. Questions of individual variation and heterogeneity of sources of similar symptom types also complicate the justification of inferences about causal responsibility for a disorder's manifestations (see Poland, in press).

Still another phenomenon complicating any inference to causal foundations and disorder types from modes of therapy or treatment is that some disorders may favorably respond to both pass through and bypass interventions. (This is to be expected, of course, given that mental disorders are based in the brain even if they are not of it.) A victim of PTSD may be favorably treated with propranolol, a beta-blocker, within hours after trauma, which may interrupt the encoding of traumatic memory. Or the disorder may abate under RET or CBT. More generally: No matter how the issue of inferring to causes/sources and disorder types from the success or failure of one or another form of therapy pans out, it must be admitted that therapeutic success or failure alone may not always or successfully distinguish mental from brain disorders. But it may help, and that is the main point being urged here. Therapeutic success or failure may serve as a platform for diagnostic insight into the categorical nature of a particular disorder.

---

[9] One consequence of the thesis that mental disorders are not brain disorders is that some uses of one and the same diagnostic word or label ("PTSD," "addiction," etc.) may identify a mental disorder and others may identify a brain disorder. A related consequence is that a condition that is a mental disorder may metamorphose into a brain disorder, if or when a neural pathology develops in consequence of the persistence of the physically harmful behavior associated with a mental disorder. The courses of some addictive behavior patterns (especially those involving chemical substances, which over time may produce a neurochemical disorder) illustrate the point.

What does it profit a person to visit a psychiatrist for visual blindness caused by extensive bilateral damage to the striate cortex of the occipital lobe or to secure the services of a neurosurgeon for suicidal ideation on the death of a spouse? Getting the right care or treatment requires knowing which sort of intervention best suits which type of disorder. Identifying the right diagnosis may be informed by appreciation of past patterns of success and failure associated with different treatments. The success or failure of various forms of therapy or treatment may contain lessons about the proper categorization of a disorder.

In a paper discussing a book by John Robinson (1919–1983), the then Bishop of Woolwich, called *Honest to God* (published in 1963) and announcing what appeared to be, at least in terms of traditional Christian theology, the bishop's personal atheism, the philosopher Alasdair MacIntyre quipped that the religious creed of the English appears to be that "there is no God and it is wise to pray to him from time to time" (MacIntyre 1963/1971, pp. 12–26). I have written this chapter as a skeptical reaction to the thesis that conditions that deserve to be classified as mental disorders can be adequately understood as disorders of the brain. I know of mental health professionals who agree with me, but still seem to wish for a creed for psychiatry like the following. *There is no brain science of mental disorder and it is wise to pay homage to it from time to time.* Truth is that if one is embracing a consistent apostasy, as I wish to do, then the second conjunct must be rejected. Not rejected a priori. Not rejected because we infallibly know that we will never have good reason to abandon a concept of mental disorder. But rejected as long as the empirical evidence for how best to explain, understand, and treat certain disorders or disturbances of mind and behavior warrants classifying them as mental and not as brain disorders or cases of neurological illness. In the study of mental disorder, deploying brain science is inescapable, for some questions about a mental disorder are, I believe, best answered in neurological terms (although absent reference to brain damage/cells gone bad as such) (on this topic see Graham 2012, 2013).[10] But paying homage to brain science as explanatorily regnant is another. The right to demand that our medical scientific understanding of a mental disorder must bottom out in some privileged set of neuroscientific descriptions has got to be empirically earned. It is not guaranteed by metaphysically physicalistic sentiment alone.

Acknowledgments

Richard Garrett, Richard Gipps, Kenneth Kendler, Robert McCauley, and Jeffrey Poland helped me with the ideas in this chapter. I am especially indebted to background work and conversations with G. Lynn Stephens.

[10] Some questions about a mental disorder are best answered in neurological terms? On the theory of mental disorder or illness that I elsewhere propose, I argue that to understand a mental disorder we need to find ways of describing conditions of mind and behavior that are (to use an expression of Donald Davidson's out of context) "in between" the operation of mindless neurological mechanisms and the fully functional reason responsiveness of persons and that combine references to each in answers to various why-questions about a mental disorder (see Davidson 1999, p. 11; see also Graham, in press).

References

Abramson, L. Y., Seligman, M., and Teasdale, J. (1978). Learned helplessness in humans. *Journal of Abnormal Psychology*, 87, 49–74.

Allman, J. M. (1999). *Evolving Brains*. New York, NY: W. H. Freeman.

American Psychiatric Association (1980). *Diagnostic and Statistical Manual of Mental Disorders, Third Edition*. Washington, DC: American Psychiatric Association.

American Psychiatric Association (1987). *Diagnostic and Statistical Manual of Mental Disorders, Third Edition, Revised*. Washington, DC: American Psychiatric Association.

American Psychiatric Association (2000). *Diagnostic and Statistical Manual of Mental Disorders, Fourth Edition*. Washington, DC: American Psychiatric Association.

Andreasen, N. C. (1984). *The Broken Brain: The Biological Revolution in Psychiatry*. New York, NY: Oxford University Press.

Andreasen, N. C. (2001). *Brave New Brain: Conquering Mental Illness in the Era of the Genome*. Oxford: Oxford University Press.

Arpaly, N. (2005). How it is not 'just like diabetes': Mental disorders and the moral psychologist. *Philosophical Issues*, 15, 282–98.

Bentall, R. (2004). *Madness Explained: Psychosis and Human Nature*. London: Penguin Books.

Davidson, D. (1999). The emergence of thought. *Erkenntnis*, 51, 1–17.

Dennett, D. C. (2009). Intentional systems theory. In B. McLaughlin, A. Beckermann, and S. Walter (Eds), *The Oxford Handbook of Philosophy of Mind*, pp. 339–50. New York, NY: Oxford University Press.

Dretske, F. (1988). *Explaining Behavior: Reasons in a World of Causes*. Cambridge, MA: MIT Press.

Graham, G. (2010). *The Disordered Mind: An Introduction to Philosophy of Mind and Mental Illness*. Abingdon: Routledge.

Graham, G. (2013). *The Disordered Mind: An Introduction to the Philosophy of Mind and Mental Illness* (Rev./2nd edn). Abingdon: Routledge.

Graham, G. (in press). Being a mental disorder. In H. Kincaid and J. Sullivan (Eds), *Psychiatric Classification and Natural Kinds*. Cambridge, MA: MIT Press.

Graham, G. and Stephens, G. L. (2007). Psychopathology: Minding mental illness. In P. Thagard (Ed.), *Philosophy of Psychology and Cognitive Science*, pp. 414–16. Amsterdam: Elsevier.

Hart, H. L. A. and Honore, A. M. (1985). *Causation and the Law*. Oxford: Oxford University Press.

Jackson, H. and McGorry, P. (2009). Psychiatric diagnoses: Purposes, limitations, and an alternative approach. In S. Wood, N. Allen, and C. Pantelis (Eds), *The Neuropsychology of Mental Illness*, pp. 178–93. Cambridge: Cambridge University Press.

Kosslyn, S. M. and Dorr, I. E. (1992). A cognitive neuroscience of Alzheimer's disease: What can be learned from studies of visual imagery? In Y. Christen and P. Churchland (Eds), *Neurophilosophy and Alzheimer's Disease*, pp. 49–59. Berlin: Springer-Verlag.

Levy, N. (2007). *Neuroethics: Challenges for the 21st Century*. Cambridge: Cambridge University Press.

Lewis, D. (1979). Scorekeeping in a language game. *Journal of Philosophical Logic*, 8, 339–59.

Litvan, I. (1996). Parkinson's disease. In J. Beaumont, P. Kenealy, and M. Rogers (Eds), *The Blackwell Dictionary of Neuropsychology*, pp. 559–63. Malden, MA: Blackwell Publishers.

MacIntyre, A. (1963). God and the theologians. *Encounter*, 21(3), 3–10. (Reprinted in MacInyre, A. (1971). *Against the Self-Images of the Age*, pp. 12–26. New York, NY: Schocken Books.)

Maslen, C., Horgan, T., and Daly, H. (2009). Mental causation. In H. Beebee, C. Hitchcock, and P. Menzies (Eds), *Oxford Handbook of Causation*, pp. 523–53. Oxford: Oxford University Press.

McCauley, R. (2007). Reduction: Models of cross-scientific relations and their implications for the psychology-neuroscience interface. In P. Thagard (Ed.), *Philosophy of Psychology and Cognitive Science*, pp. 105–58. Amsterdam: Elsevier.

Poland, J. (in press). Deeply rooted sources of error and bias in psychiatric classification. In H. Kincaid and J. Sullivan (Eds), *Psychiatric Classification and Natural Kinds*. Cambridge, MA: MIT Press.

Profet, M. (1992). Pregnancy sickness: A deterrent to maternal ingestion of teratogens. In J. H. Barkow, L. Cosmides, and J. Toobey (Eds), *The Adapted Mind: Evolutionary Psychology and the Generation of Culture*, pp. 327–65. New York, NY: Oxford University Press.

Ryle, G. (1949). *The Concept of Mind*. New York, NY: Barnes & Noble.

Stephens, G. L. and Graham, G. (2009a). Mental illness and the consciousness thesis. In S. Wood, N. Allen, and C. Pantelis (Eds), *The Neuropsychology of Mental Illness*, pp. 390–8. Cambridge: Cambridge University Press.

Stephens, G. L. and Graham, G. (2009b). An addictive lesson: A case study in psychiatry as cognitive neuroscience. In M. Broome and L. Bortolotti (Eds), *Psychiatry as Cognitive Neuroscience: Philosophical Perspectives*, pp. 203–20. Oxford: Oxford University Press.

Taylor, M. A. (1999). *Fundamentals of Clinical Neurology*. New York, NY: Oxford University Press.

Van Fraassen, B. (1980). *The Scientific Image*. Oxford: Oxford University Press.

Vogeley, K. and Newman, A. (2009). The definition and constitution of mental disorders and the role of neural dysfunctions. In S. Wood, N. Allen, and C. Pantelis (Eds), *The Neuropsychology of Mental Illness*, pp. 420–3. Cambridge: Cambridge University Press.

West, R. (2006). *Theory of Addiction*. Oxford: Blackwell Publishing.

CHAPTER 33

MENTAL DISORDER: CAN MERLEAU-PONTY TAKE US BEYOND THE "MIND–BRAIN" PROBLEM?

ERIC MATTHEWS

INTRODUCTION

If anything counts as a core problem in the philosophy of psychiatry, it must surely be the question of the nature of psychiatry itself. Is psychiatry one medical specialism among others, dealing with disorders of the mind as others deal with those of the heart or the lungs? Or are those human conditions we call "mental disorders" entirely different in character from such dysfunctions in bodily organs—so much so that they need a distinctive, non-medical, form of treatment? Actual practice in modern society expresses uncertainty in our answers to such questions. I want to argue that we are uncertain because we are unclear about the concept of "mental disorder"; and we are unclear about that concept because of a *philosophical* disagreement about the meaning of "mind" and the "mental." I also want to argue that the philosophical disagreement rests on a confusion, and to suggest a way in which that confusion could be resolved, with beneficial results for our thinking about mental disorder and for practice in its treatment.

Briefly stated, the philosophical disagreement is between rival views of the relation between mind and brain, or (as I would prefer to express it) between psychology and neuroscience. In the philosophical tradition, this dispute has been treated as a clash of two, diametrically opposed, ontologies: the view that "mind" and "brain" (or "matter" more generally) are distinct and independent "substances" ("dualism"); or the view that they are identical, that mental states and processes are completely dependent on brain states and processes, and so belong to the same "substance" ("materialism"). Part of my purpose in this chapter is to show that this way of posing the question is misleading and confusing, especially when we are trying to think about the nature of mental disorder. For it is responsible for what I contend is a damaging assumption, namely, that there is a polar opposition between what is usually called "biological" psychiatry and another, more "psychological" (often called "humanistic"), variety. I hope to show how a different model, derived from Merleau-Ponty's concept of human beings as "body-subjects" (to be explored in more detail later in the chapter), can offer a better framework, which integrates psychology and neuroscience in our conception of human beings and their ills.

THE TWO MODELS

Those who first sought, in the nineteenth century, to bring the treatment of mental disorder into the ambit of modern scientific medicine, adopted a biological model. For example, the first editor of the journal *Archives for Psychiatry and Nervous Diseases*, Wilhelm Griesinger, in his first editorial in 1867, said that "Psychiatry has undergone a transformation in its relation to the rest of medicine. This transformation rests principally on the realization that patients with so-called 'mental illness' are really individuals with illnesses of the nerves and brain" (quoted in Bentall 2004, p. 150). It is similar thinking which leads the authors of the fourth edition of the *Diagnostic and Statistical Manual of Mental Disorders* (DSM-IV), in their Introduction, to apologize for the very use of the term "mental disorder" in the title of the work, because it "unfortunately implies a distinction between 'mental' disorders and 'physical' disorder that is a reductionistic anachronism of mind/body dualism" (American Psychiatric Association 1994, p. xxi). They reject any sharp distinction between the type of disorders which they are concerned with and other medical conditions. In this way, they affirm their commitment to what is often called the "medical model" of mental disorder, according to which, as Dominic Murphy says, "psychiatry is a branch of medicine dedicated to uncovering the neurological basis of disease entities" (Murphy 2006, p. 10).

On the other hand, clinical psychologists like Richard Bentall reject explanations of severe mental disorders "in terms of abnormal brain chemistry or anatomical lesions" and view "the patient as a whole person troubled by apparently baffling problems, but also having the resources for ameliorating these problems" (Professor Aaron Beck, in Bentall 2004, p. xi). Others object to the biological model because, in treating mental disorder as brain disease, to be treated medically like bodily illness, it distracts attention from the social causes of much mental disturbance. John Sadler, for instance, reports the feminist critique of psychiatric classification as "driven by a distrust or a rejection of medicalization [which] directs attention, public resources, and responsibility away from the social causes of (in this case) women's alleged 'troubled and troubling' behavior, the social causes being the domination and exploitation of women" (Sadler 2005, p. 238). This is not to speak of those radical psychiatrists, like R. D. Laing, or anti-psychiatrists, like Thomas Szasz, who cast doubt on the orthodox psychiatric conception of "mental illness," resulting from brain pathologies, and treat bizarre behavior and experiences rather as ultimately intelligible human responses to very difficult situations. Laing says, for example, that the issues lived through by the schizophrenic "cannot be grasped through the methods of clinical psychiatry and psychopathology as they stand today but, on the contrary, require the existential-phenomenological method to demonstrate their true human relevance and significance" (Laing 2010, p. 18). Similarly, Szasz speaks of his "past efforts to analyze mental illnesses as disapproved communications, and mental treatments as rhetoric, religion, or repression, disguised as 'therapy'" (Szasz 2002, p. 115).

Writers on both sides of this argument make some apparent concessions to the other side. One defender of the biological model, Edward Shorter, for example, says:

> Yet it was not part of the biological brief to argue that all psychiatric illnesses are attributable to discreet, identifiable brain lesions. Social and psychological factors clearly play a role in the genesis of dysphoria, not merely by triggering an underlying genetic predisposition but by independently converting stress and despair into illness. (Shorter 1997, p. 287)

Nevertheless, he still sees biology as in some way fundamental. The role of social and psychological factors still tends to be regarded as subordinate: they are important in "the manifestations of mental illnesses" (Baldessarini, quoted in Shorter 1997, p. 287), but the heart of the biological approach is that mental illness is "a genetically influenced disorder of brain chemistry" (Shorter 1997, p. vii). On the other side, Bentall, for instance, accepts that biological factors may have some part to play. He takes for granted the unity of mind and brain, but argues that it is an implication of this unity "that we are likely to make more progress in understanding the biology of psychosis if we first attempt to understand the psychology" (Bentall 2004, p. 175). In a later work, he criticizes the failure of biological investigators "to consider the possibility that their findings might reflect the tribulations of life, rather than some lesion or genetic scar carried by the victim from birth" (Bentall 2009, p. 152). I take this to mean that social and psychological factors have priority, even though they may act through affecting our brain or through activating genetic predispositions. The concessions on both sides are thus *only* apparent: the core of the biological model is that neurophysiological, biochemical, and genetic explanations of mental disorder are more fundamental than psychological; and the core proposition of the opposing model is that psychology (or perhaps sociology) is the fundamental science in explaining mental disorder.

How could one argue for either model? The answer which many proponents of the biological model would give is that it alone allows psychiatry to become a truly scientific enterprise. Shorter says, "Biological psychiatry ... became able to investigate the causes and treatments of psychiatric illness by using the scientific method, a method other psychiatrists had virtually abandoned for half a century" (Shorter 1997, p. 272). The triumph of biological psychiatry is then put down to the way in which empirical scientific discoveries and hypotheses about brain structures, functioning, and biochemistry, and about genetics, have made possible striking advances in the explanation and treatment of mental disorder. Examples cited include such things as the evidence from autopsies of greater disorganization of the neurons in certain areas of the brains of patients with schizophrenia, or, from brain imaging techniques, of anatomical and physiological changes in patients with bipolar disorder or obsessive-compulsive disorder. Then there are the results of studies of the hereditability of such conditions as schizophrenia, or the ways in which discoveries about changes in levels of neurotransmitters in conditions such as depression have made possible the development of effective forms of drug treatment for such disorders.

But empirical evidence, at least on its own, can never be sufficient to establish the biological model. The point is not simply that, as Richard Bentall points out (Bentall 2004, *passim*), the alleged empirical facts cited in support are open to question and always, like any empirical claims, liable to be disproved by fresh discoveries. Nor is it only that, as Bentall rightly says, the evidence of correlations between states of the brain and the incidence of mental disorder is not sufficient to show the existence of a causal connection, or the direction of the causal relationship, if any (does the mental disorder cause the brain abnormality or vice versa?). It is rather that the biological model has to be supported by *philosophical*, rather than *empirical*, argument. Psychology, after all, is also a science, and psychological explanations of mental disorder, as Bentall's work among others shows, are also available. The kinds of empirical evidence cited are only relevant if we *first* can show that biological explanation is fundamental—that psychological explanations ought to be *reduced* to, or even replaced by, neurological explanations. Similarly, the kind of psychological approach which writers like Bentall advocate can be distinguished only if we can show that psychological explanations are *irreducible* to neurological. Questions of reducibility or irreducibility are essentially *philosophical*, rather than empirical. To show that one or another science is more "fundamental," it is necessary to show that its way of describing reality more truly fits how things actually *are*: in other words, it depends ultimately on ontology, the metaphysical account of "what there is." Roughly speaking, if psychology is irreducible to neuroscience, it is because "mind" is an essentially different kind of thing from brain; if it is reducible, it is because mind and brain are one and the same thing. In the next two sections, I shall explore these two metaphysical positions, their relevance, and the arguments which might support them: first, the reductive form of materialism, and then mind–brain dualism, which is presupposed by the claim of irreducibility.

Reductive Materialism

Reductive materialism exists in many versions, but I want to focus on two twentieth-century varieties of this thesis, which I think illustrate certain essential features of this position. Chronologically earlier is the "mind–brain identity thesis" (sometimes called "central state materialism"), proposed by such philosophers as U. T. Place and J. J. C. Smart in the 1950s. Both Place and Smart present mind–brain identity as if it were a scientific hypothesis, one that they think will be verified by future experimental evidence. Place is explicit about this: The identity of mind and brain is, he says, "a reasonable scientific hypothesis" (Place 1956/2002, p. 56), a statement of *contingent*, not *necessary*, identity, to be established by empirical research rather than logical analysis. He compares it to the hypothesis (now well established, and so regarded as more than a hypothesis) that lightning is an electrical discharge, or, as he also expresses it, that lightning is *nothing more than* an electrical discharge (Place 1956/2002, p. 58). The future development of research will, he hopes, similarly establish that consciousness is nothing more than brain processes.

But it is important to look more closely at this claim. What does it actually *mean* to say that lightning is "nothing more than" an electrical discharge, or that conscious mental activity is "nothing more than" brain processes? And how would empirical research be relevant to establishing either claim? Place's own answer (in respect of the lightning case) is that "we treat the two sets of observations [of flashes of lightning and of electrical discharges] as observations of the same event in those cases where the technical scientific observations set in the context of the appropriate body of scientific theory provide an immediate explanation of the observations made by the man in the street" (Place 1956/2002, p. 58). In this case, the motion of electrical discharges through the atmosphere is, in the context of our general scientific knowledge, sufficient to explain the visual stimulation which a human observer would report as "seeing a flash of lightning." What Place means by saying that the electrical discharges and the lightning-flashes that we see are "identical," in other words, is that the former explain the latter. But there are other possible explanations of lightning: it might, for instance, be the expression of divine anger. If Place (and most of us) reject the latter explanation in favor of that in terms of electrical discharges, it is because we accept a particular view of what *counts* as scientific evidence. Science, on this view, admits explanations which make use of physical concepts like "electrical discharge," but not those which employ theological concepts like "divine anger."

In the same way, Place's assertion of mind–brain "identity" seems to amount to the claim that there is more than a mere correlation between conscious states and brain processes: that the latter give the kind of *explanation* of the former required to fit conscious states into our modern scientific picture of the world. Smart, in the same vein, makes the point that neurophysiological explanation of our conscious processes and behavior is superior to explanations in terms of purely mental entities like thoughts and sensations, because it does not require the existence of what Herbert Feigl called "nomological danglers"—that is, roughly speaking, special laws to cover them which do not form part of the wider system of scientific laws. Smart says, "That everything should be explicable in terms of physics (together of course with descriptions of the ways in which the parts are put together—roughly, biology is to physics as radio-engineering is to electro-magnetism) except the occurrence of sensations seems to me to be frankly unbelievable" (Smart 1959/2002, p. 61). The argument, in short, is based, not on conjectures about future empirical evidence, but on the ideal of a unified science, in which all phenomena will be explained by a single, logically connected set of laws, ultimately founded on those of physics. This is the sense in which this form of materialism is "reductive."

This is made even more obvious if we consider another twentieth-century formulation of materialism, namely, the "eliminativism" or "eliminative materialism" proposed by such philosophers as Paul Churchland. Churchland sets out his definition of eliminative materialism in these words:

> Eliminative materialism is the thesis that our common-sense conception of psychological phenomena constitutes a radically false theory, a theory so fundamentally defective that both the principles and the ontology of that theory will eventually be displaced, rather than smoothly reduced, by completed neuroscience. (Churchland 2002, p. 568)

The mark of "common-sense psychology" (what he elsewhere calls "folk-psychology") is its reliance on "propositional attitudes," such as belief or desire, in its explanation of human behavior. Thus, my application for a particular job might be explained in folk-psychology by my belief that it would give me a higher salary, together with my desire to have more money. Beliefs, desires, etc. are treated as unobservable mental entities which explain the observable behavior which human beings exhibit. This is a very long-standing way of explaining human behavior, Churchland argues, but it can increasingly be seen to be defective, and has made no real advances in the thousands of years it has been in existence. In this way, it is what the philosopher of science Imre Lakatos would call a "degenerating research program"—a theory which is not a fruitful framework for understanding its field, and so ought to be abandoned in favor of something which promises greater possibilities of development.

One of the important kinds of phenomena for which folk-psychology fails to provide a satisfactory explanation, according to Churchland, is "the nature and dynamics of mental illness" (Churchland 1981/2002, p. 571). The research program which he argues ought to take over from folk-psychology is, as he says in the passage quoted, that of "completed neuroscience," which will eliminate from its ontology such entities as propositional attitudes and include only items recognized in the terminology of neuroscience, such as neurons, synapses, neurotransmitters, and the like. A statement of how this might improve our understanding of mental illness, in particular, is provided by Churchland in another work. He there rejects Freudian psychoanalysis, which he sees as deploying "the familiar prototypes of *common sense psychology*," and accuses of having a "chronically feeble explanatory and theraputic [*sic*] record." He then goes on to say:

> In confronting the entire range of psychological dysfunctions, we have done far better by looking for structural failures or abnormalities in the brain, for functional failures in its physiology, for chemical abnormalities in its metabolism, for genetic failures in its original blueprint, and for developmental hitches in its maturation. (Churchland 1995, p. 183)

What is most significant, from our present point of view, about Churchland's position is the reason why he holds it. Folk-psychology, as was said earlier, is described as a failing theory, which can offer no clear or useful explanations of psychological phenomena. It ought, in Churchland's opinion, to be replaced by one using neuroscientific concepts as soon as those concepts have been developed sufficiently by empirical research. But why is Churchland so confident that folk-psychology is bound to fail, and that neuroscience will be a more successful substitute? The answer is philosophical, not empirical. It is that folk-psychology works with a misguided dualist ontology, in which such mental entities as thoughts, belief, desires etc. have a reality independent of anything material or physical. A psychology based on neuroscience, by contrast, would operate with a superior, materialist, ontology, in which so-called "mental" entities have no reality independent of the material, or physical, entities studied by neuroscience. The superiority of this materialist ontology is that, unlike the dualist ontology on which folk-psychology is based, it makes our account of human behavior and personality coherent with the rest of science:

> If we approach *Homo sapiens* from the perspective of natural history and the physical sciences, we can tell a coherent story of his constitution, development, and behavioral capacities which encompasses particle physics, atomic and molecular theory, organic chemistry, evolutionary theory, biology, physiology, and materialistic neuroscience. (Churchland 1981/2002, p. 572)

Once again, then, we can see how this kind of materialism is held to be superior to dualism because it is supposed to make it possible to fit the facts of human behavior and experience (including the facts of *disordered* human behavior and experience) into a single unified picture of reality, rooted in physics. Human beings, the claim is, must be seen as "nothing more than" one kind of physical system, if their behavior is to be *scientifically* explained. The argument for the biological model is thus based on a philosophical conception of the world, including human beings and their behavior. The conception is that the only rationally acceptable account of things is one in which they are described and explained using concepts which are ultimately reducible to those of physics. It is only against such a metaphysical background that a purely biological approach to the explanation of mental disorder makes any sense.

MEANING AND THE PSYCHOLOGICAL APPROACH

Advocates of the psychological approach claim, as we have seen, that we cannot understand disordered attitudes or behavior in terms of brain chemistry, or anatomical lesions, or genetics, but must see them as the result of attempts by human beings to resolve baffling problems in their lives. What may be said in support of this is that most psychiatric disorders are diagnosed in terms of the way in which they affect the sufferer's subjective experience of the world, or on social functioning—his or her personal relationships, or ability to operate successfully in society, rather than in terms of the objective biological functioning of their brains and nervous systems. DSM-IV's attempt at a rough definition of "mental disorder" says:

> In DSM-IV each of the mental disorders is conceptualized as a clinically significant behavioral or psychological syndrome or pattern that occurs in an individual and that is associated with present distress (e.g., a painful symptom) or disability (i.e., impairment in one or more important areas of functioning) or with a significantly increased risk of suffering death, pain, disability, or an important loss of freedom. (American Psychiatric Association 1994, p. xxi)

This definition is offered, as was said earlier in the chapter, as part of a contention that there is no sharp distinction to be drawn between "mental" disorder and "physical" disease. But a reading of the diagnostic criteria for most of the conditions listed in DSM-IV itself suggests, at least prima facie, that there is such a distinction. The diagnoses are based on such things as "low self-esteem," "depressed mood," "anxiety about being in places from which escape might be difficult or embarrassing," "hallucinations," "delusions," "excessive emotionality," "obsessions," "abnormally elevated mood," even "childlike silliness." These are all, as the definition's own wording says, "*behavioural or psychological*" syndromes, rather than patterns of *biological* dysfunction. They are deviations, as George Graham says, from the norms of "satisfying or prudent personal activity," rather than from those of "healthy and proper brain function" (Graham 2010, p. 54). This seems, as Graham also says (p. 54) to differentiate them from conditions which are uncontroversially describable as "brain diseases," such as Parkinsonism: the *Oxford Concise Medical Dictionary* defines Parkinsonism, for instance, as "a clinical picture characterized by tremor, rigidity, slowness of movement, and postural instability" (Martin 2007, p. 533).

What is the difference between these two types of symptom? Tremor, rigidity, and the like are *objectively* observable failures of the *body* to function in *biologically* normal ways: that is, in ways which are desirable from a biological point of view, which will tend to ensure staying alive for a species-normal life span, to enable species-normal kinds and levels of physical activity, to prevent unnecessary physical disability and pain, and so on. The diagnostic signs of mental disorders given earlier, by contrast, consist in *subjectively experienced* moods, thoughts, emotions, etc., or else in *socially* abnormal patterns of behavior. The suffering which they cause consists in emotional distress, rather than physical pain, and social, rather than biological, dysfunction—an inability of the *person* to function normally in society, to form relationships, to hold down a job, or to pursue a course of study, rather than an inability of the person's *body* to stay alive for a normal span or to engage in normal physical activities. In a typical bodily disease like cancer, the disease itself directly causes death. By contrast, people with a typical mental disorder like depression may be more likely to die: but it is because they are more likely to commit suicide than other people. In other words, the direct cause of death is their own action, rather than the depression itself. (And, of course, it is possible to be depressed, even to have suicidal ideation, but not to commit suicide.) Similarly, someone with anorexia may certainly be at risk of dying: but the condition is not the *direct* cause of death. Rather, the disorder consists in being averse to eating, which results in self-starving behavior, which may result in death. But death can be prevented, for example by force-feeding, without changing the anorexic's mental condition. The connection between typical mental disorders and the increased likelihood of dying, in short, is much more indirect.

Finally, as Derek Bolton points out, the use of the phrase "clinically significant" in the DSM-IV definition is telling. "An important sign of the role of social factors is in the technical expression 'clinically significant' as applied to the conditions of interest, which turns out to refer to the fact that these are the conditions people have brought to the clinic, and thought by patient and physician to be in need of treatment" (Bolton 2008, p. 35). What makes these symptoms clinically significant, in other words, is not some objectively establishable facts about the body's ability to survive or to function according to biological norms, but the sufferer's own assessment of the depth of his or her suffering as sufficient to justify them in seeking professional help. The question of whether or not someone's emotional distress is unbearable, or someone's social relationships are satisfactory, is not one of biological fact. It can be answered only by appealing to human concepts, which may and do vary from individual to individual, and from society to society. It is a question of the *meaning* of the mental state or the behavior for the person concerned (or sometimes for those with whom that person associates).

Why is all this relevant to the explanation of mental disorder? The argument might go like this. The appropriate mode of explanation for anything depends on what kind of thing it is we want to explain. In the case of mental disorders, as the DSM-IV definition says, we are dealing with a "behavioral or psychological syndrome"—that is, with ways in which someone *acts*, or *thinks*, or *feels*, or *desires*, rather than with ways in which someone's bodily condition changes. So the question is, is the explanation of human action and psychological states of the same form as that of physical changes? There is an important tradition in philosophy which holds that these two types of explanation are indeed very different.

One way to argue for this distinction is to say that human actions and mental states can be identified as what they are only by concepts which must be understood by the subject of the mental state or the agent performing the action. Physical states, on the other hand, can be identified objectively, by such things as spatiotemporal location, physical and chemical properties, and so on. In the case of actions, the relevant concepts will be those of the *goal* which the agent has in performing the action. Two different actions, for instance, may involve identical, or almost identical, bodily movements, while being made different by their respective goals. Committing suicide is a different action from trying to cure a headache, even if both are achieved by ingesting the same pills. In the case of a mental state, like a thought, the relevant concept will be one which identifies what the thought is *about* (an "intentional" concept). Two thoughts are distinguished by what they are thoughts *about*, even if, for example, the neural processes involved in entertaining them are identical (for example, the action of calculating one's profit from a transaction is different from that of solving an abstract problem in arithmetic, even if the intellectual processes, and so presumably the neural activity, involved are the same in both cases). If so, then the explanation of the action or mental state must also, it can be argued, be different in character from that of the bodily movements, or brain processes, involved. Saying what caused someone to move his hands in such a way as to take a pill will not explain *why* he committed suicide or tried to cure his headache. To answer the latter questions, we need a *reason*. He committed suicide because he had come to the conclusion that his life was not worth living. He tried to cure his headache by taking this pill because he mistakenly thought it was an aspirin. In similar fashion, saying what caused the relevant areas of his brain to behave in the way they did when he was making these calculations will not explain why he was calculating his profits or trying to solve an arithmetical puzzle. He was calculating his profits because he wanted to see how much money he had available; he was trying to solve the arithmetical puzzle in order to show his son how good he was at mathematics.

These "reason" explanations are, it is argued, different in character from the causal explanations of muscular movements or neural processes. They essentially involve reference to a subject and his or her possession of relevant concepts. A man could not commit suicide because he felt life was not worth living unless he had the concepts of "suicide," "his life," "worth living," and so on. A man could not calculate profits in order to see how much money he had available unless he had such concepts as "profit," "money," etc. To have concepts is not identical with having processes going on in the brain, even if we human beings could not have concepts *without* certain processes going on in our brains. Having concepts necessarily involves engaging with the world outside, and in particular with other people: someone could have the concepts of "money" and "profit," for instance, only if they participated in a certain kind of economic system. This is why the explanation of the man's calculating activity cannot be reduced to the biological, chemical, electrical, etc. explanation of what is going on in his brain when he calculates. It has to be expressed in a vocabulary quite distinct from those of physiology, chemistry, and physics, and so cannot be part of a single unified system with these sciences. It works by making the man's behavior intelligible, in terms which are common to all those who share the relevant concepts. We can understand why someone should make certain calculations because he wants to work out his profits, because we know what it means to work out profits in this way, and why it should be of interest to someone to do so.

Proponents of the psychological model would argue that this can be extended to disordered behavior and experience, because it is "disordered" in terms of human norms which we share, and so can understand. If we are to understand why they deviated from those norms therefore (so the argument goes), what we need is not knowledge of the workings of their brains, but an appreciation of the kinds of reasons which may lead people to deviate in this way—which might influence us ourselves in appropriate circumstances. To quote Graham again:

> To say, for instance, that Alice and Ian are subjects of a mental disorder is to say that how they think, feel and deliberately or intentionally act are among the sources or propensity conditions of their disorders and that how they think, feel and act is *not* attributable to a neural impairment or disorder even if, or though, neural activity is involved. (Graham 2010, p. 24)

To see mentally disordered behavior in this way is thus to see it as having a certain kind of rationality, in the sense of being intelligible in essentially the same way as "normal" behavior, if perhaps requiring a greater degree of imagination than more humdrum examples. Thus,

Bentall treats mental disorders as existing "on continua with normal behaviors and experiences" (Bentall 2004, p. 115). Laing's central purpose in his work, likewise, is "to convey … that it was far more possible than is generally supposed to understand people diagnosed as psychotic" (Laing 2010, p. 11). The thesis, then, is that we can understand bizarre behavior and experience if we see it as an expression of a human attempt to grapple with particularly severe problems, because we know what it means to grapple with less severe problems of the same kind.

But this position presupposes that our *mental* life operates on different principles from the workings of a physical system like the brain. It belongs to a long-standing philosophical tradition, especially in post-Kantian German philosophy, which holds that there is a sharp distinction between the "sciences of mind" (*Geisteswissenschaften* in German) and the "natural sciences" (*Naturwissenschaften*). The sciences of mind are concerned to "understand" human actions in terms of their meaning for the agent, while the natural sciences are concerned to give "causal explanations" of the behavior of material things (including the human body and brain), in terms of universal and impersonal natural laws. But this idea of a sharp distinction between two realms of explanation surely presupposes an ontological distinction between two realms of being—"mind" and "matter": in short, a substantial dualism, of which Descartes's distinction between "mental" and "material" substance provides the classic example.

Recasting the Problem

Traditionally, as was said earlier, we are seen as presented with a stark choice between two mutually exclusive alternatives. Either we bring psychiatry into line with the rest of modern scientific medicine, by treating mental disorders as the manifestations of brain disease; or we emphasize the humanity of psychiatric patients, seeing their problems as having their roots, not in brain dysfunction but in attempts to deal with difficult situations in life (including difficulties which may have arisen long ago, in early infancy). And underlying the dispute between the two models, I have argued, is another, metaphysical, "either-or": either we accept a reductive materialism, or Cartesian dualism. But do we need to think in these "either-or" terms? One, rather unsatisfactory, attempt to escape from this way of thinking which has been proposed is the "biopsychosocial" model. This is suggested as a pragmatic compromise, in which an eclectic mix of biological, psychological and sociological explanations is allowed. But, as Nassir Ghaemi argues, the trouble with this is that it is *too* eclectic: it offers no unified theory of human nature which would enable us to weight the contributions of biological, psychological and social factors. In this way, it leads to what Ghaemi calls an "explanatory nihilism" (Ghaemi 2003, p. 82). We need rather to go deeper, to examine the views of human mentality and behavior on which the biological and psychological models are based.

Although dualism and reductive materialism are clearly opposed to each other in fundamental respects, they also have important elements in common. Both accept, above all, that in talking about human mental life we are talking about the behavior of a "thing," or "substance." The difference is only that dualists regard that thing as of a special, immaterial, kind, distinct from the rest of the universe, which is material, whereas materialists identify it with a particular sort of material thing, namely, the brain. But a second, very important, similarity follows from this: both dualism and materialism are equally reductionist in relation to the material universe. For dualists, everything which is not mental belongs to a single substance, "matter." Being all of one substance, all material things have a common essence, which Descartes defines as "extension," the property of occupying space. The laws governing the behavior of matter must therefore all ultimately be derived from those of physics, and specifically of mechanics, the science of the movement of matter from one place to another. These physical laws must also be "mechanistic" in a broader sense. Since matter is a distinct substance from mind, the description and explanation of its behavior may not employ any "mentalistic" concepts such as "meaning" or "purpose." Hence the explanation of what goes on in the material realm must be purely causal: it must consist in showing only how one physical change leads on to another, without any attempt to understand *why* (for what reason) this happens rather than that. For the materialist, there is only one realm, so that this reductionism applies to everything, including human behavior: the whole of reality is therefore to be explained in the same way, and all science forms a single, unified, system rooted in physics. But it is important to see this idea of a unified science of nature as already present in Cartesian dualism, and carried over into materialism because the latter defined itself in opposition to the dualist framework. This is why this variety of materialism has sometimes been called, and with some justification, "Cartesian materialism" (see, e.g., Gillett 2008).

The common elements between Cartesian dualism and Cartesian materialism are the source, I want to argue, of a number of misguided oppositions and assumptions which are relevant to our present topic. First, from the shared belief that "mind" is the name of a "thing" or "substance" is derived the assumption that it must be either something entirely non-material or something purely material—probably a brain. This goes with a second assumption, namely, that everything "mental" is of the same kind, sharing a common "essence"—either a different essence from everything material (if one is a dualist), or the same essence (if one is a materialist). Part of what this means is that everything mental, including mental disorders, is to be explained in the same way, either by empathetic understanding or by the laws of physical sciences such as genetics and neuroscience. Thirdly, both views share a reductionist conception of the sciences of the material world (which for the materialist, of course, contains everything which really exists, including the "mind"). It follows from this reductionism that all explanation in the physical sciences (all "causal" explanation) must take the same form. These assumptions are clearly interconnected; and they are all questionable. At their root is the assumption that the question of understanding human mental life and its relation to human existence more generally is an *ontological* one: it is the "mind–brain problem"—how does one thing called our "mind" relate to another thing called our "brain"?

I want to argue that we can think more fruitfully about mental life, and in particular about psychiatric theory, practice, and research, if we question this root assumption. Above all, we need to reject the idea that these questions are essentially ontological or metaphysical. A phenomenological approach, I shall argue, can take us further. I shall focus particularly on the phenomenological approach of the French philosopher, Maurice Merleau-Ponty (1908–1961). Phenomenology, for Merleau-Ponty, "consists in re-learning to look at the world" (Merleau-Ponty 1962, p. xx). We do this by setting aside presuppositions about how the world *must* be, derived from abstract metaphysical or scientific theories which aim to *explain* our experience of reality (the "phenomena"), and seeking simply to *describe* how reality actually presents itself to us in our pre-theoretical experience. If we do this in relation to human beings and their mental lives, we shall ask, not "What is the nature of 'mind'?" but "How do we actually encounter human beings and their thoughts, feelings, desires, wishes, etc.?" The answer to that is that we encounter them as fellow-creatures, inhabiting the same world as us and able to communicate their thoughts, feelings, desires, etc. to us, both verbally and in other ways. And we are aware of ourselves, too, as human beings like those we encounter, with our own mental lives as the thoughts, feelings, etc. which we have about things and people around us, and which we can communicate to others. Phenomenologically, therefore, what we mean by "mind" is not identifiable either with a non-material but somehow "inner" soul or self, nor with a material brain, which is literally inside our skulls. Our mental lives are, as Merleau-Ponty, following Heidegger, puts it, part of our "being-in-the-world": he would agree with the greatest of philosophers of psychiatry, Karl Jaspers, in emphasizing that "Psyche is not to be regarded as an object with given qualities but as '*being in one's own world*', the integrating of an inner and outer world" (Jaspers 1997, p. 9).

Our experience of human beings, whether in our own case or in that of the others we encounter, are for this reason "in-the-world" in a distinctive way. Inanimate beings are in the world simply as *objects*: they are located in space, and have spatial and causal relations to other objects. They have no "inner world," in Jaspers' phrase, to "integrate" with their existence in the "outer world." We do, however. We have thoughts, emotions, wishes, desires, intentions to act, and so on, all of which relate to the outside world: they are "about" the outer world in various ways. What is in this world, in this sense, has a *meaning* for us: my computer is, not just an object of metal, plastic, glass, etc. with a certain shape, color, etc., but also the means by which I can write the articles, books, and letters I want to write, can email the friends I want to contact, can get the information I want from the Internet, etc. So our relations to the things and people around us are not just spatial and causal (though they clearly are of those kinds as well), but are also relations of meaning, intentional relations. In this sense, we exist in the world as *subjects* as well as *objects* (in our case, the kind of object we are is living organisms, members of the biological species *Homo sapiens*). We are *embodied subjects* or *body-subjects*.

The hyphenation of the term "body-subject" expresses the fact that the embodiment and the subjectivity cannot be considered in isolation from each other. We can have a mental life at all only because we have functioning brains of a certain complexity, and we have the kind of mental life we do have because of the ways in which our brains, and our bodies more generally, are structured. We have a *human* mental life, the kind which belongs to members of our biological species: the desires which we have, for instance, depend on the characteristically human structures of our bodies. This does not mean that they are only what the moralists would call "carnal" desires: human beings naturally experience other kinds of desires, such as the desire for the warmth and respect which other human beings can give us, and these latter desires even help to shape the ways in which the more "carnal" desires express themselves. "In this way," Merleau-Ponty says, "the body expresses total existence, not because it is an external accompaniment to that existence, but because existence comes into its own in the body. This incarnate significance is the central phenomenon of which body and mind, sign and significance are abstract moments" (Merleau-Ponty 1962, p. 166).

Conversely, our subjectivity affects the nature of our embodiment. The fact that we are significance-giving beings makes our bodies more than merely mechanistic physical systems. The functioning of our brains, and other relevant bodily systems, needs for its full understanding an appreciation of their role in our relationship to the world around us. Having a thought, for example, such as "This book is hard to read," requires electrochemical activity in the brain, but the thought cannot be simply *identified* with this activity: rather, it is identified as the thought it is by the meaning of the words in which it is expressed. To explain the possibility of having that thought, we need to make use of the laws governing electro-chemical activity in the brain (as well as other, psychological and sociological, laws governing the acquisition of the relevant concepts). But my actual having of this thought on this occasion cannot be explained by these laws of brain activity, only by my reasons for thinking it. And at the same time, there is a sense in which the occurrence of this brain activity in having this thought can be explained by my reasons for having it: that is, it is those reasons which explain why *this* brain activity is involved in having *this* thought. In this way, our existence as subjects and as bodies is inextricably interlinked. In what may be taken as a summary of the whole idea of the body-subject, Merleau-Ponty says, "Man taken as a concrete being is not a psyche joined to an organism, but the movement to and fro of existence which at one time allows itself to take corporeal form and at others moves towards personal acts" (Merleau-Ponty 1962, p. 88).

The conclusion is, in a way, banal, but nevertheless important. It is that, when we look at what human beings are actually like ("phenomenologically"), we can see that human experience and behavior, including disordered experience and behavior, and their explanation, are more complex and subtle than is allowed for by the abstract metaphysics of "mind" and "brain." Talk about our "minds" is not talk about a single, homogeneous, thing, but about a wide variety of human meaningful interactions with their worlds, together with the capacities which make those interactions possible. Mental disorders can take a corresponding variety of forms: some, for instance, will consist, partly or wholly, in failures of capacities (the failures of memory in dementia, or of empathy in autism or in some personality disorders might be examples). Others will consist in ways of being-in-the-world which are distorted, in the sense of being deviations from normal ways of being which are distressing for the person concerned: examples might be such things as delusions, obsessive-compulsive disorder, post-traumatic stress disorder, and agoraphobia. Yet others will consist in the abnormal persistence of reactions to the world which have distressing consequences, such as mood disorders like depression.

The explanation of mental disorders (on which treatment ultimately depends) will be similarly diverse. Freeing ourselves from the assumption that we must be *either* dualists *or* reductive materialists is also freeing ourselves from accompanying oversimple views of explanation. If we examine how phenomena are *actually* explained in the various sciences, without the distorting lens of metaphysical presuppositions, we can see how absurd is the idea that the whole of "science" forms a single, unified structure, founded in physics. That idea is the product of the continuing influence of Cartesianism, even on many of those who officially reject it. In the real world, we recognize that the way in which we make phenomena intelligible depends on how we describe those phenomena; and in the case of some phenomena, especially those involving human thought, emotion and behavior, that description may be very complex and multifaceted. Some aspects of some mental disorders, for instance, the failure or absence of certain mental capacities, may be entirely explicable in terms of brain injury or disease. In other cases, brain dysfunction or neurochemistry (e.g., serotonin levels) may explain a disorder in the important sense of indicating its preconditions, or of making its persistence intelligible: but there will also be a need to understand the disordered thought-processes, emotions, and behavior as an attempt to deal with problems in the person's situation, if we are to achieve an explanation which is therapeutically useful. What is important is that Merleau-Ponty's conception of the body-subject offers the possibility of an escape from thinking that we must subscribe *either* to a biological *or* to a psychological model. More important still, perhaps, is the vision of psychiatry as requiring *both* a humanistic understanding of mental disorders as responses to human problems *and* an adequate grasp of the neurological and genetic influences on the shape of human behavior. To quote Jaspers again, "The psychiatrist as a practitioner deals with individuals, with the human being as a whole" (Jaspers 1997, p. 1).

References

American Psychiatric Association (1994). *Diagnostic and Statistical Manual of Mental Disorders, Fourth Edition*. Washington, DC: American Psychiatric Association.

Bentall, R. P. (2004). *Madness Explained: Psychosis and Human Nature*. London: Penguin Books.

Bentall, R. P. (2009). *Doctoring the Mind*. London: Allen Lane.

Bolton, D. (2008). *What is Mental Disorder?* Oxford: Oxford University Press.

Churchland, P. M. (1981/2002). Eliminative materialism and the propositional attitudes. *Journal of Philosophy*, *78*, 67–90. (Reprinted in Chalmers, D. J. (Ed.) (2002). *Philosophy of Mind: Classical and Contemporary Readings*, pp. 568–80. Oxford: Oxford University Press.

Churchland, P. M. (1995). *The Engine of Reason, the Seat of the Soul: A Philosophical Journey into the Brain*. Cambridge, MA: MIT Press.

Ghaemi, S. N. (2003). *The Concepts of Psychiatry*. Baltimore, MD: Johns Hopkins University Press.

Gillett, G. (2008). *Subjectivity and Being Somebody: Human Identity and Neuroethics*. Exeter: Imprint Academic.

Graham, G. (2010). *The Disordered Mind*. London: Routledge.

Jaspers, K. (1997). *General Psychopathology* (Volume I) (J. Hoenig and M. W. Hamilton, Trans.). Baltimore, MD: Johns Hopkins University Press.

Laing, R. D. (2010). *The Divided Self*. London: Penguin Classics edition.

Martin, E. A. (Ed.) (2007). *Oxford Concise Medical Dictionary* (7th edn.). Oxford: Oxford University Press.

Merleau-Ponty, M. (1962). *Phenomenology of Perception* (C. Smith, Trans.). London: Routledge & Kegan Paul.

Murphy, D. (2006). *Psychiatry in the Scientific Image*. Cambridge, MA: MIT Press.

Place, U. T. (1956/2002). Is consciousness a brain process? *British Journal of Psychology*, *47*, 44–50. (Reprinted in Chalmers, D. J. (Ed.) (2002). *Philosophy of Mind: Classical and Contemporary Readings*, pp. 55–60. Oxford: Oxford University Press.

Sadler, J. Z. (2005). *Values and Psychiatric Diagnosis*. Oxford: Oxford University Press.

Shorter, E. (1997). *A History of Psychiatry: From the Era of the Asylum to the Age of Prozac*. New York, NY: John Wiley and Sons, Inc.

Smart (1959/2002). Sensations and brain processes. *Philosophical Review*, *68*, 141–56. (Reprinted in Chalmers, D. J. (ed.) (2002). *Philosophy of Mind: Classical and Contemporary Readings*, pp. 60–8. Oxford: Oxford University Press.

Szasz, T. (2002). *The Meaning of Mind: Language, Morality, and Neuroscience*, Syracuse, NY: Syracuse University Press.

SECTION V

DESCRIPTIVE PSYCHOPATHOLOGY

CHAPTER 34

INTRODUCTION: DESCRIPTIVE PSYCHOPATHOLOGY

With concepts summoned and at hand, we are ready for theoretically informed descriptions of psychopathologies. This section begins with anxiety, depression, and body image disorders, and moves on through emotion and affective disorders, to delusion, thought insertion, and the fragmentation of consciousness. These phenomena call, not only for assessment and diagnosis, but also for understanding on the part of both the engaged clinician and the philosophical commentator. They also provide case studies for general philosophical questions about different levels of description and conceptualization and the relationships between them, and about the contributions to psychological understanding that are made by phenomenology, clinical expert knowledge, and the sciences of the mind.

In Chapter 35 on anxiety and phobias, Gerrit Glas distinguishes four levels of conceptualization—the level of everyday psychological understanding, and the clinical, scientific, and philosophical levels. Following a brief history of the concept of anxiety, from Hippocrates to the present day, he discusses issues that arise at the interfaces between adjacent levels. At the interface between the everyday and clinical levels of understanding, there are very general issues about the nature of clinical understanding itself and more specific questions about the patient's and the clinician's relationships to the patient's disorder and, particularly, about the way in which the disorder itself and the patient's own personality influence the patient's relationship with his disorder. At the interface between the clinical and scientific levels, there are again general issues, concerning the contributions made by clinical expert knowledge and scientific theoretical insight, and the existence of upward explanatory gaps between scientific theory and clinical phenomena. There are also questions about classification and Glas reviews recent discussions of dimensional *versus* categorical approaches, particularly as these apply to anxiety. At the interface between scientific and philosophical understanding, the major research programs—evolutionary, behavioral, cognitive—in the scientific study of anxiety come into contact with questions in the philosophy of emotion, such as whether emotions are natural kinds. Glas concludes by reviewing recent work on the subjective experience or phenomenology of emotion and commends an "embodied, embedded, and enactive" perspective.

Matthew Ratcliffe offers a phenomenological account of impaired agency in depression in Chapter 36. People with depression describe a change, a diminution, in the subjective experience or phenomenology of free will but, in order to understand this loss, we first need to characterize the normal, intact phenomenology of free will or agency. Ratcliffe argues that the experience of free will is not a quale that accompanies actions of a special kind, such as those preceded by considerable reflective decision-making. Rather, all our actions are experienced as free. Adopting the embodied, embedded, and enactive perspective, and drawing on Husserl and the notion of perceptual expectation, Ratcliffe proposes that normal perception presents possibilities, including possibilities for action, and that this perception of worldly possibility is intertwined with our experience of embodiment. Drawing on Sartre, he proposes that the experience of freedom is integral to the experienced world, shaped by our projects, and inextricable from bodily phenomenology. With this characterization of the normal sense of freedom, it is possible to interpret the change in the experience of free will that is described by people with depression as a change in their experience of the world. Their perceptual experience no longer presents a world of possibilities for action.

Completing this first trio of chapters, Katherine Morris (Chapter 37) examines body image disorders, particularly body dysmorphic disorder, anorexia nervosa, bulimia nervosa, and binge eating disorder. She focuses on attempts to understand these disorders from three perspectives: psychology and psychiatry, feminism, and phenomenology. First, Morris briefly reviews research in the "body image" tradition, where body image is conceived as individuals' own subjective experiences of their appearance, and she notes that, consistent with this conception, this research downplays social and cultural factors. Research in the "body shame" tradition, in contrast, accords a central role to social and cultural factors and, in this respect, it promises a better understanding. Second, many body image disorders exhibit a strong gender asymmetry and feminists go beyond the "body shame" tradition, to provide critiques of cultures. These critiques contribute to understanding of the social and cultural conditions in which body image disorders thrive but, in common with work in the "body image" and "body shame" traditions, they do not contribute as much to an understanding of the embodied experience of individuals suffering from these disorders. Third, that deficit is made good by phenomenological philosophers who describe body dysmorphic disorder in Sartrean terms, with particular attention to shame and alienation, and anorexia in terms of abjection. Overall, Morris judges that the body image approach is in the grip of scientism and unlikely to contribute to understanding, that the body shame approach is an improvement and provides models that shed some light on the persistence of body image disorders, and that the feminist cultural critical and phenomenological approaches are potentially complementary and together contribute to understanding of individuals with body image disorders.

In Chapter 38, Thomas Fuchs is concerned that understanding of affective disorders is impeded by the lack of an adequate account of affectivity itself. Rejecting traditional psychodynamic approaches, contemporary cognitive models, and the heritage of Cartesian dualism, he offers a phenomenological account of emotions and the field of affectivity more generally. The dominant idea is that affectivity is an ineliminable aspect of our embodied experience, giving meaning to our environment. Fuchs begins with the example of vital feelings—the feeling of being alive, the loss of which may lead to the conclusion that one has died, the Cotard delusion—and then moves on to existential feelings, which are divided into three categories. Elementary existential feelings include the feeling of being alive, and feelings of meaningfulness and significance; general existential feelings include feeling healthy or ill, strong or weak, alert or indifferent; and social existential feelings include the feeling of connectedness and the feeling of familiarity, the loss of which may lead to the conclusion that familiar people have been replaced by impostors, the Capgras delusion. The chapter continues through affective atmospheres and moods to emotions. Here, Fuchs describes four aspects of emotions: affective intentionality, which is a distinctive kind of intentionality in being evaluative; bodily resonance; action tendency; and functions and significance—emotions interrupt us, inform us, give meaning to a situation, and make us ready to act, and also have an expressive function. These aspects are brought together in an "embodied and extended" concept of emotions, in line with a general view of affects as connecting body, self, and world.

In Chapter 39 on the phenomenological approach to delusions, Louis Sass and Elizabeth Pienkos focus on what Karl Jaspers called the "true delusions" of schizophrenia. They begin by highlighting five features of the approach: the phenomenologist is interested in understanding what it is like to have a delusion; emphasizes the form, rather than the content, of the experience; appreciates the heterogeneity of delusional experience; questions the assumption that a delusion is best understood as a false belief; and recognizes the inherent difficulty in describing delusion in schizophrenia. Sass and Pienkos propose that, although Jaspers regarded true or primary delusions as un-understandable and beyond the scope of empathy, the phenomenological approach offers, not only description, but also understanding and even explanation. They begin with the delusional mood or pre-delusional state, which is characterized by feelings of change, strangeness, and elusive meaning and the sense that objects have become detached from their natural perceptual context. In this state, the patient may experience the external world both as inauthentic and as referring to himself. These changes in the patient's experience of the world are accompanied by changes in his experience of himself, his body, his thoughts, and his stream of consciousness, such as feelings of estrangement from his body. Sass and Pienkos describe how delusions of persecution, alien control, or non-existence or, as they put it, "entry into a delusional world," develop as making some sense of the patient's anomalous experience of self and world. Later in the chapter, they explore the idea of double bookkeeping—that delusions do not involve straightforwardly false claims about shared external reality and that the patient experiences his delusional world as having a status analogous to an imagined or dreamt world.

Johannes Roessler begins Chapter 40 about thought insertion by setting out an inconsistent triad, three plausible claims that cannot all be true. The first is a claim about introspective awareness: to be introspectively aware of a current episode of thinking that p is to be aware of oneself thinking that p (Transparency). The second is a claim about thought insertion: patients with the delusion of thought insertion believe that someone else is the thinker of an episode of thinking of which they are introspectively aware (Alienation). And the third is a claim about the rational intelligibility of beliefs: reports of thought insertion express rationally intelligible coherent beliefs (Intelligibility). In the philosophical literature on thought insertion, the standard response to the tension between these three claims has been to weaken Transparency by distinguishing between two concepts of the ownership of one's own thoughts. In principle, one can be introspectively aware of an episode of thinking as occurring in one's own mind without being aware that one is the agent or author of the thought. Thus, what patients believe is not beyond the bounds of rational intelligibility. Roessler rejects this standard response and, in particular, rejects recent proposals for developing a notion of agentive ownership for which Transparency would not hold. He argues that, instead of questioning Transparency, we should question the idea that schizophrenic delusions are to be understood as patients' rationally intelligible descriptions of abnormal experiences. Nevertheless, Intelligibility should not be discarded altogether and the delusion of thought insertion can be understood as the delusional transformation of a rationally intelligible precursor belief.

In Chapter 41 on the disunity of consciousness, Tim Bayne addresses the question whether consciousness is fragmented, rather than unified, in psychiatric disorders. He begins by distinguishing three aspects of the unity of consciousness: intentional, subjective, and phenomenal. Intentional unity is the integration of conscious mental states with each other; subjective unity is a subject's capacity to be aware of her conscious mental states as her own; phenomenal unity is the existence of a single total conscious state that encompasses each of a subject's conscious states at a time. Are any of these aspects of unity lost in psychiatric disorders? Bayne considers anosognosia, schizophrenia, and dissociative identity disorder. In anosognosia, the patient does not make appropriate use of available evidence to revise her belief that she can still move her arm (which is, in fact, paralyzed). This is a failure of integration or intentional unity. Since some of the available evidence is provided by her own experience of the consequences of motoric failure, it is also plausible that there is a breakdown of subjective unity. But, Bayne argues, even the phenomenon of "dim knowledge" (a patient's implicit appreciation of her impairment) does not show that anosognosia involves a breakdown of the phenomenal unity of consciousness. This pattern generalizes. Thought disorder involves a breakdown of intentional unity and it is plausible that thought insertion compromises subjective unity. But there is no reason to deny that phenomenal unity is preserved in patients with schizophrenia. Even in the case of dissociative identity disorder, there is no compelling case for the claim that it involves phenomenal disunity. Overall, even in psychiatric disorders, the phenomenal aspect of the unity of consciousness is preserved.

In the final chapter in this section, Chapter 42 on cognitive approaches to delusion, Martin Davies and Andy Egan focus on the two-factor framework for explaining delusions, which has mainly been applied to monothematic delusions of neuropsychological origin. The first factor in the etiology of a delusion is a neuropsychological deficit from which the content of the delusion arises in some plausible way. The second factor is supposed to explain why the delusional belief is not rejected, but Davies and Egan point to some unclarity surrounding its role. Does it explain why a hypothesis that is related to the neuropsychological deficit is initially adopted as a belief, rather than being rejected, or why the initially adopted belief persists, rather than being subsequently rejected? They show that it is difficult to find a role for a pathological factor in an explanation of persistence because, on standard Bayesian assumptions, persistence of an adopted belief (until new evidence is available) is the normal case. Davies and Egan do not regard this difficulty as revealing a problem for the two-factor framework, for a Bayesian approach, or for the idea that the second factor explains the persistence of the delusional belief. Instead, they recommend relaxing the standard Bayesian idealizing assumption that subjects have a single coherent assignment of credences, and allowing that newly adopted beliefs should be compartmentalized until they can be evaluated in the light of pre-existing beliefs. A newly adopted delusional belief would then be compartmentalized and could, in principle, be subsequently rejected on the grounds of its implausibility. Cognitive impairments of executive function or working memory would make critical evaluation of the belief difficult and, more dramatically, failure of compartmentalization would eliminate the very considerations in the light of which the belief was implausible.

CHAPTER 35

ANXIETY AND PHOBIAS: PHENOMENOLOGIES, CONCEPTS, EXPLANATIONS

GERRIT GLAS

INTRODUCTION

Anxiety is a central feature of many forms of psychopathology. Its phenomenology is incredibly rich and multiform. The conditions that have anxiety as their core belong to those with the highest prevalence and incidence rates. Anxiety is also a symptom of many other conditions, such as psychosis, autism, personality disorder, and mood disorder. Most importantly, however, anxiety has been interpreted as expression of who we are. Anxiety is the counterpart of what people experience when they face finitude, death, contingency, powerlessness, absurdity, and/or fundamental doubt.

Philosophical issues with respect to anxiety and its pathological variants arise at the border between everyday and clinical understanding of anxiety, between clinical and scientific approaches, and between scientific concepts and the philosophical frameworks to which they refer. These four forms of understanding can be seen as epistemic levels that each in its own way reveals aspects of anxiety in its complexity (Fig. 35.1).

The level of everyday understanding refers to anxiety in its rich variety of feelings and behavioral manifestations. The clinical level addresses the different forms of anxiety clinicians are referring to: generalized anxiety, phobia, obsession, compulsion, panic, worry, irritability, restlessness, and avoidance. The scientific way of understanding anxiety is the result of theories and hypotheses that guide clinical understanding and empirical research. At the philosophical level paradigmatic views and broad frameworks that guide scientific and clinical understanding can be discerned: anxiety as a biological dysregulation, for instance, or anxiety as expression of an inner threat, or as a result of "wrong" thinking, or as an existential feeling or attitude.

Level 1	Everyday understanding	Lay-concepts and interpretations
		Protoprofessionalized language
Level 2	Clinical understanding	Prototypes
		Multilevel explanations
		Multicausal reconstruction
Level 3	Scientific understanding	Explanatory models
		Causal pathways
		Determinants
		Statistical patterns
Level 4	Philosophical understanding	Views on causality and lawful regularities
		Paradigms
		Worldviews
		Normative issues

FIGURE 35.1 Four levels of conceptualization.

Philosophical questions arise at the interface between these levels. With respect to the first two levels (everyday understanding and clinical knowledge) there is, for instance, the issue of where to draw the boundary between the normal and the pathological, and of how to account for instances of friction between ordinary understanding and the medical view of things. At the interface between clinical and scientific approaches the question arises as to whether, and to what extent, scientific theories and models are adequate. Which aspects of the clinical picture can be explained by scientific theories and concepts, and which cannot? Between these scientific concepts and the philosophical frameworks they presuppose there is the debate about what really belongs to science and what should be regarded as metatheoretical or paradigmatic. To what extent does a particular scientific concept stand on its own and to what extent does it borrow from pre-theoretical and/or philosophical views?

In this chapter philosophical issues related to the conceptualization and explanation of pathological forms of anxiety will be discussed. The fourfold distinction just discussed will serve as a framework and as context for the questions that guide our argument. First, however, a few notes will be made about the conceptual history of anxiety and its disorders.

CONCEPTUAL HISTORY

The history of the conceptualization of anxiety does not begin with the notions of fear and anxiety, but with melancholia (Jackson 1986). For many ages anxiety was thought to be part of the much broader concept of melancholia—a term that can already be found in the *Corpus Hippocraticum*, written by Hippocrates and his pupils (fifth century BC), and that refers to the excess of black bile in conditions we now refer to as depression, agitation, or dysphoria. Black bile was one of the four humors, the other three being yellow bile, blood, and phlegm. Illness and disease were thought to be the result of an imbalance between these fluids. The fluids themselves were considered to be influenced not only by the composition of the four elements (earth, fire, water, and air) in the environment, but also by climate, the position of the planets, the moon, and the stars, the time of year, eating and drinking habits, and physical and mental efforts.

Humoral pathology was enormously influential and dominated the medical landscape up to the end of the eighteenth century. At that time, the Aristotelian teleological conception of the order of nature had already been given up for more than 150 years. Pathological anatomy had begun to expand. Doctors and scientists were fascinated by the quality of all sorts of sensory experiences. Popular notions in medical literature of that time, like irritability and tone, contributed to a preoccupation with hypersensitivity of the nervous system. The central nervous system gradually replaced the blood, the liver, and the spleen, from which, until then, melancholia was thought to originate.

The great descriptive tradition in psychopathology began, with respect to anxiety and its pathological manifestations, somewhere in the midst of the nineteenth century with descriptions of fear-related pain in the chest (Flemming 1848), agoraphobia (Benedikt 1870; Westphal 1872), irregularities of the cardiac rhythm in circumstances of war (Da Costa 1871), war neurosis (MacKenzie 1916, 1920) and the so-called effort syndrome (Lewis 1918, 1940). All these descriptions presuppose, more or less openly, the biomedical perspective, according to which medical science is advanced, first of all, by the careful description and delineation of symptoms and syndromes, and then, secondly, by the attempt to detect underlying pathophysiological mechanisms. The provisional summary of the descriptive findings—it was still too early for causal hypotheses—can be found in the sixth and later editions of Emil Kraepelin's famous handbook, in which distinctions are made that don't differ too much from contemporary classification. Kraepelin describes (spontaneous) anxiety attacks (especially nocturnal panic), anxiety related to obsessions and compulsions, social phobia, agoraphobia, and anxieties that are associated with automatic actions (Kraepelin 1899). Anxiety is not a very important topic for Kraepelin, however.

This is different for the French psychopathologist Pierre Janet, whose work is much less known but whose theories are in fact highly original and much more innovative than those of Kraepelin and his colleagues (Ellenberger 1970; Janet 1903). It is not so much the phenomenon of anxiety itself that Janet is interested in. Anxiety, in fact, belongs to the lowest level in the hierarchy of psychopathological symptoms. At the center of Janet's endeavor is a theory of the integration of different mental functions. His seminal work on obsessions and psychasthenia describes anxiety as the ultimate bodily manifestation of a "lowering of the level of mental tension." At the highest level of psychic functioning this lowering of tension is felt as a diminishment of the sense of reality (a form of chronic depersonalization) and as a feeling of incompleteness (ineffectiveness; as if actions are not followed by a message confirming their execution). Obsessions, compulsions, motor or vocal tics, and visceral anxiety are the core symptoms of this so-called psychasthenic state, together with fatigue and intolerance of effort.

One can hardly overestimate the importance of the change of perspective that took place under the influence of the ideas of Sigmund Freud. Freud was amongst the first of those who saw anxiety as the result of inner (instead of external) threat. In his conception anxiety comes in two forms, the anxiety neuroses and the so-called psychoneuroses. The anxiety neuroses are still conceived as disorders of the nervous system. Psychoneuroses like hysteria and obsessive–compulsive neurosis, however, are seen as the result of unresolved inner conflict. This conflict typically concerns sexual and aggressive drives and their forbidden expression. Anxiety becomes a signal, indicating inner danger, the inner turmoil and tension that threaten the psychic equilibrium as a result of the repression of drives. Freud's pioneering work (1895, 1926) heralded the beginning of psychotherapy and had an enormous psychological and cultural impact on the self-conception of Western citizens.

Even further went those psychopathologists, who—in the footsteps of philosophers like Blaise Pascal (1669), Sören Kierkegaard (1844/1980), and Martin Heidegger (1927)—saw anxiety as an expression of a frustrated urge for self-realization. Anxiety is no longer primarily an emotion in this approach. It is no longer the psychic indicator of concrete dangers, internal or external. Anxiety is something more comprehensive; it is the immediate expression of a disruption of the stability of personhood, the imminent destruction of vital forces that keep our mental functions together. It is the frustration of these vital forces in their urge for self-realization. At the basis of considerations such as these lie, among others, the observations of patients with brain damage by Kurt Goldstein (1929). These veterans, victims of World War I, when faced with complex tasks, displayed catastrophic reactions consisting of a wide range of physiological and psychomotor symptoms. Goldstein believed that, even in the absence of subjective feelings of fear, these reactions could best be interpreted as expressions of anxiety. The anxiety of these veterans was, strictly speaking, not a reaction to failure on certain tasks, nor an awareness of such failure; it was quite literally the actual manifestation of the failure. The powerlessness, ineffectiveness, and disruption of these people is not the result but the expression of anxiety, Goldstein hypothesized.

Views like these can also be found in the work by Arthur Kronfeld (1935) and Philipp Lersch (1964). They typically mix philosophical traditions, especially vitalism and (existential) phenomenology. Vitalists emphasize the "synthetic" power of organic forces, the inexhaustible creativity of evolution, and the mystery of the drive to individuation, understood as a combination of differentiation and integration of functions leading to individuality of the person. Existential phenomenologists consider unbiased description as crucial for psychological and philosophical understanding. They tend to interpret psychic phenomena as expressions of underlying fundamental ways of self-relating and of relating to the world. Anxiety is, according to Heidegger, a fundamental way of self-relating, indicating the impossibility of absolute openness to one's own "impossibility," i.e., impossibility of openness toward the possibility of one's own death.

These accounts are undeniably characterized by a certain eclecticism. It is, for instance, not always clear in which way the biotic forces striving for self-expression make contact with the overarching psychic structures that mediate self-relatedness and relatedness to the world. Many of these authors make use of a model which divides personality into an impersonal (biological) substructure and a personal superstructure. The substructure is described in vitalistic terms whilst the superstructure is analyzed in terms derived from existential phenomenology. In spite of the vagueness of the relationship between the subpersonal and the personal sphere, the anthropological (or existential) approach is important because of its intuitions and implicit assumptions. The anthropological (existential) approach suggests that there is a form of anxiety that is much more than just an emotion. This anxiety is not the opposite of a feeling of safety and being at home. Rather it is the opposite of the "synthetic" activity of the I, the person in its striving for wholeness and meaning. Anxiety is not an objectless form of fear, nor the result of the perception of a threatening situation. It is a fragmentation of the self, leading to the outbreak of chaotic and formless biological forces.

After 1930 the study of anxiety does not seem to have been a priority for about three decades. The relative neglect of the classification of anxiety disorders can possibly best be interpreted as a reflection of the fact that, as a rule, patients with neurotic anxiety were never hospitalized (Jablensky 1985). The situation changed in the 1950s with the emergence of psychophysiology and attempts by psychophysiologists to indicate differences between emotions in terms of differences between their peripheral physiological manifestations (Ax 1953). Furthermore, at this time, the anxiolytic effects of benzodiazepines were discovered, resulting in a flood of research into the effects of these chemicals on the central nervous system (Sternbach, 1980). It is also the decade in which Wolpe (1958) introduced systematic desensitization as a form of behavior therapy, thereby giving new impetus to the treatment of people with anxiety and phobic disorders. Roth (1959) described a form of depersonalization associated with severe anxiety and phobic phenomena, the so-called "phobic anxiety-depersonalization syndrome." Klein, finally, discovered that panic attacks in agoraphobic patients can be blocked by imipramine (Klein 1964, 1980). This heralds the beginning of an immense stream of experimental, pharmacological, clinical, longitudinal, epidemiological, genetic, and familial research into the existence and course of anxiety disorders.

Psychopharmacological and biological psychiatric research requires stringent diagnostic criteria, like the Feighner criteria (Feighner et al. 1972). These, together with the research diagnostic criteria (Spitzer et al. 1975, 1978) form the basis of the third revised edition of the *Diagnostic and Statistical Manual of Mental Disorders* (DSM-III-R; American Psychiatric Association (APA) 1980, 1987). The emphasis on descriptive precision leads to the demarcation of various forms of anxiety and to an abandonment of the concept of neurosis, which was considered too vague. Neurasthenic neurosis is discarded. Anxiety neurosis, phobic neurosis, and obsessive–compulsive neurosis are combined under the heading of anxiety disorders. Post-traumatic stress disorder, a newcomer, is added to the anxiety disorders. Anxiety neurosis is subsequently split up into panic disorder and generalized anxiety disorder, whilst phobic neurosis is divided into agoraphobia, simple phobias, and social phobia (cf. Spitzer and Williams, 1985).

In spite of the non-theoretical nature of the DSM-III, these changes indicate a fundamentally different approach to the psychopathology of anxiety. The DSM-III takes distance not only from the psychodynamic conflict model, but also from the existential tradition in which anxiety is associated with an inhibition of the urge to self-realize. This global and "deep" concept is replaced by a finely grained description and classification of more "superficial" symptoms. This change also marks the transition from a predominantly dimensional (dispositional) approach which characterizes the neurosis model, to a categorical approach to psychopathology.

It is only since 2000 that psychiatry has again begun to reconsider the relevance of dimensional models of anxiety and anxiety disorders. However, so far the diagnostic working groups of the APA do not seem to be inclined to adopt a full-blown dimensional approach, in spite of a growing body of evidence supporting this line of thinking in the psychological (Krueger 1999; Watson 2005) and epidemiological (Andrew et al. 2008; 2009) literature.

Later in this chapter we will give more detail about this discussion (see "Anxiety at the inter-face between clinical and scientific understanding" section).

ANXIETY AT THE INTERFACE BETWEEN
EVERYDAY AND CLINICAL UNDERSTANDING

Although everyone knows what anxiety is, it is nevertheless also elusive. The term "anxiety" denotes an incredible variety of manifestations. Anxiety may express itself as agitation, but also as a state of paralysis; as subtle worry without any somatic symptom but also as a storm of physical sensations without clear mental content; as behavioral avoidance, but also as thoughts or feelings without any behavioral manifestation; as a magnified form of an ordi-nary fear, but also as a nearly psychotic obsession without any basis in reality. In some cases there is a broad range of fears and worries, in other cases the preoccupation remains limited to one topic.

Clinicians have a set of prototypical cases in mind when they interview their patients. These prototypes structure the process of interviewing; they help to maintain focus; and they are partly subliminal (Dreyfus and Dreyfus 1986; Schon 1983). When clinicians hesitate about a particular diagnosis, they may consult a textbook or a clinical guideline in order to help them articulate their thoughts. Today, prototypes are to a large extent (but not entirely) molded by classification manuals such as the DSM and the *International Classification of Diseases* (ICD).

Philosophical questions at the interface between everyday and clinical understanding are primarily *epistemic*. There is first the large, in psychiatry hitherto hardly explored, area of clinical understanding itself: What is the nature of clinical knowledge, how is it structured, is clinical knowledge indeed mainly prototypical or does it consist of a mix of prototypical, dimensional, and categorical concepts? Is clinical knowledge just knowledge, or should we think of it in a much more embodied way: as a form of affective-evaluative probing and judging, based on a variety of sources? Do gut-feelings count as a form of knowledge? And if so, what is their status and epistemic legitimacy (see Stanghellini, Chapter 23, this volume).

Also of an epistemic nature is the issue of whether there are sufficient empirical and logi-cal grounds to grant a certain cluster of symptoms the status of "disorder" (Sadler 2005). The process of validation of disorders focuses on so-called validators of groups of symptoms. The guiding idea is that clustering of symptoms should not only be based on the distribu-tion of frequencies of co-occurrence of symptoms, but also on evidence about the sharing of underlying factors, or "validators" (see "Anxiety at the interface between clinical and sci-entific understanding" section for this topic). When the existence of a particular disorder has been established there is another epistemic issue: What does the disorder explain with respect to the signs and symptoms of the patient? As we have seen, current diagnostic classi-fication has shifted to a perspective that puts emphasis on reliability, objectivity, and opera-tionalization of criteria for specific disorders. Other less tangible aspects of anxiety are easily overlooked or considered to be less important. This bias toward measurement and quantifi-cation has led to a relative neglect not only of subjective aspects of the experience of anxiety (Glas 1997), but also of its layeredness. Anxiety tends to be seen as a "condition," as nothing but a group of symptoms that is characteristic for an underlying disorder or (even) brain state. However, as clinicians and psychotherapists know: patients report much more than just symptoms. They relate to their symptoms. They deny them or zoom in and develop catastrophic thoughts; they avoid facing their anxiety or persist in a helpless attitude. Anxiety itself influences the attitude of the patient and the way he or she deals with his or her anxiety. But, the extent and direction of this influence also depends on who one is, on one's background, coping skills, and personality.

To sum up, there are at least four ways of paying attention to the anxiety of the patient (see Fig. 35.2). There is, firstly, the diagnosis and treatment of signs and symptoms as expressions of a particular disorder. Then, secondly, the clinician takes into account how the patient relates to her condition, whether she faces her condition or not, and how she does this: courageous or denying; in an open or in an avoidant way, reflective or pushing for immediate relief. Thirdly, this relatedness of the patient to her mental condition is itself influenced by the disorder. Anxiety leads to a tendency to avoid a range of situations, including the situation of facing one's own anxiety. Avoiding tendencies may influence the way the patient relates to her condition. She may, for instance, deny the severity of the symptoms or she may avoid seeking help and support. Bodily symptoms may be so overwhelming that the patient feels completely powerless and paralyzed; and this of course influences the attitude toward the panic or anxiety. Similarly for depression: demoralization in depression often leads to diminishment of one's expectations about treatment and impedes self-initiated activities to counteract the depression, thereby strengthening the apathy. Fourthly, the relationship between the patient and her disorder may also be influenced by who the person is, by her biographical background, coping skills, personality traits, and worldview. The personality of the patient may be such that avoiding tendencies that are inherent to the anxiety itself, are successfully overcome. But things may also go the other way around: the personality of

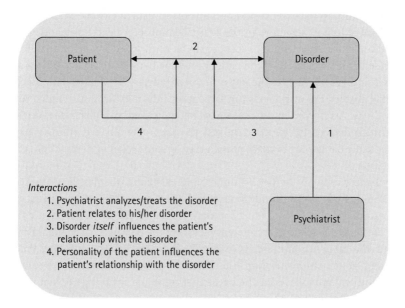

FIGURE 35.2 Interactions.

the patient may be such that even slight symptoms of anxiety lead to paralysis and lack of commitment.

A special word should be devoted in this context to so-called existential anxieties. They are a specific subset of the anxieties that are described under point 4 (Fig. 35.2). They are anxieties that have become part of one's personality, so to say, anxieties that express a basic attitude of the person. Existential anxieties are not fears *about* a certain situation; they *express* themselves *as* fundamental attitudes toward one's existence (not only toward one's anxious condition). They are expressions of the I–self relationship, not only of one's relationship with the disordered (anxious) "self," but also of one's relation with a more encompassing and biographical "self." They are, in short, not directed to one single situation but express who one is in relation toward one's existence as a whole (Glas 2003; Ratcliffe 2008, 2009).

The situation is intricate because the existential anxieties don't stand on their own in psychiatry, but usually co-occur with "psychiatric" anxieties. Panic attacks, for instance, may be mingled with more subtle and pervasive feelings of vulnerability and helplessness. These feelings can, of course, be about concrete situations in which one feels vulnerable and/or helpless. However, they may also reveal more general worries about one's existence. They express a certain "mood" about life and are fundamental forms of self-relatedness. Panic disorder may be colored by such moods. It is similar with social phobia. Avoidance of social situations may originate in a more fundamental sense of isolation or lack of presence/"being." The anxiety is in this case not *about* being isolated or *about* not being present. It is itself an *expression* of isolation and of "not being there."

Elsewhere, I have described seven of such existential anxieties. They are, respectively, anxiety related to: (1) loss of structure, (2) the facticity (the "matter of fact-ness") of one's existence, (3) lack of safety, (4) unconnectedness and isolation, (5) doubt and inability to choose, (6) meaninglessness, and (7) finitude and death (Glas 2001, 2003). The last four come close to the existential themes described by Irving Yalom: isolation (cf. 4), freedom (cf. 5), meaninglessness (cf. 6), and death (cf. 7) (Yalom 1980). The other three were added on clinical grounds. In the clinical situation one meets patients whose anxieties can be seen as expressions of lack of structure in the I–self relationship, nearly psychotic anxieties, in other words, that are experienced as losing grip on oneself (ad 1); or the anxiety that indicates a fundamental incapacity of the patient to shape her own existence (ad 2); and/or the anxiety that signifies uncontrollable physical threat (ad 3). For patients with this latter type of existential anxiety, the world feels fundamentally inhospitable, not so much socially, but physically. It feels as if everything could possibly go wrong: gas, electricity, one's housing, traffic, technical devices, the weather, the soil, the trees—literally everything is experienced as fundamentally dangerous because at the verge of some form of destruction, collapse, or sudden disaster.

Finally, anxiety may not only echo underlying existential themes. It is often also intertwined with other psychiatric conditions: mood disorder, personality problems, addiction, and/or developmental deficits. Clinical anxiety, therefore, presents us with a considerable epistemic challenge: to construe a coherent picture of the type of anxiety, the way the patient relates to it, the influence of the disturbance itself on this relationship, and the influence of personality factors on this relationship. These diagnostic deliberations should ideally be performed with an open mind for the existential color and meaning of what the patient is saying and for comorbidity with other Axis I or II disorders.

Philosophical issues at the interface of everyday and clinical understanding are not only epistemic, however, they are also *normative*. For instance, even with the rather technical and empirical study of validators one cannot entirely refrain from the use of normative points of view. Terms like genetic risk and shared familial background are only relevant insofar as they refer to abnormality, i.e., to situations that in everyday life are recognized as undesirable. In the context of psychiatric diagnosis abnormality is usually accounted for in terms the DSM mentions as criteria for disorder: subjective distress, disability (defined as impairment in one or more important areas of functioning) and risk of suffering death, pain, disability, or loss of freedom (APA 1994, p. xxi). These criteria are, after all, normative—at least, to a certain extent.

With respect to this normative aspect the key issue is not validation, but legitimacy: What kind or amount of distress, disability and/or risk is needed in order to take a group of symptoms as sign of disease, or disorder? What kind and intensity of anxiety do we consider to be "normal"? According to a widely shared way of thinking in medicine, the discussion about this issue is settled once there is a cause, a pathophysiological abnormality, leading to symptoms of the disease. However, if the definition of the cause is dependent on the definition of symptoms of the disorder, this effort is still circular and cannot avoid normative deliberations. It could, furthermore, be argued that even in cases in which the dysfunction is located at a level far from the phenomenal properties of the disorder, for instance, at a molecular biological level, normative concerns are still not out of order. Independence of definition is not the same as value-neutral definition (Stein et al. 2010; Verhoeff and Glas 2010). There may be independence between explanandum (definition of disorder) and explanans (definition of dysfunction), but still no absence of normativity in the explanans. Low levels of potassium (explanans) are, after all, low because their presence intrinsically refers to undesired (and therefore normative) consequences, like cardiac arrhythmia (explanandum) and unwanted sudden death. In psychiatry, the situation is still more difficult. In many cases causal paths are simply unknown. In other cases environmental factors interact with latent predispositions. In still other cases there is only a partial match between empirical findings and the clinical syndrome. We will not go into this more general discussion, because it is not specific for anxiety.

In a more practical sense the normative side of the distinction between level 1 (everyday experience) and level 2 (clinical knowledge) becomes apparent in the negotiations between patient and clinician. How does the medical perspective of the clinician relate to the experiential perspective of the patient? Who decides, and on what grounds, about what in the story of the patient counts as relevant and important for possible treatment? How should the clinician and the patient communicate and collaborate about what to do? Consider, for instance, the situation in which the patient does not agree with the prescription of medication because of certain side effects. What is one to do if these side effects are marginal from the perspective of the psychiatrist? What is wisdom if the weighing of these side effects by the patient is influenced by personality problems or other symptoms at the border of psychopathology (see Box 35.1)? Which perspective should precede: the possibly distorted perspective of the patient or the possibly one-sided biomedical perspective of the psychiatrist? Such questions are dealt with in the model of moral deliberation that has become known as values-based practice (Fulford 2004; Woodbridge and Fulford 2004; see also Fulford and van Staden, Chapter 26, this volume).

Box 35.1 Fear of side effects

A twenty-eight-year-old woman with panic disorder and agoraphobia has been treated with cognitive behavioral therapy (CBT) at the outpatient anxiety disorder unit of a mental hospital. Contrary to the initial expectations she does not recover: after four months she still has panic attacks; these attacks impede the homework she has to do for the CBT. She has not gone to work for almost six months. She has an administrative job at an insurance company. The psychiatrist suggests she starts taking a selective serotonin re-uptake inhibitor (SSRI). The patient refuses: she has read about antidepressants on the Internet, she doesn't like the flattening of affect she has heard of, but most of all she fears gaining weight. Her body mass index is slightly below normal (18). On closer examination there appears to exist a history of preoccupation with body image, weight, and weight gain. She even had episodes of laxative abuse ten years ago. She exercises between six and eight hours a week. She, however, does not meet DSM-IV criteria for eating disorder; even not for eating disorder not otherwise specified. This is because she does not fulfill the general criteria for mental disorder stated in the introduction of the DSM (distress, disability, and/or risk; APA 1994, p. xxi). Without the panic attacks she functions well and there are no health risks. Question: What would you do? Would you respect the wishes of the patient and exert no further pressure with respect to the use of SSRIs? Or would you try to convince her that her ideas about possible weight gain are distorted because of, say, a latent eating disorder? What legitimizes the clinician to use his or her authority as a doctor to change the patient's view of herself, her body, and her future?

Anxiety at the Interface Between Clinical and Scientific Understanding

Still other philosophical questions arise when the clinical understanding of anxiety is related to scientific theory and concept formation. To what extent do scientific theories explain clinical phenomena? Are these theories valid, reliable, and useful for clinical practice? How do these theories relate to one another? Are they compatible or contradictory? Should the clinician embrace an explanatory pluralism, and if so, what kind of pluralism are we talking about; and how does this pluralism work in clinical practice? Do we need criteria for weighing the different explanatory perspectives and for comparing them with one another; and do such criteria exist? And, what is the status of clinical (expert) knowledge compared with scientific knowledge and theoretical insight, in the practice of diagnosing and treating patients and in the organization of psychiatric care?

Many of these questions come together in discussions about the conceptual status (validity, reliability, clinical use) of the *Diagnostic and Statistical Manual of Mental Disorders* (APA 1980, 1994). This section will be limited to discussions about the DSM and especially its section on anxiety disorder.

The DSM has exerted an enormous influence on diagnosis, treatment, and the organization of care. The proponents of the third edition of the DSM (APA 1980) envisioned a large-scale endeavor that ideally would lead to greater inter-rater reliability in diagnosis and classification; and to a diminishing of, or ideally even closing the gap between, scientific research and clinical understanding. The same disorders clinicians diagnose and treat were also proposed to be the subject of study for epidemiologists, geneticists, neuroscientists, pharmacologists, and others.

In their attempt to diminish the gap between science and clinical practice the DSM task-force adopted, in the late 1960s and early 1970s, a neopositivist epistemology, i.e., a view on scientific knowledge that puts much emphasis on empirical observation, measurement, clear and distinguishable terms, and operationalization of concepts and causal hypotheses. After more than forty years, we must say that the endeavor has been quite successful with respect to its first aim (improving inter-rater reliability), but that it has failed with respect to its second one (closing the gap between science and practice). Clinicians consider the DSM-III and its successors as overly detailed and unpractical, whereas researchers complain about the reified use of classificatory terms that draw mostly artificial boundaries and, therefore, don't "carve nature at its joints." The enormous overlap between diagnostic categories has complicated epidemiological research. Whereas the evidence suggests that the distribution of symptoms can better be explained as variance on a number of underlying dimensions (see later in this section), the comorbidity between DSM categories has led to largely spurious discussions, such as whether condition X is really distinct from condition Y; or whether condition Z can better be rubricated under category A instead of under category B. Comorbidity became in other words an issue in itself, and this complicated insight into the causal background of psychiatric disorders. With hindsight it is safe to say that, with the advent of the DSM-III, diagnostic categories became fixed at too early a stage of concept formation, i.e., before the mechanisms and causal pathways that underlie the relevant psychiatric conditions were discovered and sufficiently spelled out. As a result, one particular DSM-subtype of anxiety disorder can have more than one underlying causal mechanism (agoraphobia, for instance), whereas other subtypes will probably share underlying dysfunctions and causal mechanisms with diagnostic categories from different rubrics (generalized anxiety and depression, for instance).

The DSM-III-R and DSM-IV brought some improvements in the section on anxiety disorder, mainly based on new empirical findings within the same categorical paradigm. After the DSM-IV, grossly speaking, two conceptual improvements were made. First, extensive research has been done on so-called validators of diagnostic categories. Secondly, a sophisticated discussion about the pros and cons of a dimensional compared to a categorical approach to anxiety and mood disorders has arisen.

To begin with the first: as indicated before, validators are validating factors or circumstances with respect to the existence of a certain disorder or diagnostic category. Examples are: shared genetic risk, familial background, or temperament, and early stress (these are so-called *antecedent* validators); level of physiological arousal, function of the hypothalamic–pituitary–adrenal axis, neuronal substrate, and neuropsychological profile (these are called *concurrent* validators); and course of illness and response to treatment (so-called *predictive* validators) (Andrews et al. 2009; Goldberg et al. 2009; Hettema et al. 2005; Kendell 1975 Kendler 1990). The presence of a validator gives an indication of the likelihood of the existence of a certain disorder and also in some cases suggests that certain causal pathways are involved in the genesis of the disorder.

An example of this type of research and its potential impact is provided by Goldberg et al. (2009) who report on the results of the Diagnostic Spectra Study Group of the DSM-5 Task Force. They conclude that there is strong evidence for the existence of a cluster of emotional disorders and that the strongest empirical support for this is offered by the first four validators: genetics, family history, shared risk, and temperament. Shared temperament (neuroticism), in particular, appears to be a strong validator. The authors warn, however, that higher scores on neuroticism can also be found in other clusters of disorders. Neuroticism in itself is moreover no explanation for the occurrence of anxiety and/or mood disorder (Hettema 2008). Genetic research is still in its infancy (Hettema et al. 2005). There is empirical support from twin studies, that there are two clusters of genes, corresponding with "distress" ("anxious-misery"; predominantly mental) and fear ("fear"; predominantly somatic), respectively. Neuroticism, however, is probably also determined by other genes. The same holds for depression: there are strong findings supporting the view that a significant proportion of the genetic vulnerability to depression is not determined by neuroticism (see also Hettema et al. 2006). In short, from a distance, it seems that validators establish the existence of certain clusters of disorders; however, watching more closely, there are still irregularities and inconsistencies in this picture.

With respect to the second issue, the merits and pitfalls of a dimensional over against a categorical approach to anxiety, considerable discussion has recently arisen. As has been said, DSM-III, DSM-III-R, and DSM-IV use a categorical framework. Disorders are seen as entities. The descriptions of the disorder are seen as operational definitions that require (construct) validation. This strategy ideally leads to certainty that the construct under investigation refers to an identifiable set of facts in the real world. The alternative strategy of seeing them as expressions of underlying dimensions has also been applied to anxiety and mood disorders for over forty years, initially mainly by psychologists. This approach is basically statistical and aiming at knowledge about the distribution of frequencies. Analysis of self-report questionnaires on anxiety and mood symptoms indicates, for instance, that symptom variance can be explained by loading on one or more underlying factors or dimensions. The most important of these factors appears to be a common internalizing dimension, called negative affectivity (or negative emotionality) (Mineka et al. 1998). Negative affectivity does not stand alone; research on this dimension builds on an extensive body of knowledge on the personality factor "neuroticsm," which was defined as early as the 1960s by Eysenck, and investigated by Tellegen (1985) in humans and further developed by Gray (1982, 2000). On the basis of ingenious animal studies Gray concluded not only the existence of a so-called a behavioral inhibition system (BIS), which is strongly related to neuroticism, but also the existence of a so-called behavioral activation system (BAS), related to positive affect and reward. The work of Gray (and many others since then) shows how the statistical approach can be combined with other descriptive and more causal approaches, like brain stimulation, study of brain lesions in animals, artificial chemical and pharmacological interventions in humans and animals, and molecular genetics.

Major proponents of a dimensional approach argue that dimensions like negative affectivity and neuroticism are so deeply anchored that they cannot be distinguished from personality dimensions (Brown 2007; Brown and Barlow 2009; Watson 2005; Watson et al. 2008). Therefore, they advocate an overhaul of the classification of the anxiety and mood section of the DSM and a merger between Axis I and Axis II.

To give an idea of the intricate intertwinement of conceptual and empirical issues, a little more detail will be given about the ongoing discussion. Initially Watson and others (1988) propose a two-factor model. The first, non-specific factor is negative affectivity, contributing to both anxiety and depression. The second factor, (low) positive affect, is primarily associated with depression. A few years later, the authors advocate for a tripartite model, by adding physiological arousal (hyperarousal) as third factor specifically related to anxiety disorder (Clark and Watson 1991). Negative affectivity becomes an overarching dimension including the whole spectrum of anxiety and mood disorders; low positive affect becomes a subdimension mainly related to depression; however, hyperarousal becomes a subdimension contributing to anxiety. Still later, it emerges that hyperarousal differentially loads on various anxiety disorders (i.e., mainly on panic disorder and post-traumatic stress disorder; conditions with strong somatic manifestations). Low positive affectivity also appears to load on social phobia (Watson 2005). What is new is, therefore, the recognition of a certain hierarchy between the dimensions and a regrouping of the DSM-categories along the different (sub)dimensions. The approach has gained support from larger epidemiological surveys, such as the oft-quoted reanalysis of data from the National Comorbidity Survey by Krueger (1999). Krueger distinguishes between an internalizing and an externalizing factor. The first factor is identical to the negative affectivity dimension, just discussed; whereas the latter factor shows a strong association with alcohol dependence, drug dependence, and anti-social personality disorder. As in Watson's model the internalizing factor is hierarchically located above two other factors, an "anxious-misery" dimension (highly correlating with depression, dysthymia, and generalized anxiety) and a "fear" dimension (highly correlating with all phobias and panic disorder). Broadly speaking, Krueger's findings are replicated by the Dutch NEMESIS study (Vollebergh et al. 2001) and by research among an Australian population (Slade and Watson 2006). It should, nevertheless, be noted that it is still controversial what the impact of these findings should be on the future DSM-classification of anxiety. Wittchen et al. (2009), for instance, add a cautionary note by arguing that research within the dimensional paradigm is predominantly based on factor analysis of answers on self-report measures. They argue that until findings are confirmed by results from external sources, such as genetic, physiological (biomarkers) and/or neuroimaging research, it is too early to radically change the DSM's categorical approach to anxiety.

In sum, philosophical issues at the interface between the clinical and scientific concepts of anxiety are typically related to the tension between clinical utility and scientific validity. We see this reflected in shifts in the recent history of classification of anxiety. The first three-quarters of the previous century were dominated by the dimensionality of the classical neurosis concept, which put emphasis on underlying conflicts and unconscious needs, thereby neglecting the issue of scientific validity. Later, the categorical approach of the DSM-III and subsequent editions acquired a strong foothold. This led to increase of reliability of classificatory concepts, but not to better theoretical models of anxiety. Recently, there has been a re-emergence of dimensional constructs of anxiety. These constructs are more scientifically based; however, now it is not clear whether this scientific basis is sufficient to warrant large-scale application in clinical practice.

Anxiety at the Interface Between Scientific and Philosophical Understanding

Questions at the interface between science and philosophy deal with the implicit paradigms and presuppositions underlying the scientific study of anxiety and the relation between these paradigms/presuppositions and broader issues in the philosophy of emotion.

To begin with, there are three main traditions in the current scientific study of anxiety:

1. A Darwinian, ethological tradition in which anxiety is basically viewed as a universal, biologically anchored survival response, that has become sensitive to a whole range of environmental cues via conditioning and other learning processes; generally speaking, most neurobiological research fits in this tradition (Kandel 1983, 2005; LeDoux 1996).
2. A non-unitarian, strongly empiricist, initially mainly behaviorist research tradition, which views anxiety as a theoretical term denoting the expression of the activity of different neural and/or behavioral systems (Gray 1982; Lang 1979, 1985). Most animal research is performed within this framework (Kalueff et al. 2007).
3. A cognitive research tradition that focuses on anxiety as inner experience, influenced by expectancies, (mis)interpretations, (biased) attention, and cognitive schemes (Beck et al. 1985; Rachman 1978).

Contemporary developments give the impression that these traditions are approaching one another (Lang et al. 2000). With this rapprochement, classic problems in the philosophy of emotion re-emerge. One of these problems is, whether emotions are natural kinds or the result of environmental influences. One tradition says that there is a relatively small set of six or seven basic emotions, which are universal and cross-culturally similar (Izard 1977). According to another tradition, however, emotions should be viewed as acquired behavioral responses that are susceptible to conditioning, modeling, and vicarious learning (cf. for instance the concept of learned helplessness; Seligman 1975). Current conceptualizations try to combine those two approaches by assuming the existence of fear, as a basic emotion, mediated by neural circuits in which the amygdala plays a key role. The amygdala and the circuits mediating their output are in their turn modulated by higher (or second order) circuits mediating cognitive processes, explicit memory, sensory information and motivation (Damasio 1999; LeDoux 2012). All kinds of environmental input, including peripheral feedback from the body, exert influence not only on the suppression or elicitation of fear, but also on the way fear is expressed. There is in other words the basic emotion of fear (conceptualized along the lines of tradition 1); this basic emotion is influenced by higher order systems that mediate attention, perception, cognitive processing, motivation and memory (cf. tradition 2); which in their turn give rise to feelings of anxiety (analyzed in terms of tradition 3). These feelings are accounted for as the sum total of sensory feedback from the body, mixed with second order (conscious) interpretations of what is going on in the environment and conscious awareness of one's motivational state.

From a philosophical perspective one could question whether this view, in spite of its nuance, is as radically contextual as it suggests itself to be. Are the basic emotions, after all, not just fixed, innate behavioral patterns, that are only secondarily molded by higher-order processes and environmental pressures? If so, then it has to be noted that there is empirical evidence to the contrary. Current animal research, for instance, suggests that even at the basic level of emotional responding there is more context-sensitivity than until recently has been assumed (Kalueff 2007; Pawlak et al. 2008). Developmental neurobiology and attachment theory show that the development of affect occurs in biobehavioral shifts. Each shift represents a new level of organization of the maturing brain and a new step in socioemotional development (Schore 1994). There is in other words empirical support for a more "embedded" (i.e., contextually sensitive) and developmental view on emotion, in which basic emotions are more than just invariant behavioral responses triggered by limited sets of environmental cues.

Another, related question concerns the issue of whether fear, as basic emotion (ad 1) or as sum total of a number of lower- and higher-order neural processes (ad 2), is just a theoretical construct or not. Early behaviorist theories explicitly chose for a theoretical definition of anxiety and fear. In Gray's impressive work on the neuropsychology of fear and anxiety, for instance, fear is identical to the activity of the so-called BIS. The BIS is defined in purely theoretical terms, i.e., as the neural system that transforms signals of punishment, frustrating non-reward and novelty into behavioral responses like motor inhibition, physiological arousal and increased attention (Gray 1982; for later revisions see Gray and McNaughton 2000; McNaughton and Corr 2004). Fear is identical to activity of the BIS; and is, therefore, just an explanatory, theoretical term. According to Gray this theoretical definition is necessary because otherwise fear (anxiety) runs the risk of being defined circularly as the state that is embodied by the activity of certain neural mechanisms and at the same time as the totality of behavioral and physiological manifestations of this neural activity.

Cognitive approaches are sometimes less explicit on this issue, by allowing anxiety to be part of the *explanandum* as well as the *explanans*, thereby confusing explanation and description. As a result of this confusion clinical phenomena are identified with (quasi) explanatory terms, whereas explanatory concepts are defined at a low level of abstraction, close to clinical reality. A well-known example is the so-called appraisal theory of emotion. Clark's cognitive theory of panic is a variant of this approach (Clark 1986). It suggests that anxious apprehension (or anticipatory anxiety; fear of fear) lies at the basis of panic; i.e., it is anxious apprehension that *explains* why body sensations are misinterpreted as signs of impending bodily disaster (suffocation, heart attack, losing control); whereas the term anxious apprehension is also used to *describe* states of mild anxiety that are accompanied by a wide range of body sensations. Anxious apprehension is both *explanans* and *explanandum*. Recognition of this problem has led to further distinctions in the concept of anxious apprehension; for instance, between fear of body sensations, thoughts about possible consequences of panic, and anxiety sensitivity (Chambless and Gracely 1989).

This is not the place to go into detail with respect to this subject. Cognitive theory of panic is mentioned as an example of the more general problem of finding explanatory constructs that are both independent of and sufficiently relevant to clinical practice. There is a lot of fine-grained conceptual work to do in this area, not only in the field of anxiety disorder.

Beck, in his early writings, saw theory as just an extension of common sense and clinical understanding (Beck 1976). His early cognitive theory of depression was explicitly meant to rehabilitate subjective experience and introspection. Each patient is his own researcher. The patient is not ruled by uncontrollable mechanisms; she is an actor in her own play, and she can shape both her own insufficiency and her own cure. The patient who does not understand her own depression or anxiety is not on the wrong track when she tries to make use of introspection instead of scientific explanation—for instance, in terms of subpersonal brain mechanisms, as adherents of the biomedical model would advocate for. She simply does not use introspection persistently and precisely enough (Beck 1976, pp. 6, 12–13, 47ff.). In his later work Beck deviates from this path. He explicitly states that "anxiety is not the pathological process in so-called anxiety disorders any more than the skin rash or fever represents the pathological process in yellow fever" (Beck et al. 1985, p. 191). Cognitive schemes and affective dispositions replace introspection; they become the causal mechanisms behind anxiety disorder (Beck et al. 1985, p. 86).

Beck is clearly a theorist in the third tradition. His work shows a movement toward tradition 2. Broadly speaking, this movement took place during the 1990s, with important work by for instance Barlow and collaborators. Neurobiological research (tradition 1) also began to merge with psychological theory (tradition 2), for instance in the work of LeDoux (1996, 2002) and Kandel (1983, 2005). As has been said, since 2000, there have been attempts to integrate the entire spectrum of theories (Clark and Beck 2010; LeDoux 2012).

This section will be closed by briefly discussing two recent conceptual improvements. First, Damasio's landmark study on the feeling of emotion should be mentioned. This study is important not only because of its rehabilitation of feelings (as the subjective experience of emotion), but also and even more importantly because it enriched the conceptual analysis of feeling and emotion by giving an account of what philosophers call the "first-person perspective," the awareness that it is me that has a certain feeling. Feelings are "images arising from the neural patterns which represent the changes in body and brain that make up an emotion," according to Damasio (1999, p. 280). There is, in this conception, a difference between feeling and emotion. The term emotion refers to manifest patterns of behavior and physiology together with the neural mechanisms that mediate them. "Feeling" denotes the subjective experience of emotion as such, a pre-reflective awareness of impressions from the body and one's senses. However, what we usually call feeling is something more complicated: it is "knowing that we feel," feeling of feeling, reflective awareness of one's feeling. This second-order feeling "occurs only after we build the second-order representations necessary for core consciousness" (1999, p. 280). These second-order representations come to be known only after earlier representations of body states have been integrated to give rise to a so-called proto-self.

To be precise, there is first a proto-self, an elementary awareness of oneself based on body sensations; then, there is basic feeling, the transient flux of (pre-reflective) sensations and representations of body states under the influence of current environmental challenges and demands; and thirdly, there exists the feeling of feeling, just mentioned. Core consciousness should be located at this third level of description. It consists of "representations of the relationship between the organism and the object (in this case an emotion)." So, my feeling has become my (first person) feeling because representations of organismic change that accompany my perception of an emotion eliciting situation, are related to representations of a proto-self, based on earlier body experiences. What is important from the perspective developed in this chapter is that Damasio is unfolding a *self-relational perspective* on feeling here. Feelings say something about oneself in a particular situation. They are not simply the reflection of the condition of the organism. Likewise, emotions are not just the physiological and motor output of the brain. Feelings (and emotions in their wake) say something about how one relates to a situation. Feelings require that representations of organismic change are related to representations of an elementary awareness of "self" (see also Damasio 2010).

This rehabilitation of feeling, introspection, and subjective experience is, secondly, also supported by the re-emergence of phenomenology. This has occurred in different forms. We can only briefly mention two of them here: one that has become known as *neurophenomenology*; and new approaches to so-called *existential feelings*.

Building on earlier work on autopoiesis (self-organization) Varela and co-workers defined a new paradigm for consciousness studies that put emphasis on the self-organizing features of neural networks and that saw cognition as emerging from recurrent sensorimotor couplings of body, nervous system, and environment (Varela et al. 1991). Thompson et al. (2005) explicitly formulate as the task of neurophenomenology to make progress with respect to the explanatory gap between first-person, phenomenological data, and neuroscientific data. Neurophenomenology combines descriptive phenomenology, neuroscience, and dynamical systems theory. One of the conceptual improvements is the explicit rejection of the idea that in order for an experience to be my experience, the person needs to have a (separate) consciousness of him- or herself (as Damasio sometimes seems to suggest). The me-quality of my experience is given within experience itself, it is not the result of a fusion of experiences from different sources, or of an addition afterward; it is not content, but perspective; not a tacit form of self-reflection, but self-referentiality. How is the gap closed? Basically, by looking for phenomenological categories and structural invariants of experience that can be used to identify and describe dynamical neural signatures of experience and structural invariants of brain activity (see also Thompson 2007).

With respect to the existential feelings, the work of Ratcliffe (2008, 2009) on "feelings of being" should be mentioned. Existential feelings belong to a "group of feelings that are not directed at specific objects or states of affairs within the world." They, instead, "constitute a sense of relatedness between self and world, which shapes all experience"; and they "give us a changeable sense of 'reality' and of 'belonging to the world'" (Ratcliffe 2009, p. 180). As indicated earlier, this author has written in the same vein about the existential anxieties as types of self-relatedness (Glas 2001, 2003).

The conceptual innovation is twofold. First there is a consequent rethinking of anxiety (and other feelings of being) from a self-relational (or self-referential) perspective, in an attempt to escape from both objectivistic reductionism (which views anxiety as just the physiological or motor state of an organism) and subjectivist introspectionism (that sees anxiety as merely an inner state, unconnected with the body and the world). The basic idea is simple: anxiety does say something about me and my perspective on the world, even when I am not (subjectively) aware of this. Secondly and closely connected with this: the first-person perspective is not added to an already existing, objective framework; it is wired in, from the earliest beginnings, even at a neural (biological) level. This embodied, embedded, and enactive approach needs further elucidation, but offers much promise, not only to clinical practice, but also for rethinking the conceptual basis of psychiatry as a scientific discipline.

CONCLUSION

It is no exaggeration to say that, like so many scientific disciplines, psychiatry has come under the spell of what the late R. J. Bernstein has called "Cartesian anxiety" (1983). The expression refers to the obsession with epistemic certainty in the philosophy of the social sciences. The term alludes to the mental "vertigo" that arises when the epistemic subject faces the gap between him and the world. This vertigo is Cartesian, because it is Descartes who traditionally is said to stand at the origin of the divide between mind and world.

New questions emerged as a result of this divide. How do we know there is a real world? How can we trust our knowledge? How do we assure that our models and causal hypotheses represent reality? What do we really know about human anxiety? How adequate are our models and classifications? How trustworthy are our senses and clinical intuitions? Will it ever be possible to "carve nature at its joints" or will there remain a gap between our understanding and anxiety as it "really" is? These belong to the questions that Bernstein had in mind when he coined the term Cartesian anxiety.

In answer to them mainstream psychiatry chose (neo)positivism as a solution for the anxiety. Science should stick to observable facts, search for causal mechanisms explaining these facts, and try to determine valid patterns of distribution of signs and symptoms. Today, this positivism is still highly influential though, in its classical form, philosophically outdated. Doubts have emerged about one-sided inductive (bottom-up) approaches toward scientific knowledge (Murphy 2006). Psychiatry thought that it would become a fully scientific discipline by proceeding from symptoms to categories, from categories to dysfunctions, from dysfunctions to causal mechanisms, and from these to treatment. We have seen that there are major problems with this project and we analyzed some of these problems.

We have also seen that there are alternatives. Analysis of clinical practice reveals that the clinician is not just a neutral observer, but that she is participant in a shared practice. This practice requires competencies that are based on implicit ("tacit") knowledge (Dreyfus and Dreyfus 1986). Performing a professional practice is in a way the embodiment of such implicit knowledge. The hand of the surgeon knows what to do next, just like the experienced psychotherapist almost subliminally knows how to navigate around resistance and transference reactions when talking with the patient.

This embodied, embedded, and enactive (EEE) perspective (Thompson 2007) is of course not meant to deny the importance of logical-analytical skills. There is nothing wrong with explicit procedures and analytic reflection. However, these procedures and explicit reflection take place in a context that is always already informed by implicit knowledge, which in its turn comes to expression in the affective-evaluative judgment of what is going on. This implicit affective-evaluative judgment adds a third dimension to the otherwise two-dimensional, symptom-oriented picture of the patient. The clinician no longer sees only the disorder, but the entire fabric of relations spelled out in Fig. 35.2.

We have seen that, currently, also at the scientific level there are developments aiming at convergence of subjective and objective approaches. Phenomenology, developmental and affective neuroscience, and contributions from dynamical systems theory are combined in the EEE perspective, just discussed. This perspective goes one step further than usual integrative approaches, by suggesting that the first-person perspective is not added but "wired in" within the brain.

This conclusion is especially relevant for the treatment of the anxious patient. There are forms of anxiety that are horrifying, even for the clinician. There are depths and truths in some existential anxieties that bring to silence even the most experienced therapist. There are powers in anxiety which are so strong that patients and doctors instinctively step back and look away. This is the kind of climate in which Cartesian anxiety may prosper—i.e., in which doctors are inclined to withdraw from interaction, to stick to rules and procedures, and to favor objectivism and bureaucracy. This chapter has attempted to show that there are sound clinical, scientific, as well as philosophical reasons to resist these reflexes and to strive for a richer, more mature, more relational, and intellectually more rewarding approach to anxiety.

REFERENCES

American Psychiatric Association (1980). *Diagnostic and Statistical Manual of Mental Disorders, Third Edition*. Washington, DC: American Psychiatric Association.

American Psychiatric Association (1987). *Diagnostic and Statistical Manual of Mental Disorders, Third Edition, Revised*. Washington, DC: American Psychiatric Association.

American Psychiatric Association (1994). *Diagnostic and Statistical Manual of Mental Disorders, Fourth Edition, Text Revision*. Washington, DC: American Psychiatric Association.

Andrews, G., Anderson, T. M., Slade, T., and Sunderland, M. (2008). Classification of anxiety and depressive disorders: problems and solutions. *Depression and Anxiety*, 25, 274–81.

Andrews, G., Goldberg, D. P., Krueger, R. F., Carpenter, W. T., Hyman, S. E., Sachdev, P., *et al.* (2009). Exploring the feasibility of a meta-structure for DSM-V and ICD-11: could it improve utility and validity? *Psychological Medicine*, 39, 1993–2000.

Ax, A. (1953). The physiological differentiation between fear and anger in humans. *Psychosomatic Medicine*, 15, 433–42.

Barlow, D. H. (2000). Unraveling the mysteries of anxiety and its disorders from the perspective of emotion theory. *American Psychologist*, 55, 1247–63.

Barlow, D. H. (2002). *Anxiety and its Disorders: The Nature and Treatment of Anxiety and Panic*. New York, NY: The Guilford Press.

Beck, A. T. (1976). *Cognitive Therapy and the Emotional Disorders*. New York, NY: New American Library.

Beck, A. T., Emery, G., with Greenberg, R. L. (1985). *Anxiety Disorders and Phobias. A Cognitive Perspective*. New York, NY: Basic Books, Inc., Publishers.

Benedikt, M. (1870). Über "Platzschwindel." *Allgemeine Wiener Medizinische Zeitung*, 15, 488–9.

Bernstein, R. J. (1983). *Beyond Objectivism and Relativism: Science, Hermeneutics, and Praxis*. Philadelphia, PA: University of Philadelphia Press.

Brown, T. A. (2007). Temporal course and structural relationships among dimensions of temperament and DSM-IV anxiety and mood disorder constructs. *Journal of Abnormal Psychology*, 116, 313–28.

Brown, T. A. and Barlow, D. H. (2009). A proposal for a dimensional classification system based on the shared features of the DSM-IV anxiety and mood disorder: implications for assessment and treatment. *Psychological Assessment*, 21, 256–71.

Chambless, D. L. and Gracely, E. L. (1989). Fear of fear and the anxiety disorder. *Cognitive Therapy and Research*, 13, 9–20.

Clark, D. A. and Beck, A. T. (2010). Cognitive theory and therapy of anxiety and depression: Convergence with neurobiological findings. *Trends in Cognitive Sciences*, 14, 418–24.

Clark, D. M. (1986). A cognitive approach to panic. *Behavior Research & Therapy*, 24, 461–70.

Clark, L. A. and Watson, D. (1991). Tripartite model of anxiety and depression: Psychometric evidence and taxonomic implications. *Journal of Abnormal Psychology*, 100, 316–36.

Da Costa, J. M. (1871). On irritable heart; a clinical study of a form of functional cardiac disorder and its consequences. *The American Journal of the Medical Sciences*, 71, 17–52.

Damasio, A. (1994). *Descartes' Error: Emotion, Reason, and the Human Brain*. New York, NY: Gosset/Putnam.

Damasio, A. R. (1999). *The Feeling of what Happens: Body and Emotion in the Making of Consciousness*. New York, NY: Harcourt Brace.

Damasio, A. R. (2010). *Self Comes to Mind: Constructing the Conscious Brain*. New York, NY: Pantheon Books.

Descartes, R. (1649). Les passions de l'âme. In *Oeuvres de Descartes: publiées par Charles Adam & Paul Tannery*, Tome IX [1904], pp. 13–72. Paris: Cerf [1897–1910].

Dreyfus, H. L. and Dreyfus, S. L. (1986). *Mind Over Machine. The Power of Human Intuition and Expertise in the Era of the Computer.* New York, NY: Free Press.

Ellenberger, H. (1970). *The Discovery of the Unconscious. The History and Evolution of Dynamic Psychiatry.* New York, NY: Basic Books.

Feighner, J. P., Robins, E., Guze, S. N., Woodruff, R. A., Winokur, G., and Munoz, R. (1972). Diagnostic criteria for use in psychiatric research. *Archives of General Psychiatry, 26,* 57–63.

Flemming, C. F. (1848). Über Praekordial-Angst. *Allgemeine Zeitschrift für Psychiatrie, 5,* 341–61.

Freud, S. (1895). Über die Berechtigung, von der Neurasthenie einen bestimmten Symptomenkomplex als 'Angstneurose' abzutrennen. *Gesammelte Werke*, Band *I*, 315–42.

Freud, S. (1926). Hemmung, Symptom und Angst. *Gesammelte Werke*, Band *XIV*, 111–205.

Fulford, K. W. M. (2004). Ten principles of values-based medicine. In J. Radden (Ed.), *The Philosophy of Psychiatry: A Companion*, pp. 205–34. New York, NY: Oxford University Press.

Glas, G. (1997). The subjective dimension of anxiety: a neglected area in modern approaches to anxiety? In J. A. den Boer, E. Murphy, and H. G. M. Westenberg (Eds), *Clinical Management of Anxiety; Theory and Practical Applications*, pp. 43–62. New York, NY: Marcel Dekker Inc.

Glas, G. (2001). *Angst—Beleving, Structuur, Macht.* Amsterdam: Boom.

Glas, G. (2003). Anxiety—animal reactions and the embodiment of meaning. In K. W. M. Fulford, K. Morris, J. Sadler, and G. Stanghellini (Eds), *Nature and Narrative: An Introduction to the New Philosophy of Psychiatry*, pp. 231–49. Oxford: Oxford University Press.

Goldberg, D. P., Krueger, R. F., Andrews, G., and Hobbs, M. J. (2009). Emotional disorders: cluster 4 of the proposed meta-structure for DSM-V and ICD-11. *Psychological Medicine, 39,* 2043–59.

Goldstein, K. (1929). Zum Problem der Angst. *Allgemeine ärztliche Zeitschrift für Psychotherapie und psychische Hygiene, 2,* 409–37.

Gray, J. A. (1982). *The Neuropsychology of Anxiety. An Enquiry into the Functions of the Septo-Hippocampal System.* Oxford: Oxford University Press.

Gray, J. A. and McNaughton, N. (2000). *The Neuropsychology of Anxiety. An Enquiry into the Functions of the Septo-Hippocampal System* (2nd edn). Oxford: Oxford University Press.

Heidegger, M. (1927). *Sein und Zeit.* Tübingen: Niemeyer Verlag.

Hettema, J. M. (2008). The nosologic relationship between generalized anxiety disorder and major depression. *Depression and Anxiety, 25,* 300–16.

Hettema, J. M., Neale, M. C., Myers, J. M., Prescott, C. A., and Kendler, K. S. (2006). A population-based twin study of the relationships between neuroticism and internalizing disorders. *American Journal of Psychiatry, 163,* 857–64.

Hettema, J. M., Prescott, C. A., Myers, J. M., Neale, M. C., and Kendler, K. S. (2005). The structure of genetic and environmental risk factors for anxiety disorders in men and women. *Archives of General Psychiatry, 62,* 182–7.

Izard, C. E. (1977). *Human Emotions.* New York, NY: Plenum Press.

Jablensky, A. (1985). Approaches to the definition and classification of anxiety and related disorders in European psychiatry. In A. H. Tuma and J. Maser (Eds), *Anxiety and the Anxiety Disorders*, pp. 735–58. Hillsdale, NJ: Lawrence Erlbaum.

Jackson, S. W. (1986). *Melancholia and Depression. From Hippocratic Times to Modern Times.* New Haven, CT: Yale University Press.

Janet, P. (1903). *Les Obsessions et la Psychasthenie.* Alcan: Paris.

Kalueff, A. V., Wheaton, M., and Murphy, D. L. (2007). What's wrong with my mouse model? Advances and strategies in animal modeling of anxiety and depression. *Behavioural Brain Research*, 179, 1–18.

Kandel, E. R. (1983). From metapsychology to molecular biology: explorations into the nature of anxiety. *American Journal of Psychiatry*, 140, 1277–93.

Kandel, E. R. (2005). *Psychiatry, Psychoanalysis, and the New Biology of Mind*. Arlington, VA: APA Publishing.

Kendell, R. E. (1975). *The Role of Diagnosis in Psychiatry*. Oxford: Blackwell.

Kendler, K. S. (1990). Toward a scientific psychiatric nosology. Strengths and limitations. *Archives of General Psychiatry*, 44, 451–7.

Kierkegaard, S. (1980). *The Concept of Anxiety. A Simple Psychologically Orienting Deliberation on the Dogmatic Issue of Hereditary Sin* (R. Thomte in collaboration with A.B. Anderson, Eds and Trans.). Princeton, NJ: Princeton University Press. (Original work published 1844.)

Klein, D. F. (1964). Delineation of two drug-responsive anxiety syndromes. *Psychopharmacologia*, 5, 397–408.

Klein, D. F. (1980). Anxiety reconceptualized, *Comprehensive Psychiatry*, 21, 411–27.

Kraepelin, E. (1899). *Psychiatrie. Ein Lehrbuch für Studirende und Aertzte* (sechste, vollständig umgearbeitete Auflage). Leipzig: Johann Ambrosius Barth.

Kronfeld, A. (1935). Über Angst. *Nederlandsch Tijdschrift voor Psychologie*, 3, 366–87.

Krueger, R. F. (1999). The structure of common mental disorders. *Archives of General Psychiatry*, 56, 921–6.

Lang, P. J. (1979). A bio-informational theory of emotional imagery. *Psychophysiology*, 16, 495–512.

Lang, P. J. (1985). The cognitive psychophysiology of emotion: fear and anxiety. In A. H. Tuma and J. D. Maser (Eds), *Anxiety and the Anxiety Disorders*, pp. 131–70. Hillsdale, NJ: Lawrence Erlbaum.

Lang, P. J., Davis, M., and Öhman, A. (2000). Fear and anxiety: animal models and human cognitive psychophysiology. *Journal of Affective Disorders*, 61, 137–59.

LeDoux, J. E. (1996). *The Emotional Brain*. New York, NY: Simon and Schuster.

LeDoux, J. E. (2002). *Synaptic Self: How our Brains Become Who We Are*. New York, NY: Viking.

LeDoux, J. E. (2012). Rethinking the emotional brain. *Neuron*, 73, 653–76

Lersch, P. (1964). *Aufbau der Person* (2nd edn). München: Johann Ambrosius Earth.

Lewis, T. (1918). The tolerance of physical exertion, as shown by soldiers suffering from so-called "irritable heart." *British Medical Journal*, 1(2987), 363–5.

Lewis, T. (1940). *Soldier's heart and the effort syndrome* (2nd edn). London: Shaw

MacKenzie, J. (1916). The soldier's heart. *British Medical Journal*, 1(2873), 117–19.

MacKenzie, J. (1920). The soldier's heart and war neurosis: a study in symptomatology. *British Medical Journal*, 1(3094), 491–4, 530–4.

McNaughton, N. and Corr, P. J. (2004). A two-dimensional neuropsychology of defense: fear/anxiety and defensive distance. *Neuroscience & Biobehavioral Reviews*, 28, 285–305.

Mineka, S., Watson, D., and Clark, L. A. (1998). Comorbidity of anxiety and unipolar mood disorders. *Annual Review of Psychology*, 49, 377–412.

Murphy, D. (2006). *Psychiatry in the Scientific Image*. Cambridge, MA: The MIT Press.

Pascal, B. (1669). *Pensées*. Paris: Gallimard.

Pawlak, C. R., Ho, Y.-J., and Schwarting, R. K. W. (2008). Animal models of human psychopathology based on individual differences in novelty-seeking and anxiety. *Neuroscience and Biobehavioral Reviews*, 32, 1544–68.

Rachman, S. J. (1978). *Fear and Courage*. San Franscisco, CA: W.H. Freeman & Company.

Ratcliffe, M. (2008). *Feelings of Being: Phenomenology, Psychiatry and the Sense of Reality*. Oxford: Oxford University Press.

Ratcliffe, M. (2009). Existential feeling and psychopathology. *Philosophy, Psychiatry, & Psychology*, 16, 179–94.

Roth, M. (1959). The phobic anxiety-depersonalization syndrome. *Proceedings of the Royal Society of Medicine*, 52, 587–95.

Sadler, J. Z. (2005). *Values and Psychiatric Diagnosis*. Oxford: Oxford University Press.

Schon, D. A. (1983). *The Reflective Practitioner. How Professionals Think in Action*. New York, NY: Basic Books.

Schore, A. N. (1994). *Affect Regulation and the Origin of the Self. The Neurobiology of Emotional Development*. Hillsdale, NJ: Lawrence Erlbaum Associates, Publishers.

Seligman, M. E. P. (1975). *Helplessness: On Depression, Development, and Death*. San Francisco, CA: W. H. Freeman

Slade, T., and Watson, D. (2006). The structure of common DSM-IV and ICD-10 mental disorders in the Australian general population. *Psychological Medicine*, 36, 1593–600.

Spitzer, R. L., Endicott, J., and Robins, E. (1975). *Research Diagnostic Criteria (RDC)*. New York, NY: Biometrics Research, New York State Psychiatric Institute.

Spitzer, R. L., Endicott, J., and Robins, E. (1978). Research diagnostic criteria: rationale and reliability. *Archives of General Psychiatry*, 35, 773–82.

Spitzer, R. L., and Williams, J. B. W. (1985). Proposed revisions in the DSM-III classification of anxiety disorders based on research and clinical experience. In A. H. Tuma and J. D. Maser (Eds), *Anxiety and the Anxiety Disorders*, pp. 759–73. Hillsdale, NJ: Lawrence Erlbaum.

Stein, D. J., Phillips, K. A., Bolton, D., Fulford, K.W. M., Sadler, J. Z., and Kendler, K. S. (2010). What is a mental/psychiatric disorder? From DSM-IV to DSM-V. *Psychological Medicine*, 40, 1759–65.

Sternbach, L. H. (1980). The benzodiazepine story. In R. G. Priest, U. Vianna Filho, R. Amrein, and M. Skreta (Eds), *Benzodiazepines. Today and tomorrow*, pp. 5–18. Lancaster: MTP Press Limited.

Tellegen, A. (1985). Structures of mood and personality and their relevance to assessing anxiety, with an emphasis on self-report. In A. H. Tuma and J. Maser (Eds), *Anxiety and the Anxiety Disorders*, pp. 281–706. Hillsdale, NJ: Lawrence Erlbaum.

Thompson, E. (2007). *Mind in Life. Biology, Phenomenology, and the Sciences of Mind*. Cambridge, MA: The Belknap Press of Harvard University Press.

Thompson, E., Lutz, A., and Cosmelli, D. (2005). Neurophilosophy: An introduction for neurophilosophers. In A. Brook and K. Akins (Eds), *Cognition and the Brain. The Philosophy and Neuroscience Movement*, pp. 40–97. New York, NY: Cambridge University Press.

Varela, F. J., Thompson, E., and Rosch, E. (1991). *The Embodied Mind. Cognitive Science and Human Experience*. Cambridge, MA: The MIT Press.

Verhoeff, B. and Glas, G. (2010). The search for dysfunctions. A commentary on "What is a mental/psychiatric disorder? From DSM-IV to DSM-V" by Stein et al. (2010). *Psychological Medicine*, 40(11), 1787–8.

Vollebergh, W. A., Iedema, J., Nijl, R.V., de Graaf, R., Smit, F., and Ormel, J. (2001). The structure and stability of common mental disorders: the NEMESIS study. *Archives of General Psychiatry*, 58, 597–603.

Watson, D. (2005). Rethinking the mood and anxiety disorders: a quantitative hierarchical model for DSM-V. *Journal of Abnormal Psychology*, 114, 522–36.

Watson, D., Clark, L. A., and Carey, G. (1988). Positive and negative affectivity and their relation to the anxiety and depressive disorders. *Journal of Abnormal Psychology*, 97, 346–53.

Watson, D., O'Hara, M. W., and Stuart, S. (2008). Hierarchical structures of affect and psychopathology and their implications for the classification of emotional disorders. *Depression and Anxiety*, 25, 282–8.

Westphal, C. (1872), Die Agoraphobie, eine neuropathische Erscheinung. *Archive für Psychiatrie und Nervenkrankheite*, 3, 138–61.

Wittchen, H.-U., Beesdo, K., and Gloster, A.T. (2009). The position of anxiety disorders in structural models of mental disorders. *Psychiatric Clinics of North America*, 32, 465–81.

Wolpe, J. (1958). *Psychotherapy by Reciprocal Inhibition*. Stanford, CA: Stanford University Press.

Woodbridge, K. and Fulford, K. W. M. (2004). *Whose Values? A Workbook for Values-Based Practice in Mental Health Care*. London: Sainsbury Centre for Mental Health.

Yalom, I. (1980). *Existential Psychotherapy*. New York: Basic Books.

CHAPTER 36

....

DEPRESSION AND THE PHENOMENOLOGY OF FREE WILL

....

MATTHEW RATCLIFFE

This chapter sketches a phenomenological account of impaired agency in depression. Depression, I suggest, can involve what we might call a diminished *experience of free will*. Although it is often assumed that we have such an experience, it is far from clear what it consists of. I argue that this lack of clarity is symptomatic of looking in the wrong place. Drawing on themes in Sartre's *Being and Nothingness*, I propose that the sense of freedom associated with action is not—first and foremost—an episodic "quale" or "feeling" that is experienced as internal to the agent. Rather, it is embedded in the experienced world; my freedom appears in the guise of my surroundings. This makes better sense of what people with depression consistently describe: a diminished ability to act that is inextricable from a transformation of the experienced world.

As well as illuminating an aspect of the experience of depression, I also seek to illustrate something more general: how phenomenology and psychiatry can interact in a fruitful way. Phenomenology supplies us with an interpretive framework through which to make sense of first-person reports of altered experience in psychiatric illness. Insofar as it facilitates plausible interpretations of otherwise elusive phenomena, in a way that has potential repercussions for classification and treatment, it is vindicated in the process. In addition, the commerce between phenomenology and psychiatry can involve further refinement of the former, rather than its uncritical application.

EXPERIENCE OF AGENCY IN DEPRESSION

....

People with depression often report an impaired ability to act. This not only affects actions that involve forethought or effort. Even habitual, routine, undemanding activities, such as making a cup of tea or having a shower, can seem overwhelmingly difficult and beyond one's abilities:

When I'm depressed, every job seems bigger and harder. Every setback strikes me not as something easy to work around or get over but as a huge obstacle. Events appear more chaotic and beyond my control: if I fail to achieve some goal, it will seem that achieving it is forever beyond my abilities, which I perceive to be far more meagre than I did when I was not depressed. (Law 2009, p. 355)

Given that people complain of feeling that they are no longer able to initiate action, depression seems to affect what we might call the "phenomenology of free will." Action seldom ceases altogether. However, sufferers routinely report an all-pervasive feeling of being somehow diminished, which affects all their experiences and activities: "My existence was pared away almost to nothing" (Shaw 1997, p. 27). Their activities are often experienced as somehow different, oddly mechanical, and detached. For example, in his *Autobiography*, John Stuart Mill describes how he did things "mechanistically," "by mere force of habit." Various routines persisted only because he had been "so drilled in a certain sort of mental exercise" that he could "still carry it on when all spirit had gone out of it" (1873, pp. 139–140). Hence even habitual action had lost its usual tone; it was bereft of a sense of vitality.[1]

In order to understand how depression affects the phenomenology of free will, the approach I will adopt here is to first characterize an intact experience of free will and then seek to identify what is absent, diminished, or different in depression. It seems plausible to maintain that there is some such experience. Indeed, it is arguable that this is what ultimately fuels debates over free will and determinism. A belief in libertarian free will, one might suggest, originates in an experience of free action. As Viktor Frankl remarks, most of us have an experience of free will and take for granted that it is veridical:

> Man's freedom of will belongs to the immediate data of his experience. These data yield to that empirical approach which, since Husserl's day, is called phenomenological. Actually only two classes of people maintain that their will is not free: schizophrenic patients suffering from the delusion that their will is manipulated and their thoughts controlled by others, and alongside of them, deterministic philosophers. To be sure, the latter admit that we are experiencing our will as though it were free, but this, they say, is a self-deception. (Frankl 1973, p. 14)

Experience of free will is also presupposed by recent debates concerning whether or not free will is an illusion: if we did not have an experience of free will, we could not have an illusory experience of it. For example, Libet (2004) not only assumes that we have an awareness of willing something to happen but further claims that the "conscious will to act" can be timed. However, as others have noted, it is far from clear what the alleged experience consists of (e.g., Holton 2009, p. 416). And not everyone accepts Libet's assumption that actions are experienced as initiated by "volitions." For instance, it is arguable that our phenomenology better complements "agent-causation" approaches, according to which agents rather than volitions are the causes of actions. But we can ask the same question here—is there an experience of agent causation and, if so, what does it involve? Again, the matter is unclear,

---

[1] The question of how depression affects the ability to act has not received much attention from philosophers. However, there is a recent account by Roberts (2001), which proposes that people with depression fail to act because of an inability to satisfy their desires due to loss of affect. There is a "failure to be able to achieve affective satisfaction of their desires" (2001, p. 54). A problem with this view is that people with depression not only decline to act; they also complain that action seems impossible. Realizing that one will not get any satisfaction from an action is not the same as taking that action to be beyond one's abilities.

prompting Nichols (2004, p. 491) to dismiss the idea of such an experience as "phenomeno-logically implausible."

There is thus a tension between the widespread intuition that we experience our actions as free and the elusiveness of the experience. I suggest that this tension is symptomatic of our looking in the wrong place. Our freedom is not, principally, something we experience as internal to ourselves, an episodic feeling associated with the initiation of certain actions. Instead, *all* actions (along with any feelings or "qualia" that might be associated with acting or being about to act) presuppose an experience of freedom. This experience consists simply of the world; the sense that we are free is written into the experienced world. I will show how this view facilitates a plausible interpretation of what people with depression often report: an impaired ability to act that is inextricable from "living in a different world."

Kinds of Action

What kinds of action do we experience as "free" in the relevant sense? If we can establish this much, then we will at least know where to look in order to characterize the experience. The sort of action that Libet (e.g., 2004) instructed his experimental subjects to perform—flicking a wrist without any forethought—is not a good candidate. As Lowe (2009 p. 85) points out, they were effectively asked "not to exercise their will" and instead to let the urge some-how "creep up on them unawares." Furthermore, it is arguable that free will is not simply a matter of initiating bodily movements. When one performs a goal-directed action, such as reaching for a pen, crossing the road, or drinking from a glass of water, every movement of a finger, hand, arm, or leg does not constitute a discrete free action—that would be the wrong level of description. If there is an experience of free will, it is associated with purposive activities, such as "crossing the road in order to go to the shop" (Gallagher 2006). So flicking a wrist is not a typical free action but a movement that would ordinarily contribute to such an action, which is artificially abstracted from its usual context.

Let us concede that certain behaviors contribute to actions, rather than being actions, and that others, such as flicking a wrist, may be dubious candidates for free actions. That still leaves us with many different candidate behaviors. Consider the following:

1. Thinking through a problem when there is not much as stake, deciding to do something and then doing it.
2. Making a choice that will have a significant effect upon one's life, with which various conflicting emotions are associated.
3. Performing a one-off goal-directed activity without any forethought, such as picking up a glass and drinking its contents.
4. Unreflectively performing a habitual routine, such as cleaning one's teeth in the morning.
5. Making an impulsive ostensive gesture, in order to draw a companion's attention to something exciting.
6. Expressing anger at someone.
7. Saying the word "phenomenology," rather than "experience," in a sentence where one could have used either term.

It is debatable how many different kinds of action there are and what distinguishes all of them from (a) a cluster of closely related actions, (b) an action component, and (c) a behavior that is neither an action nor an action component. The list is not intended to be exhaustive or to reflect a uniquely appropriate taxonomy of action. My aim is simply to illustrate the wide variety of actions and associated experiences. Heading to the bathroom to brush one's teeth is phenomenologically very different from deciding whether or not to marry somebody. What kinds of action are associated with an experience of freedom? Perhaps it is restricted to those that involve making a *choice*. However, it is difficult to pin down the scope of choice. Although one might restrict it to (1) and (2) in the list, it seems odd to say that I did *not* choose to clean my teeth, make a gesture, or say a word. The intuition remains that I *could have done otherwise* in these cases.

There is a simple phenomenological case against the view that our experience of freedom consists of a "magic ingredient," added only to certain kinds of action. In short, we do not experience ourselves as mechanistically determined robots that are occasionally moved by a burst of freedom, thus making a subset of our activities stand out from all others. Our experience does not incorporate a clear distinction between a subset of actions that we experience as "free" and all our other behaviors. In what follows, I will defend the view that all our actions are experienced as free. This is consistent with what people with depression describe. Their impaired ability to act encompasses not just those actions that are preceded by deliberation or choice, but even activities that are ordinarily habitual, unthinking, and effortless: "To get out of bed at midday was an ordeal" (anonymous, in Read and Reynolds 1996, p. 35).

In the next two sections, I draw first upon Edmund Husserl and then Jean-Paul Sartre, in order to argue that experience of freedom is neither an inchoate internal feeling nor an episode that accompanies some instances of action. Rather, it is an ordinarily constant background to all our activities—our choices *presuppose* that we are free to act, rather than constituting an experience of freedom. Because our actions are experienced as free even when we do not explicitly "choose" them or "will" them to occur, I refer more often to a sense of "freedom" than to "free will." And this freedom, I argue, is a way of experiencing the world.

HORIZONS

A first step toward characterizing the phenomenology of freedom is acknowledging that world-experience incorporates perception of *possibility*. A detailed case for this is made by Husserl, amongst others.[2] According to Husserl, when I perceive an object in front of me, such as a cup, I do not perceive a two-dimensional appearance and subsequently infer that there is a three-dimensional entity with various unseen properties. Rather, the cup is perceptually present to me as an *object* with various properties, even though I don't currently see all of it. How could that be? Husserl suggests that various *possible* appearances of the entity feature in my perception of what actually appears. I experience the cup *as* something with additional properties that are perceivable from different vantage points. These possibilities have variably determinate contents, such as "view me from this angle and you will see a

[2] Much the same view is later adopted and further developed by Merleau-Ponty (1962).

white handle" or "view me from this angle and you will reveal a surface that has a color and texture." Hence experience of an entity incorporates a structured system of potential experiences, along with a sense of one would have to do to reveal further features of the object. Husserl refers to this system as the entity's "horizon":

> Everywhere, apprehension includes in itself, by the mediation of a "sense," empty horizons of "possible perception"; thus I can, at any given time, enter into a system of possible and, if I follow them up, actual, perceptual nexuses. (Husserl 1989, p. 42)

A horizon is a dynamic rather than static structure. As we act, we actualize certain possibilities and reveal others, in a coherent way that involves perceptual expectations and their fulfillment (or lack of fulfillment). The horizonal structure of perception is multimodal; what is revealed to one sense incorporates an appreciation of what could be perceived by means of other senses. Husserl further adds that horizons do not consist only of self-involving possibilities. Entities also appear as perceptually and practically accessible to others who are actually or potentially present.[3] Perception therefore incorporates different *kinds* of possibility: entities can appear "perceptually accessible to me," "practically accessible to me," "perceptually accessible to others," "practically accessible to others" and as "accessible through one or more sensory modalities." However, the kinds of possibility we perceive are, I suggest, more wide-ranging than this. Husserl appreciates that, in everyday life, we do not experience entities indifferently—they present themselves as practically significant in a range of ways:

> In ordinary life, we have nothing whatever to do with nature-Objects. What we take as things are pictures, statues, gardens, houses, tables, clothes, tools, etc. These are all value-Objects of various kinds, use-Objects, practical Objects. (Husserl 1989, p. 29)

Given this, we can add that an entity might appear "easy to use," "urgently required," "well-suited to a task," "cumbersome," and so on—it is experienced in terms of its *significant* possibilities.[4] Perception of "value" is not restricted to variants of practical utility though. For example, we might perceive something as "threatening," and a threat might be perceived as imminent, distant, avoidable, or unavoidable. Hence perception incorporates a range of different *kinds* of significant possibility.[5] We can add to this Husserl's distinction between possibilities that are "enticing" and others that are not. Husserl is concerned with perceptual enticement, with the way in which perceived objects sometimes call upon us to actualize further perceptual possibilities by moving in certain ways (e.g., Husserl 2001, pp. 83–91, 196). However, it is just as plausible, in my view, to extend the point to possibilities for goal-directed action. Something could appear practically significant (e.g., useable for some task) without drawing us in or repelling us, whereas other perceived possibilities incorporate an "affective force." There is a difference between a pint of beer that says "you could drink me" and one that says "drink me now."

Husserl suggests that our ability to experience possibilities is enabled, at least in part, by our having certain kinds of bodily disposition. The body [*Leib*] is the "medium" or "organ"

---

[3] See Gallagher (2008) for a good discussion of Husserl, perception, and intersubjectivity.

[4] Of course, this is a theme that Heidegger also develops in Division I of *Being and Time* (1962).

[5] So far as I know, Husserl does not state explicitly that the horizonal structure of perception incorporates various different kinds of *significant* possibility. However, it is consistent with his work and, I think, implied by much of what he does say.

of "all perception" and thus shapes all our experiences of the world (1989, p. 61). More specifically, a sense of potential movements, which Husserl calls "kinestheses," is also a perception of the possibilities that things offer us:

> There is thus a freedom to run through the appearances in such a way that I move my eyes, my head, alter the posture of my body, go around the object, direct my regard toward it, and so on. We call these movements, which belong to the essence of perception and serve to bring the object of perception to givenness from all sides insofar as possible, *kinaestheses*. (Husserl 1973, pp. 83–84)

We can thus extract from Husserl's work the view that (a) perception incorporates various different kinds of possibility, some of which are significant to us in one way or another, and (b) perception of worldly possibility is inextricable from our bodily phenomenology. It is through the perceiving (as opposed to perceived) body that we experience our surroundings.

Elsewhere, I have argued that the contribution made by various kinds of possibility to experience can be illustrated by reflecting upon forms of anomalous experience where certain *kinds* of possibility are absent. The result is that everything looks somehow different in ways that are difficult to describe. Along with this, the overall structure of one's relationship with the world is altered (e.g., Ratcliffe 2008). For instance, everything might seem oddly intangible, altogether bereft of practical potentialities and tactual possibilities more generally. As some kinds of possibility are lost, others can become more pronounced—one's surroundings might offer only the possibility of threat. Another alteration in the space of experienced possibility involves a diminished sense of things being experientially and practically accessible to others; everything appears as "for me." In contrast, there is a form of estrangement where the world continues to offer possibilities for others, which present themselves as "impossible for me." An appreciation that experiential changes like these can occur allows one to interpret first-person reports that otherwise seem paradoxical, where everything looks exactly as it previously did and yet somehow utterly different. An example of this is what Jaspers (1963, p. 98) calls "delusional mood" or "delusional atmosphere." Even though a detailed description of what is perceptually present might incorporate exactly the same inventory of properties as before, the system of perceived possibilities has changed and things therefore *look* somehow different in a way that people struggle to articulate (Ratcliffe, in press, a).

Sartre on Freedom

If we allow that world-experience incorporates various different kinds of possibility, we can see how the experience of freedom associated with action might be integral to the experienced world. The kinds of possibility that the world incorporates include "I can." The *possibility* of my doing p or doing q is *there*, built into our surroundings. And this kind of possibility is phenomenologically distinguishable from others, such as "p might happen," "p might happen to me" or "someone else could do p." Our being presented with the "I can," along with other kinds of possibility that it can be distinguished from, is what constitutes our sense of freedom. Perhaps the best statement of such a view is that of Sartre, and I will focus upon four claims that he makes about freedom:

1. The experience of freedom involves being presented with a world that incorporates various kinds of possibility, including "I can."
2. All action is free; action preceded by reflective choice is only one kind of free action.
3. The experience of freedom is inextricable from our bodily phenomenology.
4. The fundamental project that gives meaning to all one's actions is itself a choice.

I will accept (1), (2), and (3), but reject (4). Turning first of all to (1), Sartre maintains at various points in *Being and Nothingness* that the experienced world incorporates possibilities. Consider this description of looking up at a cloudy sky and perceiving the threat of rain:

> The possible appears to us as a property of things. After glancing at the sky I state "It is possible that it may rain." I do not understand the possible here as meaning "without contradiction with the present state of the sky." The possibility belongs to the sky as threat; it represents a surpassing on the part of these clouds, which I perceive, toward rain. (Sartre 1989, p. 97)

He also indicates that the experience of being free is a matter of being presented with possibilities. When we act, we do not perceive a purely factual state of affairs, think about the discrepancy between it and some preferred situation, and then experience an internal mental state of "desire." Rather, a situation appears to us as lacking in some way and thus solicits a certain kind of action (Sartre 1989, p. 433). However, it is also clear from Sartre's account that, however much the world might call for a certain action, that action is still presented as something we *could* do, rather than something we are compelled to do.[6] Take his well-known example of walking along the edge of a precipice and feeling afraid. Sartre stresses that the fear is a way of experiencing one's surroundings; they appear as offering the "possibility of my life being changed from without." Hence the precipice also invites me to act in a certain way; it "presents itself to me *as to be avoided*" (Sartre 1989, pp. 29–30). However, moving away from the edge is not given as something I *must* do. And the revelation that nothing compels me to act in this way consists, according to Sartre, in a feeling of "anguish." However, he also maintains that I am free even when I am not *reflectively* aware of my freedom in this way. My unreflective experience of freedom consists in the simple fact of the world's offering significant possibilities that I might actualize, such as backing away from the cliff, and offering them *as* possibilities rather than inevitabilities. Action is experienced *as* the actualization of worldly possibilities, and this applies to unthinking, habitual action too: "the consciousness of man in action is non-reflective consciousness" (Sartre 1989, p. 36). One might argue that the experience of possibility is merely epistemic; it is a matter of ignorance over what will happen rather than an experience of freedom. Some of the possibilities we experience do indeed reflect lack of knowledge. However, it would be phenomenologically implausible to maintain that "I can do *p* or *q*" takes that form. The experience is quite different from "I don't know what will happen next'. Even if one knows what one will do, the relevant course

---

[6] Sartre's emphasis on how possibilities structure perception complements that of Husserl. However, he criticizes Husserl for not sufficiently acknowledging that possibilities can be clustered around an absence or lack, rather than something that is actually present (Sartre 1989, pp. 26–27).

of action presents itself as one possibility amongst others, none of which one is compelled to actualize.

For Sartre, the kinds of significance that experienced entities have are symptomatic of the kinds of projects we are already knowingly or unknowingly committed to. Insofar as I strive to be a good philosopher, a book might appear enticing, a talk interesting, a negative review of my work hurtful, and so on. Our projects thus shape not only the possibilities for action that the world offers but various other kinds of significance too. Sartre claims that even significant events that we have no control over depend—in a way—upon our freedom. A being that cared for nothing, that strove for nothing, could not be obstructed, threatened or disappointed. Things only affect us in these ways because we already have certain concerns, and we choose those concerns by choosing the projects we pursue (Sartre 1989, p. 494). Actions respond to worldly possibilities that are symptomatic of projects. These projects are symptomatic of further projects, and so on. Hence what constrains our actions is itself symptomatic of our freedom.[7]

According to Sartre, all our activities and projects, all the ways in which we find things significant, can be traced back to an original project that is chosen: "all these trivial passive expectations of the real, all these commonplace, everyday values, derive their meaning from an original project of myself which stands as my choice of myself in the world" (Sartre 1989, p. 39). I reject this last claim on phenomenological grounds.[8] All projects ultimately presuppose a structure that is not chosen. Whether it is x, y, or z that one encounters as frightening, enticing, or useful might depend upon the project one has chosen to pursue. However, in order to have any kind of project, one must have the capacity to find things significant in such ways. And that capacity is not chosen. So the ways in which we find things significant, the possibilities that they offer us, are not wholly attributable to a choice of projects. Only if one is already capable of experiencing threat can one find a specific entity threatening, and only if one already has a sense of being able to actualize possibilities in the form of "I can" is one able to have any kind of project. Hence the phenomenology of freedom does not originate in an ungrounded choice but in a modal structure (a sense of the kinds of significant possibility that entities in the world can incorporate), which is presupposed by the intelligibility of pursuing a project. And, as I will illustrate when I return to the phenomenology of depression, that structure is changeable. Although I depart from Sartre's position here, this does not preclude endorsement of his other claims. I agree with Sartre that the phenomenology of freedom is a matter of experiencing one's actions as responses to significant worldly possibilities, that freedom is not restricted to reflective choices, and that many of the possibilities we perceive are symptomatic of projects that frame our activities. Furthermore, freedom does indeed extend to some of those projects that form a habitual backdrop to our activities; people sometimes do make radical choices that change the structure of their lives.

---

[7] Sartre also acknowledges that our possibilities are shaped and thus, in some sense, "constrained" by a social world of shared meanings. However, he says that these constraints are not experienced as limits. We do not miss possibilities that were not incorporated into the experienced world to begin with (Sartre 1989, p. 531).

[8] Indeed, just about everybody who has discussed Sartre's "original choice" rejects the idea. For example, Merleau-Ponty (1962 pp. 441–453) claims that it is our "habitual being in the world" that gives things the significance they have and that the significant situation we find ourselves immersed in when we choose is not itself a choice.

For Sartre, as for Husserl, the experience of worldly possibility is essentially bodily in character. He offers a transcendental argument to the effect that having a body is a necessary condition for thought, action and choice:

> In fact if the ends which I pursue could be attained by a purely arbitrary wish, if it were sufficient to hope in order to obtain, and if definite rules did not determine the use of instruments, I could never distinguish within me desire from will, nor dream from act, nor the possible from the real. (Sartre 1989, p. 327)

If our capacities were unlimited, to wish would be to be to get, and the distinction between desire, choice and action would break down. Having a body, and thus a contingent set of capacities, is a requirement for the ability to distinguish between having, desiring, needing, willing and acting. As Sartre puts it, "the body is the contingent form which is taken up by the necessity of my contingency" (1989, p. 328); freedom requires the limitations imposed by a body but it does not require those limitations to take any specific form. The phenomenology of freedom does not implicate the body as an *object* of experience. For Sartre, our bodily capacities and dispositions manifest themselves as the system of possibilities that we take as integral to the experienced world: "the world as the correlate of the possibilities which I am appears from the moment of my upsurge as the enormous skeletal outline of all my possible actions" (Sartre 1989, p. 322). However, the specific form that this "outline" takes is not determined solely by the body. For example, Sartre says that bodily fatigue is experienced as a way in which the "surrounding world" appears, but how exactly it is experienced depends upon what projects one is committed to (1989, p. 454).

I will now apply this approach to the phenomenology of depression. Experiences of incapability in depression are, I suggest, plausibly interpreted if we accept the following:

1. The sense of freedom associated with action is principally a matter of possibilities that are integral to the experienced world.
2. The possibilities we experience reflect our projects.
3. Experience of worldly possibilities is inextricable from our bodily phenomenology.

The experience of freedom is a "way of being in the world" that is presupposed by action, rather than something attributable primarily to a kind of experienced episode that precedes certain actions.[9] Depression involves a change in the *kinds* of possibility that are integral to experience, amounting to an erosion of the experience of freedom. This change can take a number of different forms.

DEPRESSION AND FREE WILL

Most autobiographical accounts of severe depression describe a radical change in experience, thought, and activity:

> When you are in it there is no more empathy, no intellect, no imagination, no compassion, no humanity, no hope. It isn't possible to roll over in bed because the capacity to plan and

---

[9] As Merleau-Ponty (1962, p. 162) puts it, "Will presupposes a field of possibilities among which I choose."

execute the required steps is too difficult to master, and the physical skills needed are too hard to complete. […] Depression steals away whoever you are, prevents you from seeing who you might someday be, and replaces your life with a black hole. Like a sweater eaten by moths, nothing is left of the original, only fragments that hinted at greater capacities, greater abilities, greater potentials now gone. (Patient quoted by Karp 1996, pp. 24–25)

References to "stealing away whoever you are" and "preventing you from seeing who you might someday be" could be interpreted in terms of losing one or more projects that are central to one's life. Things appear significant in the ways they do partly in virtue of the possibilities that we seek to actualize through our projects. Hence, with a loss of these projects, the entities and situations we encounter do not offer what they once did or solicit action in the way they did, thus accounting for a diminished will to act. One can only look back and recall a time when the world was alive with possibilities that are now gone. The abandonment of a life-shaping project need not be self-initiated; various events can conspire to put an end to it. For example, someone's life might be dedicated to the upkeep of a rare artifact that is reduced to ashes by vandals.

Hence one way of construing the inability to act in depression is in terms of the loss, self-initiated or otherwise, of projects upon which the significance of many experienced entities and situations depends. With this, there is a diminished sense of being presented with possibilities for action. In my view, this is indeed central to some instances of diagnosed depression. However, I suggest that more severe forms, including the kind of experience described earlier, involve a different kind of loss. What is missing from experience is not simply the practical significance of however many entities. (By "practical significance," I mean a sense of (a) something's utility or functionality, combined with (b) its potential relevance with respect to a set of concerns, and/or (c) its enticing one to act in some way.) Instead, that *kind* of significance is gone from experience. It is important to distinguish two forms that this might take. In one case, a sense of there being worthwhile projects and significant scenarios remains but the world altogether ceases to entice, to draw one in. Hence there is a feeling of being unable to act, even though one retains various concerns and appreciates that certain actions are appropriate in the context of those concerns. In the other case, which I will focus on here, those concerns are absent too. So there is a more profound loss: a sense of anything being potentially relevant to any project is gone. It is not merely that one fails to experience entities as significant; one *can't*. Everything one encounters is stripped of experienced possibilities for action that it previously incorporated, and world experience as a whole is thus altered in structure. This loss is at the same time an impoverishment of freedom, of the experienced world as a realm of possibilities that might be actualized by one's activities. Such a predicament is described with remarkable clarity in the following first-person account:

It was as if the whatness of each thing—I'm no good at philosophical vocabulary—but the essence of each thing in the sense of the tableness of the table or the chairness of the chair or the floorness of the floor was gone. There was a mute and indifferent object in that place. Its availability to human living, to human dwelling in the world was drained out of it. Its identity as a familiar object that we live with each day was gone. […] the world had lost its welcoming quality. It wasn't a habitable earth any longer. […] It became impossible to reach anything. Like, how do I get up and walk to that chair if the essential thing that we mean by chair, something that lets us sit down and rest or upholds us as we read a book, something that shares our life in that way, has lost the quality of being able to do that? (Quoted by Hornstein 2009, pp. 212–213)

When all experienced entities lose their practical familiarity and cease to solicit activity, the world no longer incorporates possibilities for action. But, even here, "practical significance" at least remains intelligible. As the author goes on to say, "I never fell to that extreme, of not knowing that other ways of being existed. I always knew, through all those years, that I was trying to find my way back, that there was another way to be" (quoted by Hornstein 2009, p. 214). Even when faced with an all-pervasive loss of experienced practical significance, one might still be able to contemplate the *possibility* of one's finding things significant again and thus of pursuing some as yet unformulated project. And, even if that were gone too, one might retain an appreciation that things continue to be significant in these ways for other people. However, it is arguable that—in some cases—the loss goes so deep that the person is unable to make sense of the possibility of anything being practically significant for anyone:

> But in among the bad and worse times, there were also moments when I felt, if not hope, then at least the glimmerings of possibility. […] It was like starting from the beginning. It took me a long time, for example, to understand, or to re-understand, why people do things. Why, in fact, they do anything at all. What is it that occupies their time? What is the point of doing? During my long morning walks, I watched people hurrying along in suits and trainers. Where was it they were going, and why were they in such haste? I simply couldn't imagine feeling such urgency. I watched others throwing a ball for a dog, picking it up, and throwing it again. Why? Where was the sense in such repetition? (Brampton 2008, p. 249)

The return of "possibility" described here serves to make salient what was previously diminished or lost—a sense of what it is for someone to act purposively, to find things significant and respond to them accordingly. Activities such as playing with a ball or hurrying to a destination had become strange, without meaning.

It is important to emphasize that "practical significance" is not the only kind of experienced significance that is affected in depression. For instance, changes in the structure of interpersonal experience (although not my principal focus in this chapter) are absolutely central to some, if not all, forms of depression (Ratcliffe, in press, b). Sufferers often report an inability to relate to others, which sometimes involves a need for emotional connection that cannot be met because experiences of others fail to incorporate its possibility. In some instances, there is a pervasive sense of vulnerability that is incompatible with the possibility of emotional connection: "sufferers yearn for connection, seem bereft because of their isolation, and yet are rendered incapable of being with others in a comfortable way" (Karp 1996, p. 14). A change of this kind, involving loss of various kinds of possibility that people and the social world more usually offer, has a profound effect upon one's sense of agency. Given the extent to which the experienced world is permeated by possibilities involving other people, our sense of "practical significance" and our sense of "interpersonal possibility" are inextricable—what affects one will inevitably affect the other in some way too.

Depression not only involves the *absence* or even the *felt absence* of certain kinds of possibility from experience. Other kinds of significant possibility can become more salient. For instance, whereas only some things used to appear threatening, threat might now become something that all experienced entities offer.[10] The normal sense of being solicited to act by the world is not only lost but replaced by an all-encompassing threat before which one

---

[10]   Depression is intimately linked to anxiety, and clinical distinctions between the two are contentious. For example: "the firewall between anxiety and depression ignores the fact that the commonest form of affective disorder is mixed anxiety-depression" (Shorter and Tyrer 2003, p. 158).

is passive and helpless. The feeling of impotence that many people report is at least partly attributable to this. For example:

> At that time ordinary objects—chairs, tables and the like—possessed a frightening, menacing quality which is very hard to describe vividly in the way that I was then affected. It was as though I lived in some kind of hell, containing nothing from which I could obtain relief or comfort. (Patient quoted by Rowe 1978, pp. 269–270)

William Styron similarly complains of a pervasive change in the significance of his surroundings that began in the early stages of depression. They "took on a different tone at certain times: the shadows of nightfall seemed more somber, my mornings were less buoyant, walks in the wood became less zestful." He later describes how his "beloved farmhouse" took on "an almost palpable quality of ominousness" (2001, pp. 41–44). What we have here is not just a loss or diminution of certain kinds of experienced significance that are integral to our sense of freedom. In addition, threat, a form of significance that opposes action, becomes all-enveloping, a shape that the whole world takes on.[11] Consider the following interview excerpt:

> I lie in bed for ages dreading getting in the shower and then when I'm eventually in the shower I end up being in there for ages dreading getting out. […] The feeling of dread isn't a fear or dread about something specific happening, it's more like feeling disabled in some way, like the effort and the idea of moving onto the next thing whatever that is, feels too overwhelming. […] It's almost like I am there but I can't touch anything or I can't connect. Everything requires massive effort and I'm not really able to do anything. Like if I notice something needs cleaning or moving, it's like it's out of reach, or the act of doing that thing isn't in my world at that time … like I can see so much detail but I cannot be a part of it. I suppose feeling disconnected is the best way to describe it.[12]

There are, I think, two things going on here, working together. Experienced entities are drained of their usual significance and the world is bereft of any positive enticement for action; it no longer draws one in and thus seems distant, detached, not quite there. The bodily correlate of this is a feeling of fatigue, lethargy, and weight. In addition to this, everything is enveloped by a different kind of significance, which only certain things previously had; the world takes on the form of threat, the result being a paralyzing and inescapable sense of dread. It is debatable whether or not one could live in a world bereft of potentialities for action without at the same time having some degree of passive dread, but the two aspects of the experience can certainly vary in their salience. Despite such differences, the experiences that sufferers describe are united by a common theme. As Dorothy Rowe (1978, p. 30) notes, an experience of confinement or incarceration is reported by almost everyone:

> While different people describe their experience of depression in different ways, there is one feature that they all share. Each person describes the experience as one of being enclosed.

---

[11] Law (2009) offers the complementary view that, in depression, a change in how one perceives the world does not *cause* loss of motivation. Instead, perception incorporates motivation. He adds that the change need not simply be understood in terms of loss. Rather, something could be *added* that blocks action. An experience of the world as threat, amongst other things, might play that role.

[12] From a conference presentation by Outi Benson (SANE), entitled 'Using the Grounded Theory Method to explore Emotional Experience associated with Self-cutting" (July 2010).

Some say it is like being in a dark prison cell, some say it is like being at the bottom of a deep hole, some say it is like being wrapped in impenetrable cloth, some say it's like being enclosed by thick, soundproofed glass. The images vary, but the underlying concept is the same. The person is in solitary confinement.

This can be understood in terms of altered experience of possibilities. In the most extreme case, because the world incorporates no sense of possibilities for action by oneself or others, it also incorporates no sense of the potential for significant change. The predicament that one finds oneself in thus appears timeless and inescapable—it incorporates the sense that "this is all there is or could be." In other cases, the sense that the possibilities still exist for others but not for oneself constitutes a sense of being alienated, cut off from the social world, imprisoned. And, in those instances where a feeling of dread is salient, the only possibility for change that the world offers is the actualization of some inchoate threat before which one is passive. All of these amount, I suggest, to a diminishment of experienced freedom: loss of world is loss of will. Many sufferers describe their predicament as akin to having died; it is eternal, inescapable and involves a sense of utter estrangement from other people and from any set of potential practical concerns (e.g., Kaysen 2001, p. 32; Wurtzel 1996, p. 19).

Hence various subtly different kinds of experience might be associated with a diagnosis such as "major depression." Variables include the extent to which practical significance is lost, whether and to what extent the world appears in the guise of threat and no doubt other factors too. Here are six different kinds of experience that might be associated both with diminished agency and a diagnosis of depression, although I do not wish to rule out others:

1. A loss of some fundamental project. The world no longer offers certain possibilities for action it once did and nothing has yet replaced them. However, one does not lack an appreciation of what it *would be* for the world to have those possibilities and one also recognizes that other people retain them.[13]
2. Loss of enticing possibilities. The world might still incorporate meaningful projects but its allure is gone and it no longer solicits action.
3. A more encompassing loss, where a sense of *anything* incorporating possibilities for activity is absent from experience. One is *unable* to experience anything as practically significant.
4. An even deeper loss, involving an inability to conceive of ever regaining a sense of significant possibility in one's life. However, one retains a sense that others have meaningful possibilities. This exacerbates a feeling of being oddly cut off from them.
5. A complete absence of any sense that anything could be significant for anyone, amounting to a world that is bereft of the usual sense of freedom.
6. An all-enveloping passivity before some threat, which exacerbates the inability to act in cases where loss of practical significance is only partial.

[13] It is debatable whether or when cases of this type warrant a diagnosis of depression. A profound change in life-shaping projects is an inevitable correlate of the death of a close family member or the loss of a job to which one was dedicated. But grief and unemployment do not automatically lead to depression. However, where one fails to move on from grief or job loss, the label "depression" is more plausible. There are also cases where one "gives up" on projects that were previously central to one's life, despite there being no outward change in one's circumstances. It is similarly debatable whether and when they are attributable to "depression."

It seems plausible to suggest that (1) to (5) could all occur with some degree of (6). For example, in the case of (1), the world might still incorporate the possibility of having a shower or getting out of bed, but such activities present themselves as daunting, frightening, or even practically impossible. The world thus offers the possibility of doing *x* but at the same time incorporates a sense of *x* as impossible. All experience takes on the form "you can't," analogous to a staircase that appears climbable but at the same time too steep to climb. Hence (6) exacerbates (1). In addition, (6) surely entails a form (2), given that experiencing the world in terms of all-encompassing threat blocks any positive solicitation to act. However, it also seems that (6) is not an inevitable correlate of any of (1) to (5). Loss of practical significance is often emphasized without any reference to threat or dread, as in the earlier quotation from Hornstein (2009). Hence diminished experience of freedom in depression may come in many different degrees and forms. But common to all of these is a change in the experienced world that is, at the same time, a loss of experienced possibilities for action. Such phenomenological changes do not stop action completely. Certain habitual behaviors may continue, albeit in the context of a radically altered experience of the world and one's place in it. And one might also act in response to a sense of threat, cowering and retreating from a world that offers nothing else. But what remains is still a distortion and impoverishment of the more usual experience of freedom.

Another respect in which the phenomenology of depression complements Sartre's account of freedom is the role of bodily experience. People with depression report a wide range of bodily complaints. As Styron (2001, pp. 42–43) puts it, "I felt a kind of numbness, an enervation, but more particularly an odd fragility—as if my body had actually become frail, hypersensitive and somehow disjointed and clumsy, lacking normal coordination." He also describes how later, during recovery, he felt as though he was "no longer a husk but a body with some of the body's sweet juices stirring again" (2001, p. 75). Numerous other accounts similarly describe changes in bodily experience, and authors often remark on how difficult it is to dissociate bodily changes from changes in the world. Their testimony is thus consistent with the Sartrean view that bodily experience and worldly possibility are inextricable. A loss of worldly possibilities is at the same time a loss of vitality, and the correlate of a world that offers nothing is a cumbersome, conspicuous, awkward, and painful body (Fuchs 2005; Ratcliffe 2009).[14]

CONCLUSIONS

I propose that we employ a broadly Sartrean interpretive framework in order to illuminate alterations in the experience of freedom and agency that can occur in depression. In so far as that framework coheres with first-person testimony and makes sense of otherwise

[14] A 2011 questionnaire study, which I carried out with colleagues as part of the project "Emotional Experience in Depression: a Philosophical Study," serves to illustrate the prevalence and prominence of bodily symptoms. Of the 139 people who responded to the question "How does your body feel when you're depressed?," only two reported no bodily symptoms and two others were unsure. One or more of the words "tired," "lethargic," "heavy," and "exhausted" appeared in ninety-six of the responses, and all of the remainder included comparable complaints of lacking energy and feeling drained or fatigued.

obscure phenomena, it is itself vindicated in the process. In addition, there is the possibility of revising and refining our phenomenological account through engagement with the experience of depression. Sartre insists that even the most exceptional circumstances leave our freedom intact. For example, he writes that "the red hot pincers of the torturer do not exempt us from being free" (Sartre 1989, p. 505). However, reflection upon the experience of depression suggests that matters are more complicated than this. The structure of our experience of freedom is changeable, and it can be impoverished in a number of different ways. Through studying first-person accounts of depression, we can begin to describe some of these and, in the process, to further clarify what an intact sense of freedom consists of. This is at odds with Sartre's own view. In his *Sketch for a Theory of the Emotions* (1994), he offers an account of "melancholy," according to which the "potentialities of our world" initially remain intact but our means of actualizing them are obstructed. For example, one might lose one's car due to financial problems and thus require an alternative means of transport. He proposes that melancholy is a way of avoiding such life adjustments by "transforming the present structure of the world, replacing it with a totally undifferentiated structure" (1994, p. 44). The result is that the world altogether lacks significance and no longer solicits action. This change, he maintains, does not compromise our freedom. In fact, it is an exercise of our freedom. Even if we were to accept something along these lines, it could only account for the first of the variants I listed in the previous section, where one loses certain core projects and, with them, a range of ways in which things appeared significant. It does not accommodate (3), where one is *unable* to find anything significant, unless we maintain that the sense of inability is somehow illusory. And it does not account for variants (4) and (5) either. In these cases, it is not just that however many things lose their significance or even that one is unable to find things significant. In addition, certain *kinds* of significant possibility lose their *intelligibility*. Whereas (1) is compatible with intact freedom, cases (3) to (5) amount to an alteration in the phenomenological structure of freedom, regardless of whether or not they are accompanied by (6). Case (2) also amounts to such an alteration (albeit a less profound one), so long as we accept that the person is incapable of finding anything enticing, rather than maintaining—in line with Sartre's view—that a lack of enticement from the world is symptomatic of something chosen.

I have not addressed whether and how the impoverishment of freedom that occurs in depression differs from that associated with other kinds of psychiatric illness, and other circumstances too. For instance, the account of freedom I have sketched here can also be applied to anomalous experiences and disturbances of agency that are reported in schizophrenia. In *Autobiography of a Schizophrenic Girl* (Sechehaye 1970), a well-known autobiographical account of schizophrenia, the author—Renee—describes a profound change in experience of self and world. Madness, she says, is a "country" that is "opposed to reality," a different world (1970, p. 44). It is clear from her account that the change in her world is attributable, at least in part, to a shift in the kinds of possibility it incorporates. For instance, it is altogether bereft of practical significance: "When, for example, I looked at a chair or a jug, I thought not of their use or function—a jug not as something to hold water and milk, a chair not as something to sit in—but as having lost their names, their functions and meanings" (1970, pp. 55–56). It is in the context of this altered world that Renee experienced symptoms such as thought insertion, and was hospitalized after she followed an order from "The System" to put her hand in the fire (1970, p. 61). At one point, she describes experiencing a return of significant possibility to the world and, with it, a restoration of her sense of agency:

> When we were outside I realized that my perception of things had completely changed. Instead of infinite space, unreal, where everything was cut off, naked and isolated, I saw Reality, marvellous Reality, for the first time. The people whom we encountered were no longer automatons, phantoms, revolving around, gesticulating without meaning; they were men and women with their own individual characteristics, their own individuality. It was the same with things. They were useful things, having sense, capable of giving me pleasure. Here was an automobile to take me to the hospital, cushions I could rest on. [...] ... for the first time I dared to handle the chairs, to change the arrangement of the furniture. What an unknown joy, to have an influence on things; to do with them what I liked and especially to have the pleasure of wanting the change. (1970, pp. 105–106)

Again, we see how possibilities that are integral to the experienced world are inextricable from the capacity for action—a return of the significance of things is also a return of the sense that one can act upon them.[15] It is debatable how, precisely, the changes in freedom that characterize schizophrenia differ from those that feature in depression.[16] There clearly are differences, as severe depression involves losing the will to act, but not misattributing one's agency to someone else. Hence a task for phenomenological enquiry, through its inter-action with psychiatry and other contexts, is to refine an account of the various different forms that diminishment of freedom can take. This is not just a theoretical exercise. A better understanding of the nature of and differences between these predicaments may enhance the ability to empathize and inform therapy. Subtle phenomenological distinctions also have potential implications for pharmaceutical intervention, given the possibility of differ-ent forms of intervention proving effective for different predicaments. Furthermore, insofar as psychiatric classification systems draw upon distinctions between kinds of experience, phenomenology can inform classification. For example, it is arguable that classifications of "mental disorder" are insufficiently sensitive to the different forms that "loss of practical sig-nificance" can take. Hence, although I have only scratched the surface here, I hope that this chapter at least serves to indicate the potential fruitfulness of phenomenology in psychiatry and, indeed, psychiatry in phenomenology.

How, if at all, does any of this relate to the question of whether we are free? I have char-acterized the principal ingredient of freedom as a sense of being able to actualize, through our activities, possibilities that are experienced as belonging to the world. But the fact that we experience ourselves and the world in this way does not imply that possibilities really do reside in the world or that, when we act, we do actualize possibilities. One could maintain that, so far as the metaphysics is concerned, the phenomenology is irrelevant. Alternatively, one might attempt to formulate an argument for the reality of human freedom on the basis of phenomenology. In brief, it is arguable that, without a sense of there being worldly possibili-ties that one could actualize, one would not inhabit the kind of world that empirical enquiry

---

[15] See Sass (e.g., 2003, 2004) for a detailed account of the relationship between symptoms such as anomalous bodily experience, changes in world experience, and disorders of agency in schizophrenia. He stresses that this relationship is not causal, but instead a matter of "mutual phenomenological implication" (2003, p. 156).

[16] See Fuchs (e.g., 2005) for some comparative phenomenological work.

presupposes and attempts to characterize—one would lack the usual "sense of reality." Thus any result of empirical enquiry denying that we actualize worldly possibilities would undermine its own intelligibility. Therefore, one could not coherently deny that we have freedom in the sense I have described. This seems to be Sartre's position:

> The necessity of potentiality as a meaningful structure of perception appears clearly enough so that we need not insist on it here. Scientific knowledge, in fact, can neither overcome nor suppress the potentializing structure of perception. On the contrary science must presuppose it. (1989, p. 197)

If he is right, then most of us are free most of the time, and any attempt to maintain otherwise is ultimately self-defeating.

ACKNOWLEDGMENTS

I am grateful to Steve Burwood, Richard Gipps, Jonathan Lowe, Outi Benson, Katherine Morris, and a conference audience at the Free University of Berlin for helpful comments and suggestions. This chapter was written as part of the project "Emotional Experience in Depression: A Philosophical Study." I am very grateful to the AHRC and DFG for funding the project, and to my project colleagues in the UK and Germany for many valuable discussions.

REFERENCES

Brampton, S. (2008). *Shoot the Damn Dog: A Memoir of Depression*. London: Bloomsbury Publishing.

Frankl, V. E. (1973). *Psychotherapy and Existentialism: Selected Papers on Logotherapy*. London: Penguin Books.

Fuchs, T. (2005). Corporealized and disembodied minds: A phenomenological view of the body in melancholia and schizophrenia. *Philosophy, Psychiatry, & Psychology*, 12, 95–107.

Gallagher, S. (2006). Where's the action? Epiphenomenalism and the problem of free will. In W. Banks, S. Pockett, and S. Gallagher (Eds), *Does Consciousness Cause Behavior? An Investigation of the Nature of Volition*, pp. 109–24. Cambridge MA: MIT Press.

Gallagher, S. (2008). Intersubjectivity in perception. *Continental Philosophy Review*, 41, 163–78.

Heidegger, M. (1962). *Being and Time* (J. Macquarrie and E. Robinson, Trans.). Oxford: Blackwell.

Holton, R. (2009). Determinism, self-efficacy, and the phenomenology of free will. *Inquiry*, 52, 412–28.

Hornstein, G. A. (2009). *Agnes's Jacket: A Psychologist's Search for the Meanings of Madness*. New York, NY: Rodale.

Husserl, E. (1973). *Experience and Judgment* (J. S. Churchill and K. Ameriks, Trans.). London: Routledge.

Husserl, E. (1989). *Ideas Pertaining to a Pure Phenomenology and to a Phenomenological Philosophy: Second Book* (R. Rojcewicz and A. Schuwer, Trans.). Dordrecht: Kluwer.

Husserl, E. (2001). *Analyses Concerning Passive and Active Synthesis* (A. J. Steinbock, Trans.). Dordrecht: Kluwer.

Jaspers, K. (1963). *General Psychopathology*. Manchester: Manchester University Press.

Karp, D. (1996). *Speaking of Sadness: Depression, Disconnection, and the Meanings of Illness*. Oxford: Oxford University Press.

Kaysen, S. (2001). One cheer for melancholy. In N. Casey (Ed.), *Unholy Ghost: Writers on Depression*, pp. 38–43. New York, NY: William Morrow.

Law, I. (2009). Motivation, depression and character. In M. R. Broome and L. Bortolotti (Eds), *Psychiatry as Cognitive Neuroscience: Philosophical Perspectives*, pp. 351–64. Oxford: Oxford University Press.

Libet, B. (2004). *Mind Time: The Temporal Factor in Consciousness*. Cambridge MA: Harvard University Press.

Lowe, E. J. (2009). *Personal Agency: The Metaphysics of Mind and Action*. Oxford: Oxford University Press.

Merleau-Ponty, M. (1962). *Phenomenology of Perception* (C. Smith, Trans.). London: Routledge.

Mill, J. S. (1873). *Autobiography*. London: Longmans, Green, Reader & Dyer.

Nichols, S. (2004). The folk psychology of free will: Fits and starts. *Mind & Language, 19*, 473–502.

Ratcliffe, M. (2008). *Feelings of Being: Phenomenology, Psychiatry and the Sense of Reality*. Oxford: Oxford University Press.

Ratcliffe, M. (2009). Understanding existential changes in psychiatric illness: The indispensability of phenomenology. In M. Broome and L. Bortolotti (Eds), *Psychiatry as Cognitive Neuroscience*, pp. 223–44. Oxford: Oxford University Press.

Ratcliffe, M. (in press, a). Delusional atmosphere and the sense of unreality. In G. Stanghellini and T. Fuchs (Eds), *One Century of Karl Jaspers' General Psychopathology*. Oxford: Oxford University Press.

Ratcliffe, M. (in press, b). The structure of interpersonal experience. In D. Moran and R. Jensen (Eds), *Phenomenology of Embodied Subjectivity*. Dordrecht: Springer.

Read, J. and Reynolds, J. (Eds). (1996). *Speaking our Minds: An Anthology*. Basingstoke: Palgrave Macmillan.

Roberts, J. R. (2001). Mental illness, motivation and moral commitment. *Philosophical Quarterly, 51*, 41–59.

Rowe, D. (1978). *The Experience of Depression*. Chichester: John Wiley and Sons.

Sartre, J. P. (1989). *Being and Nothingness* (H. Barnes, Trans.). London: Routledge.

Sartre, J. P. (1994). *Sketch for a Theory of the Emotions*. (P. Mairet, Trans.). London: Routledge.

Sass, L. A. (2003). "Negative symptoms," schizophrenia, and the self. *International Journal of Psychology and Psychological Therapy, 3*, 153–80

Sass, L. A. (2004). Affectivity in schizophrenia: A phenomenological view. In D. Zahavi (Ed.), *Hidden Resources: Classical Perspectives on Subjectivity*, pp. 127–47. Exeter: Imprint Academic.

Sechehaye, M. (1970). *Autobiography of a Schizophrenic Girl*. New York, NY: Signet.

Shaw, F. (1997). *Out of Me: The Story of a Postnatal Breakdown*. London: Penguin.

Shorter, E. and Tyrer, P. (2003). Separation of anxiety and depressive disorders: Blind alley in psychopharmacology and classification of disease. *British Medical Journal, 327*, 158–160.

Styron, W. (2001). *Darkness Visible*. London: Vintage.

Wurtzel, E. (1996). *Prozac Nation: Young and Depressed in America*. London: Quartet Books.

CHAPTER 37

BODY IMAGE DISORDERS

KATHERINE J. MORRIS

The phrase "body image disorder" designates a popular rather than a psychiatric classification, in the sense that there is no *Diagnostic and Statistical Manual of Mental Disorders* (DSM) or International Classification of Diseases (ICD) category with this label. Nonetheless psychiatrists do recognize negative or distorted or disturbed body image as a diagnostic criterion or a common feature of certain disorders which do have psychiatric classifications. In both the popular and the psychiatric use, the disorders most commonly cited as involving a disturbed body image are body dysmorphic disorder (hereafter "BDD") and anorexia nervosa (hereafter "anorexia") as well as, occasionally, other "eating disorders" such as bulimia nervosa ("bulimia") and binge eating disorder ("BED"). (DSM-5 proposes to elevate BED from its inclusion under DSM-IV's "eating disorders not otherwise specified" to a disorder in its own right; in ICD-10 it is not explicitly named but would fall under "atypical bulimia nervosa.")

There are ways in which the term "body image" has been understood (as, e.g., Thompson 1990, p. 1, notes) which would count, for example, phantom limbs, anosognosia, and so-called proprioceptive blindness or loss of position and movement sense as body image disorders. (These tend to be classified as "neurological" rather than "psychiatric," but this distinction is contestable.) If one were to accept the philosopher Gallagher's widely cited distinction between "body *image*" and "body *schema*" (where the former refers to the subject's perceptual experience of his own body, his conceptual understanding of the body in general, and/or his emotional attitude toward his own body, and the latter is a "nonconscious postural model, which actively monitors body posture and movement"; Gallagher 1995, p. 226), this might justify excluding these (since they would be body schema rather than body image disorders). The decision I have taken—to exclude consideration not only of these but of psychiatric conditions other than BDD and eating disorders which might well be argued essentially to involve a disordered body schema or image, e.g., developmental coordination disorder, gender identity disorder or gender dysphoria, and hypochondriasis—is purely pragmatic. (However, since ICD-10 classifies BDD as a hypochondriacal disorder, I do touch very briefly on the last of these.)

Philosophers of psychiatry often invoke Jaspers' distinction between *explanation* and *understanding* of mental disorders. (There is of course a further issue of treatment, which will not be addressed here.) The present article focuses on understanding, and in particular on attempts to understand body image disorders by psychologists and psychiatrists, by feminist thinkers mindful of the gender imbalance in many of these disorders, and by philosophers, feminists, and anthropologists with a phenomenological bent. (I have not included a separate section on psychoanalysts and other psychotherapists, although I do quote some of their descriptions, e.g., those of Bruch, Lindner, and Orbach; and Kristeva's concept of abjection, discussed in the "The phenomenology of body image disorders" section, has roots in Lacanian psychoanalysis. Psychoanalysts and psychotherapists have their own jargon which is different from that of most phenomenologists, but insofar as they confine themselves to understanding rather than explanation, it may be said—and indeed has been said by the phenomenologists Sartre and Merleau-Ponty—that their best descriptions are ones which phenomenologists can happily embrace.) Understanding is of necessity, I would urge, multiperspectival; it does not follow, however, that all perspectives are equally illuminating, as the final section argues.

Psychological and Psychiatric Perspectives on Body Image Disorders

Very broadly, there seem to be two, albeit overlapping, traditions of body image research among psychologists and psychiatrists; these are sometimes (a little confusingly) labeled "body image" and "body shame" traditions respectively (e.g., Carr 2002, p. 99). (Although this is an over-generalization, it may help to give an initial feel for the two approaches to observe that the first is more likely to look toward drug treatment for these disorders, the second toward some sort of cognitive behavioral therapy.)

Body image research on body image disorders

The first approach distinguishes between "the 'outside view' of human appearance" and the "inside view," reserving the term "body image" for the latter (e.g., Cash 2004, p. 1). It adopts the mantra that body image is "multidimensional" (where the "dimensions" typically cited are *perceptual*, *cognitive*, *affective*, and *behavioral*); much effort is expended on developing and validating ingenious techniques and instruments (questionnaires, computer-morphed images, etc.) for measuring these dimensions. (One of the more widely used of many such instruments, the Multidimensional Body-Self Relations Questionnaire or MBSRQ, clearly announces their mantra, and it is the presupposition of the recently (2004) inaugurated journal *Body Image*.) Table 37.1 is not meant to be a definitive summary of body image research findings on body image disorders, but it should give a sense both of the *sorts* of aspects of body image that are studied and the patterns—such as they are—which emerge.

To distinguish, as the body image tradition does, between "the 'outside view' of human appearance" and the "inside view," and to focus attention solely on the latter, is to suggest that these two "views" are relatively independent. Consistent with this, social and cultural factors tend to be played down within this research tradition. Sometimes (as Bordo 1993, p. 61 notes) their relevance to eating disorders will be dismissed altogether on the grounds that only a small proportion of individuals actually develop full-blown eating disorders

Table 37.1 Body image disturbance in "body image" research

	Preoccupation with (aspects of) the body (including *weight preoccupation*)	Appearance investment (including *shape and weight concern*): how one's appearance influences one's sense of self-worth, and the importance one places on being attractive and managing one's appearance	Body dissatisfaction	Body image distortion (including *apparent size distortion*): the degree of match or mismatch between how one perceives one's own body and how it really is
BDD	Criterial	High[2]	High[4–6]	Mixed evidence[9]
Anorexia	Criterial	Partly criterial	Mixed evidence[7]	Partly criterial; mixed evidence[10]
Bulimia	Criterial	Criterial	High[4]	Mixed evidence[11]
BED	High[1]	High[1,3]	High[8]	High[12]

"Criterial" = a DSM or ICD diagnostic criterion; "partly criterial" = one of the disjuncts of a disjunctive DSM or ICD diagnostic criterion; "high" = significantly higher than gender-matched non-clinical controls.

[1] (Wilfley et al. 2000)

[2] (Phillips 2002); higher not only than controls but also than anorexia or bulimia sufferers (Hrabosky et al. 2009).

[3] (Legenbauer et al. 2011)

[4] (Cash and Deagle 1997; Ruuska et al. 2005)

[5] *Contra* the suggestion that BDD sufferers' body dissatisfaction stems from their setting peculiarly high standards of appearance for themselves, see Lambrou et al. (2011, pp. 451–452).

[6] BDD sufferers are typically very dissatisfied with just *one* of the specific areas of the body at any one time while being more or less satisfied with the others; this dissatisfaction with a specific area leads them to be dissatisfied with their appearance overall (Phillips 1996, p. 206).

[7] Contrast Cash and Deagle (1997) with Hrabosky et al. (2009); see also Sullivan (2002). This inconsistency may be in part explicable by the fact that "persistent lack of recognition of the seriousness of the current low body weight" is partly criterial for anorexia, so that an anorexic may be satisfied with and indeed take pride in her emaciated state (cf. Garner 2002).

[8] Higher than both non-obese and obese non-clinical controls (Grilo 2002).

[9] Contrast Phillips (1996, p. 203) with Lambrou et al. (2011).

[10] The partial criterion—"disturbance in the way in which one's body weight or shape is experienced" –is usually understood in terms of apparent size distortion. Thompson (1990, pp. 30–32) notes a lack of clear difference on this measure between anorexics and controls and suggests that this is in part due to the fact that non-clinical controls also tend to overestimate their size. Delinsky (2011, p. 281) notes discrepant findings, which "have been attributed to heterogeneity of assessment methods."

[11] Contrast Stice (2002) with Vocks et al. (2007).

[12] Higher than both non-obese and obese non-clinical controls (Legenbauer et al. 2011).

(e.g. Kaye et al. 2002, p. 68; see McNamara 2002 for an anthropological counter). This certainly implies that social and cultural factors are not *sufficient* to produce eating disorders, but hardly implies that they are not *relevant*.

Body shame research on body-image disorders

The second approach to an extent compensates for this limitation in the first. These researchers, while embracing the idea that body image is in *some* sense multidimensional, capture the primary dimensions with the term "biopsychosocial" (Gilbert 2002). This explicitly identifies the social as a dimension of body image; thus their theorizations draw on sociologists as well as psychiatrists and psychologists.

Much of the body image literature treats shame simply as distress or "dysphoric affect"; the body shame tradition is rather more nuanced. They make a basic distinction between *external shame* and internal (*internalized*) *shame* (e.g., Gilbert 2002). The former involves feelings that are focused on the "self as seen and judged by others" or the "self as object," and is linked to notions like *stigma* (or at least "stigma consciousness")—itself a central concept in sociology, elaborated most notably by Goffman (1963/1990)—*fear of negative evaluation*, and *social anxiety*. The latter involves feelings focused on the "self as judged by self"; it remains a socially situated concept since it is understood as involving an *internalization* of others' negative judgments (or, in Veale's (2002) usage, the application to oneself of, and the awareness of falling short of, one's *own* standards, e.g., aesthetic standards), and involves a *negative self-evaluation*. Other notions include "aesthetic identity" (e.g., Lambrou et al. 2011) which links body surveillance (viewing one's own body as an external observer) with internalized shame and "objectified body consciousness" (McKinley and Hyde 1996). These researchers see body shame as operative, in different senses and with different roles, in all body image disorders. (The following subdivisions reflect their conviction that shame operates in distinctive ways in BDD, restricting anorexia and binge eating in all eating disorders. That clear *patterns* emerge from this approach, by contrast with the lack of a clear pattern in the body image approach as exemplified in Table 37.1, is arguably a further advantage of the body shame approach.)

Body dysmorphic disorder

It is acknowledged in both research traditions that "shame is so common in BDD, it may even be intrinsic to the disorder" (Phillips 1996, p. 82); Veale describes BDD as an "extreme form of body shame" (2002, p. 267). This clearly often includes "external shame," insofar as many BDD sufferers fear negative evaluation by others (e.g., Phillips 1996, p. 142), suffer from social anxiety and avoidance (e.g., Phillips 1996, p. 138), and feel that their "defect" stigmatizes them (e.g., Phillips 1996, p. 66). There is also little doubt that many BDD sufferers judge parts of their *own* bodies negatively (e.g., Phillips 1996, p. 82; Veale 2002 suggests that internal shame is *more* characteristic of BDD than external shame). Veale (2002, pp. 273–275) develops a complex cognitive behavioral model of BDD; it begins with a "trigger," e.g., a reflection in the mirror, and integrates "processing of the self as an aesthetic object," "rumination on ugliness or 'defectiveness' and comparison to ideal," negative mood, "avoidance and safety behaviors to change or camouflage," and "mirror-checking and selective attention." Shame lies at the center of Veale's representation of the model, and many of these elements both influence and are influenced by shame.

Anorexia (restricting type)

DSM's "intense fear of gaining weight or becoming fat" (ICD-10's "dread of fatness") has been widely analyzed in the literature in terms of *control/fear of loss of control*; Goss and Gilbert (2002) analyze some of the complexities in terms of a "*shame–pride cycle*" which characterizes "restricting anorexics," i.e., those anorexics who control their weight through calorie restriction. (It could apply equally to those who use excessive exercise for weight control; Goss and Gilbert offer a different model for bingers: see later.) Fig. 37.1 summarizes this cycle.

This model certainly captures many aspects of much anorexia; however, as Goss and Gilbert note (2002, p. 221), it does not fit comfortably with historical and cross-cultural "anorexia" related to religion or asceticism (see, e.g., Huline-Dickens 2000).

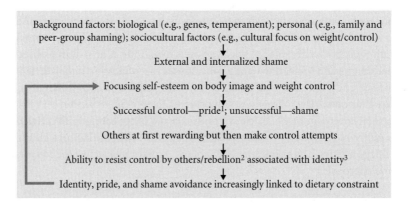

Background factors: biological (e.g., genes, temperament); personal (e.g., family and peer-group shaming); sociocultural factors (e.g., cultural focus on weight/control)
↓
External and internalized shame
↓
Focusing self-esteem on body image and weight control
↓
Successful control—pride[1]; unsuccessful—shame
↓
Others at first rewarding but then make control attempts
↓
Ability to resist control by others/rebellion[2] associated with identity[3]
↓
Identity, pride, and shame avoidance increasingly linked to dietary constraint

[1] In fact anorexia can be triggered by losing a bit of weight with dieting (Goss and Gilbert 2002, p. 39), and even by an unintentional weight loss through physical illness (Brandenburg and Anderson 2007).

[2] Hence anorexia sufferers' notorious resistance to treatment; even if detained in a medical or psychiatric ward, they frequently use trickery to avoid eating. For an autobiographical account of anorexia in which these aspects are prominent, see Krasnow (1996). Goss and Gilbert also cite anecdotal evidence on anorexia competitiveness: "restrictors can feel superior to other women in at least one respect: their ability to rigidly control their food intake" (2002, p. 240). Some anorexics criticize others who fill themselves up on salads or diet soda: "To me, this demonstrates a lack of willpower" (Krasnow 1996, p. 19).

[3] Hence there is talk of "ego syntonic resistance to feeding drives" (Kaye et al. 2002, p. 67).

FIGURE 37.1 Shame–pride cycle in restricting eating disorders. Adapted from Goss, K. and Gilbert, P. (2002). Eating disorders, shame and pride: a cognitive-behavioral functional analysis. In P. Gilbert and J. Miles (Eds), *Body Shame: Conceptualization, Research, and Treatment*, p. 242 © Brunner-Routledge, 2002 with permission.

Binge eating (bulimia, binge eating disorder, binge-purge anorexia)

Goss and Gilbert (2002) posit a "*shame–shame cycle*" for binge eating, summarized in Fig. 37.2.

This model seems to integrate many aspects of binge eating. The functions which it attributes to bingeing—e.g., to comfort or to dissociate—may be supplemented by Stice, whose "dual pathway" model of bulimia (2001) posits as the principal instigators (a) body dissatisfaction in the form of concern about one's weight and (b) subsequent dieting in the (misguided) belief that this will help to control one's weight. He suggests that the binge eating which characterizes bulimia may straightforwardly be a response to caloric deprivation as a result of dieting; alternatively, dieting requires a shift from reliance on physiological hunger and fullness cues to a cognitive control over eating behavior, which makes the individual vulnerable to bingeing at times of emotional vulnerability (Stice 2002; cf. Schaefer 2009, pp. 23ff.).

The body shame approach, in according a central role to social and cultural factors, may be thought to have some advantages over the body image research approach in allowing us to understand body image disorders. Sustained cultural critique, however, is left to feminists.

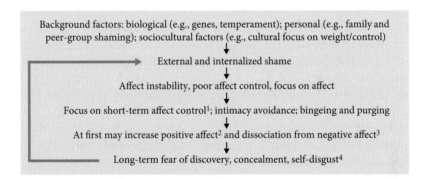

Background factors: biological (e.g., genes, temperament); personal (e.g., family and peer-group shaming); sociocultural factors (e.g., cultural focus on weight/control)
↓
External and internalized shame
↓
Affect instability, poor affect control, focus on affect
↓
Focus on short-term affect control[1]; intimacy avoidance; bingeing and purging
↓
At first may increase positive affect[2] and dissociation from negative affect[3]
↓
Long-term fear of discovery, concealment, self-disgust[4]

[1] Cf. Reindl (2002); cf. the notion of "comfort eating" or food as "self-soothing": "a way of swaddling a body that had no emotional myelin" (Orbach 2009, p. 72).

[2] For example, through self-soothing, because planning a binge can induce pride and a sense of control, and because the secrecy usually associated with binging may also give the individual "a sense of self-identity and power" (Goss and Gilbert 2002, p. 244). Purging too has its positive side, although Goss and Gilbert do not stress this: to reduce anxiety about weight gain or as a kind of emotional catharsis (Stice 2002). Some bulimics see the whole binge–purge cycle as a way of achieving control (Pope et al. 2000, p. 137).

[3] Cf. Stice (2002); bingeing often creates "an altered state of consciousness" (Pope at al. 2000, p. 137; cf. Eli 2011).

[4] For example, Pope et al. (2000, p. 136). The diagnostic criteria for BED include "eating alone because of feeling embarrassed by how much one is eating" and "feeling disgusted with oneself, depressed, or very guilty afterwards" as characteristic markers; these are also common in bulimia (see Pope et al. 2000, p. 139). Also common is a sense of loss of control: "as time passes the pride in outwitting Nature gives way to the feeling of being helplessly in the grip of a demonic power that controls their life" (Bruch 1978, p. 10).

FIGURE 37.2 Shame–shame cycle in binge eating. Adapted from Goss, K. and Gilbert, P. (2002). Eating disorders, shame and pride: a cognitive-behavioural functional analysis. In P. Gilbert and J. Miles (Eds), *Body Shame: Conceptualization, Research, and Treatment*, p. 242 © Brunner-Routledge, 2002 with permission.

FEMINIST CULTURAL CRITIQUES
AND BODY IMAGE DISORDERS

Feminists have been concerned with body image disorders for two reasons which they see as linked: firstly, many body image disorders exhibit a strong gender asymmetry (around 90% of anorexics and bulimics are female, although the asymmetry is less marked in BED, and still less in BDD); secondly, negative body image has been argued to be so prevalent in the population of women at large, i.e. those with *no* psychiatric diagnosis, in (at least) developed countries that Rodin et al., as long ago as 1985, were led to speak of a "normative discontent" with their bodies among women. (Cash (2002) casts a critical eye on the evidence for the claim of normative discontent without, however, undermining it altogether.) Feminists go beyond the notion of "thin-ideal internalization" (see, e.g., Williams et al. 2002) and ask *why* "thin" has become the ideal (Bordo 1993, p. 140), and more generally why the "grip of culture on the body" should be so obdurate that some women die from it. They go beyond taking note of the social and cultural context for body dissatisfaction and shame, and beyond diagnosis and therapy directed at individuals (or individuals' families), by providing a critique of culture.

The most famous of these critiques is Bordo's analysis of anorexia as "the crystallization of culture." Anorexia both reflects and calls our attention to "some of the central ills of our culture" (1993, p. 139). Bordo identifies three cultural currents or "axes of continuity"—the dualist axis, the control axis, and the gender-power axis—which "converge in the anorexic syndrome" (1993, p. 142). Dualism bifurcates the material body from the intellectual and volitional mind, and identifies the body as alien, as imprisoning the mind, as the enemy; the anorexic takes this to its logical conclusion, by attempting "to kill off the body's spontaneities entirely—that is, to cease to experience our hungers and desires" (1993, p. 146). The body is also that which threatens all our attempts at control; the anorexic who experiences "her life as well as her hungers as being out of control" can then get "hooked on the intoxicating feeling of accomplishment and control" (1993, p. 149). At the heart of anorexia, Bordo suggests, is "a fear and disdain for traditional female roles and social limitations" and, "more profoundly, with a deep fear of 'the Female', with all its more nightmarish archetypal associations of voracious hungers and sexual insatiability" (1993, p. 155). (Here we might note the peculiar *absence* of reference to sexual desire in many psychological and psychiatric characterizations of anorexia.) Anorexia is in part a "protest against the limitations of the ideal of female domesticity," a protest which is "not embraced as a conscious politics" but "written on the bodies of anorexic women" (1993, p. 159)—albeit a "hopelessly counterproductive" protest (1993, p. 160); cf. Orbach 1993 (and her title *Hunger Strike*).

Even feminists are not immune to "the grip of culture"; Squire notes a "dearth of material examining bulimia" in the feminist literature (2003, p. 18); Eli (2011) makes a parallel point about BED as well as the binge–purge subtype of anorexia—this is particularly surprising in view of the fact that a large percentage of restricting anorexics "cross over" either into the binge–purge type or into bulimia. Could it be that feminists, however reluctantly, *admire* restricting anorexics and their "lean masculine body of will in battle with the flabby feminine body of desire" (Squire 2002, p. 23)? "Fear of hunger is so universal that undergoing it voluntarily often arouses admiration, awe, and curiosity" (Bruch 1978, p. 3); "the iron determination with which anorexics pursue their goal of ultimate thinness, not only through food restriction but also through exhausting exercise" is "awe-inspiring to the onlooker" (Bruch 1978, p. 5; cf. Orbach 1993, p. 78). (The idea that anorexia is somehow admirable has, horrifyingly, generated "pro-anorexia" websites; see Carey 2009.) From this perspective bulimics cannot but be seen as weak and pitiful, overwhelmed by their out-of-control bodies (Squire 2003, p. 23), and the bulimic body and behavior provokes repulsion and horror (Squire 2003, p. 20), cf. Lindner's description of the contrast between his patient Laura's usual appearance (becomingly dressed, "fashionably thin" [sic], and striking-looking; 1955/1986, p. 122) and her appearance post-binge: her face "was like a ceremonial mask on which some inspired maniac had depicted every corruption of the flesh ... abomination seemed to ooze from great pores that the puffed tautness of skin revealed" (1955/1986, p. 165). Squire aims at a feminist "re-imagination" of bulimia: she urges us to see that "[t]o experience bulimia is to inhabit an intensely physical body, a body which is constantly expanding and contracting" (Squire 2003, p. 23), "a body that refuses the stubborn Cartesianism it so passionately protests against" (Squire 2003, p. 24).

There is equally a dearth of feminist literature examining BED; such an examination would have to intersect with feminist literature on obesity, given that BED sufferers (unlike either anorexics or bulimics) are typically "overweight" and thus carry all the stigma associated with "fatness": "As members of Western society, we presume to know the histories of all fat bodies ... We believe we know their desires (which must be out of control) and their will (which must be weak)"; we assume that fatness is associated with "laziness, gluttony, poor personal hygiene and lack of fortitude" (Murray 2005, p. 154); see also Heyes' (2006) nuanced study of dieting and weight-loss programs. Saguy and Gruys' study of the American media coverage of anorexia as opposed to BED found that anorexics are framed as "victims of cultural and biological forces beyond their control" while BED was denied "the status of a "real" eating disorder," instead being framed as "ordinary and blameworthy overeating" (2010, p. 247). BED too stands in need of a feminist re-imagination.

More recently, Heyes has put forward a cultural critique of "the conditions for the possibility of BDD." She notes that "with only a difference in inflection" (2009, p. 75), descriptions of a "woman who has a long-standing dissatisfaction with a particular body part, who keeps the flaws of her body always at the front of her mind, and who receives reassurance from others that she finds iteratively disappointing ('Are you *sure* I don't look fat is this?")" may be read either as a clinical description of a case of BDD or as "a trope of mainstream culture," straight out of "chick lit" (2009, p. 76). It is, she notes, "a complex epistemological task to distinguish between a normal relationship to a mirror and a pathological one," and equally difficult "to mark what should count as an 'imagined' defect or 'excessive' concern about it" (Heyes 2009, p. 90); she identifies the very attempt to demarcate such boundaries as an instance of "the crystallization of culture" (Heyes 2009, p. 77). She looks at BDD through the lens of the cosmetic surgery industry; this industry has a clear stake in normative body dissatisfaction (thus she argues that "the cosmetic surgery industry contributes to the cultivation of a culturally recognizable psychology" that differs from BDD only in degree; Heyes 2009, p. 88), but also in demarcating BDD pathology from "normal" psychology, since BDD sufferers, although they frequently seek cosmetic surgery to correct their "flaws," are seldom satisfied with the results, and may sue. Thus the drawing of a sharp boundary between BDD and women's "normative concern" about their bodies is not entirely scientifically grounded, but is motivated partly by, *inter alia*, the interests of the cosmetic surgery industry.

Feminist cultural critiques have added a great deal to our understanding of the social and cultural conditions under which body image disorders flourish and of the Foucauldian mechanisms which lie behind this; however, such analyses can tend to "eclipse phenomenology" (Heyes 2009, p. 91, n. 8)—to exclude consideration of the embodied experience of the suffering individuals who were the point of the critique. So too do both the body image and body shame research traditions, the former because it focuses on objective measurements, the latter because it situates itself within cognitive behavioral models of body image disorders, and to focus wholly on "cognitions" and "behaviors" is *eo ipso* to leave embodied experience out of account. The next section therefore sketches some contributions to the phenomenology of body image disorders.

THE PHENOMENOLOGY OF BODY IMAGE DISORDERS

Body dysmorphic disorder

BDD has been described by phenomenological philosophers (Fuchs 2003; Morris 2003) in Sartrean terms, natural enough given the prominence of shame in BDD. Sartre's well-known analysis of shame sees it as a transformation in one's being-in-the-world brought about by the "look" or "gaze" of the other, and in particular a transformation of that dimension of the body which may be called the "lived body for others."

Morris draws attention to the connections Sartre draws between shame and several further concepts that will resonate with BDD sufferers: "nausea," "alienation," and the "longing for invisibility," and also highlights the "inapprehensibility" of the body-for-others; Fuchs principally elaborates on alienation. (a) Sartre infamously refers to "the nauseous character of all flesh" (Sartre 1943/1986, p. 357), which, when mediated through the look of the other, presents my body-for-others to me as an object of disgust: "disgust with my face, disgust with my too-white flesh, with my too-grim expression, etc." (Sartre 1943/1986, p. 357)—i.e., paradigmatic BDD feelings (e.g., Phillips 1996, pp. 55, 142). (b) The look of the other alienates me from my body; Fuchs terms the apprehension of alienation "corporealization," and brings out its lived effects in the way in which "the body part concerned stands out as particularized and bulky, as a constant object of attention; it seems to be the focus of all gazes and renders spontaneous bodily performance impossible." BDD in Fuchs' view is characterized by an inability to take a "self-other metaperspective" and thus to break out of the "vicious circle of corporealization and shameful self-awareness" (2003, p. 235). (c) BDD sufferers will say, "My biggest wish is to be invisible" (Phillips 1996, p. 37). This wish may be understood either as the longing *not to be seen at all* (hence the social avoidance so common in BDD) or, more deeply, as a desire for what both Gilman (1999) and Dolezal (2010) have termed "(in)visibility," a concept which is linked to stigma. (Recall that "stigma consciousness" was linked by the body shame theorists to what they called "external shame.") Stigma is understood as "the situation of the individual who is disqualified from full social acceptance" because of "deviant" appearance or behavior, i.e., appearance or behavior which deviates from cultural norms or standards (Goffman 1963/1990, p. 9); the (in)visibility which BDD sufferers seek through their "appearance-fixing behaviors" is the full social acceptance which would allow them to "pass" as "normal" (cf., e.g., Phillips 1996, p. 66). (d) "I shall never have a concrete intuition" of my being-for-others (Sartre 1943/1986, p. 275); the well-known constant mirror-checking and reassurance-seeking of BDD sufferers may be viewed as an attempt to achieve the impossible: a concrete intuition of how they actually look to others. (Cf., up to a point, Veale 2002, pp. 274–275.)

Anorexia

Anorexia (principally of the restricting type) has been explored phenomenologically by philosophers, anthropologists, and feminist cultural critics. The primary concepts drawn upon by the philosopher Svenaeus are those of the "unhomelike" body and the "body uncanny"; the latter is the phenomenologist Zaner's term, and refers to the fact that "[i]f there is a sense in which my own-body is intimately mine, there is … an equally decisive sense in which I belong to it—in which I am at its disposal or mercy, if you will" (quoted in Svenaeus, in press). Encountering the body in the latter mode, e.g., when it is ill and has needs and demands of its own, is not unlike encountering the body as an alien creature with its own will. The feminist cultural critic Grosz (1994), the philosopher Weiss (1999), and the anthropologist Warin (2003) all draw on Kristeva's notion of abjection. (Kristeva is a feminist philosopher influenced by the psychoanalyst Lacan and the anthropologist Mary Douglas. Kristeva is not herself a phenomenologist but many phenomenologists find the concept of abjection fruitful, as it seems to point to an *essential* aspect of human reality and lived experience.) *The abject* refers to "[d]etachable, separable parts of the body—urine, faeces, saliva, sperm, blood, vomit, hair, skin, nails" which "retain something of the cathexis and value of a body part even when they are separated from the body" (Grosz 1994, p. 81); the body essentially involves the abject and hence essentially lacks stable borders. (The abject can be linked to the uncanny via the observation that bodily needs such as the need to defecate or vomit both make the body uncanny and produce the abject.) *Abjection* is the transformation of the abject into objects or horror or disgust, and the concomitant but necessarily unfulfillable desire to exclude the abject and to acquire stable borders for the body and thus the self; it is "a corporeal refusal of corporeality," as Weiss (1999, p. 90) puts it.

Anorexia, according to Svenaeus (in press), often begins with something like the Sartrean look: "being objectified as too fat by the gaze of others" may give rise to the experience of one's body being "too fat to be at home in." This bodily alienation is often reinforced by the bodily changes of puberty, when "the body takes on a strange life of its own"; these changes are paradigmatic instances of the emergence of the abject, as the borders of the body literally alter and as new forms of excreta, menstrual blood and semen, makes their appearance; both Warin (2003) and Weiss (1999, chapter 4) see anorexia as abjection, an attempt to "erase, cleanse, and even make disappear their own "dirty" and "disgusting" bodies" (Warin 2003, p. 89) and thus, impossibly, to become a stable entity. Although Gillett does not employ the framework of abjection, his interpretation of anorexia as a quest to achieve "lightness of being and resist the 'cloying nature' threatening to transform one into a lump of stuff" (2009, p. 297) could be understood from this perspective.

Svenaeus (in press) notes that "food is the major foreign thing that enters your body." Warin's study goes further: not all food is equal in the world of the anorexic. She argues (on the basis of her multisited study of a number of anorexic women) that anorexia involves not so much a "fear of fatness" (as the diagnostic criteria seem to suggest) as a fear of (the substance) *fat*, and that this is to be construed as a fear of *contamination*. Although many writers on the topic note that different types of foods are categorized by anorexics as "good" and "bad," Warin discerns in these categorizations "a hierarchy of clean and dirty foods. 'Vegetables are okay to touch—they are clean and pure'—whereas other foods [are] characterized as 'defiling', 'disgusting', 'polluting', and 'contaminating'" (Warin 2003, p. 80). Her subjects' attitudes toward food follow "primitive" ideas about contagion: some distinguished between "calorie girls" who worried about airborne contagion and "fats and oil girls" who are concerned with touch (Warin 2003, p. 84). These attitudes toward food emerge in bodily experience. "When you get that layer of grease and you can feel it on your teeth and the inside of your mouth—uugghh—some girls reckon they can feel it in their stomachs and travelling around their bodies after they've eaten it" (quoted in Warin 2003, p. 86). Thus their "fear of fat" was not in the first instance a fear of gaining weight but of allowing that most "abject" of all substances (fat "is indeterminate in form ... it seeps, infiltrates, and congeals," Warin 2003, p. 86) to transgress the boundaries of their bodies.

Although Svenaeus does not highlight this facet of "the body uncanny," he might have added that the body appears in anorexia not just as an object but, supremely, as "a creature with its own will," in virtue of its seemingly insatiable *hunger*: "I'm always hungry. I'm hungry all the time and I'm so scared that if I give into my hunger I will never stop eating, that I'll just keep eating and eating and eating and never be satisfied" (quoted in Warin 2003, p. 83; cf. Bordo 1993, p. 146; Goss and Gilbert 2002, p. 229; Schaefer 2009, p. 136). (Thus, as Gillett (2009, p. 282) points out, "anorexia" is strictly a misnomer.) If we understand anorexia in terms of abjection, we can see why hunger acquires a "negative valence" (Gillett 2009, p. 304) for the anorexic. At the same time, hunger is not to be understood merely as a physiological need; this is explored further later in this chapter.

These analyses have what are arguably advantages over those of the psychologists and psychiatrists, even apart from allowing us to understand the embodied experience of anorexia: they provide a framework which makes sense not only of anorexia but of ascetic eating disorders and the self-starvation of some religious enthusiasts. Moreover, their analyses integrate anorexia with the idea of "fear of puberty." (Again, we ought to be struck by the virtual conspiracy of silence regarding the sexual in much of the psychological and psychiatric literature.) They also offer some insight into the phenomenon (modern, but also with a long history) which has been dubbed "orthorexia nervosa": an obsession with avoiding anything but the most "pure" of foods (see Bratman and Knight 2000; strikingly, there is evidence to suggest that, unlike anorexia, orthorexia is more prevalent in men than in women and also more prevalent in less educated individuals, Donini et al. 2004).

Bingeing

We noted already that bulimia, BED, and the bingeing type of anorexia are seldom studied by feminists; they are also seldom addressed by phenomenologists. For this reason, I want to highlight the anthropologist Eli's (2011) "experience-near" description of bingeing.

("Experience-near" rather than "phenomenological" in the proper sense of the term, as she does not attempt to relate the themes she uncovers to essential aspects of human reality. Nonetheless, some of her analytical categories—"embodied strategy," "embodied metaphor"—might be valuable to phenomenologists.) Her study (based in Israel; Eli notes that the Holocaust was a reference point in some discussions of starvation) identified three major themes in her subjects' narratives: (1) "Hunger as imprisonment, binge as release." These individuals lived their bodies as their authentic selves which, in the practice of bingeing, temporarily escaped from the imprisonment of restriction. (This experiential dimension has some resonances with Squire's feminist re-imagination of bulimia.) (2) "Reconfiguring food as substance": most of Eli's subjects experienced the hunger prior to the binge not as a desire for sensory pleasure but simply the desire for fullness; the food itself became not a collection of pleasurable gustatory, tactile, and olfactory sensations but a bland substance of which the important thing was quantity, not quality. For some bingeing anorexic subjects, this reconfiguration of food was an "embodied strategy": it was important to them that they did *not* enjoy the food, because they needed this to sustain them in their anorexia. (3) "Filling up existential emptiness." Many bingers talked about an emptiness which the binge endeavored to fill; the binge had to progress to, even past, the point of discomfort because pain was an embodied experience of fullness, i.e. of the temporary banishment of the emptiness. Many narratives of eating-disordered individuals refer to such an emptiness: "I'm sure you know about the hole.... It's that hole that you tried to fill with eating disordered behaviours" (Schaefer 2009, p. 68). It would be entirely flat-footed to interpret this emptiness (only) as physiological hunger; perhaps we can adopt Gillett's (2009) language of "sliding signifiers," or Eli's notion of an "embodied metaphor," be it for an empty womb (as the psychoanalyst Lindner interprets this description of a binge: "it begins with a feeling of emptiness ... The moment I become aware of the hole opening inside I'm terrified. I want to fill it. I have to. So I start to eat ... I eat until my jaws get numb with chewing ... I get sick with eating and still I eat," quoted in Lindner 1955/1986, pp. 119–120), or "the empty space that my mum was supposed to be filling by love" (quoted in Gillettt 2009, p. 290), or a "vacancy in the soul" (Eli 2011).

SOME CRITICAL REFLECTIONS

We have looked at body image disorders from a number of perspectives, introducing each as helping to fill a gap left by the others. We need not insist that any of them is the "best" or the "right" perspective; indeed, the understanding of body image disorders is surely essentially multifaceted. However, these perspectives are in some respects in tension with one another, so more needs to be said. I will argue, first, that to the extent that psychological and psychiatric approaches are fundamentally in the grip of what the phenomenologist Merleau-Ponty (1945/2002) famously termed "the prejudice of objective thought" (and the body image approach certainly is), they obstruct rather than further understanding. I will argue, secondly, that feminist cultural critical and phenomenological approaches are at least potentially complementary, even if particular accounts appear sometimes at odds with one another, and that they together contribute positively to the task of understanding body image disordered individuals. (The potential complementarity follows once one acknowledges that "structure" and "agency," society and individual, and culture and nature are *internally related*, i.e., each half of each duality depends ontologically on the other: neither would be what it is without the other. To see them as causally interrelated, as some psychologists and psychiatrists do, requires seeing them as *externally* related.) I end by suggesting some implications of this study for psychiatry and its classifications.

Psychological and psychiatric approaches

Body image approach

The psychologists and psychiatrists who take this approach have, we might say, contributed toward a task that is dear to the hearts of philosophers: they have made important distinctions between different senses of "body image disturbance." Yet that these distinctions can be made does not entail that it makes sense to *isolate* what is thus distinguished from one another, much less that they are susceptible of quantitative measurement, as these researchers presuppose. Moreover, they sing from the same hymn-sheet in their treatment of society and culture: mostly such factors are ignored, as we have seen, but to the extent that they are not, they are given an extremely "thin" description, e.g., society and culture tend to be equated with the media and advertising (e.g., Phillips 1996, p. 182–186), their influence on the individual is frequently reduced to "thin-ideal internalization," and these studies treat the individual as externally related to society and culture, as this influence is clearly conceptualized as causal (e.g., Levine and Chapman 2011). The whole approach, we might say, is premised on a version of Merleau-Ponty's "prejudice of objective thought" which he and others have called "scientism": the idea that the world consists of atomized objects, in themselves meaningless, value-neutral and motivationally inert, which participate only in external (especially causal) relations and are subject to measurement, and that human beings, both individuals and society, are simply *part* of the world thus conceived.

A paradigm example of such scientism in operation, and its negative effects on achieving understanding, can be seen in their treatment of what they call body image distortion, i.e., the degree of match or mismatch between how one perceives one's own body and how it "really is." In line with scientism, it is presupposed (a) that how the body *really* is, is objectively describable and measurable (thereby privileging the measurable world over the experienced world) and (b) that "perceptual" and "affective" are distinct dimensions. Many ingenious methods have been used to test apparent size distortion in eating-disordered individuals. One uses silhouettes or schematic drawings ranging from "thin" to "fat"; subjects are asked to pick their actual shape from this range, and the degree of mismatch between this and their actual silhouette is a measure of degree of distortion. A variant on this is the somatomorphic matrix, where subjects are asked to adjust a computer-generated image until it matches what they believe their actual shape to be. Yet a further variation looks at "dynamic body image" (Vocks et al. 2007), premised on the observation that weight affects gait patterns; this uses point-light displays generated from walking figures and creating the illusion of a walking figure on the screen, and an individual's actual walking patterns can be distorted to correspond to a higher or lower body mass index (BMI); again individuals are asked to choose what they believe their actual gait pattern to be. What is noteworthy is that despite all the ingenuity expended on developing these techniques and instruments, the results from such studies for anorexics are mixed and inconclusive (see Table 37.1); is this not a bit surprising (even given that non-clinical controls also overestimate their size), if what is being measured is a partial diagnostic *criterion* for anorexia? We might note, first, that whatever it is that is being measured by such methods arguably often has little to do with what it is about their bodies which leads anorexics to say that they look fat, e.g., the pads of fat on the hips popularly called "love handles" (Pope et al. 2000, p. 147), or whether the tops of their thighs touch (Schaefer 2009, p. 144), or whether they are "out of proportion" (Gillett 2009, p. 285)—none of which has much to do with BMI or overall "fatness." But, secondly, to accommodate this observation by devising clever new somatomorphic matrices which vary only the size of the love handles or the proportions of the body (cf. Gardner 2011, pp. 147–148) is to miss the point. The crucial property of their bodies, the one that helps to motivate their anorexia, is a property which is not value-neutral and motivationally inert: their love handles are *too big*, the point at which their thighs touch is *horrifying*, their body's proportions are *unacceptable*. (Can psychologists and psychiatrists claim that their patients' proportions are *objectively* not *unacceptable*?) The suggestion (e.g., Carr 2002, p. 93) that this just goes to show that so-called size distortion is "affective" *rather than* "perceptual" presupposes scientistic premise (b).

These scientistic assumptions show up even more clearly in body image theorists' discussions of alleged perceptual distortion in BDD. Assumption (a)—that how the body *really* is, is objectively measurable—is the presupposition of the very definition of BDD, which refers to an "imagined" or "slight" defect in appearance, i.e., one which is not *objectively* present or which is *objectively* minimal; cf. Heyes' critique in the earlier "Feminist cultural critiques and body image disorders" section. (This is true a fortiori in ICD-10's classification of BDD as a hypochondriacal disorder, which involves the presupposition that "defects" in appearance are objectively identifiable by medics in the same way that physical diseases are.) Phillips describes a man who, "when asked to draw a picture of himself, drew only his nose—not one view of it but three! In addition, he covered all three noses with large open circles, which were the pores he perceived" (Phillips 1996, p. 204); she takes this as evidence that he perceives distortedly. But surely the patient is not implying that he sees himself as in possession of three noses! Nor is he suggesting that he perceives his pores as being, say, three centimeters across when *in fact* they are a fraction of a millimeter: his picture expresses that his pores are "*too* big" or "*disgustingly* big," to understand which, again, requires us to reject scientistic premises (a) and (b). (Here it will be said that BDD sufferers are less wont than non-clinical individuals to focus on their own face *as a whole*; thus one BDD sufferer admitted, "[m]aybe I look too closely. It's like I'm looking at my skin through a magnifying glass" (quoted in Phillips 1996, p. 207). Continuing in a scientistic vein, this is then pathologized as displaying "a bias for detail encoding and analysis rather than holistic processing," Lambrou et al. 2011, p. 451; cf. Veale 2002; Phillips 2011.)

Body shame approach

In many ways, this approach represents a substantial improvement over the body image approach. The difficulties with this approach are more subtle and also, I think, less drastic.

First, body shame researchers are very fond of flow-diagram representations of models like Figs 37.1 and 37.2 and Veale's (2002, p. 274) diagram of BDD; but there is substantial unclarity about how the arrows in these diagrams are to be understood. In some cases at least, the intended interpretation indicates some residual scientism. The very use of the word "factors" (biological, personal, sociocultural; notably, these are seen as *separate* factors), and much of the language of this literature (e.g., "give rise to," "influence") suggests that the relation between these "factors" and shame is in Figs 37.1 and 37.2 meant to be *causal* and hence external. (Again, Veale's model of BDD tells us that "Mirror gazing *activates* idealized values about the importance of appearance," Veale 2002, p. 274, italics added; what can "activate" possibly mean here?) The second arrow in Fig. 37.1 is said to represent a *choice* on the part of the individual of a way of coping with shame (Goss and Gilbert 2002, p. 243). The next arrow is more like a logical consequence, explaining what it means to "focus self-esteem on body image and weight control." I leave it to the reader to attempt interpretations of the other arrows, but they are a bit of a mishmash, and some of them suggest external relations where they don't belong.

Secondly, these analyses are described as "functional" analyses (cf. the subtitle of Goss and Gilbert 2002). The term "functional" indicates, for instance, that some behavior that looks "dysfunctional" (e.g., damaging to the person's physical health) actually has a "function" within the individual's psychology, e.g., "as a solution to problems of low self-esteem and/or as an affect control device" (Goss and Gilbert 2002, p. 225); lying behind this outlook is a therapeutic recommendation: "find the positive functions in the symptom before challenging it" (Goss and Gilbert 2002, p. 248). I take it that talk of "functions" is nothing more than a slightly more scientific-sounding way of talking about "meanings" and "values" (and, to be fair, Goss and Gilbert sometimes substitute "purpose" or "aim" for "function"; moreover, body shame theorists are very willing to embrace talk of values (e.g., Veale 2002) even if they then go on to speak of these scientistically).

Despite these weaknesses, Veale's model of BDD and Goss and Gilbert's shame–pride cycle and shame–shame cycle not only express the multifacetedness of body image disorders but offer some insight into their self-perpetuating nature and hence their persistence, as well as illuminating the different *patterns* of shame in BDD, restricting anorexia and bingeing. To that extent, the body shame theorists do contribute to the project of understanding body image disorders.

Feminist cultural critiques and phenomenology

Anthropologists are likely to complain about the lack of ethnographic "thickness" and of cultural situatedness in both feminist cultural critiques and phenomenological accounts by philosophers. Phenomenological philosophers will complain about the exclusion of embodied experience from feminist cultural critiques and may comment that many "phenomenological" anthropological contributions are not phenomenological but merely "experience-near." And feminist cultural critics may complain that phenomenological philosophers leave social structures unanalyzed and that anthropologists leave them uncriticized. By and large, however, these are sins of omission rather than commission; we might simply conclude that these perspectives each have something to contribute to a well-rounded understanding of body image disorders. Potentially more troubling is that some of these analyses appear to be incompatible with one another; I pick out two points of apparent tension in their analyses of anorexia. (No doubt there is more to be said about these, and no doubt there are others …)

1. Bordo claims that the anorexic identifies herself with her mind, sees the body as imprisoning the mind, and therefore attempts to cease to experience the body's

hunger and desire so as to escape that prison. Eli's findings appear rather different: many of her subjects apparently saw their body as their true self, and saw the mind as imprisoning the body by making it starve; bingeing was then a temporary release from that prison. Although equally dualistic, these subjects identified themselves, it seems, with opposite sides of mind/body dualism. That Eli's study was grounded in actual interviews does not explain the difference, since many actual anorexics find Bordo's analysis resonant; that Eli's study was based in Israel (whereas most of Bordo's examples are American) may possibly be relevant, but this would be a delicate matter to justify. It may also be relevant that Eli's focus is on bingeing anorexics (and other bingers) rather than restrictors: even if restricting anorexics very often cross over into bingeing, it is not impossible that this crossover is linked to a changing identification (with the body rather than with the mind); we might even try to link this with crossing over from the "shame–pride cycle" to the "shame–shame cycle." This suggestion would not refute, but simply add much-needed nuance, to Bordo's central claim that anorexia is a crystallization of culture. At the same time, one cannot help suspecting that *both* "My mind is my true self, imprisoned by my body" *and* "My body is my true self, imprisoned by my mind" are ways of giving verbal expression to experiences that are more fragmented and inchoate than either formulation captures.

2. The phenomenological analysis of anorexia in terms of abjection, especially clear in Warin's study, seems at odds not only with Bordo's analysis but with the DSM and ICD diagnostic criteria and hence much of the psychological and psychiatric literature in suggesting that anorexia is grounded not so much in a fear of becoming fat but in a fear of fat as a peculiarly abject substance, and of the body's abject status rather than its size. Anorexia on this analysis is a search not so much for a thin body as for a stable identity. In one sense, however, the tension is not fundamental: a (skeletally) thin body is the *de facto result* of this doomed search or at least of the form it takes in anorexics.

Medical anthropologists see psychiatry as part of what they call "biomedicine"; the latter term reminds us that that what we may be tempted to call just "medicine" is grounded in Western scientific biology and neurophysiology, and is as much an ethnomedicine as shamanic healing is; its "deep cultural logic" is as rooted in (dualistic, individualistic, scientistic) Western culture (Kleinman et al. 1994, p. 8) as that of shamanic healing is in the culture of Siberian and other hunter-gatherer societies. Phenomenology, as we have seen, argues that such "scientism," which pervades the body image approach in psychology and psychiatry and leaves its mark as well, although less prominently, on the body shame approach, falsifies experience and the lived world. Feminists' cultural critiques see the medical, psychological and psychiatric professions as *institutional parts* of the culture being criticized: e.g., Heyes' study amounts to an indirect critique of psychiatry, as in effect colluding with the cosmetic surgery industry (not to mention the pharmaceutical industry) to construct the specific pathology of BDD. (See also Gremillion 2003.)

None of this is, of course, to deny the very real suffering of individuals with body image disorders, although it might lead us to characterize it as "distress" rather than "disease" or "disorder." Nor is it to deny that psychological and psychiatric treatments, however situated within the deep cultural logic of biomedicine, *can* help to alleviate that suffering. It might, however, lead us to resist the notions that there is a sharp boundary between "normal" human beings and those with "disorders" and that attempts to define such boundaries are disinterested and value-free; to inquire more deeply into the social and cultural sources (perhaps even including psychiatry itself) of women's normative discontent with their bodies; and to resist the increasingly scientistic direction in which psychiatric classifications appear to be heading.

References

Bordo, S. (1993). *Unbearable Weight: Feminism, Western Culture and the Body*. Berkeley, CA: University of California Press.

Brandenburg, B. M. and Anderson, A. E. (2007). Unintentional onset of anorexia. *Eating and Weight Disorders*, 12(2), 97–100.

Bratman, S. and Knight, D. (2000). *Health Food Junkies*. New York, NY: Broadway Books.

Bruch, H. (1978). *The Golden Cage: The Enigma of Anorexia Nervosa*. Cambridge, MA: Harvard University Press.

Carey, E. (2009). Eating, food, and the female body in the media and medicine: a feminist analysis of eating disorders. *Socheolas: Limerick Student Journal of Sociology*, 1(1), 31–45.

Carr, A. T. (2002). Body shame: issues of assessment and measurement. In P. Gilbert and J. Miles (Eds), *Body Shame: Conceptualization, Research, and Treatment*, pp. 90–102. Hove: Brunner-Routledge.

Cash, T. F. (2002). A "negative body image": evaluating epidemiological evidence. In T. F. Cash and T. Pruzinsky (Eds), *Body Image: A Handbook of Theory, Research and Clinical Practice*, pp. 269–74. New York, NY: Guilford.

Cash, T. F. (2004). Body image: past, present, and future (editorial). *Body Image*, 1(1), 1–5.

Cash, T. F. and Deagle, E. A. (1997). The nature and extent of body-image disturbance in anorexia nervosa and bulimia nervosa: a meta-analysis. *International Journal of Eating Disorders*, 22, 107–25.

Cash, T. F. and Pruzinsky, T. (Eds) (2002). *Body Image: A Handbook of Theory, Research and Clinical Practice*. New York, NY: Guilford.

Delinsky, S. S. (2011). Body image and anorexia nervosa. In T. F. Cash and L. Smolak (Eds), *Body Image: A Handbook of Science, Practice, and Prevention* (2nd edn), pp. 279–87. New York, NY: Guilford.

Dolezal, L. (2010). The (in)visible body: phenomenology, feminism and the case of cosmetic surgery. *Hypatia*, 2(2), 357–75.

Donini, L., Marsili, D., Graziani, M., Imbriale, M., and Cannella, C. (2004). Orthorexia nervosa: a preliminary study with a proposal for diagnosis and an attempt to measure the dimension of the phenomenon. *Eating and Weight Disorders*, 9(2), 151–7.

Eli, K. (2011). The phenomenology of binge eating in anorexia and bulimia. Available at: <http://podcasts.ox.ac.uk>.

Fuchs, T. (2003). The phenomenology of shame, guilt and the body in body dysmorphic disorder and depression. *Journal of Phenomenological Psychology*, 33(2), 223–43.

Gallagher, S. (1995). Body schema and intentionality. In J. L. Bermúdez, A. Marcel, and N. Eilan (Eds), *The Body and the Self*, pp. 225–44. Cambridge, MA: Bradford/MIT.

Gardner, R. M. (2011). Perceptual measures of body image for adolescents and adults. In T. F. Cash and L. Smolak (Eds), *Body Image: A Handbook of Science, Practice, and Prevention* (2nd edn), pp. 146–53. New York, NY: Guilford.

Garner, D. M. (2002). Body image and anorexia nervosa. In T. F. Cash and T. Pruzinsky (Eds), *Body Image: A Handbook of Theory, Research and Clinical Practice*, pp. 295–303. New York, NY: Guilford.

Gilbert, P. (2002). Body shame: a biopsychosocial conceptualisation and overview, with treatment implications. In P. Gilbert and J. Miles (Eds), *Body Shame: Conceptualization, Research, and Treatment*, pp. 3–54. Hove: Brunner-Routledge.

Gilbert, P. and Miles, J. (Eds) (2002). *Body Shame: Conceptualisation, Research and Treatment*. Hove: Brunner-Routledge.

Gillett, G. (2009). *The Mind and its Discontents* (2nd edn). Oxford: Oxford University Press.

Gilman, S. L. (1999). *Making the Body Beautiful: A Cultural History of Aesthetic Surgery*. Princeton, NJ: Princeton University Press.

Goffman, E. (1990). *Stigma: Notes on the Management of Spoiled Identity*. London: Penguin Books. (Original work published 1963.)

Goss, K. and Gilbert, P. (2002). Eating disorders, shame and pride: a cognitive-behavioural functional analysis. In P. Gilbert and J. Miles (Eds), *Body Shame: Conceptualization, Research, and Treatment*, pp. 219–55. Hove: Brunner-Routledge.

Gremillion, H. (2003). *Feeding Anorexia: Gender and Power at a Treatment Center*. Durham, NC: Duke University Press.

Grilo, C. M. (2002). Binge eating disorder. In C. G. Fairburn and K. D. Brownell (Eds), *Eating Disorders and Obesity: A Comprehensive Handbook* (2nd edn), pp. 178–82. New York, NY: Guilford.

Grosz, E. (1994). *Volatile Bodies*. Bloomington, IN: Indiana University Press.

Hrabosky, J. I., Cash, T.F., and Veale, D., Neziroglu, F., Soll, E.A., Garner, D.M., *et al.* (2009). Multidimensional body image comparisons among patients with eating disorders, body dysmorphic disorder, and clinical controls. A multisite study. *Body Image*, 6(3), 155–63.

Heyes, C. (2006). Foucault goes to Weight Watchers. *Hypatia*, 21(2), 126–49.

Heyes, C. (2009). Diagnosing culture: body dysmorphic disorder and cosmetic surgery. *Body and Society*, 15(4), 73–93.

Huline-Dickens, S. (2000). Anorexia nervosa: some connections with the religious attitude. *British Journal of Medical Psychology*, 73, 67–76.

Kaye, W., Straher, M., and Roche, L. (2002). Body image disturbance and other core symptoms in anorexia and bulimia nervosa. In D. Castle and K. A. Phillips (Eds), *Disorders of Body Image*, pp. 67–82. Hampshire: Wrightson Biomedical.

Kleinman, A., Brodwin, P. E., Good, B. J., and DelVecchio Good, M. -J. (1994). Pain as human experience: an introduction. In M. -J. DelVecchio Good, P. E. Brodwin, B. J. Good, and A. Kleinman (Eds), *Pain as Human Experience: An Anthropological Perspective*, pp. 1–28. Berkeley, CA: University of California Press.

Krasnow, M. (1996). *My Life as a Male Anorexic*. New York, NY: Haworth.

Lambrou, C., Veale, D., and Wilson, G. (2011). The role of aesthetic sensitivity in body dysmorphic disorder. *Journal of Abnormal Psychology*, 120(2), 443–53.

Legenbauer, T., Vocks, S., Puigcerver, M. J. B, Benecke, A., Troje, N. F., and Rüddel, H. (2011). Differences in the nature of body image disturbances between female obese individuals with versus without a comorbid binge eating disorder: an exploratory study including static and dynamic aspects of body image. *Behavior Modification*, 35(2), 162–86.

Levine, M. P. and Chapman, K. (2011). Media influences on body image. In T. F. Cash and L. Smolak (Eds), *Body Image: A Handbook of Science, Practice, and Prevention* (2nd edn), pp. 100–9. New York, NY: Guilford.

Lindner, R. (1986). *The Fifty-Minute Hour: A Collection of True Psychoanalytic Tales.* London: Free Association Books. (Original work published 1955.)

McKinley, N. M. and Hyde, J. S. (1996). The objectified body consciousness scale: development and validation. *Psychology of Women Quarterly, 22,* 623–36.

McNamara, B. (2002). Disordered body image: an anthropological perspective. In D. Castle and K. A. Phillips (Eds), *Disorders of Body Image,* pp. 25–36. Hampshire: Wrightson Biomedical.

Merleau-Ponty, M. (2002). *Phenomenology of Perception* (C. Smith, Trans.). London: Routledge (Routledge Classics). (Original work in French published 1945.)

Morris, K. J. (2003). The phenomenology of body dysmorphic disorder. In K. W. M. Fulford, K. Morris, J. Sadler, and G. Stanghellini (Eds). *Nature and Narrative,* pp. 171–86. Oxford: Oxford University Press.

Murray, S. (2005). Unbecoming out? Rethinking fat politics. *Social Semiotics, 15*(2), 153–63.

Orbach, S. (1993). *Hunger Strike.* London: Penguin.

Orbach, S. (2009). *Bodies.* London: Profile Books.

Phillips, K. A. (1996). *The Broken Mirror: Understanding and Treating Body Dysmorphic Disorder.* New York, NY: Oxford University Press.

Phillips, K. A. (2002). Body image and body dysmorphic disorder In C. G. Fairburn and K. D. Brownell (Eds), *Eating Disorders and Obesity: A Comprehensive Handbook* (2nd edn), pp. 113–17. New York, NY: Guilford.

Phillips, K. A. (2011). Body image and body dysmorphic disorder. In T. F. Cash and L. Smolak (Eds), *Body Image: A Handbook of Science, Practice, and Prevention* (2nd edn), pp. 305–13. New York, NY: Guilford.

Pope, H. G., Phillips, K. A., and Olivardia, R. (2000). *The Adonis Complex.* New York, NY: Simon and Schuster.

Reindl, S. E. (Ed.) (2002). *Sensing the Self: Women's Recovery from Bulimia.* London: Harvard University Press.

Rodin, J., Silberstein, L. R., and Striegel-Moore, R. H. (1985). Women and weight: a normative discontent. In T. B. Sonderegger (Ed.), *Psychology and Gender: Nebraska Symposium on Motivation, 1984,* pp. 267–307. Lincoln, NE: University of Nebraska Press.

Ruuska, J., Kaltiala-Heino, R., Rantanen, P., and Koivisto, A. M. (2005). Are there differences in the attitudinal body image between adolescent anorexia nervosa and bulimia nervosa? *Eating and Weight Disorders, 10,* 98–106

Saguy, A. C. and Gruys, K. (2010). News media constructions of overweight and eating disorders. *Social Problems, 57*(2), 231–50.

Sartre, J. -P. (1986). *Being and Nothingness* (H. E. Barnes, Trans.). London: Routledge. (Original work in French published 1943.)

Schaefer, J. (2009). *Goodbye Ed, Hello Me.* New York, NY: McGraw-Hill.

Squire, S. (2003). Anorexia and bulimia: purity and danger. *Australian Feminist Studies, 18*(40), 17–26.

Stice, E. (2001). A prospective test of the dual pathway model of bulimic pathology: mediating effects of dieting and negative affect. *Journal of Abnormal Psychology, 110,* 124–35.

Stice, E. (2002). Body image and bulimia nervosa. In T. F. Cash and T. Pruzinsky (Eds), *Body Image: A Handbook of Theory, Research and Clinical Practice,* pp. 304–11. New York, NY: Guilford.

Sullivan, P. F. (2002). Course and outcome of anorexia nervosa and bulimia nervosa. In C. G. Fairburn and K. D. Brownell (Eds), *Eating Disorders and Obesity: A Comprehensive Handbook* (2nd edn), pp. 226–9. New York, NY: Guilford.

Svenaeus, F. (in press). Anorexia nervosa and the body uncanny: a phenomenological approach. *Philosophy, Psychology, & Psychiatry*.

Thompson, J. K. (1990). *Body Image Disturbance: Assessment and Treatment*. New York, NY: Pergamon Press.

Veale, D. (2002). Shame in body dysmorphic disorder. In P. Gilbert and J. Miles (Eds), *Body Shame: Conceptualization, Research, and Treatment*, pp. 167–82. Hove: Brunner-Routledge.

Vocks, S., Legenbauer, T., Rüddel, H., and Troje, N. (2007). Static and dynamic body image in bulimia nervosa: mental representation of body dimensions and motion patterns. *International Journal of Eating Disorders, 40*, 59–66.

Warin, M. (2003). Miasmic calories and saturating fats: fear of contamination in anorexia. *Culture, Medicine and Psychiatry, 27*, 77–93.

Weiss, G. (1999). *Body Images: Embodiment as Intercorporeality*. New York, NY: Routledge.

Wilfley, D. E., Schwartz, M. B., Spurrell, E. B., and Fairburn, C. G. (2000). Using the Eating Disorder Examination to identify the specific pathology of binge eating disorder. *International Journal of Eating Disorders, 27*(3), 259–69.

Williams, D. A., Stewart, T. M., White, M. A., and York-Crowe, E. (2002). An information-processing perspective on body image. In T. F. Cash and T. Pruzinsky (Eds), *Body Image: A Handbook of Theory, Research and Clinical Practice*, pp. 47–54. New York, NY: Guilford.

CHAPTER 38

THE PHENOMENOLOGY
OF AFFECTIVITY

THOMAS FUCHS

INTRODUCTION

The comprehension of affective disorders by today's psychiatry is still impeded by an insufficient understanding of the nature of affectivity itself. In accordance with the subordinate role of affects in the Western concept of the human being, traditional psychiatry took a primarily intellectualistic view of madness as a disturbance of the rational mind (Berrios 1985). Emotions were considered elusive mental states better reduced to either cognition or volition or ignored as epiphenomena. On this basis, for example, melancholia had to be defined as a mixture of irrationality and behavioral inhibition. Until today, the predominant psychological approaches to depression are based on cognitive models, regarding the core of the disorder as a combination of faulty information processing and distorted thinking (Beck and Alford 2009, pp. 224ff.). Consequently, cognitive behavior therapy became the generally recommended psychotherapy (Beck et al. 1979). Traditional psychodynamic approaches, for their part, regarded emotions such as anxiety or depression as mere surface phenomena that indicated the actually relevant conflicts and drives in the depths of the unconscious.[1] Thus a genuine psychopathology of affectivity is lacking until today.

Moreover, emotion theory both in philosophy and psychology still suffers from the traditional introjection of affects and feelings into an inner "psyche," separated from the body as well as from the world. Affects are generally conceived as private, "mental" phenomena that arise in the subject's mind (or brain) from a cognitive evaluation of external stimuli, whereas the objective world is actually bare of any affective qualities or meanings. From a phenomenological point of view, this picture is still a heritage of Cartesian dualism and its separation of mind and matter. In fact, we do not live in a merely physical world; the experienced

---

[1] Even at the age of seventy, Freud admitted that he was "ignorant of what an affect is" (Freud 1926, p. 132).

space around us is always charged with affective qualities. We may feel something "in the air," or we sense an interpersonal "climate," for example, a serene, a solemn, or a threatening atmosphere. Feelings befall us; they emerge from situations, persons, and objects which have their expressive features and which attract or repel us. This *affective space* is essentially felt through the medium of the *body* which widens, tightens, weakens, trembles, shakes, etc. in correspondence to the affects and atmospheres that we experience. As William James (1884) already argued, there is no emotion without bodily sensations, bodily resonance and affectability, even though the intentional aspect or directedness of emotions toward values may certainly not be disregarded.

Finally, the field of affectivity also presents an inherent difficulty to its conceptualization. The phenomena in question are generally fleeting, diffused, hardly delimitable, and even harder to describe. They vary between short-lived, intense, object-related states and longer lasting, objectless states remaining in the background of awareness. This is mirrored in the host of terms such as mood, affect, feeling, emotion, passion, or sentiment that have been variously used and defined, but still may not be neatly separated. Therefore, philosophy and psychology have often tended to subsume affects and emotions under more "tidy" mental categories such as desires, volitions, beliefs, or judgments. Recently, neurobiology has added the attempt to trace them back to physiological changes in brain activity and metabolism. However, such strategies run the risk to miss an adequate description and understanding of affective phenomena in their own right.

In this chapter, I will use the umbrella terms "affectivity," "affective states," or "affects" to denote these different phenomena. Based on the phenomenological tradition, I will give a detailed account of (1) vital and (2) existential feelings, (3) affective atmospheres, (4) moods, and (5) emotions, emphasizing their embodied as well as interaffective dimensions, with side-glances to psychopathology. My account is based on the assumption that affects are not mental states in the immanence of the subject that we project onto an otherwise indifferent sum of objects. Rather, they are modes of bodily attunement to, and engagement with, the lived world. It is only through our affectivity that we find ourselves in a meaningful environment in which persons and things matter for us, and in which we care for them as well as for ourselves. Affects are the very heart of our existence.

THE FEELING OF BEING ALIVE

At the most foundational layer of affective experience we find what may be called the *feeling of being alive*: a pre-reflective, undirected bodily self-awareness that constitutes the unnoticed background of all intentional feeling, perceiving, or acting. This continuous background feeling of the body is situated at the threshold of life and experience, between *Leben* and *Erleben* (Fuchs 2012). Most of the time, it is just taken for granted, unquestioned and pre-given; it does not require a particular cause or occasion. Nor do we feel alive in the same way as we feel angry, fearful, or happy about something. Rather, the tacit feeling of life merges in these special and changing emotions without further ado.

However, there may be states in which this feeling is heightened, intensified, or diminished. This is captured by the German term "*Befinden*" (finding oneself in a certain state), as expressed in the everyday question "How are you?" It relates to the lived body as a domain of diffuse ease or unease, relaxation or tension, freshness and vigor, or tiredness and exhaustion. These feelings with their basic polarity of *Wohlbefinden* and *Missbefinden* (well- and ill-being) may be regarded as indicators of our state of life in its ups and downs and can also be subsumed under the term *vitality.* They are centered in the lived body but also spread without borders into the environment and tinge our relationship to the world. *Wohlbefinden,* such as in freshness or vigor, lets things appear closer, more interesting, and accessible, whereas *Missbefinden,* as in fatigue or sickness, lends a monotonous or vaguely repellent coloring to the surroundings. Thus, in feelings of vitality the body functions as a *medium* of experiencing the world; its overall state imbues and pervades the experiential field as a whole.

On the neurobiological level, the feeling of being alive corresponds to Damasio's "core sense of self" that is based on continuous feedback loops between brain and body (Damasio 1995, pp. 150–151). Peripheral muscular, cardiovascular, hormonal, biochemical, and other states interact with higher brain centers (mainly thalamus, cingulate gyrus, insular and somatosensory cortex), thus serving as a basis for an elementary "feeling of life itself" (p. 207). "The somatic background feeling never subsides, though we sometimes rarely notice it, because it does not represent a particular part of the body, but the over-arching state of virtually all domains" (p. 210). Processes of life and of experience, *Leben* and *Erleben,* are thus inseparably bound to each other. Emerging from the life of the organism as a whole, the feeling of being alive may be regarded as a primary manifestation of the *embodiment* of subjectivity.

A general diminishment or a rise of vitality is found in affective disorders, i.e., in depression and mania. Schneider (1959) already emphasized the impairment of vital feelings as the hallmark of severe depression: oppression, anxiety, heaviness, exhaustion, and inhibition may be summarized as a generalized bodily constriction (Fuchs 2005a). With the loss of vitality, the lived body becomes unable to open up to the world and to disclose its potentialities. The exchange of body and environment is blocked, drive and impulse are exhausted; feelings of distance and alienation may arise. Since a diminished feeling of being alive also concerns the patient's basic self-awareness, *affective depersonalization* is a core feature of severe depression (Kraus 2002; Stanghellini 2004). It culminates in the so-called nihilistic delusion or *Cotard's* syndrome (Enoch and Trethowan 1991) where patients no longer sense their own body: taste, smell, even the sense of warmth or pain are lost. This lets them conclude that they have already died and ought to be buried. Having lost the background feeling of the body that otherwise conveys a sense of connectedness and realness to our experience, the patients may also contend that the whole world is empty or does not exist anymore. Thus, in Cotard's syndrome a severe disturbance of the basic feeling of life leads to a delusional depersonalization (Fuchs 2005a; Ratcliffe 2008, pp. 165ff.)

Existential Feelings

The feeling of being alive may be regarded as a paradigm for a number of related background feeling states that are characterized by a tacit presence of the body in the experiential field. Drawing on Heidegger's ontology of mood, Ratcliffe has termed these background states *existential feelings,* conceiving them as "both 'feelings of the body' and 'ways of finding oneself in the world'" (Ratcliffe 2008, p. 2). They include, for example, feelings of freedom, wideness, and openness, or feelings of restriction or suffocation, feelings of vulnerability or protection, uncanniness or certainty, familiarity or estrangement, reality or unreality. They do not involve the body as an object of awareness, but as a medium through which one's being-in-the world is experienced. Thus, they constitute a tacit sense of relatedness between self and world and pre-structure our experience of particular situations (Ratcliffe 2009).

Existential feelings are clearly distinct from emotions since they are not directed at specific objects or situations; thus, they lack intentional "aboutness" as well as "propositional content."[2] By contrast, there is much overlap with the concept of mood which denotes a type of existential background affect, in particular on Heidegger's account. However, existential feelings comprise a number of feeling states which are characterized by a particular relation of the embodied subject to its surrounding world (e.g., "reality," "situatedness," "connectedness," or "belonging") and which are not covered by the traditional forms of mood. Since they have largely gone unnoticed by phenomenology and psychopathology until recently, a separate term seems all the more justified.

It is important to note that background feelings are not just related to an anonymous world, but to the world that we share with others, or to the interpersonal world. In the last analysis, they are always *existential feelings of being-with*. It is primarily in our coexistence with others that we feel close or distant, familiar or alienated, open or restricted, and even real or unreal. This is also mirrored by a specific type of "social" existential feelings (see later). As I will argue later on, "*interaffectivity*" is not merely a particular section of affectivity. Rather, it is the encompassing sphere in which our emotional life is embedded from birth.

Existential feelings may be classified, though not clearly separated, into three categories (cf. Stephan and Slaby 2011):

1. *Elementary existential feelings* include the feeling of being alive, of feeling oneself, at home in one's body; the feeling of reality, the feeling of meaningfulness and significance. All these feelings are normally tacit and unquestioned; it is only in severe psychopathological states that they are disturbed or vanishing:
   - Feeling dead, having lost all affects (as in Cotard's syndrome).
   - Feeling alien to oneself, like an outside observer to one's own body, like a robot (depersonalization) (cf. also Radovic and Radovic 2002).
   - Feeling unreal, like in a dream (derealization).
   - Feeling detached from the world, experiencing a loss of all meaning or "nothingness."
   In such states, the background of taken-for-granted familiarity vanishes and is replaced by a sense of alienation from oneself and the world. Heidegger's "Angst" refers to a related existential feeling of uncanniness caused by a complete absence of all practical significances that normally connect us to the world.
2. *General existential feelings* include states of feeling healthy, fresh, strong, or, on the other hand, tired, weak, ill; feeling satisfied or empty, in harmony or disharmony with oneself; open and alert or indifferent to everything; secure or vulnerable; free

---

[2] That means, believing that *p is the case*; for example, being angry means judging "to have been wronged by another person" which is the propositional content of the anger.

or constricted, etc. Such feelings are obviously part of everyday experiences, but also of mental disorders.

3. *Social existential feelings* refer to states such as feeling at home in the world and with others, feeling welcome, familiar, connected—or feeling like a stranger, distant, disconnected, rejected, or isolated; having a sense of basic trust or feeling wary and suspicious toward others. These feelings are of major importance for psychopathology, as shown by recent concepts of delusion as being based on a loss of the basic trust and common sense which normally create a "bedrock of unquestioned certainties" in social life (Rhodes and Gipps 2008; Wittgenstein 1969). Thus, the Capgras delusion (implying the belief that spouses or other familiar persons have been replaced by impostors) may be regarded as a loss of basic familiarity with close others that leads to misperceiving their appearance as a spurious and deceitful (Ratcliffe 2008, pp. 139ff.). Similarly, the loss of basic affective connectedness to others in depression manifests itself in delusions of guilt, impoverishment or bodily decay (Fuchs, in press).

As can be seen, existential feelings comprise a host of affective states that can appear in complex blending. Although they do not feature in the usual psychiatric assessment, they are of particular importance for psychopathology. Much of what is currently conceived as belonging to higher domains of cognition, belief, or judgment—for example, the sense of reality, the sense of being oneself, paranoid ideation, even delusions—is actually based on an affective foundation, namely on the tacit background feelings of the lived body in relation to others. Disturbances of these feelings often remain unnoticed, because they manifest themselves primarily in the way the world and the others appear to the patient: "The patient is ill, that means, his world is ill" (van den Berg 1972, p. 46).

Atmospheres

Although a ubiquitous phenomenon, affective atmospheres are only rarely treated in emotion research and theory. They may be regarded as holistic affective qualities of experienced spatial and interpersonal situations, integrating their expressive features into a unitary dynamic Gestalt: for example, feeling the hilarity of a party, the sadness of a funeral march, the icy climate of a conference, the awe-inspiring aura of an old cathedral, or the uncanniness of a somber wood at night. Such atmospheric effects are evoked by physiognomic or expressive qualities of objects as well as by intermodal features of perception such as rhythm, intensity, dynamics, etc.[3] Like all affective phenomena, atmospheres are experienced through a resonance of the body (an icy atmosphere feels chilly, an uncanny situation makes one shiver or "one's hair stand on end," a tense interpersonal climate is felt as oppressive or suffocating, etc.). They appear as warm or cold, serene or melancholic, relaxed or charged, familiar or sinister, and so forth.

---

[3] These structural qualities of perception have been particularly explored by Gestalt psychology (cf. Koehler 1992) and nowadays been rediscovered by infant research as so-called "vitality affects" (Stern 1985). See also the phenomenology of affectivity in Fuchs (2000, pp. 193–217).

In comparison to existential feelings or moods, affective atmospheres are often felt more distinctly, since they are not experienced as something one carries with oneself, but rather encountered as an enveloping aura, radiating or emanating from the space or environment that one enters (cf. Anderson 2009). Thus, one feels exposed to atmospheres, drawn into them, and they are often experienced as contrasting with one's own mood which is then felt even more intensely. Insofar as the atmospheric qualities of a specific environment—in particular landscapes, architecture, interiors, and other spaces—are often experienced concordantly by many persons, they may well be regarded as objective to a certain degree. It is even possible to purposefully arrange an environment so as to emanate a certain atmosphere.

Most important for psychopathology and psychotherapy are:

1. The *personal atmospheres* which irradiate from the appearance and comportment of a person, integrating his or her physiognomy, expression, gesture, voice, posture, and comportment into a unitary impression. This is the basis for the intuitive diagnostic, for example, of depression or schizophrenia, in the latter case being captured by the well-known "praecox-feeling" (Grube 2006; Rümke 1941/1990).
2. The *interpersonal atmospheres* which arise from the interaction of two or more persons and are felt as encompassing affective climates. Whereas Western psychiatry has tended to neglect these phenomena, in traditional Japanese or Chinese psychopathology the surrounding climate and social atmospheres such as the *ki* (or *qi*) are even regarded as carriers of mental illness: *ki* means "air," "breath," but also "attunement" and "atmosphere," and thus constitutes the "in-between" from which mental disorders may take their origin (Kimura 1972/1995; Kitanaka 2012, pp. 23ff.).

Even in Western psychopathology, a classic phenomenon of schizophrenic psychopathology, namely "delusional mood" (Jaspers 1968), may be regarded as a characteristic atmosphere of perplexity, uncanniness, and enigmatic significance in which the patient senses an inexplicable change in his environment (Fuchs 2005b). A heightened sensitivity to surrounding atmospheres is also characteristic for paranoid states or social phobia and other anxiety disorders.

Mood and Attunement

Moods constitute a further layer of emotional life which permeates all current experiences and lends them a certain coloring. Typical examples are elation, euphoria, serenity, boredom, sadness, dysphoria, irritability, anxiety, or melancholy. In a first approximation, moods may be defined as global, basically evaluating (i.e., pleasant or unpleasant), but non-intentional feeling states which render a person prone to experience himself and the environment in a certain way, and to behave correspondingly. Moods are thus fundamental states of being-in-the-world that indicate "how things stand" in our life and how we are disposed to react to the present situation. In what follows, I will further elaborate this definition by describing characteristic features of mood in contrast to emotions (which are described in more detail in the next section).

1. *Duration and intensity.* Moods are sustained affective states which usually last for hours, days, or weeks; they take a gradually rising and falling course without having a definite beginning or end. In contrast, emotions are rather short-lived, episodic, and dynamic: they typically rise to a swift peak, reach a higher intensity, and fade after seconds, minutes, or hours. Thus, emotions become prominent for a short time span, whereas moods often remain in the backdrop of the experiential field and need not even be conscious (e.g., one may deny being in a dysphoric mood while other persons are aware of it; a depressive patient may have a distorted view of his situation without being able to attribute this to his altered mood).

2. *Pervasiveness.* Moods permeate and tinge the whole experiential field; they cannot be spatially localized and delimitated. "A mood assails us. It comes neither from 'outside' nor from 'inside,' but arises out of Being-in-the-world, as a way of such Being" (Heidegger 1962, p. 176). Moods are primary to the subject–object distinction, radiating through the environment and conferring concordant affective qualities on the whole situation. Thus, boredom or depression lends a dull or gloomy quality to the objects, whereas in euphoria they take on a colored and attractive expression. Hence, moods are a background through which we encounter things as mattering or not mattering. They belong to a primordial sphere of attunement of self and world, thus serving as a basis for all specifically directed intentional states.

3. *Lack of intentionality.* Moods are global states of feeling-oneself-in-the-world, without referring to certain objects, causal events, or desirable goals. In contrast, emotions are intentional in terms of being inherently motivated by, and directed toward, certain objects or events. Emotions imply an "aboutness" (joy of …, hope for …, etc.) and tend to fade once their inherent object or motive is gone. Moods may also be triggered by events or even caused by psychotropic agents, but they do not contain their cause as an inherent motive. The cheerfulness brought about by consuming alcohol is unmotivated and may only secondarily find objects to direct itself upon. It is this unspecific character of moods which has favored their interpretation in existentialist philosophy as fundamental determinants of being-there: anxiety, boredom, or depression may disclose the uncanniness, emptiness, or burden of existence *as such*.

4. *Dispositional character.* Moods render the subject prone to perceive a situation, to feel and to act in a certain way; they favor congruent and impede incongruent cognitions, emotions, and actions ("being in the mood for something"). However, whereas emotions prefigure rather specific behavior, moods imply only an unspecific directedness (e.g., an extraverted tendency in euphoria, or an introverted tendency in sadness).[4] One might also say that in moods, background feelings of

---

[4] In animals, mood states seem to determine instinctive behaviour more specifically, resulting in circumscribed phases for hunting, mating, breeding, playing, exploring, recovery, etc. On the neurobiological level, moods may be regarded as generally motivating or readiness states based on neuromodulatory and endocrine functions, the main modulating transmitters being norepinephrine (attention, impulsivity), serotonin (activation), acetylcholine (attention), and dopamine (pleasure, rewarding). For the neurobiology of moods, see e.g., Schore (1999).

the body are connected to the overall *potentialities* of a given life situation. "The mood has already disclosed, in every case, Being-in-the-world as a whole, and makes it possible first of all to direct oneself towards something" (Heidegger 1962, p. 176).

5. *Polarity.* Mood typically swings in dual polarities, the most basic being *pleasant–unpleasant*, and *high–low*. However, there are other poles derived (a) from the prevailing bodily feeling: *light–heavy*, or *tension–relaxation*; (b) from the dominating atmospheric quality: *bright–dark, familiar–uncanny,* or *exciting–dull*; (c) from the dominating tendency of movement and directedness: *centrifugal–centripetal,* or *expansive–recessive*. These opposites express fundamental polarities in the relationship of a person with his or her environment.

6. *Attunement.* The phenomenology of moods may be summarized by a short analysis of the corresponding German term *Stimmung* which implies the metaphors of orchestration, consonance, and attunement. Moods may be said to "tune" body, self, and environment to a common chord, similar to a tonality linking a series of notes to the major or minor key. First, moods imply a bodily resonance, such as feeling light and fresh in elation, or heavy and weary in depression. Therefore disturbances of bodily well-being have an immediate impact on one's mood. Second, by coloring one's whole experience, moods also imply a basic, pre-reflective self-awareness. Third, being in a mood means opening oneself toward the kinds of possibilities and projects of one's present situation. Moreover, moods are strongly influenced by surrounding atmospheres, as is best shown by the impact of music—a special carrier of atmospheric feelings. In sum, moods are comparable to a "*basso continuo*" that establishes a consonance of bodily feeling, affective self-awareness, and environmental atmosphere.

Moods are often compared to *climate* and emotion to *weather* (e.g., by DSM-IV; American Psychiatric Association 1995). However, climate may be regarded as the time integral of weather,[5] whereas emotions do not become moods, even when they persist for a longer time. A better analogy might be the relation of the *tides* (mood) to the *waves* (emotions). In any case, one's basic mood can be superimposed by emotions of congruent or (more rarely) incongruent value. Mood even has a tendency to "materialize," i.e., to elicit corresponding emotions with their according objects. Thus, a general irritability easily finds occasions for specific anger and attack; anxiety tends to become fear and thus to direct itself toward specific frightening objects. Depression notoriously facilitates guilt-feelings and self-reproaches concerning arbitrary omissions or mistakes that are recalled from autobiographical memory (Blaney 1986). Conversely, one's grief over a loss may change into an unspecific sad, wistful, or even depressed mood when the triggering event is no longer present. However, this does not mean that the intentionality or "aboutness" of emotion is only a gradual phenomenon: grief is inherently motivated and thus comprehensible for the subject in itself, whereas sadness persists even when there is no apparent motive for it. Moods are not generalized emotions but rather conditions of possibility for specifically focused emotions.

---

[5] For example, "if rain is infrequent in a region over long periods, the climate is arid" (Alpert and Rosen 1990).

EMOTIONS

Emotions may be considered the most complex phenomena of affectivity. This is mirrored by the host of different and often opposing emotion theories both in philosophy and psychology. Of the many attempts to reduce the complexity of emotions to a more simplified concept, two should be mentioned. The first focuses on their bodily component, as in the famous theory of James and Lange (James 1884), simply put: we do not shiver because we are scared of the lion, but we shiver, and *this is* what we feel as our fear. In other words, emotions are feelings of bodily changes. This counter-intuitive assumption has been widely criticized for neglecting the intentional content or "aboutness" of emotions.

On the other hand, the contrary theory seems no less one-sided: according to the currently predominant cognitive approaches (Lyons 1980; Nussbaum 2001; Solomon 1976), emotion mainly consists in an act of evaluation or appraisal of a given situation. The bodily experience of emotions is then regarded as just an additional quale without further relevance (Gordon 1987) or serving the limited purpose to assure us that an emotion is going on (Lyons 1980). Again simplified: we believe or judge the lion to be dangerous, want to run away, and *this is* our fear of him. However, belief–desire concepts of emotions have been notoriously unable to capture their experiential and phenomenal aspect. A purely cognitive or functional approach to the phenomenon loses its peculiar self-affecting character. In particular, as Downing (2000) has argued, it fails to account for the changing intensity of emotions: without referring to bodily experience (e.g., to one's increased sense of muscle tension, breath restriction, heated face, or pounding of the heart) it is virtually impossible to indicate what a more intense anger, shame, or fear should be. There are no "intensive cognitions."

In view of these difficulties, it seems advisable to follow a step-by-step approach in presenting the phenomenon. In a first approximation, we may regard emotions as affective responses to certain kinds of events of concern to a subject, implying conspicuous bodily changes and motivating a specific behavior (De Sousa 2010). This already denotes the main differences to the other affective phenomena treated so far. Accordingly, I will first consider emotions under the aspects of (1) affective intentionality, (2) bodily resonance, (3) action tendency, and (4) function and significance. Then I will try to integrate these aspects into an embodied and extended concept of emotions.

1. *Affective intentionality.* There is wide agreement among philosophers and psychologists that emotions are characterized by intentionality—they relate to persons, objects, events, and situations in the world (see e.g., De Sousa 2010; Frijda 1994; Solomon 1976). However, this intentionality is of a special kind: it is not neutral, but concerns what is particularly *valuable and relevant* for the subject. In a sense, emotions are ways of perceiving, namely attending to salient features of a situation, giving them a significance and weight they would not have without the emotion. Referring to Gibson's (1979) concept of affordances (that means, offerings in the environment that are available to animals, such as a tree being "climbable," water "drinkable," etc.), one could also speak of *affective affordances*: things appear to us as "important," "worthwhile," "attractive," "repulsive," "expressive," and so on. Without emotions, the world would be without meaning or significance; nothing would attract or repel us and motivate us to act.

Of course, this meaning-making implies an evaluative or appraising component which should not, however, be conceived in terms of propositional attitudes; otherwise, emotions could not be experienced by small children or higher animals lacking language. Moreover, this evaluation may not be regarded as a mere cognitive judgment, for in emotions, *oneself is affected*. They always imply a particular relation to the feeling subject in its very core: through emotions, I experience *how it is for me* to be in this or that situation. *It is me* who is surprised, hurt, angry, joyful, etc. Affective intentionality is thus twofold: it discloses an evaluative quality of a given situation as well as the feeling person's own state in the face of it (Slaby and Stephan 2008). To be afraid of an approaching lion (world-reference) means at the same time being afraid for oneself (self-reference). To feel envy toward another person means to begrudge her an advantage or success as well as to feel inferior and dissatisfied with oneself. Each emotion, thus, implies the two poles of feeling something and feeling oneself as inextricably bound together.

2. *Bodily resonance*. Like all other forms of affectivity, emotions are experienced through the resonance of the body, but in a far more intensive and manifold way. This includes all kinds of local or general bodily sensations: feelings of warmth or coldness, tickling or shivering, pain, tension or relaxation, constriction or expansion, sinking, tumbling, or lifting, etc. They correspond, on the one hand, to autonomic nervous activity (e.g., raised heartbeat, accelerated respiration, sweating, trembling, visceral reactions), on the other hand, to various muscular activations, bodily postures and related kinesthetic feelings (e.g., clenching one's fist or one's jaws, moving backward or forward, bending or straightening oneself, etc.). Particularly rich fields of bodily resonance are the face and the gut. Thus, for example, sadness may be felt locally as a lump in the throat, a tightening in the chest or in the belly, a tension around the eyes, a tendency to weep, or globally as a sagging tendency or a painful wave spreading through the whole body.

In sum, the body is a most sensitive "sounding-board" in which every emotion reverberates (James 1884). At the same time, these bodily feelings have an immediate repercussion on the emotion as a whole: feeling one's heart pound in fear raises one's anxiety, feeling one's cheeks burn with shame increases the painful experience of exposure and humiliation, etc. (Ekman et al. 1972). Therefore bodily feelings should not be conceived as a mere by-product or add-on, distinct from the emotion as such, but as the *very medium* of affective intentionality. Being afraid, for instance, is not possible without feeling a bodily tension or trembling, a beating of the heart or a shortness of breath, and a tendency to withdraw. It is *through* these sensations that we are anxiously directed toward a frightening situation. Our feeling body is the way we are emotionally related to the world, or in other words, affective experiences *are* bodily feelings-toward (Goldie 2000).

3. *Action tendency*. Bodily resonance of emotions is not restricted to autonomic nervous system activity or facial expression (which are in the focus of most empirical studies), but includes the whole body as being moved and moving. Fear, for example, does not only mean a raised heart beat or widely opened eyes but also the urge to break free, to flee, or to hide (Sheets-Johnstone 1999). The term "emotion" is derived from the Latin *emovere*, "to move out," implying that inherent in emotions is a potential for movement, a directedness toward a certain goal (be it attractive or repulsive) and a tension between possible and actual movement. Emotions arise

in the course of evolution when need and satisfaction are separated, as a way to bridge the resulting gap: they sustain the intentional arc of drive, desire, and action toward the desired object (Merleau-Ponty 1962). Correspondingly, Frijda (1986) has characterized emotions in terms of *action readiness*, according to the different patterns of action which they induce: approach (e.g., desire), avoidance (e.g., fear), being-with (enjoyment, confidence), attending (interest), rejecting (disgust), non-attending (indifference), agonistic (anger), interrupting (shock, surprise), dominating (arrogance), and submitting (humility, resignation).

Similarly, according to De Rivera (1977), there exist four basic emotional movements: moving oneself "toward the other" (e.g., affection, mourning), moving the other "toward oneself" (e.g., desire), moving the other "away from oneself" (e.g., disgust, anger), and moving oneself "away from the other" (e.g., fear), related to the gestures of giving, getting, removing, and escaping. These basic movements are connected to a bodily felt sense of expansion or contraction, relaxation or tension, openness or constriction, etc. In anger, for example, one feels a tendency of expansion toward an object in order to push it away from self. In affection, one feels a relaxation, opening, and emanation toward an object or person. Emotions can thus be experienced as the directionality of one's potential movement, although this movement need not necessarily be realized in physical space; they are phenomena of lived space (Fuchs 2007).

4. *Functions and significance.* On the basis of the analysis so far, the role of emotions for the individual may be determined as follows: Emotions "befall us"; they interrupt the ongoing course of life in order to inform us, warn us, tell us what is important and what we have to react upon. They (re)structure the field of relevancies and values; some of our plans, intentions or beliefs must be revised (Downing 2000). Emotions thus provide a basic *orientation* about what really matters to us; they contribute to defining our goals and priorities. At the same time, they preordain a certain scope and direction of possible responses which complement the *meaning* they give to the situation. Bodily resonance, autonomic arousal, and muscular activations make us *ready to act*: in anger we prepare for attack, in fear we tend toward flight, in shame to hide or disappear. This motivation also underlies the intentional arc that we draw in every action directed toward a desired goal. Emotion may thus be regarded as *a bodily felt recognition of a meaningful transformation of the subject's world which solicits the lived body to action.* However, even when the action tendency of emotions does not win through, they still retain an *expressive* function: by indicating the individual's state and possible action to others, they serve a communicative function in social life which will be explained below in the section on "interaffectivity."

An embodied and extended concept of emotions

We now have the necessary components that may be integrated into an embodied and extended model of emotions:

1. Emotions emerge as specific forms of a subject's bodily directedness toward the values and affective affordances of a given situation. They encompass subject and situation and therefore may not be localized in the interior of persons (be it their psyche or

their brain). Rather, the affected subject is engaged with an environment that itself has affect-like qualities. For example, in shame, an embarrassing situation and the dismissive gazes of others are experienced as a painful bodily affection which is the way the subject *feels* the sudden devaluation in others' eyes. The emotion of shame is extended over the feeling person and his body as well as the situation as a whole.

2. Emotions further imply two components of bodily resonance:
   ~ *A centripetal or affective component*, i.e., being affected, "moved," or "touched" by an event through various forms of bodily sensations (e.g., the blushing and "burning" of shame).
   ~ *A centrifugal or "emotive" component*, i.e., a bodily action readiness, implying specific tendencies of movement and directedness (e.g., hiding, avoiding the other's gaze, "sinking into the floor" from shame). In emotions, we are "*moved to move*" (Sheets-Johnstone 1999).

3. On this basis, emotions may be regarded as *circular interactions or feedback cycles* between affection, perception, and movement (cf. Fig. 38.1). Being affected by the value features or affective affordances of a situation triggers a specific bodily resonance ("affection") which in turn influences the emotional perception of the situation *and* implies a corresponding action readiness ("e-motion"). Embodied affectivity consists in the whole interactive cycle which is crucially mediated by the resonance of the feeling body.

4. Bodily resonance thus acts as the medium of our affective engagement in a situation. It imbues, taints, and permeates the perception of this situation without necessarily stepping into the foreground. In Polanyi's terms, bodily resonance is the *proximal*, and the perceived situation is the *distal,* component of affective intentionality, with the proximal component receding from awareness in favor of the distal (Polanyi 1967). This may be compared to the sense of touch which is at the same time a self-feeling of the body ("proximal") and a feeling of the touched surface ("distal"); or to the subliminal experience of thirst ("proximal") which first becomes conspicuous as the perceptual salience of water flowing nearby ("distal").

5. If the resonance or *affectability* of the body is modified in specific ways, this will change the person's affective perception accordingly. Thus, a lack of resonance will

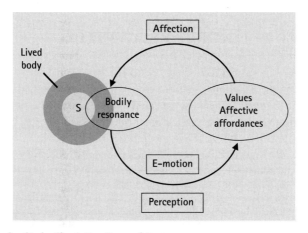

FIGURE 38.1 Embodied affectivity. S = subject.

impede the perception of corresponding affective affordances in the environment (e.g., injection of botulinum toxin in the frowning muscles impairs the understanding of negative semantic content which is normally facilitated by a slight frown; Havas et al. 2010). Conversely, increasing a certain bodily feeling favors the correlated affective perception (e.g., holding a hot cup of coffee elicits a "warmer" impression of a target person which is presented to test subjects than holding a cup of iced coffee; Williams and Bargh 2008). Thus, the different components of the affection-intention-motion cycle influence each other.

The last point is of particular psychopathological and psychotherapeutic importance, for it shows that emotions may not only be influenced by cognitive means (i.e., by changing the evaluative component of the cycle), but also by modifying the bodily resonance. It can be diminished as well as increased. The first is the case in habitual *body defenses*: When an emotion emerges, one often tends to defend against it by bodily counteraction: suppressing one's tears or cries, compressing one's lips, tightening one's muscles, keeping a stiff posture, "pulling oneself together," etc. This often happens unconsciously, as part of one's early acquired bodily *habitus* (cf. Bourdieu 1990). On the other hand, the experience of vague or diffuse emotions may be enhanced and differentiated by carefully attending to the bodily feelings and kinesthetic tendencies which these emotions imply, in order to render them accessible to verbal explication in psychotherapy.

A disturbance of bodily resonance and loss of affectability is also characteristic of severe depression. The constriction and "freezing" of the lived body in depression (Fuchs 2005a) leads to a general emotional numbness and finally to the affective depersonalization already mentioned. The deeper the depression, the more the affective qualities and atmospheres of the environment fade. The patients are no longer capable of being moved and affected by things, situations, or other persons. They complain of a painful indifference, a "feeling of not feeling," and of not being able to sympathize with their relatives any more.[6] In his autobiographical account, Solomon describes his depression as "a loss of feeling, a numbness, [which] had infected all my human relations. I didn't care about love; about my work; about family; about friends" (Solomon 2001, p. 45). Thus patients feel disconnected from the world; they lose their participation in the interaffective space that we normally share with others.

INTERAFFECTIVITY

As we have seen in the "Emotions" section, emotions imply embodied action tendencies. More specifically, in the social sphere they are characterized by various potential movements toward, or away from, an actual or implicit *other* (De Rivera 1977), i.e., they are essentially

---

[6] Schneider (1920) already pointed out that the "vital disturbances" of bodily feelings in severe depression are so intense that emotions can no longer arise. Of course, there are emotions that remain despite the loss of affectability, in particular feelings of guilt, anxiety or despair. However, these emotions show some characteristic features: (1) they do not connect, but rather separate the subject from the world and from the others; (2) their felt bodily quality is characterized by constriction and rigidity, thus corresponding to the depressive state; (3) they are embedded in the prevailing depressed mood rather than arising as independent feelings; therefore their intentional objects are just as ubiquitous as arbitrary.

relational. As such, they are not only felt from the inside, but also displayed and visible in expression and behavior, often as bodily tokens or rudiments of action.[7] The facial, gestural, and postural expression of a feeling is part of the bodily resonance that feeds back into the feeling itself, but also induces processes of *interaffectivity:* Our body is affected by the other's expression, and we experience the kinetics and intensity of his emotions through our own bodily kinesthesia and sensation. This means that in every social encounter, two cycles of affective intentionality (cf. Fig. 38.1) become intertwined, thus continuously modifying each subject's affective affordances and resonance. This complex process may be regarded as the bodily basis of *empathy* and *social understanding*.

To illustrate this (Fig. 38.2), let us assume that A is a person whose emotion, e.g., anger, manifests itself in typical bodily (facial, gestural, interoceptive, etc.) changes. He feels the anger as the tension in his face, the sharpness of his voice, the arousal in his body, etc. This resonance is an *expression* of the emotion at the same time, i.e., the anger becomes visible and is perceived as such by A's partner, B. But what is more, the expression will also produce an *impression*, namely by triggering corresponding or complementary bodily feelings in B. Thus, A's sinister gaze, the sharpness of his voice, or expansive bodily movements might induce in B an unpleasant tension or even a jerk, a tendency to withdraw, etc. (similarly, shame that one witnesses may induce embarrassed aversion, sadness a tendency to connect and console, and so forth). Thus, B not only sees the emotions in A's face and gesture, but also senses it with his own body, through his own bodily resonance.

However, it does not stay like this, for the impression and bodily reaction caused in B in turn becomes an expression for A. It will immediately affect his bodily reaction, change his

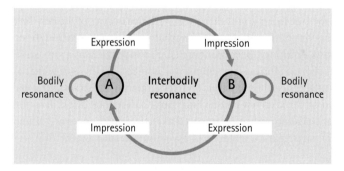

FIGURE 38.2 Interaffectivity. Adapted from *Phenomenology and the Cognitive Sciences,* *11*(2), 2012, pp. 205–236, The Extended Body: A case study in the neurophenomenology of social interaction, Froese, T., Fuchs, T., with kind permission from Springer Science and Business Media.

---

[7] According to Darwin (1872), emotional expressions once served particular action functions (e.g., baring one's teeth in anger to prepare for attack), but now accompany emotions in rudimentary ways in order to communicate these emotions to others. Evolutionary psychologists have advanced the hypothesis that hominids have evolved both with increasingly differentiated facial expressions and with sophisticated capabilities of understanding these affect displays. In any case, though strongly varying between and within cultures, emotional expression is a crucial facet of interpersonal communication in all societies; according to Ekman et al. (1972) it is based on six cross-culturally invariant emotions (happiness, sadness, fear, anger, surprise, and disgust).

own expression, however slightly (e.g., increasing or decreasing his expression of anger), and so forth. This creates a circular interplay of expressions and reactions running in split seconds and constantly modifying each partner's bodily state. They have become parts of a dynamic sensorimotor and interaffective system that connects both bodies in *interbodily resonance* or *intercorporality* (Merleau-Ponty 1964). Of course, the signals and reactions involved proceed far too quickly to become conscious as such. Instead, both partners will experience a specific feeling of being connected with the other in a way that may be termed "mutual incorporation" (Fuchs and De Jaegher 2009). Each lived and felt body reaches out, as it were, to be extended by the other. In both partners, their own bodily resonance mediates the perception of the other. It is in this sense that we can refer to the experience of the other in terms of an embodied perception, which, through the interaction process, is at the same time an embodied communication.

This can perhaps best be studied in early childhood. Emotions primarily emerge from and are embedded in dyadic interactions of infant and caregiver. Stern (1985) has shown in detail how emotions are cross-modally expressed, shared, and regulated. Infants and adults experience joint affective states in terms of dynamic flow patterns, intensities, shapes, and vitality affects (e.g., *crescendo* or *decrescendo*, fading, bursting, pulsing, effortful or easy, etc.) in just the way that music is experienced as affective dynamics. This includes the tendency to mimic and synchronize each other's facial expressions, vocalizations, postures, movements, and thus to converge emotionally (Condon 1979, Hatfield et al. 1994). All this may be summarized by the terms *affect attunement* and *interaffectivity* (Stern 1985, p. 132): The emerging affect during a joyful playing situation between mother and infant may not be divided and distributed among them. It arises from the "in-between," or from the over-arching process in which both are immersed.

Thus, affects are not inner states that we experience only individually or that we have to decode in others, but primarily *shared states* that we experience through interbodily affection. Even if one's emotions become increasingly independent from another's presence, intercorporality remains the basis of empathy: There is a bodily link which allows emotions to immediately affect the other and thus enables empathic understanding without requiring a theory of mind or verbal articulation (Fuchs and De Jaegher 2009). It is obvious that these processes of embodied interaffectivity as well as their disturbances are of major importance for psychiatry, in particular for all kinds of psychotherapeutic interaction.

Conclusion

In contrast to the common cognitivist picture in which our mental states including moods and emotions are located within our head, phenomenology regards affects as encompassing phenomena that connect body, self, and world. They emerge on the basis of a pre-reflective attunement to the current situation, indicate the current state of our relations, interests, and conflicts, and manifest themselves as sensations, motions, and expressions of the body. In this way, I have presented vital and existential feelings, affective atmospheres, moods, and emotions as embodied and extended phenomena. In all of them, the body acts as a tacit or more explicitly felt medium of our affective relation to the world. At the same time, all of them imply a pre-reflective self-awareness which links them to the core of our subjectivity.

Finally, all feelings and affects open and direct us, specifically or rather unspecifically, toward the various possibilities, tendencies, or projects of our present life situation.

As such, affectivity conveys *meaning* to our life: it is only through affects that we live in a world in which persons and things matter, that we learn what is relevant for us, and what is worth our engagement. Without affects, the world would be a place without affordances and significance; we would not even attend to anything, for nothing would attract our interest. There is no clear separation between *affection* and *cognition*, for we can only recognize what is relevant for us, i.e., what bears affective values of some sort for our life. All cognition is based on our affective participation in the world. Nor is there a clear separation between *affection* and *volition*, for we can only take action on what has already affected us, and conversely, we can only be affected by what already motivates us to act. Acting is only possible in a world of affective affordances which lend a meaningful structure to the field of possible action.

A particular emphasis has been placed in this account on the intersubjective dimension of affectivity: Even in the most basic existential background feelings of reality, belonging to and familiarity with the world, all the more in our moods and emotions, we are always related to others within a shared affective space. Our participation in this space is crucially mediated by the lived body with its affectability and resonance. Infant research demonstrates how the mutual bodily resonance of facial, gestural and vocal expression engenders our primary affective attunement to others. From birth on, the body is embedded in intercorporality, and thus becomes the medium of interaffectivity. Hence, affects are not enclosed in an inner mental sphere to be deciphered from outside, but come into existence, change, and circulate between self and other in the interbodily dialogue. This applies also to the social and moral emotions such as shame, pride, envy, or guilt feelings which imply a reflective awareness of the self-in-relation-to-others and are only called forth by social interactions in the second and third year of life. Emotions are neither individual nor unidirectional phenomena; they operate in cycles that can involve multiple people in processes of mutual influence and bonding.

The diversity of affective phenomena, in particular their frequent background character, indicate that their psychopathological significance is by no means restricted to affective disorders in the narrow sense. If affectivity is the foundation of our being-in-the-world and of our being-with-others, then in all mental disorders this basic level will also be implicated. Moreover, as I pointed out earlier, numerous disorders which at first sight appear as disturbances of thought, perception or behavior are actually based, at least to a large extent, on unnoticed background feelings that tacitly change the whole experiential field. Similarly, disorders of intersubjectivity, as in schizophrenia and autism, which are currently attributed to higher cognitive dysfunctions, i.e., a theory of mind deficit (Frith 1989, 2004), may also be conceived as more basic disturbances of pre-reflective intercorporality and interaffectivity (cf. Fuchs 2010; Gallagher 2004; Hobson 2002; Stanghellini 2004). Finally, we should not forget that in all mental disorders affectivity occurs a second time, as it were, namely as suffering *from one's own condition*. A depressive person, for example, does not only experience anxiety, inhibition, loss of drive, or lack of sleep, but also suffers from feelings of insufficiency, guilt, or despair *over* his own state. Since human beings are essentially characterized by the stance they take toward themselves, they are not only affected on the primary level of the disturbance, but they also suffer on the existential level on which they have to live and to cope with their illness.

The complexity thus indicated should caution us against neglecting the phenomenology of affectivity and its disturbances in favor of searching for their underlying processes, such as unconscious cognitive mechanisms or neurobiological dysfunctions as their alleged "real causes." First, a nuanced phenomenology is necessary for the psychiatrist to adequately understand the patient's condition and thus to build up a close therapeutic relationship. Second, affects as fundamentally motivating and meaning-bestowing experiences are indispensable for the patients to understand *themselves*. All explanations of moods and emotions in terms of underlying mechanisms, though justified for certain research purposes, risk turning our self-understanding as feeling, wishing, and intending beings into a view of ourselves as a kind of apparatus whose states can be mechanically or chemically modified like those of our cars. Third, affects are what essentially connects us to others as well as to ourselves—not primarily cognitions or knowledge about neurobiological mechanisms. Working with the patient's affects, i.e., understanding, sharing, expressing, verbalizing, clarifying, and modifying them is arguably the most important task the psychiatrist has to face. He would be ill-advised to regard all these processes as mere surface phenomena.

Affects as interpersonal experiences show that human beings are essentially relational beings, needful of others for belonging, recognition, and being themselves. To be impaired or incapacitated in participating in the interaffective space that we share with others is probably the most serious suffering which mental illness can cause to those afflicted. If the categories developed in this chapter allow for a more fine-grained and richer assessment of individual experience in disorders of affectivity, it might make a contribution to our understanding of our patients' suffering, and thus to our ability to alleviate it.

REFERENCES

Alpert, M. and Rosen, A. (1990). A semantic analysis of the various ways that the term "affect," "emotion" and "mood" are used. *Journal of Communication Disorders*, 23, 237–46.

American Psychiatric Association (1995). *Diagnostic and Statistical Manual of Mental Disorders, Fourth Edition*. Washington DC: American Psychiatric Association.

Anderson, B. (2009). Affective atmospheres. *Emotion, Space and Society*, 2, 77–81.

Beck, A. T. and Alford, B. A. (2009). *Depression: Causes and treatment*. Pennsylvania, PA: University of Pennsylvania Press.

Beck, A. T., Rush, A. J., Shaw, B. F., and Emery, G. (1979). *Cognitive Therapy of Depression*. New York, NY: Guilford Press.

Berg, J. H. van den (1972). *A Different Existence. Principles of Phenomenological Psychopathology*. Pittsburgh, PA: Duquesne University Press.

Berrios, G. E. (1985). The psychopathology of affectivity: conceptual and historical aspects. *Psychological Medicine*, 15, 745–58.

Blaney, P. H. (1986). Affect and memory: A review. *Psychological Bulletin*, 99, 229–46.

Bourdieu, P. (1990). Structures, habitus, practices. In *The Logic of Practice*, pp. 52–79. Stanford, CA: Stanford University Press.

Condon, W. S. (1979). Neonatal entrainment and enculturation. In M. Bullowa (Ed.), *Before Speech*, pp. 131–48. Cambridge: Cambridge University Press.

Damasio, A. (1995). *Descartes's Error: Emotion, Reason and the Human Brain*. London: Picador.

Darwin, C. (1872). *The Expression of Emotions in Man and Animals*. London: Murray.

De Rivera, J. (1977). *A Structural Theory of the Emotions*. New York, NY: International Universities Press.

De Sousa, R. (2010). Emotion. In E. N. Zalta (Ed.), *Stanford Encyclopedia of Philosophy* (Spring 2010 Edition). [Online.] Available at: <http://plato.stanford.edu/archives/spr2010/entries/emotion>.

Downing, G. (2000). Emotion theory reconsidered. In M. Wrathall and J. Malpas (Eds), *Heidegger, Coping, and Cognitive Science: Essays in Honor of Hubert L. Dreyfus. Vol. 2*, pp. 254–70. Cambridge, MA: MIT Press.

Ekman, P., Friesen, W. V., and Ancoli, S. (1972). *Emotion in the Human Face*. New York, NY: Pergamon.

Enoch, M. D. and Trethowan, W. H. (1991). *Uncommon Psychiatric Syndromes* (3rd edn). Bristol: John Wright.

Freud, S. (1959). Inhibitions, symptoms and anxiety. In J. Strachey (Ed.), *The Standard Edition of the Complete Psychological Works of Sigmund Freud, Volume XX*, pp. 75–176. London: Hogarth Press. (Original work published 1926.)

Frijda, N. H. (1986). *The Emotions*. Cambridge: Cambridge University Press.

Frijda, N. H. (1994). Varieties of affect: Emotions and episodes, moods, and sentiments. In P. Ekman and R. J. Davidson (Eds), *The Nature of Emotion: Fundamental Questions*, pp. 59–67. New York, NY: Oxford University Press.

Frith, C. D. (2004). Schizophrenia and theory of mind. *Psychological Medicine, 34*, 385–9.

Frith, U. (1989). *Autism: Explaining the Enigma*. Oxford: Basil Blackwell.

Froese, T. and Fuchs, T. (2012). The extended body: A case study in the neurophenomenology of social interaction. *Phenomenology and the Cognitive Sciences, 11*, 205–36.

Fuchs, T. (2000). *Leib, Raum, Person. Entwurf einer phaenomenologischen Anthropologie*. Stuttgart: Klett-Cotta.

Fuchs, T. (2005a). Corporealized and disembodied minds. A phenomenological view of the body in melancholia and schizophrenia. *Philosophy, Psychiatry, & Psychology, 12*, 95–107.

Fuchs, T. (2005b). Delusional mood and delusional perception—A phenomenological analysis. *Psychopathology, 38*, 133–9.

Fuchs, T. (2007). Psychotherapy of the lived space. A phenomenological and ecological concept. *American Journal of Psychotherapy, 61*, 432–9.

Fuchs, T. (2010). Phenomenology and psychopathology. In S. Gallagher and D. Schmicking (Eds), *Handbook of Phenomenology and the Cognitive Sciences*, pp. 547–73. Dordrecht: Springer.

Fuchs, T. (2012). The feeling of being alive. Organic foundations of self-awareness. In J. Fingerhut and S. Marienberg (Eds), *Feelings of Being Alive*, pp. 149–166. Berlin: De Gruyter.

Fuchs, T. (in press). Depression, intercorporality and interaffectivity. *Journal of Consciousness Studies*.

Fuchs, T. and De Jaegher, H. (2009). Enactive intersubjectivity: Participatory sense-making and mutual incorporation. *Phenomenology and the Cognitive Sciences, 8*, 465–86.

Gallagher, S. (2004). Understanding interpersonal problems in autism: interaction theory as an alternative to theory of mind. *Philosophy, Psychiatry, & Psychology, 11*, 199–217.

Gibson, J. (1979). *The Ecological Approach to Visual Perception*. Boston, MA: Houghton Mifflin.

Goldie, P. (2000). *The Emotions: A Philosophical Exploration*. Oxford: Clarendon Press.

Gordon, R. (1987). *The Structure of Emotions*. Cambridge: Cambridge University Press.

Grube, M. (2006). Towards an empirically based validation of intuitive diagnostic: Rümke's "praecox feeling" across the schizophrenic spectrum: preliminary results. *Psychopathology, 39*, 209–17.

Hatfield, E., Cacioppo, J., and Rapson, R. L. (1994). *Emotional Contagion*. New York, NY: Cambridge University Press.

Havas, M., Gutowski, K. A., Lucarelli, M. J., Davidson, R. J. Havas, D. A., and Glenberg, A. (2010). Cosmetic use of botulinum toxin-A affects processing of emotional language. *Psychological Science, 21*, 95–900.

Heidegger, M. (1962). *Being and Time* (J. Macquarrie and E. Robinson, Trans.). Oxford: Blackwell.

Hobson, R. P. (2002). *The Cradle of Thought*. London: Macmillan.

James, W. (1884). What is an emotion? *Mind, 9*, 188–205.

Jaspers, K. (1968). *General Psychopathology* (J. Hoenig and M. W. Hamilton, Trans.). Chicago, IL: University of Chicago Press.

Kimura, B. (1972). *Hito to Hito no Aida*. Tokyo: Kobundo. (In German: Weinmayr, E. (Trans.) (1995). *Zwischen Mensch und Mensch. Strukturen japanischer Subjektivitaet*. Darmstadt: Wissenschaftliche Buchgesellschaft.)

Kitanaka, J. (2012). *Depression in Japan: Psychiatric Cures for a Society in Distress*. Princeton, NJ: Princeton University Press.

Koehler, W. (1992). *Gestalt Psychology: An Introduction to New Concepts in Modern Psychology*. New York, NY: Liveright.

Kraus, A. (2002). Melancholie: eine Art von Depersonalisation? In T. Fuchs and C. Mundt (Eds), *Affekt und Affektive Stoerungen*, pp. 169–86. Paderborn: Schoeningh.

Lyons, W. (1980). *Emotion*. Cambridge: Cambridge University Press.

Merleau-Ponty, M. (1962). *The Phenomenology of Perception*. New York, NY: Humanities Press.

Merleau-Ponty, M. (1964). Eye and mind (C. Dallery, Trans.). In J. Edie (Ed.), *The Primacy of Perception*, pp. 159–90. Evanston, IL: Northwestern University Press.

Nussbaum, M. C. (2001). *Upheavals of Thought. The Intelligence of Emotions*. Cambridge: Cambridge University Press.

Polanyi, M. (1967). *The Tacit Dimension*. Garden City, NY: Anchor Books.

Radovic, F. and Radovic, S. (2002). Feelings of unreality: A conceptual and phenomenological analysis of the language of depersonalization. *Philosophy, Psychiatry, & Psychology, 9*, 271–9.

Ratcliffe, M. (2008). *Feelings of Being. Phenomenology, Psychiatry and the Sense of Reality*. Oxford: Oxford University Press.

Ratcliffe, M. (2009). Existential feeling and psychopathology. *Philosophy, Psychiatry, & Psychology, 16*, 179–94.

Rhodes, J. and Gipps, R. G. T. (2008). Delusions, certainty, and the background. *Philosophy, Psychiatry, & Psychology, 15*, 295–310.

Rümke, H. C. (1990). The nuclear symptom of schizophrenia and the praecox feeling. *History of Psychiatry, 1*, 331–41. (Original work published 1941.)

Schneider, K. (1920). Die Schichtung des emotionalen Lebens und der Aufbau der Depressionszustände. *Zeitschrift für die gesamte Neurologie und Psychiatrie, 59*, 281–6.

Schneider, K. (1959). *Clinical psychopathology*. New York, NY: Grune & Stratton.

Schore, A. N. (1999). *Affect regulation and the origin of the self: The neurobiology of emotional development*. Mahwah, NJ: Lawrence Erlbaum Assoc. Inc.

Sheets-Johnstone, M. (1999). Emotion and movement. A beginning empirical-phenomenological analysis of their relationship. *Journal of Consciousness Studies, 6*, 259–77.

Slaby, J. and Stephan, A. (2008). Affective intentionality and self-consciousness. *Consciousness and Cognition, 17*, 506–13.

Solomon, A. (2001). *The Noonday Demon: An Atlas of Depression*. London: Vintage Books.

Solomon, R. (1976). *The Passions*. New York, NY: Anchor/Doubleday.

Stanghellini, G. (2004). *Disembodied Spirits and Deanimatied Bodies: The Psychopathology of Common Sense*. Oxford: Oxford University Press.

Stephan, A. and Slaby, J. (2011). Affektive Intentionalitaet, existenzielle Gefuehle und Selbstbewusstsein. In J. Slaby, A. Stephan, S. Walter, and H. Walter (Eds), *Affektive Intentionalitaet*, pp. 206–29. Paderborn: Mentis.

Stern, D. N. (1985). *The Interpersonal World of the Infant: A View from Psychoanalysis and Developmental Psychology*. New York, NY: Basic Books.

Williams, L. E. and Bargh, J. A. (2008). Experiencing physical warmth promotes interpersonal warmth. *Science, 24,* 606–7.

Wittgenstein, L. (1969). *On Certainty*. Oxford: Basil Blackwell.

CHAPTER 39

....

DELUSION: THE PHENOMENOLOGICAL APPROACH

....

LOUIS A. SASS AND ELIZABETH PIENKOS

INTRODUCTION

....

The phenomenological approach to delusions focuses on delusion as a *phenomenon*, on its subjective or lived dimension. The phenomenologist is interested, first and foremost, in understanding *what it is like* to have a delusion, or, more accurately, in understanding the *variety* of ways in which one might experience delusions and the delusional world.

The term "phenomenology" derives from the Greek *phainomenon*, which means "that which shows itself in itself, the manifest" ("*das Offenbare*") and also from *logos*, which means to "let something be seen" but also "to bind together" or "gather up" (Heidegger 1996, pp. 24–25; Moran 2000, p. 229). The aim of phenomenological psychopathology is, one might say, to render manifest the manifest. It is to reveal to us (to the psychologist, psychiatrist, philosopher, etc.) how things appear to the subject or patient; and to do so in a way that clarifies, to the extent possible, the (sometimes paradoxical) coherence of the patient's world and life by showing the interdependence of different aspects and phases of her experience and expression. Phenomenology has often been characterized as "*merely* descriptive," but that is not truly the case: it offers something like "explanation" in several senses of that ambiguous term. Through clarifying the nature of the manifest, phenomenology seeks to reveal two things: (1) the *complementarity* of different aspects of the patient's experience and expression (this means showing implicatory relationships of a synchronic kind—the task of "static phenomenology") and (2) the temporal interdependence of distinct phases or stages in the *development* of the patient's lived world (here we are concerned with relationships of a diachronic kind, with understanding the intelligible unfolding of forms or structures of experiences out of earlier forms or structures—the task of "genetic phenomenology"; Sass 2010).

A second feature of the phenomenological approach is its specific emphasis on the *mode*, *manner*, or *form* of the experience in question rather than its content (Jaspers 1963, p. 93). The phenomenologist puts less emphasis on *what* is experienced or asserted by the delusional patient (or on whether his beliefs are accurate or not) than on *how* he seems to experience his delusional world or what *sorts* of reality or existence he might be ascribing to it. Martin Heidegger (1996) referred to the latter dimension of existence as "ontological," and noted the tendency of thinkers to ignore or misconstrue this more formal or encompassing dimension in favor of more object-like entities or object-oriented (what he called "ontic") modes of understanding.

For the phenomenologist, delusion is typically understood not as an individual belief that might, for example, be captured in the notion of an abnormal "framework *proposition*" (as recently discussed in analytic philosophy; Campbell 2001), but as a mutation of the *ontological framework* of experience itself. The "ontological" aspect could include a variety of aspects of the overall structure or feel of the lived-world in general, but can also refer, more specifically, to what might be called the reality-status—the quality of actuality or lack thereof (whether things seem real or unreal) that characterizes the mode of experience in question. The phenomenological approach acknowledges that the forms of human experience and understanding may not only be *diverse*, but that they will sometimes involve *radical alterations in the most basic structure* of experience—including time, space, causality, and the basic forms of self-experience or self-identity (Bovet and Parnas 1993; Parnas and Sass 2001; Rümke 1950; Sass 1992a).

A third feature of the phenomenological approach is its acute appreciation of the *potential heterogeneity* of delusional experience, that is, of the potential *variety* of orientations a "deluded" patient might have, or attitudes he might adopt, toward or within his delusional world. The very term "delusion" is highly ambiguous. As we shall see, some authors have associated delusion, at least in its primary, basic, or supposedly "true" form, with schizophrenia alone;[1] but the contemporary semantic consensus is for a broader usage that would also include forms of pathological belief or quasi-belief in manic, depressive, paranoid, and organic disorders. Certain related terms, such as "delusion-like ideas" or "overvalued ideas," are also ambiguous, without consensus on their proper usage. (These terms are used to refer to unusual beliefs or quasi-beliefs that are supposedly more understandable in light of the patient's history, emotional state, etc. (Walker 1991).)

Intimately connected with phenomenology's emphasis on subjectivity, form, and variety is a fourth trend. This involves questioning the assumption that a delusion is, in essence, a "false belief" based on *poor or faulty "reality testing."* The latter is inherent in standard conceptualizations, whose current, canonical formulation is the *Diagnostic and Statistical Manual of Mental Disorders* (DSM)-IV-TR (American Psychiatric Association 2000, p. 821) definition of delusion as "a false personal belief based on incorrect inference about external reality and firmly sustained in spite of what almost everyone else believes and in spite of what constitutes incontrovertible proof or evidence to the contrary." All who have subjected this definition to close scrutiny (e.g., Munro 2000; Spitzer 1990) have found it utterly

---

[1] Binswanger believed that the problem of schizophrenia reached its culmination in the problem of delusion. Schneider said that schizophrenia was the delusional illness in the strict sense of the term (Ey 1996, p. 204).

inadequate and even misleading, though few have suggested alternative formulations. Some patients with pure paranoid psychosis or affective psychoses may fit this homogenizing definition fairly well. It is often noted, however, that deluded patients with schizophrenia sometimes do not *act* as if their delusions were or implied normal truth claims. Eugen Bleuler (1911/1950, p. 378), coiner of the term "schizophrenia," spoke here of "double bookkeeping" or "double recognition," giving the example of a patient who insisted that his psychiatrist had been misdirecting his mail but then would ask the psychiatrist to be so kind as to post his next letter. Some phenomenologists have tried to distinguish between the more "ontic" or "empirical" delusions that seem to involve something like mundane truth claims, and that may not involve major transformations in the horizons or background of experience; versus the ontological or autistic/solipsistic ones that operate in another realm, and that may not correspond to usual conceptions of "beliefs" at all (Parnas 2004; Sass 1992a).

A fifth and final feature of the phenomenological approach is an appreciation of the *inherent difficulty of describing or conceptualizing delusion*, especially in schizophrenia. The normal use of standard language assumes the usual horizons of experience, which provide a semantic background for our comprehension. It follows that experiences involving alteration of the fundamental frameworks of experience can be difficult to describe—whether for patient, therapist, or phenomenological theorist. One patient felt defeated in her attempt to describe what her past delusions were like: "I can resort to bizarre metaphors, but I can't even in the grossest, roughest way communicate that state of mind" (Aviv 2010, p. 46).

The first phenomenological psychopathologist, Karl Jaspers, believed that the defining feature of schizophrenia and of "true" delusion (which for him meant schizophrenic), was in fact its incomprehensibility, an utter recalcitrance to psychological comprehension or empathic understanding on the part of normal individuals (Walker 1991). This placed the essence of schizophrenic delusion beyond the purview of phenomenological investigation. Most subsequent phenomenologists have rejected this extreme position. They do however emphasize the bizarre nature of this condition, which seems to deviate from normalcy in radical fashion. Accordingly, phenomenologists are generally suspicious of any account that downplays the discordant or alien qualities of schizophrenic delusion. They also tend to assume that discussing such phenomena may demand some creativity in the use of language, and some tolerance (even appreciation) of modes of description that can seem aberrant or even paradoxical in nature.

Some analytic philosophers writing on delusion have focused on one or another way of defining the word "belief." Some insist, for example, that since the patient may not act on his delusion, he must merely *believe* that he *believes* (when in fact he is only "imagining" his psychiatrist's malevolent tendencies; e.g., Currie 2000). Other analytic philosophers (Bortolotti 2009, p. 175) reply that such patients *do* in fact "believe," noting that we speak of normal individuals as "believing" even when they fail to act on their beliefs (e.g., I may believe in the recycling of garbage, but fail to carry it out in my actual daily life). From a phenomenological standpoint there can seem something idle or academic about these debates: the more interesting questions concern not semantics or conceptual analysis but the nature of the subjective attitudes or orientations that underlie and, presumably, explain these anomalous modes of experience and action (Sass 2004a).

In the pages to follow, we offer an introduction to the phenomenological approach to delusion in which these points will be illustrated. Since schizophrenia has received by far the greatest amount of attention within phenomenology, we will focus on this condition, with only a few words about other disorders. Although the neurobiological correlates of delusional experience is obviously a topic of great interest, it lies beyond the scope of the present article.[2]

We will discuss three overlapping themes that have been central in phenomenological discussion of this condition or set of conditions: (1) the famous "delusional mood"; (2) altered ipseity or self-experience and its role in delusion formation ("*ipseity*" is synonymous with minimal self, core self, or the *cogito*, referring to the basic, pre-reflective sense of existing as a unified and vital *subject* of experience); and (3) the ontological or reality-status of the schizophrenic delusional mood, including double bookkeeping and related phenomena. We begin, however, with a few words on Jaspers' decisive formulation of the notion of delusion. It is his synthesis that crystallized previous notions and set the agenda for subsequent work.

Jaspers on Delusion

As already noted, Jaspers (1963) considered "true" delusion to be specific to schizophrenia. He offered the following account:

> The term delusion is vaguely applied to all false judgments that share the following external characteristics to a marked, though undefined, degree: they are held with an *extraordinary conviction*, with an incomparable, *subjective certainty*; there is an *imperviousness* to other experiences and to compelling counter-argument; their content is *impossible*. (p. 95–96)

Jaspers did not, however, think that these features went to the heart of the matter. The characteristic conviction, certainty, imperviousness, and impossibility were "symptoms" or associated features ("external characteristics") rather that true "criteria" of delusion—or, at least of what he considered the *true* delusion of the schizophrenic sort. To investigate delusion, says Jaspers (1963, p. 96), it is necessary to learn about "the primary experience traceable to the illness," of which the incorrect judgment is merely a secondary product. For it is the particular *form* of true or "primary" delusion that largely distinguishes it from other types of belief or quasi-belief—which he lists as "normal belief," the "overvalued idea," and the "delusion-like idea." In contrast with these, primary delusion is a direct and unmediated experience that, he says, is *un*-understandable in light of previous experiences or beliefs. Perhaps most importantly, it entails what Jaspers (1963, p. 97) calls "a change in the totality of understandable connections," a change in the entire organizing personality or mode of consciousness of the patient.

Jaspers' account of "primary" or "true delusion" has a somewhat paradoxical air: he claims, at the same time, that we must discern a distinctly anomalous mode of experience (the "primary experience traceable to the illness") *and* recognize that the experience in question is, in some crucial sense, *un*-understandable to normal or non-schizophrenic individuals. Jaspers' very ability to identify and describe these decisive transformations

---

[2] See Gerrans (in press) for a sophisticated overview and critique of current cognitive-neuroscientific research on delusion. Gerrans sees his emphasis on the heightening or dominance of the "default system" as congruent with the emphasis in Sass (1994) on schizophrenic delusion as involving withdrawal from normal, world-oriented forms of belief.

(his description of delusional mood is particularly vivid and evocative) might make one question the sharpness of this distinction between the comprehensible (e.g., mere delusion-like ideas) and the incomprehensible (the "true" delusions of schizophrenia), with which we supposedly are unable to empathize.[3] This, at least, would seem the implicit assumption of most subsequent writers in phenomenological psychopathology. Some of the latter have, in fact, offered phenomenological accounts of the two types of global change that Jaspers considered most incomprehensible: namely, delusional mood and disturbance of the core self, ipseity, or "cogito."

We turn now to these two experiential transformations, after which we will reflect further on their contribution to delusion formation.

Delusional Mood

The period before the crystallization of a delusional belief is a well-recognized clinical phenomenon that has been called, variously, the delusional mood (*Wahnstimmung*), delusional atmosphere, or pre-delusional state. Occurring most notably in schizophrenia, this psychological state is typically characterized by feelings of strangeness and tension and a sense of tantalizing yet ineffable meaning. "The environment," writes Jaspers (1963, p. 98), "is somehow different—not to a gross degree—perception is unaltered in itself but there is some change which envelops everything with a subtle, pervasive and strangely uncertain light." Scenes or even objects may seem to have lost their usual qualities of coherence or usefulness; things may stand forth as strange, surreal, or suggestive entities. These feelings of uncanny and ineffable change in one's surroundings are coupled with a kind of unbearable tension and confusion sometimes combined with exaltation (Fuentenebro and Berrios 1995, p. 253). In this state, "Every detail and event takes on an excruciating distinctness, specialness, and peculiarity—some definite meaning that always lies just out of reach, however, where it eludes all attempts to grasp or specify it" (Sass 1992b, p. 52). "Something is happening, but I don't know what it is," the patient will say (Conrad 1958/1997, p. 102; Jaspers 1963, p. 98).

Both Jaspers and Schneider suggest that delusions and delusional perceptions often arise out of this mood or mindset, as attempts to make sense of the confusion and the feelings of unidentified significance (Jaspers 1963, p. 98). Typically these ideas have a delusional quality, but they serve to make a certain sense out of the perceptual alterations. (See Box 39.1.)

Two later psychiatrists, Paul Matussek and Klaus Conrad, brought phenomenology together with Gestalt psychology, thereby combining the method of empathy with an analysis of "psychological structure." Matussek (1987, p. 90) described the pre-delusional transformation as involving a "loosening of the natural perceptual context" that allows "individual perceptual components" to float free of any standard anchoring in common-sense unities or scenes; this, in turn, opens the way to attributions of exaggerated or peculiar significance, or to the bringing together of isolated elements into relationships of delusional significance that may be kaleidoscopic but can also become rigidified. For the patient R., "A dog, a horse, and an old lady were no longer just objects among many others within a certain natural

---

[3] Even the possibility of *description* might be taken to imply a certain coherence and understandability. Such would be the implication of the Davidsonian and Wittgensteinian positions.

Box 39.1 Vignette 1

A patient noticed the waiter in the coffee-house; he skipped past him so quickly and uncannily. He noticed odd behavior in an acquaintance which made him feel strange; everything in the street was so different, something was bound to be happening. A passer-by gave such a penetrating glance, he could be a detective. Then there was a dog who seemed hypnotized, a kind of mechanical dog made of rubber … Something must be going on; the world is changing, a new era is starting. Lights are bewitched and will not burn; something is behind it. A child is like a monkey; people are mixed up, they are imposters all, they all look unnatural. The house-signs are crooked, the streets look suspicious; everything happens so quickly. The dog scratches oddly at the door. "I noticed particularly," is the constant remark these patients make, though they cannot say why they take such particular note of things nor what it is they suspect. First they want to get it clear to themselves.

(Jaspers 1963, *General Psychopathology*, p. 100)

perceptual context, but specially accentuated elements against a more or less meaningless background" (Matussek 1987, p. 90). Lifted out of context they "acquire a certain 'weighting' … [and] become as it were, 'framed'" (pp. 90, 95).

Matussek describes this mindset as a distinctive combination of passivity with activity. The patient experiences a fixed gaze or general rigidity of perception that can be difficult to interrupt; indeed he may feel "held captive" by the object. Yet he also has an exaggerated capacity or ability to *focus* his attention, and may indeed take "pleasure" in doing so. This rigid perception (*Wahrnehmungstarre*) may be *elicited* by the isolated object in the decontextualized perceptual field, but the staring also plays a role in *transforming* the perceptual field: "the perception of an object can change purely as a result of prolonged gazing"—from a staring that it is difficult for normal individuals to sustain (p. 94). One patient stared at a swinging cord of a light-switch so intently that, after a time, he came to feel that not the cord but the wall and background were moving back and forth; and this lead, in turn, to the thought that the world was coming to an end (p. 93). (See also Boxes 39.2 and 39.3.)

In *Die Beginnende Schizophrenie* (1958/1997), the German psychiatrist Klaus Conrad describes several stages in the development of delusion, each involving a global alteration in

Box 39.2 Vignette 2

Day is breaking. This is the hour of the enigma.… One bright winter afternoon I found myself in the courtyard of the palace at Versailles. Everything looked at me with a strange and questioning glance. I saw then that every angle of the palace, every column, every window had a soul that was an enigma. I had a presentiment that this was the way it must be, that it could not be different. An invisible link ties things together, and at that moment it seemed to me that I had already seen this palace, or that this palace had once, somewhere, already existed. Why are these round windows an enigma? … They have a strange expression.

(Giorgio de Chirico, the proto-surrealist artist (and a person with strikingly schizotypal or schizoid features), describes a state of mind that seems to involve the "delusional mood." In Jean, M. (Ed.) (1980), *The Autobiography of Surrealism*, pp. 8–9; discussed in Sass 1992b, *Madness and Modernism*, chapter 2)

Box 39.3 Vignette 3

I remained quiet, unmoving, my gaze fixed on a spot or a gleam of light. But behind this wall of indifference, suddenly a wave of anxiety would come over me, the anxiety of unreality. My perception of the world seemed to sharpen the sense of the strangeness of things. In the silence and immensity, each object was cut off by a knife, detached in the emptiness, in the boundlessness, spaced off from other things. Without any relationship with the environment, just by being itself, it began to come to life. It was there, facing me, terrifying me.

(Renée, in Sèchehaye 1951, *Autobiography of a Schizophrenic Girl*, p. 57)

the structure of experience. The first of these he terms the *trema*—a term of theatrical jargon that refers to the stage-fright before the play begins. There is a sense that something is in the offing. Most commonly the patient feels a sense of threat and associated anxiety, depression, inhibition, and indecisiveness (Conrad 1958/1997, pp. 93, 105–106), but there may also be anticipatory excitement, exaltation, manic-like euphoria, or ecstasy. Despite some difficulties with concentration, there is no clouding of consciousness but rather a hyper-vigilance and sense of being hyper-awake and hyper-aware (pp. 230, 249). The patient attributes these changes to the external world and searches for clues to render the new unpredictable changes more comprehensible. What follows is the *apophany*, during which the delusion takes form. "*Apophany*" comes from a Greek word meaning "to become visible or apparent," and is meant to emphasize the feeling of revelation that is central to this second phase.

In the *apophany* the patient shifts from a general sense of change and unease into feelings of revelation or recognition that may involve various degrees of clarity or certainty. Typically the patient experiences the world as somehow false, inauthentic, or insinuating, and as referring somehow to himself: "I have the feeling that everything turns around me" (p. 161). Conrad uses the term *anastrophe* (literally: a turning-back or turning-inward), to capture this self-referential or self-observing quality—a form of "hyper-reflexivity" (Sass 1992b) that he considered "extraordinarily important" (Conrad 1958/1997, p. 165). There is an intimate complementarity between *apophany* and *anastrophe*, which are two sides of the same coin. Changes in the perceived environment (e.g., the sense of things being false or planned) elicit reflection and inhibit spontaneous engaged activity; yet these changes themselves can only occur in the presence of a reflexive or self-conscious turning inward toward the self (pp. 165–166), of a veritable "spasm of reflexion" that accompanies all *apophany* and persists throughout the delusional period (pp. 167, 199). Conrad notes as well that the patient, unlike the normal individual, seems unable to engage in the personal "Copernican Revolution" that would relativize her self-consciousness: she is unable to stand *outside* her own self-consciousness and recognize the egocentric distortion it can impose.

The delusional mood seems fraught with apparent contradiction: the patient is hyper-self-conscious yet also *lacking* in self-consciousness—or, at least, in the type that might release him *from* his self-consciousness. The patient is the center of the world and everything relates to him, yet he is no longer the meaning-giving center of his universe in the sense that objects have lost their pragmatic, user-relative status as tools or objects of his goals and desires. The patient is a victim of his own way of experiencing the world yet is somehow "detached and alienated from his own perceiving" (Fuchs 2005, p. 136). All these paradoxes are exacerbated if we now turn from the external world and toward the patient's experience of his own consciousness, body, and thoughts.

SELF-DISTURBANCE AND DELUSION

We have focused so far on altered experience of the external world—the central theme of classical accounts of delusional mood. But as Conrad (1958/1997, p. 193) points out, there is also an *apophany* of "*internal* space" that affects the experience of one's own body, feelings, and stream of consciousness and that leads as well to the development of delusions. Although this may be less obvious in early or pre-morbid phases of schizophrenia, it is an inevitable accompaniment: self and world are complementary poles of experience; changes in one are inconceivable without concomitant changes in the other. (See Boxes 39.4 and 39.5.)

The mutations of self-experience characteristic of schizophrenia are clearly described in classical phenomenological psychiatry. "The remarkable things about the particular phenomenon," writes Jaspers, "is that the individual, though he exists, is no longer able to feel he exists.

Box 39.4 Vignette 4

These thoughts go on and on. I'm going over the border. My real self is away down—it used to be just at my throat, but now it's gone further down. I'm losing myself. It's getting deeper and deeper. I want to tell you things, but I'm scared. My head's full of thoughts, fears, hates, jealousies. My head can't grip them; I can't hold on to them. I'm behind the bridge of my nose—I mean my consciousness is there. They're splitting open my head—oh, that's schizophrenic, isn't it? I don't know whether I have these thoughts or not. I think I just made them up last time in order to get treated.

(Quote from patient, in Laing 1960, *Divided Self*, p. 151)

Box 39.5 Vignette 5

And then something odd happens. My awareness (of myself, of him, of the room, of the physical reality around and beyond us) instantly grows fuzzy. Or wobbly. I think I am dissolving. I feel—my mind feels—like a sand castle with all the sand sliding away in the receding surf. What's happening to me? This is scary, please let it be over! I think maybe if I stand very still and quiet, it will stop.... This experience is much harder, and weirder, to describe than extreme fear or terror. But explaining what I've come to call "disorganization" is a different challenge altogether. Consciousness gradually loses its coherence. One's center gives way. The center cannot hold. The "me" becomes a haze, and the solid center from which one experiences reality breaks up like a bad radio signal. There is no longer a sturdy vantage point from which to look out, take things in, assess what's happening. No core holds things together, providing the lens through which to see the world, to make judgments and comprehend risk. Random moments of time follow one another. Sights, sounds, thoughts, and feelings don't go together. No organizing principle takes successive moments in time and puts them together in a coherent way from which sense can be made. And it's all taking place in slow motion.

(Saks 2007, *The Center Cannot Hold*, pp. 12–13)

Descartes' 'cogito ergo sum' (I think therefore I am) may still be superficially cogitated but it is no longer a valid experience" (Jaspers 1962, p. 122; see also Berze and Gruhle 1929; Ey 1996). "I feel strange," "My heart is displaced," "I am a dead leaf or a spiral of smoke," the patient may say (Ey 1996, p. 206). These mutations have been formulated recently as an alteration of minimal or core self or "*ipseity*" (of the basic sense of existing as a unified and vital *subject* of experience) that has two complementary facets: hyper-reflexivity and diminished self-affection (Sass 2010; Sass and Parnas 2003). Whereas "hyper-reflexivity" describes the way in which experience that would normally be tacit emerge into the focus of awareness, where they are experienced as objects *separate* from the self-as-subject, diminished self-affection describes the diminished sense of existing *as* an experiencing consciousness or lived body.

The Examination of Anomalous Self Experiences (EASE) (Parnas et al. 2005), an interview format developed for use with self-disordered patients, divides these phenomena into several domains including the following:

1. Disturbed "Cognition and Stream of Consciousness," typified by hyper-reflexive experiences of one's own thinking as objectified and having acoustic qualities (e.g., "thoughts aloud").
2. Disturbed "Self-Awareness and Presence," typified by feelings of non-existence or lack of self-affection (patient feels like a vacuum or a mere thing, e.g., like a refrigerator).
3. Disturbed "Bodily Experiences," typified by somatic estrangement (feeling that one's body is alien or does not "hang together").
4. Disturbed "Demarcation," typified by confusion as to whether one's thoughts or feelings belong to oneself rather than to an interlocutor or bystander.

Klaus Conrad (1958/1997, p. 211) describes these anomalies of self-experience as involving an inner *apophany* that is strictly comparable, and complementary, to the outer-directed *apophany* of "delusional mood." It is part of the "reflexive spasm" of "*anastrophe*": a "permanent reflection" or "permanent reflexivity" whereby the patient has a constant self-consciousness of his own actions. (Recall that *anastrophe* means "turning back" or "inversion.") This hyper-reflexive "turning backward" toward the self is incompatible with more spontaneous, world-directed forms of activity.

In *Die Beginnende Schizophrenie*, Conrad describes the progression from more subtle to more blatant alterations of inner space. Mild sonorization of thoughts may occur, and grow more intense until the thoughts can seem fully audible. This may lead to the sense of one's own thoughts being diffused outward; eventually they may no longer be felt to belong to oneself, and may even, in some cases, seem to belong to someone else (Klosterkoetter et al. 2001). Subtle bodily sensations, of nervous or electric-like tension, turn eventually into blatant feelings of passivization, often involving delusions of being controlled from without. Conrad (1958/1997, p. 211) describes these as involving a hyper-reflexive awareness of bodily sensation that would not normally be in the focus of attention—e.g., postural pressures, the feeling of one's clothes against the body or sensations of heat and cold—and that may lead, over time, to experiences and beliefs of being subject to external control. An intriguing example of this progression is described in a classic article by Victor Tausk and later analyzed by Sass (1992b). The patient Natalija's illness began with mild experiences of estrangement from herself and culminated in a full-blown delusion involving a sense of

---

Box 39.6 Vignette 6

The patient is Miss Natalija A., thirty-one years old, formerly a student of philosophy. She declares that for six and a half years she has been under the influence of an electrical machine made in Berlin ... It has the form of a human body, indeed, the patient's own form, though not in all details ... The truck has the shape of a lid, resembling the lid of a coffin and is lined with silk or velvet ... She cannot see the head—she says that she is not sure about it and she does not know whether the machine bears her own head ... The outstanding fact about the machine is that it is being manipulated by someone in a certain manner, and everything that occurs to it happens also to her. When someone strikes this machine, she feels the blow in the corresponding part of her own body ... The inner parts of the machine consist of electric batteries, which are supposed to represent the internal organs of the human body. Those who handle the machine produce a slimy substance in her nose, disgusting smells, dreams, thoughts, feelings, and disturb her while she is thinking, reading or writing. At an earlier stage, sexual sensations were produced in her through manipulation of the genitalia of the machine.

(Tausk 1919, pp. 519–520, discussed in Sass 1992b, *Madness and Modernism: Insanity in the Light of Modern Art*, pp. 217–218)

---

being controlled by a distant "influencing machine" that determined her every thought, sensation, and movement (Box 39.6). The machine itself resembled Natalija's own body and, in particular, her lived or subjective body (e.g., there was no head, as this would not be seen by the person herself), and can be read as an externalized representation of her own hyper-reflexive alienation, a crystallization of the *apophany* of her inner space under conditions of the "reflexive spasm." Natalija's influencing machine delusion emblematizes the linkage between hyper-reflexive *apophany* of inner space and the loss of a sense of possession or control of one's own bodily experience.

DEVELOPMENT OF DELUSIONS

We have described several ways in which the overall framework or structuring of experience, both "inner" and "outer," can be altered in schizophrenia. These include loosening of perceptual context, framing of isolated elements, and promiscuous linkages between decontextualized elements; also a sense of being at the center of things, the target of all glances and messages coming from without; and finally a kind of alienating introspection in which personal thoughts, feelings, or bodily sensations that would normally be inhabited or tacitly lived become the targets of one's own focus of attention. (One may wonder, incidentally, to what extent these constitute a heterogeneous set of features, and to what extent they derive from or reflect some central disruption; the notion of ipseity disturbance (Sass 2010; Sass and Parnas 2003) is one hypothesis re such a *trouble génerateur*.)

In the previous two sections we have treated delusional mood and self-disturbances separately. Usually, however, both are involved, at least to some extent, and prodromal patients frequently complain of both self-disorders and indescribable alterations of the perceptual world (Møller and Husby 2000). It seems likely, in any case, that these several features would jointly contribute to the development of delusions in a variety of ways.

Matussek (1987, p. 94) stresses the importance of decontextualization and the framing of isolated features for "apperception of delusional significance" and the generation of delusional beliefs. The destabilization of normal perceptual context precedes the development of true delusions and prepares the ground for entry into a delusional world. The very salience or framing of particular objects (or features of objects) may, in itself, suggest that something of particular importance or "weighting" is being indicated: it conveys an aura of having intensified "symbolic content" (p. 95). By isolating and fixing the impression, this framing may contribute to the "firmness and incorrigibility of the delusional content" (p. 96). The delusional significance remains rooted in perception, however, and can thus be "experienced directly as inherent in the object," as if rooted in sensory experience (p. 98). "The schizophrenic who experiences the meaning of 'innocence' in the white bark of a birch tree does not 'perceive' the color of the bark as a symbol of innocence, but sees incorporated in the white bark a very definite quality, namely that of innocence" (Matussek, 1987, p. 98).

Disembedding from everyday context allows unusual significances readily to emerge; objects or meanings are now free to link up with other, isolated features or meanings floating outside any standard or practical context. "One is much clearer about the relatedness of things, because one can overlook the factuality of things. They don't exist so one has nothing to do with them," said one patient, who reported a sense of having special, revelatory access to meanings ignored by others: "Out of these perceptions comes the absolute awareness that my ability to see connections had been multiplied many times over" (Matussek 1987, p. 96). Patients may feel "specially blessed with powers of insight" or "in possession of special powers of understanding the world" (p. 97). The isolation of particular qualitative features may be sufficiently intense, for example, as to make two persons who share a characteristic seem to the patient to be simply identical (p. 100). There may be a tendency to emphasize "more abstract properties of the perceptual world," (p. 103) as with the patient R., for whom the dog and foal seemed to be saying that the surrounding environment was somehow "rooted in nature and primordial in character" (p. 97).

The abstract or universal meanings and linkages of delusional experience need not have a paranoid cast. They can, however, easily take on such qualities—whether as a natural consequence of disconcerting environmental change in the context of normal human anxiety and self-concern, or due to the exaggerated schizophrenic self-referentiality of *anastrophe*. Because of the general feeling of uncanny particularity and overall strangeness (in which nothing is random; everything is "just so"), together with the sense of things being directed toward oneself, persons, situations, and objects can easily be interpreted (apperceived) as artificial, manufactured, manipulated, or somehow conspiratorial. Paranoid delusions may help to make a kind of rational sense out of what would otherwise be experienced as a disturbing, and otherwise inexplicable, change in the very foundations of the perceptual world. In this sense the crucial feature of a given delusion may not be its specific content but its ability simply to offer *some* meaning that is able to resolve the generalized, yet often excruciating, tension of the external *apophany*, with its torturous sense of things being "just so" or bristling with strange, cosmic, intentional significance (Sass 1992b, p. 61). The internally driven self-alienation or self-fragmentation inherent in the *apophany* of inner space can lead to still other forms of delusions common in schizophrenia, especially those that involve experiencing oneself as some kind of monster or in which one's thoughts or body parts are alienated or even controlled or taken over by an alien being.

Self-consciousness itself seems to play a generative role in fostering experiences that, in turn, form the basis of delusions of self-alienation, alien control, and non-existence. The "more I focus on my thoughts," said one woman with schizophrenia, "the more it feels like they don't actually belong to me ... It physically feels like my head is just completely hollow." The very process of over-focusing on one's thoughts seems to have an externalizing effect, transforming internal mental threads into something felt to be distanced and alien (Sass 1992b, chapter 7). Another woman with schizophrenia believed that many of her symptoms stemmed from "this constant questioning of what my true self is—even though that sounds really cheesy" (Aviv 2010, pp. 40, 44): "I think too much about every action I take. Like 'I'm moving my hand right now! That's so magical!'"

These various modes are not mutually exclusive and may sometimes combine. Consider the typically schizophrenic form of auditory hallucination (usually involving delusion as well) in which the patient hears a voice describing, or two voices discussing, her own ongoing behavior, often in a critical tone. "Now he's walking down the road, now he's reached the corner and he's wondering which way to turn; now he's looking at that girl's legs, the filthy so and so," the patient may hear (Sass 1992b, p. 231). Here, it seems, we have both kinds of *anastrophe*, of the self-conscious stepping-back described by Conrad: that associated with *external apophany* (the patient is himself the target or object of all attention felt to be coming from *without*), and also that associated with *internal apophany* (the voice heard in auditory hallucinations have been shown to involve the patient's *own* vocal chords, but experienced by him as external). It is understandable, as well, that a person who experiences change in the overall structure of the world, the self, or self-world relationships will be inclined to develop delusions that have a distinctively ontological, metaphysical, or otherwise encompassing cast. We see, then, that the various forms of delusional or quasi-delusional tendencies characteristic of schizophrenia—paranoid/self-referential, ontological/metaphysical, or involving themes of influence, omnipotence, or bodily transformation—can all be seen as rooted in overall mutations of the structure of experience that both underlie and, in a pathogenetic sense, precede the development of frank delusions. What is altered is not an isolated belief or framework proposition but the overall lived background or horizon of the whole life-world, thought-world, and lived body. These formal or structural changes set up the conditions for delusion, and the delusional content will frequently reflect these alterations of form—as we have seen with both self-referential delusions and the influencing machine. In this sense, phenomenological description does help us to understand, in some sense to explain (Sass 2010), the nature and development of delusions, and in fact to comprehend some of the very features that are at the heart of schizophrenic "bizarreness" (Cermolacce et al. 2010). But what, then, shall we say about Jaspers' original criterion for the definition of schizophrenia—un-understandability or incomprehensibility?

Comprehensibility

Jaspers draws a distinction between "static" and "genetic" understanding (Jaspers 1963, pp. 27, 307). Lack of *static* understandability refers to the sheer recalcitrance to empathy, for a normal person, of a given experience or state of mind. Examples here would be the loss in schizophrenia of the sense of ownership of one's own experience and also the uncanny way in which (in "delusional percept") a psychotic person may experience a given sensory perception as being immediately imbued with some profound meaning. Jaspers believed it was simply impossible for a normal individual to empathize with such experiences. A lack of *genetic* understandability refers to the difficulty of grasping through empathy how one "psychic event" (Jaspers 1963, p. 307) emerges from another—as when, in schizophrenia, an apparent emotional reaction arises or an action is undertaken that bears little apparent relation to circumstances.[4]

Jaspers and Conrad certainly recognized that the *content* of schizophrenic delusional beliefs will typically involve understandable elements: preoccupation with Nazis may, for example, be understandable in relation to past life circumstances, ideas concerning an influencing machine in relation to alterations of the experience of action (Conrad 1958/1997, p. 285). But, at least in the case of the primary or "true" delusions of schizophrenia, there is always, they claim, an aspect or element that remains incomprehensible—for instance, the nature of the *conviction* concerning the Nazis or the quality of the experiential alterations that *give rise* to the delusional elaboration. In this sense either the delusion's mode of existence or its genesis remains (in their view) "totally outside the categories of comprehensibility" (Conrad 1958/1997, p. 131).

Jaspers formulated his position in the early twentieth century, under the influence of the *Erklaren/Verstehen* distinction propounded by Dilthey and Weber. More recently this distinction, at least in its classical form, has been questioned, and certain more recent notions have been applied to schizophrenia. These latter include the philosopher Donald Davidson's claim that logical coherence is a prerequisite for the very attribution of mind or mental ("intentional") states (see Campbell 2001), and also the Wittgensteinian notion that language turns nonsensical when it is, without acknowledgment and without the provision of alternative paradigms of sense, applied too far outside its standard usage in descriptive or practical contexts (Read 2001). Both positions can be interpreted to imply that schizophrenia is incomprehensible—whether because schizophrenic thinking is fundamentally incoherent or because schizophrenics tend to speak in ways that are simply incompatible with the requirements of any legitimate "language game."

But the phenomenological account offered above concerning outer and inner *apophany/anastrophe* (delusional mood and self-disturbance) seems to go a long way toward rendering delusional experience comprehensible in some psychological, phenomenological, and even empathetic way. We can see how paranoid, ontological, influence-related, bodily, and solipsistic delusions might develop on the basis of the overall structural or horizonal changes associated with the delusional mood and ipseity disturbance. This corresponds to what Jaspers referred to as genetic understandability.

Both Jaspers (1963) and Conrad (1958/1997) insist, however, that the *apophanic* experience *itself* remains un-understandable, both in itself and in its contribution to delusional development; but the point seems debatable. Various accounts offer either abstract descriptions or revelatory analysis that do allow a degree of empathic comprehension—e.g., the use of Gestalt psychology by Matusssek (1987) and of such analogies as modernist self-consciousness, psychological introspectionism, and philosophical solipsism by Sass (1992b, 1994). Grasping the inner *apophany* and loss of ipseity may be especially challenging. Still, it seems unnecessary (and contrary to the teaching of both hermeneutic

---

[4] The action, for example, may not appear to fit into any sensible practical syllogism.

phenomenology and Wittgenstein) to hold that empathic comprehension is an either-or issue—a matter either of perfect co-living and empathic/intellectual grasp or a form of incomprehension that is absolute and unsurpassable (Sass 2003). At least some degree of understanding, both static and genetic, may well be possible, and it seems arbitrary to deny this on some a priori ground.

We see, in fact, that phenomenology offers not only description but also *explanation* in several senses of that commodious term (Sass 2010); and several of these refute the idea that schizophrenic delusions are somehow utterly incomprehensible or un-understandable phenomena. Some forms of explanation are non-causal, demonstrating relations of phenomenological implication, as is the case of *expressive* relationships between the content of a delusion and underlying changes in the structure of experience. Thus Natalija's influencing machine is emblematic of a paradoxical yet real aspect of schizophrenic reality: simultaneously expressing the sense of bodily alienation, of being passively controlled, and of being the solipsistic center of the universe.[5] Absolute power and absolute passivity seem to go together in schizophrenia, like two sides of the same coin (Conrad 1958/1997; Sass 1992b chapter 11).

Other forms of phenomenological explanation involve something closer to causal or quasi-causal relations (akin to what Husserl (1989, p. 227) called "motivational relationships" or even "motivational causality") concerning the development of symptoms over time. Some of these relationships are "consequential," involving psychological transformations whereby one state leads naturally to the next: thus prolonged staring (which is not, of course, a purely volitional phenomenon) can, by its very nature, contribute to the fragmentation of the perceptual field and, if directed to one's body, to the sense of separation from one's own corporeal being. Other forms of phenomenological explanation are "compensatory" in the sense of postulating understandable defensive (thus motivated) reactions to what is occurring on a more primary plane.[6]

Two (of many) possibilities relevant to this compensatory aspect of delusion-formation are: (1) the need to provide some explanation for experiential changes that would otherwise seem utterly random or monstrous, and (2) the wish to escape an intolerable reality by entering a world felt to be safer or more satisfying. The first is exemplified by certain paranoid delusions as well as by Natalija's influencing machine (which can thus be explained in both expressive and compensatory terms). The second is exemplified not only by rather

---

[5] Conrad (1997) states that complex delusional elaboration of this sort can be understood as the product of the reasoning mind attempting to make sense out of, or somehow to justify, the experiential alterations suffered on a more basic level. This may sometimes be the case. But the mind can also conjure up such symbolic forms of self-expression in a spontaneous, almost quasi-automatic fashion—as demonstrated by Silberer's (1951) classic studies of 'auto-symbolic' phenomena during the transitional hypnagogic and hypnapompic periods of falling asleep of waking up, when the mind spontaneously creates images of its own current functioning.

[6] Compensatory processes need not, of course, be consciously directed or purely volitional in nature. Further, as they become increasingly habitual, they become automatized and thereby shed a degree of *unconscious* goal-directedness. Also it is also important to avoid thinking of defensive psychological reactions as being somehow *created* by, or purely in the service of, defensive purposes. Schizophrenic derealization or subjectivization, for example, may often be exploited for defensive purposes (i.e., escape from the feeling of real threat). But its very possibility or availability can be a more *direct* manifestation of an underlying ipseity disturbance that may well have neurobiological roots.

"ontic" or "empirical" delusions, such as one patient's belief that he is a brilliant scientist, of world-historical importance, but also (and more tellingly, for the phenomenologist) by more ontological transformations—as with certain chronic and withdrawn patients who may experience themselves as the godly center or support of the universe, and whose delusions may afford escape into a solipsistic world of unreality that is serenely cut off from any possibility of worldly competition, risk, or suspense (e.g., Adolf Wölfli's delusional memories of sublime cosmic journeying; Sass 2004b). The presence of motivations such as these should not, however, be generalized. Delusions can also be excruciating or horrifying; and these hardly seem defensive or compensatory.

We have been concerned with alterations in the quality of objects and events, and with the experience of one's own thinking and bodily sensations. In the next two sections we turn to an aspect of experience that is crucial in schizophrenic delusion but remains poorly understood and under-described: with challenges to (what Husserl (1983) called) the "natural attitude" itself, namely, to the very sense of encountering an objective or shared world and thus to the world's full ontological status in the full sense of that term.

Double Bookkeeping

One of the most puzzling aspects of delusion, at least in schizophrenia, is the question of the experienced reality-status of the delusional beliefs or quasi-beliefs at issue.[7] Standard definitions imply that delusions involve claims about external or public reality that happen to be false, but it is not always obvious that this is truly the case. Jaspers (1963, pp. 105–106) spoke of "the specific schizophrenic incorrigibility," but stated:

> we should look at *what* it is that is actually incorrigible.... Reality for [the patient] does not always carry the same meaning as that of normal reality.... Hence the attitude of the patient to the content of his delusion is peculiarly inconsequent at times. .. Belief in reality can range through all degrees, from a mere play with possibilities via a double reality—the empirical and the delusional—to unequivocal attitudes in which the delusional content reigns as the sole and absolute reality.

But even when delusion reigns as "sole and absolute," it is not clear that it is experienced within anything like the "natural attitude." Telling illustrations of these aspects can be found in the case of Daniel Paul Schreber, perhaps the most famous patient in the history of psychiatry.

In his memoirs, Schreber (1988), who suffered from paranoid schizophrenia, describes an elaborate delusional world consisting of "souls" and "gods" and of "nerves" and "rays" that seem to span the cosmos, to connect him with God and, often, to monitor or control his thoughts and actions. He speaks of being transformed into a woman, of losing his stomach and having it reappear repeatedly, and of foreign beings inhabiting his consciousness and controlling his thoughts. But though Schreber clearly took these delusional realities very seriously indeed (his revelations, he claims, afforded him "deeper insight than [that available to] all other human beings" (p. 7)) and is (in some sense) confident of their truth value

---

[7] For extensive discussion of this issue, see Sass (in press).

("I have come infinitely closer to the truth than human beings who have not received divine revelation" (p. 41))—still he does not seem to have ascribed to them the kind of reality-status or ontological weight of something objectively real, or in which he could be said fully to believe—at least in the standard sense of that term. This is apparent in his description of being transformed into a woman.

As Schreber explains in the memoir, his feminization occurred when he stood before a mirror looking at himself while stripped to the waist and wearing feminine jewelry. As he stared at his own torso, he would feel the approach of "the rays," which constitute an important center of consciousness in his delusional world, and then, he explains, "my breast gives the impression [*Eindruck*] of a pretty well-developed female bosom" (p. 207). Attentive reading makes it clear the Schreber is *not* describing an actual anatomical change, but something more like a way of seeing or construing an unchanged physical reality: "Naturally hairs remain.... on my chest ... ; my nipples also remain small as in the male sex" (p. 207). Indeed, he even speaks of getting "the undoubted *impression* of a female trunk—especially when the illusion [*Illusion*] is strengthened by some feminine adornments" (p. 26). Typically Schreber does *not* make claims about the external or interpersonally shared world, claims that could be supported or refuted by evidence independent of the experience itself. His delusional beliefs are frequently described in a way that gives them a coefficient or accent of subjectivity—as when he says not "I am a scoffer at God" or "I am given to voluptuous excesses," but I am "represented" [*dargestellt*] as one of these things' (p. 27). (See Box 39.7.)

We see, then, that the delusions of at least this classic case lack the kind of straightforward objective or intersubjective referentiality that would seem to be implied by the standard "poor reality testing" formula, with its use of such terms as "false," "incorrect," and "absurd." What is suggested, rather, is something akin to Bleuler's (1911/1950, p. 378) double book-keeping or double registration, where the patient experiences the delusional reality as existing in a different ontological domain from that of everyday reality. This, perhaps, is what Sophie, a woman diagnosed with schizophrenia, is referring to when she states: "I often feel that many of my aberrant pseudo-perceptions feel the way they do because I am actually perceiving them taking place in a parallel reality that only partially overlaps with this one."[8] Sophie was well aware of the difficulty of describing this aspect of her delusional experiences, and complained of the incomprehension of virtually all the doctors and therapists whom she had known. (See Box 39.8.)

Box 39.7 Vignette 7

I have to confirm the first part (a) of this [Dr. Weber's] statement, namely that my so-called delusional system is unshakable certainty, with the same decisive "yes" as I have to counter the second part (b), namely that my delusions are adequate motive for action, with the strongest possible "no." I could even say with Jesus Christ: "My Kingdom is not of this world"; my so-called delusions are concerned solely with God and the beyond; they can therefore never in any way influence my behavior in any worldly matter...

(Schreber 1988, *Memoirs of My Nervous Illness*, pp. 301–302)

---

[8] All quotations from Sophie are taken from emails written to the first author in 2010 and 2011. We are very grateful for her contribution.

Box 39.8 Vignette 8

I often feel that many of my aberrant pseudo-perceptions feel the way they do because I am actually perceiving them taking place in a parallel reality that only partially overlaps with this one. She continues:

  For instance I can feel absolutely certain that space and time (and hence physical reality) no longer or never did exist, and yet understand that in order to get to a psychiatry appointment I have to walk down the street, get on the train, and so on (in other words, physically navigate or move through the "objective" world). Or I can feel certain, even as I am talking to my psychiatrist, that I killed him five minutes earlier (fully aware that he is sitting a few feet from me talking). The strangeness is that both "beliefs" exist simultaneously and seem in no way to impinge on one another (nor have I ever figured out any way of consciously reconciling them)—which is not to say that the very simultaneity isn't rather deeply disturbing (it is, and it often drives me to self-consciously engage with and elaborate on the delusional in order to escape this painful contradiction).

(Sophie)

Schreber (1988, p. 28) too was acutely conscious of the difficulty of conveying the precise nature of his experiences and the likelihood of being misunderstood by his readers or other interlocutors: "Again it is extremely difficult to describe such changes in words because matters are dealt with which lack all analogies in human experience and which I appreciated directly only in part with my mind's eye [*mit meinem geistigen Auge*]." "To make myself at least somewhat comprehensible I shall have to speak much in images and similes, which may at times perhaps be only *approximately* correct" (p. 28).

Various phenomenologists (Blankenburg 1971; Tatossian 1997) have suggested an affinity between this fundamental stance or orientation and the nature of phenomenological "bracketing" or the phenomenological "reduction" itself, which is the key methodological move of Husserlian phenomenology. In phenomenological bracketing one sets aside the objectivist claims of the "natural attitude" in order to isolate an immanent realm of pure experiencing, a realm from which doubt can presumably be expunged and within which "apodictic" or absolute certitude can be achieved. Another affinity (neither, of course, is an exact parallel) is with the experiential stance or modality of imagination. As philosopher Edward Casey (2000) points out in *Imagining: A Phenomenological Study*, the imaginary realm or modality is characterized by a felt discontinuity or delimitation from other psychological acts, such as perception and memory. It implies as well a certain "unexplorability": the imagined object, insofar as it exists at all, is given all at once, without a backside or hidden depth. The imagined object or event is also self-evident in the sense of being non-corrigible (non-falsifiable, non-verifiable) and apodictic: containing a kind of indubitable presence and certainty: hence "I cannot doubt that what I imagine is appearing to me precisely as it presents itself to me" (Casey 2000, p. 98).

Drawing these parallels may help to explain a feature of many schizophrenic delusions that might otherwise seem strange and even nonsensical: the characteristic combination of what Jaspers (1963) called "certitude" with "inconsequentiality"—and especially the seemingly odd fact that it is often the delusion about which the patient is *most certain* with regard to which he is *least likely* to act. If one imagines that the delusion is believed in the context of something like a (subjectively maintained) natural attitude, this makes no sense—for surely one ought to act in relation to that whose existence one most assumes. But if the delusion is felt to be true only *for me*, in my mind's eye and for me alone (or, at least, only for me and my *delusional* others), then the contradiction is resolved: One need hardly seek evidence for an experience (akin in this sense to the imaginary) that makes no claim with regard to objective or normal intersubjective reality; and one will hardly take action *in actuality* with regard to what one knows to exist in a purely virtual realm. This provides a phenomenological way of accounting for at least some instances of the famous "double bookkeeping" of which Bleuler spoke. The patient who insists he is God or Napoleon, yet willingly sweeps the floor, would presumably recognize that this God-status is purely subjective—only a kind of imaginary truth, holding within his own mind's eye world, and therefore irrelevant to the daily routine of life on the hospital ward.[9, 10] Indeed the very unreality of the delusional world may, in fact, be the feature that most recommends it, providing the deepest motivation for dwelling in the delusional realm (see Sartre regarding the "morbid dreamer" in Sass 1992b).

The status of the imaginary is not of course *identical* to that of delusion. (The experience of delusion may be closer to that of dreams than to imagination, but here too there are important differences.) For the normal individual, and even for the artist or writer (except perhaps in the throes of creative trance), the imaginary realm remains *subordinated* to the primacy of the natural attitude. As a result, the "suspension of disbelief" characteristic of imaginary or aesthetic experience is never complete enough to allow the imaginary to become the dominant realm—to eclipse "reality" and replace it with something else.

The standard explanations for *why* such an eclipse often does occur in schizophrenia point to a supposed cognitive deficiency, some inability to monitor external reality or the boundary between the internal and the external world, probably due to a loss of rational faculties rooted in dysfunction of the frontal lobes. But there are problems with such explanations.[11] These include evidence that not the rational capacity but something closer to practicality and common sense is what is most disturbed in schizophrenia (Owen et al. 2007). Also, the most deluded patients with schizophrenia tend to be those whose thinking is more logical (namely, those with *paranoid* as opposed to disorganized or hebephrenic schizophrenia).

It may be more apt to emphasize the importance of the overall or ontological nature of the experiential change—a change that transforms the immediacy of the perceptual world itself and in a totalizing way that alters the very coordinates of reality and possibility. Also important is the role of an attitude or orientation, namely, an autistic stance that fails or refuses (most probably, a combination of failure and refusal) to accept the organizing horizon of intersubjectivity and the natural attitude. The mark of delusion in schizophrenia may be the fact that such persons find it natural to put more or at least equal faith in their own private experiences rather than in the shared, objective world. Unlike the normal person, who

---

[9] Cognitive scientists tend to base their models of delusion formation on formal logic and notions about scientific discovery (e.g., Coltheart et al., 2011). But once belief (the so-called doxastic model) is not assumed, then notions from aesthetic or imaginative experience may seem equally or more relevant.

[10] Incidentally, after his cogent critique of standard views, Manfred Spitzer (1990) suggests an alternative definition of delusion as involving "statements about external reality which are uttered like statements about a mental state, i.e., with subjective certainty and incorrigible by others" (p. 147). Spitzer does not, however, take the next, phenomenological step of suggesting that delusions may, in some sense, actually be *experienced* by the patient as if they were akin to subjective contents of his or her own mind.

[11] Jaspers (1963, p. 97) recognized this long ago: "For any true grasp of delusion, it is most important to free ourselves from this prejudice that there has to be some poverty of intelligence at the root of it."

only sojourns in the imaginary, the individual with schizophrenia does not have the same, unshakeable faith in the public, the objective, and the ordinary. Sophie, at least, rejects ignorance or intellectual incapacity as the source of her perspective: "I cannot count the number of times I've been told 'but Sophie, X is impossible' and all I ever want to say in response is 'yes, I am perfectly capable of appreciating why you think X is impossible, but your conceptual or metaphysical constraints are simply not mine.'" All this goes some way toward explaining the *acceptance* and *persistence* of delusional ideas—the fact that apparently absurd notions, once they occur, are not rejected, as would be the case for a person operating within a normal intersubjective framework and with a standard "belief evaluating system" (Coltheart et al. 2011, p. 293). Perhaps the most useful analogy is the dream-state—in which one turns away from practical and shared reality in favor of a largely passive witnessing of a private realm that lacks normal constraints of time, space, and identity.

DOUBLE EXPOSURE

The notion of poor reality-testing generally implies that the patient takes the imaginary for real, that he *believes* in his imaginary objects with essentially the same form of belief as we address to our surrounding world (i.e., adopting the doxastic or "natural attitude"). This may well capture the condition of *some* schizophrenia patients at least *some* of the time, perhaps especially in the case of the more world-oriented paranoid delusions. The notion of double bookkeeping implies, by contrast, that the patient recognizes the essential unreality of his delusional world and thus of the distinction between the imaginary and the real. This seems to approximate the condition of certain chronic patients for whom delusional reality can afford reliable escape from both the content and the form of the real (Wölfli; e.g., Sass 2004b). But often, one must recognize, things are not so clear-cut, nor so potentially reassuring for the deluded person.

The parallel realities may in fact be difficult to distinguish one from another. The patient may feel uncertain as to which track he is on, or may sense that the different tracks intersect or even fuse with each other in unanticipated ways. There is the possibility, in fact, that rather than double bookkeeping, the patient will experience something more like a kind of photographic *double exposure*: a merging of two perspectives on reality akin to the famous "contamination" response on the Rorschach test—with all the potential for confusion this implies. As Sophie states: "often I feel like a big part of the problem is precisely that I lose my conceptual (metaphysical and experiential) grasp of what reality is, was, or should be." "Isn't the general (unconscious) confusion of perception, fantasy, memory, and imagination simply a ubiquitous part of each and every delusion?" she asks. (See Boxes 39.9 and 39.10.)

But it would be wrong to assimilate this confusion to the poor reality-testing notion as this is usually understood (e.g., DSM's "false [belief] about external reality"). What actually occurs may, in fact, involve less a sense of everything being *real*, an object of standard belief, than of everything being somehow *unreal*; there may even be a breakdown of the very distinction between real and unreal, in which everything seems uncertain or somehow unhinged. We have seen, after all, that derealization can affect not only a separate delusional realm of fantasies, but also the experience of one's *actual* body, thoughts, and surrounding world. Schreber (1988), for instance, experienced *actual* people in his asylum as what he

---

Box 39.9 Vignette 9

Whenever I took my eyes off them [the hospital guards], they disappeared. In fact, everything at which I did not direct my entire attention seemed not to exist. There was some curious consistency in the working of my eyes. Instead of being able to focus on one object and retain a visual awareness of being in a room, a visual consciousness of the number of objects and people in that room, all that existed was directly in my line of vision.

(F. Peters, in Landis 1964, *Varieties of Psychopathological Experience*, p. 90)

Box 39.10 Vignette 10

The term coexistence is not meant to imply a literal or qualitatively symmetrical "doubling" of phenomena—i.e., it's not like literally seeing both a distorted chair and normal chair at the same time (or as somehow superimposed on each other). Instead a single chair may seem perceptually distorted and yet if one checks oneself one realizes that it really isn't (somehow it appears radically changed and perfectly normal at the same time but the former apperception is considerably more vague, amorphous and/or "unbookable").

(Sophie)

---

called the "fleeting-improvised men"—beings who only existed when he laid eyes on them (this also relates to what Schreber calls the "wasp miracle"); this could lend just about everything a certain tinge of unreality. Given this nearly *universal* derealization, it is understandable that the very distinction between realms might come into question.

As already noted, the experience of unreality can serve defensive purposes, perhaps akin to the derealization characteristic of depersonalization disorder and post-traumatic stress disorder. It would not, however, be an entirely willful or teleological product, but also the product of a basic ipseity disturbance that is partly grounded in neurobiological factors: Without a foundational sense of existing as a subject, seat, or locus of consciousness, whatever manifests itself within consciousness will readily seem unreal.[12]

Still, to speak of this as a universal subjectivizing or even derealization also has some potential to be misleading. We must recognize that whereas *some* of the features of "the real" may be absent in certain delusional states (such as the sense that events are consequential and, in some sense, irreversible), others may be present (e.g., the sense that I cannot control delusional objects or situations). Equally important is the fact that such terms as "subjective" or "objective," "real" or "unreal" can hardly retain their usual meanings if one enters a world in which the basic ontological coordinates have changed. In such a world, *all* objects can be experienced in quasi-dreamlike fashion, more as figments or projections than as independent entities persisting through time—thus eliminating the very contrast that normally gives "real" its meaning. Or, stranger still, one can experience one's own experience as somehow belonging to another being, thus as subjective yet alien at the same time. (Consider

---

[12] There is nothing unusual about such tendencies. Psychological defenses typically involve exploitation of propensities (such as a particular cognitive style) that are inherently present on a more foundational, perhaps temperamental fashion (Shapiro 1965). (See footnote 6.)

Schreber's experience of a "seeing" or representing of the femininity of his own torso—a "seeing" that is somehow not his own, even though it is he himself who stand before the mirror doing the staring.) The very meaning of certain unavoidable terms will change when one countenances possibilities of this kind. For how can we say that Schreber's rays and nerves, or his feminized torso, are experienced as either "subjective" *or* "objective," "real" *or* "unreal"? As Sophie writes: "There's a sense in which the law of contradiction—that something can't be X and not X at the same time—has ceased to matter … What I know and what I believe no longer coincide and I can't make them."

There is a technique, used by both Heidegger and Derrida, of writing certain metaphysical terms—words such as subjective, objectivity, or real—while simultaneously crossing them out. This, it seems, is no vain conceit, but almost a requirement for any serious attempt to understand the realm of "true" delusions.

In summary, we have seen that, even within schizophrenia alone, there are multiple and sometimes overlapping ways in which reality may be experienced, including both double bookkeeping and the confusion of double exposure. It seems that delusions, at least in schizophrenia, can frequently involve a mode of experience that is distinct and even, in some sense, *sui generis*. This does not however place them beyond all psychological understanding. One may not be able fully to grasp precisely what it is like to experience one's body mutating or being destroyed, then snapping back to normalcy, or of the world being destroyed yet persisting just the same. Still, one can have inklings, and one can pursue certain analogies; and in doing so approach closer to an understanding than if one had never made the effort in the first place.

A note on treatment: The application of the phenomenological approach to the treatment of delusions cannot, of course, be a purely armchair or anecdotal enterprise, but requires exploration of particular psychotherapeutic strategies and, ultimately, the demonstration of efficacy through empirical means. Still, on theoretical grounds certain implications are suggested. If a particular delusion is not "believed" by the patient in quite the normal manner, but is the consequence or expression of a generally altered mode of being, then one might wonder about the appropriateness of therapeutic techniques (e.g., Kuipers et al. 1997, p. 321) that focus on getting the patient to evaluate the truth value of (and ultimately to refute) such a belief by using argument and evidence that presuppose the natural attitude. Such an approach might be useful with empirical or ontic delusions that fit the poor reality-testing formula. It would seem less to the point in the case of the more ontological or autistic/solipsistic delusions often found in schizophrenia.[13]

DELUSIONS IN OTHER CONDITIONS

The delusions of pure paranoid psychosis ("delusional disorder") have been presumed, by most phenomenologists, to involve a more straightforward condition of belief (e.g., Parnas 2004). Certainly the content of pure paranoid delusion is less likely to include cosmic or

---

[13] One might argue, as well, that the success such techniques seem to have could have more to do with the general way in which such conversation brings the patient into a different, more intersubjective overall orientation, than with the actual processes of refutation per se.

bizarre themes, but rather assertions of an "ontic" or "empirical" kind about real-world beings—e.g., about a malevolent enemy with nefarious intent. Also, the pure paranoid patient seems more likely to engage in actions premised on this kind of normal belief, characteristic of the "natural attitude." All this suggests that the ontological complexities discussed above may not apply in the case of such patients, and that their delusions may fit more directly into the poor-reality-testing formula.[14] But a feature of many such delusions suggests that matters could be slightly more complicated: the fact that paranoid patients (like most delusional patients) tend to avoid putting themselves into situations where their delusional claims could be disproven or refuted (Munro 2000, pp. 655, 664). Does this suggest that they too have a subtle, perhaps background inkling of the unreality or special nature of what they so assertively claim to be the case? (Such avoidance could be related to the fact that a paranoid delusion can serve defensive purposes: despite its frightening nature, it may have a powerful organizing effect, helping the patient avoid an even more frightening sense of chaos or the unknown.) Perhaps the pure paranoid psychotic has a somewhat more qualified form of belief than has been typically assumed, albeit more literal than in the case of schizophrenic double-bookkeeping or subjectivization. Some would suggest that such complex, even contradictory orientations toward the same belief are, in fact, rather common even in normal persons (Manonni 2003).

Another major type of delusion is that of patients with affective psychosis. Such delusions are generally assumed to be but manifestations or consequences of emotions (elation or excitement, shame or despair) that, though exaggerated, are normal in their essential nature and can be tied in with the obvious existential concerns and preoccupations of such individuals—that is, that can be "comprehend(ed) vividly enough as an exaggeration or diminution of known phenomena," in Jaspers' words (1963, p. 577). The manic has delusions of heroic accomplishment, while the melancholic focuses on themes of poverty, illness, death, disgrace, incapacity, or low self-worth (Kraus 1991). Also, affective delusions do not seem to involve the sort of apodictic certitude found in schizophrenia, and appear to bear a more direct relationship to action, even if the behavioral inhibition in severe depression can make this difficult to discern. But here too some further exploration would seem appropriate. It is well known, e.g., that extreme depression (melancholia) typically involves a movement *beyond* sadness or any other recognizable emotion, and seemingly beyond any hint of investment in the social world or interest in the opinions of others—into what seems a void-like realm in which the very existence of self, society, or external world can come into question. This can involve forms of disturbed self-experience somewhat akin to schizophrenia, and that may motivate all-encompassing delusions that may be held with a certainty that can seem impenetrable.

The final set of delusions to be considered are the so-called "monothematic delusions" characteristic of certain neurological conditions. Such delusions are circumscribed in their content, referring to a rather specific *aspect* of experience and without being elaborated in the way that the persecutory, grandiose, or bizarre delusions of schizophrenia or paranoia

---

[14] The psychiatrist Müller-Suur (1950) asked his paranoid and schizophrenic patients how certain they were about their delusions. Whereas paranoiacs believed in their basic experience (*Grunderlebnis*) with a relative certainty, schizophrenia patients claimed to be absolutely certain (100% certainty; as certain as that $2 \times 2 = 4$) about their delusions, even when these delusions seemed absurd to the listener. Müller-Suur describes the delusional certainty of schizophrenics as something that is "suffered"—that is, registered passively, akin to feeling a sensation—whereas the paranoid's was "achieved" or "hard-earned" (presumably, by the seeking of evidence).

may be. Best known are the Capgras delusion, in which the patient thinks that a loved one, such as a family member or spouse, has been replaced by an imposter, and the Cotard delusion, in which the patient claims that he himself is dead.

The delusions have been a major focus of study in cognitive neuroscience and analytic philosophy. Cognitivist explanations typically view the delusions as a disorder of belief, roughly in accordance with the poor-reality-testing formula (they are called "doxastic"). Typically they are explained as a form of false belief that results from a fundamental disorder in perceptual or emotional processing (e.g., Capgras delusion resulting from a disturbance in the affective circuit of visual perception) as well as from some cognitive dysfunction at the level of belief formation that prevents the false belief (e.g., my wife is an imposter or robot) from being rejected despite its apparent absurdity (Coltheart et al. 2011).

Although a phenomenological approach need not reject many elements of the these accounts, it would attempt to look beyond the disturbance as a belief or statement of belief and explore the underlying, abnormal *mode* of experience that might lead to the morbid statement. Ratcliffe (2004) notes, for example, that Capgras patients experience changes not just in their perception of their spouse, but also as a more *general* view of the world. He cites reports in which such patients describe general feelings of unreality or strangeness in relation to the world, which "suggest that certain affects are not *just bodily* [i.e., related to physical sensation] but also structure world experience in some way" (p. 31). Ratcliffe (2008) speaks in particular of "existential feelings" or "feelings of being": In Capgras the "sense of existence and of things 'being what they are,' which 'invades' or 'pounces' on one, is stripped away, leaving a world whose sense of being is diminished or absent" (p. 39). To explain the predicament of the Cotard patient, Ratcliffe draws on Heidegger's description of *Angst*, a mood that breaks apart the "meaning-giving background," leaving a sort of nothingness, as "an absence of ordinary existence-sense" (Heidegger, in Ratcliffe 2004, p. 40). It is not that the Cotard patient *infers* or *believes* that he no longer exists; rather he is responding to an immediate and overall "*experience of nihilation or effacement*" (p. 41).

CONCLUSION

We have offered an overview of the phenomenological approach to delusions, with almost exclusive focus on the so-called "true delusions" of schizophrenia. First we surveyed some distinctive features of the phenomenological approach, including its emphasis on formal qualities of experience and its questioning of standard assumptions about delusions as erroneous belief (the doxastic view or the "poor reality-testing" formula). Then we described the altered modalities of world-oriented and self-oriented experience that precede and ground delusions: the outer and inner *apophany* of "delusional mood" and ipseity-disturbance. We considered the classic question of the understandability or comprehensibility of schizophrenic delusion and the related issue of wish-fulfillment and rationalizing motives. We touched upon the crucial but mysterious and neglected issue of the reality-status of delusions, with critical discussion of derealization, double bookkeeping, and double exposure. Finally we mentioned the rather different kinds of delusions characteristic of paranoid psychosis, affective psychoses, and monothematic organic conditions. We noted some uncertainties about how these latter should be understood—uncertainties that suggest the need to expand phenomenological explorations beyond the domain of schizophrenia.

Acknowledgments

For helpful comments on this chapter, we thank Nev Jones, Brian McLaughlin, Philip Gerrans, Matthew Ratcliffe, and Richard Gipps.

References

American Psychiatric Association (2000). *Diagnostic and Statistical Manual of Mental Disorders, Fourth Edition, Text Revision*. Washington, DC: American Psychiatric Association.

Aviv, R. (2010). Which way madness lies: Can psychosis be prevented? *Harper's Magazine*, December, 35–46.

Berze, J. and Gruhle, H. W. (1929). *Psychologie der Schizophrenie*. Berlin: Julius Springer.

Bleuler, E. (1950). *Dementia Praecox or the Group of Schizophrenias* (J. Zinkin Trans.). New York, NY: International Universities Press. (Original work published 1911.)

Bortolotti, L. (2009). *Delusions and Other Irrational Beliefs*. Oxford: Oxford University Press.

Blankenburg, W. (1971). *Der Verlust der Naturlichen Selbstverstandlichkeit: Ein Beitrag zur Psychopathologie Symptomarmer Schizophrenien*. Stuttgart: Ferdinand Enke Verlag.

Bovet, P. and Parnas J. (1993). Schizophrenic delusions: A phenomenological approach. *Schizophrenia Bulletin*, 19, 579–97.

Campbell, J. (2001). Rationality, meaning, and the analysis of delusion. *Philosophy Psychiatry, & Psychology*, 8, 89–100.

Casey, E. (2000). *Imagining: A Phenomenological Study*. Bloomington, IN: Indiana University Press.

Cermolacce, M., Sass, L., and Parnas, J. (2010). What is bizarre in bizarre delusions: A critical review. *Schizophrenia Bulletin*, 34, 667–79.

Coltheart, M., Langdon, R., and McKay, R. (2011). Delusional belief. *Annual Review of Psychology*, 62, 271–98.

Conrad, K. (1997). *La Esquizofrenia Incipiente* (J. M. Belda and A. Rabano, Trans.). Madrid: Fundación Archivos de Neurobiología. (Original work published in German: Conrad, K. (1958). *Die Beginnende Schizophrenie: Versuch einer Gestatlanalyse des Wahns*. Stuttgart: Georg Thieme Verlag.)

Currie, G. (2000). Imagination, delusion, and hallucination. *Mind & Language*, 15, 168–83.

Cutting, J. and Shepherd, M. (Eds) (1987). *The Clinical Roots of the Schizophrenia Concept*. Cambridge: Cambridge University Press.

Ey, H. (1996). *Schizophrénie: Études Cliniques et Psychopathologiques*. Les Plessis-Robinson: Synthelabo.

Fuchs, T. (2005). Delusional mood and delusional perception—A phenomenological analysis. *Psychopathology*, 38, 133–9.

Fuentenebro, F. and Berrios, G. (1995). The predelusional state. *Comprehensive Psychiatry*, 36, 251–9.

Gerrans, P. (in press). *The Measure of Madness. Philosophy and Cognitive Neuropsychiatry*. Cambridge, MA: MIT Press.

Heidegger, M. (1996). *Being and Time* (J. Stambaugh, Trans.). Albany, NY: State University of New York Press.

Husserl, E. (1983). *Ideas Pertaining to a Pure Phenomenology and to a Phenomenological Philosophy: First Book* (F. Kersten, Trans.). Dordrecht: Kluwer.

Husserl, E. (1989). *Ideas Pertaining to a Pure Phenomenology and to a Phenomenological Philosophy: Second Book: Studies in the Phenomenology of Constitution* (R. Rojcewicz and A. Schuwer, Trans.). Dordrecht: Kluwer.

Jaspers, K. (1963). *General Psychopathology* (J. Hoenig and M. Hamilton, Trans.). Chicago, IL: University of Chicago Press.

Jean, M. (Ed.) (1980). *The Autobiography of Surrealism*. New York, NY: Viking.

Klosterkoetter, J., Hellmich, M., Steinmeyer, E. M., and Schultze-Lutter, F. (2001). Diagnosing schizophrenia in the initial prodromal phase. *Archives of General Psychiatry*, *58*, 158–64.

Kraus, A. (1991). Der melancholische Wahn in identitätstheoretischer Sicht. In W. Blankenburg (Ed.), *Forum der Psychiatrie: Wahn und Perspektivität*, pp. 81–9. Stuttgart: Ferdinand Enke Verlag.

Kuipers, E., Garety, P., Fowler, D., Dunn, G., Bebbington, P., Freeman, D., *et al.* (1997). London-East Anglia randomised control trial of cognitive-behavioural therapy for psychosis, I: Effects of the treatment phase. *British Journal of Psychiatry*, *171*, 319–27.

Laing, R. D. (1960). *The Divided Self: An Existential Study in Sanity and Madness*. Harmondsworth: Penguin.

Landis, C. (1964). *Varieties of Psychopathological Experience*. New York, NY: Holt, Rinehart & Winston.

Manonni, O. (2003). I know well but all the same. In M. A. Rothenberg, D. A. Foster, and S. Zizek (Eds), *Perversion and the social relationship*, pp. 62–91. Durham NC: Duke University Press.

Matussek, P. (1987). Studies in delusional perception. In J. Cutting and M. Shepherd (Eds), *The Clinical Roots of the Schizophrenia Concept*, pp. 89–104. Cambridge: Cambridge University Press.

Møller, P. and Husby, R. (2000). The initial prodrome in schizophrenia: Searching for naturalistic core dimensions of experience and behavior. *Schizophrenia Bulletin*, *26*, 217–32.

Moran, D. (2000). *Introduction to Phenomenology*. New York, NY: Routledge.

Munro, A. (2000). Persistent delusion symptoms and disorders. In M. Gelder, J. López-Ibor, and N. Andreasen (Eds), *New Oxford Textbook of Psychiatry*, pp. 651–76. Oxford: Oxford University Press.

Müller-Suur, H. (1950). Das Gewissheitsproblem beim schizophrenen und beim paranoischen Wahnerleben. *Fortschritte der Neurologie, Psychiatrie under ihrer Grenzgebiete*, *18*, 44–51.

Owen, G., Cutting, J., and David, A. S. (2007). Are people with schizophrenia more logical than healthy volunteers? *British Journal of Psychiatry*, *191*, 453–4.

Parnas, J. (2004). Belief and pathology of self-awareness: A Phenomenological contribution to the classification of delusions. *Journal of Consciousness Studies*, *11*, 148–61.

Parnas, J., Møller, P., Kircher, T., Thalbitzer, J., Jansson, L., Handest, P., *et al.* (2005). EASE: Examination of Anomalous Self Experience. *Psychopathology*, *38*, 236–58.

Parnas, J. and Sass, L. (2001). Self, solipsism, and schizophrenic delusions. *Philosophy, Psychiatry, & Psychology*, *8*, 101–20.

Ratcliffe, M. (2004). Interpreting delusions. *Phenomenology and the Cognitive Sciences*, *3*, 25–48.

Ratcliffe, M. (2008). *Feelings of Being*. Oxford: Oxford University Press.

Read, R. (2001). On approaching schizophrenia through Wittgenstein. *Philosophical Psychology*, *14*, 449–75.

Rümke, H. C. (1950). Significance of phenomenology for the clinical study of sufferers of delusion. In F. Morel (Ed.), *Psychopathologie des Délires* (papers from *Congrés International de Psychiatrie*), pp. 174–209. Paris: Hermann.

Saks, E. (2007). *The Center Cannot Hold: My Journey Through Madness*. New York, NY: Harper & Row.

Sass, L. (1992a). Heidegger, schizophrenia, and the ontological difference. *Philosophical Psychology*, 5, 109–32.

Sass, L. (1992b). *Madness and Modernism: Insanity in the Light of Modern Art, Literature, and Thought*. New York, NY: Basic Books.

Sass, L. (1994). *The Paradoxes of Delusion: Wittgenstein, Schreber, and the Schizophrenic Mind*. Ithaca, NY: Cornell University Press.

Sass, L. (2003). Incomprehensibility and understanding: On the interpretation of severe mental illness (reply to Rupert Read). *Philosophy, Psychiatry, & Psychology*, 10, 125–32.

Sass, L. (2004a). Some reflections on the (analytic) philosophical approach to delusion. *Philosophy, Psychiatry, & Psychology*, 11, 71–80.

Sass, L. (2004b). Affectivity in schizophrenia: A phenomenological perspective. *Journal of Consciousness Studies*, 11, 127–47.

Sass, L. (2010). Phenomenology as description and as explanation. In S. Gallagher and D. Schmicking (Eds), *Handbook of Phenomenology and the Cognitive Sciences*, pp. 635–54. Berlin: Springer Verlag.

Sass, L. (in press). Delusion and double bookkeeping. In G. Stanghellini and T. Fuchs (Eds), *One Century of Karl Jaspers' General Psychopathology*. Oxford: Oxford University Press.

Sass, L. and Parnas, J. (2003). Schizophrenia, consciousness, and the self. *Schizophrenia Bulletin*, 29, 427–44.

Schreber, D. P. (1988). *Memoirs of My Nervous Illness* (I. Macalpine and R. Hunter, Trans.). Cambridge, MA: Harvard University Press.

Sèchehaye, M. (1951). *Autobiography of a Schizophrenic Girl*. New York, NY: Grune and Stratton.

Shapiro, D. (1965). *Neurotic Styles*. New York, NY: Basic Books.

Silberer, H. (1951). Report on a method of eliciting and observing certain symbolic hallucination-phenomena. In D. Rapaport (Ed.), *Organization and Pathology of Thought: Selected Sources*, pp. 195–207. New York, NY: Columbia University Press.

Spitzer, M. (1990). On defining delusions. *Comprehensive Psychiatry*, 31, 377–97.

Tatossian, A. (1997). *La Phénomémologie des Psychoses*. Paris: Imprimerie Desseaux.

Walker, C. (1991). Delusion: What did Jaspers really say? *British Journal of Psychiatry*, 159, 94–103.

CHAPTER 40

THOUGHT INSERTION, SELF-AWARENESS, AND RATIONALITY

JOHANNES ROESSLER

Thought insertion raises two kinds of philosophical issues: general issues concerning the interpretation of what some diagnostic systems in psychiatry call bizarre delusions, and specific issues concerning the nature of self-awareness and its pathologies. The basic philosophical puzzle generated by the delusion, I suggest, may be put in the form of an inconsistent triad that brings together both kinds of concerns.

> *Transparency:* To be introspectively aware of a current episode of thinking that p is to be aware of oneself thinking that p.
>
> *Alienation:* Patients with the delusion of thought insertion believe that someone else is the thinker of an episode of thinking of which they are introspectively aware.
>
> *Intelligibility:* Reports of thought insertion express rationally intelligible, coherent beliefs.

Let me start by going over the apparent inconsistency between the three claims. Consider an example of thought insertion: "Thoughts are put into my mind like 'Kill God.' It is just like my mind working, but it isn't. They come from this chap, Chris. They are his thoughts." Transparency—or its natural extension to the case of thoughts in the imperative mood—suggests that insofar as the patient is introspectively aware of an episode of thinking "Kill God" he is aware of *himself* thinking "Kill God." His introspective awareness cannot settle the question of *what* is being thought without simultaneously settling the question of *who* is thinking it, viz. he himself. Then if the patient nevertheless believes that someone else is the thinker of the episode in question, as Alienation maintains, this would not just be an eccentric or mildly irrational belief, on a par with ideas such as telepathy. Rather the belief would be manifestly inconsistent with the content of the patient's introspective knowledge. This interpretation would scupper any prospects for attempting to make rational sense of the delusion, as demanded by Intelligibility.

The standard view in the recent philosophical literature on thought insertion is that reflection on the delusion should lead us to discard, or at least modify, Transparency. This view goes back to two pioneering papers published in the 1990s, by Stephens and Graham

(1994) and by John Campbell (1999). They propose different versions of what I will call the two-concept view. Commonsense psychology, they claim, recognizes two distinct concepts of ownership of a thought, "introspective" and "agentive" ownership (my terminology, not theirs). Given that these are distinct concepts, one may coherently acknowledge one's "introspective ownership" of an episode of thinking while simultaneously questioning or denying that one is the "agent" of the episode. This, according to the standard view, is what patients are doing. As far as this core element of the delusion is concerned, the delusion involves a perfectly coherent belief. Moreover, two-concept theorists standardly argue that it is possible to make sense of a patient's acquisition of the belief by adverting to their highly unusual inner experience, perhaps involving an impaired sense of agency. This does not mean that proponents of the standard view will accept Intelligibility without qualification. They are not committed to the simple scheme "abnormal experience/rational belief." They may concede, for example, that patients' tendency to attribute the thinking in question to other individuals and to invoke abstruse mechanisms of "transmission," or even just their apparent inability to appreciate the implausibility, all things considered, of their denial of "agentive ownership," reflects a disorder of rationality, in addition to disturbed inner experience. However, these are relatively minor qualifications. The standard view does endorse Intelligibility at least on this minimal reading: the core of the delusion—the denial of ownership of an episode of thinking—is a coherent belief that is open to reason-giving explanation; patients' abnormal inner experience provides them at least with a prima facie reason for denying "agentive ownership."

I started by distinguishing two kinds of issues raised by thought insertion, to do with the interpretation of "bizarre" delusions in general, and with the nature of self-awareness in particular. I want to suggest that on both counts the standard view faces serious problems. In the first half of the chapter I focus on self-awareness. The standard view insists that self-awareness exhibits a certain explanatory structure, which in turn yields a substantive explanation of the kind of alienation voiced in reports of thought insertion. I want to argue that recent attempts to identify some such structure have been unsuccessful. I shall also suggest that there are good reasons to think that the search for it is futile, and that Transparency resists revision (second and third sections, "Inner speech" and "Making sense"). In the fourth section ("Empirical versus autistic-schizophrenic delusions") I present independent reasons for thinking that it is Intelligibility that should be modified. On the "historical" analysis of thought insertion to be explored in the last section ("Thought insertion and its history"), interpreting the delusion requires paying close attention to its prehistory in the prodromal phase of schizophrenia. On this account, the truth in Intelligibility is this: Reports of thought insertion express attitudes that *originate in* rationally intelligible, coherent beliefs.

TRANSPARENCY

I am going to use the notion of introspective awareness in a fairly non-committal way. To speak of introspective awareness of episodes of thinking, as I understand the notion, does not commit one to the view that introspection is a special source of knowledge, let alone one that involves some quasi-perceptual awareness of inner objects. Introspective awareness of an event may just be a matter of having a distinctive kind of propositional knowledge of the occurrence of the event—knowledge, at a first pass, that is non-inferential and non-observational. We can take transparency in an equally low key. The basic idea is that when you enjoy introspective awareness of an episode of thinking, the question of who is doing the thinking is "transparent to" the question of what is being thought. That is, insofar as your introspective awareness provides an answer to the latter question, the first question is settled—you are committed to a *self*-ascription of the episode.

The idea is familiar from discussions of "immunity to error through misidentification." For Transparency suggests that a certain kind of question, and a certain kind of error, would not be rationally intelligible. Consider Wittgenstein's well-known remark in the *Blue Book* (I've adapted the example):

> There is no question of recognizing a person when I say "I think it will rain." To ask "Are you sure that it's *you* who are thinking it will rain?' would be nonsensical. Now, when in this case no error is possible, it is because the move which we might be inclined to think of as an error, a "bad move," is no move of the game at all.[1]

If Wittgenstein is right, then thought insertion, construed on the lines of Alienation, involves a belief that is not an error or a "bad move" but no move at all. This is what the two-concept view denies. Two-concept theorists agree that it would be "no move at all" to question one's *introspective* ownership of a current episode of thinking, perhaps by asking "Is this episode occurring in *my* mind?" After all, they hold that introspective awareness of an episode is a necessary and sufficient condition for ownership in the "introspective" sense. But they insist that "*I think*" is naturally used to talk about ownership in the "agentive" sense. And when it comes to "agentive" ownership, they claim, we should reject Transparency.

Here is how Stephens and Graham put the idea:

> There may well be a sense of the verb *to think* in which the statement "I am the subject in whom the thought occurs" necessarily entails "I think the thought." We contend, however, that the verb also has a sense in which "I think a thought" indicates not that I am the subject in whom the thought occurs but that I am the agent of the thought. It is this sense of *to think* that is relevant to understanding thought insertions. And when *to think* is used in this agentive sense the above entailment fails to hold. (Stephens and Graham 1994, p. 6)

And here is a series of quotations from John Campbell:

> At the very least, these reports by patients show that there is some structure in our ordinary notion of the ownership of a thought which we might not otherwise have suspected.
>
> [T]he schizophrenic has introspective knowledge of a thought of which he does not recognize himself to be the agent.
>
> The content of the schizophrenic's illusion is that he has first-person knowledge of token thoughts which were formed by someone else. (Campbell 1999, pp. 610, 619, 620)

What does it mean to be the "agent of a thought"? A phrase commonly used in the literature as a more familiar-sounding variant is "*author* of a thought." We know what is meant

---

[1] See Wittengstein (1958, p. 67; Wittgenstein's example is "I have toothache.")

by authorship of books or peace plans, and it seems unproblematic to speak of someone's authorship of a thought in just this sense. Note, though, that in the familiar sense, the term applies to types, not tokens. It is books that have authors, not individual copies of books. In the context of thought insertion, therefore, the term "authorship" is not particularly useful: it's obscure what, if anything, the phrase "author of a *token* thought" might mean. This raises a further question. Are there such things as *token thoughts*? If seven members of the audience think the lecture is soporific, how many thoughts are we talking about? The natural answer, I suppose, is "one thought." Could we say, in addition, that seven thoughts "occurred"? No doubt we could—Stephens and Graham, for example, use this construction in the earlier quotation. But that usage is arguably uncommon in ordinary parlance.[2] Moreover, it breeds confusion. What is the relation between a thought someone is thinking and a thought that is "occurring"? The natural answer is that the former is the *content* of an episode of thinking, whereas the latter is the episode of thinking itself. Stephens and Graham tend to conflate the two notions: their wording suggests that when someone thinks a thought, that very thought is something that "occurs." Partly to avoid the risk of equivocation, I prefer the cumbersome phrase "episode of thinking" to "token thought."[3]

How, then, should we understand the notion of "agentive" ownership? On what I'll call the explanatory model, A is the subject of an episode of thinking, in the "agentive" sense, if the episode is *intelligible* in terms of A's propositional attitudes. Stephens and Graham offer a version of this model, as does Campbell. More recent work in the two-concept tradition tends to exploit the idea that thinking involves acts of inner speech: "agentive" ownership of an episode of thinking, on this model, is a matter of being the *agent of an act of inner speech* involved in, or identical with, the episode (Byrne 2011; Jones and Fernyhough 2007; Langland-Hassan 2008). The question whether some version of either—or perhaps both—of these models can be sustained is a major issue in the philosophy of mind. It amounts to nothing less than the question of whether to think is to act, a question that can only be properly addressed in the context of a discussion of an even larger subject, viz., the question of what *actions* are. Fortunately, for my purposes here it will not be necessary to address these big issues head-on. For the question I want to press concerns not so much the notion of "agentive" ownership as such but rather its relation to the putatively distinct and independent notion of "introspective" ownership. What I want to challenge is the assumption that it's possible to be introspectively aware of the content of an episode of thinking without being aware of being the agent of the episode. If the assumption is invalid, Transparency holds for both "introspective" and "agentive" ownership. Indeed no useful purpose will be served by distinguishing the two notions. I begin with the inner speech model. In the "Making sense" section I review the explanatory model.

---

[2] Should this lead us to challenge Alienation? That is, should we question the near-universal assumption that patients use the word "thought" to refer to an episode of thinking? I think the matter is certainly less clear-cut than advocates of the standard view tend to assume. I return to the issue in the last section.

[3] Another reason is the following. Is the thought shared by the seven thinkers adequately understood as a type of which the seven episodes of thinking are tokens? I doubt that it is. The type in question would have to be a type of *event*, but that is arguably not how we think of thoughts when we think of them as things we think or have. For illuminating critical discussion of the application of the type-token distinction to the (in some ways analogous) case of beliefs: see Steward (1997, chapter 4).

Inner Speech

Inner speech involves both agency and sensory phenomenology. This dual nature might inspire the following proposal. If you were to enjoy an experience with the distinctive phenomenology of inner speech without any awareness of performing an act of inner speech, you would be introspectively aware of an episode of thinking without being aware that it is you who is doing the thinking. You might then consistently, and intelligibly, affirm, say, that the thought "Kill God" is being entertained in your mind while denying that it is you who is thinking "Kill God."

I think the most promising way to develop this proposal would be on the following lines. To say something in "inner speech" is to *imagine* saying something. This is not the same as imagining *hearing* anyone say something. Yet it involves a distinctive, and distinctively elusive, kind of auditory phenomenology. For as part of the imaginative project one imagines the auditory experience attendant on the imagined utterance. On the basis of that phenomenology, it might be said, you may recognize that an episode of *thinking* is occurring, even as you lack any awareness of the activity of imagining saying something. In an illuminating paper that provides the most detailed formulation of the "inner speech model" I'm aware of, Peter Langland-Hassan puts the idea as follows: "Because the sensory character of inner speech is not nearly as rich as that of actual speech perception, an act of inner speech is usually phenomenologically distinguishable *as inner speech* partly due to this paucity of sensory character" (2008, p. 393).

One worry about this proposal is that the various kinds of sensory phenomenology relevant here may not actually exhibit any such "Humean" gradation. Note that to identify an experience as an act of inner speech you would need to recognize it not only as one of *imagining* rather than *hearing* (or hallucinating) speech, but also as one of imagining a *performance* rather than an *observation* of a speech act.[4] Especially in the case of the latter pair, it's not clear that its members are clearly discriminable on the basis of their differential "paucity of sensory character."

More importantly, I think it's evident that we don't actually rely on the character of the sensory phenomenology involved in inner speech to recognize that the experience is an episode of *thinking*. Rather, we know that an episode of thinking is occurring in virtue of the way we know *what* is being thought. Consider first the case of hearing someone else say "Kill God." In that case, to know what thought is being expressed you may, and normally need to, listen to what he is saying. At the very least, auditory attention is a possible source of knowledge of the content and type of the utterance. Next suppose you imagine hearing someone

---

[4] I think a third distinction is relevant too, between acts of inner speech that constitute episodes of thinking and acts of inner speech that do not. If I ask you to imagine saying "2 + 2 = 5," your act of inner speech would not be naturally characterized as a case of thinking that 2 + 2 = 5. The point here is not that thinking requires *belief*. As Hampshire reminds us, "there are countless thoughts that occur to me, and that pass through, or that linger, in my mind, and of these only a small minority constitute beliefs" (Hampshire 1965, p. 97–98). The distinction we need is a more subtle one. One suggestion might be that episodes of thinking aim to express views that are least serious contenders for beliefs. If Hampshire is right, Byrne's "epistemic rule" for self-ascribing thoughts—"If the inner voice says that p and p, believe that you are thinking that p" (2011, p. 121)—is too restrictive.

else say "Kill God." In that case, your knowledge of the content and type of the imagined utterance will have no perceptual basis. You will normally have non-observational knowledge of what it is you are imagining. However, it is part of the imaginative project that the imagined experience is one that, in the imagined situation, would provide you with a possible source of knowledge of the content and type of the imagined speech act. Moreover, in the case of relatively spontaneous, "unbidden" imaginings it may be for the subject as if she came to know which speech act she is imagining by listening. Compare and contrast the case of imagining *saying* "Kill God." In this case, you have non-observational knowledge of the type and content of the imagined speech act; and you are not imagining an experience that could provide you with a source of such knowledge—whether in the imagined or indeed in the real situation. The project of finding out what one is thinking by "listening" to one's own inner speech is arguably just as fraught with difficulty as the project of finding out what one is saying by listening to one's own current outer speech. (See O'Shaughnessy 1963.)

I think few would be prepared to deny the existence of some such epistemic "asymmetry" or deny that we have non-observational knowledge of the content of any episode of thinking of which we are introspectively aware.[5] It seems to me, though, that once this point is granted, the idea of introspective awareness of a thought without awareness of being its thinker is beginning to look like a chimera. What is involved in having non-observational knowledge of what one is saying in inner speech? The natural answer is that such knowledge reflects the fact that acts of inner speech are intentional actions and as such performed "knowingly." Following Anscombe we might call this kind of knowledge "knowledge in intention." What makes the proposal so natural is that it explains why we not only don't have to "listen" to what we are saying in inner speech but don't need any other method of *finding out* about the content of what we are saying either: the standpoint we occupy in relation to our own actions is that of practical rather than theoretical reason.[6] You might say that much of our thinking is spontaneous. (It wouldn't be much use if it weren't.) It would be quite mistaken, though, to assume that spontaneous actions cannot be intentional, at least in a broad sense of "intentional." They may involve spontaneously acquired intentions rather than premeditated ones. So they may not be intentional if that is taken to imply prior intent. But they can still be voluntary actions, performed "knowingly" (albeit without *fore*knowledge), in virtue of one's possession of "knowledge in intention." Intentions, though, have a first-personal content, and could not play their distinctive causal and rational role without having a first-personal content.[7] So your knowledge "in intention" of the content of an act of inner speech is knowledge of what you yourself are imagining saying. If the act constitutes an episode of thinking, you know what it is *you* are thinking. If introspective awareness of an episode of thinking that p involves "knowledge in intention" of the content of an act of inner

---

[5] For an exception, see Byrne (2011). Central to Byrne's account are two assumptions: "One can know what one thinks by hearing one's outer speech. Likewise, one can know what one thinks by "hearing" one's inner speech" (2011, p. 115). Byrne assumes, further, that "inwardly speaking about x" is a matter of "auditorily imagining words that are about x." What these assumptions have in common, in my view, is that they misrepresent us as observers of our own current mental activities.

[6] See Anscombe (1957). The concept of "knowledge in intention" can and should arguably be detached from the theoretical elaboration it receives in Anscombe's hands. See Wilson (2000) and Roessler (2010) for discussion.

[7] For illuminating discussion of this point, see Campbell (1994, chapter 5).

speech that p, then such introspective awareness just is awareness of *oneself* silently saying, and thinking, that p. Transparency would be vindicated.

Admittedly my discussion of the inner speech model has been somewhat schematic. Real thinking is a more multifarious matter than imagining saying things. For example, it often involves imagining conversations with others. Sometimes it is far from clear whether one imagines saying something or imagines listening to someone else saying something. I doubt, though, that a more life-like analysis would make a difference to the point that matters in the current context. For even if we sometimes think in the guise of others, or indeed in an indeterminate guise, we know what is being thought in virtue of doing the imagining involved in the thinking. Advocates of the inner speech model may seek to devise an alternative account of introspective knowledge of the content of an episode of thinking, on which such knowledge need not be first-personal. I've argued that appeal to sensory phenomenology would be insufficient. It might be said that the explanation should instead appeal to non-sensory, "cognitive" phenomenology. There is no space here to pursue this, but I think the basic problem is that no method of "finding out," whether it be sensory or otherwise, can deliver knowledge "from within" of what is being thought.

I would like to end this section by drawing attention to an alternative proposal Langland-Hassan makes in the paper already cited. He suggests that "some reports of voices [i.e., auditory-verbal hallucinations] may be reports of *the very same phenomenon* that others report as inserted thoughts" (2008, p. 373, my emphasis). The idea is that thought insertion may reflect an unusual auditory phenomenology that does "not fall neatly into any preexisting category" (p. 373). It seems to me that intuitively this is a more promising way to try to secure an explanatory role for patients' auditory phenomenology. But note that the proposal amounts to a wholesale revision of the standard view of thought insertion. It denies that the delusion arises from ordinary introspective awareness of episodes of thinking. If this denial is correct, our inconsistent triad would be a less serious problem than the standard view makes out. The obvious solution would be to reject Alienation. There would be no need to develop a two-concept theory of thought ownership, or to modify Transparency. The weakness of the proposal, though, is that it remains mysterious why (some) patients should describe a certain kind of *auditory* phenomenology in terms of thoughts, rather than in terms of voices.

MAKING SENSE

Thoughts can be judged in some sense "alien" if they are not intelligible in terms of one's concerns, beliefs, and values. Stephens and Graham think that if a thought were alien, it would, in one sense, not be one's own thought. They compare this with the case of a wayward bodily movement (2000, pp. 153–154). Suppose you feel your arm going up without any sense of raising your arm. You would presumably acknowledge that your arm went up but quite intelligibly, and perhaps correctly, deny that you raised it. (Patients with anarchic hand syndrome find themselves in just this predicament.)

But what would be the analog of the proprioceptive experience of one's arm going up? Suppose advocates of the explanatory model accept my suggestion of the previous section. Suppose they grant that to encounter a thought in one's own mind involves "agentive" self-awareness in the minimal sense that it involves an awareness of (oneself) saying something in inner speech. Still, they might insist that this anemic sense of "agentive" (i.e., introspective) ownership contrasts with the more full-blooded sense in which I am the agent of only those episodes of thinking that are intelligible in terms of my concerns, beliefs, and values. Would this be a stable combination of views? I think not. If thinking involves "knowledge in intention" of what one is saying in inner speech, finding oneself saddled with an alien, unintelligible thought would not be akin to feeling one's arm going up. It would more be like finding oneself raising one's arm, without any sense of why one might have done this. For one thing, one would certainly be aware of *oneself* thinking something, rather than merely of an episode of thinking occurring in one's mind. For another, one would be aware not just of the occurrence of an event but of having an *attitude*—the intention to say something in inner speech—that finds expression in the event.[8] Indeed one would presumably be aware of the attitude as one's own, supposing that one's own first-person intentions are easily apprehended as one's own.

Now it seems to me that as a matter of fact this account is entirely consonant with the way we ordinarily think about thoughts judged to be "alien." The cellist Pablo Casals reports that when his left hand was badly injured during a mountaineering trip on Mount Tamalpais, his first thought was: "Thank goodness, I'll never have to play again." The datum, for Casals, was that he found himself thinking this thought, or equivalently, that the thought occurred to him. The question whether the thought could be understood in terms of his attitudes was not, for Casals, a question that had any bearing on the ownership of the episode of thinking. His own later interpretation was that the thought probably reflected his long struggle with stage fright. But he did not take this to mean that the thought was probably his own. The example also highlights a second problem facing the explanatory model. We are normally aware of our thinking as our own concurrently and effortlessly, without engaging in the construction of an autobiographical narrative that might render the occurrence of the thought intelligible. Stephens and Grahams' version of the explanatory model represents awareness of ownership as an implausibly high-level, reflective matter.[9]

[8] Importantly, acts of inner speech that constitute episodes of *thinking* are informed by further intentions, such as, perhaps, the intention to express a view worth considering. (See footnote 4.)

[9] See Gerrans (2001) for helpful discussion of this problem. In Campbell's theory, the task of determining whether an episode of thinking reflects the subject's "long-standing dispositional states" devolves upon a subpersonal mechanism whose operation is said to result in an occurrent "sense of ownership." This is hard to square with the possibility of cases where finding *oneself* thinking something presents one with an interpretative puzzle, as illustrated in the Casals example. There is also a more basic problem. Why should the question whether an episode of thinking is caused by one's "long-standing dispositional states" have any bearing on one's ownership of the episode? Campbell's answer turns on the idea that the owner, and "agent," of a token thought is the person "producing" or "forming" it or "bringing it into existence" (see especially Campbell 2002), where this, in turn, is thought to be a matter of the token thoughts being produced by the person's long-standing dispositional states. Now "being the effect of a propositional attitude" is not sufficient for "being something that has an agent." (A headache may be brought on by a complex combination of propositional attitudes but it is not clear what it would mean to be the agent of a headache.) If a "token thought" is to be something that has an agent, the attitudes producing it would presumably have to include an *intention* to produce a (certain kind of) "token thought." But in that case, ownership could be secured simply in virtue of having a *proximal* intention to think something now. Intelligibility in terms of one's "long-standing dispositional states" would be quite irrelevant to the issue of ownership.

Explanatory theorists, then, should reject the view that thinking involves an awareness of saying things in inner speech. They need a conception of thinking on which there can be such a thing as a primitive, wholly "non-agentive" introspective encounter with an episode of thinking in one's own mind—somewhat analogous to a proprioceptive experience of one's arm going up. The crucial disanalogy, it seems to me, is that in the introspective case, there is awareness of the intentional *content* of the episode. The content of the episode is determined by the attitudes finding expression in that episode. So it is hard to see how one can be aware "from within" of the content of the episode, without enjoying an awareness "from within" of the attitudes expressed in it.

EMPIRICAL VERSUS AUTISTIC-SCHIZOPHRENIC DELUSIONS

If Transparency is resistant to revision, the natural course to adopt is to probe Intelligibility. This, according to some psychiatrists, is what we should have done in the first place. The idea that schizophrenic delusions are to be interpreted as rational descriptions of abnormal experiences, according to these psychiatrists, falsifies the nature and depth of the disturbance of the normal state of consciousness in schizophrenia. I want to look at a recent elaboration of this view by Josef Parnas and his collaborators. I then state what I take to be the two major challenges confronting the task of revising Intelligibility. In the final section I argue that these challenges can be met by taking into account the *prehistory* of the delusion.

Parnas's view of what he calls "autistic-schizophrenic" (or "bizarre") delusions is best understood by way of the contrast he draws with "empirical" delusions. Empirical delusions generally "comply with a normative view of natural causality" (give or take some idiosyncrasies), they tend to be about everyday matters (such as that one's home is infested with insects), and they reflect concerns that often "caricature human desires familiar to most of us, e.g., becoming rich, starting a software company in order to compete Microsoft out of business" and so forth (Parnas 2004, p. 155). Furthermore, empirical delusions are like ordinary beliefs in being "attached to the intersubjective world": patients frequently and sometimes passionately try to convince others of the correctness of their delusions. It's not unusual for them to produce supporting evidence during consultations with their psychiatrist. In contrast, not only is the content of autistic-schizophrenic delusions far removed from everyday concerns (as thought insertion illustrates), but they are "intersubjectively disengaged," partly in that patients tend not to argue for their delusions. Indeed they can be puzzled by the request for supporting reasons. To a patient with schizophrenia, Parnas suggests, a delusion is given with the same kind of "experiential evidence" we would normally associate with avowals of pain (2004, p. 158). When asked about their reasons, these patients may feel the way most of us would feel if asked "What makes you think you have a headache?"

In the case of empirical delusions, there can be no doubt that patients know what they are talking about. The patient who thought her home was infested with insects, for example, was remarkably resourceful in explaining away unwelcome evidence. Still, her conception of what evidence was *relevant* to her claim was intact, reflecting her undiminished grasp of the content of her belief. In the case of autistic-schizophrenic delusions, the question whether patients really know what they are saying is at least a natural question to ask. For their conception of what counts as relevant evidence appears to bear no intelligible relation to the content of the delusion. It certainly seems to bear no such relation in cases where patients are mystified by the very idea that their claims might stand in need of supporting evidence. But even in cases where justifying reasons are provided, patients' views of what counts as a good reason reflect at best an idiosyncratic understanding of what they are saying.[10]

Parnas's view may be put by saying that in the light of this disconnection between evidence and content we should abandon the quixotic project of making rational sense of the delusion. To pursue that project is to falsify the phenomenon. It is to mistake an autistic-schizophrenic delusion for an empirical delusion. That is not to say that such delusions are ununderstandable. On Parnas's view, schizophrenia is a "disorder of consciousness." It involves a fundamental transformation and disturbance of the normal state of consciousness, affecting both the "presence" of the world in perceptual experience and patients' awareness of themselves and others as subjects of experience and action.[11] This "phenomenological" interpretation, Parnas argues, secures "a degree of coherence, and, in contrast to Jaspers' view, a certain understandability of the psychotic symptoms" (Parnas et al. 2002, p. 135).

But can the phenomenological interpretation furnish an explanation of *why* patients come to (e.g.,) believe in thought insertion? For advocates of the standard view, this question is critical. Thought insertion is a delusion shared by numerous patients with schizophrenia. This can be no coincidence. The way to establish that it is not is to discover some common causal factor accounting for patients' acquisition of the delusion. At this point, the "phenomenological" interpretation faces a dilemma, corresponding to two ways of thinking about the explanatory relation between the altered state of consciousness and individual psychotic symptoms. On the first model, we should think of the altered state of consciousness as *constituted* by the symptoms. This would not necessarily deprive the state of any explanatory role. For, as Brian O'Shaughnessy (another thinker steeped in the phenomenological tradition) has argued, a state of consciousness and its constituent properties may be *mutually dependent*. The state may be constituted by the co-presence of the properties; at the same time the constituents may depend on the state of consciousness they help to constitute. To illustrate, O'Shaughnessy maintains that being disposed to attend to perceived objects or events is a constitutive element of the state of waking consciousness. At the same time, he argues that the ability to exercise that disposition depends on the presence of the other (mutually dependent) constituents of the state of waking consciousness, such as "occurrent rationality," self-knowledge, intentional activity, and so on.[12] There is a sense, on this account, in which being in the state of waking consciousness explains one's possession of the individual abilities that co-constitute the state. Note, though, that the account owes whatever explanatory force it has to O'Shaughnessy's careful

---

[10] Compare Parnas's example of a patient who sought to demonstrate that he was Jesus Christ by appeal to these facts: "he felt himself a kind of anonymous being—he did not feel that any predicates really applied to his void," and "Jesus was also without predicates, because God cannot be said to have mundane features or predicates" (2004, p. 159).

[11] For a particularly helpful formulation of the view, see Parnas and Sass (2001).

[12] See O'Shaughnessy (2000, chapters 2 and 3).

and detailed analyses of the ways in which the co-constituents of the state of consciousness depend on each other. Parnas and Sass offer no analogous account of any putative explanatory relations amongst psychotic symptoms—say, of the ways in which thought insertion might depend on the altered "presence of the world" in perceptual experience. In any case, a natural thought here is that this whole model looks promising only in connection with psychological abilities or dispositions, rather than particular beliefs. This brings us to the second conception of the explanatory relation between the altered state of consciousness and psychotic symptoms. One might think of a state of consciousness as something that affects the way we perceive things. For example, if you are in a blind rage, you may perceive the recalcitrance of a gadget as a provocation, hence as a good reason to hit it. On this model, though, the state of consciousness affects what we do or believe by affecting our conception of what we have *reason* to do or believe. Appeal to the state of consciousness would work in tandem with a reason-giving explanation, rather than providing an alternative style of explanation.

We can call this the explanatory challenge. The worry is that the phenomenological interpretation renders delusions inexplicable. If we are interested in the reason *why* patients believe that thoughts are being inserted in their minds, we really have no alternative but to look into patients' reasons *for* holding that belief. Appeal to an altered state of consciousness cannot replace this style of explanation. Nor does it seem plausible that a non-psychological explanation—e.g., in terms of biological factors—alone could adequately account for the acquisition of a belief with a particular kind of content.

Discarding Intelligibility is problematic for another, deeper reason. If reports of delusions are meaningful statements, patients must grasp the meaning of the terms they are using. But grasp of the meaning of a term is inseparable from the disposition to use the term rationally. This raises the question whether autistic-schizophrenic delusions, in Parnas's sense, are *possible*. On the face of it, they are not. If there is a real disconnection between the content of the delusion and patients' conception of the relevant evidence this would simply mean that patients have lost their grip on the meaning of the terms they are using. This is what John Campbell has described as "the basic philosophical problem raised by delusions." The problem is that "since we have to ascribe meaning in such a way as to make the subject rational, we end up having no way in which to formulate the content of the subject's delusion." We face the prospect of having to think of the delusion as "'empty speech' masquerading as belief" (Campbell 2001, p. 91).

It is to avert this unacceptable consequence that the standard view insists that an apparent disconnection between content and evidence must reflect an insufficiently sensitive interpretation. For example, it may initially strike us as unintelligible how inner experience, however unusual, could be taken to suggest that someone else is controlling the thinking going on in one's head. But once we learn to distinguish between "introspective" and "agentive" ownership, we realize that there is a perfectly intelligible justificatory link between a certain abnormal inner experience and at least one element of the content of the delusion. In the end we have no choice but to interpret apparently bizarre delusions as disguised empirical delusions.

In view of the two challenges, explanatory and semantic, I think simply *discarding* Intelligibility is not an option. But I want to argue that contrary to the standard view, Intelligibility can and should be modified, along these lines: reports of thought insertion express attitudes that originate in rationally intelligible, coherent beliefs.

THOUGHT INSERTION AND ITS HISTORY

Schizophrenic patients' preoccupation with the themes that form the subject matter of their delusions does not suddenly spring into existence with the onset of psychosis. Understanding a delusion such as thought insertion may require charting its development from some non-delusional "precursor." As Parnas and Sass remark, "one cannot comprehend the delusional transformation in schizophrenia unless the subtler, fundamental features, *predating* the onset of psychosis, are also taken into account" (2001, p. 102). They provide the following richly suggestive example in which a patient describes his state of mind during the prodromal phase of schizophrenia:

> I bypass a window display of a shop in which there are exposed bicycles and bicycle parts; [in a wheel] all the metal spokes cross each other in sharp angles before they reach the axle ... the axle turns around with the spokes. No, it is not the axle that rotates; it is the bar, a piece of steel. The axle does not exist; it is just a mathematical line, perpendicular to the plane of the wheel that is determined by the spokes, by forty straight lines. However, this is not necessary either: Only two lines are needed to determine a flat surface. And the circumference? $2\pi r$ is the expression for the length of the felloe, or more precisely, for the theoretical circumference, outlined by this inexact circle (i.e., the felloe). Are we able to conceive of an ideal line by paying attention to the lines in nature? Is Spencer's claim that mathematics originates from experience and induction correct? ... These associations ... would not seem to me as sick if I were able to master them, like someone who calmly reflects on the matters he is working with, contemplating some professional problems. But when I am thinking in this way, without being able to stop it ... I have no mastery over the course of these ideas ... it seems to me *as if it is not me* who generates them. (Hesnard 1909, p. 146; translation and italics by Parnas and Sass 2001, p. 108)

The patient does not believe that he is not generating the ideas troubling him, let alone that they are generated by someone else. Nor is it plausible to interpret him as putting forward the claim that he is not generating them as an epistemic possibility—something for which there is good evidence, as when you remark "it looks as if it's going to rain." A more illuminating comparison may be with this claim: "it looks as if the sun is sinking into the sea." One way to interpret this claim is as an implicitly comparative use of "look." (See Martin 2010.) The way things look is said to be relevantly similar to a look that might lead someone who was ignorant of astronomy to think the sun was something that could, and did, sink into the sea. To make that claim, obviously, is not to say that the sun *is* something that could conceivably sink into the sea. Similarly the patient's description may amount to the claim that his state of mind was such as might lead one to think one wasn't generating the thoughts one was thinking. One doesn't have to regard it as a genuine possibility that certain ideas occurring to one may not be generated by oneself for it to help describe one's state of mind.[13]

I think this point may help to illuminate what is surely the most puzzling feature of thought insertion, the nature of the causal relation invoked in the delusion. Thoughts are said to be inserted or "put" into one's mind by others, rather as if they were physical objects.

---

[13] Parnas and Sass speak of a description of the altered state of consciousness at the "'as if' metaphorical level" (2001, p. 109).

The two-concept view holds that this peculiar causal judgment represents, or at least arises from, an unusual application of an entirely commonsensical idea—the idea that a (token) thought is something that has an agent. On this interpretation, it would be natural to expect that prior to the onset of psychosis and delusion, patients might describe their state of mind by saying "when I am thinking in this way it seems to me as if it is not I who is thinking." It is admittedly hazardous to try to reach general conclusions from a single case. But at least the example quoted by Parnas and Sass points toward a suggestive alternative interpretation. The patient says "it seems to me as if it is not me who *generates* these ideas." On the face of it, the notion of ideas being generated—whether by oneself or anyone else for that matter—is not one that forms part of ordinary commonsense psychological explanatory practice. The question of who is generating the ideas that occupy me is not one we ordinarily face, or would find it easy to make sense of. Patients' concern with what (or who) is "generating" their thoughts may have its origin not in the familiar notion that thoughts have thinkers but in a notion that is as unfamiliar as the state of mind it is intended to articulate—a state of mind in which it seems to one that one's thinking resists "mastery" and lacks its normal intelligibility, being a matter of mere "associations," and in which, therefore, it is for one as if one's thoughts or ideas were something that had an utterly perplexing causal explanation and, perhaps connectedly, were something rather like a physical thing.[14]

At this point let's return to the two challenges of the previous section. On the current proposal, the task of explaining thought insertion has to be divided into two parts or stages: an account of the acquisition of the "precursor" belief and an explanation of its transformation into a delusion. This analysis promises to meet the explanatory challenge by tracing the content of the delusion, at least in part, to the perfectly intelligible way in which patients are disposed to describe their state of mind before the onset of the psychosis. This would account for the fact that thought insertion is a delusion shared by numerous patients. It would even be true that the explanation of that fact requires an element of reason-giving explanation, as defenders of Intelligibility insist. But in addition, the explanation would appeal to the "delusional transformation" of the belief. It claims that with the onset of psychosis patients' altered state of consciousness leads them to take at face value the idea of an utterly unusual, quasi-mechanical explanation of their thinking, previously invoked within the scope of "it seems to me as if." The disconnection between content and evidence, highlighted earlier, may reflect patients' tendency to adopt the same posture toward the content of the delusion as, previously, toward the content of the "precursor" belief, treating it as a matter on which they enjoy first-person authority.

But given that disconnection between content and evidence, are we not forced to conclude that patients no longer understand the terms they are using? How can we interpret reports of the delusion as expressive of a real belief when it seems doubtful that patients grasp the content of that belief?

Parnas sometimes characterizes autistic-schizophrenic delusions as "metaphorical thematizations" of patients' altered state of consciousness (2004, p. 160). One might take this

---

[14] This would suggest that a "historical" analysis of thought insertion should modify not just Intelligibility but Alienation as well. The theme of the stream of consciousness assuming physical characteristics is familiar from other schizophrenic delusions, such as "thought pressure." One patient reported, prior to the onset of psychosis, feeling as if "his consciousness consisted of multiple emanating sources, […] each 'pulsating' at its own pace" (Parnas and Sass 2001, p. 108).

to mean that even during the psychotic phase patients are perfectly aware that what they are saying is not literally true, and merely intend it to convey a sense of the strangeness of their state of consciousness. So the delusion would turn out to be a coherent, rationally intelligible belief after all. Now there is some support for the idea that, "at some level," patients do retain a proper sense of reality. For example, Parnas mentions the "double bookkeeping" characteristic of schizophrenic delusions, the fact that patients' intentional activities are not always influenced by their delusions. Still, I doubt that a straightforward "metaphorical" interpretation is what Parnas has in mind. I take it "metaphorical thematization" is meant to suggest that that the delusion *develops* out of a (broadly) metaphorical description of patients' experience. The canonical statement of Parnas's view may be that bizarre delusions are "*distorted metaphors*" (Cermolacce et al. 2010, p. 10, my emphasis).

A more plausible response to the semantic challenge is to acknowledge that patients' conceptual abilities are impaired, but to suggest that impaired conceptual abilities can sustain impaired beliefs—viz., delusions. The standard theorist's bugbear, that unless Intelligibility is correct reports of delusions turn out to be "empty speech," cannot be taken seriously. Or rather, it poses a serious threat only if we accept a certain kind of instrumentalism about propositional attitudes. If the correctness of an attribution of a belief consists in its usefulness in the context of the enterprise of rational prediction and explanation, the very idea of a belief that is impaired, in that its basis and consequences are somewhat out of step with its content, makes no sense. But that is not how we ordinarily think of propositional attitudes. The idea that an attitude may fail to play its proper rational-explanatory role, due to the subject's state of consciousness, is arguably one that is familiar to commonsense psychology.[15] True, autistic-schizophrenic delusions involve something more serious than a temporary failure to make proper use of one's intellectual powers. But there are two reasons to think that patients' conceptual abilities have not faded away completely. One is that even during the psychotic phase all their propositional attitudes are not suddenly turned into delusions. As Louis Sass observes, "it is remarkable to what extent even the most disturbed schizophrenics may retain, even at the height of their psychotic periods, a quite accurate sense of what would generally be considered to be their objective or actual circumstances" (1994, p. 21). The force of the second reason depends on the intuitive plausibility of a "historical" account of thought insertion. It seems compelling that there is some continuity between the content of the "precursor" belief and that of the delusion—that the latter is a *distortion* of the former. And that continuity implies the persistence of the relevant conceptual abilities. In O'Shaughnessy's words, "insanity arises upon the ground of sanity: an inherently impossible cognitive representation of the world must be a distortion of an already acquired viable representation" (2000, p. 150).

Acknowledgments

Previous versions of this chapter were presented at workshops and seminars in Copenhagen, Birmingham, London, and Warwick. I'm very grateful to participants for their suggestions

---

[15] O'Shaughnessy's searching analysis of the state of drunkenness provides an illustration (see O'Shaughnessy 2000, chapter 3).

and criticism. I'd also like to thank Richard Gipps for extremely helpful comments on the penultimate draft.

References

Anscombe, E. (1957). *Intention*. Oxford: Blackwell.

Byrne, A. (2011). Knowing that I am thinking. In A. Hatzimoysis (Ed.), *Self-Knowledge*, pp. 105–24. Oxford: Oxford University Press.

Campbell, J. (1994). *Past, Space, and Self*. Cambridge, MA: MIT Press.

Campbell, J. (1999). Schizophrenia, the space of reasons, and thinking as a motor process. *The Monist, 82*, 609–25.

Campbell, J. (2001). Rationality, meaning, and the analysis of delusion. *Philosophy, Psychiatry, & Psychology, 8*, 89–100.

Campbell, J. (2002). The ownership of thoughts. *Philosophy, Psychiatry, & Psychology, 9*, 35–9.

Cermolacce, M., Sass, L., and Parnas, J. (2010). What is bizarre in bizarre delusions? A critical review. *Schizophrenia Bulletin, 34*(6), 667–79.

Gerrans, P. (2001). Authorship and ownership of thoughts. *Philosophy, Psychiatry, & Psychology, 8*, 231–7.

Hampshire, S. (1965). *Freedom of the Individual*. London: Chatto and Windus.

Hesnard, A. L. M. (1909). *Les troubles de la personalité dans les étas d'asthénie psychique. Étude de psychologies clinique*. Thése de medicine. Bordeaux: Université de Bordeaux.

Jones, S. R. and Fernyhough, C. (2007). Thought as action: Inner speech, self-monitoring, and auditory verbal hallucinations. *Consciousness and Cognition, 16*, 391–9.

Langland-Hassan, P. (2008). Fractured phenomenologies: Thought insertion, inner speech, and the puzzle of extraneity. *Mind & Language, 23*, 369–401.

Martin, M. (2010). What's in a look? In B. Nanay (Ed.), *Perceiving the World*, pp. 160–225. Oxford: Oxford University Press.

O'Shaughnessy, B. (1963). Observation and the will. *Journal of Philosophy, 60*(14), 367–92.

O'Shaughnessy, B. (2000). *Consciousness and the World*. Oxford: Oxford University Press.

Parnas, J. (2004). Belief and pathology of self-awareness. *Journal of Consciousness Studies, 11*, 148–61.

Parnas, J., Bovet, P., and Zahavi, D. (2002). Schizophrenic autism: clinical phenomenology and pathogenic implications. *World Psychiatry, 1*, 131–6.

Parnas, J. and Sass, L. (2001). Self, solipsism, and schizophrenic delusions. *Philosophy, Psychiatry, & Psychology, 8*, 101–20.

Roessler, J. (2010). Agents' knowledge. In T. O'Connor and C. Sandis (Eds), *A Companion to the Philosophy of Action*, pp. 236–44. Chichester: Wiley-Blackwell.

Sass, L. (1994). *The Paradoxes of Delusion*. Ithaca, NY: Cornell University Press.

Stephens, G. L. and Graham, G. (1994). Self-consciousness, mental agency, and the clinical psychopathology of thought insertion. *Philosophy, Psychiatry, & Psychology, 1*, 1–12.

Stephens, G. L. and Graham, G. (2000). *When Self-Consciousness Breaks. Alien Voices and Inserted Thoughts*. Cambridge, MA: MIT Press.

Steward, H. (1997). *The Ontology of Mind*. Oxford: Clarendon Press.

Wilson, G. J. (2000). Proximal practical foresight. *Philosophical Studies, 99*, 3–19.

Wittgenstein, L. (1958). *The Blue and Brown Books*. Oxford: Blackwell.

CHAPTER 41

THE DISUNITY OF CONSCIOUSNESS IN PSYCHIATRIC DISORDERS

TIM BAYNE

INTRODUCTION

Philosophers have often held that the unity of consciousness is one of its deep and perhaps essential features. However, since the late nineteenth century many theorists have argued that various psychiatric conditions reveal the unity of consciousness to be a merely contingent feature of consciousness—a feature that may characterize consciousness in its normal manifestations, but one that can also be lost in the context of pathology. This chapter examines the case for such claims. As we will see, whether the unity of consciousness does indeed break down in the context of any particular psychiatric disorder depends not only on just what that disorder involves but also on how we conceive of the unity of consciousness. There are multiple ways in which conscious states can be unified with each other, and any particular psychiatric disorder might involve a loss of some aspects of the unity of consciousness but not others. Indeed, there may be a case for thinking that there is a certain form of the unity of consciousness that is not lost in any psychiatric disorder.

This chapter is structured as follows. I begin in the following section by identifying some of the central forms of the unity of consciousness. I then turn to examine the case for thinking that these unities may break down in the context of certain psychiatric disorders. Although a great number of psychiatric disorders could be considered in this context, I restrict my attention to just three conditions: anosognosia, schizophrenia, and dissociative identity disorder.

THE UNITIES OF CONSCIOUSNESS

Three aspects of the unity of consciousness stand out as being of particular relevance to the investigation of psychiatric disorders.

The first of these aspects concerns the intentional structure of consciousness. We can say that a subject's conscious states are intentionally unified to the extent that they are integrated with each other (Shoemaker 1996). Normal conscious experience involves high degrees of intentional unity. Within perception, we typically experience perceptual features as bound together in the form of perceptual objects, and we experience those objects as located within a unitary space. Within thought, a subject's beliefs, desires, and intentions typically "hang together," such that their beliefs are largely consistent with each other, their intentions do not generally undermine each other, and their desires and intentions are intelligible in light of their beliefs. We can say that a subject whose conscious states are only very weakly integrated with each other in these ways suffers from a breakdown in the intentional unity of consciousness.

A second conception of the unity of consciousness concerns self-consciousness. According to David Rosenthal, the "so-called unity of consciousness consists in the compelling sense we have that all our conscious mental states belong to a single conscious subject" (2003, p. 325). We can think of this as the *subjective* unity of consciousness. Subjective unity requires not only that the subject be aware of their own conscious states, but also that they be aware of these states *as* their own states. There are a number of ways in which we might give this general idea some precision. We could say that a subject's consciousness is subjectively unified just in case they are aware of each of their conscious states as their own states, but it is unclear whether we are normally aware of each of our states as our own, even in an "implicit" or "pre-reflective" sense. With this in mind, we can give the subjective conception of the unity of consciousness a Kantian spin, and say that a subject enjoys subjective unity just in case they possess the capacity to be aware of each of their experiences as their own. Subjects who have lost the capacity to be aware of their conscious states as their own can be said to suffer from a breakdown in the subjective unity of consciousness.

Intentional unity and subjective unity capture important aspects of the unity of consciousness, but there is a third aspect of the unity of consciousness that must also be recognized. Consider any two experiences that you are currently enjoying—say, an auditory experience of traffic and a visual experience of these words. These two experiences will, I suggest, possess a *conjoint experiential character*. There is something it is like to hear traffic, there is something it is like to see words on a page, and there is something it is like to enjoy both of these experiences together as the components, parts, or elements of a single conscious state. Let us call this kind of unity—sometimes dubbed "co-consciousness"—*phenomenal unity* (Bayne 2010; Bayne and Chalmers 2003; Dainton 2000/2006; Tye 2003).

Phenomenal unity is implicit in many references to the "stream" or "field" of consciousness. What it is for a pair of simultaneous experiences to occur within a single stream of consciousness or phenomenal field *just is* for them to possess a conjoint phenomenal character—for there to be something it is like for the subject in question not only to have each experience but to have them *together*. By contrast, simultaneous experiences that occur within distinct phenomenal fields do not share a conjoint phenomenal character. To say that a subject's consciousness is unified in this sense of the term is to say that all of the conscious states that they enjoy at the time in question are phenomenally unified with each other. A subject whose consciousness is phenomenally unified will have a single total conscious state that "subsumes" every one of their conscious states and captures precisely what it is like to be that subject at that time (Bayne and Chalmers 2003). By contrast, creatures who suffer from a breakdown in the phenomenal unity of consciousness will lack any such state.

We have identified three aspects of "the" unity of consciousness: an aspect that concerns the intentional integration and coherence of the subject's conscious states; an aspect that concerns the subject's capacity to self-ascribe their conscious states; and an aspect that concerns the phenomenal unity (or "co-consciousness") that holds between conscious states. I turn now to the question of which of these three aspects of the unity of consciousness might be lost in the context of psychiatric disorders.

ANOSOGNOSIA

> It was now completely astonishing, that the patient did not notice her massive and later complete loss of her ability to see ... When she was asked directly about her ability to see, she answered in a vague, general way, that it is always so, that one sees better in youth. She assured in a calm and trustful way that she saw the objects that were shown to her, while the everyday examination proved the opposite. (Anton 1899, p. 93; Trans. David et al. 1993, p. 267)

Anton called this impairment "soul blindness" (Seelenblindheit), but it was a term coined by Babinski some 15 years later, "anosognosia,"—literally, lack of knowledge of impairment— that stuck. (Curiously, Anton's own name is reserved for a particular form of anosognosia, namely anosognosia for blindness.) Anosognosia can occur in the context of any number of deficits; it is possible to be anosognosic for paralysis, deafness, aphasia (difficulty producing meaningful speech), and prosopagnosia (the inability to recognize faces). Indeed, anosognosia can take different forms even within each of these domains, for patients can be unaware of their physical impairment and/or its behavioral consequences and/or those changes in their own conscious states that result from either the impairment itself or its consequences.

Some of these aspects of anosognosia can be seen in the following interview with an eighty-year-old woman who was anosognosic for paralysis to the left side of her body due to a right-hemisphere stroke.

Examiner:	Where are we?
C.C.:	In the hospital.
Examiner:	Which hospital?
C.C.:	Santa Orsola.
Examiner:	Why are you in the hospital?
C.C.:	I fell down and bumped my right leg.
Examiner:	What about your left arm and leg? Are they all right?
C.C.:	Neither well nor bad.
Examiner:	In which sense?
C.C.:	They are aching a bit.
Examiner:	Can you move your left arm?

C.C.:   Yes, I can.
Examiner: [The examiner puts her right index finger in C.C.'s right visual field.] Can you
             touch my finger with your left hand. [C.C. does not move.]
Examiner: What happens?
C.C.:   It happens that I am very good.
Examiner: Have you touched my finger?
C.C.:   Yes.

Later in the interview:

Examiner: Could you clap your hands?
C.C.:   I am not at the theatre.
Examiner: I know. But we just want to see whether you are able to clap your hands.
[C.C. lifts her right arm and puts it in the position for clapping, perfectly aligned with the
     trunk midline, moving it as if it were clapping against the left hand. She seems perfectly
     satisfied with the performance.]
Examiner: Are you sure that you are clapping your hands? We did not hear any sound.
C.C.:   I never make any noise. (Berti et al. 1998, pp. 28–29)

Although memory problems may play *a* role in accounting for anosognosia, it is implausible
to suppose that anosognosia can be fully explained by appealing to impairments of memory.
Not only does C.C. claim that she *could* move her arm and that she *had* moved her arm,
she also claimed that she *was moving* her arm despite the fact that it was immobile. C.C.'s
impairments were not restricted to memory but seem to have affected her ability to become
aware of her ongoing behavior.

Anosognosia clearly involves certain kinds of impairments to the unity of consciousness.
Most fundamentally, it involves a certain kind of breakdown in the intentional unity of consciousness. A patient may fail to use her awareness of what she is (or is not) doing in order to
update her conception of what general capacities for action she has (or doesn't have). Such
failures of updating are not unique to patients with anosognosia—indeed, we are all prone to
them—but they are particularly striking in the context of anosognosia. In part these failures
are so striking in anosognosia because they are domain specific. In general, patients do not
seem to have global difficulties in integrating various items of knowledge with each other,
but appear instead to have local difficulties in updating particular facets of their model of
the world. This feature of anosognosia is reflected in the fact that a patient with multiple
impairments may be anosognosic for some of their impairments but not others (Marcel
et al. 2004).

Anosognosia also appears to involve a certain kind of breakdown in the unity of subjectivity (Nikolinakos 2004). Although patients self-ascribe their conscious states when they
are aware of them, they seem often to be unaware of at least some portion of their conscious
states, either overlooking experiences that they have or failing to notice that they no longer
enjoy the kinds of experiences that they once did. Not only was C.C. (the anosognosic
patient described earlier) unaware of the fact that she was not clapping, she seems to have
been unaware of the nature of her own experiential states, for had she been aware of the
fact that she wasn't experiencing herself as clapping then—so the thought goes—she would
surely have been aware of the fact that she wasn't clapping. More generally, one might think
that the fact that one was (say) hemiplegic or blind ought to be apparent—indeed, manifestly apparent—to anyone with normal introspective abilities.

In response to this proposal, one might argue that the sensory impairments implicated in anosognosia are "never phenomenally immediate but instead must be discovered by observation and inference" (Levine 1990, p. 234). Perhaps patients are unaware of their impairments not because their introspective capacities have been disrupted, but because the missing perceptual content has been replaced by internally generated experiences that "mimic" the kinds of states that the patient expects to have in the environment in which they find themselves. Consider the following dialogue between a physician and H.S., a forty-six-year-old woman who was anosognosic for complete cortical blindness.

Examiner:	(Moves a bunch of small keys, producing a sound): I am holding an object. Do you have any idea what it might be?
H.S.:	Could that be a key?
Examiner:	(Silently moves the keys beneath the table): What does it look like?
H.S.:	On top there is a big ring, and it has a dark key-bit.
Examiner.	Do you see the key well?
H.S.:	I am seeing that it is a key.
Examiner.	(Opens and shuts scissors): Do have any idea what that might be?
H.S.:	Are those scissors?
Examiner:	Do you see them?
H.S.:	Only vaguely. I guessed a little.
Examiner:	(Silently hides the scissors beneath the table): What can you see of these scissors?
H.S.:	Upside are the handles where you take them, and below them is the part for cutting.
Examiner:	Are you seeing this?
H.S.:	Yes. (Goldenberg et al. 1995, p. 1378)

Quite reasonably, Goldenberg and colleagues suggest that H.S. had mistaken her internally generated imagery experience of the keys for normal perceptual experience. The objects that she described seeing were either the kinds of objects likely to be encountered in the environment in which she found herself, or—as in the scenario described here—suggested by what the patient was aware of via other sensory modalities (such as audition). Arguably, H.S.'s blindness was not apparent to her because the missing perceptual experience had been filled-in by visual imagery, perhaps in a manner akin to the way in which the blind-spot is filled in by the mechanisms responsible for perceptual completion.

But the imagery hypothesis does face objections. Consider the fact that C.C. *admits* that she's not making any sound when she "claps." Even if she has experiences of intentionally moving her arms, she does not appear to experience the sound of herself clapping, and surely this ought to have alerted C.C. to the fact that something was amiss if her introspective faculties were operating normally. Similarly, one might have thought that the evident failure of H.S.'s visual experiences to support successful agency ought to have led her to wonder whether these experiences were perceptual states or internally generated imagery states. So, even allowing for the fact that involuntarily generated imagery might plug some of the experiential gaps created by the patient's impairments, other gaps would appear to remain, and one would expect these to be noted by a subject with intact introspective capacities.

What about the phenomenal unity of consciousness? Might patients with anosognosia have experiences that are not phenomenally unified with each other within the context of a single stream of consciousness? Bisiach and Berti speculate that in anosognosia "different mental states or events, although being individually endowed with phenomenal quality, are kept separate from one another" (1995, p. 1338; see also Marcel 1993).

The main argument for thinking that anosognosia might involve phenomenal disunity—indeed, the only argument that I know of—involves an appeal to the fact that patients often appear to possess some kind of *implicit* appreciation of the proposition with respect to which they are anosognosic. This phenomenon is known as "dim" or "clouded" knowledge. For example, a patient with hemiplegia who denies that there is anything wrong with him might acknowledge that he does not possess the full suite of behavioral capacities that he once did. Another hemiplegic patient may insist that there is nothing wrong with her, but acknowledge that the examiner would be unable to perform certain tasks had he or she been affected by the same impairment. When asked to account for his inability to perform a task, a patient might provide a justification that suggests that he has some awareness of his deficit. For example, he might explain his inability to move his arm by insisting that "it has a cold" (Vuilleumier 2004).

How might dim knowledge support the claim that the phenomenal unity of consciousness breaks down in anosognosia? The idea, I think, is this. We can explain why the patient has explicit awareness of some facts but only implicit awareness of other facts by supposing that her conscious states are distributed between two (or more) streams of consciousness. Most of her conscious states occur within the context of a primary stream, the contents of which are available for explicit forms of cognitive and behavioral control (verbal report, belief revision, and so on). But the patient also has a secondary stream of consciousness, a stream whose contents are able to exert only indirect (or "implicit") influence on thought and action.

Although this proposal is intriguing it does face a number of objections. One problem is that it is unclear why conscious states that are "kept separate" from the rest of the subject's conscious states would play only a restricted role in cognitive and behavioral control. Prima facie, one would expect the contents of consciousness to be available to the same forms of cognitive and behavioral control whether or not they are isolated from the rest of the subject's conscious states.

But if dim knowledge does not involve a secondary stream of consciousness, what does it involve? That depends, I suspect, on the kind of dim knowledge in question. Some patients exhibit dim knowledge of their impairment in the sense that they seem to be aware of certain aspects of it but not others. For example, a patient might seem to be oblivious of the impairment itself but aware of its behavioral consequences. This kind of dim knowledge involves a loss of intentional unity, and does not seem to be particularly difficult to account for, at least in broad outline. The patients simply have not "put two and two together." They are aware of one fact about themselves (say, that they can no longer walk to the store), but not other facts (that one of their legs is weak). Of course, the facts of which they are unaware are intimately related to the facts of which they are aware—someone who is aware that they cannot walk to the store ought to wonder why this is the case—but the phenomenon of failing to draw out the implications of what one accepts is not unfamiliar.

In other cases of dim knowledge, however, the patient appears to be both aware and also unaware of one and the same fact. For example, a patient might appear to be aware of his impairment when required to produce a verbal report of it but not when required to engage in certain kinds of non-verbal behavior. Can this kind of dissociation be explained without appealing to a breakdown in the phenomenal unity of consciousness?

I think so. In fact, a plausible explanation can be constructed by drawing on Bisiach's suggestion that the contents of consciousness are "probe-dependent" (Bisiach 1992). Consider a patient who is anosognosic for unilateral visual neglect due to right-hemisphere damage. There is evidence that the severity of neglect can be modulated by the kinds of tasks that one requires the patient to perform. For example, patients may manifest more neglect when pointing with their ipsilesional hand than when pointing with their contralesional hand. This may occur because pointing with the contralesional hand activates sensory-motor circuits within the damaged hemisphere and thus improves contralesional discrimination (Ricci and Chatterjee 2004, p. 91). But if the severity of the patient's neglect can be modulated by task demands, it is also possible that the severity of the patient's unawareness of their neglect can also be modulated by task demands. Suppose, for example, that the patient relies on right-hemisphere circuits in order to be aware of their neglect. In that case, asking the patient to say whether or not they have neglect might itself inhibit awareness of the neglect, for the requirement to produce a verbal report might "suck" neural activity from the right hemisphere and transfer it to the left hemisphere. By contrast, patients might be more likely to be aware of their neglect when carrying out tasks—such as pointing with the left hand—that involve right-hemisphere activity.

If this account is on the right track, then it is possible that at no point does the patient have experiences that are not phenomenally unified with each other. Rather, what might appear to be a breakdown in the phenomenal unity of consciousness is really just a manifestation of the fact that the patient's awareness of her deficit fluctuates depending on the kinds of tasks in which she is engaged and the ways in which she is probed. In sum, although anosognosia may involve breakdowns in the intentional and subjective unity of consciousness, there is little reason to think that it also involves a breakdown in the phenomenal unity of consciousness.

Schizophrenia

Another psychiatric syndrome that is frequently said to involve a breakdown in the unity of consciousness is schizophrenia. The disease takes its name from the Greek for "splitting of the psyche" and one of its earliest commentators, Ernst Kraepelin (1896), considered the loss of the unity of consciousness to be one of its core features. Whether or not that claim can be sustained, there is certainly reason to think that various aspects of the unity of consciousness are severely compromised in the context of two of schizophrenia's so-called "positive symptoms": thought disorder and thought insertion.

Thought disorder involves an impairment in the patient's ability to structure their thoughts and actions around goals—to keep themselves "on track." The cognitive and perceptual focus of patients is guided by associations and irrelevant stimuli that capture their attention, rather than by the logic of the task that they have set themselves. Attention is "sticky," and cannot be easily moved from one stimulus to another. As one patient remarked:

> The mind must have a filter which functions without our conscious thought, sorting stimuli and allowing only those which are relevant to the situation at hand to disturb consciousness. And this filter must be working at maximum efficiency at all times, particularly when we require a high degree of concentration. What happened to me ... was a breakdown of the

filter, and a hodge-podge of unrelated stimuli were distracting me from things which should have had my undivided attention. (MacDonald 1960, p. 218)

The filter this patient describes is selective attention (Anscombe 1987; Gray et al. 1991). Whereas attention is normally tuned to be sensitive to stimuli that are either intrinsically salient or important to the subject, in thought disorder the patient's attention is drawn to mundane matters—a stray remark, a vase, or the pattern on some brickwork. The patient may initially be confused as to why she is attending to a trivial stimulus, and in order to make sense of her own behavior she may come to believe that it *is* significant, that it possesses a hidden meaning that is manifest only to her. Thought disorder involves a breakdown in the intentional unity of consciousness insofar as the patient's goals are not able to guide their behavior effectively. Although the causes of this breakdown are to be found in pathologies of pre-conscious processes, its effects are manifest in the structure of the patient's experience.

Although striking, the breakdown in conscious unity seen in thought disorder is not radically foreign, for we are all familiar with difficulties in screening out distracting information. Thought insertion, by contrast, involves forms of mental fragmentation that are rather more alien (Mullins and Spence 2003). Karl Jaspers characterized the phenomenon as follows:

> Patients think something and yet feel that someone else has thought it and in some way forced it on them. The thought arises and with it a direct awareness that it is not the patient but some external agent that thinks it. The patient does not know why he has this thought nor did he intend to have it. He does not feel master of his own thoughts and in addition he feels in the power of some incomprehensible external force. (Jaspers 1963, pp. 122–123)

Mellor provides an oft-cited example of a patient who claimed that the thoughts of Eamonn Andrews, a well-known TV presenter from the 1960s, were entering her mind. "There are no other thoughts there, only his.... He treats my mind like a screen and flashes his thoughts into it like you flash a picture" (Mellor 1970, p. 17).

Such statements provide us with a rudimentary sketch of the phenomenon, but going beyond this sketch leads us immediately into controversy. The literature contains two rather different conceptions of what it is that patients with thought insertion mean when they claim that certain thoughts are "not their own." According to the first conception, patients are to be understood as denying that thoughts of which they are introspectively aware—thoughts that occur in their stream of consciousness—are theirs. This account is implicit in Freud's description of thought insertion as a condition in which "portions of [the patient's] mental life—his perceptions, thoughts, and feelings—appear alien to him and as not belonging to his own ego" (Freud 1962, p. 13). Call this the *no-subjectivity* account of thought insertion. A rather different conception of thought insertion conceives of patients as meaning to deny only that they are the *agents* of the thoughts in question (Campbell 1999; Gallagher 2000; Stephens and Graham 2000). Understood in this way, we should take "the thoughts of Eamonn Andrews" to refer to the thoughts that Eamonn Andrews *produces*, not the thoughts that Eamonn Andrews *has*. We might call this the *no-agency* account of thought insertion. Underlying this debate about what patients with thought insertion mean by their statements is a parallel debate about the kind of phenomenology that they have: does thought insertion involve a loss of the sense of subjectivity or "my-ness" that is said to ordinarily accompany conscious thought, or does it involve only a loss of the sense of agency?

The verbal reports of patients with thought insertion do not clearly favor one of these two models over the other. Although some of what patients say suggests that a sense of passivity lies at the root of the patient's experience—one patient says that his mind is being treated like a screen; another patient that thoughts are put into his mind—other expressions of thought insertion suggest that patients deny not only authorship of the relevant thoughts but ownership over them as well. Nor do cognitive neuropsychiatric models of thought insertion enable us to decide between these two accounts. At present, both the no-subjectivity and the no-agency accounts appear to provide us with viable conceptions of what patients might mean in denying that certain thoughts are "their own"; indeed, it is possible that both proposals contain some truth (Roessler, Chapter 40, this volume).

Leaving to one side the question of which of these two models might best capture thought insertion, let us consider what implications each model might have for the unity of consciousness. The no-subjectivity account, if true, would appear to show that the unity of subjectivity is not an essential feature of human consciousness. By this I don't mean merely that it would show that it is possible to have conscious states of which one was not introspectively aware—arguably, we needn't look to pathologies of consciousness for examples of that phenomenon—but that it would show that it is possible to have conscious states that one could not recognize *as* one's own states. Even when patients are introspectively aware of the relevant thoughts, they are not aware of them as their own.

In response, a critic might argue that even if patients with delusions of thought insertion don't recognize some of their conscious states as their own it doesn't follow that they have lost the *capacity* to recognize those states as their own. What has gone wrong in thought insertion, our imagined critic continues, is simply that the patient refuses to exercise this capacity in the way that they should. There may be something to this line of thought, but we might also ask why our critic is so sure that the patient retains the capacity to recognize the thoughts in question as their own. Certainly the mere fact that patients retain the capacity to recognize some of their thoughts as their own does not imply that they have retained the capacity to recognize each of their thoughts as their own.

Unlike the no-subjectivity model, the no-agency model of thought insertion allows that patients retain the unity of subjectivity. However, even on the no-agency model, thought insertion involves some kind of disruption to the unity of self-consciousness. After all, a creature with a fully unified self-conception will normally be able to track which of its mental events it is responsible for and which are brought about by external agents or events. An impairment in the ability to recognize one's own agency may not be as striking as an impairment in the ability to recognize one's own subjectivity, but it nonetheless represents a radical departure from the coherence and integrity that self-consciousness normally underwrites. Although they emphasize different aspects of that unity, both the no-subjectivity and no-agency models conceive of thought insertion as compromising in some fundamental manner the unity that self-consciousness normally brings with it.

What about phenomenal disunity? Are there reasons to think that patients suffering from thought disorder and thought insertion might have suffered from a breakdown in the phenomenal unity of consciousness? Not that I know of. The forms of disunity within consciousness just discussed can be fully accounted for without supposing that patients have simultaneous experiences that are not phenomenally unified ("co-conscious") with each other. There is something apt in Krepelin's description of the "schizophrenic mind" (to use a dangerous phrase) as "an orchestra without a conductor," but there is no reason to deny that the notes produced by this orchestra occur within the context of a single phenomenal field, just as they do in the context of unimpaired states of consciousness.

DISSOCIATIVE IDENTITY DISORDER

Perhaps the clinical syndrome most closely associated in the popular mind with breakdowns in the unity of consciousness is dissociative identity disorder (DID), also known as multiple personality disorder (MPD). In order to qualify for a diagnosis of DID a person must have two or more distinct identities or personality states. These identities—or "alters" as they are also known—"each have their own relatively enduring pattern of perceiving, relating to and thinking about the environment and the self" (American Psychiatric Association 2004). Alters take turns directing the behavior of the multiple, and while a particular alter is "out" the multiple's behavior will generally be guided only by the memories, beliefs, plans, and other intentional states associated with it.

Although one can find reports of what might now be classified as cases of multiplicity in the eighteenth century (Carlson 1981), serious interest in dissociation dates from the late nineteenth century, with theorists such as Alfred Binet and Théodule Ribot on one side of the Atlantic and William James and Morton Prince on the other side all arguing that the phenomenon demonstrates that consciousness is not necessarily unified. After 1915 multiplicity enjoyed a dramatic decline, but by the 1970s it was back in the form of "multiple personality disorder," a change of name that was in part prompted by an increase in the average number of personality states manifested by "multiples." Although multiple personalities were not unknown in the late nineteenth and early twentieth century the norm was two, and the condition was often referred to as "double consciousness." Reports of duality are now infrequent, and the typical multiple is said to have between five to ten personality states, with some multiples reported to have hundreds of personalities.

Multiplicity involves a rather radical breakdown in the intentional unity of consciousness. Whereas the conscious beliefs, intentions, and desires of a normal subject enjoy a large degree of coherence with each other, this is not the case in contexts of multiplicity. Although each alter may have its own reasonably coherent conception of the world, the conception of one alter may depart in radical ways from that of its co-alters. Alters may be unaware of the very existence of their fellow alters, and even when they are aware of them they will often fail to identify with—and may even attempt to thwart—their projects.

Multiples not only have distinct and autonomous conceptions of the world, they also have distinct and autonomous *self*-conceptions. In one alter state a patient might believe, correctly, that she is an adult woman, but in another alter state she might believe that she is a young man or even a child. Importantly, this lack of a unitary self-conception permeates the patient's experience of her own mental life. In a phenomenon known as "inter-alter access," an alter may take itself to be directly aware of the thoughts of a fellow-alter. The patient will say such things as "That's not my thought, it's hers."

Inter-alter access appears to involve a breakdown in the unity of subjectivity, for it looks as though the patient is failing to recognize her own conscious states *as* her own states. One could, however, attempt to resist this view by suggesting that in the relevant sense a multiple's conscious states do not belong to a single subject of experience but are instead distributed between distinct subjects of experiences. Following Dennett and Humphrey, one might argue that "the grounds for assigning several selves to [a multiple] can be as good as—indeed the same as—those for assigning a single self to a normal human being" (Dennett and Humphrey 1998, p. 54). I myself would be inclined to resist the urge to reify alters in this way. Rather than thinking of alters as bona fide selves, I suggest that we should instead think of them as personality "states" or "files" that share control of the multiple's thought and action between them. The multiple might *think* that she has (or is) multiple selves, but in this regard she would suffer from what Putnam et al. (1986) describe as the "delusion of separateness." We might liken the multiple to an individual who is massively self-deceived, not in the sense that she is deceived *by* herself—although that may indeed be true—but in the sense that she is deceived *about* herself (Heil 1994). With this in mind, I think we have good reason to retain the prima facie plausible view that multiplicity involves a breakdown in the unity of subjectivity.

Might multiplicity also involve a loss of the phenomenal unity of consciousness? Although discussions of multiplicity often seem to presuppose an affirmative answer to this question there are few explicit defenses of this view. Perhaps the most thorough treatment of this issue is to be found in Stephen Braude's book *First-Person Plural*. Braude's view is rather nuanced. Although he holds that alters have their own streams of consciousness—indeed, that they are independent loci of *self*-consciousness (1995, p. 78ff.)—he also argues that multiples have a single, underlying self, what he describes as a "Kantian ego." I will leave the Kantian components of Braude's view to one side, and focus on his arguments for the view that multiples have simultaneous conscious states that occur within distinct streams of experience.

Braude's first argument appeals to the way in which multiples "switch" between alter states:

> One can actually observe and clearly identify the participants in the struggle. For example, as two alters vie for executive control, the multiple's face might shift rapidly between the distinctive features of each. Even more importantly, the clear personality shifts on the subject's face often reflect the alters' idiosyncratic contributions to the conflict. For example, one personality might show anger, tension or confusion, and the other might display amusement and contempt. And those dispositions can be exhibited in a manner characteristic of the respective personalities. (Braude 1995, pp. 67–68)

Even if switching lives up to Braude's description of it—see Hacking (1995) for a rather different picture—one might argue that the conflict Braude describes is merely an exaggerated form of the struggle for emotional control with which many of us are familiar and which is fully consistent with possession of but one stream of consciousness. Consider a person who has been deeply insulted in a context in which anger is not an appropriate emotion to manifest. One might witness a "struggle" between distinct emotional states being played-out on their face as they attempt to regain control of their emotions. Perhaps inter-alter conflict is in some sense "deeper" than this, but it is not clear to me that it is deeper in any way that might bring with it phenomenal disunity.

A second line of thought that Braude provides has its roots in a common account of the etiology of multiplicity according to which the victim deals with the pain of abuse by creating other personalities to whom it can be transferred. Braude suggests that switching could play this role only if alters qualify as independent loci of consciousness:

> Switching personalities enables a multiple to cope with exhaustion, pain, or other impairments to normal or optimal functioning. For example, if A is tired or drugged, B can emerge fresh

or clear-headed. When in pain, A can switch to an anesthetic personality. Or, personalities can keep passing the pain to each other in turn, switching when the persistent pain becomes intolerable. (Braude 1995, p. 45)

An initial objection to this argument is that pains are not the sorts of things that can be transferred between subjects of experience. Even if pains are transferable, we have no conception of *how* they might be passed from one alter to another, nor is it clear how the multiple could be better off by transferring pain between alters, for wouldn't she herself still be in pain irrespective of which of her alters "had" the pain?

These questions can be answered by supposing that the personality states or files to which alters correspond are not to be thought of as distinct subjects of experience, but are instead best understood as "schemas"—networks of intentional states that govern an organism's responses to particular environments (Bower 1994; Silberman et al. 1985). Schemas are not unique to multiples; in fact, they play a role in explaining many features of normal behavioral interaction. Switches between one schema and another can be triggered by changes in one's environment, as when a teacher takes on a pedagogical persona upon entering a classroom. They can also be endogenously elicited, as when one adopts a certain mood state in order to cope more effectively with a challenging situation. On this picture of things, what it is for one alter to "transfer" its pain to another is just for the multiple to switch from one behavioral schema with another. We can understand how switching might be of benefit to the multiple, for some behavioral schemas might be more effective than others in dealing with noxious stimuli. But although we have made sense of the idea that alters can "transfer" their pains, we have also deflated any ambitions that the argument might have had for establishing phenomenal disunity. On this view, the "transfer" of a pain from one alter to another involves nothing more than a single stimulus being processed within the context of distinct behavioral schemas, rather than the migration of a token experience from one stream of consciousness to another.

A final argument for the view that multiples have multiple streams of consciousness appeals to a certain interpretation of inter-alter access—the phenomenon in which alters appear to be directly aware of the thoughts of their fellow alters. Braude presents inter-alter access as a kind of telepathy, as if alters who enjoy it are "able to peek into a private room of experiences, or access or 'read' a stream of experiences distinct from their own" (Braude 1995, p. 82). On this view, alters have introspective (or, if you like, "quasi-introspective") access to two kinds of mental states: their own and those of their fellow alters. Not only might an alter be aware of what other alters are thinking, it can also—so the thought goes—be aware of *which* particular alter is thinking each of the various thoughts to which it has "quasi-introspective access."

This conception of inter-alter access raises some awkward questions. How might introspection tag thoughts as the thoughts of particular alters? Why might such a mechanism have evolved? Would the existence of such a mechanism undermine the warrant that introspectively based beliefs normally enjoy? We might be forced to accept the telepathic model even in the face of these challenges if it were the only game in town, but it isn't. In fact, there are two alternatives to telepathy.

One alternative to the telepathic account holds that reports of inter-alter access are confabulations—"mere hallucinations"—of mental states (Stephens and Graham 2000). The introspective state that the multiple is reporting might be real enough, but its mental target might be a mere figment of the multiple's imagination. Support for this proposal is provided by the fact that alters can be created in hypnotic contexts as merely intentional entities (Harriman 1942; Kampman 1976; Merskey 1992). Here, as elsewhere, fiction may give rise to fact: alters might begin life as purely intentional entities but thereafter acquire a degree of reality as the multiple begins to live out her fantasy.

A second alternative to the telepathic account holds that in inter-alter access multiples are aware of genuine mental states, but these states are their own rather than those of some other subject of experience. Just as individuals who experience thought insertion mistake their own thoughts for those of someone else, so too—this proposal runs—individuals who experience multiplicity mistake their own thoughts for those of someone else. (The difference between the two conditions is that in thought insertion the subject represents the thought as having an "external" source, whereas in inter-alter access the thought is represented as having its source "within" the patient.) This proposal receives some support from the fact that the line between inter-alter access on the one hand and the schizophrenic symptoms of thought insertion and auditory hallucination on the other is far from sharp (David et al. 1996). In fact, studies have found that cohorts of patients who had received a diagnosis of dissociative identity disorder had *higher* levels of first-rank symptoms of schizophrenia—notably thought insertion—than cohorts of patients who had been diagnosed as suffering from schizophrenia (Kluft et al. 1987; Ross et al. 1990; Steinberg et al. 1994; see also Bliss et al. 1983). These studies may not show what many take them to show—namely, that many individuals with multiplicity are falsely diagnosed with schizophrenia—but they do indicate that the distinction between auditory hallucinations and thought insertion on the one hand and inter-alter access on the other is not easily drawn. Given that we have little hesitation in regarding auditory hallucinations and thought insertion as involving the failure to identify one's mental states as one's mental states, perhaps we should say precisely the same thing about so-called "inter-alter access." In sum, although multiplicity involves quite radical breakdowns in the unity provided by the intentional and subjective structure of consciousness, the case for thinking that it also involves breakdowns in the phenomenal unity of consciousness has not yet been made (Clark, Chapter 53, this volume).

CONCLUSION

We have seen that there is a great deal of truth in the oft-made claim that certain psychiatric disorders involve some kind of breakdown in the unity of consciousness. In anosognosia the patient may suffer both from an inability to update their beliefs in the way that they should, and from an inability to track the contents of their own conscious states in the ways that they ought to. In schizophrenia we see a disruption to the intentional unity of consciousness in thought disorder and a disruption to the integrity of self-consciousness in thought insertion. Multiplicity presents us with an even more profound impairment to the unity of self-consciousness, for here the patient labors under the delusion that he or she is (or "harbors") multiple subjects of experience. In varying ways, then, each of these syndromes presents us with notable departures from the coherence and integration that consciousness—particularly *self*-consciousness—normally displays.

But despite these disruptions there is one aspect of the unity of consciousness that appears to remain intact in each of these disorders: as best one can tell, the experiences of patients continue to occur within a single phenomenal field. Changing the metaphor, we might say that patients appear to retain a single stream of consciousness. The intentional structure of that stream may be fundamentally disrupted, but its singularity—the fact that patients retain but one conscious perspective on the world—appears to remain unscathed in even the most profound psychiatric disorders.

ACKNOWLEDGMENTS

I am grateful to Martin Davies and Richard Gipps for their very helpful comments on a previous version of this chapter. This chapter was written with support from the European Research Council (ERC Grant No. 313552: "The Architecture of Consciousness"), for which I am very grateful.

REFERENCES

American Psychiatric Association (2004). *Diagnostic and Statistical Manual of Mental Disorders, Fourth Edition, Text Revision.* Washington, DC: American Psychiatric Association.

Anscombe, R. (1987). The disorder of consciousness in schizophrenia. *Schizophrenia Bulletin*, 13(2), 241–60.

Anton, G. (1899). Uber die Selbstwahrnehmung der Herderkrankungen des Gehirns durch den Kranken bei Rindenblindheit und Rindentaubheit. *Archiv fur Psychiatrie und Nervenkrankheiten*, 32, 86–127.

Bayne, T. (2010). *The Unity of Consciousness.* Oxford: Oxford University Press.

Bayne, T. and Chalmers, D. (2003). What is the unity of consciousness? In A. Cleeremans (Ed.), *The Unity of Consciousness: Binding, Integration and Dissociation*, pp. 23–58. Oxford: Oxford University Press.

Berti, A., Làdavas, E., Stracciara, A., Giannarelli, C., and Ossola, A. (1998). Anosognosia for motor impairment and dissociations with patients' evaluation of the disorder: Theoretical considerations. *Cognitive Neuropsychiatry*, 3(1), 21–44.

Bisiach, E. (1992). Understanding consciousness: Clues from unilateral neglect and related disorders. In A. D. Milner and M. D. Rugg (Eds), *The Neuropsychology of Consciousness*, pp. 113–39. London: Academic Press.

Bisiach, E. and Berti, A. (1995). Consciousness in dyschiria. In M. S. Gazzaniga (Ed.), *The Cognitive Neurosciences*, pp. 1131–340. Cambridge, MA: MIT Press.

Bliss, E. L., Larson, E. M., and Nakashima, S. R. (1983). Auditory hallucinations and schizophrenia. *The Journal of Nervous and Mental Disease*, 171(1), 30–3.

Bower, G. (1994). Temporary emotional states act like multiple personality. In R. M. Klein and B. K. Doane (Eds), *Psychological Concepts and Dissociative Disorders*, pp. 207–234. Hillsdale NJ: Lawrence Erlbaum Associates.

Braude, S. (1995). *First-Person Plural* (2nd rev. edn). Lanham, MD: Rowman and Littlefield.

Campbell, J. (1999). Schizophrenia, the space of reasons, and thinking as a motor process. *The Monist*, 82(4), 609–25.

Carlson, E. (1981). The history of multiple personality in the United States. I. The beginnings. *The American Journal of Psychiatry*, *138*, 666–8.

Dainton, B. (2000). *Stream of Consciousness: Unity and Continuity in Conscious Experience* (New edn. published 2006). London: Routledge.

David, A., Owen, A. M., and Förstl, H. (1993). An annotated summary and translation of "On the self-awareness of focal brain diseases by the patient in cortical blindness and cortical deafness," by Gabriel Anton (1989). *Cognitive Neuropsychiatry*, *10*, 263–72.

David, A., Kemp, R., Smith, L., and Fahy, T. (1996). Split minds: Multiple personality and schizophrenia. In P. W. Halligan and J. C. Marshall (Eds), *Method in Madness: Case Studies in Cognitive Neuropsychiatry*, pp. 123–46. Hove: Psychology Press.

Dennett, D. and Humphrey, N. (1998). Speaking for ourselves. In D. Dennett (Ed.), *Brainchildren*, pp. 31–57. Cambridge, MA: MIT Press.

Freud, S. (1962). *Civilization and its discontents* (J. Strachey, Trans.). Boston, MA: Norton.

Gallagher, S. (2000). Self-reference and schizophrenia: A cognitive model of immunity to error through misidentification. In D. Zahavi (Ed.), *Exploring the Self: Philosophical and Psychopathological Perspectives on Self-experience*, pp. 203–43. Amsterdam: John Benjamins.

Goldenberg, G., Müllbacher, W., and Nowak, A. (1995). Imagery without perception: A case study of anosognosia for cortical blindness. *Neuropsychologia*, *33*, 1373–82.

Gray, J. A., Rawlins, J. N. P., Hemsley, D. R., and Smith, A. D. (1991). The neuropsychology of schizophrenia. *Behavioural and Brain Sciences*, *14*, 1–84.

Hacking, I. (1995). *Rewriting the Soul: Multiple Personality and the Sciences of Memory*. Princeton, NJ: Princeton University Press.

Harriman, P. L. (1942). The experimental production of some phenomena related to multiple personality. *Journal of Abnormal and Social Psychology*, *37*, 244–55.

Heil, J. (1994). Going to pieces. In G. Graham and G. L. Stephens (Eds), *Philosophical Psychopathology*, pp. 111–34. Cambridge, MA: MIT Press.

Jaspers, K. (1963). *General Psychopathology* (J. Hoenig and M. W. Hamilton, Trans. from the German 7th edn). Manchester: Manchester University Press.

Kampman, R. (1976). Hypnotically induced multiple personality: An experimental study. *International Journal of Clinical and Experimental Hypnosis*, *24*, 215–27.

Kluft, R. P. (1987). First-rank symptoms as a diagnostic clue to multiple personality disorder. *American Journal of Psychiatry*, *144*, 293–8.

Kraepelin, E. (1896). *Psychiatrie* (4th edn). Leipzig: J. A. Barth.

Levine, D. N. (1990). Unawareness of visual and sensorimotor defects: A hypothesis. *Brain and Cognition*, *13*, 233–81.

MacDonald, N. (1960). The other side: living with schizophrenia. *Canadian Medical Association Journal*, *82*, 218–21.

Marcel, A. (1993). Slippage in the unity of consciousness. In G. R. Bock and J. Marsh (Eds), *Experimental and Theoretical Studies of Consciousness*, pp. 168–79. Chichester: John Wiley and Sons,

Marcel, A., Tegnér, R., and Nimmo-Smith, I. (2004). Anosognosia for plegia: Specificity, extension, partiality and disunity of bodily awareness. *Cortex*, *40*, 19–40.

Mellor, C. H. (1970). First rank symptoms of schizophrenia. *British Journal of Psychiatry*, *117*, 15–23.

Merskey, H. (1992). The manufacture of personalities: The production of multiple personality disorder. *British Journal of Psychiatry*, *157*, 327–40.

Mullins, S. and Spence, S. (2003). Re-examining thought insertion. *British Journal of Psychiatry*, *182*, 293–8.

Nikolinakos, D. D. (2004). Anosognosia and the unity of consciousness. *Philosophical Studies*, *119*, 315–42.

Putnam, F. W., Guroff, J. J., Silberman, E. K., Barban, L., and Post, R. M. (1986). The clinical phenomenology of multiple personality disorder: Review of 100 recent cases. *Journal of Clinical Psychiatry*, *47*, 285–93.

Ricci, R. and Chatterjee, A. (2004). Sensory and response contributions to visual awareness in extinction. *Experimental Brain Research*, *157*, 85–93.

Rosenthal, D. (2003). Unity of consciousness and the self. *Proceedings of the Aristotelian Society*, *103*, 325–52. (Reprinted in Rosenthal, D. (2005). *Consciousness and Mind*, pp. 339–63. Oxford: Clarendon Press.)

Ross, C. A., Miller, S. D., Reagor, P., Bjornson, L., Fraser, G. A., and Anderson, G. (1990). Schneiderian symptoms of multiple personality disorder and schizophrenia. *Comprehensive Psychiatry*, *31*(2), 111–18.

Shoemaker, S. (1996). Unity of consciousness and consciousness of unity. In *The First-Person Perspective and Other Essays*, pp. 176–97. Cambridge: Cambridge University Press.

Silberman, E. K., Putnam, F. W., Weingartner, H., Braun, B. G., and Post, R. M. (1985). Dissociative states in multiple personality disorder. *Psychiatry Research*, *15*, 253–60.

Steinberg, M., Cicchetti, D., Buchanan, J., Rakfeldt, J., and Rounsaville, B. (1994). Distinguishing between multiple personality disorder (dissociative identity disorder) and schizophrenia using the structured clinical interview for DSM-IV dissociative disorders. *Journal of Nervous and Mental Diseases*, *182*(9), 495–502.

Stephens, G. L. and Graham, G. (2000). *When Self-Consciousness Breaks*. Cambridge, MA: MIT Press.

Tye, M. (2003). *Consciousness and Persons*. Cambridge, MA: MIT Press.

Vuilleumier, P. (2004). Anosognosia: The neurology of beliefs and uncertainties. *Cortex*, *40*, 9–17.

CHAPTER 42

······································

DELUSION: COGNITIVE APPROACHES—BAYESIAN INFERENCE AND COMPARTMENTALIZATION

······································

MARTIN DAVIES AND ANDY EGAN

Delusions in individuals with schizophrenia are personal-level phenomena and no account of delusion could be complete unless it included a rich phenomenological description of individuals' experience of their delusions (Sass and Pienkos, Chapter 39, this volume). Cognitive approaches aim to contribute to our understanding of delusions by providing an explanatory framework that extends beyond the personal level to the subpersonal level of information-processing systems (Cratsley and Samuels, Chapter 27, this volume). At other subpersonal levels, contributions are also offered by neurobiological, neurocomputational, and psychopharmacological approaches.[1]

There are questions to be asked about the relationships between these different subpersonal levels (for example, about the relationship between the level of cognitive psychology and the level of neurobiology; Gold and Stoljar 1999). There are also questions about the relationship between the personal level, where description extends to phenomenology and normativity and where there are distinctive practices of rationalizing explanation, and subpersonal levels of mechanistic description and explanation. According to one extreme view of this relationship, all that is literally true at the personal level can be recast in the terms favored by the sciences of the mind. According to the opposite extreme, what is distinctive

······································

[1] The distinction between personal and subpersonal levels of description was introduced by Dennett (1969). The personal level of description is the folk psychological level at which we describe people as experiencing, thinking subjects and agents. It includes descriptions of conscious mental states as such and descriptions of normative requirements of rationality, for example. Personal-level descriptions figure in explanations in which actions are rationalized in terms of mental states such as beliefs and desires. Subpersonal levels, in contrast, are suited to the mechanistic descriptions and explanations of the objective sciences of the mind, such as information-processing psychology and neurobiology. (For discussion, see Davies 2000; Shea, Chapter 62, this volume.)

and important at the personal level is independent from the sciences of the mind. But inter-mediate options, between reduction and independence, are available (interlevel interaction without reduction; Davies 2000). It is a familiar point that there seems to be an explana-tory gap between the objective sciences of the mind and the subjective character of con-scious experience (Levine 1983; Nagel 1974). But it would be an overreaction to this point to maintain that the science of color vision, for example, could contribute nothing at all to our understanding of the normal or impaired experience—the "what it is like"—of seeing colors. In a similar way, we can agree that phenomenological description is essential while maintaining that cognitive psychology and cognitive neuroscience can contribute to our understanding of personal-level phenomena, including personal-level pathologies (such as addiction or hearing voices; Shea, Chapter 62, this volume).

Cognitive approaches to understanding delusions have focused first, not on the elabo-rated polythematic delusional systems or worlds of some individuals with schizophrenia, but on monothematic delusions—islands of delusion in a sea of apparent normality—and particularly, on monothematic delusions of neuropsychological origin. A starting point for understanding monothematic delusions is provided by Maher's (1974, 1988, 1992) anoma-lous experience hypothesis: a delusion arises as a normal response to an anomalous experi-ence. The methodology of cognitive approaches has been that of cognitive neuropsychiatry (David 1993; Halligan and David 2001); that is, the application of the methods of cognitive neuropsychology to psychiatric disorders. Thus, it has been assumed that the anomalous experience that figures in Maher's proposed etiology of delusions is the product of a neuro-psychological deficit (Coltheart 2007, p. 1047):

> The patient has a neuropsychological deficit of a kind that could plausibly be related to the content of the patient's particular delusion—that is, a deficit that could plausibly be viewed as having prompted the initial thought that turned into a delusional belief.

Maher himself shares the assumption that "[t]he origins of anomalous experience lie in a broad band of neuropsychological anomalies" (1999, p. 551) but, as we see in the quota-tion from Coltheart, cognitive approaches allow that Maher's anomalous conscious expe-rience might not always be essential. In some cases, the route from neuropsychological deficit to delusional belief might be wholly hidden from consciousness so that the delu-sional belief is "the first delusion-relevant event of which the patient is aware" (Coltheart et al. 2010, p. 264).

Because the neuropsychological deficit is supposed to be related to the content of the delusion in some plausible way, the type of deficit (and anomalous experience, if any) will vary from delusion to delusion. The type of deficit may also vary between individuals with the same delusion if different deficits can prompt the same "initial thought." Thus, cogni-tive approaches need to document types of neuropsychological deficit (and perhaps also types of experience) that could plausibly give rise to each of a variety of monothematic delusions, such as: Capgras delusion—"This [the subject's wife] is not my wife. My wife has been replaced by an impostor" (Capgras and Reboul-Lachaux 1923; Edelstyn and Oyebode 1999), Cotard delusion—"I am dead" (Cotard 1882; Young and Leafhead 1996), Fregoli delusion—"I am being followed around by people who are known to me but who are unrec-ognizable because they are in disguise" (Courbon and Fail 1927; de Pauw et al. 1987; Ellis et al. 1994), mirrored-self misidentification—"The person I see in the mirror is not really me" (Breen et al. 2000a, 2001a), somatoparaphrenia—"This [the subject's left arm] is not my arm" (Bottini et al. 2002; Halligan et al. 1995), and the delusion of alien control—"Other people can control the movements of my body" (Frith 1992; Frith and Done 1989).

Candidate neuropsychological deficits have been proposed as factors in the etiology of each of these delusions and others. But, in each case, there are examples of individuals who have the proposed deficit but not the delusion. The conclusion that is drawn from this dissociation is that there must be some additional factor or factors implicated in the etiology of delusions. In this chapter, we shall be concerned with the *two-factor* cognitive neuropsychological approach to understanding delusions (for early expositions, see e.g., Davies and Coltheart 2000; Davies et al. 2001; Langdon and Coltheart 2000; for recent reviews, see e.g., Aimola Davies and Davies 2009; Coltheart 2007, 2010; Coltheart et al. 2011; McKay 2012).

Before moving on, we shall illustrate the proposal of a neuropsychological deficit as a first factor, and the dissociation argument for a second factor, in the widely discussed case of Capgras delusion. We shall draw on important early work in cognitive neuropsychiatry (Ellis and Young 1990), which in turn built on a well-supported model of normal face processing (Bruce and Young 1986). In the Bruce and Young model, information about known faces is stored in face recognition units (FRUs), one for each known face. When a known face is seen, one FRU will be activated to a high level and biographical information stored in a corresponding personal identity node (PIN)—such as information about the person's occupation—will be accessed, as will the person's name. An important functional difference between FRUs and PINs is that only a seen face will activate an FRU, whereas a PIN can be accessed from the person's seen face or heard voice, or in other ways.

In some individuals with severely impaired face recognition (prosopagnosia), skin conductance responses continue to discriminate between familiar and unfamiliar faces—there is covert recognition (Tranel and Damasio 1985, 1988; see also Bauer 1984). So, although the primary face-recognition system is damaged in these individuals, there must be a preserved connection between an early stage of face processing (the FRUs) and the autonomic nervous system. Ellis and Young (1990) proposed that the neuropsychological deficit in Capgras delusion is the mirror image of the deficit in prosopagnosia with covert recognition. In Capgras delusion, the primary face-recognition system is intact but the connection between the FRUs and the autonomic nervous system is damaged. Normally, the seen face of a loved one, such as the spouse, causes activity in the autonomic nervous system and the experience of the loved one's face has a strong affective component. But now, with the connection between the face-recognition system and the autonomic nervous system disrupted, this component of the experience is missing.

Ellis and Young's proposal about the neuropsychological deficit and anomalous experience in Capgras delusion made a clear empirical prediction that the skin conductance responses of individuals with Capgras delusion would not discriminate between familiar and unfamiliar faces. This prediction was subsequently confirmed in four studies using photographs of familiar (famous or family) faces and unfamiliar faces (Brighetti et al. 2007; Ellis et al. 1997, 2000; Hirstein and Ramachandran 1997)—an "exemplary vindication" of the new discipline of cognitive neuropsychiatry (Ellis 1998). Thus, it is plausible that a neuropsychological deficit, disconnection of the primary face-recognition system from the autonomic nervous system, is a factor in the etiology of Capgras delusion. But there is a dissociation between this deficit and the delusion. There are individuals (patients with damage to ventromedial regions of frontal cortex; Tranel et al. 1995) whose skin conductance responses do not discriminate between familiar and unfamiliar faces, but who do not have Capgras delusion (or any other delusion). There is also a report of an individual who (following temporal lobe surgery for relief of epilepsy) had an anomalous "Capgras-like" experience of her mother—"she was different, something was different about her ... you can look different by, you know, doing your hair or whatever, but it wasn't different in that way ... it didn't feel like her" (Turner and Coltheart 2010, pp. 371–372)—but did not have the Capgras delusion.[2] Thus there must be a second factor in the etiology of Capgras delusion—presumably, in cases of neuropsychological origin, a second deficit.

THE TWO-FACTOR FRAMEWORK
FOR EXPLAINING DELUSIONS

Coltheart (2007 p. 1044) has proposed that, in order to explain any delusion, we need to answer two questions. First, where did the delusion come from? Second, why does the patient not reject the belief? The leading idea of the two-factor framework for explaining delusions (Coltheart 2007, 2010; Coltheart et al. 2011) is that the two factors will provide answers to these two questions.

> The first question is always: *where did the delusion come from?*—that is, what is responsible for the *content* of the delusional belief? The second question is always: *why does the patient not reject the belief?* ...—that is, what is responsible for the *persistence* of the belief? (Coltheart 2007 p. 1044)
>
> Factor 1 is what is responsible for the belief having occurred to the person in the first place ...: this factor determines the *content* of the delusional belief. Factor 2 is responsible for the failure to reject the hypothesis despite the presence of (often overwhelming) evidence against it ... this factor determines the *persistence* of the delusional belief. (Coltheart 2010, p. 18)
>
> The first question is, what brought the delusional idea to mind in the first place? The second question is, why is this idea accepted as true and adopted as a belief when the belief is typically bizarre and when so much evidence against its truth is available to the patient? (Coltheart et al. 2011, p. 271)

The two-factor framework has provided explanations (at least in outline) of a range of delusions including those that we have already mentioned and also anosognosia for motor impairments (Aimola Davies and Davies 2009; Aimola Davies et al. 2009; Davies et al. 2005). It has been proposed that the second factor is the same in all cases of delusion (or at least in all cases of delusion of neuropsychological origin) and that it consists in an impairment of normal processes of belief evaluation, associated with pathology of right lateral prefrontal cortex (e.g., Coltheart et al. 2011, p. 285). The nature of the putative task of belief evaluation suggests that the second factor could be an impairment of executive function or working memory (or both), consistent with its proposed neural basis (Aimola Davies and Davies 2009). But the cognitive nature and neural basis of the second factor have not been specified as precisely as the nature and basis of putative first factors.

---

[2] This patient was studied by Nora Breen and Mike Salzberg.

Adoption and persistence: Two options for the two-factor framework

It is important to notice that the three quotations listed earlier leave open two possible interpretations of the second question (that is, the question to which the second factor is supposed to provide an answer). In the third quotation, the second question is about *adoption* of the delusional belief. But it is possible initially to adopt a belief and then, on reflection, to reject it. Sometimes we initially believe what we see and then realize that we are subject to an illusion or we initially believe what we are told and then realize that our informant is unreliable. In the case of a delusional belief we can ask why the belief, once adopted, is not subsequently rejected. Why is it "firmly sustained" (American Psychiatric Association 2000, p. 821), why does it *persist*? This is more like the version of the second question that is posed in the first two quotations.

Explaining a delusion requires answers to both the adoption question and the persistence question. In principle, it might turn out that two factors (two pathologies or departures from normality) are needed to answer the adoption question and that a third factor is needed to answer the persistence question. That would, of course, be incompatible with the two-factor framework, but compatible with a less specific multi-factor framework. An exactly-two-factor account must say either:

(A) that no pathology or departure from normality beyond the first factor is needed to answer the adoption question and the second factor answers the persistence question;

or else:

(B) that two factors are needed to answer the adoption question and no additional pathology or departure from normality is needed to answer the persistence question.

(In principle, it might be that option (A) is correct for some delusions and option (B) for others.)

According to option (A), we should expect each dissociation of the "first deficit without delusion" form (e.g., ventromedial frontal damage without Capgras delusion; Tranel et al. 1995) to be a case in which the delusional belief is initially adopted, but does not persist. According to option (B), we should expect each dissociation to be a case in which the first deficit is present, but the delusional belief is not even initially adopted. This presents a potential problem for option (A) because there is no evidence that patients with ventromedial frontal damage, for example, initially adopt the Capgras delusion but subsequently reject it (nor is there evidence that this is not the case; see Coltheart et al. 2010, p. 281 and McKay 2012, pp. 341–342, for discussion).

On the other hand, there are reports of individuals who, after recovering from a delusion, still feel the attraction of the belief that they now reject. For example, a patient (HS) who had recovered from anosognosia reported that the idea that he could move his paralyzed limbs still seemed credible even though he was able to reject it (Chatterjee and Mennemeier 1996, p. 227):

> E: What was the consequence of the stroke?
> HS: The left hand here is dead and the left leg was pretty much.
> HS: (later): I still feel as if when I am in a room and I have to get up and go walking … I just feel like I should be able to.
> E: You have a belief that you could actually do that?
> HS: I do not have a belief, just the exact opposite. I just have the feeling that sometimes I feel like I can get up and do something and I have to tell myself "no I can't."

Turner and Coltheart describe a patient in the early stages of recovery from Capgras delusion (2010, p. 371):

> I've started going through it, and seeing what could possibly happen and what couldn't happen. That was wrong, that couldn't happen. Even though it has happened it couldn't. Mary couldn't suddenly disappear from the room, so there must be an explanation for it.… And then I worked it out and I've wondered if it's Mary all the time. It's nobody else.

In summary, the standard examples of deficit without delusion, which figure in the dissociation argument for a second factor, are potentially problematic for option (A) and fit option (B) better. But the examples of recovery from delusion fit option (A) well, on the assumption that the recovery resulted from remission of the second factor. Thus, not only the cognitive nature and neural basis of the second factor, but also—and even more importantly—its role in the etiology of delusions, requires further specification.[3]

Bayesian approaches

One of the aims of cognitive neuropsychology is to understand disorders of cognition in terms of theories or models of normal cognition. Cognitive impairments are understood in terms of damage to one or more components of the normal cognitive system. When the methods of cognitive neuropsychology are applied to delusions—pathologies of belief— what is required is an information-processing model of the normal formation, evaluation, and revision of beliefs. Thus, one of the problems faced by cognitive neuropsychiatry—in comparison with the cognitive neuropsychology of face recognition, for example—is that we do not have an articulated, still less a computationally implemented, model of normal believing. Indeed, there may be reasons of principle why it is difficult to understand believing in terms of the computational theory of mind (Fodor 1983, 2000; see Cratsley and Samuels, Chapter 27, this volume, on Fodorian pessimism).

More than twenty-five years ago, Hemsley and Garety suggested a strategy for making progress in the absence of a model of normal believing (1986, p. 52): "A normative theory

---

[3] In this chapter, we shall be defending a version of option (A), but we do not offer a resolution of the potential problem associated with option (A). In the specific case of the ventromedial frontal patients, it might be suggested that they do not initially adopt the Cagras delusion because they do not, in fact, have exactly the same neuropsychological deficit as Capgras patients (see Ellis and Lewis 2001). That suggestion provides a response to the potential problem for option (A) but at the price of removing the standard dissociation argument for a second factor.

of how people *should* evaluate evidence relevant to their beliefs can provide a conceptual framework for a consideration of how they do *in fact* evaluate it." Their specific proposal was to begin from a probabilistic analysis of hypothesis evaluation and then to investigate whether individuals with delusions deviate from the normative Bayesian model. In pursuing this strategy and interpreting its results, it is important to distinguish the normative from the normal; it is important not to forget that, as Hemsley and Garety put it, there is "'normal' deviation from the prescriptive model" (p. 55).

Recently, the Bayesian approach has been married with the neuropsychological deficit approach in continuing development of the two-factor framework for explaining monothematic delusions (Coltheart et al. 2010; McKay 2012). A second body of work has adopted a Bayesian approach—and, specifically, the theoretical framework of predictive coding and prediction error signals, in which neural processing aims to minimize prediction error or "free energy" (Friston 2005, 2009, 2010; Friston and Stephan 2007)—to delusions in schizophrenia (Corlett et al. 2009; Fletcher and Frith 2009).[4] In this chapter, we shall focus on the Bayesian two-factor approach to explaining monothematic delusions and on the idea that delusions arise through a process of Bayesian inference or updating.

Bayesian inference

On a Bayesian approach, probabilities are updated on the basis of evidence, E, so that the new or *posterior* probability of a hypothesis, H, is equal to the old or *prior* conditional probability of H given E. This updating procedure is known as *simple conditionalization*. By Bayes' theorem, the conditional probability, $P(H|E)$, can be further unpacked to give:

Simple conditionalization:

$$P'(H) = P(H|E) = P(H) \cdot P(E|H)/P(E).$$

(Here, P' is the new distribution of probabilities.) The notions of prior and posterior probabilities are relative. The prior probability of H is prior only to the evidence E; it already takes account of antecedently available evidence—today's priors are yesterday's posteriors. In simple conditionalization, the evidence is treated as certain: $P'(E) = 1$. A more general updating procedure, Jeffrey conditionalization (Jeffrey 1965/1983), allows that the evidence may be less than certain, so that $P'(E) < 1$.[5]

The posterior probability of a hypothesis, H, updated on the basis of evidence E by simple conditionalization, is proportional to the prior probability of H, $P(H)$, and to the probability of E given H, $P(E|H)$, also known as the *likelihood* of H on E. The likelihood provides a measure of how well H predicts E. In this chapter, we shall usually be more interested in the balance of probabilities between two competing hypotheses than in the precise probability of each hypothesis. If we are considering two hypotheses, H_1 and H_2, then the ratio

---

[4] See Frith (2007, chapters 4 and 5) for an accessible introduction to the predictive coding approach and Corlett et al. (2007, 2009) for prediction error and delusion. See also Shea (Chapter 62, this volume) for discussion of prediction error signals.

[5] In Jeffrey conditionalization, the probability of H is updated to:
$$P'(H) = P(H|E) \cdot P'(E) + P(H|\text{not-E}) \cdot P'(\text{not-E}).$$

of posterior probabilities (the posterior odds) is the product of two other ratios, the ratio of prior probabilities (the prior odds) and the likelihood ratio:

Bayes ratio formula:

$$\frac{P'(H_1)}{P'(H_2)} = \frac{P(H_1|E)}{P(H_2|E)} = \frac{P(H_1)}{P(H_2)} \cdot \frac{P(E|H_1)}{P(E|H_2)}$$

Thus, on a Bayesian approach, the balance of probabilities between two candidate hypotheses, updated on the basis of evidence E, depends on (*a*) how probable each hypothesis is in the light of available evidence other than E—given by the prior probability $P(H_i)$—and (*b*) how well each hypothesis predicts the evidence—given by the likelihood $P(E|H_i)$.

In the next two sections, we shall review two versions of the Bayesian two-factor approach (Coltheart et al. 2010; McKay 2012) in some detail. One section is about the initial adoption of a delusional belief and the other is about the persistence of the belief. Before moving on, however, we note that there are complex and difficult issues surrounding the relationship between, on the one hand, Bayesian inference or updating and, on the other hand, abductive inference or inference to the best explanation (Lipton 2004).

Coltheart et al. (2010) sketch two models of abductive inference, the logical empiricist model based on an understanding of explanation as logical implication and the Bayesian model based on a probabilistic account of explanation (p. 271): "the hypothesis H explains observations O to the degree *x* just in case the probability of O given H is *x*." They adopt a Bayesian model of abduction, but we are not committed to the view that Bayesian inference is a model of inference to the best explanation. One reason is that the likelihood, $P(E|H)$, is not in general a good measure of how well a hypothesis H explains evidence E. A hypothesis about barometer readings (e.g., the barometer is falling) does not explain weather patterns (e.g., a storm is coming), however high the likelihood (that is, the probability of the weather patterns given the barometer readings) may be. Rather, causation and explanation run in the opposite direction, from weather patterns to barometer readings (van Fraassen 1980, p. 104).

More generally, Lipton's account of inference to the best explanation takes account, not only of whether a candidate explanatory hypothesis is the most probable given the available evidence, but also of whether it exhibits explanatory virtues such as parsimony, scope, depth, unifying disparate phenomena, and making new predictions. The question then arises whether it could ever be rational to accept an explanation because of its virtues, if an alternative explanation was more probable (van Fraassen 1989). Lipton (2004) aims to neutralize this concern about the relationship between inference to the best explanation and Bayesianism by suggesting that explanatory virtues are a guide to probability, but we take no stand on that issue.

In our discussion of delusions and Bayesian inference, it will be the standard Bayesian apparatus of probability assignments, likelihoods, and updating that bears the theoretical load. The notion of explanatory virtue will play only a peripheral role, in that it may influence the psychological accessibility of hypotheses. It is true that some of the literature that we shall engage with is couched in terms of inference to the best explanation. But this seems to be largely inessential and, because of the issues that we have just mentioned, potentially distracting. Most or all of the theoretical work in explaining the adoption and persistence of delusional beliefs in terms of Bayesian *abductive* inference could be done just as well by talking about Bayesian inference *simpliciter*, thereby sidestepping those complex and difficult issues.

Bayes in the Two-Factor Framework:
Adoption of the Delusional Belief

Coltheart and colleagues (2010) propose that the answer, in outline, to the question where a delusion came from is that it arose through a process of Bayesian inference. In principle, this might be a process of inference carried out consciously by the person with the delusion, but Coltheart and colleagues focus on the case of unconscious inferential processes. To illustrate their approach, Coltheart and colleagues provide a worked example of how Bayesian inference could lead from a neuropsychological deficit to the initial onset of Capgras delusion.

From deficit to delusional belief: Capgras delusion

Suppose that, as the result of a stroke, a patient suffers disconnection of the primary face processing system from the autonomic nervous system (while the two disconnected systems themselves remain intact). Before the patient suffered the stroke, the appearance of his wife caused activation of the face recognition unit for the wife (FRU_W), which normally led to activation, not only of the corresponding personal identity node (PIN_W), but also of the autonomic nervous system. As a result of the learned association between the appearance of the patient's wife and activation of his autonomic nervous system, the appearance of his wife generated an unconscious prediction of activity in the autonomic nervous system, and this prediction was reliably fulfilled. Following the stroke, some things remain the same and some things are different. When the patient sees his wife, the face recognition unit FRU_W and the personal identity node PIN_W are still activated, and activity in the autonomic nervous system is still predicted. But, because of the disconnection, the prediction is not fulfilled. The abnormal absence of the predicted autonomic activity, resulting from the neuropsychological deficit (disconnection), stands in need of explanation.

The aim of the Bayesian approach is to show that a delusional hypothesis may be initially adopted as a belief as a result of Bayesian inference or updating on the basis of abnormal data, D (in this case, the absence of activity in the autonomic nervous system). Consequently, the next stage of Coltheart and colleagues' (2010) worked example involves two competing hypotheses. One is the true hypothesis, H_W, that the woman that the patient sees in front of him, who looks like the patient's wife and says that she is the patient's wife is, indeed, his wife. The other is the delusional hypothesis, H_S, that the woman is not the patient's wife but a stranger.[6]

What needs to be shown is that the ratio of posterior probabilities, $P(H_S|D)/P(H_W|D)$, could favor the stranger hypothesis, H_S, over the wife hypothesis, H_W. The Bayes ratio formula tells us that this ratio is equal to the product of the ratio of prior probabilities and the

---

[6] Coltheart et al. (2010) do not consider hypotheses that are incompatible with both H_W and H_S, such as the hypothesis H_A, that the person that the patient sees in front of him is aunt Agatha, or the hypothesis H_B, that the person that the patient sees in front of him is Bob the bank teller. As a result of this simplification, H_S is treated as the negation of H_W.

likelihood ratio. So, how might the balance between those two ratios favor H_S over H_W? The prior probabilities, $P(H_W)$ and $P(H_S)$, are prior only to the to-be-explained abnormal data D. They take account of antecedently available evidence including, in particular, the evidence that the woman that the patient sees in front of him looks just like his wife and says that she is his wife. Consequently, the probability that the woman is the patient's wife is much higher than the probability that she is a stranger and the ratio $P(H_S)/P(H_W)$ is correspondingly low. In contrast, Coltheart and colleagues say, the likelihood ratio, $P(D|H_S)/P(D|H_W)$ is high: "It would be highly improbable for the subject to have the low autonomic response [D] if the person really was his wife, but very probable indeed if the person were a stranger" (2010, p. 277).

According to the worked example, then, the ratio of prior probabilities favors the wife hypothesis, H_W, but the likelihood ratio favors the stranger hypothesis, H_S. Whether the ratio of posterior probabilities favors H_W or H_S depends on the relative values of these ratios and, specifically, on whether the likelihood ratio is sufficient to outweigh the ratio of prior probabilities. Suppose, for example, that the prior probabilities favored H_W in the ratio 100:1 but the likelihoods favored H_S in the ratio 1000:1. Then the posterior probabilities would favor H_S in the ratio 10:1. If these were the only two hypotheses to consider, their probabilities would be $P(H_S) = 0.91$ and $P(H_W) = 0.09$. Thus, Bayesian inference might lead from the abnormal data D to the assignment of a high probability to the hypothesis that the woman who looks just like the patient's wife and also claims to be the patient's wife is not his wife but a stranger, and so an impostor. Equally, if the prior probabilities favored H_W in the ratio 100:1 but the likelihoods favored H_S only in the ratio 10:1, then the posterior probabilities would be reversed: $P(H_S) = 0.09$ and $P(H_W) = 0.91$.

Coltheart et al. suggest that the likelihood ratio does outweigh the ratio of prior probabilities (2010, p. 278):

> The delusional hypothesis provides a much more convincing explanation of the highly unusual data than the nondelusional hypothesis; and this fact swamps the general implausibility of the delusional hypothesis. So if the subject with Capgras delusion unconsciously reasons in this way, he has up to this point committed no mistake of rationality on the Bayesian model.[7]

One difficulty in evaluating this suggestion about Bayesian inference is that it is somewhat unclear which probabilities are to figure in the worked example. Are they supposed to be, for example, realistic probabilities or the patient's subjective probabilities (credences)? As we shall see later (in the "Bayesian inference in a perceptual module" section), there are problems with each of these options. But the main point here is that if Coltheart and colleagues' suggestion is correct then the disconnection of the patient's face processing system from the autonomic nervous system is the only pathology or departure from normality that need be implicated in the processes leading up to the initial onset of Capgras delusion. Consequently, the role for a second factor in the etiology of the delusion must lie beyond that point, in an impairment of post-onset belief evaluation that explains the persistence of the delusion. This is option (A) (see "Adoption and persistence" section).

---

[7] Coltheart and colleagues move from the fact that the delusional hypothesis, H_S, provides a much more convincing explanation of the data than the wife hypothesis, H_W, does to the claim that the likelihood ratio strongly favors H_S. It is worth noting, however, that explanatoriness is not always a good indicator of likelihood. From the fact that a hypothesis, H, utterly fails to explain evidence, E, it does not follow that the likelihood, $P(E|H)$, is close to zero.

Biased Bayesian inference

McKay (2012) challenges Coltheart and colleagues' (2010) description of the unconscious inferential processes that lead up to the initial onset of the delusional belief. The general point that Coltheart and colleagues make is that the superior explanatory (better: predictive) potential of the stranger hypothesis can outweigh the prior odds in favor of the wife hypothesis. McKay objects that the prior probability of the stranger hypothesis in their worked example ($P(H_S) = 0.01$) is "unrealistically high" (2012, p. 339). A more realistic estimate would give a ratio of prior probabilities that would much more strongly favor the wife hypothesis and would be much more difficult for the likelihood ratio to outweigh.[8]

The exact value of $P(H_S)$ is, of course, a point of detail. But the moral that McKay (p. 340) draws is that, with a realistic distribution of prior probabilities, unbiased Bayesian inference would not lead from abnormal data to the onset of delusional belief. Specifically, the likelihood ratio in Coltheart and colleagues' worked example (999:1 in favor of H_S) would be insufficient to outweigh a realistic ratio of prior probabilities favoring H_W. Unbiased updating of probabilities gives weight to both the prior probabilities and the likelihoods of competing hypotheses. Actual updating departs from the normative Bayesian model if it discounts either of these components in the Bayes ratio formula. McKay proposes that, if updating is to lead to the onset of Capgras delusion, there must be a departure from the normative Bayesian model. If posterior probabilities are to favor H_S over H_W then prior probabilities must be discounted to increase the relative weight given to likelihoods.[9]

Once again, it is difficult to evaluate this proposal because it is unclear how we are to understand the probabilities that are supposed to figure in the worked examples. But we set aside issues of interpretation for the time being (see "Bayesian inference in a perceptual module" section) in order to highlight a clear and important point of contrast between McKay (2012) and Coltheart et al. (2010). According to McKay, the disconnection of the patient's face processing system from the autonomic nervous system is *not* the only pathology or departure from normality that is implicated in the processes leading up to the onset of Capgras delusion (McKay 2012, p. 345): "the second factor in delusion formation comprises a bias towards explanatory adequacy." Here, we should recall that a bias or other deviation from the normative Bayesian model might be normal (Hemsley and Garety 1986). But if McKay's proposed updating bias does amount to a departure from normality then, in order for his account to remain within the exactly-two-factor framework, no additional pathology

[8] McKay points out, in effect, that if Coltheart et al.'s (2010) proposed prior probability, $P(H_S) = 0.01$, were correct then one should expect that one time in a hundred, an encounter with a person who looked just like one's spouse and claimed to be one's spouse would be an encounter with a stranger (impostor). He suggests that a more realistic prior probability for H_S would be two orders of magnitude lower; that is, of the order of 0.0001. (McKay's proposal is $P(H_S) = 0.00027$.)

[9] In a case of comparison between two hypotheses, if the ratio of prior probabilities were 1:1 then the ratio of posterior probabilities would be equal to the likelihood ratio. So an updating bias in favor of likelihoods can be implemented by treating the ratio of prior probabilities as being closer to 1:1 than it really is. This could be achieved by treating the absolute magnitude of the logarithm of the prior odds as being closer to zero than it really is (by subtraction, so that the logarithm would approach zero linearly, or by division, so that the logarithm would approach zero asymptotically). Conversely, a reduction in the absolute magnitude of the logarithm of the likelihood ratio would implement an updating bias in favor of prior probabilities. See McKay (2012, pp. 350–352) for a different, and more general, way of implementing these biases.

should be needed to answer the persistence question. This is option (B) (see "Adoption and persistence" section).

Bayes in the Two-Factor Framework: Persistence of the Delusional Belief

The Capgras patient believes that the woman who looks like his wife and says that she is his wife is really a stranger; his wife has been replaced by an impostor.[10] We have been considering two Bayesian answers to the question how this belief came to be adopted. Now we turn to the question why, given that this belief has been initially adopted, it is not subsequently rejected when evidence and implausibility count against it. One possible form of answer to this question is that there is a separate impairment of post-adoption belief evaluation—as in option (A). The other is that no additional pathology or departure from normality is needed to explain the delusional belief's persistence once it has been adopted—as in option (B).

Two accounts of persistence

Coltheart and colleagues (2010) envisage that, after adopting the delusional belief, the patient will be presented with new evidence, N, that is better explained (predicted) by the wife hypothesis than by the stranger hypothesis. Friends and relatives assure the patient that the woman he believes to be an impostor is really his wife, the woman knows many things about the patient's life, and she arrives home from his wife's place of employment, driving his wife's car, wearing his wife's clothes, and carrying his wife's briefcase with his wife's initials in gold lettering.

So there should be a new round of Bayesian updating of probabilities. The new prior probabilities are $P'(H_S) = P(H_S|D)$, and $P'(H_W) = P(H_W|D)$ and, because the delusional belief has been adopted, the ratio of new prior probabilities favors H_S (perhaps in the ratio 10:1). In contrast, the likelihood ratio, $P'(N|H_S)/P'(N|H_W)$, favors H_W. For example, friends and relatives would be more likely to give such assurances if the woman were the patient's wife than if she were a stranger. If the likelihood ratio is sufficient to outweigh the ratio of prior probabilities then, according to the normative model, the ratio of posterior probabilities, $P'(H_S|N)/P'(H_W|N)$, should favor H_W over H_S and the delusional belief should be rejected on the basis of the new evidence N. However, the delusion persists. According to Coltheart and colleagues (2010), this persistence is to be explained by the second factor, which is some kind of impairment—to be specified—in the evaluation of already adopted beliefs in the light of new evidence.

---

[10] The proposition, H_S, that the woman that the patient sees in front of him is a stranger is strictly speaking distinct from the proposition that the woman is an impostor—that is, a stranger who looks like the patient's wife and says that she is the patient's wife. But since probabilities have already been updated to take into account the evidence that the woman that the patient sees in front of him looks like his wife and says that she is his wife, the stranger hypothesis and the impostor hypothesis have the same probability and we can elide the distinction between them.

It is crucial to this account of persistence as being explained by a second factor that, according to the normative Bayesian model, the delusional belief, H_S, *should* be rejected on the basis of the new evidence N. This, in turn, depends on the claim that the likelihood ratio, $P'(N|H_S)/P'(N|H_W)$, favors H_W strongly enough to outweigh the ratio of prior probabilities, which favors of H_S. There is a potential problem for the account here. An estimate of the likelihood ratio, and particularly an estimate of $P'(N|H_S)$, depends on what exactly the new evidence N is taken to be.

On a Bayesian approach, evidence—such as the new evidence, N—is a proposition. Suppose, for example, that a trusted friend of the patient asserts that the woman who looks just like the patient's wife *is* the patient's wife. Is the evidence, N, the proposition *that the woman is the patient's wife* (essentially, the proposition H_W) or the proposition *that the trusted friend asserted that the woman is the patient's wife*? On the first (more committed) interpretation, the likelihood, $P'(N|H_S)$, is low; in fact it is zero (or very close to zero). But on the second (more cautious) interpretation, $P'(N|H_S)$ might be quite high and almost as high as $P'(N|H_W)$: even a trusted friend may be taken in by a very good impostor.[11] The potential problem for Coltheart and colleagues' explanation of persistence is that, on the more cautious interpretation of what the evidence is, the likelihood ratio might not favor H_W strongly enough to outweigh the ratio of prior probabilities. (We shall consider the more committed interpretation shortly; see "Rejecting evidence" section.) If the ratio of posterior probabilities still favors H_S rather than H_W then, of course, there is no need for a second factor (a pathology or departure from normality) to explain the persistence of the delusional belief.

On McKay's (2012) account, in contrast to that of Coltheart et al. (2010), there are already two factors involved in the answer to the question how the delusional belief came to be initially adopted (the neuropsychological deficit and the updating bias in favor of likelihoods). But we still need an answer to the question why the belief is not subsequently rejected when there is so much evidence against it. Is a *third* factor needed in order to explain the persistence of the delusion?

Our discussion (two paragraphs back) of Coltheart and colleagues' (2010) account suggests that there may be no need for an additional factor to explain persistence and this is, indeed, McKay's (2012) view. He agrees that, after the initial adoption of the delusional belief, there will be new evidence that counts in favor of the wife hypothesis and against the stranger hypothesis. But he points out that much of this new evidence (e.g., trusted friends say that the woman is the patient's wife) is similar in kind to evidence that was taken into account in the previous prior probabilities of the competing hypotheses (e.g., the woman herself says that she is the patient's wife). The patient's evidential situation remains very similar to the situation that led to the initial adoption of the delusional belief and so the same processes of updating (processes biased in favor of likelihoods—McKay's second factor) will lead to similar posterior probabilities. Thus, McKay says (2012, p. 343): "if the

---

[11] For some other pieces of new evidence, there will be similar, though less dramatic, differences in likelihood estimates depending on what exactly the evidence is taken to be. Suppose, for example, that the woman is carrying what is in fact the wife's briefcase. Is the evidence, N, the proposition *that the woman is carrying the wife's briefcase* or the proposition *that the woman is carrying a briefcase that looks just like the wife's*? However, the distinction between more committed and more cautious interpretations of what the evidence is might not extend smoothly to all pieces of new evidence (e.g., the fact that the woman is able to give correct accounts of many past events involving the patient and his wife). Different kinds of new evidence require more discussion than they can receive here.

neuropsychological data that stimulate the stranger hypothesis are so salient that they can compensate for the low prior probability of that hypothesis, then supplementary testimony from friends and clinicians will be powerless to overwhelm those data."

Diagnostic evidence, similar evidence, and "unfalsifiability"

Consider just a subset of the evidence against the Capgras patient's delusional belief: the evidence that the woman that the patient sees in front of him looks just like his wife and says that she is his wife. This evidence is predicted by the patient's impostor hypothesis no less than by the true hypothesis, H_W. The evidence is not *diagnostic* between the two hypotheses—it cannot shift the prior balance of probabilities toward H_W, because the likelihood ratio is 1:1. In this limited way, the Capgras patient's hypothesis is similar to skeptical hypotheses (such as Descartes's evil demon hypothesis) in being "unfalsifiable." The evil demon hypothesis, or the "brain in a vat" hypothesis, is not falsified by the evidence of my senses, "Here is one hand, and here is another" (Moore 1939), because a perceptual experience as of hands is predicted by the skeptical hypothesis no less than by the external world hypothesis. (It is important to note that, on a Bayesian approach, this unfalsifiability depends on the evidence being the cautious proposition *that I am having a perceptual experience as of hands* rather than the committed proposition *that I have hands*.)

It is only a small set of evidence (only the evidence that the woman looks just like the patient's wife and says that she is his wife) that is utterly unable to shift the balance of probabilities toward H_W. But, as we have just seen, the value of a larger set of evidence is diminished because accepted evidence makes other similar evidence more probable. It is improbable that a trusted friend should assert, concerning a stranger, that she is the patient's wife. But it is not so improbable that a trusted friend should assert, concerning a stranger who looks just like the patient's wife and says that she is his wife (an impostor, and a good impostor at that), that she is the patient's wife. So, although the evidence of the trusted friend's testimony is somewhat better predicted by the wife hypothesis, H_W, it does not favor H_W very strongly—arguably not strongly enough to outweigh the ratio of prior probabilities in favor of H_S. It is for this reason that McKay's (2012) account and, equally, our reservations about Coltheart et al.'s (2010) account, seem plausible. It is difficult to identify a role for a pathology or departure from normality that would distinctively explain the persistence of a delusional belief after its initial adoption had been accounted for—that is, a role for a second factor according to option (A).

Coltheart and colleagues' view is, of course, that they have identified such a role. So let us consider their example (2010, p. 279) again.[12]

---

[12] Coltheart and colleagues say (2010, p. 282): "subjects are impaired at revising preexisting beliefs on the basis of new evidence relevant to any particular belief." McKay interprets this as a Bayesian proposal that the second factor is an updating bias in which likelihoods are discounted to increase the relative weight given to prior probabilities. Against the proposal, he objects that it is hard to see how the delusional belief would ever have been adopted if a bias in favor of prior probabilities were in place. With such a bias, the patient would have updated his credences much more conservatively on the basis of the unexpected absence of activity in the autonomic nervous system (McKay 2012, section 3.3). This is an interesting objection, but we set it aside here and consider a strand in Coltheart et al.'s (2010) account of the second factor that is rather different from the idea of a general bias in favor of prior probabilities.

Rejecting evidence

The patient has adopted the delusional belief and the ratio of new prior probabilities, $P'(H_S)/P'(H_W)$, favors H_S. But now, new evidence N is presented, and the likelihood ratio, $P'(N|H_S)/P'(N|H_W)$, favors H_W. If the likelihood ratio is sufficient to outweigh the ratio of prior probabilities then the delusional belief should be rejected—but it persists. We pointed to a potential problem for Coltheart and colleagues' explanation of persistence in terms of a second factor. On the more cautious interpretation of which proposition the evidence is, the likelihood ratio might not favor H_W strongly enough to outweigh the ratio of prior probabilities. In fact, we suggested that the likelihood $P'(N|H_S)$ might be only slightly lower than $P'(N|H_W)$.

Coltheart and colleagues (2010) go on to say that, before the new evidence is actually presented, the patient should attach a low credence to the evidence proposition. In the normative model, the prior probability of N is given by:

$$P'(N) = P'(N|H_S) \cdot P'(H_S) + P'(N|H_W) \cdot P'(H_W).^{13}$$

If, as Coltheart et al. say, $P'(N|H_S)$ and $P'(H_W)$ are both low, then $P'(N)$ is also low: the patient should not expect N to be true. We suggested, however, that $P'(N|H_S)$ is not low and that the prior probability of N might be quite high. (This is what diminishes N's evidential value.)

The potential problem that we saw for Coltheart and colleagues' explanation of persistence disappears if we read them as adopting the more committed interpretation of the evidence (e.g., taking N to be the proposition *that the woman is the patient's wife* rather than the proposition *that the trusted friend asserted that the woman is the patient's wife*). On that interpretation (as the "more committed" terminology suggests), the prior probability, $P'(N)$, and the likelihood, $P'(N|H_S)$, are lower—as Coltheart et al.'s account requires. Consequently, it is more plausible that the likelihood ratio outweighs the ratio of prior probabilities so that the ratio of posterior probabilities favors H_W over H_S. It is also more plausible that, normatively, the delusional belief should be rejected on the basis of the new evidence, N. Why, then, does the delusional belief persist? Coltheart and colleagues answer this question as follows (2010, pp. 279–280):

> What the deluded Capgras subject seems to be doing here is ignoring or disregarding any new evidence that cannot be explained by the stranger hypothesis. It is as though he is so convinced of the truth of the stranger hypothesis by its explanatory power that his conviction makes him either disregard or reject all evidence that is inconsistent with that hypothesis, or at least cannot be explained by the hypothesis.... it seems as if the new information does not even enter the deluded subject's belief system as data that need to be explained.

It is striking that there is nothing evidently Bayesian about this answer to the persistence question.[14]

---

[13] This is an instance of the total probability theorem. We follow Coltheart et al. (2010, p. 280) in assuming (for simplicity) that hypotheses inconsistent with both H_S and H_W, such as the aunt Agatha hypothesis and the Bob the bank teller hypothesis, have probability zero (equivalently, that H_W is the negation of H_S).

[14] There are two other notable features of this quotation. First, the answer that it gives to the persistence question seems to be completely different from the answer quoted in footnote 12 (Coltheart et al. 2010, p. 282; also quoted by McKay 2012, p. 343). Second, it does not seem to describe any impairment of information processing.

One important idea behind Coltheart and colleagues' account of how the Capgras patient goes wrong is that, "it is reasonable in suitable circumstances to accept the evidence of one's senses and the testimony of others" (2010, p. 281; see also p. 275). It is clear that, on their view, it would be reasonable for the Capgras patient to accept as evidence, and update his credences on the basis of, not just the cautious proposition *that the trusted friend asserted that the woman is the patient's wife* but also the committed proposition *that the woman is the patient's wife*. But Coltheart and colleagues also accept that "it is sometimes reasonable to reject information that cannot be explained by the hypothesis that one is committed to" (p. 280). For example, if a trusted friend and distinguished scientist tells you that, in a tunnel under Switzerland and Italy, particles travel faster than the speed of light, it might be reasonable not to accept the proposition that particles travel faster than the speed of light as evidence—not to update all your credences on that proposition. So when is it reasonable to accept and when is it reasonable to reject, the evidence of perception and testimony?

As we noted earlier, Coltheart and colleagues draw attention to the fact that, in the case of the Capgras patient, the prior probability of the new evidence in favor of the wife hypothesis is low (on the more committed interpretation of which proposition the evidence is). But low prior probability is not supposed to be sufficient to make rejection reasonable (2010, p. 281; emphasis added):

> Capgras subjects are so much *in the grip of the stranger hypothesis* that they refuse to accept the evidence of their senses and the testimony of others. They fail to incorporate the new data into their belief systems *when it is reasonable to do so*.

No explicit account is offered of what conditions, in addition to low prior probability, need to be met if rejection of evidence is to be reasonable. Furthermore, there seems to be a suggestion—depending on what being in the grip of a hypothesis amounts to—that the real problem is the patient's initial adoption of (assignment of a high credence to) the impostor hypothesis. But, if persistence flows from adoption without additional pathology or departure from normality, then there is no need for a second factor.

Even if we step back from any suggestion that there is no need for a second factor, it remains the case that Coltheart and colleagues have provided no distinctively Bayesian answer to the persistence question.[15]

---

[15] There is, in fact, a fairly natural Bayesian answer to the specific question about the conditions under which acceptance or rejection of evidence (that is, evidence on the committed interpretation) is reasonable. Acceptance of (assignment of a high credence to) a committed evidence proposition, E^+ (e.g., *that the woman is the patient's wife*), is reasonable if the probability of E^+ given E^-, $P'(E^+|E^-)$, is high, where E^- is the corresponding cautious evidence proposition (e.g., *that a trusted friend asserted that the woman is the patient's wife*). Similarly, rejection of (assignment of a low credence to) E^+ is reasonable if $P'(E^+|E^-)$, is low. This will be so if there is a proposition, E^*, inconsistent with E^+, such that $P'(E^*|E^-) > P'(E^+|E^-)$—that is, if a proposition that is inconsistent with E^+ has a higher probability than E^+ given E^-.

Evidently, however, that Bayesian proposal would take us back to the earlier potential problem for Coltheart and colleagues' (2010) account. Rejection of the committed evidence proposition, E^+ (e.g., *that the woman is the patient's wife*), *would* be reasonable because there is a proposition, H_S, inconsistent with E^+ (= H_W), such that $P'(H_S|E^-) > P'(E^+|E^-)$, where E^- is the corresponding cautious evidence proposition (e.g., *that a trusted friend asserted that the woman is the patient's wife*). The reason for this is that the prior probability of H_S ($P'(H_S)$) is substantially higher than the prior probability of E^+ (= $P'(H_W)$), while the likelihood $P'(E^-|H_S)$ is only slightly lower than $P'(E^-|E^+)$ (= $P'(E^-|H_W)$).

Interim summary

We have considered two recent Bayesian developments of the two-factor framework for explaining delusions. There is a fairly clear disagreement between the two accounts over whether, in addition to the first neuropsychological deficit, a second pathology or departure from normality figures in the explanation of the initial adoption of the delusional belief. Coltheart et al. (2010) say that unbiased Bayesian inference could lead to the onset of Capgras delusion, whereas McKay (2012) says that a bias in favor of likelihoods at the expense of prior probabilities would be required. But we have not been able to identify a role for a further factor (a second factor in Coltheart et al.'s account, a third factor in McKay's) that would explain the persistence of the belief, once it had been adopted. When we adopt a Bayesian approach to the adoption question, persistence of the newly adopted belief appears to be the normal case—and even the normatively correct case.

   The lesson that we draw from this is not that there is something wrong with the two-factor framework for explaining delusions, nor that there is something wrong, specifically, with the proposal that the second factor answers the persistence question—option (A). Our view is that the Bayesian approach does not reveal how post-adoption belief evaluation goes wrong in individuals with delusions because it provides no account at all of evaluation of beliefs, once they have been adopted and before new evidence becomes available, even in healthy individuals. In the next section, we argue that the problem lies, not with the Bayesian approach as such, but with a standard idealizing assumption.

Belief Evaluation and
the Fragmented Mind

If we conceive of believing as a binary (on/off) matter, so that each proposition is either believed or not believed, then the normative ideal for an individual's system of beliefs seems to require a single consistent set of beliefs (propositions for which believing is *on*) that guide action in all contexts. If we adopt a Bayesian approach and conceive of believing as a graded matter, so that each proposition is assigned a credence (subjective probability), then the ideal for a system of beliefs seems to require a single coherent distribution of credences that guide action in all contexts.

   Notoriously, we fall short of these supposed ideals. Actual belief systems are fragmented or compartmentalized. Individual fragments are consistent and coherent but fragments are not consistent or coherent with each other and different fragments guide action in different contexts. We hold inconsistent beliefs and act in some contexts on the basis of the belief that P and in other contexts on the basis of the belief that not-P. Frequently we fail to put things together or to "join up the dots." It can happen that some actions are guided by a belief that P and other actions are guided by a belief that if P then Q, but no actions are guided by a belief that Q because the belief that P and the belief that if P then Q are in separate fragments. For example, some people are described as having their philosophical beliefs and their religious beliefs in separate compartments. David Lewis describes himself as having once had fragmented beliefs about the geography of Princeton. According to one fragment, Nassau Street ran north-south and was parallel to the railway track; according to another fragment, the railway track ran east-west and was parallel to Nassau Street (Lewis 1982, p. 436).

It is natural to assume that fragmentation is a consequence of our limited information-processing resources and that consistency and coherence across a single web of belief, though practically unattainable, is indeed the ideal. Fragmentation allows inconsistency and it allows failure to believe the consequences of our beliefs. But fragmentation also brings a benefit: it allows us to undertake reflective, critical evaluation of our own beliefs after their initial adoption.

Limits on belief evaluation imposed by consistency and coherence

It is a datum that sometimes we initially adopt a belief (assign a high credence to a proposition), subsequently reflect on the matter and, on the basis of other things that we already know and believe, without any new evidence, reject the belief (assign a lower credence to the proposition). As we shall now explain, this kind of critical reflection involves a departure from the supposed norm of a single consistent and coherent web of belief (Egan 2008).

The limits that are imposed on belief evaluation by the supposed normative ideals are particularly clear in the case of binary (on/off) belief. No consistent system of belief includes both P and $not\text{-}P$, or all or P, Q, and *at least one of P and Q is false*. No consistent system includes all of P, *my belief that P was formed by method M*, and *every belief formed by method M is false*. And no consistent system includes beliefs, P, Q, R, … formed on the basis of perception, *those are all the beliefs that I have formed on the basis of perception*, and *at least one of the beliefs that I have formed on the basis of perception is false*. Obviously, if you are a consistent binary believer then you will never be in a position to reject an already adopted belief on the grounds that it is inconsistent with other things that you believe. Thus, the ideal of a single consistent system of binary belief excludes rejection of a belief on the basis of evaluation (without new evidence) after the belief has been adopted. The ideal requires that evaluation of a hypothesis should always precede adoption of the hypothesis as a belief.

In the case of graded belief, similar limits are imposed by the supposed ideal of a single coherent assignment of credences. No coherent assignment of credences includes both P and $not\text{-}P$ amongst the propositions assigned a credence greater than 0.5. No coherent assignment includes P and Q amongst the propositions assigned a credence greater than 0.9 and assigns a credence greater than 0.2 to *at least one of P and Q is false*. And no coherent assignment includes P, Q, R, … amongst the propositions assigned a credence greater than 0.9 and assigns a credence greater than 0.2 to *at least half of the those propositions, P, Q, R, …, are false*. If you are a coherent graded believer and you assign a credence greater than 0.9 to some propositions then, provided that you are well informed about your own credences, you cannot assign a credence greater than 0.2 to *half of the propositions to which I assign a credence greater than 0.9 are false*.[16]

The general situation is that, if you are a coherent graded believer then you will never be in a position to reject an already adopted belief (reduce the high credence that you have assigned to a proposition) on the grounds that it is not coherent with other things that you

---

[16] For the general theorem, see Egan and Elga (2005).

believe (the assignment of high credences to other propositions). If you have assigned a high credence to *P*, and *Q* is evidence against *P* (the conditional probability of *P* given *Q* is low) then, because your assignment of credences is coherent, you will not have assigned a high credence to *Q*. On a Bayesian approach, there is no place for post-adoption (that is, post-updating) belief evaluation, without new evidence.

Compartmentalization and Spinozan belief formation

A fragmented belief system and, specifically, a belief system in which newly adopted beliefs were compartmentalized, would escape the limits imposed by the ideal of a single consistent and coherent system. Assignments of credences that were not coherent with each other could be separated and, specifically, a new assignment of a high credence to a proposition could be separated from a prior assignment of credences with which it was not coherent. By retaining the prior credences, such compartmentalization would allow the possibility of post-adoption belief evaluation, even without new evidence. It might be suggested that, although our belief systems are in fact fragmented in various ways, earlier evaluation of candidates for belief is always preferable to the post-adoption evaluation that compartmentalization allows. But, as we explain in the next few paragraphs, default or prepotent doxastic responses to incoming information, particularly from perception, may leave little, if any, opportunity for early evaluation of candidates for belief.

In a series of papers, Gilbert and colleagues (Gilbert 1991; Gilbert et al. 1990, 1993) have contrasted Cartesian and Spinozan views of belief and have presented experimental results in support of the Spinozan view.[17] Each view of belief can be summarized in terms of two stages, a representation stage and an assessment stage. On the Cartesian view, the representation stage involves *comprehension*. A hypothesis is first grasped and then, in a separate assessment stage, the hypothesis is either *accepted* as true and adopted as a belief, or else *rejected* as false. On the Spinozan view, in contrast, the representation stage involves both comprehension and *acceptance* (Gilbert 1991, p. 107): "People believe in the ideas they comprehend, as quickly and automatically as they believe in the objects they see." Then, in the separate assessment stage, the already adopted belief is either *certified* or else *unaccepted*.

Consider, for example, a case of belief based on perception, such as my belief that there is a pencil on the desk in front of me. The Cartesian view is that the representational content of my perceptual experience *as of* there being a pencil on the desk is first grasped as a hypothesis, which is then assessed. Such an assessment might consider the explanatory potential of the hypothesis—whether the hypothesis that there is a pencil on the desk explains my having an experience as of there being a pencil on the desk—and how probable the hypothesis is in the light of other available evidence. Whatever the exact nature of the assessment, its outcome is that the hypothesis is either accepted—I adopt the belief that there is a pencil on the desk—or else rejected—I do not believe my eyes. The Spinozan view, in contrast, is that comprehension and acceptance are inseparable. There is no gap between grasping how the experience represents the world to be and believing that the world is that way. On the basis of the perceptual experience, I automatically adopt the belief that there is a pencil on the

---

[17] We shall not discuss the relationship between the two views that Gilbert describes and the historical philosophers for whom they are named.

desk. Assessment is still separate from comprehension and so it follows this initial acceptance. The outcome of the assessment is that the already adopted belief is either certified and
retained or else unaccepted in "a deliberate revision of belief" (1991, p. 108).

Gilbert assumes that assessment, whether Cartesian or Spinozan, is demanding of cognitive resources and that if resources are depleted or in use elsewhere then the pre-assessment
state of the system will be revealed. He finds the Spinozan view to be supported by a range
of empirical findings (see Gilbert 1991, for a review) including results from his own
experiments (Gilbert et al. 1990, 1993). As Gilbert explains the logic of these experiments,
"resource-depleted Cartesians should be uncertain, uncommitted, but not persuaded,"
whereas the results indicate that "resource depletion facilitate[s] believing" (1991, p. 111).
Belief based on perception seems to be the most promising case for the Spinozan view but
Gilbert's results also suggest that the view may be correct for belief based on heard testimony and read text, even when individuals are forewarned that some of what they hear or
read is not true.

Spinozan belief formation, by definition, excludes assessment or evaluation of hypotheses
before they are adopted as beliefs. If belief systems were required to be consistent and coherent, then Spinozan belief formation would also exclude post-adoption belief evaluation
without new evidence—acceptance would preclude assessment. The reason is that automatic
adoption of an antecedently implausible belief would, given consistency and coherence,
eliminate the very considerations in the light of which the belief was implausible. So there
would be no basis for reflective, critical evaluation of the newly adopted belief. Spinozan
belief formation would be consistent with post-adoption belief evaluation, however, if newly
adopted beliefs were to be compartmentalized, at least until evaluation (Gilbert's assessment) had been undertaken. We assume that these compartmentalized beliefs would guide
action in some, but not all, contexts.

Prepotent doxastic responses, compartmentalization, and belief evaluation

We have said that it is a datum that beliefs are sometimes evaluated after they have been initially adopted and we have shown that a fragmented belief system in which newly adopted
beliefs were compartmentalized would allow post-adoption belief evaluation, even without
new evidence. As we have just seen, this is important for the Spinozan view of belief formation, which places evaluation (assessment) after adoption (acceptance). The claim that belief
is the default or prepotent doxastic response to perceptual experience (Davies et al. 2001,
p. 153) allows that the prepotent response might sometimes be inhibited; so it is not quite
as strong as the claim that belief formation based on perception is Spinozan.[18] Nevertheless,
on this near-Spinozan view the default case will be that there is no assessment before acceptance; reflective evaluation will have to follow initial adoption of the belief. Evidently, if
beliefs that are newly adopted on the basis of perceptual experience are compartmentalized then the near-Spinozan view is consistent with post-adoption belief evaluation. To the

[18] Hasson et al. (2005) argue that the relationship between comprehension and acceptance is more
complex than the Spinozan view allows.

extent that belief is also the prepotent doxastic response to heard testimony or read text, a similar argument will apply.

On a Bayesian approach, the near-Spinozan view is that, in the default case, a high credence is automatically assigned to a proposition that specifies how a perceptual experience presents or represents the world as being (e.g., the proposition *that there is a pencil on the desk in front of me*). The ideal of a single coherent distribution of credences would require that all other credences should be automatically updated (presumably by simple conditionalization or Jeffrey conditionalization). Compartmentalization separates the assignment of a high credence to the perception-based proposition from the prior assignment of credences and the two assignments coexist *pro tem*. Thus the prior credences remain available to figure in subsequent evaluation of the high credence that was initially assigned to the perception-based proposition.

With some understanding of how—thanks to compartmentalization—there could be post-adoption belief evaluation in healthy individuals, we can return to the explanation of delusions. The two-factor framework for explaining delusions is also a three-stage framework (Aimola Davies and Davies 2009; Aimola Davies et al. 2009). At the first stage there is a neuropsychological deficit, the first factor, which is supposed to be related to the content of the delusional belief in some plausible way. There is then a second stage that leads from the neuropsychological deficit to the initial adoption of the delusional belief. Finally, there is the third, post-adoption, stage of persistence rather than rejection of the delusional belief.

How Did the Patient Come to Adopt the Belief?

Coltheart's first question is, "Where did the delusion come from?" (2007, p. 1044). One kind of answer to this question simply cites the first factor; the answer specifies the neuropsychological deficit from which the delusion's content is supposed to have arisen in some plausible way. In the case of Capgras delusion, the deficit is disconnection of the primary face processing system from the autonomic nervous system. But a neuropsychological deficit is not a belief and an answer to the adoption question must specify, not only the neuropsychological deficit, but also the route from the deficit to initial adoption of the delusional belief—the second stage in the two-factor/three-stage framework.

Abnormal data and anomalous experience

The framework allows for considerable variation in the second stage. For example, this stage might be hidden from consciousness to a greater or a lesser extent. As we have already seen, Coltheart and colleagues commend the view that the processing that leads up to onset of the delusion is wholly unconscious, so that the delusional belief itself is "the first delusion-relevant event of which the patient is aware" (2010, p. 264).

On a Bayesian account of the kind that we have been considering, there must be, near the beginning of the second stage, evidence or data from which Bayesian inference leads to initial adoption of the delusional belief. On Coltheart and colleagues' account, the starting point for Bayesian inference leading to the Capgras delusion is abnormal data; namely, the absence of activity in the patient's autonomic nervous system. Importantly, this absence of autonomic activity is assumed *not* to be available to consciousness (2010, p. 264): "people are not conscious of the activities of their autonomic nervous systems, and so a man would not be conscious of a failure of his autonomic nervous system to respond when he encountered his wife." There is a good theoretical reason behind this assumption (Coltheart 2005). If the autonomic activity that is normally produced in response to a familiar face were available to consciousness then patients suffering from prosopagnosia, but with covert recognition, should be able to use their experience of autonomic activity to discriminate familiar from unfamiliar faces. But such patients are unable to do this (Tranel and Damasio 1985, 1988).[19]

We assume, with Coltheart and colleagues (2010), that neither autonomic activity produced by familiar faces, nor the absence of autonomic activity, is available as such to consciousness. But this does not rule out the possibility that the abnormal absence of autonomic activity—itself unavailable to consciousness—should lead to an anomalous experience that would be causally antecedent to the adoption of the delusional belief. Indeed, Coltheart suggests just such a possibility, beginning from an important idea about information processing (2005, p. 155): "It is a general principle of cognitive life that we are continually making predictions, on the basis of what we currently know about the world, concerning what will happen to us next." Sometimes we engage in the conscious mental activity of making predictions and then learning whether our predictions are fulfilled. But prediction and the comparison of predictions with actual outcomes are also ubiquitous features of unconscious information processing. Coltheart says (2005, p. 155): "Only when a prediction fails does consciousness get involved; the unconscious system makes some kind of report to consciousness to

---

[19]   Garry Young has suggested that the results of a study by Greve and Bauer (1990) lend support to the view that autonomic activity does "pervade consciousness" in the form of a "sense of preference" (Young 2008, p. 868; see also 2007). Greve and Bauer presented a prosopagnosic patient with pairs of unfamiliar faces. One face in each pair had previously been exposed five times (for 500 msec each time), following trials of a task in which verbal personality descriptors were presented. When asked to select the face that he liked best, the patient chose the previously exposed face from 70% of the pairs. This is certainly an interesting finding and Young's proposal that "there was something-it-was-like ... for [the patient] to prefer one face over the other" (2008, p. 868) is plausible. But the finding does not support the proposal that this "sense of preference" was underpinned by activity in the patient's autonomic nervous system. Greve and Bauer (1990) report no data on skin conductance responses and they explicitly attribute the patient's preference responses, not to autonomic activity, but to perceptual fluency (Mandler 1980; Whittlesea 1993). They also tentatively suggest that the patient may have a deficit in forming new FRUs and that the more fluent processing of the briefly exposed face stimuli may have been independent of their status as faces.

Although Greve and Bauer's (1990) results do not support Young's claim that autonomic activity is available to consciousness as a sense of preference, we speculate that the results may indirectly raise a question about Coltheart's (2005) argument that autonomic nervous system responses to faces are *not* available to consciousness. It is plausible that, when a previously exposed face was presented to the patient in Greve and Bauer's study, information about perceptual fluency was, in some way, available to consciousness (e.g., as a sense of preference) although the patient was not able to make use of information about fluency to identify the face as previously exposed. By analogy, it might be suggested, the fact that prosopagnosic patients are not able to use information about autonomic activity to discriminate familiar from unfamiliar faces does not absolutely exclude the possibility that information about autonomic activity is, in some way, available to consciousness.

instigate some intelligent conscious problem-solving behavior that will discover what's wrong." Thus, in the case of the Capgras patient, what happens is (2005, p. 155): "the unconscious system predicting that when the wife is next seen a high autonomic response will occur, detecting that this does not occur, and reporting to consciousness, 'There's something odd about this woman.'"

Maher makes a very similar suggestion about the consequences for conscious experience of the unconscious operation of prediction and comparison systems (1999, p. 558):

> Survival requires the existence of a detector of changes in the normally regular patterns of environmental stimuli, namely those that are typically dealt with automatically. The detector functions as a general non-specific alarm, a "significance generator," which then alerts the individual to scan the environment to find out what has changed.

Maher's (1999) and Coltheart's (2005) suggestions converge on the idea that, as the result of a neuropsychological deficit and the subsequent operation of a comparator system, the Capgras patient's experience of his wife is anomalous, characterized by a sense of significance and change.

In summary: From a starting point of abnormal data, the processing that leads to the initial adoption of the delusional belief might be wholly hidden from consciousness. Alternatively, unconscious processes might lead to an anomalous experience that is causally antecedent to the delusional belief.

Explanation or endorsement

There are two importantly different ways in which an anomalous experience might figure in the etiology of a delusion (Davies et al. 2001). On the first (explanation) option, the content of the delusion is not encoded in the anomalous experience. For example, the content of the experience might be: "This woman looks just like my wife but there is something different or odd about her." The content of the delusion itself arises first as the content of an explanatory hypothesis that is then adopted as a belief. This is the account given by Maher (1974, p. 103):

> [T]he explanations (i.e. the delusions) of the patient are derived by cognitive activity that is essentially indistinguishable from that employed by non-patients, by scientists, and by people generally.... [A] delusion is a hypothesis designed to explain unusual perceptual phenomena.

It is clear that, on the explanation option as Maher conceives it, the project of explaining the anomalous experience is a project of the person. If explanation proceeds by Bayesian inference, then this is personal-level inference. We shall understand the explanation option in Maher's way.

On the second (endorsement)[20] option, the content of the delusion is encoded in the anomalous experience. Thus, a state in which the content of the delusion is present is "the first delusion-relevant event of which the patient is aware." The anomalous experience is

---

[20] The terminology of "endorsement" comes from Bayne and Pacherie (2004). Descriptions of the explanation *versus* endorsement options, with varying terminology, are also given by Davies and Coltheart (2000), Fine et al. (2005), Aimola Davies and Davies (2009), Langdon and Bayne (2010), and Turner and Coltheart (2010).

not the delusional belief itself, but the belief would arise as the prepotent doxastic response to the experience (or, on the Spinozan view, would be adopted automatically on the basis of the experience). Although the endorsement option is distinct from Coltheart and colleagues' (2010) view that the delusional belief *itself* is the first conscious delusion-relevant event, both agree that no conscious personal-level reasoning is involved in the stage leading to onset of the delusion (see Turner and Coltheart 2010, p. 368).

The explanation and endorsement options are distinct. But it is important to observe that the distinction between them is *not* that one allows, while the other excludes, the possibility that Bayesian inference figures in the etiology of the delusion. It is entirely consistent with the endorsement option that the anomalous experience encoding the content of the delusion is the product of perceptual processes that are well described as unconscious subpersonal-level Bayesian inference.

Bayesian inference in a perceptual module

In our earlier discussion of the processes leading up to initial adoption of the delusional belief (see "Bayes in the two-factor framework: Adoption of the delusional belief" section), we noted that it is somewhat unclear which probabilities are supposed to figure in the worked examples of Coltheart and colleagues (2010) and McKay (2012). Are they supposed to be realistic probabilities or the patient's credences, for example? McKay challenges Coltheart et al.'s account on the grounds that their proposed prior probability for the stranger hypothesis, $P(H_S) = 0.01$, is "unrealistically high" (2012, p. 339) and offers a much lower estimate. But he accepts their estimate of the likelihood ratio as favoring H_S in the ratio 999:1. This acceptance is puzzling because it seems clear that realistic values for the likelihoods, $P(D|H_S)$ and $P(D|H_W)$, would be identical. The seen face of a woman who looked just like the patient's wife would activate FRU_W in the same way as the seen face of the patient's wife would; and it would cause the same activity in the autonomic nervous system. So a realistic likelihood ratio would be 1:1 and no amount of discounting prior probabilities (which favor H_W) would produce posterior probabilities favoring H_S.

It may seem more natural to interpret the probabilities in the worked examples as the patient's own credences but this, too, is problematic. First, the worked examples (so interpreted) are far from intuitive if, as Coltheart and colleagues explicitly maintain, activity in the patient's autonomic nervous system is not available to the patient's consciousness. How are we to understand a credence such as $P(D|H_W)$ if the patient knows nothing of autonomic activity as such and does not even experience autonomic activity? Second, waiving this first concern, suppose that the patient assigns a low conditional credence to there being no activity in his autonomic nervous system given that the woman he sees in front of him is his wife and a high conditional credence to there being no activity in his autonomic nervous system given that the woman is not his wife but looks just like his wife. The only way for the patient's credences $P(D|H_W)$ and $P(D|H_S)$ coherently to come apart in the way described is for the patient to assign high credences to hypotheses according to which the autonomic nervous system is not just responsive to qualitative inputs from visual perception via the FRUs, but also directly sensitive to facts about the identity of the person perceived.

Our suggestion is that the probabilities in Bayesian inference that starts from the abnormal data, D (the absence of activity in the patient's autonomic nervous system), should be conceived as probabilities assigned by a subpersonal-level unconscious information-processing system or perceptual module.[21] The module's probabilities may not be realistic, because a module has only limited information about how the world (including the module itself) really works. And the module's probabilities may not be coherent with personal-level credences because modules are, at least to some extent, informationally encapsulated (Fodor 1983). Processes in a module do not draw on all that the person knows or believes and so we sometimes experience what we, at the personal level, know to be perceptual illusions. It is also because of this relative independence of the probability distributions of perceptual systems from a person's credences that we can learn from experience (Fodor 1989).

Let us return to Coltheart and colleagues' (2010) and McKay's (2012) worked examples, now conceived as examples of Bayesian inference within a perceptual module. Fodor says that the function of modules is "to so represent the world as to make it accessible to thought" (1983, p. 40) and that the outputs of modules "are typically phenomenologically salient" (p. 87). So we assume that, although the Bayesian inference begins from data that are not available to personal-level consciousness, the results of the inference will determine the content of an experience that presents or represents the world as being a certain way.

A module that is dedicated to processing information about faces will have a limited representational "vocabulary" and the hypotheses that it can "consider" will be correspondingly restricted. We assume, for the purposes of the example, that these include, not only hypotheses about whose face a presented face qualitatively looks like, but also hypotheses about who the presented person *is*; for example, that the person is the patient's wife (H_W), or aunt Agatha (H_A), or Bob the bank teller (H_B), or that the person is somebody unfamiliar (H_S). From some initial distribution, the probabilities of these hypotheses are updated on the basis of input information about the qualitative appearance of the presented face; specifically, the face looks just like the face of the patient's wife. After this updating, $P(H_W)$ is much greater than $P(H_S)$. Since these are probabilities assigned by a module performing a specific computational task on the basis of limited information, we do not assume that they are wholly realistic.

It is important that, at the processing stage we are considering, the module generates predictions about levels of activity in the autonomic nervous system from hypotheses about the identity of the person whose face is presented. From the hypothesis H_W, the module generates the prediction that there will be a high level of autonomic activity. From H_A or from H_B, the prediction is that there will be a low level of autonomic activity, somewhat above baseline. And from H_S, the prediction is that there will be no autonomic activity above baseline. We assume that the generation of these predictions is based on past associations—perhaps

---

[21] Attributions of credences to persons are standardly explained in terms of dispositions to accept (or regard as fair) bets at specified odds. Information-processing systems or modules do not engage in betting behavior but simply produce outputs that are available to other systems. A description of a system as engaging in Bayesian inference or updating is to be understood as a putative account of the computations being carried out by the system. As such it is answerable to the system's input–output dispositions and to such evidence as may be available concerning intermediate stages of the computation (Shea 2012; Chapter 62, this volume).

between activation of one or another PIN, or none, and levels of autonomic activity.[22] So we do not expect that the predictions will be based on information about how the module itself actually works. Specifically, we do not expect that the predictions will take into account that autonomic activity is caused by activation of a FRU and that if a stranger's face looks just like a known face then it will activate the same FRU, and cause the same autonomic activity, as the known face would.

We can regard the module's predictions as manifesting its estimates of conditional probabilities. If D is the absence of autonomic activity then the module's likelihoods, $P(D|H_W)$ and $P(D|H_S)$, will favor (H_S) over (H_W)—just as in Coltheart et al.'s (2010) and McKay's (2012) examples. These likelihoods are unrealistic but they are not the likelihoods of the person within whom the module resides (the patient).

The main point of disagreement between Coltheart and colleagues and McKay was over the question whether the disconnection of the patient's face processing system from the autonomic nervous system is the only pathology or departure from normality that need be implicated in the processes leading up to the onset of the Capgras delusion (see "Biased Bayesian inference" section). McKay argued that, given realistic estimates of prior probabilities, an updating bias in favor of likelihoods at the expense of prior probabilities was needed in order to answer the adoption question. He proposed that this bias is the second factor in the two-factor framework. When we consider Bayesian inference in a perceptual module, the question whether prior probabilities—or, indeed, likelihoods—are realistic is less pressing. Also, because modules are, to some extent, informationally encapsulated, it is of their nature to discount personal-level prior probabilities and to be biased in favor of likelihoods. Earlier, we recalled Hemsley and Garety's (1986) remark about normal deviation from the normative model. Now, as we consider information processing in a perceptual module, this remark seems even more to the point. In perceptual processing, a bias in favor of likelihoods may well be entirely normal.

From anomalous experience to delusional belief

We have described, in a speculative spirit, how information processing in a perceptual module could lead from abnormal data (absence of autonomic activity as the consequence of a neuropsychological deficit) to the stranger hypothesis, H_S, being favored over the wife hypothesis, H_W. We assumed that the favored hypothesis would determine the content of an experience that presents or represents the world as being a certain way. This would be an experience as of a woman who qualitatively looked just like the patient's wife but was not really her (was really a stranger). An anomalous experience is not yet a belief, but the delusional belief, "This woman looks just like my wife (and says that she is my wife) but is not my wife," would arise as the prepotent doxastic response to this experience. There

---

[22] In the model of face processing proposed by Ellis and Lewis (2001), an integrative device has access to information from PINs and from affective responses to familiar stimuli in the autonomic nervous system (see also Breen et al. 2000b, 2001b; Lewis and Ellis 2001). Such a device could, in principle, learn associations, generate predictions, and compare predicted and actual autonomic activity. In a more comprehensive account, we should also consider predictions about the voice and the gait, for example, of the person putatively identified.

are two points to notice about this answer to the adoption question. First, no conscious personal-level reasoning is involved in the stage leading to adoption of the delusional belief. Second, the original neuropsychological deficit seems to be the only pathology or departure from normality that is essential to the answer—in line with option (A) (see "Adoption and persistence" section).

It might be objected against this answer that it assumes a controversial position in the philosophy of perception; namely, that properties of being numerically identical to, or distinct from, a particular individual (e.g., the property of being numerically distinct from the patient's wife) are represented in perceptual experience. It is true that the question of which properties of objects are represented in perceptual experience is important and much debated (e.g., Bayne 2009; Hawley and Macpherson 2010; Siegel 2010) and that this has sometimes been offered as an objection to an endorsement account of the Capgras delusion (Coltheart 2005). We find the endorsement option attractive but, to conclude this section on the adoption question, we briefly consider the possibility that hypotheses like H_W and H_S do not figure in perceptual processing and that the content of the delusion is not encoded in an anomalous experience.

This returns us to the explanation option described by Maher (1974, 1999) and Coltheart (2005). The Capgras patient's experience presents or represents a woman who qualitatively looks just like his wife. There is nothing anomalous about that. But, on the basis of past associations between the qualitative appearance of a presented face and the level of activity in the autonomic nervous system, an unconscious subpersonal-level mechanism predicts a high level of autonomic activity. Because the patient's primary face processing system has been disconnected from the autonomic nervous system, this prediction is not fulfilled and a prediction error signal is generated. Consequently, the patient's experience of the woman who is, in fact, his wife is suffused with a feeling of heightened significance, it cries out for explanation in terms of something different or odd in the immediate environment and particularly in the woman perceived.

The prepotent doxastic response to this experience is to believe something like, "This woman looks just like my wife but there is something different or odd about her." But this underdescribes the way in which the belief is permeated by the sense of significance and the urgent demand for explanation and interpretation. We assume that the cognitive processes that are engaged by a situation like that of the Capgras patient are not reflective and unbiased processes of Bayesian inference to the most probable hypothesis all things considered, but more encapsulated and biased processes of inference to the first (most accessible) hypothesis to predict the anomalous experience well enough (that is, with a high enough likelihood on the evidence of the anomalous experience).[23] The accessible hypotheses are not restricted by the limited representational vocabulary of a perceptual module. But the sense that there is something different or odd about the woman that the patient sees in front of him demands attention and explanation. What is it that has changed? In this situation, it may be that the most accessible hypothesis that answers this question and predicts the sense

---

[23] Coltheart et al. (2011, pp. 283–284) observe, in effect, that C.S. Peirce's notion of abduction was close to this idea of inference to the first hypothesis with a high enough likelihood. Peirce's characterization of abduction considered as an inference was: The surprising fact, C, is observed. But if A were true, C would be a matter of course. Hence, there is reason to suspect that A is true. (See Psillos 2009, for a recent review.)

that there is something different or odd about the woman is that, although she looks just like the patient's wife and says that she is the patient's wife, she is not really his wife but a stranger, and so an impostor.[24]

In a Cartesian—rather than Spinozan or near-Spinozan—spirit, Coltheart et al. (2011, p. 284) say:

> The propositions yielded by abductive inference are not beliefs, but rather are hypotheses or candidates for belief. For any such proposition to be adopted as a belief, it must be submitted to, and survive, a belief-evaluation process, and it is here that plausibility has a critical role.

In contrast, we conjecture that there is a prepotent doxastic tendency toward acceptance of a hypothesis that arises in the way that we have just described; that is, as the first hypothesis to predict (and perhaps also explain) a highly salient piece of evidence.[25] This prepotent tendency would correspond to a cognitive imperative of explanatory adequacy, as the prepotent response to perceptual experience corresponds to the cognitive imperative of observational adequacy. On the explanation option, as on the endorsement option, the delusional belief arises as a prepotent doxastic response and, in both cases, the processes leading to initial adoption of the belief discount personal-level prior probabilities and are biased in favor of likelihoods. The difference between the two cases is just that, while the endorsement option involves encapsulated and biased subpersonal-level perceptual processes of Bayesian inference, the explanation option involves encapsulated and biased post-perceptual processes of Bayesian inference. Compartmentalization of the newly adopted belief allows prior probabilities to be taken into account in subsequent belief evaluation, in accordance with the third cognitive imperative of conservatism (Aimola Davies and Davies 2009; Stone and Young 1997).

Why Does the Belief, once Adopted, Persist Rather Than Being Rejected?

Coltheart's second question is, "Why does the patient not reject the belief?" (2007, p. 1044). As we have noted (see "Adoption and persistence" section), this question can be interpreted in two ways. On one interpretation, the question asks why the patient adopts the hypothesis as a belief, rather than rejecting it (Coltheart et al. 2011). On a second interpretation, it asks why the patient, having initially adopted the belief, does not subsequently reject it (Coltheart 2007, 2010). On the first interpretation, Coltheart's second question is the adoption question; on the second interpretation, it is the persistence question.

---

[24] This somewhat encapsulated inference to the first hypothesis to predict or explain a salient piece of evidence is analogous to somewhat encapsulated inference to the first relevant enough interpretation of an utterance, as proposed by Sperber and Wilson's relevance theory of pragmatics (Sperber and Wilson 1986/1995, 2002; Wilson and Sperber 2012). We do not commit ourselves to the thesis that the mind is modular through and through (Carruthers 2006; Sperber 2001) but we acknowledge that informational encapsulation does not provide a straightforward criterion for separating perception from cognition (see Shea, in press).

[25] In the section entitled "Bayesian inference" we allowed that explanatory virtue might influence the psychological accessibility of hypotheses.

The distinction between these two interpretations of Coltheart's second question led us to two options for the role of the second factor in the two-factor framework. According to option (A), no pathology or departure from normality beyond the first factor (neuropsychological deficit) is needed to answer the adoption question and the second factor answers the persistence question. Thus, the role of the second factor is to explain a failure of post-adoption belief evaluation. According to option (B), two factors are needed to answer the adoption question and no additional pathology or departure from normality is needed to answer the persistence question. Thus, the role of the second factor is to explain the transition from the first neuropsychological deficit to the initial adoption of the delusional belief. On our reading, Coltheart et al. (2010) adopt option (A) while McKay (2012) adopts option (B)—as, it seems, do Coltheart et al. (2011).

On option (B), it is plausible to propose that the cognitive nature of the second factor is that of a bias; specifically, an updating bias in favor of likelihoods at the expense of prior probabilities. (What is not so clear is whether the bias amounts to a pathology or departure from normality. Might it just be a bias within the normal range, so that option (B) would appeal to only one pathological factor?) We were not able, however, to find a role for a second factor of the kind specified by option (A). This would be an impairment that would explain the persistence of the delusional belief once it had been adopted. Given the implausibility of the belief, why is it not rejected, even before new evidence becomes available? On a Bayesian approach, there seems to be no role for such an impairment because, once a belief has been adopted, persistence is the normal, and even normatively correct, case.

We do not regard that difficulty as revealing a problem for the two-factor framework, for a Bayesian approach, or for option (A). Rather, it reflects the fact that, given the standard idealizing assumption of a single coherent assignment of credences, Bayesian belief evaluation can only be updating of credences by conditionalizing on new (that is, post-adoption) evidence. Our view (see "Belief evaluation and the fragmented mind" section) is that we should relax the standard idealizing assumption and allow that the assignment of a high credence to a proposition in accordance with the cognitive imperative of observational or explanatory adequacy can be compartmentalized, so that prior credences remain available to figure in subsequent belief evaluation. We suggest that compartmentalization should normally be triggered whenever belief formation is near-Spinozan. The reason for this suggestion is that near-Spinozan belief formation ensures that belief adoption precedes evaluation. In such cases, compartmentalization allows the prior assignment of credences to be protected, at least until belief evaluation has been undertaken. Without compartmentalization, the prior credences would be automatically updated by conditionalization on the proposition newly assigned a high credence, with the result that critical belief evaluation would be impossible.[26]

Now that we have seen how post-adoption belief evaluation could be possible in principle, we can ask how it could be impaired.

---

[26] It might be that compartmentalization should not be triggered when it is not required; for example, when the newly assigned credence coincides with the prior credence assigned to that proposition. But equally, if compartmentalization were triggered in such a case, it would be short-lived as belief evaluation and subsequent integration would be trivial.

Bayesian belief evaluation and cognitive resources

The Capgras patient has initially adopted the belief that the woman who looks just like his wife and claims to be his wife is not really his wife but a stranger. The content of the delusional belief has arisen in one or other of two plausible ways (endorsement or explanation) from an anomalous experience that arose, in turn, from a neuropsychological deficit by processes of Bayesian inference in a perceptual module. On either option, the processes that led up to initial adoption of the delusional belief were (we assume) normal, but were at least somewhat encapsulated and correspondingly biased in favor of likelihoods at the expense of prior probabilities. Thanks to compartmentalization of the delusional belief, the patient's prior credences have been preserved and are, in principle, available for reflective, critical evaluation of the newly adopted belief. But belief evaluation is demanding of cognitive resources (Gilbert 1991).

In their seminal contribution to the philosophy and psychology of delusion, Stone and Young describe (1997, p. 349): "a tension between forming beliefs that require little readjustment to the web of belief (conservatism) and forming beliefs that do justice to the deliverances of one's perceptual systems" and they propose that, in delusion, the balance between these cognitive imperatives "goes too far towards observational [or explanatory] adequacy as against conservatism." Our account is broadly consistent with that proposal and we agree that belief evaluation will involve control or management of these potentially competing imperatives. More specifically, critical evaluation of the delusional belief in the light of prior credences will require some inhibition of the prepotent tendencies corresponding to the imperatives of observational and explanatory adequacy. The patient will need to step back from his initial adoption of the delusional belief and say (paraphrasing patient HS, described by Chatterjee and Mennemeier 1996, p. 227), "Sometimes I feel like my wife has been replaced by an impostor and I have to tell myself 'no she hasn't.'"

Critical evaluation of the delusional belief will also require that the patient achieve a better understanding of his real situation. As the patient described by Turner and Coltheart said (2010, p. 371):

> I've started going through it, and seeing what could possibly happen and what couldn't happen.... there must be an explanation for it.... The lady knows me way back. She could say things that happened 40 years ago, and I wonder where she gets them from. And then I worked it out and I've wondered if it's Mary all the time.

This "going through it" and "working it out" requires, not only executive processes of control and inhibition, but also working memory resources for the maintenance and manipulation of information. Impaired executive function or working memory could figure in an answer to the persistence question (Aimola Davies and Davies 2009).

These suggestions about the cognitive resources that are demanded by the task of belief evaluation do not yet amount to a proposal about the nature of the evaluation. The obvious proposal on a Bayesian approach would be that it is an assessment based on prior probability and likelihoods.[27] The question for such an evaluation is whether there is a proposition, C^*, that is inconsistent with the Capgras delusion proposition and is more probable than

---

[27] This evaluation would assess whether the probability of the committed Capgras delusion proposition, C^+, given the evidence on which its adoption as a belief was based, is high or low (see footnote 15).

(continued)

the delusion proposition given the anomalous experience on the basis of which the delusional belief was initially adopted (by endorsement or explanation). Informally, and departing somewhat from the Bayesian approach, one might ask whether there is an alternative to the impostor hypothesis that provides a better explanation of the patient's anomalous experience.

There is, of course, an obvious candidate for such a proposition, C*. The patient has suffered a stroke, resulting in disconnection of his primary face processing system from his autonomic nervous system; and this neuropsychological deficit has led to the anomalous experience of his wife. This proposition can, in principle, be recognized as having a higher posterior probability than the Capgras delusion proposition because the patient's prior credences remain available. They have not been updated by conditionalization on the compartmentalized delusion proposition. Nevertheless, for several reasons, the patient's path to a correct understanding of his situation may be difficult.

First, even if the patient accepts that he has had a stroke and appreciates that a stroke can have many debilitating consequences, the probability of an anomalous experience of the relevant kind given only that the patient has had a stroke is not especially high. The probability of such an experience given that the patient has had a stroke resulting in disconnection of his primary face processing system from his autonomic nervous system is much higher. But the patient may not realize that a stroke can have this consequence and, even if the patient knows about the possibility of disconnection, it may be far from self-evident to him how such disconnection would be manifested in experience.[28] Second, from the point of view of the Capgras patient, once the delusional belief has been initially adopted, the question of interest is not why he is having this anomalous experience (the question answered by C*), but why his wife has been replaced by a stranger (Hohwy and Rosenberg 2005, p. 155):

> The brain pathology hypothesis would only be relevant if the patient could accept that what needs explaining is the mere experience that it is as if the spouse looks like a stranger; it is not relevant if what needs explaining is the real occurrence of a stranger looking like the spouse.

Third, on the explanation option, the feeling of heightened significance that suffuses the experience of the patient's wife cries out for explanation in terms of change in the environment, not change in the patient's brain (such as a stroke).

It is plausible that, if the patient suffered from impaired executive function or working memory, these difficulties in reaching a correct understanding of his situation would be

---

C^+ that the woman who looks just like the patient's wife and claims to be his wife is not really his wife but a stranger.

The evidence proposition would be a more cautious proposition describing the patient's experience. On the endorsement option, this would be the proposition:

C^-_{end} that the patient has a perceptual experience as of the woman who looks just like his wife and claims to be his wife not really being his wife but being a stranger.

On the explanation option, it would be the proposition:

C^-_{exp} that the patient has a perceptual experience (an experience suffused with a feeling of significance and change) as of the woman who looks just like his wife and claims to be his wife having something different or odd about her.

The probability of C^+, given the evidence on which its adoption as a belief was based, will be low if there is a proposition, C^*, inconsistent with C^+, such that $P'(C^*|C^-_{end}) > P'(C^+|C^-_{end})$ in a case of endorsement, or such that $P'(C^*|C^-_{exp}) > P'(C^+|C^-_{exp})$ in a case of explanation.

[28] Here we are indebted to Ryan McKay.

exacerbated. Even without such impairments, it seems plausible that the patient might need some assistance in understanding his situation.

Failure of compartmentalization

Compartmentalization of a newly adopted belief allows post-adoption belief evaluation and we have suggested that it should normally be triggered whenever belief formation is near-Spinozan. It is of some interest to compare our suggestion about compartmentalization with a proposal by Turner and Coltheart that an unconscious checking system "tags" thoughts "that require extra conscious checking" (2010, p. 357). The presence of a tag has phenomenal and functional consequences. It "gives rise to the experience of doubt" and the tagged thought is "referred to the conscious evaluation system for further work" (p. 357). Failure of the unconscious checking system results in "absence of doubt" and "a subjective feeling of conviction" (pp. 358, 360). The untagged thought is able to "bypass the conscious evaluation system, and ... directly affect speech and other behaviour" (p. 358).

There are certainly points of similarity between the compartmentalization and tagging ideas. Compartmentalization is primarily functional and we have not suggested any phenomenology associated with it. But we do not rule out the possibility that it might be accompanied by a sense that evaluation is called for. Also, although belief evaluation is demanding of cognitive resources and not automatic, it is plausible that, in healthy individuals whose cognitive resources are not engaged elsewhere, newly adopted and compartmentalized beliefs are normally subject to evaluation—as on Gilbert's (1991) Spinozan view. However, unlike Turner and Coltheart's tagging, compartmentalization does not preclude guidance of action. A notable advantage of Spinozan or near-Spinozan belief formation—adoption before evaluation—is that it allows early action, though at the cost of occasional action on the basis of unreliable information (Egan 2008). When the near-Spinozan view is combined with compartmentalization, we expect beliefs that are adopted, but not yet evaluated, to guide action in some, but not all, contexts.

On Turner and Coltheart's (2010) account, absence of a tag allows beliefs to guide action without having been evaluated but, even when the unconscious checking system fails, conscious belief evaluation is still possible and may be externally prompted or initiated. The consequences of failure of compartmentalization are more dramatic, for it is compartmentalization that allows post-adoption belief evaluation even without new evidence. Without compartmentalization, initial adoption of a delusional belief would, given consistency and coherence, eliminate the very considerations in the light of which the belief should be rejected. There would be no basis for reflective, critical evaluation of the delusional belief. This is particularly clear in the case of antecedently available considerations but, as we have seen (see "Diagnostic evidence, similar evidence, and 'unfalsifiability'" section), the value of new evidence that is similar to evidence that has already been accepted is also diminished. This is the basis for McKay's (2012) view that no additional pathology or departure from normality is needed to explain the delusional belief's persistence once it has been adopted.

When we adopt a Bayesian approach, with the standard idealizing assumption of a single coherent assignment of credences, persistence seems to be the normal, and normatively correct, consequence of adoption of the delusional belief. Once we shift to the view of the mind as fragmented, and of compartmentalization as normal, compartmentalization of newly adopted beliefs allows post-adoption belief evaluation. So there is a role for a pathology or departure from normality that would distinctively explain the persistence of a delusional belief—even after its initial adoption had been accounted for. We have suggested that impaired executive function or working memory might play that role. Impaired executive function might prevent the patient from stepping back from his initial adoption of the delusional belief; and impaired working memory might not allow the patient to work out the consequences of his prior beliefs. Failure of compartmentalization takes us closer to the supposed normative ideal of a single coherent assignment of credences. But now it appears as a departure from normality and as another possible explanation of persistence. Failure of compartmentalization allows updating of credences by conditionalizing on the newly adopted belief (that is, on the proposition newly assigned a high credence) and thus eliminates the considerations on which reflective, critical evaluation of that belief should be based.

Conclusion

The leading idea of the two-factor framework for explaining delusions is that two factors in the etiology of delusions provide answers to two questions. First, where did the delusion come from? Second, why does the patient not reject the belief? Answers to the first question have been provided for a range of monothematic delusions, mainly of neuropsychological origin. These answers have a common form: they specify a neuropsychological deficit that is supposed to be related to the content of the delusion in some plausible way. The particular answers inevitably differ from delusion to delusion and may differ between patients with the same delusion.

The second question can be interpreted in more than one way. Interpreted as the adoption question, it asks why a delusional hypothesis that is related to the neuropsychological deficit was adopted as a belief, rather than being rejected. Interpreted as the persistence question, it asks why the initially adopted belief persists, rather than being subsequently rejected. The adoption question and the persistence question both need answers but the fact that there are two interpretations of the second question indicates that there is some unclarity about the role of the second factor in the two-factor framework. In fact, while it has been proposed that the second factor is the same in all cases of delusion of neuropsychological origin, the role, cognitive nature, and neural basis of the second factor have not been well specified (see Coltheart et al. 2010, p. 282).

In the second and third sections of this chapter, we reviewed two Bayesian developments of the two-factor framework (Coltheart et al. 2010; McKay 2012). The two accounts disagree about the processes that lead from the first factor (neuropsychological deficit) to the initial adoption of the delusional belief. According to Coltheart and colleagues, no departure from normality other than the first factor is implicated in the processes leading to adoption of the belief and they take this to be a vindication of "Maher's basic contention that delusional beliefs *arise* via rational inferential responses to highly unusual data" (2010, p. 277; emphasis added). In contrast, McKay argues that a second factor in the form of an updating bias is required.

The inevitable consequence of this difference is that the two accounts also disagree over the role of the second factor in the etiology of delusions. Coltheart et al. say that the second factor is not needed to answer the adoption question but is needed to answer the persistence question—option (A). But we were unable to discover a role in a Bayesian account for a pathological factor that would distinctively explain the persistence of a delusional belief after its initial adoption had been accounted for. McKay says that the second factor is needed to answer the adoption question and that no additional departure from normality is needed to answer the persistence question—option (B).

In the central section of the chapter, we showed that, with the standard Bayesian idealizing assumption of a single coherent assignment of credences in place, Bayesian belief evaluation could only be updating of credences by conditionalizing on new evidence. There is no place for evaluation of a newly adopted belief on the basis of pre-existing considerations. We argued for a relaxation of the idealizing assumption in order to allow compartmentalization of newly adopted beliefs, so that prior credences would remain available to figure in subsequent belief evaluation.

In the fifth and sixth sections, we returned to the adoption and persistence questions. We proposed an answer to the adoption question in terms of Bayesian inference within an unconscious information-processing system or perceptual module. On our account, the results of the inference process determine the content of an experience. The initial adoption of the delusional belief is a prepotent doxastic response to that experience, on the endorsement option, or the result of a prepotent doxastic tendency to accept an accessible hypothesis that predicts the experience, on the explanation option (see "From anomalous experience to delusional belief" section). We suggested that compartmentalization should normally be triggered whenever belief formation is near-Spinozan. Thus delusional beliefs would normally be compartmentalized, in line with the oft-remarked circumscription of monothematic delusions. In answer to the persistence question, we argued that evaluation of a delusional belief would normally be a difficult task that might require assistance. The difficulties would be exacerbated by impairments of executive function or working memory (or both) and a more dramatic explanation of persistence would be provided by failure of compartmentalization itself.

ACKNOWLEDGMENTS

Our debt to the papers by Max Coltheart, Peter Menzies, and John Sutton (2010) and Ryan McKay (2012) will be evident on almost every page of this chapter. MD also acknowledges intellectual debts to Max Coltheart extending over thirty years. AE would like to thank Adam Elga, in particular, for informing and improving his thinking about compartmentalization and Spinozan belief formation. We are grateful to Richard Gipps, Matthew Parrott, and Nicholas Shea for comments on, and conversations about, an earlier version.

REFERENCES

Aimola Davies, A. M. and Davies, M. (2009). Explaining pathologies of belief. In M. R. Broome and L. Bortolotti (Eds), *Psychiatry as Cognitive Neuroscience: Philosophical Perspectives*, pp. 285–323. Oxford: Oxford University Press.

Aimola Davies, A. M., Davies, M., Ogden, J. A., Smithson, M., and White, R. C. (2009). Cognitive and motivational factors in anosognosia. In T. Bayne and J. Fernández (Eds), *Delusion and Self-Deception: Affective Influences on Belief Formation*, pp. 187–225. Hove: Psychology Press.

American Psychiatric Association (2000). *Diagnostic and Statistical Manual of Mental Disorders, Fourth Edition, Text Revision*. Washington, DC: American Psychiatric Association.

Bauer, R. M. (1984). Autonomic recognition of names and faces: A neuropsychological application of the Guilty Knowledge Test. *Neuropsychologia, 22,* 457–69.

Bayne, T. (2009). Perception and the reach of phenomenal content. *Philosophical Quarterly, 59,* 385–404.

Bayne, T. and Pacherie, E. (2004). Bottom-up or top-down? Campbell's rationalist account of monothematic delusions. *Philosophy, Psychiatry, & Psychology, 11,* 1–11.

Bottini, G., Bisiach, E., Sterzi, R., and Vallar, G. (2002). Feeling touches in someone else's hand. *NeuroReport, 13,* 249–52.

Breen, N., Caine, D., and Coltheart, M. (2000b). Models of face recognition and delusional misidentification: A critical review. *Cognitive Neuropsychology, 17,* 55–71.

Breen, N., Caine, D., and Coltheart, M. (2001a). Mirrored-self misidentifiation: Two cases of focal onset dementia. *Neurocase, 7,* 239–54.

Breen, N., Caine, D., Coltheart, M., Hendy, J., and Roberts, C. (2000a). Towards an understanding of delusions of misidentification: Four case studies. *Mind & Language, 15,* 74–110.

Breen, N., Coltheart, M., and Caine, D. (2001b). A two-way window on face recognition. *Trends in Cognitive Sciences, 5,* 234–5.

Brighetti, G., Bonifacci, P., Borlimi, R., and Ottaviani, C. (2007). "Far from the heart far from the eye": Evidence from the Capgras delusion. *Cognitive Neuropsychiatry, 12,* 189–97.

Bruce, V. and Young, A. W. (1986). Understanding face recognition. *British Journal of Psychology, 77,* 305–27.

Capgras, J. and Reboul-Lachaux, J. (1923). L'illusion des "sosies" dans un délire systématisé chronique. *Bulletin de la Société Clinique de Médicine Mentale, 2,* 6–16.

Carruthers, P. (2006). *The Architecture of the Mind: Massive Modularity and the Flexibility of Thought*. Oxford: Oxford University Press.

Chatterjee, A. and Mennemeier, M. (1996). Anosognosia for hemiplegia: Patient retrospections. *Cognitive Neuropsychiatry, 1,* 221–37.

Coltheart, M. (2005). Conscious experience and delusional belief. *Philosophy, Psychiatry, & Psychology, 12,* 153–7.

Coltheart, M. (2007). Cognitive neuropsychiatry and delusional belief. *Quarterly Journal of Experimental Psychology, 60,* 1041–62.

Coltheart, M. (2010). The neuropsychology of delusions. *Annals of the New York Academy of Sciences, 1191,* 16–26.

Coltheart, M., Langdon, R., and McKay, R. (2007). Schizophrenia and monothematic delusions. *Schizophrenia Bulletin, 33,* 642–7.

Coltheart, M., Langdon, R., and McKay, R. (2011). Delusional belief. *Annual Review of Psychology, 62,* 271–98.

Coltheart, M., Menzies, P., and Sutton, J. (2010). Abductive inference and delusional belief. *Cognitive Neuropsychiatry, 15,* 261–87.

Corlett, P. R., Frith, C. D., and Fletcher, P. C. (2009). From drugs to deprivation: A Bayesian framework for understanding models of psychosis. *Psychopharmacology, 206,* 515–30.

Corlett, P. R., Krystal, J. H., Taylor, J. R., and Fletcher, P. C. (2009). Why do delusions persist? *Frontiers in Human Neuroscience*, 9(12), 1–9.

Corlett, P. R., Murray, G. K., Honey, G. D., Aitken, M. R. F., Shanks, D. R., Robbins, T. W., *et al.* (2007). Disrupted prediction-error signal in psychosis: Evidence for an associative account of delusions. *Brain*, 130, 2387–400.

Cotard, J. (1882). Du délire des négations. *Archives de Neurologie*, 4, 152–70, 282–95.

Courbon, P. and Fail, G. (1927). Syndrome d' "illusion de Frégoli" et schizophrenie. *Bulletin de la Société Clinique de Médecine Mentale*, 20, 121–5.

David, A. S. (1993). Cognitive neuropsychiatry. *Psychological Medicine*, 23, 1–5.

Davies, M. (2000). Interaction without reduction: The relationship between personal and sub-personal levels of description. *Mind and Society*, 1, 87–105.

Davies, M., Aimola Davies, A. M., and Coltheart, M. (2005). Anosognosia and the two-factor theory of delusions. *Mind & Language*, 20, 209–36.

Davies, M. and Coltheart, M. (2000). Introduction: Pathologies of belief. *Mind & Language*, 15, 1–46.

Davies, M., Coltheart, M., Langdon, R., and Breen, N. (2001). Monothematic delusions: Towards a two-factor account. *Philosophy, Psychiatry, & Psychology*, 8, 133–58.

de Pauw, K. W., Szulecka, T. K., and Poltock, T. L. (1987). Frégoli syndrome after cerebral infarction. *Journal of Nervous and Mental Diseases*, 175, 433–8.

Dennett, D. C. (1969). *Content and Consciousness*. London: Routledge & Kegan Paul.

Edelstyn, N. M. J. and Oyebode, F. (1999). A review of the phenomenology and cognitive neuropsychological origins of the Capgras syndrome. *International Journal of Geriatric Psychiatry*, 14, 48–59.

Egan, A. (2008). Seeing and believing: Perception, belief formation and the divided mind. *Philosophical Studies*, 140, 47–63

Egan, A. and Elga, A. (2005). I can't believe I'm stupid. *Philosophical Perspectives*, 19, 77–94.

Ellis, H. D. (1998). Cognitive neuropsychiatry and delusional misidentification syndromes: An exemplary vindication of the new discipline. *Cognitive Neuropsychiatry*, 3, 81–90.

Ellis, H. D. and Lewis, M. B. (2001). Capgras delusion: A window on face recognition. *Trends in Cognitive Sciences*, 5, 149–56.

Ellis, H. D., Lewis, M. B., Moselhy, H. F., and Young, A. W. (2000). Automatic without autonomic responses to familiar faces: Differential components of covert face recognition in a case of Capgras delusion. *Cognitive Neuropsychiatry*, 5, 255–69.

Ellis, H. D., Whitley, J., and Luauté, J. P. (1994). Delusional misidentification: The three original papers on the Capgras, Fregoli and intermetamorphosis delusions. *History of Psychiatry*, 5, 117–46.

Ellis, H. D. and Young, A. W. (1990). Accounting for delusional misidentifications. *British Journal of Psychiatry*, 157, 239–48.

Ellis, H. D., Young, A. W., Quayle, A. H., and de Pauw, K. W. (1997). Reduced autonomic responses to faces in Capgras delusion. *Proceedings of the Royal Society: Biological Sciences*, B264, 1085–92.

Fine, C., Craigie, J., and Gold, I. (2005). Damned if you do, damned if you don't: The impasse in cognitive accounts of the Capgras delusion. *Philosophy, Psychiatry, & Psychology*, 12, 143–51.

Fletcher, P. C. and Frith, C. D. (2009). Perceiving is believing: A Bayesian approach to explaining the positive symptoms of schizophrenia. *Nature Reviews Neuroscience*, 10, 48–58

Fodor, J. A. (1983). *The Modularity of Mind*. Cambridge, MA: MIT Press.

Fodor, J. A. (1989). Why should the mind be modular? In A. George (Ed.), *Reflections on Chomsky*, pp. 1–22. Oxford: Blackwell.

Fodor, J. A. (2000). *The Mind Doesn't Work That Way*. Cambridge, MA: MIT Press.

Friston, K. (2005). A theory of cortical responses. *Philosophical Transactions of the Royal Society: Biological Sciences, 360*, 815–36.

Friston, K. (2009). The free-energy principle: A rough guide to the brain? *Trends in Cognitive Sciences, 13*, 293–301.

Friston, K. (2010). The free-energy principle: A unified brain theory? *Nature Reviews Neuroscience, 11*, 127–38.

Friston, K. and Stephan, K. E. (2007). Free-energy and the brain. *Synthese, 159*, 417–58.

Frith, C. D. (1992). *The Cognitive Neuropsychology of Schizophrenia*. Hove: Lawrence Erlbaum Associates.

Frith, C. D. (2007). *Making Up the Mind: How the Brain Creates Our Mental World*. Oxford: Blackwell Publishing.

Frith, C. D. and Done, D. J. (1989). Experiences of alien control in schizophrenia reflect a disorder in the central monitoring of action. *Psychological Medicine, 19*, 359–63.

Gilbert, D. T. (1991). How mental systems believe. *American Psychologist, 46*, 107–19.

Gilbert, D. T., Krull, D. S., and Malone, P. S. (1990). Believing the unbelievable: Some problems in the rejection of false information. *Journal of Personality and Social Psychology, 59*, 601–13.

Gilbert, D. T., Tafadori, R. W., and Malone, P. S. (1993). You can't not believe everything you read. *Journal of Personality and Social Psychology, 65*, 221–33.

Gold, I. and Stoljar, D. (1999). A neuron doctrine in the philosophy of neuroscience. *Behavioral and Brain Sciences, 22*, 809–69.

Greve, K. W. and Bauer, R. M. (1990). Implicit learning of new faces in prosopagnosia: An application of the mere-exposure paradigm. *Neuropsychologia, 28*, 1035–41.

Halligan, P. W. and David, A. S. (2001). Cognitive neuropsychiatry: Towards a scientific psychopathology. *Nature Reviews Neuroscience, 2*, 209–15.

Halligan, P. W., Marshall, J. C., and Wade, D. T. (1995). Unilateral somatoparaphrenia after right hemisphere stroke: A case description. *Cortex, 31*, 173–82.

Hasson, U., Simmons, J. P., and Todorov, A. (2005). Believe it or not: On the possibility of suspending belief. *Psychological Science, 16*, 566–71.

Hawley, K. and Macpherson, F. (Eds) (2010). *The Admissible Contents of Experience*. Oxford: Wiley-Blackwell.

Hemsley, D. R. and Garety, P. A. (1986). The formation and maintenance of delusions: A Bayesian analysis. *British Journal of Psychiatry, 149*, 51–6.

Hirstein, W. and Ramachandran, V. S. (1997). Capgras syndrome: A novel probe for understanding the neural representation of the identity and familiarity of persons. *Proceedings of the Royal Society: Biological Sciences, B264*, 437–44.

Hohwy, J. and Rosenberg, R. (2005). Unusual experiences, reality testing and delusions of alien control. *Mind & Language, 20*, 141–62.

Jeffrey, R. (1965). *The Logic of Decision*. New York, NY: McGraw-Hill. (2nd edn, Chicago, IL: University of Chicago Press, 1983.)

Langdon, R. and Bayne, T. (2010). Delusion and confabulation: Mistakes of perceiving, remembering and believing. *Cognitive Neuropsychiatry, 15*, 319–45.

Langdon, R. and Coltheart, M. (2000). The cognitive neuropsychology of delusions. *Mind & Language, 15*, 184–218.

Levine, J. (1983). Materialism and qualia: The explanatory gap. *Pacific Philosophical Quarterly, 64*, 354–61.

Lewis, D. (1982). Logic for equivocators. *Noûs, 16*, 431–41.

Lewis, M. B. and Ellis, H. D. (2001). A two-way window on face recognition: Reply to Breen et al. *Trends in Cognitive Sciences*, 5, 235.

Lipton, P. (2004). *Inference to the Best Explanation* (2nd edn). London: Routledge.

Maher, B. A. (1974). Delusional thinking and perceptual disorder. *Journal of Individual Psychology*, 30, 98–113.

Maher, B. A. (1988). Anomalous experience and delusional thinking: The logic of explanations. In T. F. Oltmanns and B. A. Maher (Eds), *Delusional Beliefs*, pp. 15–33. Chichester: John Wiley and Sons.

Maher, B. A. (1992). Delusions: Contemporary etiological hypotheses. *Psychiatric Annals*, 22, 260–8.

Maher, B. A. (1999). Anomalous experience in everyday life: Its significance for psychopathology. *The Monist*, 82, 547–70.

Mandler, G. (1980). Recognizing: The judgment of previous occurrence. *Psychological Review*, 87, 252–71.

McKay, R. (2012). Delusional inference. *Mind & Language*, 27, 330–55.

Moore, G. E. (1939). Proof of an external world. *Proceedings of the British Academy*, 25, 273–300. (Reprinted in G. E. Moore (1959). *Philosophical Papers*, pp. 127–50. London: Allen and Unwin.)

Nagel, T. (1974). What is it like to be a bat? *Philosophical Review*, 83, 435–50. (Reprinted in T. Nagel (1979). *Mortal Questions*, pp. 165–80. Cambridge: Cambridge University Press.)

Psillos, S. (2009). An explorer upon untrodden ground: Peirce on abduction. In D. M. Gabbay, S. Hartmann and J. Woods (Eds), *Handbook of the History of Logic, Volume 10: Inductive Logic*, pp. 117–51. Amsterdam: Elsevier BV.

Shea, N. (2012). Reward prediction error signals are meta-representational. *Noûs*, DOI: 10.1111/j.1468-0068.2012.00863.x.

Shea, N. (in press). Distinguishing top-down from bottom-up effects. In S. Biggs, M. Matthen, and D. Stokes (Eds), *Perception and Its Modalities*. Oxford: Oxford University Press.

Siegel, S. (2010). *The Contents of Visual Experience*. Oxford: Oxford University Press.

Sperber, D. (2001). In defense of massive modularity. In E. Dupoux (Ed.), *Language, Brain, and Cognitive Development: Essays in Honor of Jacques Mehler*, pp. 47–57. Cambridge, MA: MIT Press.

Sperber, D. and Wilson, D. (1986). *Relevance: Communication and Cognition* (2nd edn, 1995). Oxford: Blackwell Publishing.

Sperber, D. and Wilson, D. (2002). Pragmatics, modularity and mind-reading. *Mind & Language*, 17, 3–23.

Stone, T. and Young, A. W. (1997). Delusions and brain injury: The philosophy and psychology of belief. *Mind & Language*, 12, 327–64.

Tranel, D. and Damasio, A. R. (1985). Knowledge without awareness: An autonomic index of facial recognition by prosopagnosics. *Science*, 228, 1453–4.

Tranel, D. and Damasio, A. R. (1988). Non-conscious face recognition in patients with face agnosia. *Behavioural Brain Research*, 30, 235–49.

Tranel, D., Damasio, H., and Damasio, A. R. (1995). Double dissociation between overt and covert recognition. *Journal of Cognitive Neuroscience*, 7, 425–32.

Turner, M. and Coltheart, M. (2010). Confabulation and delusion: A common monitoring framework. *Cognitive Neuropsychiatry*, 15, 346–76.

van Fraassen, B. C. (1980). *The Scientific Image*. Oxford: Oxford University Press.

van Fraassen, B. C. (1989). *Laws and Symmetry*. Oxford: Oxford University Press.

Whittlesea, B. W. A. (1993). Illusions of familiarity. *Journal of Experimental Psychology: Learning, Memory, and Cognition, 19*, 1235–53.

Wilson, D. and Sperber, D. (2012). *Meaning and Relevance*. Cambridge: Cambridge University Press.

Young, A. W. and Leafhead, K. M. (1996). Betwixt life and death: Case studies of the Cotard delusion. In P. W. Halligan and J. C. Marshall (Eds), *Method in Madness: Case Studies in Cognitive Neuropsychiatry*, pp. 147–71. Hove: Psychology Press.

Young, G. (2007). Clarifying "familiarity": Phenomenal experiences in prosopagnosia and the Capgras delusion. *Philosophy, Psychiatry, & Psychology, 14*, 29–37.

Young, G. (2008). Capgras delusion: An interactionist model. *Consciousness and Cognition, 17*, 863–76.

SECTION VI

ASSESSMENT AND DIAGNOSTIC CATEGORIES

CHAPTER 43

INTRODUCTION: ASSESSMENT AND DIAGNOSTIC CATEGORIES

In the opening seconds of a psychiatric interview, the clinician is confronted with a myriad of philosophical-methodological questions: How to start? What kind of relationship do I want to develop with this person? How can I be sure that the information I gain from this relationship will be true? Am I to believe my own observations or the patient's report of her own experiences? What kinds of information are important, and which marginal? How do I draw the line between existential, normal distress and psychopathology? For that matter, how do I characterize or interpret this person's experience? What does science have to offer the unique ordeal of this person? This list could go on and on. For better and for worse, the psychiatric assessment process is enshrined in a series of highly stylized and traditional structures—the history, examination, adjunctive studies, and diagnostic formulation to be brief—which enable a clinician to not be frozen by a crisis of philosophical overload. However, every one of the fundamental metaphysical, pragmatic, ethical, and even aesthetic questions that philosophy can pose to psychiatry can have direct and indirect impacts on the clinician's tasks of helping, healing, caring, and curing.

The challenge of the philosophy of psychiatry, however, is not just reserved for psychiatrists, as the practice of psychiatry, the science of psychiatry, and the phenomena of psychopathology pose their own sets of myriad challenges to philosophers. From this standpoint, the philosophy of psychiatry overlaps with intellectual territories of philosophy of science, hermeneutics, phenomenology, narrative theory, epistemology, philosophy of mind—again the list is long. The ten essays which make up this section illustrate many of these challenges, particularized into a dynamic interaction between clinical problems and philosophical problems.

In Chapter 44, the psychologist/philosopher team of Jeffrey Poland and Barbara Von Eckardt address one of the fundamental and important questions faced by clinicians and clinical scientists: how to "map" the domain of mental illness, a domain which is metaphysically and ethically complex. They frame their task by offering an evaluative triad of challenges to any mapping scheme: such schemes should be *empirically adequate*, *conceptually adequate*, and *foundationally* (concerning metaphysical assumptions) *adequate*. This triad of evaluation becomes a template for their lucid and systematic working-through of the adequacy of several approaches to mapping mental illness. Most of their effort is focused upon the *Diagnostic and Statistical Manual of Mental Disorders* (DSM)-IV and the emerging DSM-5 effort, which they find wanting. They then illustrate how some alternative conceptual systems for classifying mental distress tally up against their evaluative triad, including the US National Institute of Mental Health's Research Domain Criteria (RDoC) neuroscience-directed system, as well as the connectivity-analysis approach of Buckholtz and Meyer-Lindenberg. What emerges in Poland and Von Eckardt's conclusions is that the context of use of classificatory systems is crucial, because of the unavoidable trade-offs of value and aptitude to context. What emerges as especially problematic for DSM efforts is that system's "all-things-to-all-people" objectives, trying to make a universally valid diagnostic system which satisfies the needs of scientific, administrative, clinical, and educational contexts.

While Poland and Von Eckardt address value commitments in mapping domains of mental illness, John Sadler, in Chapter 45, addresses the influence of values in the development of diagnostic systems as well as in the particular kinds of evaluations that frame diagnostic criteria and diagnostic categories. He summarizes a philosophical method for values-analysis in psychiatric discourses, and then demonstrates the utility of this method for key issues in current DSM categories, framing recent work in this area from other authors. He then addresses, in more detail, sample areas of controversy in the ongoing DSM-5 effort as examples of the ongoing vitality of this method.

In Chapter 46, Matthew Broome, Paolo Fusar-Poli, and Philipe Wuyts use another DSM-5 controversy, concerning the proposed category of attenuated psychotic disorder, as one of several examples of the general conceptual and ethical issues posed by considerations of "prodromal" phases of psychosis. They introduce a continuum concept of psychosis, with early signs and symptoms posing conceptual and ethical challenges. The conceptual challenges revolve around the limiting sets of assumptions provided when the neuroscience, brain-centered model of psychosis is used, over against more intersubjective, phenomenological conceptions of psychotic illnesses. The ethical challenges are posed by the idea of preventive treatment during prodromal stages of illness—treatments which at this phase are unproven, have substantive toxicities of their own, and may inflict social stigma upon individuals who may never have a full-blown psychotic illness.

Using the clinical phenomenon of mania as his focus, Nassir Ghaemi (Chapter 47) elegantly combines two agendas: one, to describe contemporary thought on the phenomenology of manic conditions, and two, to apply this thinking critically to traditional psychoanalytic and social-constructionist conceptions of mania as a reaction to depressive illness. Setting aside traditional conceptions of mania as a mood disorder, Ghaemi instead formulates it as a disorder fundamentally characterized by psychomotor activation, creativity, and insight. He subsequently criticizes the idea of mania being environmentally reactive, at least in the traditional psychodynamic sense as a reaction against depressing life events, citing key sources from the history of psychiatry, as well as empirical research to support his formulation.

Peter Hobson points out in Chapter 48 that autistic disorders offer challenges to both psychiatrists and philosophers. He provides a thorough consideration of theory of mind and situationist theories of autism, drawing upon the philosophical work of Wittgenstein, Buber, Merleau-Ponty, Sartre, and others in the process. Hobson's chapter is an exercise in the mutual benefit between philosophy of mind, on the one hand, and developmental psychology and psychopathology, on the other. Hobson shows how philosophical theory can generate testable hypotheses about development; as well as developmental psychology's aptitude to challenge philosophical theories of mind. In this regard, Hobson shows how philosophy is an essential tool in interpreting scientific facts generated by empirical science.

An expert in old-age (geriatric) psychiatry, Julian Hughes uses clinical topics of dementia and Alzheimer's disease as foils to explore the epistemic notion of essentialism in psychiatry in Chapter 49. Essentialism, the ideal of the invariant concept, is problematic in multiple ways for Hughes. One way is that fuzzy concepts with vague boundaries, like "dementia," when released into common lay use, become reified and presumed to be much sharper concepts than they prove to be, given proper scrutiny. Hughes finds no sharp boundaries between aging processes and "dementia," leading him to question the ethics of using the latter term. The "edges" of the Alzheimer concept are framed by value considerations, not sharp epistemic boundaries. Hughes sees the clinical challenge of aged people as how to regard them as "being-with" rather than formulating how to "do-to."

In Chapter 50, the problem of essentialism raised by Hughes is explored by Walter Sinnott-Armstrong and Hanna Pickard with regard to the concept of addiction. As still another fuzzy but clinically crucial concept, the authors suggest that the kind of definition of addiction that is needed is a "precising" definition—one that is not excessively stipulative to restrict application unduly, but one which avoids the "vagueness of common usage." They then consider a series of concepts of addiction, starting with that of DSM-IV-TR, finding its polythetic structure (different sets of independent diagnostic criteria can be met, yielding non-uniform populations) inadequate to the "precising" challenge. They then consider in detail three core features which reflect common usage but offer potential for a precising definition: appetites, control, and harm. For Sinnott-Armstrong and Pickard, although variability exists in severity of appetite for drugs, ability to control use, and degrees of harm, these three frameworks for the concept offer the potential for practical criteria to address boundaries of diagnosis and treatment, particularly when the particular concept of use of addiction concept is specified.

Chapter 51 is a frank personal memoir, as well as commentary on "memoir," by philosopher Owen Flanagan, inspired by his own addiction and recovery experience. One of the many things memoir teaches us, and Flanagan, is the myriad ways the habit of drinking interweaves with one's sense of self—indeed, personal identity—not the least of which is one's sense of "feeling safe in the world." Philosophy and narrative are one of the ways which sufferers and their would-be helpers can help each other navigate, understand, and overcome such harrowing existential situations.

In Chapter 52, Peter Zachar and Robert Krueger approach the fuzzy concept of personality disorder(s) from the standpoint of a historical and philosophical analysis of validity for these conditions. Zachar and Krueger frame the issue of personality disorders alongside the problem of characterizing "personality" in normal psychology, including the latter's relationship to the older notion of "self." They frame their discussion about the conceptual validity of personality disorders from three standpoints: (1) What role do values and moral evaluations play in personality disorder concepts? (2) What determines whether a personality is disordered? (3) Is "personality" causally substantive, or simply an epiphenomenon of other causal factors? Particularly for the third set of considerations, Zachar and Krueger break new ground, inviting scholars to explore this difficult area with them.

The phenomena of multiple personality disorder/dissociative identity disorder have fascinated philosophers for over two decades, making this topic one of the most generative problem areas in the philosophy of psychiatry. Stephen R. L. Clark makes it easy to see why. In Chapter 53, the concluding chapter in this section, Clark explores both reciprocities of the philosophy of psychiatry vis-à-vis these conditions: what philosophy has to offer psychiatry in comprehending these uncommon but perplexing conditions, and what psychiatry has to offer philosophical theories of personal identity. It turns out these conditions are problematic for both groups of scholars! Clark reviews perspectives of both psychiatric theories of dissociation as well as philosophical theories of personal identity, showing us in the process a model for bilateral scholarship in the field.

....

CHAPTER 44

MAPPING THE DOMAIN OF MENTAL ILLNESS

....

JEFFREY POLAND AND BARBARA VON ECKARDT

The domain of mental illness is a face of the domain of human functioning, which includes phenomena involving individual life problems, distress, disability, deviance, failures to perform social functions, and maladaptation, in which mental and behavioral capacities are centrally involved. This is not a formal definition, but rather an informal way to specify a human domain of interest. This domain is a target of scientific research, clinical practices of various forms, social practices (e.g., law, business, social policy, education, affiliations, etc.), and substantial personal interest. Such purposes and interests call out for informed means of conceptualization and intervention, although it should not be assumed that one approach will effectively serve all contexts equally well.

In this chapter, we consider how best to conceptualize and "map" the domain of mental illness for scientific research purposes. Our discussion will have two major parts. First, drawing on previous publications (Poland et al. 1994, in press; Von Eckardt 1993) we will provide a more detailed description of the domain of mental illness and clarify why the traditional, psychiatric, *Diagnostic and Statistical Manual of Mental Disorders* (DSM)-based research approach is inadequate. Second, we will turn to the main task of this chapter, which is to explore alternative approaches to the study of mental illness. Here we will consider the current National Institute of Mental Health (NIMH) Research Domain Criteria (RDoC) initiative and several recent examples of mental illness research, detailing their strengths, weaknesses, and lessons. We'll conclude with some recommendations for how research concerning the domain of mental illness might be productively pursued.

MAPPING THE DOMAIN OF MENTAL ILLNESS

....

With respect to scientific research, what we call "mapping a domain" is simply the activity of carrying out a research program that targets a pre-theoretically conceived class of phenomena (e.g., mental illness as described at the start of this chapter). A research program is a strategic plan for answering certain basic questions about a target domain, in accordance with a set of substantive and methodological assumptions concerning, respectively, the domain and the methods most likely to yield answers to the basic questions. Scientists are said to "map a domain" in the sense of discovering what the phenomena in that domain "really" are and how they relate to each other in causal and other ways (cf. Von Eckardt 1993). We take DSM-based research, NIMH's RDoC initiative, and recent approaches to mental illness within neuroscience all to be concerned with mapping the domain of mental illness.

For the purposes of this chapter, we take a research approach's "fitting a domain" to be critical in whether it can adequately conceptualize and map its domain. This relation of fitting a domain involves three important components. First is the *empirical adequacy* of the approach: How successful is it in answering the questions it is concerned to address and what is its promise for answering those questions in the future? Second is the *conceptual adequacy* of the approach: Does it have the resources for representing and managing the features of the target domain? Successful mapping of a domain requires representational power sufficient for identifying and systematically integrating important features and relationships within that domain. Third is the *foundational adequacy* of the approach: How sound are its substantive and methodological assumptions? Are its substantive assumptions (e.g., that mental illnesses are brain diseases) true or at least plausible? Are its methodological assumptions (e.g., that research concerning mental illness should be pursued in ways comparable to the rest of medicine) pragmatically useful and productive? These three adequacy criteria will be central to our following evaluations.

THE DOMAIN OF MENTAL ILLNESS

One final preliminary step needs to be taken. We need to flesh out the informal characterization of the domain of mental illness given earlier. On the basis of a pre-theoretical understanding of the domain along with findings from both the basic sciences of human functioning and research targeting mental illness, it is possible to identify a number of general features of mental illness, features that are widely acknowledged and that place considerable demands on any scientific research approach targeting this area of human functioning. Here is a quick survey:[1]

- *Ambiguity*: features in the domain of mental illness can be derived from many different causal processes.
- *Hierarchical organization*: human biological systems consist of many levels of organization ranging from low-level genetic, biochemical, and neuroanatomical to high-level cognitive, behavioral, and sociocultural. These levels are also present in mental illness.
- *Multidimensionality*: the state or condition of a person with mental illness at a time consists of features and processes of many different sorts, within and across levels of organization.

---

[1] The following draws on Poland (in press), which provides a more extended discussion of the features of the domain of mental illness. See also Spaulding et al. (2003).

- *Interactivity and context sensitivity*: the features and processes of mental illness are typically interactive with each other and, hence, each is sensitive to the context in which it is embedded.
- *Dynamics*: the features and processes of mental illness evolve over time at various time scales along varying trajectories, and they can exhibit phase dependence and a variety of distinctive causal patterns.
- *Perspective and agency*: individuals suffering mental illness are persons who are agents and who have a first-person perspective on themselves, the world, their past, and their future.
- *Normativity*: the identification of conditions as problematic, deviant, maladaptive, dysfunctional, diseased, distressing, or disabling presupposes background norms, values, or interests that may be theoretical, personal, social, or of some other sort.
- *Normal and abnormal conditions and processes*: although there may be conditions or processes in mental illness that violate some specified norms, there are also conditions and processes that are normal by the same or different standards.
- *Relational and non-relational problems*: the kinds of problems that people with mental illness can suffer can be both non-relational (i.e., conditions of the individual) and relational (i.e., conditions involving relationships between an individual and other people or between an individual and some aspect of the non-personal environment).
- *Individual variability*: individuals suffering a mental illness vary widely and tend to exhibit relatively unique combinations of problems, functional profiles, embedding contexts, and causal processes.

Such features, abstractly conceived, demarcate the broad contours of the domain of mental illness. Of course, substantial inquiry and elaboration are required to flesh out how each of these features is concretely manifested by the various phenomena in the domain; this is where scientific research and various other forms of relevant inquiry (e.g., the philosophical analysis of normativity) enter the picture.[2]

WHY A DSM-BASED APPROACH IS INADEQUATE[3]

In 1980, the American Psychiatric Association published the third edition of its *Diagnostic and Statistical Manual of Mental Disorders* (American Psychiatric Association 1980); since that time, there have been three revisions issuing in the current version, DSM-IV-TR (American Psychiatric Association 2000). The DSM lays out a categorical scheme comprised of several hundred categories of mental disorder; each is conceived as a harmful dysfunction that can be identified on the basis of *atheoretical*, *polythetic* diagnostic criteria framed in

---

[2] Although our focus will be on research programs in cognitive neuroscience, the range of the relevant sciences and other forms of inquiry necessary for understanding the domain of mental illness is potentially quite broad, including other areas of neuroscience, psychology, relevant social sciences, and certain types of philosophical analysis.

[3] The following discussion of the DSM approach to research draws on Poland et al. (1994) and Poland (in press).

terms of clinically salient features or other characteristics (e.g., of history or context) read-ily determined by the clinician. The idea that mental disorders can be identified in terms of "atheoretical" criteria (i.e., in terms not referring to either pathology or etiology) is a core assumption of the approach. The employment of criteria drawing on clinical phenomenol-ogy[4] and other pre-theoretically conceived characteristics is supposed to make the criteria better operationalized and, hence, better suited for the purpose of increasing diagnostic reli-ability (cf. Blashfield 1984). Such increases in reliability were believed to be a necessary con-dition for pursuing research that would eventually "validate" the diagnostic categories. The employment of "polythetic" criteria (i.e., disjunctive criteria) reflects the idea that mental disorders can manifest themselves in various ways across individuals with the same disor-der. Another important feature of the DSM taxonomy is that it presupposes a form of *indi-vidualism* requiring that mental disorders are non-relational (i.e., conditions that are of the individual and that do not involve any relations to the social or non-social environment). Thus, even though atheoretically conceived, each disorder is assumed to involve a putative (but unspecified) biological, psychological, or behavioral dysfunction of the individual, a dysfunction that manifests itself in terms of the signs and symptoms specified by the diag-nostic criteria.

In addition to the DSM categorical scheme, with its associated assumptions, the DSM-based approach to research currently includes three other important commitments:

C1. One system of classification can and should serve both research and clinical purposes, because such an arrangement will best serve the goal of translating scientific research into clinical practice.
C2. Control over the process of developing and revising the DSM system of classification should rest firmly in the hands of the American Psychiatric Association.[5]
C3. Mental health practices ought to be medicalized.

The significance of this last commitment is substantial. The *medicalization* of contempo-rary mental health practice[6] typically manifests itself in the following ways.

Regarding the *disciplinary identity* of psychiatry, psychiatry is a branch of medicine, psy-chiatrists are physicians concerned with treating medically ill patients who suffer from men-tal illnesses, and all psychiatric practices should be based on biomedical scientific evidence and knowledge.

Regarding the *domain of mental illness*, mental illnesses are distinct from normal func-tioning and are neither moral failings nor problems in living encountered in the normal course of life; rather, they are brain diseases that involve a "pathophysiology" (i.e., genetic, molecular, cellular, or biochemical pathology or abnormal neural circuitry and functioning) which develops as the result of an "etiology" (i.e., genetic or other biological vulnerabilities interacting with environmental and experiential triggers).

---

[4] In this context, the term "phenomenology" is used in a narrow sense referring to aspects of the clinical presentation of individuals.
[5] This is the case even though the system is employed by a wide range of mental health professionals who engage in a variety of forms of mental health practice and work in a wide range of mental health contexts.
[6] See Klerman (1978) for a classic statement of the medicalization of psychiatric practice, a statement dubbed "the neo-Kraepelinian credo." See also Blashfield (1984).

Regarding *clinical practice*, as in other areas of medicine, psychiatric practice involves physicians diagnosing and treating patients for diseases in a context shaped by medical roles, identities, statuses, authority, and relationships. Psychiatrists know how to diagnose these diseases using the diagnostic criteria found in the DSM. Psychotropic drugs are typically the first line of treatment for these brain diseases since they treat biochemical dysregulations, restore functionality to neural circuitry, and reduce symptoms. Mental illness should be viewed and treated like any other disease.

Regarding *research practice*, as in other areas of medicine, research practices in psychiatry are based on modern scientific knowledge, technologies, and methodologies (e.g., genomics, statistics, risk analysis, neuroimaging) and approach the study of brain diseases in ways comparable to research concerning cancer and cardiovascular disease. Central research questions concern the pathophysiology and etiology of mental illnesses, the reliability and validity of diagnostic categories and associated criteria, and biological and psychosocial treatments for these brain diseases. Combined with the DSM category scheme as well as C1–C3, this medicalized approach to research has resulted in a research practice in which DSM categories are routinely used as independent or dependent variables, and for sampling and subject grouping purposes; typical investigations examine such diagnostically defined groups with respect to pathology, etiology, response to intervention, demographics, etc.

How has this research approach fared over the past three decades? It is now widely acknowledged that the research program structured by the DSM and its associated commitments has serious problems. Specifically, DSM-based research programs have not yielded the sorts of robust results hoped for by the authors of DSM-III in 1980 (cf. Andreasen 2007; Hyman 2010; Insel and Cuthbert 2010; Kendell and Jablensky 2003; Kendler et al. 2009; Regier et al. 2009). While reliability statistics associated with some DSM categories of mental disorder are better than those of their predecessors, DSM researchers have produced a relatively weak research record of findings that tend to be negative, inconsistent, non-replicable, weak, non-specific, or uninterpretable. As a result, the categories exhibit substantial problems of construct and predictive validity, lack of precise phenotypic definition, and widespread heterogeneity and comorbidity. Consequently, no firm consensus has emerged on the basic questions at which the research is aimed (e.g., validation of the categories, identification of underlying dysfunctions/pathophysiology associated with each category, identification of the etiology of each, etc.). In other words, DSM-based research has failed to satisfy the standard of empirical adequacy.

This failure provides strong evidence that the available conceptual resources of the DSM approach do not properly line up with the domain. The reason why is not a mystery. Given both the character of the DSM approach (e.g., its atheoretical, polythetic, and phenomenological criteria, and its categorical structure) and its failure to produce well-confirmed models associated with each category, there are insufficient conceptual resources for identifying and managing the features of the domain of mental illness.[7] As a result, it is virtually guaranteed that there will be heterogeneity (including "process heterogeneity") at all levels of analysis within categorical groupings.[8] And, given the dynamic interactivity and context sensitivity of

[7] An atheoretical categorical approach to classification, for example, has limited resources for representing multiple dimensions of variation characteristic of individuals who are classified.

[8] Such heterogeneity has been confirmed by various literature reviews associated with specific diagnostic categories. For example, see Heinrichs (2001) for a review of research bearing on heterogeneity in schizophrenia. And, see later for references to research concerning heterogeneity in attention-deficit/hyperactivity disorder (ADHD).

processes in the domain of mental illness, this heterogeneity will lead to uncontrolled sources of systematic and unsystematic error that will undermine research and reveal the categories to be artificial impositions on the domain that are lacking in empirical or theoretical integrity (i.e., they are non-natural kinds lacking in validity). Alternatively put, the DSM categories fail the standard of conceptual adequacy (cf. Poland in press; Poland et al. 1994).

Finally, there are also problems of foundational adequacy, which provide further understanding of why DSM-based research has been non-progressive, namely, that the DSM has been highly tuned to a specific form of clinical practice shaped by the assumptions and commitments outlined earlier (e.g., individualism, medicalization, American Psychiatric Association control, one system for clinical and research purposes). Two points are worth mentioning in this regard. First, in the DSM development process, which is firmly controlled by the American Psychiatric Association, DSM diagnostic criteria and categories have been tailored to serve specific clinical needs and constraints (e.g., the training of psychiatrists, the forms of standard psychiatric practice, the contextual features of such forms of practice, etc.). As a consequence, many of the decisions regarding what categories to include/exclude and what criteria to employ (e.g., symptom cutoffs) are based not on relevant science, but rather on perceptions of clinical utility and, in some cases, political considerations.[9] This arguably reflects an inappropriate intrusion of pragmatic and political considerations on decisions that affect scientific research practice. And, it signals a source of some of the problems exhibited by the research approach: viz., the classification system, rather than being tuned to the demands of research concerning the domain of mental illness, is tuned to the proprietary needs, interests, and constraints associated with a specific clinical guild. This suggests the need for some sort of insulation of basic research from such proprietary considerations.

Second, the commitments to the following substantive and methodological assumptions discussed earlier are suspect: that the domain of mental illness consists (entirely) of individualistically conceived mental disorders (individualism), that the domain of mental illness consists (entirely) of brain diseases that involve a "pathophysiology" which develops as the result of an "etiology" (medicalization of the domain), that mental illnesses are distinct from normal functioning (medicalization of the domain), that one classification system can effectively serve both clinical and research purposes (C1), and that DSM categories are appropriate targets of scientific investigation (nature of traditional psychiatric research practice). Such assumptions reflect many of the clinical biases that shaped the DSM[10] and are not vindicated by the research program that they inform: i.e., the non-progressiveness of the approach does not provide support for either their truth or their pragmatic utility. Hence the approach has questionable foundational adequacy.

The bottom line is that the commitments that have shaped the current DSM-IV-TR and the conventional forms of psychiatric research practice based upon it (viz., commitments to individualism, C1–C3, and the importance of tuning the DSM to a specific form of clinical practice) have led to a classification scheme and associated research program that provide a

[9] For example, see Kirk and Kutchins (1992) for a discussion of the processes associated with the development of DSM-III; and see Rounsaville et al. (2002, p. 1) and Kendler et al. (2009, p. 1) for the importance of utility in clinical psychiatric practice for the crafting of DSM criteria.

[10] See Blashfield (1984) for extensive discussion of how the neo-Kraepelinian movement in psychiatry shaped the DSM approach to classification and the research practices based upon it.

very poor map of the domain of mental illness, a map that, in turn, undermines the pursuit of research purposes. This result combined with the deep entrenchment and dominance of this form of research practice mean that, currently, a severe crisis in mental health research practice exists. Such a crisis calls out for an effective response that will break the grip of the DSM approach on research and free up resources for more scientifically grounded research agendas.

As we shall see later, there are encouraging signs that the grip of the DSM framework is being loosened; however, we shall also see that researchers are finding it difficult to divest themselves of the DSM completely. This is most clear in the case of the DSM-5 revision process currently being overseen by the American Psychiatric Association. This process is, on our view, a non-starter for effectively responding to the crisis and guiding research in more productive directions and toward adequate maps of the domain of mental illness. More specifically, there is every indication[11] that the DSM-5 will consist of virtually all of the "grandfathered through"[12] clinical categories codified in DSM-III and its successors, categories based on clinical tradition not scientific research. The changes introduced in DSM-5 (e.g., dimensional scales,[13] metastructure of the categorical system,[14] revised definition of mental disorder, revised criteria for some categories, addition/deletion of some categories) are simply more products of the same approach and biases that informed prior DSMs and, hence, a propagation of substantially the same problematic categories, assumptions, and commitments. Since those categories, assumptions, and commitments are constitutive of a research approach lacking in empirical, conceptual, and foundational adequacy, the DSM-5 is very unlikely to provide a better map of the domain of mental illness than DSM-IV.

ALTERNATIVE APPROACHES TO
MENTAL ILLNESS RESEARCH

In the light of the now widely acknowledged problems with the DSM-based approach, several alternatives are being pursued. We will begin by looking at one general strategic

---

[11] See the DSM-5 website at <http://www.dsm5.org> for materials concerning the proposals for revision of DSM-IV. See also Kendler et al. (2009) for the official guidelines for making changes to the DSM; such guidelines are essentially quite conservative.

[12] The term here refers to the fact that categories of mental disorder in DSM-III were introduced on the basis of "expert" clinical judgment and political negotiations, rather than rigorous science, and that subsequent revisions of the DSM (III-R, IV, V) have allowed such categories to be retained despite the fact that there continues to be no sound scientific basis for doing so. See Kirk and Kutchins (1992), and Poland (2001, 2002).

[13] Although the measurement of dimensions of functioning is an important component of a more progressive approach to mapping the domain of mental illness, the DSM-5 scales and approach are too limited and problematic to yield substantial improvement over DSM-IV. See Frances (2010) for discussion of some of the problems.

[14] See Andrews et al. (2009) and Bernstein (2011) for a description of this idea, which concerns grouping existing DSM categories into clusters based on similarities and targeting those clusters for research purposes. However, given the problems of validity and heterogeneity of individual DSM categories, it is likely that these clusters will exhibit similar problems.

initiative aimed at shifting research funding away from projects that employ DSM categories and "develop[ing], for research purposes, new ways of classifying mental disorders based on dimensions of observable behavior and neurobiological measures" (NIMH 2011): viz., NIMH's RDoC initiative.

The NIMH RDoC initiative

RDoC (NIMH 2011) represents an important step forward in attempting to shift the course of mental health-related research. This initiative is explicitly premised on an acknowledgment of the shortcomings of DSM categories for the purposes of scientific research (Cuthbert and Insel 2010; Insel and Cuthbert 2010), and its immediate aim is to encourage and fund research proposals that do not rely on the DSM. More specifically, it calls for proposals that are focused on various units of analysis (genes, molecules, cells, circuits, physiology, behavior, self-reports) in specific research domains (e.g., functional domains such as negative valence systems, positive valence systems, cognitive systems, systems for social processes, arousal/regulatory systems), without employing DSM categories. The initiative further emphasizes the value of investigating each functional domain with respect to a wide range of constructs (e.g., with regard to cognitive systems: perception, attention, working memory, declarative memory, language, cognitive control) and the importance of selecting subjects broadly, specifically, in ways that cross-cut the traditional DSM categories. The ultimate aim is to build a research base that will underwrite a new classification system based on behavioral neuroscience and that will promote new approaches to treatment (especially, but not exclusively, drugs, surgery, and stimulation technologies) (cf. Insel, et al. 2010).

What are the strengths of this initiative? In addition to explicitly acknowledging the serious shortfall of DSM-based research and the need for a new approach to classification, it promotes the importance of tuning research concerning mental illness to basic science and of focusing on specific domains of human functioning taken to be highly relevant to mental health and illness (NIMH 2011). It also acknowledges the importance of taking into account many (but not all) of the features of the domain of mental illness. For example, by not targeting DSM categories, focusing on several domains of functioning, and addressing each of these at many levels of analysis, the research approach has considerable promise for managing the features of ambiguity, multidimensionality, hierarchical organization, interactivity/context sensitivity, and individual variability. In addition, the initiative recognizes the importance of sampling subjects in a broad way in order to create more representative and more meaningful samples. They suggest, for example, identifying subjects for a study by including all patients presenting for treatment at a given type of facility or all patients who meet a particular neurobehavioral criterion, such as patients who show significant activation in a specified brain area on a neuroimaging task. All of these changes constitute a substantial improvement over the DSM approach and underwrite greater promise for enhancing the empirical adequacy of mental illness research.

However, the current implementation of RDoC also exhibits several limitations that will likely compromise its effectiveness as both an engine for providing better maps of the domain of mental illness and for providing a better response to the extant crisis in mental health research practice. Specifically, the initiative is, on our view, too closely tied to the traditional psychiatric clinical tradition and its commitments to medicalization. It, thus, presumes a form of pathology-oriented individualism for all forms of mental illness that focuses on brain disease and appears to privilege lower-level genetic and neurophysiological (as opposed to computational/representational, personological, or sociocultural) levels of analysis and physical forms of intervention (e.g., drugs).[15] There is, thus, a risk that the role of normal processes,[16] relational problems, personal agency, and social processes in mental illness will be neglected, and that the sorts of research projects that will be funded will be inappropriately restricted and not representative of the full range of scientific investigations relevant to understanding the various features of the domain of mental illness.

In sum, then, relative to our standards of adequacy, RDoC promises to give rise to more sophisticated neuroscientific and genetic research, and, hence, enhanced empirical adequacy. However, current descriptions of the initiative suggest that it may still suffer important limitations with respect to its conceptual and foundational adequacy.

Two case studies

In the remainder of this chapter, we will examine two case studies of recent research targeting the domain of mental illness to underscore some of the points previously discussed and to extract certain lessons that may be useful in developing a better, alternative approach to basic research on mental illness. We'll see that although headway is being made in developing important new conceptual resources, particularly, in how to describe patient populations and how to theorize about deficits, researchers are still strongly tied to the DSM categories and traditional, psychiatric commitments to medicalization.

Case 1: Subtypes of ADHD

We will begin by focusing on two examples concerned with identifying subtypes of so-called "ADHD" and with managing the well-established heterogeneity of that category.

The first example (Fair et al. 2012) applies graph theoretical techniques to data derived from a battery of neurocognitive measures administered to both a sample of ADHD children and to a sample of typically developing children (TDC). The measures employed involve tasks thought to assess capacities implicated in ADHD (e.g., inhibition, working memory, arousal/activation, response variability, temporal information processing, memory span, processing speed). The central idea was to identify subtypes of individuals in both the TDC cohort and the ADHD cohort based upon characteristic neurocognitive profiles as identified by the battery. The results of this study were as follows: (a) there were four well-defined neurocognitive profiles in the TDC cohort that identified four distinct neurocognitive subtypes; (b) there were six well-defined neurocognitive profiles in the ADHD cohort that identified six distinct neurocognitive subtypes (NB: there were two pairs of profiles that were substantially similar though distinct, leading to four main subtypes.); (c) the variation by subtypes within the ADHD cohort was embedded in the variation by subtype within

---

[15] See Insel (2010) for a clear statement of this sort of emphasis within the RDoC initiative.

[16] NIMH (2011) notes that insofar as RDoC is conceived as a dimensional system, it will span the range from normal to abnormal. This is, however, a quite different way to include normality than our feature of normal/abnormal as characterized earlier.

the TDC cohort; (d) the ADHD status of any given individual was more readily identifiable when subtypes were taken into account. The authors conclude that the use of graph theory applied to neurocognitive profiles has substantial promise for managing the heterogeneity of diagnostic categories, for identifying subtypes that may correspond to neurocognitive circuitry subtypes comprising the varying pathophysiology of ADHD, and for improving clinical diagnostic accuracy.

A second related approach (Durston et al. 2011) hypothesizes that three different neuro-cognitive circuits, the functioning of which can be measured by a battery of neurocognitive tasks, underlie three distinct subtypes of ADHD manifested by characteristic neurocog-nitive profiles and clinical symptoms. More specifically, and building on a review of the ADHD research literature, Durston et al. argue that whereas ADHD has been conceived as a disorder of cognitive control implicating dysfunctions of the prefrontal cortex (Barkley 1997), evidence suggests that this model is too simple and that three separable circuits serv-ing distinct neurocognitive functions are implicated in ADHD. They argue further that dysfunctions in those circuits give rise to distinct neurocognitive deficits which, in turn, manifest as symptoms in the clinic: (a) dorsofronto-striatal dysfunction gives rise to cogni-tive control deficits, (b) orbitofronto-striatal dysfunction gives rise to reward processing deficits, and (c) fronto-cerebellar dysfunction gives rise to timing deficits. The hypothesis on offer is that these three circuits and related dysfunctions underlie three distinct types of ADHD and that these three types can be distinguished in terms of distinct neurocognitive profiles based on task batteries that tap the three relevant neurocognitive functions realized by the circuitry.

In commenting on the significance of their approach, Durston et al. (2011, p. 1182) envision a pathway of future research that improves upon past research programs based exclusively on psychiatric diagnosis by introducing subtypes of those categories (in this case ADHD) associated with a neurobiological substrate (viz., circuit dysfunctions) and a neurocognitive assessment approach that enables identification of the subtypes and the representation of individual differences in cognitive function associated with those circuit dysfunctions. Such an approach is supposed to open up new possibilities for understanding both the neurobiology and the etiology of psychiatric disorders.

These two examples represent some of the strategies for research concerning mental ill-ness that have been pursued in recent years. For our purposes, they exhibit a variety of both strengths and limitations that provide the basis for lessons concerning how to productively pursue such research. At the top of the list of strengths for both examples is not only the recognition that traditional DSM categories (e.g., ADHD) exhibit problems of heterogene-ity that compromise their value for research purposes but also an attempt to manage this heterogeneity for research purposes. As discussed earlier, such categories, which are atheo-retical and based upon clinical diagnostic criteria and practices, mask important differences across individuals, and, hence, introduce uncontrolled sources of systematic and unsystem-atic error that undermine the interpretability of research findings. In both examples, the strategy is to expand the available conceptual resources to help manage this heterogeneity. These conceptual resources include the introduction of multivariate functional profiles, in the first example, and hypothesized neural circuits, in the second. Such strategies create the possibility of improving management of individual variability in the domain of mental ill-ness, providing a representation of dimensions of functioning and the context of such func-tioning, assisting in resolving the causal ambiguity of clinical phenomenological features (e.g., by clarifying multiple pathways to a clinical feature), and assisting in the interpretation of task performance data (e.g., by representing multiple sources of possible influence on task performance).

A further strength of the first example is the strategy of sampling and studying both identified clinical populations and typical (normal) populations. Although Fair et al. (2012) pursue this strategy to better manage the heterogeneity of ADHD, it has a much broader significance. In particular, various pathologies (deficits, impairments) can only be understood against a background understanding of non-pathological functioning. Only if variation in "normal" functioning is understood and the sources of individual and group differences in such functioning are identified and quantified, can meaningful talk of abnormality proceed. More importantly, the domain of mental illness includes normal processes, involved in the production of suffering, disability, or other sorts of problems, which are essential to an understanding of an individual's particular form of mental illness (e.g., normal learning processes). Hence, a scientific investigation of normal functioning is an essential component of a well-balanced research approach to mental illness.

These examples involve strategies (viz., multidimensional profiles, neurocognitive circuitry, sampling and investigation of normal individuals, management of individual variation) that improve the conceptual adequacy of the research approach and enhance its prospects for empirical adequacy. Despite these strengths, both examples exhibit (actual or potential) limitations. First, in both cases, the research continues to be too closely tied to the DSM category of ADHD. In our two examples, the category was used for sampling and subject grouping, for selecting tasks to tap important functions, and for projecting hypotheses regarding relevant circuitry. In addition, the aim of both research projects was to better manage the "problem of heterogeneity in ADHD," a problem that exists only if the category is taken seriously. However, given its atheoretical character and its problems of validity and heterogeneity, the category is too artificial to be taken seriously, and hence it is too artificial to serve such critical research functions as problem definition, sampling and subject grouping, task selection, and hypothesis formation.

A second limitation is that both examples show indications of commitment to the medicalization of ADHD and its associated disease model with a consequent focus on individual pathology and a search for its pathophysiology and etiology.

Finally, the functional profiles identified in the two examples are arguably insufficiently broad and balanced to serve the important functions such profiles should serve, namely, manage the features of the domain of mental illness. If such profiles are supposed to help identify important cognitive functions and associated circuits (as they are in the two examples), then it is important to have a survey of the broader neurocognitive context, on the basis of performance on a broad range of tasks, in order to represent sources of interactive influence and hence to more effectively identify distinct neurocognitive functions and more complex cognitive capacities (cf. Badre 2011). In addition, as already noted, the employment of tasks relevant to putative dysfunctions in ADHD is a dubious basis for task selection, given the artificial nature of that category; better, perhaps, is to focus on specific symptoms or specific measurable neurocognitive differences and to develop task batteries designed to probe those differences, their neurocognitive basis, and sources of individual and group differences. Finally, assessment of neurocognitive strengths and weaknesses requires a broad functional profile representing possible sources of variation in functioning. Task performance data can be reflective of many sources of individual differences beside a putative deficit in the target function. Without such sufficiently broad functional profiles, task performance data is potentially uninterpretable.

With respect to our first case study, the bottom line is that, while recognizing the problems of DSM categories like ADHD, both examples still take the category much too seriously in their research and import dubious foundational assumptions. Nonetheless, each expands the conceptual resources to enable better management of some of the features of the domain.

Case 2: The human "connectome" and mental illness

Our second case study of current research focuses on brain connectivity and its functional significance. The approach is partially expressed by Buckholtz and Meyer-Lindenberg (2012) as follows:

> What makes a brain a brain is its ability to flexibly create, adapt, and disconnect networks in a manner that permits efficient communication within and between populations of neurons, a feature that we call connectivity. The panoply of cognitive, affective, motivational and social processes that underpin normative human experience requires precisely choreographed interactions between networked brain regions. Aberrant connectivity patterns are evident across all major mental disorders, suggesting that breakdowns in this interregional choreography lead to diverse forms of psychological dysfunction. (p. 990)

As they understand it, "connectivity" is used to refer broadly to information flow, relatively local circuitry, and interactivity between regions and circuits. Researchers have employed both functional connectivity approaches (i.e., correlational, model-free approaches that concern functional relations but do not permit directional/causal inferences) and effective connectivity approaches (i.e., explicitly causal, model-based approaches that identify mechanisms of directional influence). According to Buckholtz and Meyer-Lindenberg, whereas functional connectivity approaches are useful for discovery of networks and may allow for specification of heritable system parameters suggesting genetic constraints on inter-regional synchronization, effective connectivity approaches identify mechanisms of directional influence that provide the basis for more powerful causal inferences and explanations and that permit specification of how embedding contexts can moderate causal influences. Both approaches have promise for research aimed at clarifying how aspects of mental illness are manifestations of variations in, and disruptions of, system level circuits and their interactions.

Researchers who recognize the limitations of a DSM category-based approach often attempt to respond to one or another problematic feature of that approach. In our previous case study, the focus was on the heterogeneity problem with respect to the clinical category ADHD. In the current example, the focus is on the problem of comorbidity. As Buckholtz and Meyer-Lindenberg (2012) note:

> Comorbidity between mental disorders is the rule rather than the exception, invading nearly all canonical diagnostic boundaries. In fact, covariation among psychiatric diagnoses is so prevalent, and so extensive, that it alone belies the artificial nature of phenomenologically based categorical classification. (p. 996)

In this context, "comorbidity" is defined relative to categories of mental disorder: two categories exhibit comorbidity if they share common features in their symptomatic manifestations (e.g., schizophrenia and bipolar illness exhibit comorbidity because each is associated with similar cognitive deficits).[17] Such shared features are said by Buckholtz and Meyer-Lindenberg (2012) to be "transdiagnostic." The question these researchers address is: "Why do categorically distinct clinical disorders exhibit common transdiagnostic features?"

In affirming the idea that connectivity analyses can contribute to an understanding of the etiology and pathology of mental illness, Buckholtz and Meyer-Lindenberg (2012) propose that the pathology of mental illness involves (inter alia) brain circuit dysfunctions that characteristically manifest themselves in specific cognitive deficits that are observed in the clinic as symptoms. The fact that a brain circuit can be involved in multiple cognitive domains helps explain why diverse psychiatric disorders can exhibit common deficits and symptoms (comorbidity). More specifically, transdiagnostic patterns of dysconnectivity underlie transdiagnostic patterns of psychiatric symptoms and hence such patterns of dysconnectivity explain why categorical mental disorders exhibit comorbidity. At the heart of this proposal is the core idea that common symptoms arise from common circuit dysfunction (see their figure 1; Buckholtz and Meyer-Lindenberg 2012, p. 991). They cite four examples of cognitive circuitry that fit well with their proposal: brain networks for attention and cognitive control, for affective arousal and regulation, for reward and motivation, and for social cognition.

Complementing this framework for understanding the pathology of mental illness is an etiological proposal that genetic and environmental risk factors induce susceptibility to broad domains of psychopathology because they disrupt connectivity circuits that subsequently give rise to cognitive deficits and clinical symptoms. Evidence for this hypothesis is marshaled by a review of various studies concerning a range of genetic variants (e.g., *COMT*, *DRD2*) associated with various mental disorders as well as with connectivity disruptions and related cognitive impairments.

How does this research approach and specific set of hypotheses fare with respect to our standards for mapping the domain of mental illness? Like Fair et al. (2012), in addition to recognizing the limitations of DSM categories for research, Buckholtz and Meyer-Lindenberg (2012) aim to expand the conceptual resources available for identifying and managing features of the domain of mental illness. Their focus on connectivity in the brain is important because connectivity mediates the existence of both (1) well-defined, functionally specific circuits that underlie human capacities and (2) contextual influences within the brain. It is, thus, an essential conceptual resource for representing capacities within a multidimensional, hierarchically organized system that manifest the context sensitivity and interactivity characteristic of human functioning. With respect to the first, circuits constitute both the realization of higher-level psychological functions and an intermediate level that can be decomposed biologically. With respect to the second, circuits are, typically, embedded in larger contexts; and circuits, typically, interact with other circuits.

Further, connectivity analyses enable the decomposition of complex cognitive capacities, the analysis of task performance (e.g., by allowing a broad survey of systemic contributions to task engagement), the disambiguation of behavioral features (e.g., by specifying multiple pathways that can lead to some high level characteristic) and a judgment as to whether an

---

[17] The term "comorbid" is also more typically used to refer to individuals who suffer from multiple forms of disorder: i.e., comorbidity involves the concurrent occurrence of categorically distinct disorders in a given individual. Although related, the two senses of "comorbidity" are not equivalent.

impairment will lead to a clinical symptom (e.g., by specifying the presence or absence of compensatory processes).

All of this constitutes the promise of the connectivity approach. However, Buckholtz and Meyer-Lindenberg's implementation suffers from several weaknesses, some of which they themselves acknowledge. First, the focus on isolated circuits (e.g., prefrontal cortex-striatal, cortical-limbic, default mode network) is too narrow (as they acknowledge) and not adequately responsive to issues raised by context sensitivity and interactivity (e.g., issues concerning the assignment of functions, the interpretation of task performance data, the manifestation of impairments, and the disambiguation of clinical features). Such issues reinforce the methodological importance of multidimensional functional profiles for research purposes, as was noted in our first case study.

Second, although Buckholtz and Meyer-Lindenberg (2012) discuss the importance of environmental risk factors and influences in the context of genetic vulnerability to mental illness, their discussion substantially underestimates the importance of higher levels of analysis when studying how individuals are embedded in extra-individual contexts. Psychosocial and other social processes are potentially quite relevant to the understanding of mental illness but are not adequately understood simply as risk factors for disease or modulators of disease. Further, there is no mention of how the connectome relates to a person-level perspective and personal agency in Buckholtz and Meyer-Lindenberg's discussion, nor an explicit recognition that mental illness is partially constituted by normal processes.[18] Finally, there appear to be some residual influences of the psychiatric clinical tradition associated with the DSM that inform the research program Buckholtz and Meyer-Lindenberg (2012) envision. Although their focus on the comorbidity of psychiatric diagnostic categories is important both for understanding some of the reasons such categories are artificial and flawed and for motivating a focus on connectivity, it outruns its utility if it suggests that the comorbidity problem is worth serious attention for, like heterogeneity, comorbidity only exists given the DSM categories.

A further influence of the psychiatric clinical tradition is manifested by an apparently exclusive focus both on pathology and on genetic etiological models (p. 999). Such a focus, as manifested in part by a concern with the goal of a nosology of mental illness, belies a disease model of mental illness that may seriously underestimate the importance of normal functioning for understanding mental illness. At a minimum, the context in which problems of connectivity occur includes any number of "normal" processes that are part of the constitution of an individual's relatively unique form of mental illness. In addition to playing a role in the production of deficits and "symptoms," such normal processes may lead to compensatory processes that offset the effects of some impairment or that are designed to solve problems posed by impairments, and such processes may lead to an individual taking actions designed to reshape their context and redirect their energies toward life goals and interests despite various problems they might experience. Thus, normal processes can be essential components of what leads to symptomatic manifestations or they can be essential to how an individual engages their life problems or they may be aspects of a person's "strengths" that can be recruited in treatment or rehabilitation efforts. Research programs

---

[18] These two omissions are not necessarily flaws in the connectome approach but they do exist in Buckholtz and Meyer-Lindenberg's (2012) study.

directed toward understanding mental illness must, of necessity, take normal processes into account.

What emerges from this concern about pathology and normality is the question of how researchers manage issues of normativity with respect to mental illness. A simplistic disease model should be rejected, if for no other reason than such models have not been empirically vindicated by the DSM-based research record and they are typically vaguely conceived and do not address problems concerning the relevant norms that are presupposed. Instead, researchers can and should address questions of individual and group differences with respect to important aspects of human biological systems; and such differences should be quantitatively studied (e.g., with measures both of statistical variation and of the significance of different cutoff points).

The earlier discussion suggests that the research program identified by Buckholtz and Meyer-Lindenberg (2012) involves several potentially important steps toward a more empirically adequate research program concerned with the domain of mental illness. The focus on connectivity, especially model-based effective connectivity, promises to enhance conceptual adequacy by revealing important circuits and pathways related to mental illness. This promise complements the important promise provided by the employment of broad, multidimensional profiles suggested by our first case study. However, as with that other study, the proposal of Buckholtz and Meyer-Lindenberg (2012) displays remnants of the problematic clinical tradition that has shaped the current crisis; such remnants should be abandoned. In particular, basic research is best conceived if it abandons ideological commitments to disease models and recognizes the importance of effectively managing the normativity of mental illness: for basic research this means attempting to address individual and group differences without the application of problematic prescriptive norms, be they moral, social, or personal.

LESSONS AND OUTLOOK

In the light of this discussion, a number of lessons suggest themselves. First, in basic research, researchers should divest completely of the DSM categories, with their atheoretical focus on clinical phenomenology, as well as distance themselves from the clinical tradition of psychiatric diagnosis and the related commitment to medicalization with its focus on pathology, its privileging of low levels of analysis, and its employment of medical research strategies. Any of these will need to earn re-entry into basic research (i.e., their fit with the domain will need to be demonstrated not presupposed.) Such divestment and distancing is warranted by the shortcomings in empirical, conceptual, and foundational adequacy of the DSM-based research approach.

Second, we suggest a different strategic approach for mental health research practices, one that incorporates what seems right in the RDoC initiative, but that is free of problematic commitments and assumptions. Specifically, we think a "firewall" should be created between basic scientific research[19] on human functioning, on the one hand,

---

[19] Basic research here includes the study of typical functioning as well the study of normal variation, individual and group differences, and atypical functioning.

and research programs directly relevant to specific forms of clinical (and other) practice focused on mental illness, on the other. Creation of such a firewall will permit the possibility of developing multiple maps of the domain, each appropriate to the specific agendas, purposes, interests, and values of research and the clinic, respectively. Basic research programs would, thereby, be freed up to create a scientifically rigorous and plausible representation of important causal structure in the domain of mental illness as well as an understanding of how human persons and agents are embodied and embedded in that causal structure: viz., a basic map of the domain. Clinically relevant research programs would also be freed up to build on that basic map in accord with their own needs (viz., specific interests, purposes, values, and social commitments that shape different forms of clinical practice.)

Third, research paradigms should be developed that incorporate the various ideas identified in our discussion of the case studies, including novel approaches to sampling, a background of typical functioning and individual variation, multivariate functional profiles that are sufficiently broad and balanced, and model-based research designs that focus on neurocognitive architecture (e.g., neurocognitive circuitry, the landscape of connectivity within which circuitry is realized, etc.) And, such paradigms should be extended in ways that are further responsive to the features of the domain of mental illness: model-based research designs that allow inclusion of the broad contextual (neural/psychological) processes in which function-based circuits are embedded, extensive study of sources of individual and group differences (prior to normative evaluation), utilization of a broad range of relevant sciences so as not to privilege genetics and neuroscience (while granting their importance as appropriate), and appropriate attention to personal perspective and agency, social and cultural contexts, higher-order social processes, relational and non-relational problems. These sorts of investigation will expand the conceptual and foundational adequacy of mental illness research and, thereby, enhance its promise for empirical adequacy.

These lessons and suggestions represent an alternative pathway for research concerning mental illness that arguably should supersede the still prevalent DSM-based approach. Currently, a crisis exists in mental illness research: traditional psychiatric research practice exhibits profound problems while at the same time this practice and the DSM framework on which it is based are deeply entrenched (Poland in press; Poland et al. 1994) Recent developments in mental illness research, of the sort discussed in this chapter, suggest that the entrenchment of the DSM framework, at least with respect to research practice, is beginning to become dislodged. This is good news. However, currently ongoing research efforts also reveal how difficult it is for researchers to eliminate the conceptual hold of the DSM framework (including the category scheme and various accompanying commitments) entirely. The lessons outlined here may assist in further breaking this hold to some extent.

Acknowledgments

Thanks to Michael Frank and Thomas Wiecki for helpful conversations concerning the issues discussed in this chapter.

References

American Psychiatric Association (1980). *Diagnostic and Statistical Manual of Mental Disorders, Third Edition*. Washington, DC: American Psychiatric Association.

American Psychiatric Association (2000). *Diagnostic and Statistical Manual of Mental Disorders, Fourth Edition, Text Revision*. Washington, DC: American Psychiatric Association.

Andreasen, N. C. (2007). The DSM and the death of phenomenology in America. *Schizophrenia Bulletin*, *33*(1), 108–12.

Andrews, G., Goldberg, D. P., Krueger, R. F., Carpenter, W. T., Hyman, S. E., Sachdev, P., *et al.* (2009). Exploring the feasibility of a metastructure for DSM-V and ICD-11: Could it improve utility and validity? *Psychological Medicine*, *39*(12), 1993–2000.

Badre, D. (2011). Defining an ontology of cognitive control requires attention to component interactions. *Topics in Cognitive Science*, *3*, 217–21.

Barkley, R. (1997). Behavioral inhibition, sustained attention, and executive functions: Constructing a unifying theory of ADHD. *Psychological Bulletin*, *121*, 65–94.

Bernstein, C. (2011). Metastructure in DSM-5 process. *Psychiatric News*, *46* (5), 7.

Blashfield, R. (1984). *The Classification of Psychopathology*. New York, NY: Plenum Press.

Buckholtz, J. and Meyer-Lindenberg, A. (2012). Psychopathology and the human connectome: Toward a transdiagnostic model of risk for mental illness. *Neuron*, *74*, 990–1004.

Cuthbert, B. and Insel, T. (2010). Classification issues in women's mental health: Clinical utility and etiological mechanisms. *Archive of Women's Mental Health*, *13*, 57–9.

Durston, S., van Belle, J., and de Zeeuw, P. (2011). Differentiating frontostriatal and fronto-cerebellar circuits in attention-deficit hyperactivity disorder. *Biological Psychiatry*, *69*, 1178–84.

Fair, D., Bathula, D., Nikolas, M., and Nigg, J. (2012). Distinct neuropsychological subgroups in typically developing youth inform heterogeneity in children with ADHD. *Proceedings of the National Academy of Sciences of the United States of America*, *109*(17), 6769–74.

Frances, A. (2010). Rating scales: DSM5 bites off far more than it can chew. *Psychiatric Times*, May 7.

Heinrichs, R. W. (2001). *In Search of Madness*. New York, NY: Oxford University Press.

Hyman, S. (2010). The diagnosis of mental disorders: The problem of reification. *Annual Review of Clinical Psychology*, *6*, 155–79.

Insel, T. and Cuthbert, B. (2010). Research domain criteria (RDoC): Toward a new classification framework for research on mental disorders. *American Journal of Psychiatry*, *167*(7), 748–50.

Insel, T., Cuthbert, B., Garvey, M., Heinssen, R., Pine, D. S., Quinn, K., *et al.* (2010). Research domain criteria (RDoC): Toward a new classification framework for research on mental disorders. *American Journal of Psychiatry*, *167*(7), 748–51.

Kendell, R. and Jablensky, A. (2003). Distinguishing between the validity and utility of psychiatric diagnoses. *American Journal of Psychiatry*, *160*(1), 4–12.

Kendler, K., Kupfer, D., Narrow, W., Phillips, K., and Fawcett, J. (2009). *Guidelines for Making Changes to DSM-V*. [Online.] (Revised October 21, 2009.) Available at: <http://www.dsm5. org/ProgressReports/Documents/Guidelines-for-Making-Changes-to-DSM_1.pdf>.

Kirk, S. and Kutchins, H. (1992). *The Selling of DSM: The Rhetoric of Science in Psychiatry*. New Brunswick, NJ: Aldine de Gruyter.

Klerman, G. (1978). The evolution of a scientific nosology. In J. Shershow (Ed.), *Schizophrenia: Research and Practice*, pp. 99–121. Cambridge, MA: Harvard University Press.

National Institute of Mental Health (2011). *NIMH Research Domain Criteria (RDoC)*. [Online.] Available at: <http://www.nimh.nih.gov/research-funding/rdoc/nimh-research-domain-criteria-rdoc.shtml>.

Poland, J. (2001). Review of *DSV-IV Sourcebook, Volume 1. Metapsychology, Spring*. Available at: <http://metapsychology.mentalhelp.net/poc/view_doc.php?type=book&id=557>.

Poland, J. (2002). Review of *DSV-IV Sourcebook, Volume 2. Metapsychology, Spring*. Available at: <http://metapsychology.mentalhelp.net/poc/view_doc.php?type=book&id=996&cn=394>.

Poland, J. (in press). Deeply rooted sources of error and bias in psychiatric classification. In H. Kincaid and J. Sullivan (Eds), *Psychiatric Classification and Natural Kinds*. Cambridge, MA: The MIT Press.

Poland, J., Von Eckardt, B., and Spaulding, W. (1994). Problems with the DSM approach to classifying psychopathology. In G. Graham and G. L. Stephens (Eds), *Philosophical Psychopathology*, pp. 235–260. Cambridge, MA: The MIT Press.

Regier, D., Narrow, W., Kuhl, E., and Kupfer, D. (2009). The conceptual development of DSM-V. *American Journal of Psychiatry*, 166(6), 645–50.

Rounsaville, B., Alarcón, R., Andrews, G., Jackson, J., Kendell, R., and Kendler, K. (2002). Basic nomenclature issues for DSM-V. In D. Kupfer, M. First, and D. Regier (Eds), *A Research Agenda for DSM-V*, pp. 1–29. Washington, DC: American Psychiatric Association Press.

Spaulding, W., Sullivan, M., and Poland, J. (2003). *Treatment and Rehabilitation of Severe Mental Illness*. New York, NY: Guilford Press.

Von Eckardt, B. (1993). *What Is Cognitive Science?* Cambridge, MA: The MIT Press.

CHAPTER 45

VALUES IN PSYCHIATRIC DIAGNOSIS AND CLASSIFICATION

JOHN Z. SADLER

INTRODUCTION

The philosophical analysis of values in psychiatric diagnosis and classification serves as an apt entry point into the philosophy of psychiatry because, as will be described in this chapter, virtually every major division of academic philosophy (epistemology, ontology, aesthetics, ethics, etc.) offers a path into value considerations in this psychiatric domain. When the contemporary consideration of the philosophy of values in psychiatric diagnosis/classification was introduced by K. W. M. Fulford in the 1980s, the field of Anglo-American psychiatry was still operating within a de facto positivist/logical-empiricist ideology, where psychiatric categories were considered objective, value-neutral concepts which were aimed toward an ideal of correspondence mapping onto brain structure and function (see Faust and Miner 1986; Gorenstein 1992; Grove et al. 1991; Margolis 1994; Robins and Barrett 1989; Sadler 2005; Schwartz and Wiggins 1986). In the scholarship following Fulford's lead in the ensuing two decades, not only has philosophical understanding of the value-content of diagnosis and classification expanded, the recognition of the value-ladenness of psychiatric categories and the processes in developing them has increasingly come to be accepted by the psychiatric mainstream (Frances 1994; Frances et al. 1991, 1995; Fulford 2002; Fulford et al. 2005; Spitzer 2001).

This chapter is organized into four main sections. The first section defines and introduces core concepts such as values, psychiatric diagnosis and classification, and their significance to a philosophy of psychiatry. The second section reviews some of the core philosophical contributions to the study of values in psychiatric diagnosis and classification. The third section then presents some examples of the kinds of value considerations that manifest in this area of psychiatry, as well as considering a few examples of the current literature and debate in the field. The chapter concludes with conclusions and a discussion of questions and areas worthy of further discussion and analysis.

WHAT ARE VALUES?

A value is a particular property of things, that is, a predicate. Drawing from Hilary Putnam (1981, 1990a, 1990b), values-as-predicates present particular logical properties. In addition to the aforementioned aspect of value as a property, a value is a kind of judgment, opinion, or disposition. As a kind of disposition, values are linked to human action—are "action-guiding." When I hear a piece of music that I like, I want to hear it again. If I hate another piece of music, I may avoid it in the future. In either the positive or negative evaluation, action is guided. Because the properties (symptoms, signs) of illness are built upon the assumption that illness is something to be avoided, the values typically associated with descriptions of mental illness involve negative values—concepts like "dysfunction," "incapacity," "suffering," and the like. If I am suffering it is (usually) a negatively-valued state of affairs that I would like to avoid, reverse, or otherwise get rid of. Finally, values also have a social function, in that we typically praise or blame objects that embody this or that value. If John acts unethically, I will appraise his behavior as blameworthy. The operative concept of "value" can be summarized here as "values are attitudes or dispositions which are action-guiding and subject to praise or blame" (Sadler 1997, 2005).

With a little reflection, one can see that any sentence's meaning—including diagnostic criteria for a mental disorder, or a principle used in developing a classification of mental disorders—can be scrutinized for these action-guiding, blameworthy/praiseworthy features, revealing the value-content of the sentence (Sadler 1997, 2005).

Why be concerned with psychiatric diagnosis/classification?

For those philosophers who are not familiar with contemporary psychiatric diagnostic classification of mental disorders, today two prevailing systems are used in educational, clinical, administrative, and research settings: the World Health Organization's International Classification of Disease—Clinical Modification for Mental and Behavioural Disorders (ICD-10; World Health Organization 1992; see also <http://www.cms.gov/Medicare/Coding/ICD10/2013-ICD-10-CM-and-GEMs.html>) and the American Psychiatric Association's (APA's) *Diagnostic and Statistical Manual of Mental Disorders, Fourth Edition, Text Revision* (DSM-IV-TR; APA 2000). These two manuals are intended to provide a systematic and comprehensive set of diagnostic categories for mental health professionals worldwide; the ICD has the international imprimatur of the World Health Organization, while the DSM is popular worldwide as it is viewed as the representing the cutting-edge of the field (Frances et al. 1995). The importance of these diagnostic manuals stems from their widespread use in clinical settings, and the spread of their nomenclature into popular culture as well as the popular imagination. The DSM and ICD frame the concepts of mental illness for the world, and in this capacity function as de facto public policy about mental disorders, through setting the conceptual-linguistic terms of the policy discussion (Sadler 2002, 2005).

For reasons that space does not permit me to recount, the DSMs have, much more than the ICD, been controversial in their ambitions and delivery, and have often served as anchor points for many social, moral, and philosophical criticisms of psychiatry in general (Beutler and Malik 2002; Bracken and Thomas 2005; Caplan 1995; Cooper 2007; Gaines 1992; Horwitz 2002; Kirk and Kutchins 1992; Kutchins and Kirk 1997; Murphy 2005; Radden 1994, 1996; Sadler 2002, 2005; Sadler et al. 1994; Zachar 2000). Rather than discussing these issues here, I will simply mention a few of the more prominent points of controversy, and use later sections to show how an analysis of the values in these manuals can shed light on the controversies. In no particular order of importance, and with some sample references included:

1. Blurring of ordinary human foibles and psychopathology (Horwitz 2002; Horwitz and Wakefield 2007; Lane 2008). In more philosophical terms, these issues revolve around the appropriateness of the normative judgments made through psychiatric diagnosis.
2. Medicalization, or the transforming of human problems into medical problems (Conrad 2007; Sadler et al. 2009). This issue has many ramifications, including criticisms of the proliferation of DSM categories (Horwitz 2002; Kirk and Kutchins 1992; Kutchins and Kirk 1997), undue influence of the pharmaceutical industry on DSM architects (Cosgrove and Krimsky 2012; Cosgrove et al. 2006), medical imperialism, or the marginalizing of non-medical accounts of psychopathology (Bergin 1991; Beutler and Malik 2002; Schacht and Nathan 1977), and ethnocentrism—biomedical reformulations of social deviance (Davis 1996, 1998; Gaines 1992).
3. Metaphysical objections. This group of criticisms also casts a wide net, including various attributions of reductionism, including the DSMs' marginalizing of narrative understandings of mental illness (Sadler 2005), a focus on psychopathology as residing "in" the individual, as opposed to larger family/social contexts (First 2006b; Kaslow 1993, 1996), gender bias (Broverman and Broverman 1970; Broverman et al. 1972; Caplan 1995) or the lack of a developmental perspective in understanding psychopathology (Achenbach 1995; Bemporad and Schwab 1986; Jensen et al. 2006).
4. Attributions of an overly politicized DSM process. The nature of mental disorder, dealing as it does with thoughts and behaviors, is prone to political meanings, which correspondingly confounds efforts to describe and classify mental disorder (Sadler 2002, 2005). Since the early 1960s the political contents of psychiatry have been debated, including political values in the DSMs (Sadler 2002, 2005; Schacht 1985a, 1985b; Spitzer 1981; Szasz 1960, 1961) and accusations of jockeying for dominance in the mental health field (Caplan 1995).
5. Critiques of DSM science. The quality of DSM science, or lack of it, for DSM categories has been a recurrent theme in the literature. Good summaries are included in Beutler and Malik (2002), Cooper (2007), Hyman (2002, 2007), Murphy (2005), Sadler (2002, 2005), and Zachar (2000).

Brief overview of this chapter

The next section sketches the philosophical context for considerations of values in psychiatric diagnostic classification. I review an historical zeitgeist in Western psychiatry, of logical empiricism as applied to the diagnostic classification of mental disorders. I then briefly consider Fulford's adaptation of the value theory of R. M. Hare and J. Austin's ordinary language philosophy, which proved to be influential in developing analytical-philosophy approaches to values in psychopathology. This material leads to Sadler's elaboration of a method for identifying values in psychiatric discourse. In the following (third) section, this method is elaborated with some examples from the DSM literature. The concluding section considers a few of the many unexplored opportunities for the analysis of value in psychiatric diagnostic classification.

Philosophical Value Theory in Understanding Diagnostic/Nosological Values

Background

Mid-twentieth-century psychiatry in the West was characterized by many transitions, not the least of which was a rethinking of the scientific basis for psychiatry (Healy 1997, 2002; Wallace 1994). The alienation of psychiatry from medicine as a whole was blamed on the influx of psychoanalytic thought in the post-World War II era, and the limitations of this approach for the treatment of serious mental illness, over time, bred discontent in academic psychiatry. By the dawn of the psychopharmacology era in the 1950s, Western psychiatrists were looking for a more robust scientific basis for their field, and like much of the science of the time, found (or more likely, happened upon) the logical empiricist thought that had gained traction in the then-contemporary philosophy of science. The logical empiricist theory of science, emphasizing an ideal of value-free theory, a minimum of inference, the articulation and promulgation of the hypothetico-deductive method, and strict theoretical logics (Proctor 1991; Salmon 1989) was perhaps exemplified best by Carl G. Hempel's explication of logical empiricism in the diagnostic classification of psychopathology in 1965 (Hempel 1965; Sadler et al. 1994). For historical reasons (see, for instance, Wallace 1994), by the 1980s a significant gap had emerged in Western psychiatric theory, where the combined factors of progressive social change and the suspicion of psychiatric authority, disappointment over the limited successes of psychopharmacology, and a theory gap in clinical science and clinical practice (from the marginalizing of psychoanalysis) led to an intellectual setting responsive to a renaissance for philosophy in psychiatry. Philosophy offered a set of methods, conceptual tools, and insights that at once could be critical and rigorous, while still maintaining a pro-science, pro-patient, pro-psychiatry, and pro-theory stance for the field, offering new substance for a field that had become impoverished of theory (Wallace et al. 1997).

Fulford on value terms

A formative figure in the philosophy of psychiatry, K. W. M. (Bill) Fulford's work, beginning in the late 1980s, provided key theoretical elements in deepening the appreciation of, and academic engagement with, the manifestations of values in psychiatric discourse, and particularly, diagnostic discourse. Fulford's work laid out key logical properties of value terms, examining key concepts in psychiatry and medicine like "disease," "dysfunction," "illness," and the like, and sketching out their logical structures in practical use by clinicians (Fulford 1989, 1991, 1994, 1999, 2001, 2002a, 2002b). Through this analysis, he provided the key insight that some kinds of value judgments implicit in medical concepts could approximate facts in their uniform social appraisals (e.g., most everyone agrees that having a broken leg is bad for you), while other kinds of value judgments, especially many of those in psychiatry, lack the uniform social appraisals typical of general medicine (e.g., some aspects of manic euphoria and increased energy are desirable for some, problematic for others). Through these insights Fulford set the stage for a collaborative, rigorous discourse among philosophers and psychiatrists to consider and debate the practical, ethical, and scientific importance of various values in the mental health field.

Sadler on value heuristics and values analysis

The American psychiatrist John Z. Sadler had come to know Bill Fulford in the late 1980s through the transcontinental founding of the journal *Philosophy, Psychiatry, & Psychology*. Sadler, who had been up to that time steeped in the continental existential/phenomenological tradition, was intrigued by Fulford's work on the "logic of value terms." Sadler's work with Osborne Wiggins and Michael Alan Schwartz on *Philosophical Perspectives on Psychiatric Diagnostic Classification* (Sadler et al. 1994) had generated a fascination with the philosophical issues in diagnosis and classification of psychopathology. Sadler, however, was troubled by the lack of a philosophical method to discover or excavate values in discourses. He wanted to find out how one could identify values in human discourse, and the philosophy of the time had only limited theory in this regard. Sadler's interest in these issues led to philosophical work to develop a method for identifying values in discourses. At the time, the identification of values in bioethics and philosophy of medicine was simply intuited and methodologically implicit; Sadler was concerned that reliance on intuition alone would not make for a rigorous analysis of how values "operated" in complex discourses such as those surrounding the DSMs. Fulford's work on value terms offered a crystallizing insight: that values were concepts whose meaning could illuminate disagreements, ambiguities, and controversies, but this work was limited by the lack of a systematic approach to identifying values in discourses. What was needed was a heuristically-useful definition of "value" that could be applied to the discourses of psychiatric diagnosis, or, for that matter, any other discourse. By using the Austinian/Wittgensteinian methods of examining how words are used in discourses, Sadler could then examine texts for how terms/concepts/words and more complex semantics in DSM discourse would tally up against a heuristic definition of value (as action-guiding and praise/blameworthy).

Sadler discovered his heuristic definition of value through Harvard logician Hilary Putnam's work on ethics and value theory (Putnam 1981, 1990a, 1990b). Putnam argued that values were descriptors or conditions which (a) were action-guiding and (b) were subject to praise or blame (Sadler 1997). As action guides, values were not definitive; but they did have some causal or motivating power. As "descriptors," values often describe other things or states of affairs, for example: a *threatening* hallucination, or an *ineffectual* committee meeting. Importantly, value terms could be "thin," a concept whose meaning is narrowly evaluative (like *good* or *worst*), as well as "thick," an evaluative concept intertwined with factually-descriptive meaning, as in the aforementioned *threatening* or *ineffectual*. Including conditions as values is important because the semantic meaning of a term or sentence may not be reflected by the independent lexical meaning of any of the sentence's terms. This aspect reveals the Austinian influence (Austin 1962) of the importance of illocutionary meaning in sentences—that is, the meaning of the sentence is only revealed by an analysis of the context of use. In Sadler's work, he uses the example "John will do anything to get a grant" as an example. Here there is no Fulfordian value term, thick or thin. However, in the conventional use of this sentence, the speaker is condemning John as unethical or ruthless in conduct (Sadler 1997, 2005). Briefly put, the values of discourses could be revealed through an analysis of semantics and pragmatics that denoted the action-guiding and praise/blame-worthy element of meaning.

This heuristic definition of value could then be applied to any sentence or discourse to evaluate the value(s) that are embodied in the discourse. Sadler went on to describe various manifestations of values in discourses—value "commitments," "entailments," and "consequences," which need not concern us here in this brief chapter, but more meticulous arguments are found in the original publications (Sadler 1997, 2005). What is of keen interest for the analysis of values in discourses is Sadler's "descriptive dimension" of values, which plots out the kinds of values one encounters in discourses against the major branches of philosophy: e.g., aesthetic values, epistemic values, ethical values, ontological values, and pragmatic values. These dimensions of value semantics are not monolithic, but rather fluid and multivalent. For example, *clarity*, depending on the context of usage, can be simultaneously an aesthetic, practical, and epistemic value: "Professor Jones was moved by the *clarity* of his student's elaboration of the use of philosophical methods on the problem of involuntary psychiatric treatment." Table 45.1 describes each dimension, its domain, and sample value terms. In the next section, each of these dimensions will be applied to sample issues in psychiatric diagnostic classification.

Some Values in Diagnosis

and Classification

As noted earlier, these descriptive kinds of values may disclose aspects of evaluative meaning, and often, perhaps usually, overlap with other descriptive value types in nosological discourse. So in the examples to follow, some will demonstrate best examples of singular values behind psychiatric diagnosis/classification, while others will exemplify combinations of value types. For detailed philosophical discussions of these methods, see Sadler (1997, 2005).

An additional note should also clarify what aspects of diagnostic classification can be addressed through this method. The most obvious places to look for value commitments or entailments are the categories and diagnostic criteria themselves. Various kinds of evaluations emerge when considering the values underlying diagnostic categories and diagnostic criteria. A second place to look is in the processes in developing the diagnostic classification. In Sadler's *Values and Psychiatric Diagnosis* (2005) an extensive set of considerations

Table 45.1 Sadler's dimensions of value: domain and sample value terms

Dimension	Domain	Sample value terms
Aesthetic values	Form and beauty	*Beautiful, elegant, magisterial*
Epistemic values	Knowledge claims	*Lucid, coherence, precision, simplicity*
Ethical values	"The good," morality, virtue	*Autonomy, discretion, sordid, courage*
Ontological values	Human nature; being; existence	*Reification, reductionism, dread*
Pragmatic values	Utility; usefulness	*Efficient, powerful, awkward*

Adapted from Sadler (1997, 2005).

of the values behind the choices made in building the DSMs are presented in detail. These kinds of values begin with considerations of scientific and clinical practice-related values and then extend into the political, cultural, and even religious values that provide the social background "priorities" for constructing the DSMs or ICDs. From this standpoint the utility of values analysis for historical studies is evident.

In these examples, what becomes evident is the potential for value conflict in psychiatric discourse about diagnosis and classification—and the elements of such value conflict teased apart by values analysis. Often the values in conflict are apparent to participants in the discourse, though perhaps too often the value commitments and entailments involved in the dispute are presupposed or buried in cultural-ontological assumptions. By identifying ontological values, which are often the most deeply presupposed and "invisible," clarification and the opportunity for resolution of the value conflict becomes possible.

Aesthetic values

Starting with perhaps the most infrequent type of value encountered in DSM-related discourse, aesthetic values are likely among the most commonly presupposed of the value commitments and entailments found in said discourse. Additionally, the place where aesthetic values might play a prominent role is least likely to be brought to public attention. That place is in the design, editing, and preparation of the diagnostic manual. While concerns for stylistic *clarity* and *elegance* of layout and prose are hopefully present in the preparation of diagnostic criteria, to the degree that they do, they introduce aesthetic considerations to the preparation and composition of the DSM manuals. The DSM-IV was open about its interest in providing a "helpful" manual for clinical practice (APA 2000, p. xxiii), but while *helpfulness* in this context is undoubtedly a pragmatic value, one can argue where *elegant* and *lucid* prose (in the aesthetic sense) leaves off and *helpful* prose begins. From this perspective, the fusion of aesthetic values and pragmatic values is analogous to the fusion of *functional utility* and the *pleasing curves* of contemporary industrial design. Few would argue that *clunky, stilted* prose contributes to *helpfulness*! In regard to the deepness of presupposition with aesthetic values, we can understand this because of the habit of experienced authors in editing for elegance, ease of reading, and clarity of style. The adaptive and aesthetic values of habits long-ago inculcated are not evident to ordinary reflection, yet operate as action guides nonetheless, and perhaps, even more powerfully compared to a premeditated embrace of a particular value.

A consideration of aesthetic values in framing diagnostic concepts and criteria was offered in a 2002 paper by David Veale and Christina Lambrou. They discuss DSM-IV Body Dysmorphic Disorder (BDD) as reflecting an exaggerated aesthetic sense in patients with this condition. BDD is a condition where the patient has excessive, and impairing, preoccupation with defects in personal appearance. BDD is a bane for cosmetic plastic surgeons because the patient is never satisfied with the aesthetic results of their surgery. The authors hypothesize and provide some supportive evidence that BDD is a combination of an enhanced aesthetic sensibility and emotional tenor, combined with a distorted body image reminiscent of Anorexia Nervosa.

Epistemic values

Epistemic values are values involved in knowledge claims or implemented in theories of knowledge. As such we might expect epistemic values to be extensively explored in the philosophy of science, but this was not the case until well into the latter half of the twentieth century. Thomas Kuhn offered a groundbreaking discussion of values as involved in scientific theory choice. In his 1977 paper "Objectivity, value judgment, and theory choice," set in an era when logical empiricism's dominance was fading, Kuhn considered the difficulties in providing a rational basis for scientists to select one competing scientific theory over another. No mathematical formulae or stepwise logic could dictate scientists' choice of one theory over another, a realization that led Kuhn to reconsider the social influence of like-minded scientific communities in the second edition of *The Structure of Scientific Revolutions* (Kuhn 1979). The outcry of his colleagues, along with their accusations of Kuhn advocating a "mob psychology," was the motivation for Kuhn to explore the role of values in scientific theory choice. The steps to his argument cannot be duplicated here, but suffice to say Kuhn concluded that differential investment in various properties of theories, like *simplicity, prediction, coherence,* and *instrumental efficacy* were what guided (not determined) scientists' theory choices. Such properties Kuhn identified as values.

In a 1996 paper describing epistemic values in the context of psychiatric nosological disputes about DSM-IV personality disorders, Sadler analyzed a set of values that came to bear upon the debate over whether personality psychopathology should be conceptualized as a category (an either-or entity with more-or-less crisp boundaries) which was the traditional DSM approach. Diagnostic criteria using the categorical approach could either be met, or not, making diagnostic judgment a binary. In contrast, the dimensional approach to personality diagnosis plotted personality disorders at extremes of continuously variable traits which all people possess in greater or lesser degree. In using his methods of values analysis, Sadler found textual evidence in this debate's literature for a variety of terms which evaluate the quality of knowledge—epistemic values—terms such as *coherence, consistency, comprehensiveness, fecundity, simplicity, instrumental efficacy, originality, relevance,* and *precision.* In his analysis, Sadler noted that some epistemic values were presented as more characteristic of one theoretical approach (for example, dimensional diagnosis was more *consistent*), while the same (dimensional) approach would falter when considered against other epistemic values (for example, the dimensional approach's *clinical utility*, its user-friendliness for practicing clinicians, could be another variety of *instrumental efficacy*). These kinds of epistemic value conflicts could then be considered against more broad practical, theoretical, and social interests or values. For example, at the time, the DSMs' prevailing value was that the diagnostic classification system be useful for clinical practice. In the case of DSM-IV, the categorical approach prevailed largely because of the importance of instrumental efficacy for clinical diagnosis. Today, Michael First has trumpeted the crucial importance of "clinical utility" in the DSMs (First 2005a, 2005b, 2006a). Of course, considerations of clinical utility also blend into the domain of pragmatic values to be discussed later.

Interestingly, the issue of categorical versus dimensional personality diagnosis is still being debated for the upcoming DSM-5, with the DSM-5 Personality Disorders work group promulgating a complex hybrid system utilizing elements of categories and dimensions. This step is out of respect for the more extensive scientific evidence for personality dimensions, while recognizing the need for clinical utility. These proposals (which are yet to be finalized for DSM-5) were prompted by the diagnostic problem of comorbidity of personality disorder categories (the same individual meeting criteria for multiple personality disorder categories) in prior, DSM-IV era, clinical research (see <http://www.dsm5.org/PROPOSEDREVISIONS/Pages/PersonalityandPersonalityDisorders.aspx>, accessed July 9, 2012).

Today's DSM-5 controversy involves criticism of the unruly complexity of the draft personality diagnostic structures, undermining the epistemic virtue of *simplicity* and *instrumental efficacy* which had been prevailing values for DSM-IV, in an effort to improve the diagnostic comorbidity problem (see Frances 2010; Skodol et al. 2011).

A perhaps more vivid and ongoing DSM-5 debate concerning epistemic values addresses novel approaches to the science of the DSM introduced by the DSM-5 Task Force. A debate initiated by Robert Spitzer, past Chair of the DSM-III Task Force, accused the DSM-5 Task Force of non-transparency and a closed scientific process because of new confidentiality agreements that DSM-5 work group members were required to sign (Spitzer 2008). Alarcón (2009) provides an overview, and the extensive debate is documented online in the *Psychiatric Times* website and blog (<http://www.psychiatrictimes.com>). The DSM-5 Task Force, at the lead of Michael First, developed the first online documentation system for DSM development, enabling the DSM-5 leaders to make a claim toward the "most open" DSM process ever. However, what has resulted from the combined silence of DSM committees through the confidentiality agreement, and the APA-controlled content on the <http://www.DSM-5.org> website, has been a shift in the DSM debate away the professional/scientific journals and into the online environment. What this means for the epistemic values of *openness* to peer criticism, *transparency* of data, *data-sharing*, and related social-epistemic values in the scientific process (Longino 1990) remains to be seen.

Ethical and moral values

Like other descriptive types of values, ethical and moral values find their way into the discourse in three prevailing domains: (1) around the process of developing diagnostic classifications, (2) the terms of diagnostic criteria, and (3) the use of the diagnostic system. Of paradigmatic interest in the latter is use of the DSM outside of Western biomedical-native settings (e.g., in endemic traditional cultures) (Alarcon et al. 2009). In spite of the rich academic opportunities presented by culturally-different communities, philosophical deliberation upon the cross-cultural ethics of developing psychiatric diagnostic classification systems has been, perhaps surprisingly, a neglected area in the philosophical scholarship around values in psychiatric diagnosis and classification. If this domain of inquiry could be summarized by a single question—"What makes up a morally-justifiable process for classifying mental disorders for cross-cultural use?"—then the answers in the literature are rather limited, and typically commingled about concerns for epistemic values (What makes for a good science of psychiatry?) and pragmatic values (What makes for greater utility of diagnosis in clinical practice?).

Sadler (2002, 2005) provides for some discussion in this domain, noting the moral elements in the "politics" of DSM development, relevant to domain 1, as well as exploring in some detail the ethics of promulgating mental disorder categories derived from Western normative cultural assumptions for health and pathology (see especially his 2005), relevant to domain 3. These latter normative assumptions about health are also situated in ontological values (see later), which in turn are situated within the larger cosmology of the resident culture.

According to Sadler, the core difficulty in promulgating DSM/Western diagnostic categories in other cultures is the problem of cross-cultural validity. Cross cultural validity is the degree to which a diagnostic category, developed within culture A, applies accurately, fairly, and completely to individuals within cultures B, C, D, and so on. What makes cross-cultural validity a tough problem for nosologists is the potential differences in judgments about normativity of behavior, as well as the translation of one pathological concept into terms that make sense to the "recipient" culture with their variant cosmologies and ontological assumptions (see also Gaines 1992). A full discussion of cross-cultural validity and its components is far beyond the space limitations of this short chapter, but is reviewed in Kleinman et al. (1996) and Sadler (2005). For the purposes of this section on ethical/moral values in classification, some discussion about the ethics of the use of DSM categories in non-Western, traditional cultures will illuminate the ethical values embedded in diagnostic process.

Perhaps the core Western biomedical assumption underlying use of DSM categories in other cultures is the idea that DSM mental disorders converge upon a *universal* and core pathological process, the clinical presentation of which is only elaborated by cultural differences between peoples, while the core disorder remains *essential*. This assumption of disorder universalism and essentialism can provide for a moral hubris that DSM categories are not only harmless, but helpful to non-Western traditional cultures. So for Sadler (2005) the first step in an ethics of DSM use in other cultures is a questioning of disorder *essentialism* and *universalism*, a recognition of the limitations of DSM categories in cross-cultural settings, and the potential dangers of using those categories in such settings. In their function as advisors to DSM-IV, Kleinman and colleagues (1996) addressed a number of cautionary suggestions regarding use of DSM categories in other cultural settings. These included more research on use of DSM categories and criteria in different ethnic and cultural groups, a recognition of cultural "idioms of distress" (culturally-specific health and distress complaints), the significance of dissociation phenomena across cultures, and appropriate use of language interpreters, to name only a few of this group's important suggestions.

The problem of cross-cultural validity plays out in settings where symptoms of Western mental disorder are described by the endemic culture as responses to moral wrongdoing, spiritual or religious transitions, or supernatural phenomena. Intervening with Western diagnosis and treatment may have adverse and often unforeseeable consequences (Gaines 1992; Kleinman 1996).

Among the core ethical dangers in using DSM categories in other cultures is the potential for naively labeling culturally-normative behavior as pathological, and then imposing potentially socially-disruptive Western treatments into an otherwise stable, but traditional, social network. Moreover, diagnosing a patient, at least in Western biomedical settings, implies an obligation to offer treatment. In traditional, developing countries settings, DSM-relevant treatments may not, and likely are not, available on any sustained basis, a problem which has been raised by trend toward performing clinical trials by Western pharmaceutical companies in developing countries, where a "necessary" treatment become unavailable for the study population once the clinical trial ends (Petryna 2007).

However, ethical and (particularly) moral values often define the kinds of evaluations specific to DSM categories and diagnostic criteria. Frankena (1973) made an early distinction between moral (relating to the good and wrongfulness) and non-moral (other kinds of) values. That is to say, some of the evaluations made in diagnostic categories and criteria are moral in meaning rather than "medical"; between moral value judgments and non-moral value judgments. For instance, consider "formal thought disorder," a particular kind of disorganized thinking characteristic of people with schizophrenia. What is undesirable about having a formal thought disorder is not that it is morally offensive, but that it compromises a person's ability to process their interactions with the world accurately. In this sense, formal thought disorder is an impairment leading to faulty knowledge and therefore an epistemic impairment. However, consider the case of a patient with pedophilia, who has erotic arousal to children and engages in molesting behavior. Based upon prevailing cultural norms in the United States, "pedophilia" then represents, at least in part, a moral failing, and the evaluation of pedophilic behavior and experience as wrongful makes the diagnostic construct pedophilia one that is *morally* value-laden (Sadler 2008; for a more detailed discussion see Sadler, Chapter 29, this volume).

So some categories of mental disorder, by the nature of the kind of evaluations they make (describing this or that aspect of experience and behavior as disordered), can be laden with moral value-judgments of the kind Frankena described. In his 2005 elaboration of this issue, Sadler proposed the "Moral Wrongfulness Test" (MWT) as an analytic tool in identifying psychiatric categories/criteria as potentially morally value-laden (Sadler 2005, pp. 213–224). The MWT poses a question to diagnostic criteria: "Would a substantial portion of people of this culture, when considering the behavior or experience described in this criterion, conclude that the behavior or experience is 'morally wrong?'" (p. 213). The potential answers in response to the MWT may be culturally relative, and the test is intended to provoke careful conceptual consideration about whether such a moral value-judgment is warranted or justifiable.

The relative importance of, weight of, and ethical justification for moral evaluations in categories of personality disorder has captured interest in the philosophy of psychiatry through a series of publications by Louis Charland (2006, 2010), Peter Zachar and Nancy Potter (2010a, 2010b, Potter 2009), Zachar and Krueger (Chapter 52, this volume), Hanna Pickard and Steve Pearce (2009), Pickard (Chapter 66, this volume), and Sadler (2009, in press, Chapter 29, this volume). The philosophical interest in these disorders has centered around the DSM "Cluster B" personality disorders, including Antisocial Personality Disorder, Narcissistic Personality Disorder, and Borderline Personality Disorder (American Psychiatric Association 2000) These authors wrestle with the issue of the moral content of personality disorders in theory and in practice. How much, if any, moral content is justifiable in diagnostic concepts that are intended for clinical use? Do disturbances in moral conduct qualify as a component of, or even the definition of, mental disorders? If so, what are the practical and ethical ramifications of providing medical treatment with its own moral "agenda" (intentional or accidental)? These questions are defining for psychiatry as a moral practice, as well as of complex social significance. The focus of this discussion has considered the legitimacy of these personality disorders as diagnostic categories, as well as considered the moral significance of complex "thick" value terms such as *impulsivity* used in diagnostic criteria (Potter 2009).

Ontological values

Simultaneously the most obscure and among the most determinative of values at work in psychiatric diagnosis and classification, some elaboration of the meaning of "ontological values" is warranted before giving examples. Consider ontological values as those values which are connected to the veneration, intentional or presupposed, of particular viewpoints of "the way things are"—the nature of being and existence; or what constitutes "human nature." While ontological values can manifest in several ways (see Sadler 2005 for more detail), the most common manifestation of ontological values is through their "entailments"—presuppositions about the nature of being that are expressed in discourses indirectly through being encumbered, tied-up with, or necessarily associated with something—in the sphere of this discussion, that something being mental disorders.

The best way to understand entailed ontological values is through example. With the DSMs' medical identity, a certain set of assumptions can be identified as DSM categories being presented as "disorders" and inevitably likened to physical diseases like pneumonia or myocardial infarction. When Western physicians formulate disease concepts, certain assumptions come into play. Prominent among these is that (Western, biomedical) diseases are natural phenomena, subject to the laws of Nature and having an identity as a manifestation of Nature. In the case of human pneumonia, that natural manifestation is the accumulation of bacteria and a bodily inflammatory response in a particular region of the lung, leading to fever, malaise, cough, and perhaps shortness of breath. (Contrast the metaphysical standpoint of pneumonia as a punishment from God for one's sins, or the result of a hex placed upon the patient by a witch.) Sadler dubbed this particular "entailed ontological value" as "disease naturalism" (2005, pp. 92–94) and made a case that the DSMs presuppose disease naturalism in building their categories of disorder. What makes disease naturalism evaluational is that it is a preferred and presupposed way of viewing the world—hence the action-guiding quality for ontological values. Perhaps a simple example of this "valorization" of one's ontological standpoint is betrayed by the reaction of disease-naturalistic scientists and philosophers to contemporary strains of hermeneutic/narrative oriented psychoanalytic theory. Because this psychoanalytic theory is not naturalistic, at least not in the narrow sense of current neuroscience, it is prone to dismissal, as threatening, dangerous, or irrelevant by bioscientists possessing disease-naturalistic assumptions (Sadler 2005).

Why entailed ontological values are obscure is because they govern, in ordinary as well as technical life, our taken-for-granted assumptions about the way the world works. Perhaps more importantly in the setting of a medical/scientific community, ontological values are conceptual building blocks for careers—one invests one's life into a research program and trajectory, a method of doing psychiatry, a way of making sense of patients' experiences. Such psychological investment makes entailed ontological values difficult to change—they become wrapped up in the person's identity and played out into details like grant support, collegial communities, and personal investments of time and effort. Ontological values are not changed like a suit of clothes.

In Sadler's (2005) analysis of the DSMs for common entailed ontological values, he identified six important entailed ontological values redolent throughout DSM thinking: (1) empiricism, (2) hyponarrativity, (3) individualism, (4) naturalism, (5) pragmatism, and (6) traditionalism. While space here does not permit a detailed elaboration of each, a brief sketch can suffice, followed by an example of entailed ontological values embodied in a contemporary DSM-5 debate which was ongoing at the time of this writing.

DSM empiricism is very close to scientific empiricism: the belief or assumption that genuine and reliable knowledge is best derived by our perceptual experiences, rather than reflection, divine revelation, or some other supernatural means to knowledge. Indeed, major points of debate throughout the late twentieth century concern the adequacy of DSM empiricism as noted earlier. On the other hand, the DSM authors devote a lot of effort to presenting and explaining the scientific-empirical basis for the DSMs (for examples, see Frances et al. 1995; Kupfer et al. 2002; Millon 1991).

DSM hyponarrativity refers to the marginalizing of the narrative, life-story perspective (McHugh and Slavney 1998) by the DSM nomothetic system of identifying mental disorders through identifying the shared features of psychopathology in populations of patients. The DSMs prefer syndrome to story, and the absence of patient stories in the DSM has had some interesting implications for the philosophical anthropology of the DSMs (see Charland 2004; Tekin 2011).

The DSM definition of mental disorder specified, in each addition since DSM-III, that mental disorders occur *in an individual* (APA 1980, 1987, 1994, 2000; Stein et al. 2011). This despite that family (systems) therapy, a substantial discipline within mental health care, is based upon the contrasting ontological values-commitment that at least some mental disorders are embodied by multiple persons through familial interactions (Denton 1989, 1990, 1997; First 2006b; Kaslow 1993, 1996). Hence the idea that the current model DSMs value ontological "individualism," the idea that mental disorders are metaphysically resident within individual people.

Other than DSM (disease) naturalism, DSM pragmatism is perhaps the most openly recognized ontological value in the DSMs—being mentioned in the justification for the DSM-IV-TR in the first paragraph of its Introduction: "Our highest priority has been to provide a helpful guide to clinical practice" (APA 2000, p. xxiii). DSM pragmatism is not based upon American philosophical pragmatism (though there may be important areas of overlap), but rather on a practical orientation to the primordial tasks of medicine: diagnosing and treating patients. The pragmatic ontological values that can be found in the DSM texts, concepts like *user-friendliness, brevity, clarity, facilitating research, improving the collection of clinical information*, among others, all refer to the practical chores of the working doctor and investigator. Indeed, at least as framed by the DSM-IV-TR Introduction, the ontological value of *pragmatism* may represent the prevailing value in the DSMs. Sadler raised the question in his 2005 book that perhaps one or another set of values should be of the highest priority, such as enabling excellent patient care.

The last substantive DSM ontological value identified by Sadler is "traditionalism," referring to the close relationship between most of the common DSM categories and the mental disorders of classical psychiatry: DSM bipolar disorder née manic-depressive insanity, DSM schizophrenia née dementia praecox, DSM major depressive disorder née melancholia, etc. However, DSM traditionalism is not simply, or even primarily, a nod to the history of psychiatry. It is a commitment to the continuity of psychiatric nomenclature and recognition of the investment of educators, clinicians, and administrators in entrenched clinical concepts. Indeed, some of the pushback around the frequent revision of the DSMs stems in part to the disruptive fallout from breaking away from commonly used categories of disorder (Zimmerman 1988, 1991).

DSM-5 proposal for (pedo)hebephilic disorder—a case study in the clash of values

At the time of this writing, representing the April 22, 2012 update of the <http://www.dsm5.org> posting of proposed disorders, the American Psychiatric Association offered the following modification of DSM-IV-TR Pedophilia, renaming it "Pedophilic Disorder":

> Pedophilic Disorder
>   A. Over a period of at least 6 months, an equal or greater sexual arousal from prepubescent or early pubescent children than from physically mature persons, as manifested by fantasies, urges, or behaviors.
>   B. The individual has acted on these sexual urges, or the sexual urges or fantasies cause marked distress or impairment in social, occupational, or other important areas of functioning.
>   C. The individual must be at least 18 years of age and at least 5 years older than the children in Criterion A.
>
> Specify type:
>   Classic Type—Sexually Attracted to Prepubescent Children (Tanner Stage 1)
>   Hebephilic Type—Sexually Attracted to Early Pubescent Children (Tanner Stages 2–3)
>   Pedohebephilic Type—Sexually Attracted to Both
>
> Specify type:
>   Sexually Attracted to Males
>   Sexually Attracted to Females
>   Sexually Attracted to Both
>
> Specify if:
>   In a Controlled Environment
>   In Remission (No Distress, Impairment, or Recurring Behavior for Five Years and in an Uncontrolled Environment).

This proposed diagnosis has been among the most controversial proposals issued by the DSM-5 workgroups, generating a number of impassioned commentaries in the literature and online, beginning with the launch of the proposed diagnosis in March 2011. Of specific interest for discussion here is the "(Pedo)Hebephilic Type" which adds pubescent children to a category that previously limited paraphilic interest to prepubescent children, the latter now dubbed the "Classic Type." The "Tanner stages" mentioned in the criteria are well-established medical criteria for staging the onset of puberty and sexual maturity. The criteria for girls and boys sequence the development of secondary-sex characteristics in five stages, progressing from prepubertal to adult. Of interest here are the first three stages: Stage 1, pre-adolescent, (example: no pubic hair); Stage 2, involving development of sparse, long slightly pigmented, downy pubic hair; and Stage 3, involving darker, coarser, curly pubic hair. The Tanner stages also specify changes for girls' breast development and boys' genital changes, body hair, and other secondary sex characteristics. The Tanner stages address an admittedly fluid set of phenotypic traits that develop slowly over time; making the boundaries between stages blurry rather than sharp (Marshall and Tanner 1969, 1970).

The core of the debate about the Hebephilic Type of Pedophilia is simply about whether inclusion as an official category of mental disorder in DSM-5 is warranted, justified, or acceptable. Key articles referred to for this example include Blanchard (2010a, 2010b, 2010c, 2011), First (2010), Frances and First (2011), Franklin (2010), Green (2010), Hinderliter (2011), Kramer (2011), Sadler (2008), Wakefield (2011), and Wollert and Cramer (2011). Because the focus of this handbook is philosophical rather than clinical, the following brief discussion sketches how the methods of values analysis can be applied to a scientific-clinical debate about the classification of psychopathology. The following subsections will list selected considerations in the controversy around Hebephilia and identify the characteristic values that are driving the viewpoint. The intention here is illustrative and not "conclusive" in supporting or refuting the inclusion of Hebephilic Disorder as a category. Moreover, the analysis does not pass judgment on the accuracy or validity of claims made, only identifies guiding values "behind" them. The issues at hand are listed in a stepwise order to facilitate understanding of the larger issues.

Failure to follow DSM-5 Research Agenda methodology

Richard Kramer is a frequent spokesperson for the B4U-Act organization, which is a US advocacy group for public education and mental health services for individuals who are sexually attracted to minors (<http://b4uact.org/news/20110725.htm>). In an October 2010 letter to the *Archives of Sexual Behavior*, Kramer provides a four-point critique of the Hebephilic Disorder proposal, referring to the DSM-5 leadership's white papers on the Research Agenda for DSM-5 (APA 2010a, 2010b, 2010c, 2010d, 2010e, 2010f). Kramer's critiques overlap with many of the comments to follow, so the focus here will be on his most unique contribution to the discourse. That unique contribution is the accusation that APA disregarded its own guidance to DSM-5 committees regarding a valid and effective DSM-5 developmental process.

Briefly, Kramer argues that the DSM-5 workgroup on Paraphilias disregarded APA's own guidance about formulation and use of research findings. Points made address the: (a) lack of a developmental perspective on normal and pathological sexual desire; (b) disregard of APA's recommendations to address "problematic diagnostic questions" (Kramer 2011 p. 233) of which he argues paraphilias are a premier example; (c) disregard of APA's own recommendation to include diverse clinical and scientific perspectives, noting disciplines which could offer perspective, but are absent from committees (specifically psychology, sexology, evolutionary biology, ethology, anthropology, sociology); and (d) disregard for APA guidance on "representing patient and family groups" (p. 233) and noting most research in this area draws upon the skewed sample of correctional populations. Kramer concludes that

"The APA and the paraphilias subworkgroup have an intellectual and ethical responsibility to promote valid research and to counter rather than reinforce false stereotypes" (p. 234).

What kinds of values are involved in this short excerpt? Of novel interest in this critique is the focus on the failed professional/scientific responsibilities of the DSM (sub) workgroup over and against the APA guidance offered in the 2010 white papers. What is philosophically interesting here is the nesting of epistemic, ontological, ethical, and pragmatic values under a rubric of professional/scientific obligation. It indicates that guiding values for a DSM enterprise can be submerged into policy recommendations; requiring systematic excavation to understand the values-play.

An overview of this excavation can be sketched. Kramer's concluding statement embraces several values-types, referring back to the components of his argument. He invokes epistemic values over his concerns for diverse scientific perspectives, the utilization of developmental and social sciences, and scientifically adequate study populations. He invokes ethical values by noting the stigma of paraphilias; unjustified in the face of invalid categories. He invokes pragmatic values in citing the failure to address paraphilias as nosologically problematic categories, and implying a limited applicability of current research given the skewed correctional population upon which the proposed categories are built. Finally, he invokes ontological values by raising questions about the normative status of desire for pubescent children (discussed in more detail later).

Distinction of paraphilias from paraphilic disorders

The current draft criteria for Pedophilia in the <http://www.dsm5.org> website modify previous DSMs by distinguishing Pedophilia from a Pedophilic Disorder. This change applies to all of the disorders previously identified as Paraphilias (disorders involving "atypical" erotic interests). The reason for the changes are described on the website as reflecting the difference between atypical sexual interests, which may be non-pathological (e.g., Pedophilia) and atypical sexual interests which manifest distress and/or impairment, which then qualifies them as a disorder (e.g., Pedophilic Disorder) (see <http://www.dsm5.org/ProposedRevision/Pages/proposedrevision.aspx?rid=186#>).

The response from the workgroup subcommittee is apparently intended as a response to concerns from the sexology and other communities that prior DSMs were pathologizing harmless sexual diversity (in the case of consenting adults). The curious maintenance of a non-pathological Pedophilia category in a DSM is defended as the need to have a non-pathological category for research comparisons:

> This approach leaves intact the distinction between normative and non-normative sexual behavior, which could be important to researchers, but without automatically labeling non-normative sexual behavior as psychopathological. An additional advantage of this approach is eliminating certain logical absurdities in the DSM-IV-TR. In that version, for example, a man could not be identified as having transvestism—however much he cross-dressed and however sexually exciting that was to him—unless he was unhappy about this activity or impaired by it. (<http://www.dsm5.org/ProposedRevision/Pages/proposedrevision.aspx?rid=186#>, accessed July 21, 2012)

The interest in maintaining a distinction for research purposes implies epistemic values involving controlled research designs and valid comparison groups, while the specification of distress and impairment in the Disorder categories can be construed as a response to the negative ethical values of invalid stigmatizing raised by Kramer in the prior subsection. As will be seen later, this change may also be related to ontological values concerning the nature of human sexuality.

Patient prevarication

The context of American classification of individuals with pedophilic desire is largely framed by the forensic setting. In the United States, the molestation of minors is one of, and perhaps the most, despised of crimes, and the stigma of child molesters and "pedophiles" is one of the greatest encountered in psychiatry (Frances and First 2011; Zonana et al. 1999). Many US jurisdictions have laws severely penalizing and regulating individuals committing sex offenses, and many states have "sexual predator laws" which provide for harsh preventive measures: severe sentencing, preventive incarceration and involuntary hospitalization for offenders completing sentences, public registries of sex offenders, and regulations against convicted offenders living in neighborhoods close to children (Zonana et al. 1999). In considering the diagnosis of paraphilic disorders involving illegal transgressions against others, US psychiatry has a fundamental epistemological problem, in that the usual assumptions that patients will be *truthful* in their responses to psychiatric interviewing is lost, as the expectation is that "patients" will deny, minimize, and lie in order to avoid the severe consequences of diagnosis, even absent criminal implications (Blanchard 2010a; Frances and First 2011; Zonana et al. 1999). Tools and techniques for finding more conclusive knowledge of the pedophilic patient's sexual interests, activities, and behaviors are highly valued and universally sought in the quest of epistemic *certainty*.

Use in forensic settings

This background of prevaricating paraphilic patients and the undermining of a fundamental epistemic assumption of medical examinations—patients by and large tell the truth—set the stage for psychiatrists' wariness of diagnosis of any alleged or convicted sex offender. In their 2011 paper, Frances and First, along with legal scholars such as Karen Franklin (2010) warn of the potential abuse of paraphilic diagnosis in forensic settings as a tool for prosecutors to frighten and sway juries into guilty verdicts and more severe sentencing. Franklin also warns that diagnoses such as Hebephilia can potentially be misused to seclude and involuntarily treat individuals for a disorder that may be invalid and unjustified.

From this brief summary, the epistemic concern about diagnostic validity is evident; as evidenced by Frances and First's concern about poor diagnostic reliability given not just the prevarication problem but the problem of normative sexual desire (see "Normative status of arousal to pubescent children" section) with Hebephilia. These authors are also concerned about ethical lapses of inappropriate treatment and restriction of civil liberties, as "unconstitutional preventive detention" (Franklin 2010, p. 765).

Normative status of arousal to pubescent children

As early as 1996, anthropologist Dona Davis warned DSM-IV committees about the wide cultural variability of normative sexual desire, sexual social practices, and individual sexual behavior (Davis 1996, 1998). A major focus of the antagonism to DSM-5 Hebephilia and Hebephilic Disorder is centered on this variability. In addition, another concern involves lines of evidence supporting the idea that sexual desire by (primarily) men for pubescent females is a normal expression of erotic desire in Western industrialized countries, not an "atypical" sexual interest as implied by DSM hebephilic categories. Frances and First (2011) describe several studies, including both criminal and non-offender populations, that indicate low interest ratings in prepubescent children, with pubescent and older adolescents being similar to young adults in erotic interest by adult men. These concerns about the ubiquity of non-clinical, non-offending men showing interest in pubescent age children was also shared by Franklin (2010), Green (2010), and Wakefield (2011) in their reviews. Several of these authors appeal to everyday cultural evidence manifested by commercial advertising, such as teenagers' sexualized portrayal in fashion advertisements, ubiquitous in Western culture; and the variable minimum legal ages of consent for sexual activity, which vary considerably from country to country, from twelve (Mexico) to twenty (Tunisia) (see <http://www.avert.org/age-of-consent.htm>).

These considerations are good examples of entailed ontological values, the culturally-specific assumptions about what it means to be human—in this case, in the sexuality arena. As discussed earlier, the deeply assumed nature of entailed ontological values plays out in the domain of morality (adding ethical meaning to the values as well), where desire for pubescent children may be cast as heinous by fundamental religious groups, and more tolerated by other more sexually "liberal" groups. These customs held by various groups also illuminate the arbitrariness of age-based cutoff points for whether desire for a youth is acceptable or not, raising the pragmatic interest of age-based limits for these legal considerations. However, these group differences about what is normative and tolerable diminish when the discussion is not about desire, but sexual action, where many opinions converge around the unacceptability of sexual engagement of children by adults.

Inadequate scientific research base

Much of the debate around the proposed inclusion of a Hebephilic Disorder concept in DSM-5 has focused upon a variety of problems with the scientific research base. For clarity's sake, these criticisms can be grouped into the following headings: (a) undue influence of a single research group; (b) questionable research design and use of statistics; (c) a feeble epidemiological basis for the proposed category.

Franklin (2010) provides a history of the development of the University of Toronto's Law and Mental Health program within the Centre for Addiction and Mental Health (CAMH), instituted by sexologist Kurt Freund, pioneer of phallometry (measurement of erectile arousal through volumetric displacement technology) and developing one of the most important centers for the study of sexual disorders and sex offenders. Ray Blanchard PhD, until recently the Head of Clinical Sexology Services in the Law and Mental Health Program at CAMH, has served as the premier scientific advocate for the Hebephilia/Hebephilic Disorders taxons. The remarkable, and largely singular, success of Blanchard's group in providing an extensive research base for paraphilias has been, according to his critics, been excessively dependent upon a forensic/correctional population. Such a skewed population ignores, according to critics like Kramer (2011), the substantial numbers of non-offending individuals the B4U-ACT group represents, representing an epidemiological hole in the data about "minor-attracted persons" and thus limiting the generalizability of the Toronto group's research findings.

First (2011), on a related theme, describes the limitations of the data from the Blanchard group and argues that these investigators mis- or overinterpret their research findings in defense of a proposal to use numeric thresholds of molestation offenses ("victim counts") as a diagnostic criterion. First was primarily concerned that the studies presented did not apply to the clinical settings characteristic of DSM users. Blanchard in turn responded with the intent to refute First's criticisms (Blanchard 2010) and later provided "anthropological" data that defended the idea of the reproductive inferiority of pubescent matings (Hames and Blanchard 2012).

From another scientific perspective, Wollert and Cramer (2011) criticize the Toronto group's use of victim counts-as-criterion from another standpoint, that of research design and use of statistics. The details of their critique, as well as Blanchard's (2011) response, are too technical for a detailed values analysis here.

From a values-analytic perspective, the points of these abbreviated criticisms and responses is to illustrate the importance of epistemic values such as *adequate sampling* (Kramer's points about sampling bias in a correctional sample), *appropriate selection and use* of statistical analysis (Wollert and Cramer's and First's critiques and Blanchard's response), and the *overgeneralization* of research findings into a different population and setting (First).

Conceptual validity and strength of arguments

Weighing in on the hebephilic disorder debate from his own perspective of mental disorders being "harmful dysfunctions," Jerome C. Wakefield (1992, 2011) argues that, citing Nagle (1969) and echoing similar points of Dona Davis mentioned earlier, that desire for and even sexual activity with pubescent children is too culturally and historically common to warrant classification as a disorder. For Wakefield, mental disorders must be harmful and involve disturbances in "biologically designed/naturally selected" functions (2011, p. 198), and for Wakefield the ubiquity of sexual desire and activity with pubescent children across cultures and history curtail the argument about hebephilia as a harmful dysfunction. (As an aside, Wakefield's (2011) and Hames and Blanchard's (2012) reproductive competitiveness argument appear to have been too contemporaneous for Wakefield to include in his analysis, which would have been interesting.)

Citing the APA's posted rationale for including hebephilia concepts to DSM-5:

> There are four reasons for replacing Pedophilia with Pedohebephilic Disorder. These reasons are: (a) Hebephilia (the erotic preference for pubescents) is similar to pedophilia in that both involve sexual attractions to persons who are physically quite immature, (b) Many men do not differentiate much or at all between prepubescent and pubescent children and offend against both, (c) Many hebephilic patients are getting DSM diagnoses anyway—they are diagnosed as pedophilic under a very liberal definition of prepubertal child, or they are diagnosed with Paraphilia NOS (Hebephilia) and (d) This would harmonize with an ICD definition of Pedophilia: "A sexual preference for children, boys or girls or both, usually of prepubertal or early pubertal age." (Wakefield 2011 p. 205, quoting the <http://www.dsm5.org> website; internal citations omitted)

Wakefield then attacks these arguments as "remarkably weak" (p. 205), finding, (for example) the (a) argument being a simile rather than an argument: "This is about as valid an argument as saying that both dyslexia and illiteracy involve difficulties [in] reading, thus illiteracy should be considered a disorder" (Wakefield p. 205).

How might we consider the values involved in Wakefield's viewpoints? His notion of "conceptual validity" appears to be used in an epistemic sense—validity referring to a characteristic that accurately captures a descriptive feature of the world. He invokes evolved biological mechanisms as (likely) an epistemic as well as ontological benchmark for his analysis. The epistemic value-content here resides in the view that finding biological mechanisms are a way of knowing the truth of psychopathology. The ontological values come in through the valorization of evolutionary biology as defining the nature of being human and as the metaphysical benchmark for psychopathology. Finally, his concern for the quality of arguments certainly represents epistemic interests—while leaving open the question of whether Wakefield thinks the inelegance of the arguments offered raise an aesthetic value-aspect to his critique.

Unanswered Questions

The descriptive analysis of values in psychiatric discourses provides an opportunity for philosophical research of both intellectual and practical merit. The analysis of value commitments and entailments in psychiatric diagnosis and classification is at its very beginnings, and the field is wide open for philosophical inquiry. From this chapter's very brief discussion, several lines of potential further interest emerge; to mention a few: (a) further exploration of the aesthetic-values realm; (b) the interplay of ontological values in the framing of psychiatric diagnostic concepts; and particularly (c) exploring the kinds of interactions between all values in shaping nosology development, diagnostic categories, and diagnostic practice. Moreover, at present only a minority of DSM or ICD categories have been studied intensively; the hundreds of mental disorder categories currently identified in these manuals offer opportunities for philosophical study for years, even decades, to come.

References

Alarcón, R. D. (2009). Inside the DSM-V process: Issues, debates, and reflections. *Psychiatric Times*, 26(7). Available at: <http://www.psychiatrictimes.com/dsm-5/content/article/10168/1426119>.

Alarcón, R. D., Becker, A. E., Lewis-Fernández, R., Like, R. C., Desai, P., Foulks, E., *et al.* (2009). Issues for DSM-V: The role of culture in psychiatric diagnosis. *Journal of Nervous & Mental Disease*, 197(8), 559–60.

American Psychiatric Association (1980). *Diagnostic and Statistical Manual of Mental Disorders, Third Edition*. Washington, DC: American Psychiatric Association.

American Psychiatric Association (1987). *Diagnostic and Statistical Manual of Mental Disorders, Third Edition, Revised*. Washington, DC: American Psychiatric Association.

American Psychiatric Association (1994). *Diagnostic and Statistical Manual of Mental Disorders, Fourth Edition*. Washington, DC: American Psychiatric Association.

American Psychiatric Association (2000). *Diagnostic and Statistical Manual of Mental Disorders, Fourth Edition, Text Revision*. Washington, DC: American Psychiatric Association.

American Psychiatric Association (2010a). *Current Activities: Report of the DSM-5 Task Force (March 2009).* [Online.] Available at: <http://www.dsm5.org/ProgressReports/Pages/CurrentActivitiesReportoftheDSM-VTaskForce(March2009).aspx>.

American Psychiatric Association (2010b). *Definition of a Mental Disorder.* Available at: <http://www.dsm5.org/ProposedRevisions/Pages/proposedrevision.aspx?rid=465>.

American Psychiatric Association (2010c). *DSM-5: The Future of Psychiatric Diagnosis.* Available at: <http://www.dsm5.org/Pages/Default.aspx>.

American Psychiatric Association (2010d). *DSM-V Planning Conference Series Monographs.* Available at: <http://www.psych.org/MainMenu/Research/DSMIV/DSMV/DSMRevisionActivities/DSM-V-Monographs.aspx>.

American Psychiatric Association (2010e). *Phase 1: A Research Agenda for DSM-V: White Paper Monographs.* Available at: <http://www.psych.org/MainMenu/Research/DSMIV/DSMV/DSMRevisionActivities/ResearchonDiagnosis.aspx>.

American Psychiatric Association (2010f). *Phase 2: Refining the Research Agenda for DSM-V: NIH Conference Series.* Available at: <http://www.psych.org/MainMenu/Research/DSMIV/DSMV/DSMRevisionActivities/ResearchPlanningatHigherMagnification.aspx>.

Bemporad, J. R. and Schwab, M. E. (1986). The DSM-III and clinical child psychiatry. In T. Millon and G. L. Klerman (Eds), *Contemporary Directions in Psychopathology: Toward the DSM-IV*, pp. 135–50. New York, NY: Guilford.

Bergin, A. E. (1991). Values and religious issues in psychotherapy and mental health. *American Psychologist, 46*(4), 394–403.

Beutler, L. E. and Malik, M. L. (2002). *Rethinking the DSM: A Psychological Perspective.* Washington, DC: American Psychological Association.

Blanchard, R. (2010a). The DSM diagnostic criteria for pedophilia. *Archives of Sexual Behavior, 39*(2), 304–16.

Blanchard, R. (2010b). The specificity of victim count as a diagnostic indicator of pedohebephilia. *Archives of Sexual Behavior, 39*, 1245–52.

Blanchard, R. (2011). Misdiagnoses of pedohebephilia using victim count: A reply to Wollert & Cramer (2011). *Archives of Sexual Behavior, 40*(6), 1081–8.

Bracken, P. and Thomas, P. (2005). *Postpsychiatry.* Oxford: Oxford University Press.

Broverman, I. K., Broverman, D. M., Clarkson, F. E., Rosenkrantz, P. S., and Vogel, S. R. (1970). Sex-role stereotypes and clinical judgments of mental health. *Journal of Consulting & Clinical Psychology, 34*, 1–7.

Broverman, I. K., Vogel, S. R., Broverman, D. M., Clarkson, F. E., and Rosenkranz, P. S. (1972). Sex-role stereotypes: a current appraisal. *Journal of Social Issues, 28*, 59–78.

Caplan, P. J. (1995). *They Say You're Crazy: How the World's Most Powerful Psychiatrists Decide Who's Normal.* Reading, MA: Addison-Wesley.

Charland, L. C. (2004). A madness for identity: Psychiatric labels, consumer autonomy, and the perils of the internet. *Philosophy, Psychiatry, & Psychology, 11*(4), 335–49.

Charland, L. C. (2006). The moral nature of the cluster B personality disorders. *Philosophy, Psychiatry, & Psychology, 20*(2), 119–28.

Charland, L. C. (2010). Medical or moral kinds. Moving beyond a false dichotomy. *Philosophy, Psychiatry, & Psychology, 17*(2), 119–25.

Conrad, P. (2007). *The Medicalization of Society.* Baltimore, MD: The Johns Hopkins University Press.

Cooper, R. (2007). *Psychiatry and the Philosophy of Science.* Montreal: McGill-Queen's University Press.

Cosgrove, L. and Krimsky, S. (2012). A comparison of DSM-IV and DSM-5 Panel members financial associations with industry: A pernicious problem persists. *PLoS Medicine*, *9*(3), e1001190.

Cosgrove, L. Krimsky, S., Vijayaraghavan, M., and Schneider, L. (2006). Financial ties between DSM-IV panel members and the pharmaceutical industry. *Psychotherapy and Psychosomatics*, *75*, 154–60.

Davis, D. L. (1996). Cultural sensitivity and the sexual disorders in DSM-IV: Review and assessment. In J. E. Mezzich, A. Kleinman, H. Fabrega, and D. Parron (Eds), *Culture and Psychiatric Diagnosis: A DSM-IV Perspective*, pp. 191–211. Washington, DC: American Psychiatric Press.

Davis, D. L. (1998). The sexual and gender identity disorders. *Transcultural Psychiatry*, *35*(3), 401–12.

Denton, W. H. (1989). DSM-III—R and the family therapist: Ethical considerations. *Journal of Marital & Family Therapy*, *15*(4), 367–77.

Denton, W. H. (1990). A family systems analysis of DSM-III—R. *Journal of Marital & Family Therapy*, *16*(2), 113–25.

Denton, W. H., Patterson, J. E., and Van Meir, E. S. (1997). Use of the DSM in marriage and family therapy programs: Current practices and attitudes. *Journal of Marital & Family Therapy*, *23*(1), 81–6.

Faust, D. and Miner, R. A. (1986). The empiricist and his new clothes: DSM-III in perspective. *American Journal of Psychiatry*, *143*(8), 962–7.

First, M. B. (2005a). Clinical utility: A prerequisite for the adoption of a dimensional approach in DSM. *Journal of Abnormal Psychology*, *114*, 560–4.

First, M. B. (2005b). Keeping an eye on clinical utility. *World Psychiatry*, *4*(2), 87–8.

First, M. B. (2006a). Beyond clinical utility: Broadening the DSM-V research appendix to include alternative diagnostic constructs. *American Journal of Psychiatry*, *163*(10), 1679–81.

First, M. B. (2006b). Relational processes in the DSM-V revision process: Comment on the special section. *Journal of Family Psychology*, *20*(3), 356–8.

First, M. B. (2010). DSM-5 proposals for paraphilias: Suggestions for reducing false positives related to use of behavioral manifestations. *Archives of Sexual Behavior*, *39*, 1239–44.

Frances, A. (2010). The DSM-5 personality disorders – great intentions, unusable result-way too cumbersome and complex. *Psychology Today Blog, DSM5 in Distress*, March 18. Available at: <http://www.psychologytoday.com/blog/dsm5-in-distress/201004/the-dsm5-personality-disorders-great-intentions-unusable-result>.

Frances, A., and First, M. B. (2011). Hebephilia is not a mental disorder in DSM-IV-TR and should not become one in DSM-5. *Journal of the American Academy of Psychiatry and the Law*, *39*, 78–85.

Frances, A. J., First, M. B., and Pincus, H. A. (1995). *DSM-IV Guidebook: The Essential Companion to the Diagnostic and Statistical Manual of Mental Disorders, Fourth Edition*. Washington, DC: American Psychiatric Press.

Frances, A. J., First, M. B., Widiger, T. A., Miele, G. M., Tilly, S. M., Davis, W. W., *et al.* (1991). An A to Z guide to DSM-IV conundrums. *Journal of Abnormal Psychology*, *100*(3), 407–12.

Frankena, W. K. (1973). *Ethics* (2nd edn). Englewood Cliffs, NJ: Prentice-Hall.

Franklin, K. 2010. Hebephilia: Quintessence of diagnostic pretextuality. *Behavioral Sciences & the Law*, *29*, 751–68.

Fulford, K. W. M. (1989). *Moral Theory and Medical Practice*. Cambridge: Cambridge University Press.

Fulford, K. W. (1991). Evaluative delusions: Their significance for philosophy and psychiatry. *British Journal of Psychiatry Supplement, 14*, 108–12.

Fulford, K. W. M. (1994). Closet logics: Hidden conceptual elements in the DSM and ICD classification of mental disorders. In J. Z. Sadler, O. P. Wiggins, and M. A. Schwartz (Eds), *Philosophical Perspectives on Psychiatric Diagnostic Classification*, pp. 211–32. Baltimore, MD: The Johns Hopkins University Press.

Fulford, K. W. (1999). Nine variations and a coda on the theme of an evolutionary definition of dysfunction. *Journal of Abnormal Psychology, 108*(3), 412–20.

Fulford, K. W. (2001). 'What is (mental) disease?': An open letter to Christopher Boorse. *Journal of Medical Ethics, 27*(2), 80–5.

Fulford, K. W. (2002a). Values in psychiatric diagnosis: Executive summary of a report to the Chair of the ICD-12/DSM-VI Coordination Task Force (dateline 2010). *Psychopathology, 35*(2–3), 132–8.

Fulford, K. W. M. (2002b). Report to the Chair of the DSM-VI Task Force from the Editors of *Philosophy, Psychiatry, & Psychology*. Contentious and noncontentious evaluative language in psychiatric diagnosis (dateline 2010). In J. Z. Sadler (Ed.), *Descriptions and Prescriptions: Values, Mental Disorders, and the DSMs*, pp. 323–62. Baltimore, MD: The Johns Hopkins University Press.

Fulford, K. W., Broome, M., Stanghellini, G., and Thornton, T.(2005). Looking with both eyes open: Fact and value in psychiatric diagnosis? *World Psychiatry, 4*(2), 78–86.

Gaines, A. D. (1992). From DSM-I to III-R; Voices of self, mastery and the other: A cultural constructivist reading of U.S. psychiatric classification. *Social Science & Medicine, 35*(1), 3–24.

Gorenstein, E. E. (1992). *The Science of Mental Illness*. New York, NY: Academic Press.

Green, R. (2010). Hebephilia is a mental disorder? *Sexual Offender Treatment, 5*(1). Available at: <http://www.sexual-offender-treatment.org>.

Grove, W. M., Andreasen, N. C., McDonald-Scott, P., Keller, M. B., and Shapiro, R.W. (1981). Reliability studies of psychiatric diagnosis. Theory and practice. *Archives of General Psychiatry, 38*(4), 408–13.

Hames, R. and Blanchard, R. (2012). Anthropological data regarding the adaptiveness of hebephilia. *Archives of Sexual Behavior, 41*(4), 745–7.

Healy, D. (1997). *The Antidepressant Era*. Cambridge, MA: Harvard University Press.

Healy, D. (2002). *The Creation of Psychopharmacology*. Cambridge, MA: Harvard University Press.

Hempel, C. G. (1965). Fundamentals of taxonomy. In *Aspects of Scientific Explanation and Other Essays in the Philosophy of Science*, pp. 137–54. New York, NY: Free Press.

Horwitz, A. V. (2002). *Creating Mental Illness*. Chicago, IL: University of Chicago Press.

Horwitz, A. V. and Wakefield, J. C. (2007). *The Loss of Sadness: How Psychiatry Transformed Normal Sorrow into Depressive Disorder*. New York, NY: Oxford University Press.

Hyman, S. E. (2002). Neuroscience, genetics, and the future of psychiatric diagnosis. *Psychopathology, 35*(2–3), 139–44.

Hyman, S. E. (2007). Can neuroscience be integrated into the DSM-V? *Nature Reviews Neuroscience, 8*(9), 725–32.

Jensen, P. S., Knapp, P., and Mrazek, D. A. (2006). *Toward a New Diagnostic System for Child Psychopathology: Moving Beyond the DSM*. New York, NY: The Guilford Press.

Kirk, S. A. and Kutchins, H. (1992). *The Selling of the DSM: The Rhetoric of Sicence in Psychiatry*. Hawthorne, NY: Aldine de Gruyter.

Kaslow, F. W. (1993). Relational diagnosis: An idea whose time has come? *Family Process*, *32*, 255–9.

Kaslow, F. W. (1996). *Handbook of Relational Diagnosis and Dysfunctional Family Systems*. New York, NY: John Wiley & Sons.

Kleinman, A. (1996). How is culture important for DSM-IV? In J. E. Mezzich (Ed.), *Culture and Psychiatric Diagnosis: A DSM-IV Perspective*, pp. 15–25. Washington, DC: American Psychiatric Press.

Kramer, R. (2011). APA guidelines ignored in development of diagnostic criteria for pedohebephilia. *Archives of Sexual Behavior*, *40*, 233–5.

Kuhn, T. S. (1977). Objectivity, value judgment, and theory choice. In *The Essential Tension*, pp. 320–9. Chicago, IL: University of Chicago Press.

Kuhn, T. S. (1979). *The Structure of Scientific Revolutions* (2nd edn). Chicago, IL: University of Chicago Press.

Kupfer, D., First, M. B., and Regier, D. (2002). *A Research Agenda for DSM-V*. Washington, DC: American Psychiatric Press.

Kutchins, H. and Kirk, S. A. (1997). *Making us Crazy: The Psychiatric Bible and the Creation of Mental Disorders*. New York, NY: The Free Press.

Lane, C. (2008). *Shyness: How Normal Behavior Became a Sickness*. New Haven, CT: Yale University Press.

Longino, H. E. (1990). *Science as Social Knowledge: Values and Objectivity in Scientific Inquiry*. Princeton, NJ: Princeton University Press.

Margolis, J. (1994). Taxonomic puzzles. In J. Z. Sadler, O. P. Wiggins, and M. A. Schwartz (Eds), *Philosophical Perspectives on Psychiatric Diagnostic Classification*, pp. 104–28. Baltimore, MD: Johns Hopkins University Press.

Marshall, W. A. and Tanner, J. M. (1969). Variations in the pattern of pubertal changes in girls. *Archives of Disease in Childhood*, *44*, 291–303.

Marshall, W. A. and Tanner, J. M. (1970). Variations in the pattern of pubertal changes in boys. *Archives of Disease in Childhood*, *45*(239), 13–23.

Murphy, D. (2005). *Psychiatry in the Scientific Image*. Cambridge, MA: MIT Press.

Nagel, T. (1969). Sexual perversion. *The Journal of Philosophy*, *66*(1), 5–17.

Pearce, S. and Pickard, H. (2009). The moral content of psychiatric treatment. *British Journal of Psychiatry*, *195*, 281–2.

Petryna, A. (2007). Clinical trials offshored: on private sector science and public Health. *BioSocieties*, *2*, 21–40.

Potter, N. N. (2009). *Mapping the Edges and the In-Between: A Critical Analysis of Borderline Personality Disorder*. Oxford: Oxford University Press.

Proctor, R. N. (1991). *Value-Free Science? Purity and Power in Modern Knowledge*. Cambridge, MA: Harvard University Press.

Putnam, H. (1981). Fact and value. In *Reason, Truth, and History*, pp. 127–49. New York, NY: Cambridge University Press.

Putnam, H. (1990a). Beyond the fact/value dichotomy. In *Realism with a Human Face*, pp. 135–41. Cambridge, MA: Harvard University Press.

Putnam, H. (1990b). The place of facts in a world of values. In *Realism with a Human Face*, pp. 142–62. Cambridge, MA: Harvard University Press.

Radden, J. (1994). Recent criticism of psychiatric nosology: A review. *Philosophy, Psychiatry, & Psychology*, *1*(3), 193–200.

Radden, J. (1996). Lumps and bumps: Kantian faculty psychology, phrenology, and twentieth-century psychiatric classification. *Philosophy, Psychiatry, & Psychology*, *3*(1), 1–14.

Sadler, J. Z. (1996). Epistemic value commitments in the debate over categorical vs. dimensional personality diagnosis. *Philosophy, Psychiatry, & Psychology*, 3, 203–22.

Sadler, J. Z. (1997). Recognizing values: A descriptive-causal method for medical/scientific discourses. *Journal of Medicine and Philosophy*, 22(6), 541–65.

Sadler, J. Z. (2002). *Descriptions and Prescriptions: Values, Mental Disorders, and the DSMs*. Baltimore, MD: Johns Hopkins University Press.

Sadler, J. Z. (2005). *Values and Psychiatric Diagnosis*. Oxford: Oxford University Press.

Sadler, J. Z. (2008). Vice and the diagnostic classification of mental disorders: A philosophical case conference. *Philosophy, Psychiatry, & Psychology*, 15(1), 1–17.

Sadler, J. Z. (in press). *Vice and Psychiatric Diagnosis*. Oxford: Oxford University Press.

Sadler, J. Z., Jotterand, F., Lee, S. C., and Inrig, S. (2009). Can medicalization be good? Situating medicalization within bioethics. *Theoretical Medicine and Bioethics*, 30, 411–25.

Sadler, J. Z., Wiggins, O. P., and Schwartz, M. A. (Eds) (1994). *Philosophical Perspectives on Psychiatric Diagnostic Classification*. Baltimore, MD: Johns Hopkins University Press.

Salmon, W. and Kitcher, P. (Eds) (1989). *Four Decades of Scientific Explanation*. Minneapolis, MN: University of Minnesota Press.

Schacht, T. and Nathan, P. E. (1977). But is it good for psychologists? Appraisal and status of DSM-III. *American Psychologist*, 32(12), 1017–25.

Schacht, T. E. (1985a). DSM-III and the politics of truth. *American Psychologist*, 40(5), 513–21.

Schacht, T. E. (1985b). Reply to Spitzer's "Politics-science dichotomy syndrome." *American Psychologist*, 40(5), 562–3.

Schwartz, M. A., and Wiggins, O. P. (1986). Logical empiricism and psychiatric classification. *Comprehensive Psychiatry*, 27(2), 101–14.

Skodol, A. E., Bender, D. S., Morey, L. C., Clark, L. A., Oldham, J. M., Alarcon, R. D., *et al.* (2001). Personality disorder types proposed for DSM-5. *Journal of Personality Disorders*, 25(2), 136–9.

Spitzer, R. L. (1981). The diagnostic status of homosexuality in DSM-III: A reformulation of the issues. *American Journal of Psychiatry*, 138(2), 210–15.

Spitzer, R. L. (2001). Values and assumptions in the development of DSM-III and DSM-III-R: An insider's perspective and a belated response to Sadler, Hulgus, and Agich's 'On values in recent American psychiatric classification.' *The Journal of Nervous and Mental Disease*, 189(6), 351–9.

Spitzer, R. L. (2008). DSM-V: Open and transparent? *Psychiatric News*, 43(14), 26.

Stein, D. J., Phillips, K. A., Bolton, D., Fulford, K. W., Sadler, J. Z., and Kendler, K. S. (2010). What is a mental/psychiatric disorder? From DSM-IV to DSM-V. *Psychological Medicine*, 40(11), 1759–65.

Szasz, T. S. (1960). The myth of mental illness. *American Psychologist*, 15, 113–18.

Szasz, T. S. (1961). *The Myth of Mental Illness: Foundations of a Theory of Personal Conduct*. New York, NY: Hoeber-Harper.

Tekin, S. (2011). Self-concept through the diagnostic looking glass: Narratives and mental disorder. *Philosophical Psychology*, 24(3), 357–80.

Veale, D. M. and Lambrou, C. (2002). The importance of aesthetics in body dysmorphic disorder. *CNS Spectrums*, 7(6), 429–31.

Wakefield, J. C. (1992). Disorder as harmful dysfunction: a conceptual critique of DSM-III-R's definition of mental disorder. *Psychological Review*, 99(2), 232–47.

Wakefield, J. C. (2011). DSM-5 proposed diagnostic criteria for sexual paraphilias: Tensions between diagnostic validity and forensic utility. *International Journal of Law and Psychiatry*, 34, 195–209.

Wallace, E. R. (1994). Psychiatric nosology: An historico-philosophical overview. In J. Z. Sadler, O. P. Wiggins, and M. A. Schwartz (Eds), *Philosophical Perspectives on Psychiatric Diagnostic Classification*, pp. 16–86. Baltimore, MD: Johns Hopkins University Press.

Wallace, E. R., Radden, J. H., and Sadler, J. Z. (1997). The philosophy of psychiatry–who needs it? *Journal of Nervous and Mental Disease*, 185(2), 67–73.

Wollwert, R. and Cramer, E. (2011). Sampling extreme groups invalidates research on the paraphilias: Implications for DSM-5 and sex offender risk assessments. *Behavioral Sciences & the Law*, 29, 554–65.

World Health Organization (1992). *The ICD-10 Classification of Mental and Behavioural Disorders: Clinical Descriptions and Diagnostic Guidelines*. Geneva: World Health Organization.

Zachar, P. (2000). *Psychological Concepts and Biological Psychiatry: A Philosophical Analysis*. Amsterdam: J. Benjamins.

Zachar, P. and Potter, N. N. (2010a). Personality disorders: Moral or medical kinds—or both? *Philosophy, Psychiatry, & Psychology*, 17(2), 101–17.

Zachar, P. and Potter, N. N. (2010b). Valid moral appraisals and valid personality disorders. *Philosophy, Psychiatry, & Psychology*, 17(2), 131–42.

Zimmerman, M. (1988). Why are we rushing to publish DSM-IV? *Archives of General Psychiatry*, 45(12), 1135–8.

Zimmerman, M. (1990). Is DSM-IV needed at all? *Archives of General Psychiatry*, 47(10), 974–6.

Zonana, H., Abel, G., Bradford, J., Hoge, S., Metzner, J., Becker, J., *et al.* (1999). *Dangerous Sex Offenders: A Task Force Report of the American Psychiatric Association*. Washington, DC: American Psychiatric Association.

CHAPTER 46

CONCEPTUAL AND ETHICAL ISSUES IN THE PRODROMAL PHASE OF PSYCHOSIS

MATTHEW BROOME, PAOLO FUSAR-POLI,

AND PHILIPPE WUYTS

INTRODUCTION

Our focus in this chapter is to address some of the philosophical issues that arise in the scientific and clinical study of the prodromal phase of psychosis (Bortolotti and Broome 2009; Broome and Bortolotti 2009). We will discuss issues from both metaphysics and philosophy of science as well as those related to phenomenological approaches and clinical ethics. A clear challenge arises in considering how models of a continuum of psychosis and of schizophrenia as a neurodevelopmental disorder can be reconciled with a scientific understanding of the prodrome as a discrete constellation of signs and symptoms. Given the importance of psychopathology in the delineation of "prodromal" or "ultra-high-risk" (UHR) states, there may be wider classification concerns regarding the status of the "at-risk" syndrome, and its place in psychiatric classifications.

In addition to these more scientific and metaphysical concerns, clinical and research work on the prodromal stage of psychosis also highlights ethical concerns. Demarcating a mental disorder and applying therapeutic interventions, based solely on risk estimation, should not be carried out lightly.

The Neurodevelopmental Model of Schizophrenia and the Historical Development of Prodromal Research

It has been apparent for over two decades that there is a developmental component to schizophrenia (Broome et al. 2005b). In its simple form, the neurodevelopmental model postulates that genes involved in the development of the neural apparatus and/or environmental insults in early life lead to aberrant brain development, which in turn predisposes to the later onset of schizophrenia (Bullmore et al. 1998; McDonald et al. 1999; Murray and Lewis 1987). However, more recent formulations incorporate the role of social factors such as urban upbringing, social isolation, and migration (Boydell et al. 2004; Morgan et al. 2007), and point to an interaction between the biological and psychological in a cascade of increasingly deviant development (Howes et al. 2004; van Os et al. 2010).

Although early symptoms of schizophrenia have long been recognized (Sullivan 1994), the term "prodromal" was first introduced by Mayer-Gross in 1932 (Mayer-Gross 1932). However it formally appeared in PubMed literature only about twenty years ago in a pioneering work by Huber and Gross who, influenced by Mayer-Gross' observations, first described basic symptoms (BS) in the 1960s and initiated the first prospective early detection study in the 1980s (Huber and Gross 1989). In the late 1980s, Häfner et al. for the first time examined the prodrome on a representative population of 232 patients with schizophrenia admitted for the first time from a large catchment area in the ABC (Age, Begin and Course of Schizophrenia) study (Häfner et al. 1992a, 1992b, 1993, 1998; Riecher et al. 1989). These authors showed that in 73% of all cases the disorder began with a prodromal phase, which lasted on average five years (Häfner et al. 1993, 1998). In the early 1990s, Jackson and McGorry started reliability studies to assess first-episode subjects via a semistructured interview in order to determine the presence or absence of prodromal symptoms (Jackson et al. 1994). On the basis of this early work, Yung and colleagues set up the first clinical service for potentially prodromal individuals, began investigating the predictive validity of the prospectively defined "at-risk mental state, ARMS" criteria, developing the first UHR psychometric instrument (Yung et al. 1996, 2003, 2004). In the following years, in the USA, Miller and McGlashan (Miller et al. 1999) developed a similar psychometric instrument for quantitatively rating symptom severity for patients at UHR for psychosis (McGlashan et al. 2010). In Europe, the further development of the BS approach for identifying those at high risk (HR) was largely grounded in the diagnostic validation of a scale for the assessment of basic symptoms (Klosterkötter et al. 1996) as implemented by the investigations of Klosterkötter and colleagues (Bechdolf et al. 2012; Ruhrmann et al. 2010; Schultze-Lutter et al. 2012). One point to bear in mind is that some groups sought to predict schizophrenia (such as Klosterkötter and colleagues), whereas others sought to predict the first episode of a functional psychosis (Yung, McGorry, and the Melbourne group).

In parallel, initial prospective studies of children at risk for developing schizophrenia, before the onset of a first episode (Hartmann et al. 1984, 1985; Watt and Lubensky 1976; Watt et al. 1979), suggested that no gross prototypical behavioral abnormalities could be identified in subjects that would go on to develop schizophrenia in a later stage of life, even though Hartmann et al. concluded simultaneously "that each of the minor (behavioral) abnormalities involves information on one or several separate aspects of a single underlying vulnerability that is simply manifested more clearly in some sorts of behaviour in one case and other sorts in other cases" (Hartmann et al. 1984, p. 1055; Cannon et al. 1990; Jorgensen and Parnas 1990; Jorgensen et al. 1987; Mednick et al. 1987; Parnas 1986, 1999; Parnas and Handest 2003; Parnas and Jorgensen 1989; Sass and Parnas 2003). Such behaviors included: male aggressiveness and female introversion in school (Watt 1978; Watt et al. 1979); difficulties in interpersonal relations, anxiety, neophobia, and flat affect in males (Hartmann et al. 1984); defective emotional rapport, eccentricity, formal thought disorder in HR pre-schizophrenia subjects (Sass and Parnas 2003); and neuromotor disturbances in early life (Rosso et al. 2000).

Other studies show that children who later develop schizophrenia were more likely than peers to show subtle developmental delays and cognitive impairments; they also tend to be solitary and socially anxious (Cannon et al. 2002; Jones et al. 1994). Some evidence suggests that individuals destined to develop schizophrenia fail to learn new cognitive skills as they enter adolescence, thus appearing to show a relative decline compared with their peer group (Fuller et al. 2002). In addition to traditional neurocognitive measures, recent evidence has suggested deficits in social cognition domains in subjects at risk for psychosis (Fett et al. 2011; Thompson et al. 2011a). Impairments in social cognition are a core feature of psychosis, ranging from: (a) deficits in theory of mind (ToM; Bora et al. 2009), which refers to one's ability to comprehend the intentions of others; (b) deficits in social perception and social knowledge (Sergi et al. 2009), both of which refer to the ability to use social cues (e.g., gestures) and apply social rules to a complicated situation; and (c) emotion processing deficits in expression and recognition of facial and prosodic affect (Marwick and Hall 2008). The combination of neurocognitive and emotional deviance increases the likelihood of developing minor quasi-psychotic symptoms: indeed a prospective study in Dunedin, New Zealand, showed pre-schizophreniform individuals to be more likely to manifest such symptoms as early as age eleven years (Cannon et al. 2002; Poulton et al. 2000). It is postulated that in those destined to develop psychosis, the strength, frequency, and associated distress of the odd ideas and experiences increases, and at some ill-defined point, the individual crosses a threshold into the pre-psychotic or prodromal phase (Broome et al. 2005b).

The Continuum of Psychosis

A problem when considering unusual experiences in people without a diagnosis of a psychotic illness, and whether to view such experiences as part of a prodromal phase or not, is the existence of such experiences in those who are not distressed, nor help-seeking, and may not develop a psychiatric illness. It is now clear that not only many children but also a proportion of the general adult population experience brief or isolated psychotic phenomena without coming into contact with psychiatric services (Johns and van Os 2001). For example, in the Dunedin cohort, 25% of the entire population reported having experienced isolated or transient delusions or hallucinations at the age of twenty-six years though only 3.7% met criteria for a schizophreniform illness.

Van Os found a median prevalence rate of around 5% and a median incidence rate of around 3% psychotic symptoms and experiences in the general population (van Os et al. 2009), demonstrating rates much higher than those recognized for clinically significant non-affective psychotic disorder. Another study by the van Os group demonstrated that patients with borderline personality and cluster C personality disorders reported paranoid reactivity and hallucinatory reactivity to daily life stress (Glaser et al. 2010).

Such findings have suggested to some that psychosis is distributed on a continuum and that psychotic phenomena may be present in healthy individuals, in people suffering from non-psychotic mental health disorders, and patients suffering from psychotic disorders. However, the continuum approach has been criticized, both methodologically and conceptually (David 2010; Lawrie et al. 2010), with a growing awareness that we may need to develop a thicker conception of psychosis and psychotic disorder that is less reliant on the presence of positive psychotic symptoms, such as hallucinations and delusions (Murray and Jones 2012), and hence marks a move away from the Schneiderian conception of schizophrenia introduced in the third edition of the *Diagnostic and Statistical Manual of Mental Disorders* (DSM-III).

EARLY DETECTION AND PREVENTION STRATEGIES

However, developing the important work of colleagues in Melbourne, Yale, and Cologne, over the last decades, several research groups have identified clinical characteristics of young people thought to be at UHR of developing frank psychosis and have published measures and semi-structured interviews to assess risk of psychosis (Klosterkötter et al. 2001; McGlashan et al. 2001; Miller et al. 1999, 2002, 2003; Morrison et al. 2004; Yung et al. 1998a, 1998b, 2003, 2004). Typically, individuals in the prodromal phase are described as experiencing cognitive dysfunction as the earliest detectable anomaly, followed by attenuated "negative" symptoms such as decreased motivation and socialization (Cornblatt et al. 2002). Later, positive psychotic symptoms develop but are not sufficient in intensity or duration to meet formal criteria for frank psychotic illness. Measures have been developed based upon those later psychotic experiences as well as the earlier cognitive and negative symptoms.

Broadly, two sets of criteria have been used to diagnose the HR state: the UHR and BS criteria. The UHR criteria have been the most widely applied in the literature to date (Broome et al. 2005a; Carr et al. 2000; Cornblatt et al. 2003; McGlashan et al. 2006; Ruhrmann et al. 2003; Ruhrmann et al. 2010; Simon et al. 2006; Yung et al. 2006) and demarcate the later stage of the prodromal phase, dominated by positive symptoms. Inclusion requires the presence of one or more of: attenuated psychotic symptoms (APS), brief limited intermittent psychotic symptoms (BLIPS), or trait vulnerability plus a marked decline in psychosocial functioning (Genetic Risk and Deterioration Syndrome: GRD) and unspecified prodromal symptoms (UPS). Different interview measures have been developed to assess UHR features and to determine if individuals meet criteria: the Comprehensive Assessment of At Risk Mental State (CAARMS), the Structured Interview for Prodromal Symptoms (SIPS) including the companion Scale of Prodromal Symptoms (SOPS), the Early Recognition Inventory for the Retrospective Assessment of the Onset of Schizophrenia (ERIraos), and the Basel Screening Instrument for Psychosis (BSIP).

BS are anomalous subjective experiences of different domains including perception, thought processing, language and attention that are distinct from classical psychotic symptoms, in that they are independent of abnormal thought content and reality testing and insight into the symptoms' psychopathological nature is intact (Schultze-Lutter 2009). BS, which have been studied prospectively in several studies (Bechdolf et al. 2012; Klosterkötter et al. 2001; Ruhrmann et al. 2010; Schultze-Lutter et al. 2007b; Ziermans et al. 2011), were originally assessed using the Bonn Scale for the Assessment of Basic Symptoms (BSABS; Klosterkötter 1997) and, more recently, the Schizophrenia Proneness Instrument, Adult Version (SPI-A; Schultze-Lutter et al. 2007a) and Child & Youth version (SPI-CY; Schultze-Lutter and Koch 2010). A special version for children and adolescents seemed necessary to make allowance for developmental issues and a distinct clustering of symptoms in this age group (Schultze-Lutter et al. 2012).

Because the UHR and BS criteria relate to complementary sets of clinical features, with the BS perhaps identifying an earlier prodromal state, and the UHR criteria reflecting a somewhat later phase (Keshavan et al. 2011; Klosterkötter et al. 2011) there is an increasing tendency for centers to use both when assessing HR subjects (Fusar-Poli et al. 2008).

In addition to HR symptoms, people who meet criteria for HR in help seeking populations usually present with other clinical concerns. Many have comorbid diagnoses, in particular anxiety, depression, and substance use disorders that are clinically debilitating (Broome et al. 2005a, 2012a; Woods et al. 2009; Yung et al. 2008). High levels of negative symptoms, significant impairments in academic performance and occupational functioning, and difficulties with interpersonal relationships as well as substantially compromised subjective quality of life (Bechdolf et al. 2005) are often observed (Addington et al. 2008; Lencz et al. 2004; Velthorst et al. 2010; Yung et al. 2008). The experience of HR symptoms per se is also associated with a marked impairment in psychosocial functioning (Velthorst et al. 2010) which appears as a core feature of the HR state (Seidman et al. 2010). Social impairment is a predictor of longitudinal outcome (Fusar-Poli et al. 2009; Velthorst et al. 2010) and tends to be resistant to treatment, both pharmacological and psychosocial (Cornblatt et al. 2012). It is also reflected by a considerably decreased subjective quality of life (Bechdolf et al. 2005; Ruhrmann et al. 2008).

Despite concerns about the lack of prediction of putative high risk measures, in a recent meta-analysis of about 2500 HR subjects, using both measures detailed earlier, it was shown that there was a mean transition risk, independent of the psychometric instruments used, of 18% at six months of follow-up, 22% at one year, 29% at two years, and 36% after three years (Fusar-Poli et al. 2012a). Most of the subjects converting to psychosis will develop a schizophrenia spectrum disorder (Fusar-Poli et al. 2012b). The outcome of the non-converters is poorly investigated. Hence, the measures do seem to have some predictive validity.

However, and returning to our discussion of the continuum model of psychosis, if one accepts psychosis as a dimension, then the "at-risk mental state" is likely to cover a segment of it, and the point of transition to a frank psychotic illness, based on frequency and intensity of certain symptoms, can be seen as somewhat arbitrary. This relates to the first concern we outlined earlier: the "UHR" or ARMS could be viewed as being a segment of the continuum coupled with help-seeking, decline of function and/or distress. Hence, this group could be a very heterogeneous population clinically: identified and grouped by the presence of attenuated psychotic symptoms and help-seeking or distress, but where they may vary widely is in actual risk for schizophrenia or other mental illness. Addressing this point, van Os and colleagues suggest a "Psychosis Proneness-Persistence-Impairment Model," whereby transitory subclinical psychotic experiences can become persistent, and eventually of clinical significance, if "at-risk" individuals are exposed to additional environmental risk factors (van Os 2009). Van Os and Delespaul (2005) point out that the highest transition rates occur in those "at-risk" populations which have been most highly selected, and that the process of screening and referral into these populations makes a major contribution to the success of researchers in identifying individuals at such high risk of transition.

Indeed, the predictive accuracy of ARMS criteria depends on the prevalence of the at-risk mental state in the population sampled and thus the population from which the sample is drawn (Thompson et al. 2011b). To date, transition rates have largely been derived from clinical samples of help-seeking subjects who were engaged by specialized early intervention services. These individuals are often referred to these services because of a suspicion that they are at risk for psychosis and thus would be expected to have relatively high base rates of an ARMS, and hence may not be representative of a community, epidemiological sample. Further, how these clinical samples access such services can vary: services can vary between university clinics seeing a population who have passed through many other assessments, to others that are closer to primary care. The prevalence of the ARMS in community samples is still unknown, and it is probable that there are individuals in the community who would meet ARMS criteria but do not seek clinical help. As such, the predictive value of the ARMS criteria may be considerably lower than estimated.

Another potential factor suggesting that the predictive value of the ARMS is influenced by the sampling method is reflected by the declining transition rates of the ARMS over recent years (Yung et al. 2007). This may be explained by the fact that clinical services are detecting ARMS individuals and providing them with care at an earlier stage than in the past (Yung et al. 2007). As a given centre for this group becomes more established, and referrers and the local community become more familiar with the ARMS, it is likely that subjects with ARMS features may be detected and referred earlier, and hence, for the reasons given earlier, the measure, based on attenuated positive symptoms, may be less predictive. Further, even if a subset of this group are genuinely at risk of developing schizophrenia, these individuals are presenting at an earlier stage of the prodrome, and there may be a relatively longer period before transition to psychosis not currently captured in the existing follow-up studies (Yung et al. 2007).

Thus, to summarize, the bald application of ARMS criteria to the general population may have much less predictive power than in a clinic to which individuals suspected of being in a pre-psychotic phase have been specially referred. The reason for this loss of power is the evidence already discussed, namely, that pathways, distress, help seeking, and persistence may also impact on predictive power as well the fact that the commonest outcome of subclinical psychotic symptoms in a general population is remission (Hanssen et al. 2005). On this account, the clinical population is different from the general population not just in the level of psychotic psychopathology, but rather in the prevalence of additional factors that lead to those symptoms being persistent and distressing. These factors are those variables that, although not captured in existing taxonomies, distinguish a neurodevelopmental disorder like schizophrenia from a collection of positive psychotic symptoms. This point returns to an earlier comment: the work on the prodromal phase, and the continuum of psychosis, has forced psychiatry and mental health research to think about a conception of psychotic disorder and of schizophrenia that is less dependent on positive psychotic symptoms: arguably this could be seen as a retreat from the Schneiderian first rank systems approach towards one that, in a more Kraepelinian manner, stresses the significance of clinical course, outcome, general functioning, and neuropsychological performance.

To improve the predictive power of at-risk criteria, the strategy of "sample enrichment" is utilized by most prodromal services to increase their ability to predict transition in an at-risk population. This can lead to the assumption that such enhanced predictive power may be falsely attributed to the psychopathological measure employed, or the symptoms measured, rather than the sampling method (van Os and Delespaul 2005); thus, as noted earlier, the high predictive value may be consequent upon how the patients that make up a prodromal service are selected, rather than their psychopathology or underlying physiological characteristics. On this hypothesis, pathways into services may carry greater predictive power than mental state abnormalities. This is not necessarily because those so detected are any less at risk, but rather that the greater proportion of those in the general population who would meet "at-risk" criteria for developing psychosis will never make it through the various selection procedures that account for the sample enrichment.

However, such epidemiological criticisms may be more valid for some services than others, which have fewer "filters" between the person experiencing early psychotic symptoms and the clinician (Broome et al. 2005a). This is an obvious example of the more general problem we have discussed: findings from cohort, epidemiological, and clinical at-risk studies have not yet been fully integrated. Thus, neurodevelopmental theorists have struggled to explain what converts a developmentally impaired or socially isolated adolescent with odd ideas and experiences into a psychotic individual. Similarly, it is not yet wholly clear what differentiates an individual in the community who experiences hallucinations and holds delusional beliefs but never sees a psychiatrist, from the individual who reaches a specialized clinic for those at risk of psychosis where he/she is considered as prodromal. The work of Hanssen et al. (2005) suggests that the intensity of the experiences is important but so too, they suggest, is depression. Escher et al. (2002) also believe that the coexistence of affective disturbance is a major factor in determining whether young people who experience minor psychotic symptoms will progress to psychotic disorder.

This shift away from a brain- and symptom-based conception of clinical high risk, to one that recognizes the important role of epidemiology and pathways through services, has important theoretical ramifications in how we conceptualize mental illness. Contrary to the prevailing ideology in the DSM-IV, disorders are determined, at least in part, by a series of epidemiological factors and selection filters, by health behaviour of the individual and society, and by the beliefs and attitudes of health and legal professionals. On this conception, disorders can only be understood in relation to their place within the wider society and health system, rather than as free-standing nosological entities. Such a position is further supported by evidence indicating that the definition of "psychosis threshold" within the HR research is somewhat arbitrary (Yung et al. 2010b). The intensity, frequency, and duration of psychotic experiences in HR subjects appear to vary along continua, and defining transition to frank disorder involves making a quantitative distinction between a symptom severity that corresponds to one of two categories (psychosis and non-psychosis; Nelson et al. 2011; Winton-Brown et al. 2011). For example, in the two commonly used instruments used to assess HR subjects, CAARMS and SIPS transition criteria are weighted towards positive psychotic symptoms (Fusar-Poli and Borgwardt 2007). As a result, HR subjects may develop severe negative symptoms or functional impairments, which we may wish to see as part of a disorder, yet still be categorized as not having made a transition to psychosis (Yung et al. 2010b). Based on these considerations, we would suggest, as with the creators of the CAARMS instrument, that the threshold between being at risk and having a frank episode of psychosis is, if not entirely arbitrary, unlikely to be successfully demarcated using narrow clinical, biological, or psychological criteria—but might rather be related to help-seeking, distress, and the wider context, ecology, and response of health services (Raballo et al. 2011).

The Phenomenological Prodrome
of Schizophrenia

Another criticism of the ARMS approach, which looks at attenuated positive symptoms, is grounded in principles and concepts based on the continental European tradition of phenomenological psychopathology (Broome et al. 2012b; Jaspers 1959/1997; Nelson et al. 2009a, 2009b; Nelson and Yung 2009, 2011; Raballo and Nelson 2010; Raballo et al. 2011a; Ratcliffe and Broome 2012).

Instead of screening for the presence of positive symptomatology of psychosis in order to detect people in the prodromal phase of schizophrenia, as with the UHR model discussed earlier, this alternative approach considers the presence of "clinically significant signs" which can be very distinct from psychotic-like experiences and which may have no direct relation with positive symptoms as such. It is posited that these signs signify the presence of vulnerability for the development of schizophrenia particularly, rather than psychosis broadly.

Authors of the European Prediction of Psychosis Study (EPOS) have recently suggested a two-step risk assessment approach to more closely select those at increased risk of transition to schizophrenia. In this model, help-seeking individuals are screened using both the CAARMS and COGDIS scale, the latter based on the BSABS (Ruhrmann et al. 2010).

The "basic symptoms" and BSABS have been developed conducting longitudinal prospective investigation of experiential anomalies of patients with schizophrenia. As discussed briefly already, "basic symptoms" are subtle, anomalous subjective experiences in the domains of affect, perception, cognition, action, and the body (Ebel et al. 1989; Gross 1989). The authors argue that these may be present in every stage of the illness, even during the prodromal phase. These phenomena are called "basic symptoms" because they are understood as direct phenomenological consequences of the underlying pathogenesis of the disorder. The BS have been operationalized in the BSABS, a semi-structured interview, later translated in English in a brief version, as the Schizophrenia Proneness Inventory for Adults, SPI-A (Schultze-Lutter et al. 2007a).

Klosterkötter and colleagues have demonstrated in the Cologne Early Recognition (CER) Project that the BSABS is excellent at identifying a population with increased risk of developing schizophrenia (Klosterkötter et al. 2001). Their study was remarkable as it was the first to demonstrate how subtle anomalies of subjective experiences can herald a first episode of psychosis long before attenuated positive symptoms are present; it therefore represents a distinct strategy to the earlier-described ARMS and UHR approach.

This interest in BS links back to research throughout the twentieth century into the phenomenology of schizophrenia. Since the very beginning of the schizophrenia concept, its prototypical psychopathological features have been extensively described and referred to as disturbances in the "subjective experiential world" and in "the sense of self" of affected subjects by European psychiatrists. Kraepelin used the metaphor of "orchestra without a conductor" to describe the "loss of inner unity" and fragmentation of consciousness that he found so typical for the psychopathology of what he then called "dementia praecox." However, references to disturbances of cognition, consciousness and sense of self were very common in the description of schizophrenic psychopathology in the writings of nearly all prominent classic schizophrenia researchers (Kraepelin 1896). Bleuler, for example, observed that "splitting of the self" ("*Ich-spaltung*") and loss of sense of agency (the feeling of being in control of one's own actions) were central features in the psychopathology of affected subjects (Raballo et al. 2011b); he coined the term "schizophrenia," joining the Ancient Greek *skhizein* "to split" and *phrēn* "mind," to highlight what he saw as its core features. Berze proposed that a subtle alteration of self-consciousness ("primary insufficiency": a pervasive experience of diminished transparency and affectability of awareness) was the primary disorder of schizophrenia (Bleuler 1911/1968; Schultze-Lutter et al. 2007a). Thus, disturbances in the basic structural aspects of 'self awareness' and 'subjectivity' were already noted at the conception of the notion of schizophrenia. Expressions used by European phenomenologists, such as "loss of vital contact with reality" (Parnas 2011), "global crisis of common sense" or "loss of natural evidence" (Broome et al. 2012b), and "loss of ego boundaries" (Broome et al. 2012b) refer to a defective attunement between the self and the outside world. This "lack of attunement" corresponds to what Minkowski called "schizoidia" (Broome et al. 2012b).

Remarkably, the specificity of this psychopathological core is hardly recognizable in any single behavioral disturbance; rather, it is the overall picture that attains some prototypical value, what was later reflected in the notion of the "Gestalt" of schizophrenia. A "Gestalt" refers to a salient unity or intrinsic organization of diverse phenomenal features, based on reciprocal part–whole interactions. Parnas suggests that grasping the notion of the core of schizophrenia in a theoretically adequate manner requires a background theory on the nature of mental life; "a mental state should not be isolated but interpreted as an aspect, a trace of the whole of which it originates"... "Every anomalous mental state contains an imprint of more basic experiential alterations that transpire phenomenally in the single symptoms, shaping them and founding as such the specificity of the overall underlying Gestalt of Schizophrenia" (Parnas 2011, pp. 1123, 74; Wuyts and Parnas 2011).

The Dutch psychiatrist Rümke coined the term "praecox gefühl" ("praecox feeling") referring to the experience of a skilled clinician coming in contact with this "lack of attunement" when assessing someone suffering from schizophrenia. He noted that the praecox feeling surrounds all symptoms of schizophrenia and is evoked due to a lack of directedness and affective attunement of the patient towards other people and the world beyond. According to Rümke, the praecox feeling is the essential "colouration of schizophrenia" (Broome et al. 2012b).

Examination of Anomalous Self-Experience

Drawing from phenomenological psychopathology tradition, descriptions from patients suffering from schizophrenia and empirical research using BSABS, Parnas and colleagues have developed the "Examination of Anomalous Self-Experience" (EASE; Parnas 2005; Parnas and Handest 2003; Parnas et al. 2005). The EASE is a semi-structured interview with a specific focus on disturbances in the structure of self-awareness and consciousness. The term "structural" refers to enduring and enabling conditions that make a normal deployment of cognition and affectivity possible. To such conditions belong pre-reflective self-awareness, comprising the first-person perspective, sense of one's enduring living presence and the transparency and availability of consciousness as a medium and a source. Temporality, embodiment and the intentionality of consciousness are other such structural conditions (Jansson and Parnas 2007; Parnas 2005, 2011; Parnas et al. 2005; Raballo and Parnas 2011; Sass and Parnas 2003). These disturbances are not explicit in the focus of thematic attention but constitute the overall background of awareness. The EASE instrument should be deployed to establish a dynamic dialogue with the patient, exploring his or her subjective experiential world and attempting to describe disturbances in the different domains of consciousness such as "hyper-reflexivity" (or excessive awareness of one's own mental activities which accordingly become objects of interest in their own right, rather than affording a normal transparent cognitive access to the outer world) and disturbances of "ipseity" (or the sense of self) in detail.

The EASE contains five different domains:

1. *Cognition and stream of consciousness.* A normal sense of consciousness as continuous over time, flowing, inhabited by one subject and introspectively transparent (immediately or directly given) in a non-spatial way.

2. *Self-awareness and presence.* A normal sense of being (existence) involves automatic unreflected self-presence and immersion in the world (natural, automatic, self-evident). This phenomenological concept of presence implies that in our everyday transactions with the world the sense of self and sense of immersion in the world are inseparable, "Subject and object are two abstract moments of a unique structure which is *presence*" (Merleau-Ponty 1962/2002, p. 430).

3. *Bodily experiences.* A normal sense of psychophysical unity and coherence, a normal interplay or oscillation of the body as "lived from within" as a subject or soul (non-spatial, spiritual "Leib") and of the body as an object (spatial and physical "Körper"). In other words, our bodily experience is neither of an object nor of a pure subject. It is simultaneously both.

4. *Demarcation/transitivism.* Loss or permeability of self-world boundary. These disorders are closely linked to disorders of self-awareness and presence, but are listed separately because of their more articulated symptomatic nature.

5. *Existential reorientation.* The patient experiences a fundamental reorientation with respect to his general metaphysical worldview and/or hierarchy of values, projects and interests. Basically, the experiences of anomalies in self-awareness are enacted and existentially expressed.

In a study using a population sample and comparing schizophrenia spectrum conditions (schizophrenia and schizotypal personality disorder), other mental conditions and a control group, Raballo demonstrated a specific aggregation of "self-disorders" in the schizophrenia spectrum conditions (Raballo et al. 2011b, p. 349). Furthermore, previous research has demonstrated that disorders of self-experience can discriminate individuals suffering from residual schizophrenia spectrum disorders from individuals suffering from bipolar disorder and from patients with various non-schizophrenia spectrum diagnoses (Parnas et al. 2003; Parnas and Handest 2003).

In another study, Parnas and colleagues demonstrated that self-disorders and perplexity remain stable over a five-year period in people suffering from schizophrenia and as such can be suggested to be trait-like features of the schizophrenia spectrum vulnerability. It is therefore concluded that these features might be important prognostic indicators for identifying those subjects in the prodromal phase (Parnas et al. 2011). That such disturbances are present and can be assessed in adolescents at risk (according to CAARMS criteria) has recently been demonstrated by Nelson, who showed that basic self-disturbance predict psychosis onset in the UHR group, using the EASE interview in a two-step approach (Nelson et al. 2012).

The Prodrome and Continuum of Psychosis: Brief Summary

Recent interest in the prodromal phase of psychotic disorders has re-ignited the debate on the construct validity of psychotic disorders in general and schizophrenia in particular. When based merely on operationalized criteria, predominant attention on positive symptomatology has been shown limited success in discriminating those help-seeking individuals at risk of developing psychosis from other help-seeking individuals. It is now acknowledged that psychotic-like experiences are abundant also in the general population and in people suffering from non-psychotic mental health disorders and that "psychosis" is a fluctuating state, its features changing in time and severity and its presence not necessarily linked to an underlying psychotic disorder such as schizophrenia. On the other hand, even as schizophrenia is still characterized by episodes of severe psychosis, it is a neurodevelopmental disorder with an often slow and gradual course and coming to expression only when the interplay of genetic vulnerability and environmental risk factors allows its progression. The phenomenological tradition argues that subtle alterations in the subjective experiential world such as self-disorders, hyper-reflectivity, and perplexity signify the first features of a development towards schizophrenia, long before its prototypical symptomatology reveals itself.

Clinical and Ethical Implications

We have seen that the prodromal phase of psychosis may represent a segment of a heterogenous sample of those with psychotic experiences within the general population, with some cases progressing to frank psychosis. However, a significant proportion resolve spontaneously, and many do not experience distress or seek help. So how do we as clinicians judge when and to whom we should target intervention? Furthermore, what kind of intervention would be appropriate, acceptable, and effective?

The principle of early intervention in psychosis is now widely accepted. However, early detection and intervention in individuals with ARMS is a more controversial area, but one that has generated an enormous amount of research interest and investment. While targeting interventions with the purpose of preventing or delaying the onset of psychosis is hugely appealing, a number of authors have highlighted ethical and clinical concerns (Cornblatt et al. 2002; McGlashan et al. 2001; McGorry et al. 2001; McGuire 2002; Warner 2005). These concerns focus on the validity of the ARMS criteria and the related problem of "false positives"; this clinical problem relates seamlessly to the more conceptual issues discussed earlier.

Even in research trials there is huge variability in transition rates from ARMS to psychosis. For example, in the original PACE trial using the UHR criteria there was a transition rate of 35–40% over twelve months. However, other research groups using the same or similar criteria have reported twelve-month transition rates of as many as 54% in the PRIME clinic at Yale University and as little as 15% in the CARE clinic in San Diego. In the original PACE clinic, a significant reduction in transition rates over time has also been observed, with a six-month transition rate of only 9.2% being reported in 2007 (Haroun et al. 2006; Miller and McGlashan 2000; Miller et al. 2002; Yung et al. 1998b, 2003, 2007). This may be a positive effect due to treatments being more effective at the very early stages of illness or a negative "dilution effect" due to finding more "false positives" (see later). As we have already discussed, it is also likely that when criteria used to detect at-risk individuals are applied to less highly selected populations, false positive rates will be much higher. It could be argued that the tools used are not yet well enough refined, relying on arbitrary cutoff points to select those at risk of developing psychosis. Yet, this does not fit with the conceptualization of psychosis being a dimensional variable, with varying degrees of risk of developing a psychotic illness in the "at-risk" population, and such risk possibly being attributable to environmental factors. Currently the instruments used rely on the presence of subclinical features of psychosis, or "state and trait" markers, to the exclusion of important environmental variables. As such the presence of attenuated positive symptoms may be epiphenomenal to the risk, i.e., they are merely markers for other causal processes that convey the risk.

Implications for Treatment

of the Prodrome

Even if positive symptoms were markers of risk, then there would still be a question of whether treating them with antipsychotics will have a role in averting onset of the disorder. However, if they are not good markers of risk, and as such, even less likely to be on the causal path, then it is even less likely that treating them symptomatically with antipsychotics will ameliorate the risk of developing a psychotic disorder or schizophrenia. An alternate causal account needs to be developed which in turn may inspire use of alternate pharmacological agents (Amminger et al. 2010) or perhaps, given the arguments detailed earleir, thinking about causality in a more public health and epidemiological manner (Campbell 2009), where the precise internal pathophysiology of the condition may be in doubt, may enable efficacious political and social interventions (Campbell 2009; van Os and Delespaul 2005; van Os and Linscott 2012). Examples where changes in public policy could affect major mental illness incidence may include addressing social inequality, cannabis use, migrants' experience of racism, and urban deprivation.

More concretely, there is concern about the potential harmful consequences of over-treatment and stigmatization of individuals identified as being at risk, who will never develop a psychotic illness (Warner 2005). These are the so-called "false positive" at-risk individuals—i.e., those who are not prodromal for psychosis ultimately, but meet at-risk criteria cross-sectionally. This may be for the reasons already detailed. Also, where antipsychotics are used as an intervention, there is a risk of iatrogenic dopamine sensitization, symptom rebound on drug withdrawal (Warner 2005) and brain changes. Despite these concerns, in the proposed revisions for DSM-5 (<http://www.dsm5. org/ProposedRevisions>) there is a new category referred to as "Attenuated Psychotic Symptoms Syndrome" (Carpenter and van Os 2011; Fusar-Poli and Yung 2012; Tandon and Carpenter 2012) that is suggested for inclusion or as part of the Appendix (Yung et al. 2012). This construct is largely based upon attenuated positive symptoms, as discussed earlier and, like the measures used to assess the "at-risk mental state," may pick out a group that merges with those members of the normal population who have unusual experiences—and hence also relies on the possibly false assumption that the risk of psychotic disorder is best indexed by the presence of certain symptoms. Arguably, the DSM-5 proposal conflates a "risk syndrome" with the earliest signs of the disorder, a *forme fruste*, in linking their category with the retrospective abnormalities seen in cohorts with the disorder. Although detection of those at risk of psychosis is an important ethical, scientific, and clinical duty, reifying this research program into a DSM-5 category may have the problematic consequence of over-identification of people as at risk, missing those who are genuinely likely to develop psychosis, and offering needless or, indeed, harmful interventions to those whose outcome may be benign. Diagnostic creep may occur resulting in lowering of the high threshold and subsequent reduction in transition rate (Yung et al. 2010a). Ironically, the codification of the HR may actually reduce research in the area (Drake and Lewis 2010) as it may give a false degree of comfort with the current definition. A further ethical concern is the tension between reassurance and normalization of the unusual experiences with the follow-up and monitoring present in HR services, and genuine appreciation of risk.

Further, we have to be aware of iatrogenic harms, even if unforeseen and unintended. The monitoring and care offered to those with unusual experiences may itself, through its impact on anxiety, appraisals, etc., have the paradoxical effect of increasing, rather than decreasing, the rate of transition in an at-risk group if not delivered in services of certain levels of skill and expertise. Expanding clinical awareness and service delivery may lead to this and other unwanted outcomes, one of which may be how the criminal justice systems decides to treat an offender who demonstrates the Attenuated Psychotic Symptom Syndrome: will it be viewed as a mental disorder, with all the attendant consequences to both the patient, the courts, and the clinicians? Or will the court just interpret it as a state of increased risk to development of psychotic disorders (Broome et al. 2010)?

Furthermore, how much information should clinicians who work in early detection share with their patients deemed to be at risk? Should clinicians consider whether patients have a right not to know their prognosis (Bortolotti and Widdows 2011)? Given that no specific treatments have been demonstrated to alter clinical course, one could argue that there may be no positive benefit in knowing. Further, there are the possible harms of self-stigmatization and fear from the potential diagnosis. Unlike in seemingly analogous states, such as screening for cancer, the difference in psychosis is that such negative affects may themselves be of causal relevance in the development of psychosis, as noted earlier. Hence, the monitoring and support of early detection services, if not handled sensitively and carefully, may have the unwanted outcome of making the individual more depressed and anxious, and that in turn may lead to a greater intensity and frequency of their psychotic symptoms, change in the way they appraise them, and ultimately a greater chance of transition to an episode of frank psychosis.

Possible Solutions and
Future Directions

Supporters of early detection and intervention argue that in spite of the high false positive rate, those identified are by definition help seeking and in need of some form of care, whether or not they go on to develop a psychotic or non-psychotic disorder (McGorry 2008). They also argue that the risk of lack of or delayed care, in terms of clinical and functional outcomes, far overshadows the theoretical one of premature labeling and overtreatment (McGorry 2008). Further, it seems clear that those clients, even if they do develop a psychotic illness, may have a better outcome after having been through early detection services (Valmaggia et al. 2009).

Contemporary classifications (such as DSM-IV or the International Classification of Disease, tenth revision (ICD-10)) offer criteria for rather stable conditions (e.g., schizophrenia), but do not consider early phases of psychosis. However, the diagnosis of a psychotic disorder is based on the presence of characteristic symptoms, and it is well known that the presence of such symptoms varies during its course and treatment (McGorry et al. 2009; Salvatore et al. 2009; Whitty et al. 2005). The clinical staging model, which has been widely used in somatic medicine but virtually ignored in psychiatry, provides a coherent clinicopathological framework which can restore the utility of diagnosis and promote early intervention. Such staging defines the progression of the disease in time and helps us determine where a person lies along the course of the illness. The staging indicates both increasing risk of disorder, with unspecific conditions at the initial stages and more define clinical-diagnostic profiles at the later stages (Raballo and Laroi 2009), and parallel changes in processes thought to underpin the development of the disorder.

At least four stages have now been identified: first a premorbid phase with endophenotypic vulnerability traits and risk factors but no significant psychosocial impairment; second, an early prodromal phase with anomalous subjective experiences, initial psychosocial impairment, deterioration of quality of life and inter-peer performance; third, a late prodromal phase of subthreshold attenuated psychotic symptoms and/or brief, limited, intermittent psychosis (this phase would map onto that captured by most measures to determine the prodrome); fourth, a phase with full-blown prolonged psychotic symptoms which may develop into schizophrenia (Raballo and Laroi 2009).

The advantages of considering a clinical staging model are substantial. A stratification of interventions could be developed for conditions not considered in the available diagnostic classifications. It offers a progression through at-risk mental states which could lead to a spectrum of phase-specific treatments, providing earlier, safer, and more effective clinical interventions with potential to clarify the biological basis of psychiatric disorders, minimize stigma and re-organize mental health care (McGorry et al. 2006, 2009; Raballo and Laroi 2009). Yung and McGorry advocate the use of clinical staging so that treatment can be tailored according to the stage of illness, preventing overtreatment and reducing stigma (McGorry 2008; Yung et al. 2007). This would allow for a period of observation, monitoring, and treatment of comorbid disorders (such as depression, anxiety, and substance misuse disorders).

Conclusions

There has been an increasing move away from studying solely discrete, categorical psychotic illnesses towards a continuum model of psychosis. Our view would be that psychosis as a psychopathological state, characterized by hallucinations and delusions, should be seen in a continuum, while schizophrenia should be seen as a neurodevelopmental disorder, primarily characterized by recurring states of psychosis, but also by other features. This view also impacts upon the status of the prodromal phase or at-risk mental state. There is a tension between it being seen both as a syndrome and collection of mental state abnormalities, if a somewhat fuzzy category, and as a region of the psychosis continuum with somewhat arbitrary borders. The danger lies in the assumption that categorical phenomena are more likely to have discrete pathophysiology (Broome 2006) when in fact it may be that there is a rich diversity of variables to be examined that serve as risk factors for a given individual progressing along the continuum to frank psychosis, particularly in the latter stages from at risk to first episode. As such, risk factors are proximal markers or causes that may be useful as predictors or as targets for therapeutic intervention. Related to these issues is a narrower research question of whether focusing on the at-risk phase is worthwhile in understanding psychosis. The epidemiological data (an der Heiden and Häfner 2000) suggests that the vast majority of those who develop a psychotic disorder go through a prodromal phase. However, this phase is currently characterized in different ways, with some groups studying the prodromal phase of psychosis, others the prodrome of schizophrenia, and with others distinguishing between an early and late prodromal phase or attenuated negative and attenuated positive syndrome.

In the light of these complications, some researchers propose a return to the phenomenological psychopathology of early 20th century continental psychiatry. It is proclaimed that the vast range of anomalous subjective experiences and symptoms of psychotic disorders are in fact various expressions of one central underlying disturbance, directly related to the pathophysiology of the disorder, i.e. the fundamental alteration in the structure of self-awareness (the 'Gestalt'). We have also noted several of the important clinical and ethical issues that arise in both indentifying and intervening in this HR group, and how these are now cast sharply into focus with the inclusion of the risk syndrome in the draft DSM-5.

Acknowledgments

The authors would like to thank Dr. Richard Gipps for his helpful comments on earlier drafts of the chapter.

References

Addington, J., Penn, D., Woods, S. W., Addington, D., and Perkins, D. O. (2008). Social functioning in individuals at clinical high risk for psychosis. *Schizophrenia Research*, *99*(1–3), 119–24.

Amminger, G. P., Schäfer, M. R., Papageorgiou, K., Klier, C. M., Cotton, S. M., Harrigan, S. M., *et al.* (2010). Long-chain omega-3 fatty acids for indicated prevention of psychotic disorders: a randomized, placebo-controlled trial. *Archives of General Psychiatry*, *67*(2), 146–54.

an der Heiden, W. and Häfner, H. (2000). The epidemiology of onset and course of schizophrenia. *European Archives of Psychiatry and Clinical Neuroscience*, *250*(6), 292–303.

Bechdolf, A., Pukrop, R., Köhn, D., Tschinkel, S., Veith, V., Schultze-Lutter, F., *et al.* (2005). Subjective quality of life in subjects at risk for a first episode of psychosis: a comparison with first episode schizophrenia patients and healthy controls. *Schizophrenia Research*, *79*(1), 137–43.

Bechdolf, A., Wagner, M., Ruhrmann, S., Harrigan, S., Putzfeld, V., Pukrop, R., *et al.* (2012). Preventing progression to first-episode psychosis in early initial prodromal state. *British Journal of Psychiatry*, *200*(1), 22–9.

Bleuler, E. (1968). *Dementia Praecox or the Group of Schizophrenias* (J. Zinkin, Trans.). New York, NY: International Universities Press. (Original work published 1911.)

Bora, E., Yucel, M., and Pantelis, C. (2009). Theory of mind impairment in schizophrenia: meta-analysis. *Schizophrenia Research*, *109*(1–3), 1–9.

Bortolotti, L. and Broome, M. (2009). The future of scientific psychiatry. In M. Broome and L. Bortolotti (Eds), *Psychiatry as Cognitive Neuroscience: Philosophical Perpsctives*, pp. 365–75. Oxford: Oxford University Press.

Bortolotti, L. and Widdows, H. (2011). The right not to know: the case of psychiatric disorders. *Journal of Medical Ethics*, *37*(11), 673–6.

Boydell, J., van Os, J., McKenzie, K., and Murray, R. M. (2004). The association of inequality with the incidence of schizophrenia—an ecological study. *Social Psychiatry and Psychiatric Epidemiology*, *39* (8), 597–9.

Broome, M. R. (2006). Taxonomy and ontology in psychiatry: A survey of recent literature. *Philosophy, Psychiatry, & Psychology*, *13* (4), 303–19.

Broome, M. and Bortolotti, L. (Eds) (2009). *Psychiatry as Cognitive Neuroscience: Philosophical Perspectives*. Oxford: Oxford University Press.

Broome, M. R., Bortolotti, L., and Mameli, M. (2010). Moral responsibility and mental illness: a case study. *Cambridge Quarterly of Healthcare Ethics*, *19*(2), 179–87.

Broome, M. R., Day, F., Valli, I., Valmaggia, L., Johns, L. C., Howes, O., *et al.* (2012a). Delusional ideation, manic symptomatology and working memory in a cohort at clinical high-risk for psychosis: A longitudinal study. *European Psychiatry*, *27*(4), 258–63.

Broome, M. R., Harland, R., Owen, G. S., and Stringaris, A. (Eds) (2012b). *The Maudsley Reader in Phenomenological Psychiatry*. Cambridge: Cambridge University Press.

Broome, M. R., Woolley, J. B., Johns, L. C., Valmaggia, L. R., Tabraham, P., Gafoor, R., et al. (2005a). Outreach and support in South London (OASIS): implementation of a clinical service for prodromal psychosis and the at risk mental state. *European Psychiatry, 20*, 372–8.

Broome, M. R., Woolley, J. B., Tabraham, P., Johns, L. C., Bramon, E., Murray, G. K., et al. (2005b). What causes the onset of psychosis? *Schizophrenia Research, 79*(1), 23–34.

Bullmore, E. T., Woodruff, P. W., Wright, I. C., Rabe-Hesketh, S., Howard, R. J., Shuriquie, N., et al. (1998). Does dysplasia cause anatomical dysconnectivity in schizophrenia? *Schizophrenia Research, 30*(2), 127–35.

Campbell, J. (2009). What does rationality have to do with psychological causation? Propositional attitudes as control variables and as mechanisms. In M. Broome and L. Bortolotti (Eds), *Psychiatry as Cognitive Neuroscience: Philosophical Perspectives*, pp. 137–49. Oxford: Oxford University Press.

Cannon, M., Caspi, A., Moffitt, T. E., Harrington, H., Taylor, A., Murray, R. M., et al. (2002). Evidence for early-childhood, pan-developmental impairment specific to schizophreniform disorder: results from a longitudinal birth cohort. *Archives of General Psychiatry, 59*(5), 449–56.

Cannon, T. D., Mednick, S. A., and Parnas, J. (1990). Antecedents of predominantly negative- and predominantly positive-symptom schizophrenia in a high-risk population. *Archives of General Psychiatry, 47*(7), 622–32.

Carpenter, W. T. and van Os, J. (2011). Should attenuated psychosis syndrome be a DSM-5 diagnosis? *American Journal of Psychiatry, 168*(5), 460–3.

Carr, V., Halpin, S., Lau, N., O'Brien, S., Beckmann, J., and Lewin, T. (2000). A risk factor screening and assessment protocol for schizophrenia and related psychosis. *Australian and New Zealand Journal of Psychiatry, 34*(Suppl), S170–80.

Cornblatt, B., Lencz, T., and Obuchowski, M. (2002). The schizophrenia prodrome: treatment and high-risk perspectives. *Schizophrenia Research, 54*(1–2), 177–86.

Cornblatt, B. A, Carrión, R. E., Addington, J., Seidman, L., Walker, E. F., Cannon, T. D., et al. (2012). Risk factors for psychosis: Impaired social and role functioning. *Schizophrenia Bulletin, 38*(6), 1247–57.

Cornblatt, B. A., Lencz, T., Smith, C. W., Correll, C. U., Auther, A. M., et al. (2003). The schizophrenia prodrome revisited: a neurodevelopmental perspective. *Schizophrenia Bulletin, 29*(4), 633–51.

David, A. S. (2010). Why we need more debate on whether psychotic symptoms lie on a continuum with normality. *Psychological Medicine, 40*(12), 1935–42.

Drake, R. J. and Lewis, S. W. (2010). Valuing prodromal psychosis: what do we get and what is the price? *Schizophrenia Research, 120*(1–3), 38–41.

Ebel, H., Gross, G., Klosterkötter, J., and Huber, G. (1989). Basic symptoms in schizophrenic and affective psychoses. *Psychopathology, 22*(4), 224–32.

Escher, S., Romme, M., Buiks, A., Delespaul, P., and van Os, J. (2002). Independent course of childhood auditory hallucinations: a sequential 3-year follow-up study. *British Journal of Psychiatry, Supplement, 43*, s10–8.

Fett, A. K., Viechtbauer, W., Dominguez, M. D., Penn, D. L., van Os, J., and Krabbendam, L. (2011). The relationship between neurocognition and social cognition with functional outcomes in schizophrenia: a meta-analysis. *Neuroscience and Biobehavioural Reviews, 35*(3), 573–88.

Fuller, R., Nopoulos, P., Arndt, S., O'Leary, D., Ho, B. C., and Andreasen, N. C. (2002). Longitudinal assessment of premorbid cognitive functioning in patients with schizophrenia through examination of standardized scholastic test performance. *American Journal of Psychiatry*, 159(7), 1183–9.

Fusar-Poli, P., Bechdolf, A., Taylor, M. J., Bonoldi, I., Carpenter, W. T., Yung, A. R., *et al.* (2012b). At risk for schizophrenic or affective psychosis? A meta-analysis of ICD/DSM diagnostic outcomes in individuals at high clinical risk. *Schizophrenia Bulletin*, doi: 10.1093/schbul/sbs060.

Fusar-Poli, P., Bonoldi, I., Yung, A. R., Borgwardt, S., Kempton, M., Barale, F., *et al.* (2012a). Predicting psychosis: a meta-analysis of evidence. *Archives of General Psychiatry*, 69(3), 220–9.

Fusar-Poli, P. and Borgwardt, S. (2007). Integrating the negative psychotic symptoms in the high risk criteria for the prediction of psychosis. *Medical Hypotheses*, 69(4), 959–60.

Fusar-Poli, P., Borgwardt, S., and Valmaggia, L. (2008). Heterogeneity in the assessment of the at-risk mental state for psychosis. *Psychiatric Services*, 59(7), 813.

Fusar-Poli, P., Byrne, M., Valmaggia, L., Day, F., Tabraham, P., Johns, L., *et al.* (2009). Social dysfunction predicts two years clinical outcomes in people at ultra high risk for psychosis. *Journal of Psychiatric Research*, 44(5), 294–301.

Fusar-Poli, P. and Yung, A. R. (2012). Should attenuated psychosis syndrome be included in DSM-5? *Lancet*, 379(9816), 591–2.

Glaser, J. P., van Os, J., Thewissen, V., and Myin-Germeys, I. (2010). Psychotic reactivity in borderline personality disorder. *Acta Psychiatrica Scandinavica*, 121(2), 125–34.

Gross, G. (1989). The 'basic' symptoms of schizophrenia. *British Journal of Psychiatry, Supplementum*, 7, 21–5; discussion 37–40.

Häfner, H., Maurer, K., Löffler, W., an der Heiden, W., Munk-Jørgensen, P., Hambrecht, M., *et al.* (1998). The ABC Schizophrenia Study: a preliminary overview of the results. *Social Psychiatry and Psychiatric Epidemiology*, 33(8), 380–6.

Häfner, H., Maurer, K., Löffler, W., and Riecher-Rössler, A. (1993). The influence of age and sex on the onset and early course of schizophrenia. *British Journal of Psychiatry*, 162, 80–6.

Häfner, H., Riecher-Rössler, A., Hambrecht, M., Maurer, K., Meissner, S., Schmidtke, A., *et al.* (1992a). IRAOS: an instrument for the assessment of onset and early course of schizophrenia. *Schizophrenia Research*, 6(3), 209–23.

Häfner, H., Riecher-Rössler, A., Maurer, K., Fätkenheuer, B., and Löffler, W. (1992b). First onset and early symptomatology of schizophrenia. A chapter of epidemiological and neurobiological research into age and sex differences. *European Archives of Psychiatry and Clinical Neuroscience*, 242(2–3), 109–18.

Hanssen, M., Bak, M., Bijl, R., Vollebergh, W., and van Os, J. (2005). The incidence and outcome of subclinical psychotic experiences in the general population. *British Journal of Clinical Psychology*, 44(Pt 2), 181–91.

Haroun, N., Dunn, L., Haroun, A., and Cadenhead, K. S. (2006). Risk and protection in prodromal schizophrenia: ethical implications for clinical practice and future research. *Schizophrenia Bulletin*, 32, 166–78.

Hartmann, E., Milofsky, E., Vaillant, G., Oldfield, M., Falke, R., and Ducey, C. (1984). Vulnerability to schizophrenia. Prediction of adult schizophrenia using childhood information. *Archives of General Psychiatry*, 41(11), 1050–6.

Hartmann, E., Mitchell, W., Brune, P., and Greenwald, D. (1985). Vulnerability to schizophrenia: childhood indicators predict adult outcome. *Psychopharmacology Bulletin*, 21(3), 503–8.

Howes, O. D., McDonald, C., Cannon, M., Arseneault, L., Boydell, J., and Murray, R. M. (2004). Pathways to schizophrenia: the impact of environmental factors. *International Journal of Neuropsychopharmacology*, 7(Suppl 1), S7–S13.

Huber, G. and Gross, G. (1989). The concept of basic symptoms in schizophrenic and schizoaffective psychoses. *Recent Progress in Medicine*, 80(12), 646–52.

Jackson, H. J., McGorry, P. D., and McKenzie, D. (1994). The reliability of DSM-III prodromal symptoms in first-episode psychotic patients. *Acta Psychiatrica Scandinavica*, 90(5), 375–8.

Jansson, L. B. and Parnas, J. (2007). Competing definitions of schizophrenia: what can be learned from polydiagnostic studies? *Schizophrenia Bulletin*, 33(5), 1178–200.

Jaspers, K. (1997). *General Psychopathology* (J. Hoenig and M.W. Hamilton, Trans.). Baltimore, MD: Johns Hopkins University Press. (Original work published 1959.)

Johns, L. C. and van Os, J. (2001). The continuity of psychotic experiences in the general population. *Clinical Psychology Review*, 21(8), 1125–41.

Jones, P., Rodgers, B., Murray, R., and Marmot, M. (1994). Child development risk factors for adult schizophrenia in the British 1946 birth cohort. *Lancet*, 344(8934), 1398–402.

Jorgensen, A. and Parnas, J. (1990). The Copenhagen High-Risk Study. Premorbid and clinical dimensions of maternal schizophrenia. *Journal of Nervous and Mental Disease*, 178(6), 370–6.

Jorgensen, A., Teasdale, T. W., Parnas, J., Schulsinger, F., Schulsinger, H., and Mednick S. A. (1987). The Copenhagen high-risk project. The diagnosis of maternal schizophrenia and its relation to offspring diagnosis. *British Journal of Psychiatry*, 151, 753–7.

Keshavan, M. S., DeLisi, L. E., and Seidman, L. J. (2011). Early and broadly defined psychosis risk mental states. *Schizophrenia Research*, 126(1–3), 1–10.

Klosterkötter, J., Ebel, H., Schultze-Lutter, F., and Steinmeyer, E. M. (1996). Diagnostic validity of basic symptoms. *European Archives of Psychiatry and Clinical Neuroscience*, 246 (3), 147–54.

Klosterkötter, J., Gross, G., Huber, G., Wieneke, A., Steinmeyer, E. M., Schultze-Lutter, F. (1997). Evaluation of the Bonn Scale for the Assessment of Basic Symptoms—BSABS as an instrument for the assessment of schizophrenia proneness: A review of recent findings. *Neurology, Psychiatry and Brain Research*, 5, 137–50.

Klosterkötter, J., Hellmich, M., Steinmeyer, E. M., and Schultze-Lutter, F. (2001). Diagnosing schizophrenia in the initial prodromal phase. *Archives of General Psychiatry*, 58(2), 158–64.

Klosterkötter, J., Schultze-Lutter, F., Bechdolf, A., and Ruhrmann, S. (2011). Prediction and prevention of schizophrenia: what has been achieved and where to go next? *World Psychiatry*, 10(3), 165–74.

Kraepelin, E. (1896). *Psychiatrie*. Leipzig: Barth.

Lawrie, S. M., Hall, J., McIntosh, A. M., Owens, D. G., and Johnstone, E. C. (2010). The 'continuum of psychosis': scientifically unproven and clinically impractical. *British Journal of Psychiatry*, 197(6), 423–5.

Lencz, T., Smith, C.W., Auther, A., Correll, C. U., and Cornblatt, B. (2004). Nonspecific and attenuated negative symptoms in patients at clinical high-risk for schizophrenia. *Schizophrenia Research*, 68(1), 37–48.

Marwick, K. and Hall, J. (2008). Social cognition in schizophrenia: a review of face processing. *British Medical Bulletin*, 88(1), 43–58.

Mayer-Gross, W. (1932). Die Klinik der Schizophrenie. In O. Bunke (Ed.), *Handbuch der Geisteskrankheiten* (Vol. IX), pp. 293–578. Berlin: Springer.

McDonald, C., Fearon, P., and Murray, R. (1999). Neurodevelopmental hypothesis of schizophrenia 12 years on: data and doubts. In J. L. Rapoport (Ed.), *Childhood Onset of "Adult" Psychopathology*, pp. 193–220. Washington, DC: American Psychiatric Press.

McGlashan, T. H., Miller, T. J., and Woods, S. W. (2001). Pre-onset detection and intervention research in schizophrenia psychoses: current estimates of benefit and risk. *Schizophrenia Bulletin, 27*(4), 563–70.

McGlashan, T. H., Walsh, B. C., and Woods, S. W. (2010). *The Psychosis-Risk Syndrome: Handbook for Diagnosis and Follow-Up*. New York, NY: Oxford University Press.

McGlashan, T. H., Zipursky, R. B., Perkins, D., Addington, J., Miller, T., Woods, S. W., *et al.* (2006). Randomized, double-blind trial of olanzapine versus placebo in patients prodromally symptomatic for psychosis. *American Journal of Psychiatry, 163*(5), 790–9.

McGorry, P. (2008). Head to head. Is early intervention in the major psychiatric disorders justified? Yes. *British Medical Journal, 337*, a695.

McGorry, P. D., Hickie, I. B., Yung, A. R., Pantelis, C., and Jackson, H. J. (2006). Clinical staging of psychiatric disorders: a heuristic framework for choosing earlier, safer and more effective interventions. *Australian and New Zealand Journal of Psychiatry, 40*(8), 616–22.

McGorry, P. D., Nelson, B., Amminger, G. P., Bechdolf, A., Francey, S. M., Berger, G., *et al.* (2009). Intervention in individuals at ultra high risk for psychosis: a review and future directions. *Journal of Clinical Psychiatry, 70*(9), 1206–12.

McGorry, P. D., Yung, A., and Phillips, L. (2001). Ethics and early intervention in psychosis: keeping up the pace and staying in step. *Schizophrenia Research, 51*(1), 17–29.

McGuire, P. K. (2002). Prodromal intervention: the need for evaluation. *Journal of Mental Health, 11*, 469–70.

Mednick, S. A., Parnas, J., and Schulsinger, F. (1987). The Copenhagen High-Risk Project, 1962–86. *Schizophrenia Bulletin, 13*(3), 485–95.

Merleau-Ponty, M. (2002). *The Phenomenology of Perception* (C. Smith, Trans.) London: Routledge. (Original work published 1962.)

Miller, T. J. and McGlashan, T. H. (2000). Early identification and intervention in psychotic illness. *Connecticut Medicine, 64*(6), 339–41.

Miller, T. J., McGlashan, T. H., Rosen, J. L., Cadenhead, K., Cannon, T., Ventura, J., *et al.* (2003). Prodromal assessment with the structured interview for prodromal syndromes and the scale of prodromal symptoms: predictive validity, interrater reliability, and training to reliability. [Erratum appears in *Schizophrenia Bulletin* 2004; *30*(2), following 217]. *Schizophrenia Bulletin, 29*(4), 703–15.

Miller, T. J., McGlashan, T. H., Rosen, J. L., Somjee, L., Markovich, P. J., Stein, K., *et al.* (2002). Prospective diagnosis of the initial prodrome for schizophrenia based on the Structured Interview for Prodromal Syndromes: preliminary evidence of interrater reliability and predictive validity. *American Journal of Psychiatry, 159*(5), 863–5.

Miller, T. J., McGlashan, T. H., Woods, S. W., Stein, K., Driesen, N., Corcoran, C. M., *et al.* (1999). Symptom assessment in schizophrenic prodromal states. *Psychiatric Quarterly, 70*(4), 273–87.

Morgan, C., Kirkbride, J., Leff, J., Craig, T., Hutchinson, G., McKenzie, K., *et al.* (2007). Parental separation, loss and psychosis in different ethnic groups: a case-control study. *Psychological Medicine, 37*(4), 495–503.

Morrison, A. P., French, P., Walford, L., Lewis, S. W., Kilcommons, A., Green, J., *et al.* (2004). Cognitive therapy for the prevention of psychosis in people at ultra-high risk: randomised controlled trial. *British Journal of Psychiatry, 185*, 291–7.

Murray, G. K. and Jones, P. B. (2012). Psychotic symptoms in young people without psychotic illness: mechanisms and meaning. *British Journal of Psychiatry, 201*(1), 4–6.

Murray, R. M. and Lewis, S. W. (1987). Is schizophrenia a neurodevelopmental disorder? *British Medical Journal (Clinical Research Ed.)*, 295(6600), 681–2.

Nelson, B., Fornito, A., Harrison, B. J., Yücel, M., Sass, L. A., Yung, A. R., *et al.* (2009a). A disturbed sense of self in the psychosis prodrome: linking phenomenology and neurobiology. *Neuroscience and Biobehavioral Reviews*, 33(6), 807–17.

Nelson, B., Sass, L. A., Thompson, A., Yung, A. R., Francey, S. M., Amminger, G. P., *et al.* (2009b). Does disturbance of self underlie social cognition deficits in schizophrenia and other psychotic disorders? *Early Intervention in Psychiatry*, 3(2), 83–93.

Nelson, B., Thompson, A., and Yung, A. R. (2012). Basic self-disturbance predicts psychosis onset in the ultra high risk for psychosis "prodromal" population. *Schizophrenia Bulletin*, 38(6), 1277–87.

Nelson, B., Yuen, K., and Yung, A. R. (2011). Ultra high risk (UHR) for psychosis criteria: are there different levels of risk for transition to psychosis?. *Schizophrenia Research*, 125(1), 62–8.

Nelson, B. and Yung, A. R. (2009). Psychotic-like experiences as overdetermined phenomena: when do they increase risk for psychotic disorder? *Schizophrenia Research*, 108(1–3), 303–4.

Nelson, B. and Yung, A. R. (2011). Should a risk syndrome for first episode psychosis be included in the DSM-5? *Current Opinion in Psychiatry*, 24(2), 128–33.

Parnas, J. (1986). Risk factors in the development of schizophrenia: contributions from a study of children of schizophrenic mothers. *Danish Medical Bulletin*, 33(3), 127–33.

Parnas, J. (1999). From predisposition to psychosis: progression of symptoms in schizophrenia. *Acta Psychiatrica Scandinavica, Supplementum*, 395, 20–9.

Parnas, J. (2005). Clinical detection of schizophrenia-prone individuals: critical appraisal. *British Journal of Psychiatry, Supplementum*, 48, s111–12.

Parnas, J. (2011). A disappearing heritage: the clinical core of schizophrenia. *Schizophrenia Bulletin*, 37(6), 1121–30.

Parnas, J. and Handest, P. (2003). Phenomenology of anomalous self-experience in early schizophrenia. *Comprehensive Psychiatry*, 44(2), 121–34.

Parnas, J., Handest, P., Saebye, D., and Jansson, L. (2003). Anomalies of subjective experience in schizophrenia and psychotic bipolar illness. *Acta Psychiatrica Scandinavica*, 108(2), 126–33.

Parnas, J. and Jorgensen, A. (1989). Pre-morbid psychopathology in schizophrenia spectrum. *British Journal of Psychiatry*, 155, 623–7.

Parnas, J., Møller, P., Kircher, T., Thalbitzer, J., Jansson, L., Handest, P., *et al.* (2005). EASE: Examination of anomalous self-experience. *Psychopathology*, 38(5), 236–58.

Parnas, J., Raballo, A., Handest, P., Jansson, L., Vollmer-Larsen, A., and Saebye, D. (2011). Self-experience in the early phases of schizophrenia: 5-year follow-up of the Copenhagen Prodromal Study. *World Psychiatry*, 10(3), 200–4.

Poulton, R., Caspi, A., Moffitt, T. E., Cannon, M., Murray, R., and Harrington, H. (2000). Children's self-reported psychotic symptoms and adult schizophreniform disorder: a 15-year longitudinal study. *Archives of General Psychiatry*, 57(11), 1053–8.

Raballo, A. and Laroi, F. (2009). Clinical staging: a new scenario for the treatment of psychosis. *Lancet*, 374(9687), 365–7.

Raballo, A. and Nelson, B. (2010). Unworlding, perplexity and disorders of transpassibility: between the experiential and the existential side of schizophrenic vulnerability. *Psychopathology*, 43(4), 250–1.

Raballo, A., Nelson, B., Thompson, A., and Yung, A. (2011a). The comprehensive assessment of at-risk mental states: from mapping the onset to mapping the structure. *Schizophrenia Research*, 127(1–3), 107–14.

Raballo, A. and Parnas, J. (2011). The silent side of the spectrum: schizotypy and the schizotaxic self. *Schizophrenia Bulletin*, *37*(5), 1017–26.

Raballo, A., Saebye, D., and Parnas, J. (2011b). Looking at the schizophrenia spectrum through the prism of self-disorders: an empirical study. *Schizophrenia Bulletin*, *37*(2), 344–51.

Ratcliffe, M. and Broome, M. (2012). Existential phenomenology, psychiatric illness and the death of possibilities. In S. Crowell (Ed.), *Cambridge Companion to Existentialism*, pp. 361–82. Cambridge: Cambridge University Press.

Riecher, A., Maurer, K., Löffler, W., Fätkenheuer, B., an der Heiden, W., and Häfner, H. (1989). Schizophrenia—a disease of young single males? Preliminary results from an investigation on a representative cohort admitted to hospital for the first time. *European Archives of Psychiatry and Neurological Sciences*, *239*(3), 210–12.

Rosso, I. M., Bearden, C. E., Hollister, J. M., Gasperoni, T. L., Sanchez, L. E., Hadley, T., *et al.* (2000). Childhood neuromotor dysfunction in schizophrenia patients and their unaffected siblings: a prospective cohort study. *Schizophrenia Bulletin*, *26*(2), 367–78.

Ruhrmann, S., Paruch, J., Bechdolf, A., Pukrop, R., Wagner, M., Berning, J., *et al.* (2008). Reduced subjective quality of life in persons at risk for psychosis. *Acta Psychiatrica Scandinavica*, *117*(5), 357–68.

Ruhrmann, S., Schultze-Lutter, F., and Klosterkötter, J. (2003). Early detection and intervention in the initial prodromal phase of schizophrenia. *Pharmacopsychiatry*, *36*(Suppl 3), S162–7.

Ruhrmann, S., Schultze-Lutter, F., Salokangas, R. K., Heinimaa, M., Linszen, D., Dingemans, P., *et al.* (2010). Prediction of psychosis in adolescents and young adults at high risk: results from the prospective European prediction of psychosis study. *Archives of General Psychiatry*, *67*(3), 241–51.

Salvatore, P., Baldessarini, R. J., Tohen, M., Khalsa, H. M., Sanchez-Toledo, J. P., Zarate, C. A. Jr, *et al.* (2009). McLean-Harvard International First-Episode Project: two-year stability of DSM-IV diagnoses in 500 first-episode psychotic disorder patients. *Journal of Clinical Psychiatry*, *70*(4), 458–66.

Sass, L. A. and Parnas, J. (2003). Schizophrenia, consciousness, and the self. *Schizophrenia Bulletin*, *29*(3), 427–44.

Schultze-Lutter, F. (2009). Subjective symptoms of schizophrenia in research and the clinic: the basic symptom concept. *Schizophrenia Bulletin*, *35*(1), 5–8.

Schultze-Lutter, F., Addington, J. and Rurhmann, S. (2007a). *Schizophrenia Proneness Instrument, Adult version (SPI-A)*. Rome: Giovanni Fiorito Editore.

Schultze-Lutter, F., Klosterkötter, J., Picker, H., Steinmeyer, E. M., and Ruhrmann, S. (2007b). Predicting first-episode psychosis by basic symptoms criteria. *Clinical Neuropsychiatry*, *4*(1), 11–22.

Schultze-Lutter, F. and Koch, E. (2010). *Schizophrenia Proneness Instrument, Child and Youth version (SPI-CY)*. Rome: Giovanni Fioriti Editore s.r.l.

Schultze-Lutter, F., Ruhrmann, S., Fusar-Poli, P., Bechdolf, A., Schimmelmann, B. G., and Klosterkötter, J. (2012). Basic symptoms and the prediction of first-episode psychosis. *Current Pharmaceutical Design*, *18*(4), 351–7.

Seidman, L. J., Giuliano, A. J., Meyer, E. C., Addington, J., Cadenhead, K. S., Cannon, T. D., *et al.* (2010). Neuropsychology of the prodrome to psychosis in the NAPLS consortium: relationship to family history and conversion to psychosis. *Archives of General Psychiatry*, *67*(6), 578–88.

Sergi, M. J., Fiske, A. P., Horan, W. P., Kern, R. S., Kee, K. S., Subotnik, K. L., *et al.* (2009). Development of a measure of relationship perception in schizophrenia. *Psychiatry Research*, *166*(1), 54–62.

Simon, A. E., Dvorsky, D. N., Boesch, J., Roth, B., Isler, E., Schueler, P., *et al.* (2006). Defining subjects at risk for psychosis: a comparison of two approaches. *Schizophrenia Research, 81*(1), 83–90.

Sullivan, H. S. (1994). The onset of schizophrenia. 1927. *American Journal of Psychiatry, 151*(6 Suppl), 134–9.

Tandon, R. and Carpenter, W. T. (2012). DSM-5 status of psychotic disorders: 1 year prepublication. *Schizophrenia Bulletin, 38*(3), 369–70.

Thompson, A., Nelson, B., and Yung, A. R. (2011b). Predictive validity of clinical variables in the "at risk" for psychosis population: international comparisons with results from the North American Prodrome Longitudinal Study. *Schizophrenia Research, 126*(1–3), 51–7.

Thompson, A. D., Bartholomeusz, C., and Yung, A. R. (2011a). Social cognition deficits and the "ultra high risk" for psychosis population: a review of the literature. *Early Intervention in Psychiatry, 5*(3), 192–202.

Valmaggia, L. R., McCrone, P., Knapp, M., Woolley, J. B., Broome, M. R., Tabraham, P., *et al.* (2009). Economic impact of early intervention in people at high risk of psychosis. *Psychological Medicine, 39*(10), 1617–26.

van Os, J. (2009). A salience dysregulation syndrome. *British Journal of Psychiatry, 194*(2), 101–03.

van Os, J. and Delespaul, P. (2005). Toward a world consensus on prevention of schizophrenia. *Dialogues in Clinical Neuroscience, 7*(1), 53–67.

van Os, J., Kenis, G., and Rutten, B. P. (2010). The environment and schizophrenia. *Nature, 468*(7321), 203–12.

van Os, J. and Linscott, R. J. (2012). Introduction: The extended psychosis phenotype—relationship with schizophrenia and with ultrahigh risk status for psychosis. *Schizophrenia Bulletin, 38*(2), 227–30.

van Os, J., Linscott, R. J., Myin-Germeys, I., Delespaul, P., and Krabbendam, L. (2009). A systematic review and meta-analysis of the psychosis continuum: evidence for a psychosis proneness-persistence-impairment model of psychotic disorder. *Psychological Medicine, 39*(2), 179–95.

Velthorst, E., Nieman, D. H., Linszen, D., Becker, H., de Haan, L., Dingemans, P.M., *et al.* (2010). Disability in people clinically at high risk of psychosis. Br J *Psychiatry, 197*(4), 278–84.

Warner, R. (2005). Problems with early and very early intervention in psychosis. *British Journal of Psychiatry, Supplement, 48*, s104–7.

Watt, N. F. (1978).Patterns of childhood social development in adult schizophrenics. *Archives of General Psychiatry, 35*(2), 160–5.

Watt, N. F., Fryer, J. H., Lewine, R. R., and Prentky, R. A. (1979). Toward longitudinal conceptions of psychiatric disorder. *Progress in Experimental Personality Research, 9*, 199–283.

Watt, N. F. and Lubensky, A. W. (1976). Childhood roots of schizophrenia. *Journal of Consulting & Clinical Psychology, 44*(3), 363–75.

Whitty, P., Clarke, M., McTigue, O., Browne, S., Kamali, M., Larkin, C., *et al.* (2005). Diagnostic stability four years after a first episode of psychosis. *Psychiatric Services, 56*(9), 1084–8.

Winton-Brown, T. T., Harvey, S. B., and McGuire, P. K. (2011). The diagnostic significance of BLIPS (Brief Limited Intermittent Psychotic Symptoms) in Psychosis. *Schizophrenia Research, 131*(1–3), 256–7.

Woods, S. W., Addington, J., Cadenhead, K. S., Cannon, T. D., Cornblatt, B. A., Heinssen, R., *et al.* (2009). Validity of the prodromal risk syndrome for first psychosis: findings from the North American Prodrome Longitudinal Study. *Schizophrenia Bulletin, 35*(5), 894–908.

Wuyts, P. and Parnas, J. (2011). Het onderzoek van de verstoorde zelfbeleving (Examination of anomalous self-experience, Nederlandstalige versie), 11–12. Belgische Schizofrenie Liga.

Yung, A. R., McGorry, P. D., McFarlane, C. A., Jackson, H. J., Patton, G. C., and Rakkar, A. (1996). Monitoring and care of young people at incipient risk of psychosis. *Schizophrenia Bulletin*, 22(2), 283–303.

Yung, A. R., Nelson, B., Stanford, C., Simmons, M. B., Cosgrave, E. M., Killackey, E., *et al.* (2008). Validation of "prodromal" criteria to detect individuals at ultra high risk of psychosis: 2 year follow-up. *Schizophrenia Research*, 105(1–3), 10–17.

Yung, A. R., Nelson, B., Thompson, A. D., and Wood, S. J. (2010a). Should a risk syndrome for psychosis be included in the DSM-V? *Schizophrenia Research*, 120, 7–15.

Yung, A. R., Nelson, B., Thompson, A., and Wood, S. J. (2010b). The psychosis threshold in ultra high risk (prodromal) research: is it valid? *Schizophrenia Research*, 120, 1–6.

Yung, A., Phillips, L., and McGorry, P. D. (1998a). Can we predict the onset of first episode psychosis in a high risk group? *International Clinical Psychopharmacology*, 13(Supplement), S23–S30.

Yung, A. R., Phillips, L. J., McGorry, P. D., McFarlane, C. A., Francey, S., Harrigan, S., *et al.* (1998b). Prediction of psychosis—A step towards indicated prevention of schizophrenia. *British Journal of Psychiatry*, 172, 14–20.

Yung, A. R., Phillips, L. J., Yuen, H. P., Francey, S. M., McFarlane, C. A., Hallgren, M., *et al.* (2003). Psychosis prediction: 12-month follow up of a high-risk ("prodromal") group. *Schizophrenia Research*, 60(1), 21–32.

Yung, A. R., Philips, L. J., Yuen, H. P., and McGorry, P. D. (2004). Risk factors for psychosis in an ultra high-risk group: Psychopathology and clinical features. *Schizophrenia Research*, 67 (2–3), 131–42.

Yung, A. R., Stanford, C., Cosgrave, E., Killackey, E., Phillips, L., Nelson, B., *et al.* (2006). Testing the ultra high risk (prodromal) criteria for the prediction of psychosis in a clinical sample of young people. *Schizophrenia Research*, 84(1), 57–66.

Yung, A. R., Woods, S. W., Ruhrmann, S., Addington, J., Schultze-Lutter, F., Cornblatt, B. A., *et al.* (2012). Whither the attenuated psychosis syndrome? *Schizophrenia Bulletin*, 38(6), 1130–4.

Yung, A. R., Yuen, H. P., Berger, G., Francey, S., Hung, T. C., Nelson, B., *et al.* (2007). Declining transition rate in ultra high risk (prodromal) services: dilution or reduction of risk? *Schizophrenia Bulletin*, 33(3), 673–81.

Ziermans, T. B., Schothorst, P. F., Sprong, M., and van Engeland, H. (2011). Transition and remission in adolescents at ultra-high risk for psychosis. *Schizophrenia Research*, 126, 58–64.

CHAPTER 47

UNDERSTANDING MANIA AND DEPRESSION

S. NASSIR GHAEMI

INTRODUCTION

In this chapter, I will try to give a conceptual understanding of mania and depression that extends from its phenomenology to its biology and to its role in diagnosis. The main thread of this discussion will be as follows: Mania, as part of manic-depressive illness (MDI), may be intrinsically tied to the experience of depression. The two may not be separable, both clinically and biologically. Mania is not, primarily, driven by mood; it is driven by a speeding up of bodily and mental states: psychomotor activation. Mania is not understandable primarily by life events; they can trigger the timing of an episode, but their causal role extends no further. Since mood is not the central feature of mania, the stereotype of the euphoric happy state is epiphenomenal, and, though relevant to a person's experience, not central to the state biologically or diagnostically. In contrast, creativity is a more central feature of mania, and especially when mild as in hypomania or hyperthymic temperament, mania can be quite useful, productive, and beneficial—both for the individual and society. Our greatest heroes often have mania. Another central aspect to the phenomenology of mania is lack of insight: those who have mania are not Cartesian philosophers; they have little awareness of the reality of their experience. In contrast to these aspects of understanding mania, I am critical of two common approaches: the Freudian view that mania is an epiphenomenon of depression, and the postmodernist view that mania (like all psychopathology) is mainly social construction. In sum: to understand mania, we should understand and appreciate psychomotor activation, creativity, and lack of insight. Further, we should appreciate the diagnostically central role of mania to all mood illnesses, and the biological basis for both its causation and its treatment.

THE IRRELEVANCE OF LIFE EVENTS

Let's begin with "normal" happiness. This tends to be seen as contextual: if I win the lottery, I'm happy. Good things happen; one feels happy. Psychiatrists call this "normal mood reactivity": the ability to react normally to good or bad news with happier or sadder mood, respectively. The problem with this definition, though it is not in itself false, is that abnormal happiness and abnormal depression also often, in fact usually, have a context. This is because of the split-brain nature of our minds: we provide rationalized contexts for everything that we feel (Gazzaniga 1998). But the feeling comes first, the rationalization comes later. As described later in this chapter, the feeling is always right, the rationalization often wrong.

In the era prior to the third edition of the *Diagnostic and Statistical Manual of Mental Disorders* (DSM-III), moods were distinguished based on these supposed causes (Shorter 2007). Depression was "reactive," caused by some painful experience in the environment, and thus not biological; or it was "endogenous," occurring without any environmental cause, and thus biological. We now know this is untrue: many depressive periods that are part of diseases like MDI are triggered, though not caused, by some life event; their deeper cause is a biological susceptibility.

Although this concept has long been debated in relation to depression, it has not been discussed in relation to happiness. Yet we have all tended to implicitly use this same commonsense, though mistaken, notion: if someone is happy "because" x and y happened, then that happiness is normal. Only if nothing in the world has happened, and someone is inexplicably happy, do we consider that he or she might be manic.

The Girlfriend Test

A good example of this kind of assumption is found in a recent study of German psychologists, to whom researchers gave two vignettes of a person with severe depression and another person with mania (Bruchmuller and Meyer 2009). The cases were set up so as to clearly meet DSM-IV definitions of a major depressive episode and a manic episode. The psychologists were asked to diagnose the cases as major depression, mania, or neither. Ninety-five percent of them correctly diagnosed the case of DSM-IV-defined major depression; only 38% of the psychologists diagnosed the case of mania correctly (53% saw it as depression!). The researchers put in a wrinkle: half of the vignettes for the case of mania stated that the male patient (who had happy mood, decreased need for sleep, increased activity level, increased talkativeness, and impulsive behavior) had just started a new relationship with a girlfriend; the other half of the vignettes for the case of mania said nothing about any external trigger. In the girlfriend case, the correct diagnosis of mania dropped to 23%; in the non-girlfriend case, it rose to 60%.

Girlfriends, especially new ones, tend to make men happy. However, most men do not become manic upon obtaining a new girlfriend, nor, according to rather good scientific research, should anyone become manic unless that person has a strong genetic susceptibility to bipolar disorder (Bienvenu et al. 2011).

The point is that getting a girlfriend does not cause: distractibility, decreased need for sleep, grandiosity, flight of ideas, increased goal-directed activities, pressured speech, and impulsive risk-taking behavior—along with euphoric or irritable mood, lasting one week or longer, as a change from baseline behavior, repeatedly once per year throughout life, as is the course of bipolar disorder.

Having a girlfriend or not is irrelevant to determining whether a person is experiencing a manic episode; yet most of us think this way, naturally, as with the psychologists in that study. This may be common sense. But it is not scientific sense. Science indeed is about learning when and why to reject common sense. Common sense is frequently erroneous, and certainly should not be presumed regularly veracious.

THE IRRELEVANCE OF MOOD

The earlier discussion might seem unconvincing to some who think that having a girlfriend might cause euphoria and some of the described symptoms. But one response is to pay attention to the issue of *recurrence*: this is central, even essential, to the concept of bipolar disorder. A manic episode does not happen just once; it almost always is part of recurrent episodes that happen over and over again, on average once yearly in bipolar disorder. So the issue is not: Can I explain a theoretical single manic episode by having a girlfriend? But rather: Can I explain a manic episode every year by having a girlfriend every year?

The centrality of recurrence—which was the hallmark of MDI in Kraepelin's view—shows us an aspect of bipolar disorder that is misunderstood by the majority of persons who have it, or treat it, or don't have it and don't treat it: mood doesn't matter. Mood is not central to the concept of bipolar disorder, nor is mood central to the concepts of mania and depression. We are misled by the designation "mood disorders" into thinking that these illnesses are primarily illnesses of mood. They are not. The phenomenological core of mania (and depression) is not mood; for mania, it is psychomotor activation—the speeding up and increasing of one's physical and mental states (Cassano et al. 2012). (For depression, the phenomenological core is psychomotor retardation—the slowing down of one's body and mind.) When one is psychomotorically activated, the mood tends to change: it becomes labile, and sometimes (though not usually) euphoric. When one is psychomotorically retarded, similarly, the mood tends to do down (but not always). In other words, mood is not the driver of the process; it is the driven.

ECSTASY

Despite the fact that abnormal mood is not central to mania, many prior studies of the topic have focused on the extreme happiness, or ecstasy, that happens with mania. One view is to see such extreme moods as emotions that totally take over one's mind: all of one's thoughts and feelings are imbued with happiness. In contrast, normal happiness might be more partial: we are happy about this or that, but not in a general or absolute sense about everything. This was the view of psychiatrist Willy Mayer-Gross in a doctoral dissertation he wrote under the supervision of Karl Jaspers (Wolff 2000). The philosopher William James called the absolute experience of happiness "ecstasy" and the psychologist Kay Jamison refers to it as "exuberance." To provide examples, James turns to the experience of patients with mania (including himself) and the rapturous experiences of religious mystics. Here is an example from James, reporting the experience of a mystic:

> Last night was the sweetest night I ever had in my life. I never before, for so long a time together, enjoyed so much of the light and rest and sweetness of heaven in my soul, but without

the least agitation of body during the whole time … all night I continued in a constant, clear, and lively sense of the heavenly sweetness of Christ's excellent love, of his nearness to me, and of my dearness to him; with an inexpressibly sweet calmness of soul … I seemed to myself to perceive a glow of divine love dome down from the heart of Christ in heaven into my heart in a constant stream, like a stream or pencil of sweet light … I appeared to myself to float or swim, in these bright, sweet beams, like the moats swimming in the beams of the sun … It was pleasure, without the least sting, or any interruption. It was sweetness which my soul was lost in; it seemed to be all that my feeble frame could sustain. (Mayer-Gross 2000, p. 300)

It could be that this kind of complete mind-filling euphoria is behind the mystical experience of union with the outside world. Everything seems the same as me, and I seem a part of everything around me, because the parts of me have disappeared inside this mind-saturating experience of ecstasy. The self dissolves in the outside world.

Another kind of abnormal happiness is not characterized, as is ecstasy, by a complete overtaking of the mind. This next kind of happiness is abnormal not because it is absolute but because it is not "real." We are not realistically happy because good things are going on around us; we are just happy inside our minds, and then we project that happiness onto the outside world. Our happiness does not extend over the whole world, the abstract universe, God, but rather to concrete objects, engendering a sense of jubilation that pushes one to express it, either in words or actions. Here is a mid-nineteenth-century description:

I was lifted up by soft clouds, it was as if with every passing minute my mind was freed from its fetters, and inexpressible delight and gratitude entered my heart … A wholly new, celestial life began within me … My ideas surged forward so that I now contradicted what I had enthusiastically proclaimed just an hour before. But I was indescribably cheerful and seemed transfigured … I was in an enviable state at the time, such as I had always wished for. In truth, I experienced a foretaste of heaven within my soul …. The world and humanity smiled at me, I longed for action so that I could start life anew … My voice suddenly became light and clear, I sang all the time … every face appeared to me unrecognizably more beautiful … I wanted to make the whole world happy through my own self-sacrifice and to resolve all conflicts. (Mayer-Gross 2000, p. 302)

Emotions sublimes, the French psychologist Pierre Janet (1903) called it, combined with a push to action. This experience, which is typical of a manic episode, is so pleasurable that it contradicts our association of disease with suffering. Writes one person with the condition:

I do not know why I use the term illness, because subjectively I have never felt better. Sometimes I thought my vigour and productivity had doubled; it seemed to me that I knew and understood everything; my imagination gave me endless joy. (Mayer-Gross 2000, p. 302)

Nor is this heightened potency merely emotional; it is also physical, especially sexual: one's muscles feel stronger, Janet wrote; one's sexual drive is heightened, libido surges, sex is pleasurable, frequent, and varied in its fulfillment.

Beyond Euphoria

A pleasurable disease, you might think, this mania. Yet as pleasure is most closely allied to pain, so is this extreme happiness easily tipped over into anger and dysphoria. If after all,

I am so intelligent, why does the rest of the world not recognize it? I should be able to reach the president, for instance; he needs to hear from me, since I know more than all others around him. But he doesn't respond to my phone calls. If I'm smart, and the rest of the world doesn't realize it, then others must be stupid. When my pleasure collides with the world's reality, love quickly turns to hate, and joy to rage.

It is for this reason that most manic episodes involve anger, and not just pure euphoria. This is one reason why manic episodes are not unalloyed experiences of rapture. This is what the manic-depressive poet Robert Lowell had in mind when he commented that depression is a burden to oneself, mania a burden to one's friends.

And then there is the unavoidable psychological law of gravity that whoever is granted access to that kind of high must at some point come down, and fast: the price of mania is depression.

And then the worst, and unfortunately common outcome: the energy and power of mania, and the moods and climate of depression, mixed together:

> On occasion, these periods of total despair would be made even worse by terrible agitation. My mind would race from subject to subject, but instead of being filled with the exuberant and cosmic thoughts that had been associated with earlier periods of rapid thinking, it would be drenched in awful sounds and images of decay and dying: dead bodies on the beach, charred remains of animals, toe-tagged corpses in morgues. During these angry periods I became exceedingly restless, angry, and irritable, and the only way I could dilute the agitation was to run along the beach or pace back and forth across my room like a polar bear at the zoo. (Jamison 2004, p. 45)

There are many varieties of abnormal types of happiness, it seems, and they are not all happy ones.

These mixed states are not an exception but the rule. Most manic symptoms occur while mixed with some depression symptoms. Instead of the stereotype of pure euphoria, the core of mania seems to be *impulsivity with heightened energy*. Sometimes a classic triad of symptoms is mentioned: euphoric mood, flight of ideas, and hyperactivity. This triad gets closer to the syndrome, with the proviso that euphoric mood is present, and flight of ideas absent, in a minority of cases. If I had to pick out a central feature of mania, present in most cases, I would say mood lability along with decreased need for sleep. Mood lability appears to be central to the manic experience: it is not that one is simply euphoric; euphoria tends to alternate rapidly with irritability, anxiety, and even depressive mood.

As described previously, recent research shows that "psychomotor activation" is the central feature of mania which distinguishes it from depression (Cassano et al. 2012). It is a state of excitement, which can be reflected not just as euphoria, but also marked agitation and irritability and anxiety. A key problem in understanding mania in the past has been the tendency to conflate it with euphoria, such as in the girlfriend case with which this chapter began.

CREATIVITY

Another way of thinking about mania, besides focusing on the mood of euphoria, is to consider its cognitive impact: an enhancement of creativity. Certainly there is an association but the nature of that association is unclear. I think one approach would be to see manic creativity as the ability to think quickly and tangentially, especially with visual imagery. I will now try to explain this claim.

One definition of creativity is "divergent thinking"—generating many potential solutions to a problem. Standard tests of creativity measure this feature: the usual ways of solving a problem already being known, creativity is measured by unusual solutions. For instance, one kind of divergent thinking test asks a person "to think of many different and unusual uses for a common item, such as a tin can or a brick." Other tests include word association tests (like the Adjective Check List) where persons who make more unusual associations are thought to be more creative, or tests of visual creativity (like the Barron–Welsh Art Scale), where partially drawn visual figures need to be completed, and more unusual and asymmetrical visual completions are interpreted as more creative. Think of a classic manic symptom: flight of ideas. One's thoughts seem to literally fly in many different directions; they may or may not make sense, but they certainly get around. Divergent thinking is a daily experience in mania. Manic people are also hyperactive; they think quickly, talk rapidly, and need little sleep; they write much; they draw, plan, propose, implement.

It could also be that the divergent thinking model has its terms reversed. Creativity may have to do, not with *solving* problems, but with *finding* the right problems to solve. Creative scientists, for instance, sometimes discover problems that others did not imagine. Their solutions aren't as novel as their recognition that those problems existed to begin with. Newton's theories left most physicists untroubled until a young Zurich Patent Office employee realized they did not work when applied to light; Albert Einstein asked questions that had not yet been asked—new questions replaced old solutions (Mansfield and Busse 1981). Creativity may be about identifying problems, not solving them.

Most of the evidence to support the link between mania and creativity is of the biographical and historical variety. An exception is a study where *visual*, but not *verbal*, creativity was found to be similar in persons with bipolar disorder—when feeling well, not manic or depressed—versus "creative controls" (art school and creative writing graduate students) (Srivastava et al. 2010). This finding, in the only experimental study so far, may be uniquely meaningful: a special knack for *visual* creativity may be an essential feature of creative success. Jamison writes about literally "seeing" new ideas during mania, and physicist Richard Feynman directly links creativity, even in abstract science, to vision (Feynman 1988):

> "When I'm teaching some esoteric technique such as integrating Bessel functions ... I see equations, I see the letters in colors—I don't know why. As I'm talking, I see vague pictures of Bessel functions ... with light-tan j's, slightly violet-bluish n's, and dark brown x's flying around. And I wonder what the hell it must look like to the students." Albert Einstein commented similarly: "Combinatory play seems to be the essential feature in productive thought.... the psychical entities which seem to serve as elements in [this] thought ... are of visual and some of muscular type.... Conventional words or signs have to be sought for laboriously only in a secondary stage." (Simonton 1994, p. 96)

If one is a little manic, one can make these connections more effectively than if one is completely normal. This link was recognized by another great physicist, Neils Bohr. Once, when the physicist Wolfgang Pauli was presenting a new theory of electron spin, Bohr responded from the audience: "We are all agreed that your theory is crazy. The question which divides us is whether it is crazy enough to have a chance of being correct. My own feeling is that it is not crazy enough" (Simonton 1994, p. 101).

Einstein mentioned playfulness, another feature of mania. Manic people sometimes seem child-like, euphoric, giddy, silly. A sense of play, a childish willingness to experiment and just have fun, is an important aspect of creativity. Feynman is again a good resource, describing how he made his greatest discovery (Feynman 1985, p. 173):

> When it came time to do some research, I couldn't get to work. I was a little tired; I was not interested; I couldn't do research! This went on for what I felt was a few years.... I simply couldn't get started on any problem.... Then I had another thought: Physics disgusts me a little bit now, but I used to *enjoy* doing physics. Why did I enjoy it? I used to *play* with it. I used to do whatever I felt like doing—it didn't have to do with whether it was important for the development of nuclear physics, but whether it was interesting and amusing for me to play with.... So I got this new attitude. Now that I am burned out and I'll never accomplish anything, I've got this nice position at the university teaching classes which I rather enjoy, and just like I read the *Arabian Nights* for pleasure, I'm going to play with physics, whenever I want to, without worrying about any importance whatsoever.

A week later, while eating lunch, Feynman saw someone throw a cafeteria plate in the air; he noticed how the red central medallion rotated faster than the plate wobbled; he thought up a complex equation for the faster central rotation versus the peripheral wobbling, showing a twofold mass-to-acceleration relation in the plate. Upon hearing the equation, a colleague said: "Feynman, that's pretty interesting, but what's the importance of it? Why are you doing it?" (p. 174).

According to Feynman:

> His reaction didn't discourage me; I had made up my mind I was going to enjoy physics and do whatever I liked. I went on to work out equations of wobbles. Then I thought about how electron orbits start to move in relativity. Then there's the Dirac Equation in electrodynamics. And then quantum electrodynamics. And before I knew it (it was a very short time) I was 'playing'—working, really—with the same old problem that I loved so much, that I had stopped working on.... It was effortless. (p. 174)

This playing eventually earned Feynman a Nobel Prize in Physics. (Feynman also had a healthy libido, stopping at strip clubs on his lunch break; and was impulsive, getting into fights at bars on academic conference trips, though, to my knowledge, he was not psychiatrically diagnosed or treated.)

HYPOMANIA

The phenomenon of hypomania, which basically reflects mild manic symptoms, needs separate attention. How one defines "mild" is, of course, the problem. Some authors make rather silly statements, such as the notion that psychiatry is pathologizing happiness. Happiness is quite different from hypomania in a very simple way, as a major proponent of the bipolar spectrum concept, Hagop Akiskal, once commented (personal communication, 2009): hypomania is recurrent, happiness is not.

This quip has a meaning that I would venture to say many, if not most, interested parties do not understand. Many commentators begin with DSM, as if the world did not exist before 1980. The concept of MDI, for one hundred years, was about recurrence, not mania or hypomania or depression (Goodwin and Jamison 2007). MDI meant recurrent mood episodes, usually depressive, sometimes manic or hypomanic. It is an illness of recurrence, with cycles. These cycles consist of mania or hypomania followed by depression, or the reverse (less commonly), but rarely if ever just mania alone, or hypomania alone, or even depression alone.

Thus, in the original MDI concept dating to Kraepelin, it is meaningless to talk about mania or hypomania or depression in isolation. They are all linked. It doesn't matter whether or not hypomania is pathological or needs treatment; what matters is that it is part of the cycling into and out of mood episodes, mostly depressive, that is very harmful and needs treatment. One has to treat the cycles, not just the mania or hypomania or depression in isolation, if the illness itself is to be treated. That is what mood stabilizers do.

DSM-III moved away from this traditional view of MDI, and it separated out mania and depression, encouraging interpretations along those lines, treating parts of the illness in isolation. But that is only one way of looking at MDI, or bipolar disorder as it was transformed in DSM-III. One could return to the Kraepelinian model and see the illness as one of recurrence, not polarity.

This perspective is important for addressing those who criticize the concept of hypomania as a pathologization of happiness. Such critics seem to assume that if a definition is in DSM it is inherently a pathologization, in the sense of being very harmful, or needing treatment, or representing disease (the usual definitions of pathology). Yet, the plethora of adjustment "disorders" are not pathological, do not represent disease, and often don't need treatment—although they are in DSM. Why should the presence of a diagnosis imply treatment? Many diagnoses in medicine are terminal and have no treatment. Many are self-limiting (adenovirus pharyngitis—also known as the common cold) and do not require treatment.

Hypomania is unique in that it is one of the few, perhaps only, DSM Axis I conditions which do not have significant dysfunction as a definitional criterion. In the introduction to DSM-IV, in the general definition of mental disorder, it is claimed that mental disorders involve symptoms with either subjective distress or functional impairment or an "important loss of freedom." Hypomania involves little to no subjective distress, no functional impairment, and no apparent loss of freedom. In fact, usually one's functioning is enhanced. In this sense, hypomania in isolation does not meet DSM definitions of a mental disorder. This is another reason why its proper understanding cannot happen in isolation; hypomania is only relevant because it doesn't happen in isolation; it is followed by depression; it might even cause depression.

Another aspect to the debate has to do with whether we are certain we are faced with hypomania. The history of the term may help us. Originally, for much of the twentieth century, it just meant manic symptoms that were not severe enough to require hospitalization. Hypomania meant non-hospitalized mania. Readers may appreciate that the criteria for hospitalization differed quite widely in 1900 in Munich in a German state mental hospital, in 1940 in upstate New York in a state mental hospital, in 1970 in New York City at a private hospital using private insurance, and in 1995 in Los Angeles using a health maintenance organization (HMO). In 1900 Germany, one had to be quite psychotic and severely dysfunctional with mania to be placed in a state institution, with no treatment available beyond custodial care, which might mean staying institutionalized for years or even decades. In 1970 New York, with private insurance and no managed care hand-slappers, one could enter the hospital for a few months with moderate manic symptoms, receive lithium, and be cured. In 1995 Los Angeles, with the HMO making the decisions, one to two weeks was all one would receive, and most manic episodes were treated outside hospitals. Recognizing the rising threshold for hospitalization in the 1990s, DSM-IV defined hypomania based on absence of severe functional impairment. In Europe, where capitalism did not control health care as much as in the USA, the International Classification of Disease, tenth revision (ICD-10) did not use the same criterion. A change in functioning from normal was emphasized instead (also in DSM-IV), but absence of functional impairment is not part of the ICD-10 definition of hypomania.

One could argue the question of functional impairment forever. For example, in the early 1990s, my colleagues and I had a case of a businesswoman, who had recently gone to a conference out of state, and engaged in a one-night stand. She had not used condoms. She never knew the man previously, never saw him again; she did not usually engage in such behaviors. Prior to going to the conference, she had experienced a decreased need for sleep, increased energy, racing thoughts, and increased talkativeness, along with a mood that was higher than normal. All these symptoms were different from her normal baseline sleep, energy, and behavior, and they had persisted for over a week. In prior years, she had experienced numerous manic symptoms as described here, lasting for weeks, and numerous clinical depressive episodes (meeting standard DSM definitions) lasting about one to two months. When she returned, and we discussed the case at our bipolar clinic, three experienced clinician/ researchers wondered whether the diagnosis should be type II or type I bipolar disorder. Much seemed to hinge on whether or not she had engaged in "safe" sex. She had not used a condom on the occasion of her one-night stand, during a time when HIV was not yet treatable. One of the three clinicians thought that this impulsive decision was markedly dysfunctional, and put her at serious risk of potentially terminal disease, thus making the episode a full manic, not hypomanic, episode. A second clinician disagreed and thought the risk of serious disease from one episode of unprotected sex low enough so as not to meet the standard of *marked* functional impairment, and thus the diagnosis would be hypomania. The third clinician could not make up his mind.

In a sexually liberated society, such as some Scandinavian countries for instance, this case might seem like hypomania at best. In sexually repressed countries, like some Arab countries for instance, it would like seem like mania. America, with its puritan past and liberal present, is torn in the middle.

Besides the value judgments inherent in assessing marked functional impairment, the problem of hypomania is complicated by the reality of hyperthymic personality. Originally popularized by Ernst Kretschmer in the early twentieth century as a mild version of mania (just as dysthymia was a mild version of depression, and schizothymia a mild version of schizophrenia) (Kretschmer 1970), hyperthymia did not make it into DSM-III and beyond and thus has been relatively ignored by modern psychiatry. Yet a number of studies in the past two decades suggest that it can indeed be validly and reliably identified not only in persons with bipolar disorder, but in persons with unipolar depression, and indeed in persons who have no mood disorder (Kesebir et al. 2005). Hyperthymic personality does appear to be overrepresented, though, in families of people with bipolar disorder. In fact, some genetic data suggest it might be the most common phenotypic variant of bipolar illness. In a typical family tree, many people will have hyperthymia or cyclothymia or dysthymia, some may be diagnosable with unipolar depression, a few will be diagnosable with type II bipolar disorder, and one or two persons may have full-blown type I bipolar disorder. This type of familial transmission is consistent with the evidence from twin studies that the genetic predisposition to bipolar disorder involves many genes that add up to cause the disease. If only a few of those genes are present, one might have hyperthymic temperament; more might lead to unipolar depression; even more to recurrent hypomania and depression; and even more to full mania.

Hyperthymic temperament is, then, constant hypomania, not as an illness, but as one's biological temperament, genetically reflective of a mild predisposition to bipolar disorder. As noted, some people only have hyperthymic temperament, and no depressive episodes ever. Such persons generally do not seek or get psychiatric treatment; they tend to be quite productive and successful, becoming wealthy businessmen, or esteemed academics, or famous politicians. (I have separately tried to show that Presidents Franklin Roosevelt and John Kennedy seem likely to have had hyperthymic personalities; Ghaemi 2011.) Commonly, though, people with hyperthymic temperament have intermittent clinical depressive episodes. In our current nosology, they are diagnosed with major depressive disorder (MDD), just as those who have depression with no hyperthymic temperament. It appears to matter if one's temperament is hyperthymic, though; such persons are more likely to experience antidepressant-induced mania, and they may be less responsive in general to antidepressants. One might think of the relation of hyperthymia to depression this way: constant low-level hypomanic symptoms are not dysfunctional by themselves at any one time; but over a long period of time, like the dripping of Chinese water torture, they add up and can lead to problems in life, often ending in depression. I have seen numerous highly successful businessmen, who appear to have been hyperthymic for decades, without any depression, and then, at some point in their fifties or sixties, they experience recurrent depressive episodes. Those depressive episodes fail to respond to antidepressants but then respond to mood stabilizers like lithium or valproate.

There is another aspect to hyperthymia which is harmful. If you add up all the harm caused by low-grade mild manic symptoms over a lifetime, they probably add up to as much harm as a few severe manic episodes of short duration. In other words, the drip–drip–drip of Chinese water torture in hyperthymia eventually equals the effects of a sudden brief flood of mania. At any one time, the hyperthymic person is functional, even super-functional. But over time, there is a toll to be taken by all that workaholism, the focus on productivity, the roving sexual eye, the self-centeredness. Marriages rarely last in such persons; divorce is the rule; infidelity common; fortunes made and lost; reputations ruined.

Another issue with hypomania is the resistance to identifying it if it is brief; there is a wish to ignore it if it only lasts hours to days. Indeed, this reluctance has taken on the characteristics of a fixation, seen in the personal opinions of the head of DSM-IV (Frances 2010), that there is something sacrosanct about the four-day cutoff for the diagnosis of hypomania. This criterion was entirely arbitrary, with no scientific basis whatsoever. It was based on the general notion held by the leaders of DSM-IV that psychiatric diagnoses should not be excessively easy to make. Since, using the criteria as they were, a DSM-III-R psychiatric disorder could be identified in about one-quarter of the general population (Kessler et al. 2005), the makers of DSM-IV were concerned about adding to that number, and thus opening themselves further to the standard criticism about "pathologization." One leader of DSM-IV told me that he preferred a one-week criterion; my understanding is that the bipolar clinicians and researchers on the task force preferred two days based on their own experience. A compromise of four days became the rule, and for two decades it has been defended against all scientific evidence otherwise. In fact, based on a very large forty-year prospective study, the average hypomanic episode lasts two to three weeks (Wicki and Angst 1991). (Interestingly, this same study was used in DSM-III to make radical changes in diagnostic definitions of psychotic and mood disorders; yet the leaders of DSM-IV ignored it.) Thus, at one level, this debate about the minimal threshold is irrelevant. On the other hand, in that study, Angst and colleagues assessed the validity of different diagnostic threshold based on the standard validators of psychiatric diagnosis: symptoms, family history, course of illness, and treatment effects (Robins and Guze 1970). If definitions produce different results based on those validators, then it can be claimed that those definitions are identifying different disorders. If definitions produce the same results on those validators, then those definitions identify the same disorder. This is standard practice in psychiatric epidemiology. Angst's group showed that the diagnostic threshold of one to three days of hypomania produced the same results on the four diagnostic validators as the diagnostic threshold of four days or longer, or even one week or longer (Wicki and Angst 1991). In other words, the duration of hypomania does not identify different conditions. Two days of hypomania certainly seems to validly identify a hypomanic episode.

A linguistic clarification: I speak of "manic" symptoms, not hypomanic symptoms, as many commonly do, because there are no such things as hypomanic symptoms. All such symptoms are manic symptoms; hypomania refers to an episode definition, as does mania. If one has a few manic symptoms, and not severely, then one can speak of a hypomanic episode. If one has more manic symptoms, and more severely, then one speaks of a manic episode. But technically, we should be clear that the symptoms are always manic symptoms, just as depressive symptoms are always depressive, even if they should fail to meet major depressive episode criteria. One does not speak of "hypodepressive" symptoms. I think this reluctance to use the word "manic" and to append "hypo" when it is inappropriate reflects stigma against bipolar disorder, and the general reluctance of patients and clinicians to diagnose this condition. When they diagnose it, they still want to make it as mild as possible. Thus, many patients that meet type I bipolar definitions are called type II; and the type II patients are labeled cyclothymic; and then cyclothymics are called normal.

This brings us to an important cultural implication: our culture values manic, and deprecates depressive, symptoms. We value people who are highly energetic; they get more done. Who is the successful academic? The person who publishes the most. Citation count is the measure of academic merit; how many papers did you publish? We don't ask: What did you discover? When people are introduced to give lectures, we are impressed by how many articles were published, by how much money in research grants were obtained, by how many awards have been received. Quantity is the touchstone of modern success: we value productivity above all else. And yet, there's something missing. Gore Vidal once commented that he hated all those men of many accomplishments who have accomplished so little of value. Lincoln would not pass the muster of quantitative accomplishments so valued today, Vidal said. We don't value the slowed down but often rigorous thinking characteristic of depression, the kind of thinking that Jefferson described in George Washington, whose thinking was said to be slow in operation but sure in conclusion. He was diffident, Jefferson said, always doubtful of himself (Flexner 2003). This is depression, not hypomania, and, no matter how much lip service we now pay to Washington and Lincoln, modern Western culture hates depression and loves mania (though we prefer to call it "hypo").

Recently I was visited by a professor of philosophy. She had experienced severe recurrent depressive periods, lasting about a month, which clearly met definitions of clinical depression. She also described constant manic symptoms of high energy, high productivity, high libido, low sleep requirements, rapid and creative thinking, and talkativeness. My hypomania, she said forthrightly, has served me well; I've published thirty books, I was chair of philosophy in Prague, I've been a respected professor in Chicago for three decades. Except for repeated sexual escapades outside her marriage, she had not engaged in harmful activities to any marked degree, and those activities had not been episodic and beyond her normal baseline personality, as part of DSM or ICD defined hypomanic episodes. This is why she was never officially diagnosed with "bipolar disorder"; she did not have *episodes* of hypomania, alternating with depression. She was *always* hypomanic, and experienced episodes of severe depression. In other words, she had hyperthymic personality, along with severe recurrent depression. This is not hypomania, according to the writers of DSM and ICD. But it is MDI, according to Emil Kraepelin and his way of thinking about that condition. It is hyperthymic personality, as described earlier.

There may be another aspect to this kind of case: it may be no coincidence that recurrent severe depression happens in people with hyperthymic personality. It could be that hyperthymic personality in fact *causes* depression. This is the view of the prominent Italian/Greek mood expert, Athanasios Koukopoulos. Calling it the "primacy of mania," his view is that *mania causes depression* (Koukopoulos and Ghaemi 2009); and, put more strongly, depression *never* happens without mania (either pre-existing or coexisting with the depression symptoms). Koukopoulos defines mania broadly, the way it existed before the big bang of 1980 (DSM-III). Prior to that date, mania was conceived as a general psychopathological state of excitation: this excitation could be thought of as elevated energy and mood (as in the current DSM/ICD definitions), but it also involved the excitation seen with agitation or anxiety. Psychomotor agitation and psychological anxiety are, obviously, the most non-specific psychiatric symptoms. They can be found in many psychiatric conditions; in the DSM/ICD approach they are found in anxiety disorders, but also in MDD, in many personality disorders, and in some psychotic disorders. Contemporary psychiatrists have lost sight of the fact that before 1980, those symptoms were viewed as manic symptoms. This is the way mania was conceived by Pinel in the early nineteenth century, and by Kraepelin in the early twentieth century. When Kraepelin wrote about MDI, he meant not just euphoric mania with increased energy; he also meant irritability with marked psychomotor agitation and anxiety, even in the absence of increased energy or flight of ideas or decreased need for sleep or increased talkativeness or any other core features of DSM-III defined mania. This is what Koukopoulos is trying to resurrect, the broad notion of mania involving not just increased energy, but also marked anxiety and agitation.

If one accepts such a broad definition of mania, then the claim made by Koukopoulos is that depressive symptoms are always accompanied by, or preceded by, mania, defined as marked anxiety or agitation or euphoria/increased energy (the key word is "or" not "and"). For instance, the classic manic-depressive cycle is a standard manic episode followed by a depressive episode. This is the most common sequence of a cycle of bipolar disorder (often labeled M-D-I, for mania followed by depression followed by an interval of normality). A substantial minority of cycles are the reverse, however: a depressive episode followed by a hypomanic episode (more commonly than full mania; labeled D-M-I). This would seem to contradict the primacy of mania thesis. Koukopoulos' view is that in such cases, the depressive episode is mixed with manic symptoms: such patients tend to be highly agitated, anxious, irritable, impulsive, labile in mood, and even sometimes have frank manic symptoms like increased energy, decreased need for sleep, flight of ideas, and hypersexuality. This kind of mixed depression is quite different from melancholia, where there is no anxiety or agitation or irritability or lability: instead there is marked anhedonia with severe psychomotor retardation. Koukopoulos' thesis would predict that the D-M-I pattern would not begin with a pure melancholic depression, but rather with a mixed depression.

Another potential counterexample to the primacy of mania thesis would be so-called unipolar depression. It appears that commonly depressive episodes happen by themselves, without any swing into mania or hypomania, as defined by Karl Leonhard in his concept of unipolar depression (Leonhard 1957), and now codified in DSM as MDD. Koukopoulos' view is that this interpretation of unipolar depression is superficial, because it ignores the important role of temperament. In other words, it matters what such patients are like in between their depressive episodes. What are the euthymic intervals like? Often they are not euthymic; instead such patients have abnormal temperaments which are essential mild variants on depression or mania, like dysthymia or cyclothymia or hyperthymia. When patients have hyperthymia or cyclothymia, they have manic symptoms, constantly, in between their clinical depressive episodes. Thus Koukopoulos sees those depressive episodes as the result of the manic symptoms that are present as part of patients' temperaments. Dysthymia is not characterized by having manic symptoms, but it often has notable anxiety, associated with irritability and agitation. Thus, in MDD, the majority of patients have abnormal temperaments with manic symptoms, broadly defined, and those manic symptoms could again be seen as necessary for the occurrence of episodic depression. The mechanism of how mania produces depression is, in Koukopoulos' view, biological: neuronal excitement leads to neuronal depression, i.e., excitotoxicity occurs.

Koukopoulos' primacy of mania thesis is exactly the reverse of the standard Freudian theory of mania. Freud wrote very little about mania, and only one major paper on melancholia. (And that paper was written hastily to pre-empt an article by a young student of Freud, Victor Tausk, who himself likely had manic-depression; Tausk committed suicide soon thereafter, and the story was hushed up by the psychoanalytic community for half a century until discovered by the historian Paul Roazen in his classic work, *Brother Animal* (Roazen 1969).) Freud's view was that mania was a reaction to depression, a flight from depression; this view has been repeated without much profundity for almost a century now. Traditional psychoanalysis has thus seen mania as a superficial phenomenon which, when stripped of its external symptoms, is to be revealed as depression once more. Hence only depression really matters, not mania. The originality of Koukopoulos' thesis is to suggest that depression may be the superficial experience, and mania the profound one.

LACK OF INSIGHT

Another key feature to understanding mania is the problem of insight. Those who see mania or hypomania as inherently "good" do not appear to attend to this problem. We found that about one-half of patients in the throes of a severe acute manic episode deny that they are experiencing manic symptoms (Ghaemi and Rosenquist 2004). They are, to put it mildly, not entirely aware of what is happening. They are not psychotic; they don't have delusions or hallucinations. Lack of insight has been clearly shown to be a different phenomenon than psychosis (Amador and Anthony 2004). Instead, it seems that part of the nature of some illnesses, like mania, is the fact that patients don't appreciate that they are ill.

This fact, well proven for mania as well as schizophrenia and some other conditions (Amador and Anthony 2004), has important conceptual consequences. One of these is that one cannot rely on the patient's self-report. The manic patient is the opposite of Descartes' subject: his clear and distinct ideas are clearly and distinctly false to others. The autonomy of the self is not present; the self is sick and doesn't realize it is sick. And this lack of insight is present not only in severe mania, but in mild mania or hypomania. In fact, insight seems even more impaired in hypomania than in mania (Ghaemi and Rosenquist 2004).

Such considerations make many of us uncomfortable, partly because of deeply felt (though not necessarily explicit) philosophical assumptions about the nature of happiness. The problem of mild mania or hypomania highlights how the assessment of insight depends on the clinician's diagnostic certainty; if the clinician is not certain (or worse, is mistaken) about the patient's diagnosis, then there is no way to be certain whether the patient has insight into the diagnosis. In an important paper, Moore and colleagues (Moore et al. 1995) relate the concept of insight in "mild" mania to ethical conceptions of well-being. They describe a manic patient who, when manic, does not wish to be married, leaves his family, spends money generously, and generally enjoys himself. When not manic, he regrets many of those behaviors, but he is not sure which "person" he is: the manic care-free person, or the not-manic responsible person. Thus, he vacillates between taking and not taking medication. The authors indicate that the perspective of the patient when manic may be as acceptable and deserving of respect as the perspective of the patient when not-manic; this is based on a desire-fulfillment theory of well-being, where the autonomous individual has the right to determine his/her well-being based on the satisfaction of whatever desires that person possesses. Other perspectives, such as hedonism (or simple pursuit of pleasure) might also be used to justify mania. Another viewpoint, which perhaps comes most naturally to clinicians, assumes that manic patients are not expressing their true desires due to a biological infirmity, and thus their perspective when manic is not representative of either their true wishes or their best interests. Moore and associates cast doubt on this clinical perspective as excessively paternalistic and disrespectful of patient autonomy.

At one level, the case just presented is not really a case of hypomania, nor even "mild" mania, but simply mania. In this case, the patient clearly has social dysfunction in relation to his marriage and his friendships, and this dysfunction is more than mild, since it is placing his marriage in serious jeopardy. So we might say that the patient should take lithium to allow him to function well in his usual, average, "normal," "healthy" state. This average state is defined by how he is most of the time, outside of his brief manic or depressive episodes. Further, one could argue that he is not "himself" in the manic state, that his agency is impaired by his manic illness, and thus he is exercising his free will only in his non-manic state. All these considerations would argue for treatment with lithium.

However, the philosophical considerations raised by Moore and colleagues would indeed hold for a case of true hypomania. Imagine the same case without any significant dysfunction in the hypomanic state. The case would have to be rewritten, the spousal conflict would have to be minimal, but seen in that manner, it would be ethically less confusing. Many would agree that treatment for hypomania, in isolation, is not necessary. But the problem of insight raises another issue: in making judgments about this question, the hypomanic or manic person's views are not the last word.

PRAGMATIC ASSUMPTIONS

Many of those who are critical of diagnosing mania or hypomania seem concerned mainly on pragmatic grounds: they don't want drugs to be given. It wouldn't matter what we think about mania or hypomania in a pure intellectual ether; one could have any opinion one wanted there. It seems to matter because people don't want "powerful" drugs like neuroleptics or lithium or mood stabilizers to be given. In the case of hypomania, in particular, such concerns are raised; if we need to diagnose bipolar disorder type II to treat its depression, then we should do so; but hypomania itself should not be treated.

These attitudes contain a multitude of assumptions, as readers may sense at this point of this discussion. If the primacy of mania thesis is valid, then the concerns are nonsensical. If we recognize that bipolar disorder is an illness of recurrence, not polarity—in other words if hypomania and depression cannot be isolated, but always occur as a cycle—then again the concern is vacuous.

Mania, hypomania, depression—even anxiety, agitation, and irritability—are of a piece. They can be distinguished, and yet they cannot be isolated. That seems to be just the way the human mind is, unless we take a purely social constructionist view that doubts the biological reality of conditions like mania or depression, a postmodernist assumption that underlies many of the views of contemporary critics, as discussed in detail elsewhere (Dennett 2000; Ghaemi 2009).

SUMMARY

Mania is a mental state centrally characterized by psychomotor activation, creativity, and lack of insight. It is biologically based, and primarily characterized by psychomotor activation, with mood changes being secondary and epiphenomenal. Mania may be diagnostically central to all mood illnesses, including depressive conditions. Mania enhances creativity, and in its milder forms, such as cyclothymic or hyperthymic temperaments, has many positive aspects, reflected in social benefits and historical achievements. Lack of insight impairs the self-understanding of the person with manic symptoms, and is an important clinical problem. Psychoanalytic and postmodernist approaches fail to appreciate these important features of mania.

References

Amador, X. F. and Anthony, D. S. (2004). *Insight and Psychosis* (2nd edn). Oxford: Oxford University Press.

Bienvenu, O. J., Davydow, D. S., and Kendler, K. S. (2011). Psychiatric 'diseases' versus behavioral disorders and degree of genetic influence. *Psychological Medicine*, *41*(1), 33–40.

Bruchmuller, K. and Meyer, T. D. (2009). Diagnostically irrelevant information can affect the likelihood of a diagnosis of bipolar disorder. *Journal of Affective Disorders*, *116*(1–2), 148–51.

Cassano, G. B., Rucci, P., Benvenuti, A., Miniati, M., Calugi, S., Maggi, L., *et al.* (2012). The role of psychomotor activation in discriminating unipolar from bipolar disorders: a classification-tree analysis. *Journal of Clinical Psychiatry*, *73*, 22–8.

Dennett, D. (2000). Postmodernism and truth. In J. Hintikka, S. Neville, E. Sosa, and A. Olsen (Eds), *Proceedings of the Twentieth World Congress of Philosophy* (Volume 8), pp. 93–103. Charlottesville, VA: Philosophy Documentation Center.

Feynman, R. (1985). *Surely You're Joking, Mr. Feynman!* New York, NY: Bantam.

Feynman, R. (1988). *What Do You Care What Other People Think?* New York, NY: Bantam.

Flexner, J. T. (2003). *George Washington: The Indispensable Man*. Newtown, CT: American Political Biography Press.

Frances, A. (2010). The first draft of DSM-V. *British Medical Journal*, *340*, c1168.

Ghaemi, S. N. (2009). *The Rise and Fall of the Biopsychosocial Model: Reconciling Art and Science in Psychiatry*. Baltimore, MD: Johns Hopkins University Press.

Ghaemi, S. N. (2011). *A First-Rate Madness: Uncovering the Links between Mental Illness and Leadership*. New York, NY: Penguin Press.

Ghaemi, S. N. and Rosenquist, K. J. (2004). Insight in mood disorders: An empirical and conceptual review. In X. Amador and A. David (Eds), *Insight and Psychosis*, pp. 101–18. Oxford: Oxford University Press.

Gazzaniga, M. S. (1998). The split brain revisited. *Scientific American*, *279*(1), 50–5.

Goodwin, F. K. and Jamison, K. R. (2007). *Manic Depressive Illness* (2nd edn). New York, NY: Oxford University Press.

Jamison, K. R. (2004). *An Unquiet Mind: A Memoir of Moods and Madness*. New York, NY: Vintage Books.

Janet, P. (1903). *Les Obsessions et la Psychasthenie, Volume 1*. Paris: Ancienne Librairie Germer Baillière.

Kesebir, S., Vahip, S., Akdeniz, F., Yuncu, Z., Alkan, M., and Akiskal, H. (2005). Affective temperaments as measured by TEMPS-A in patients with bipolar I disorder and their first-degree relatives: a controlled study. *Journal of Affective Disorders*, *85*(1–2), 127–33.

Kessler, R. C., Demler, O., Frank, R. G., Olfson, M., Pincus, H. A., Walters, E. E., *et al.* (2005). Prevalence and treatment of mental disorders, 1990 to 2003. *New England Journal of Medicine*, *352*(24), 2515–23.

Koukopoulos, A. and Ghaemi, S. N. (2009). The primacy of mania: a reconsideration of mood disorders. *European Psychiatry*, *24*(2), 125–34.

Kretschmer, E. (1970). *Physique and Character*. New York, NY: Cooper Square Publishers.

Leonhard, K. (1957). *The Classification of Endogenous Psychoses* (R. Berman, Trans.). New York, NY: Irvington.

Mansfield, R. and Busse, T. (1981). *The Psychology of Creativity and Discovery*. Chicago, IL: Nelson-Hall.

Mayer-Gross, W. (2000). The translation: "The Phenomenology of Abnormal Emotions of Happiness". *Philosophy, Psychiatry, & Psychology*, *7*(4), 298–309.

Moore, A., Hope, T., and Fulford, K. W. M. (1995). Mild mania and well-being. *Philosophy, Psychology, & Psychiatry, 1*, 166–91.

Roazen, P. (1969). *Brother Animal*. New York, NY: Knopf.

Robins, E. and Guze, S. B. (1970). Establishment of diagnostic validity in psychiatric illness: its application to schizophrenia. *American Journal of Psychiatry, 126*, 983–7.

Shorter, E. (2007). The doctrine of the two depressions in historical perspective. *Acta Psychiatrica Scandinavica Supplementum, 433*, 5–13.

Simonton, D. (1994). *Greatness: Who Makes History and Why*. New York, NY: Guilford Press.

Srivastava, S., Childers, M. E., Baek, J. H., Strong, C. M., Hill, S. J., Warsett, K. S., *et al.* (2010). Toward interaction of affective and cognitive contributors to creativity in bipolar disorders: a controlled study. *Journal of Affective Disorder, 125*(1–3), 27–34.

Wicki, W. and Angst, J. (1991). The Zurich Study: Hypomania in a 28-to 30-year-old cohort. *European Archives of Psychiatry and Clinical Neuroscience, 240*, 339–48.

Wolff, S. (2000). The phenomenology of abnormal emotions of happiness: A translation from the German of William Mayer-Gross's doctoral thesis. *Philosophy, Psychiatry, & Psychology, 7*, 295–7.

CHAPTER 48

AUTISM AND THE PHILOSOPHY OF MIND

R. PETER HOBSON

INTRODUCTION

Over thirty years of life as an autism researcher, I have harbored the idea (fanciful though it is) that I have been pursuing practical philosophy. In order to understand the nature and development of autism, we need to draw on philosophy to establish an appropriate conceptual framework within which to set our psychological theorizing. From a complementary perspective, the phenomena of autism may show us how far our current ways of thinking about psychological issues—for example, the nature of and basis for understanding minds, or the relations among cognition, conation, and affect, or the structure of social emotions and the self, or the mechanisms of communication and thought—are at best limited and often inadequate. In this contribution, therefore, I shall attempt to flesh out the significance of autism for philosophy, as well as the importance of philosophy for understanding autism.

Of course this overview will not be comprehensive. For instance, considerations from autism are relevant for philosophical discussions of ethics and aesthetics, but I shall not address these topics. Instead, I shall concentrate on themes that fall within the domain of philosophy of mind. In some places I shall begin with phenomena of autism and then introduce philosophical writings, and elsewhere I shall begin with philosophy and show its relevance for autism. I hope that what this strategy lacks in consistency will be offset by something else: the approach embodies the view that there is and should continue to be two-way traffic between the disciplines of philosophy and the developmental psychopathology of autism.

A final note by way of introduction: What is autism? Autism is a syndrome, which is neither more nor less than a constellation of clinical features that tend to occur together. The clinical features include profound difficulties in engaging and communicating with other people, limitations in flexible and creative thinking, and stereotyped forms of behavior such as rituals or preoccupations that are often decidedly odd. There are diverse causes of autism, both from a biological (etiological) viewpoint and from the perspective of developmentally unfolding psychological dysfunction (psychopathogenesis). So, too, children with autism may follow different pathways as they get older, and in some cases may even partly grow out of autism (e.g., see Hobson and Lee, 2010, for the case of children with autism who are congenitally blind). This means that one needs to be cautious about thinking of autism as an "it" that some children and adults "have." Even this fact has a philosophical dimension, insofar as it reminds us to be circumspect about the dangers of being trapped or misled by the concepts we employ.

Theory of Mind

When he published the paper in which the syndrome of autism was first described, Kanner (1943) launched a tradition of clinical writing (e.g., Bosch 1970; Ricks and Wing 1975; Scheerer et al. 1945) that vividly portrays how children with autism are limited in their emotional engagement with, and understanding of, other people. Then toward the end of the 1980s, two lines of research from experimental psychology propelled these children's social difficulties into the limelight of psychological and philosophical debate.

The greatest impact came from a study by Baron-Cohen et al. (1985), who employed a test designed by Wimmer and Perner (1983) to reveal that children with autism have difficulty in taking into account another person's false beliefs. In this experiment, a doll called Anne witnessed another doll called Sally placing a marble in a basket. Sally left the scene, and while she was away Anne transferred the marble from Sally's basket into her own box, where it was hidden from view. When Sally returned, the experimenter asked the critical "belief question": "Where will Sally look for her marble?" The results were that 85% of typically developing and Down syndrome children indicated that Sally would look in her basket, but only 20% of children with autism did so. All sixteen children with autism who responded incorrectly pointed to where the marble really was. In a companion study, Baron-Cohen et al. (1986) tested participants' abilities to order sequences of pictures according to a storyline, and again, children with autism found difficulty in ordering stories that involved figures being surprised. Moreover, in recounting the stories, they rarely used mental state terms such as want, believe, and know.

At roughly the same time, colleagues and I (e.g., Hobson 1986; Weeks and Hobson 1987) began to publish a series of papers that pointed to the children's limited ability to recognize and interpret facial and other bodily expressions of emotion (reviewed in Hobson 1991a). In theoretical writings (e.g., Hobson 1989, 1990a, 1993a), I considered how the findings might reflect impairments in affectively configured interpersonal relations that are foundational for broader difficulties in the children's interpersonal understanding and thinking processes.

These studies prompted a flurry of empirical research on "social cognition" among children with autism that continues to the present day. I shall not review this research, because for the present purposes, our foremost concern is to consider how the studies have been interpreted. Most important from a philosophical perspective, we need to explore whether the concepts that have been deployed are adequate to the task of interpreting and explaining the results—and whether findings from autism point to strengths and weaknesses in alternative philosophical positions. What is striking here, is that much contemporary discussion is divorced from what had once been mainstream in developmental psychology, namely a preoccupation with what Piaget (1972) called genetic epistemology. Genetic epistemology explores the conditions that allow for the possibility of knowledge and its development. It would have seemed natural for developmentalists to analyze the kinds of social experience that underpin young children's knowledge of people's minds, so that one might pinpoint what is lacking in the case of children with autism. In the event, the dominant mode of theorizing took a different, computational turn.

The title of the first study by Baron-Cohen et al. (1985) that I have already described was entitled: "Does the autistic child have a 'theory of mind'?" The expression "theory of mind" had been adopted from a paper by Premack and Woodruff (1978), who wrote (p. 515):

> In saying that an individual has a theory of mind, we mean that the individual imputes mental states to himself and to others (either to conspecifics or to other species as well). A system of inferences of this kind is properly viewed as a theory, first, because such states are not directly observable, and second, because the system can be used to make predictions, specifically about the behavior of other organisms.

This way of thinking about interpersonal understanding—that it must involve inferences because mental states are not directly observable, and that its primary role is to make predictions—became widespread among developmental psychologists who took Theory of Mind (now further reified by the introduction of two capital letters) as the psychological domain concerned with the acquisition and deployment of mental state concepts.

Even here, it was not clear that acquiring mental state *concepts* was set center-stage. Much theoretical discussion concerned representations and especially representations *of* representations, and there was a bias toward conceiving of such representations in the context of computationally formal information-processing models. Little attention was given to the content of the concept of "belief," and little effort expended in explicating quite what it means to hold a belief. Correspondingly, questions about a range of prerequisites for acquiring such concepts, or understanding such commitments, were mostly neglected. In addition, representing "belief" and "false belief" were taken as paradigmatic for understanding representational mental states, even though it was yet to be established how far a grasp of other mental states such as intentions, feelings, and wishes either conformed to this model, or might provide its developmental underpinnings.

The seminal approach of Leslie (e.g., 1987, 1991) may be taken to exemplify the style of Theory of Mind theorizing with what Leslie called the "computational metaphor." Leslie's terminology evolved over time, but essentially, he posited that an innate "decoupling mechanism" is responsible for children's ability to achieve metarepresentation. This he considered to be a particular form of internal representation that consists of the following parts: an agent (typically, a person), an informational relation (e.g., pretend, think, or believe), an anchor (often in the form of a prop for the play), and a decoupled expression which comprises a primary veridical representation of the world that is no longer tied to the reality it represents (e.g., a child representing mother as pretending that a cup contains water in an imaginary, playful context). Leslie supposed that the metarepresentational capacity determines "the human mind's ability to characterize and manipulate its own attitudes to information" (Leslie 1987, p. 416). The "decoupling mechanism" is innate; it does not develop through social experience; it has nothing to do with feelings; and it leads to (rather than derives from) the ability to recognize the nature of mental states. This scheme maps on to

Leslie's explanation of autism, insofar as he attributed impairments in symbolic play and "theory of mind" among children with autism to an absence or malfunction of the decoupling mechanism and to difficulties in forming and/or processing metarepresentations. He adopted the position (e.g., in Leslie 1991) that these individuals' affective disorder and impairment in social and communicative behavior are secondary consequences of the basic cognitive deficit.

Theory of Mind theorizing attracted advocates from the realms of philosophy (see, for example, contributions to Carruthers and Smith 1996). Yet as we shall see, there are philosophical reasons for seeking a different kind of theory about the nature and developmental psychopathology of interpersonal understanding and knowledge of minds.

For a long time the most popular alternative to Theory of Mind theorizing was the "simulation" approach. Simulationists were represented by both developmental psychologists (e.g., Harris 1989), and philosophers (e.g. Goldman 2006; Gordon 1996). As Gordon (1996) pointed out, there are two kinds of simulation theory. According to one of these, one first recognizes one's own mental states and then infers, on the basis of an assumed similarity or analogy, that the person simulated is in similar states. Another emphasizes imaginative transformation into the position of the other, but does not require recognition of one's own mental states as such, nor possession of concepts of mental states simulated. The crux of the simulationist position is that much of the cognitive-computational processing posited to underlie Theory of Mind is not only unnecessary, but also misplaced as characterizing the most basic and developmentally primitive form of social understanding. This orientation is shared with other psychologists (e.g. Hobson 1993b) and philosophers (e.g., Gallagher 2001) who would reject other tenets of simulation theory—in particular, the suggestion that "imaginative transformation" is basic to interpersonal understanding—and who aim to provide a third, distinctive account of how we arrive at knowledge of persons with minds. The remainder of this contribution explores philosophical, psychological, and specifically autism-related considerations that point the way to such alternatives to "theory theory."

The Argument from Analogy

The first step in this third approach was to dispense with the idea that we arrive at knowledge of other minds through processes of inference, and in particular, through drawing analogies from what one knows from a first-person perspective. One reason that developmental psychologists such as Harris (1989), Perner (1990), Tomasello (1999), and Meltzoff (2002) were attracted to this idea was a difficulty in seeing how it could be otherwise. For example, Leslie (1987, p. 422) wrote as follows: "It is hard to see how perceptual evidence could ever force an adult, let alone a young child, to invent the idea of unobservable mental states."

I shall not dwell on the arguments against such positions that have been mounted by Scheler (1954) as well as Wittgenstein and his followers, for the reason that developmentalists including myself have attempted to distil the reasoning elsewhere (Hobson 1991b, 1993a, 1993b: and Hobson 2008a, on the wider relevance of Wittgenstein to autism). In summary, Wittgenstein's (1958) attack on the very concept of a private language undermines the assumption that all by oneself and without the possibility of correction by others (already experienced as others), one would be able to identify a given mental state as the same when this recurs within one's own experience, and then go on to ascribe it to other people. Even if this were possible, moreover, and if—implausibly—one could develop the mental equipment to formulate and apply analogy prior to engaging with the mental states of other people, still one would lack an adequate basis for such analogical reasoning. Other people would seem very *unlike* oneself unless already, one could apprehend in some way that they have subjective states of mind. Prior to the application of analogy, one might suppose, "human things" in the environment could be perceived to have bodily characteristics like one's own, but they would appear to lack what is to the forefront of one's own subjective experience, namely the having-of-experience itself. As Wittgenstein (1958, section 302) noted:

> If one has to imagine someone else's pain on the model of one's own, this is none too easy a thing to do: for I have to imagine a pain which I *do not feel* on the model of the pain which I *do feel.*

If we were to adopt the premises from which the argument from analogy proceeds, young children (as well as we adults) would need to ascribe minds not to persons but to *bodies* that conveyed no sense of subjective, emotional life. Noticing that other bodies are like one's own would give little clue that they might instantiate persons with minds. These considerations undermine notions dear to simulationists, namely that one might begin with knowledge of one's own mental states and use analogy, or alternatively apply some form of (preconceptual) imagination, in order to ascribe similar states to other people.

THE PRIMACY OF PERSONAL RELATIONS

An alternative starting point is with what Hamlyn (1974) called "natural reactions of persons to persons." In *Philosophical Investigations*, Wittgenstein (1958, p. 178) argued for the epistemological primacy of relatedness in our dealings with people: "My attitude towards him is an attitude towards a soul. I am not of the *opinion* that he has a soul." Malcolm (1962, p. 92) explicated how the bedrock for explaining our understanding of other people does not lie in what we believe, and concluded with a quotation from Wittgenstein (1958, p. 226):

> As philosophers we must not attempt to justify the forms of life, to give reasons for *them*—to argue, for example, that we pity the injured man because we believe, assume, presuppose, or know that in addition to the groans and writhing, there is pain. The fact is, we pity him! "What has to be accepted, the given, is—so one could say—*forms of life.*"

Or as Martin Buber (1937/1984, p. 18) wrote: "In the beginning is relation."

If we do not infer the existence of mental states, then how do we begin to appreciate the subjective lives of others? Wittgenstein's (1980, vol. II, section 570) response is that we apprehend feelings *in* the expressions of other people:

> "We *see* emotion."—As opposed to what?—We do not see facial contortions and *make the inference* that he is feeling joy, grief, boredom. We describe a face immediately as sad, radiant, bored, even when we are unable to give any other description of the features.—Grief, one would like to say, is personified in the face. This is essential to what we call "emotion."

There is something primitive about our capacity to apprehend another person's feelings as that person's feelings, through our perception of what is expressed in the person's "facial contortions." The reason that these are not mere contortions is that when we see a smile, for example, we apply a special kind of perception—what might be called feeling perception— that entails we have an affective response to what we see (or at least, entails that we have had, or have the capacity to have had, such responses). Merleau-Ponty (1964, p. 146) expressed similar ideas from a phenomenological perspective: "Sympathy ... is the simple fact that I live in the facial expressions of the other, as I feel him living in mine."

The upshot is our engagement with other people is such that it provides direct access to other people with their own subjective life. This being so, then we can ask: Is this also the case for children with autism? A body of evidence (e.g., as summarized in Hobson 2002) suggests that these children are limited in what they perceive in, and experience through, the bodily expressed emotions of other people. If this is so, then might *this* account for their limitations in so-called Theory of Mind—as well as for a range of their cognitive as well as social deficits?

Acquiring the Concept of Persons-With-Minds

A preliminary, philosophical matter is to consider what is involved in acquiring a concept of any kind, because this will be important when we come to examine what is involved in acquiring mental state concepts. Malcolm (1962, p. 92) writes: "If we want to understand any concept we must obtain a view of the human behavior, the activities, the natural expressions, that surround the words for that concept." The same is true if we want to understand how concepts are acquired. Hamlyn (1978) argued that to have a concept of X is to know what it is for something to be an X. "What something is" (as we conceive it) depends on its relations to us. Just as one could not have the concept of a clutch in a car without a grasp of what it means to drive a car, so one could not arrive at a concept of persons without standing in relations that are fitting to persons, namely relations that involve mutual feelings. The critical thing is that if one always experienced and treated people as things, one would not master the concept of "person."

Elsewhere (Hobson 1993a) I have described the clinical case of a young adult with Asperger syndrome, a form of autism, who was unable to grasp the concept of "friend." The reason was that he had scant experience of friendship, and especially of sharing activities and experiences in ways that make friendship what it is. In Malcolm's terms, he did not engage in the human behavior, the activities, and the natural expressions that surrounded words for the concept of friend. In Hamlyn's terms, he did not know what it is for someone to be a friend, in that he lacked experience of the engagements that friendship entails. In this respect, he did not fully share a "form of life" (Wittgenstein) in which friendships plays a natural role.

Here we return to how relations between embodied people embedded in a shared world are critical for interpersonal understanding (including so-called Theory of Mind). The vital importance of such relations for acquiring concepts of mind becomes especially clear through the philosophy of Strawson (1959, pp. 101–102), who insisted on "the primitiveness of the concept of a person … a type of entity such that *both* predicates ascribing states of consciousness *and* predicates ascribing corporeal characteristics, a physical situation, etc. are equally applicable to a single individual of that single type." To acquire such a concept one needs to relate to persons *as* persons—and only subsequently does a child come to distinguish the "mental" dimension that such relations entail.

Now one might wonder whether Theory of Mind theorists were arguing for necessary rather than sufficient conditions for a child to come to represent other people and other people's representations. Something like Leslie's decoupling mechanism might simply operate within a broader set of developmental processes that contribute to mental state understanding. There are two points to make here. Firstly, Theory of Mind theorists would need to find a place for these other factors, and show how they interact with supposed computational mechanisms. Secondly, developmental psychopathology might reveal how the story of evolving interpersonal relations can *explain* the origins of symbolic representations and the acquisition of concepts of mind, and indeed explain the process of "decoupling" thoughts from the objects of those thoughts, so that thoughts become objects of further thought in their own right.

As we shall see, there is such a developmental story, and one of its themes is how the distancing of thought from the objects of thought is intimately connected with the differentiation between self and other people (Werner and Kaplan 1963/1984).

Self and Other

Until recently, and with notable exceptions (e.g., Barresi and Moore 1996; Hobson 1990b), much theorizing about Theory of Mind has proceeded with little reference to "self" and "other." This is curious, given that concepts of mind entail concepts not just of persons, but of self and others to whom minds are ascribed. More than this, such concepts can be used with first-, second-, and third-person meanings. We need to understand how this can be.

In the literature on autism, there has been occasionally intense but mostly inconsistent concern with the children's experience of themselves in relation to others. One focus has been the oft-reported confusions that are observed in the children's use of the personal pronouns "I" and "you." De Villiers and de Villiers (1974) point out that "I" and "you" are words that can only be understood by "nonegocentric" individuals who recognize the context of the relationship between the speaker and the addressee, and who have grasped reciprocal roles in discourse. Do children with autism understand speaker–addressee relations—and if not, why not?

An especially rich perspective on self–other relations drawing upon European phenomenological writings was that offered by Bosch in a book entitled *Infantile Autism* (1970) and subtitled (in translation): *A Clinical and Phenomenological-Anthropological Investigation Taking Language as a Guide.* This forewarns of the density of Bosch's writings, steeped as it is in the tradition of Husserl's phenomenological philosophy. In attempting to delineate "the particular mode of existence of an autistic child" (Bosch 1970, p. 3), Bosch illustrates how the child often seems to lack a sense of possessiveness as well as self-consciousness and shame, to be delayed in "acting" on others by demanding or ordering, and to be missing something of the "'self-involvement', the acting with, and the identification with the acting person" (p. 81). Bosch interprets the autistic child's delay in using "I" and "you" with reference to such "paths to the 'I' in language" (p. 64). He also suggests that "counter-attack or defense is impossible because the child has no experience of attacking or defensive relationship with others" (p. 99). Perhaps most prescient of all, he emphasizes that "delay occurs in the constituting of the other person as someone in whose place I can put myself … [and] … in the constituting of a common sphere of existence, in which things do not simply refer to me but also to others" (p. 89).

It will be clear that Bosch sets self–other awareness in the context of a rich array of self–other attitudes and relations. He also stresses three things I highlighted earlier, namely the significance of engagement with the attitudes of others, the ability to move in perspective through others, and the experience of a shared world. It is notable that Bosch refers to "the identification with the acting person." This notion of identification is one that colleagues and I have explored over recent years, insofar as it seems to characterize a process that is both critical for self-other connectedness and differentiation, *and*, in its relative absence among individuals with autism, critical for explaining the pathogenesis of autism. If, as G. H. Mead (1934) explicated, the origins not only of self-reflective awareness but also symbolic thinking are to be found in a human capacity to take the role of other persons, then failures in identification might explain much about the cognitive as well as social deficits of individuals with autism.

ON IDENTIFYING WITH OTHERS

Something like identification appears in the writings of philosophers concerned with how we understand people. Consider how Wittgenstein (1980, vol. I, section 920) wrote, "One may also say: 'He made *this* face' or 'His face altered like *this*', imitating it—and again one can't describe it in any other way."

Or again, moving away from the face to whole-body expressions, Wittgenstein (1980, vol. I, section 1066) stated:

> "I see that the child wants to touch the dog, but doesn't dare." How can I see that? - Is this description of what is seen on the same level as a description of moving shapes and colours? Is an interpretation in question? Well, remember that you may also *mimic* a human being who would like to touch something, but doesn't dare.

There is something basic about the ability to transpose what one perceives in the expression of someone else, to one's own bodily expression and activity. This fact is relevant for understanding what the expression means. If one could not do this, then one would fail to understand something important about what is expressed. Wittgenstein appears to be highlighting something about self-other relations, in that "*this* face" begins as his and ends up as mine, yet in some sense it is the same facial expression. Or in the case of the hesitant gesture, the fact that one *may* mimic the gesture gives us a clue to how we understand gestures as witnessed.

I suggest that Wittgenstein's example captures the process of "identifying with" someone, that is, assimilating the stance of someone else so that it becomes a potential stance for oneself. This explains how one could mimic, even if one does not explicitly do so. Taking up Wittgenstein's approach, Hampshire (1976) explored how something like identification (he calls it "the primitive faculty of imitation") provides a psychological bridge between people, or as he expresses it, "a necessary background to the communication of feeling" (p. 73):

> In direct dealings with men, and outside the context of fiction, we perceive, and react to, the physiognomy of persons almost as immediately as to the full behaviour of which the facial expression is the residue ... And we can show that we have perceived it by adopting the same expression in imitation, without trying to reproduce, item by item, the physical features of the face or posture of another. (pp. 78–79)

This leads on to the conditions that make first-, second-, and third-person ascriptions of given mental states so natural (Strawson 1959). In particular, there are forms of first-person state that encompass second- and/or third-person stances. Or to put this differently, second- and third-person states (or more accurately, states closely allied to these) can become a part, and potentially a differentiated part, of first-person experience. So, from a phenomenological perspective, Merleau-Ponty (1964, pp. 118, 145) wrote:

> In perceiving the other, my body and his are coupled, resulting in a sort of action which pairs them [*action à deux*]. This conduct which I am able only to see, I live somehow from a distance. I make it mine; I recover [*reprendre*] it or comprehend it ... Mimesis is the ensnaring of me by the other, the invasion of me by the other; it is that attitude whereby I assume the gestures, the conducts, the favorite words, the ways of doing things of those whom I confront ... [it] is the power of assuming conducts or facial expressions as my own.

If, as colleagues and myself have proposed (e.g., Hobson et al. 2006, 2007), the propensity to identify with the attitudes of others is specifically diminished among children with autism, then one can begin to understand why they are limited in the capacity to share experiences and engage in joint attention, as well as to move through other-person-centered perspectives. Is there evidence for or against this account in the children's limited experience and expression of other-person-centered relational states?

Social Emotions

One area in which there is an emphasis on specifically emotional aspects of self-other relations, is that of so-called "social emotions" such as empathy, concern, shame, guilt, embarrassment, pride, jealousy, and envy. Many philosophers take a rather grown-up and often cognitively slanted view of what such emotions entail. For example, here is Taylor (1985, pp. 1–2) writing about so-called self-conscious emotions:

> The interest of the emotions of self-assessment, for the philosopher at least, lies primarily in the nature and complexity of the beliefs involved ... Over a wide range of emotions ... beliefs are constitutive of the emotional experience in question.

The predominance of cognitive perspectives on emotion has prompted Goldie (2000), in his philosophical study of *The Emotions*, to criticize "the over-intellectualization of emotion" (p. 11) in philosophical writings. Goldie illustrated his objection thus: "What really comes first is the emotional response itself—the feeling of fear towards the snake—and not the thought that its bite is poisonous and the thought that poison would harm me" (p. 45). A similar form of reasoning may be relevant for social emotions, because the capacity to have thoughts or hold beliefs may not be a prerequisite for complexly structured emotions. As Frijda (1993) has suggested, "even emotions like anger, guilt, and shame, that have cognitively complex definitions, can result from rather elementary stimulus constellations, and through rather elementary appraisal processes" (p. 374).

Research in autism suggests that affected children have specific limitations in expressing (and probably, experiencing) other-person-centered emotions such as concern, guilt, and embarrassment (e.g., Hobson et al. 2006; J. A. Hobson et al. 2009), whereas other emotional states such as jealousy or ill-focused responsiveness to the moods of others are relatively spared. One part of what it means to identify with someone else is that one is affectively engaged with and cares about the other person's feelings *as* the other's. A specific deficit in identifying with others promises to explain why children with autism show signs of being aware when they are being observed, but little sign of being affected by and engaged with the attitudes of particular embodied other people, for example in embarrassment or shame. Moreover, they show a (relative) failure to be moved to take an "alter" stance toward themselves, and thereby achieve reflective self-awareness.

There is a further implication of this theoretical approach. Consider how in *Being and Nothingness*, Sartre (1956, p. 350) described shame as a *source* of self-awareness, rather than the outcome of cognitively elaborated self-reflective thoughts:

> *I am that Ego;* I do not reject it as a strange image, but it is present to me as a self which I *am* without *knowing* it; for I discover it in shame and, in other instances, in pride. It is shame or pride which reveals to me the Other's look and myself at the end of that look. It is the shame or pride which makes me *live*, not *know* the situation of being looked at.

Note that here, Sartre considers what shame "reveals to me"—where the emotional state is primary. Therefore certain emotional states, perhaps configured through processes of identification, may underpin rather than result from increasingly sophisticated forms of self-awareness.

THE DEVELOPMENT OF
COMMUNICATION AND THOUGHT

The account I have outlined is one in which the capacity for thinking arises out of particular forms of human communication. Many children with autism only partly comprehend how communication, including language, functions. Most important here is the fact that language is the most exquisite means of expressing a speaker's attitude both to the listener, and to whatever is being talked about. Autistic children are (relatively) insensitive to the infinite variety of ways that language embodies a speaker's psychological orientation to the listener and to the topic(s) of conversation. One underlying reason is that they fail to understand how people have a set of intentions-in-speaking, a repertoire of speech acts (Searle 1969), and how speakers select from a limitless set of co-referential expressions the one(s) that captures the particular aspects of meaning that are to be communicated or thought about. At root is a fundamental limitation in comprehending what it means for a person to have a range of psychological attitudes to other people, to things, and to events, and moreover to have a variety of communicative motives and attitudes in speaking at all. Difficulties of these kinds infect some meanings more than others: deictic terms such as personal pronouns which shift meaning according to speaker–listener roles are especially vulnerable, so are metaphors. Echolalia is one notable instance of the failure to adjust linguistic forms according to speaker–listener perspectives. Yet the problems are ubiquitous—all utterances convey nuances of "speaker's meaning" that will be lost on autistic individuals.

No wonder, then, that children with autism face developmental obstacles when it comes to thinking. David Hamlyn (1978, p. 76) has captured what it means to think, thus:

> For a thought to be a genuine thought it must be about something, and something else must be thought about that something; so that there is in that thought something corresponding to the distinction between subject and predicate that becomes explicit in language itself.

Therefore the development of thinking involves a distancing between attitudes and the objects of those attitudes, in an individual's minds. How might that distancing come about?

The developmental story is one that begins with one-to-one engagement between an infant and other people, then opens out into triangular situations of joint attention in which the infant is engaged with the other person's engagement with a shared world. In the phenomena of social referencing (Sorce et al. 1985), for example, infants are moved by the perceived attitudes of another person as this is directed at objects and events in a visually specified, shared environment. If a caregiver manifests fear toward an object, the infant may be affected in such a way that the infant, too, comes to be wary of the object. The critical thing here is that the child is drawn into such sharing and co-orientation before he or she *understands* (or "represents") what it is to have and relate to person-anchored perspectives— and more than this, such non-conceptual and non-inferential role-taking places the child in a position to acquire such understanding and to develop concepts of self and other with their own takes on reality over the coming months of life. Elsewhere I have argued that this in turn is critical for the one-and-a-half year-old to be able to grasp that there are alternative descriptions-for-persons under which objects and events can fall, and with this, to acquire the ability to engage in symbolic play (Hobson 2000). The power of symbols in communication is well captured by Ogden and Richards (1923/1985, p. 11): "When we hear what is said, the symbols both cause us to perform an act of reference and to assume an attitude which will, according to circumstances, be more or less similar to the act and the attitude of the speaker."

The picture of development in autism is the negative image of this story. Affected children are very restricted in the degree to which they show "sharing" forms of joint attention and social referencing (e.g., Charman et al. 1997; Sigman et al. 1992), they are delayed and probably atypical in developing playful, creative symbolic play (Hobson et al. 2008) and, as we have seen, limited in understanding the psychological perspectives of other people.

Theory of Mind theorizing has paid special attention to the importance of understanding (or in the case of children with autism, not-understanding) beliefs, rather than perspectives in general. What does one acquire in acquiring the concept of "belief." It is one thing to have attitudes toward the world and to construe objects and events this way or that; it is another to recognize that there is a correct or true state of affairs, a reality that one needs to respect and concerning which one may be in error. To acquire a concept of belief, one needs first to have grasped what it means to assume a perspective, and then to appreciate that there is a particular perspective that is not merely a matter of taste or personal choice, but one that has a status beyond that of any individual person's take on the world—namely, that which is true of reality. So to understand what it is to hold a belief, is to understand what everyone would assent to if they were in the right position to make a judgment about the state of affairs in question (and not, for example, waylaid by misleading appearances). In my view, children with autism have such difficulty in acquiring this concept because their difficulty in shifting among person-centered perspectives undermines both their grasp of what is means to hold a perspective and, beyond this, what it means to claim that any given perspective is true of reality.

Finally, it is important to remember that thought is never completely emancipated from feeling and action. According to the present account, thought develops *out of* relations with the world that have affective as well as cognitive aspects (where aspects are very different from components; Hobson 2008b). This is in keeping not only with Vygotsky's (1962, p. 8) suggestion that "every idea contains a transmuted affective attitude toward the bit of reality to which it refers," but also the philosophical view elaborated by Warnock (1976, p. 171):

> If we are successfully imagining something, then, this is what we are doing: either by means of physical or non-physical analogues we are calling up the sense or significance of something which is not present to us in fact. It is for us affectively as if the absent object were present.

Moreover, as G. H. Mead (1934) and Werner and Kaplan (1963/1984) explicated, the achievement of self-reflective awareness and the ability to think about self and other appears to be one side of a coin, of which the other face is the ability to grasp how symbols can function as the means to thought. One could not think about self and other without symbols, but one could not achieve the requisite ability to use symbols without the appropriate kind of differentiation between symbolic vehicles and their referents. Each entails a grasp of what it means to take alternative person-anchored perspectives on a shared world.

Therefore we can see how and why in the syndrome of autism, specific impairments in affectively configured forms of interpersonal engagement are associated with characteristic atypicalities in symbolic play and thinking, as well as in the children's experiences of self and other.

FINAL REFLECTIONS

I have illustrated the potential value of mutual influence between research in developmental psychopathology, and specifically in autism, and studies in the philosophy of mind. Already these two domains have provided reciprocal stimulation and enrichment in theoretical perspective. In conjunction, they promise to change how we conceive the relations among perception and knowledge, body and mind, emotion and cognition, and self and other. Together they allow a penetrating analysis of the nature of and bases for concepts of persons and minds, the origins of symbolic representation, and more broadly, the role of interpersonal engagement in human understanding. Research on autism may do more than give us new facts about typical as well as atypical development. It may also prompt us to reconfigure the concepts in terms of which those facts are framed.

ACKNOWLEDGMENTS

I am very grateful to the Tavistock and Portman NHS Trust and the Center for Advanced Study in the Behavioral Sciences, Stanford, for allowing me the sabbatical during which this article was completed.

REFERENCES

Baron-Cohen, S., Leslie, A. M., and Frith, U. (1985). Does the autistic child have a "theory of mind"? *Cognition, 21*, 37–46.

Baron-Cohen, S., Leslie, A. M., and Frith, U. (1986). Mechanical, behavioural and Intentional understanding of picture stories in autistic children. *British Journal of Developmental Psychology, 4*, 113–25.

Barresi, J. and Moore, C. (1996). Intentional relations and social understanding. *Behavioral and Brain Sciences, 19*, 107–54.

Bosch, G. (1970). *Infantile Autism* (D. Jordan and I. Jordan, Trans.). New York, NY: Springer-Verlag.

Buber, M. (1937). *I and Thou* (R. G. Smith, Trans.) (2nd edn 1958). Edinburgh: Clark.

Carruthers, P. and Smith, P. K. (Eds) (1996). *Theories of Theories of Mind*. Cambridge: Cambridge University Press.

Charman, T., Swettenham, J., Baron-Cohen, S., Cox, A., Baird, G., and Drew, A. (1997). Infants with autism: An investigation of empathy, pretend play, joint attention, and imitation. *Developmental Psychology, 33*, 781–9.

de Villiers, P. A. and de Villiers, J. G. (1974). On this, that, and the other: Nonegocentrism in very young children. *Journal of Experimental Child Psychology, 18*, 438–47.

Frijda, N. H. (1993). The place of appraisal in emotion. *Cognition and Emotion, 7*, 357–87.

Gallagher, S. (2001). The practice of mind: Theory, simulation or primary interaction? *Journal of Consciousness Studies, 8*, 83–108.

Goldie, P. (2000). *The Emotions*. Oxford: Clarendon.

Goldman, A. I. (2006). *Simulating Minds*. Oxford: Oxford University Press.

Gordon, R. M. (1996). 'Radical' simulationism. In P. Carruthers and P. K. Smith (Eds), *Theories of Theories of Mind*, pp. 11–21. Cambridge: Cambridge University Press.

Hamlyn, D. W. (1974). Person-perception and our understanding of others. In T. Mischel (Ed.), *Understanding Other Persons*, pp. 1–36. Oxford: Basil Blackwell.

Hamlyn, D. W. (1978). *Experience and Growth of Understanding*. London: Routledge & Kegan Paul.

Hampshire, S. (1976). Feeling and expression. In J. Glover (Ed.), *The Philosophy of Mind*, pp. 73–83. Oxford: Oxford University Press.

Harris, P. L. (1989). *Children and Emotion*. Oxford: Blackwell.

Hobson, J. A., Harris, R., García-Pérez, R., and Hobson, R. P. (2008). Anticipatory concern: A study in autism. *Developmental Science, 12*, 249–63.

Hobson, R. P. (1986). The autistic child's appraisal of expressions of emotion. *Journal of Child Psychology and Psychiatry, 27*, 321–42.

Hobson, R. P. (1989). Beyond cognition: A theory of autism. In G. Dawson (Ed.), *Autism: Nature, Diagnosis, and Treatment*, pp. 22–48. New York, NY: Guilford Press.

Hobson, R. P. (1990a). On acquiring knowledge about people and the capacity to pretend: Response to Leslie. *Psychological Review*, 97, 114–21.

Hobson, R. P. (1990b). On the origins of self and the case of autism. *Development and Psychopathology*, 2, 163–81.

Hobson, R. P. (1991a). Methodological issues for experiments on autistic individuals' perception and understanding of emotion. *Journal of Child Psychology and Psychiatry*, 32, 1135–58.

Hobson, R. P. (1991b). Against the theory of ʻTheory of Mind'. *British Journal of Developmental Psychology*, 9, 33–51.

Hobson, R. P. (1993a). *Autism and the Development of Mind*. Hove: Erlbaum.

Hobson, R. P. (1993b). The emotional origins of social understanding. *Philosophical Psychology*, 6, 227–49.

Hobson, R. P. (2000). The grounding of symbols: A social-developmental account. In P. Mitchell and K. J. Riggs (Eds), *Reasoning and the Mind*, pp. 11–35. Hove: Psychology Press.

Hobson, R. P. (2002). *The Cradle of Thought*. London: Macmillan (Reprinted 2004, New York, NY: Oxford University Press.)

Hobson, R. P. (2008a). Wittgenstein and the developmental psychopathology of autism. *New Ideas in Psychology*, 2, 243–57.

Hobson, R. P. (2008b). Interpersonally situated cognition. *International Journal of Philosophical Studies*, 6, 377–97.

Hobson, R. P., Chidambi, G., Lee, A., and Meyer, J. (2006). Foundations for self-awareness: An exploration through autism. *Monographs of the Society for Research in Child Development*, 284(71), 1–165.

Hobson, R. P., and Lee, A. (2010). Reversible autism in congenitally blind children? *Journal of Child Psychology and Psychiatry*, 51, 1235–41.

Hobson, R. P., Lee, A., and Hobson, J. A. (2007). Only connect? Communication, identification, and autism. *Social Neuroscience*, 2, 320–35.

Hobson, R. P., Lee, A., and Hobson, J. A. (2008). Qualities of symbolic play among children with autism: A social-developmental perspective. *Journal of Autism and Developmental Disorders*, 39, 12–22.

Kanner, L. (1943). Autistic disturbances of affective contact. *Nervous Child*, 2, 217–50.

Leslie, A. M. (1987). Pretense and representation: The origins of "Theory of mind." *Psychological Review*, 94, 412–26.

Leslie, A. M. (1991). The Theory of Mind impairment in autism: Evidence for a modular mechanism of development? In A. Whiten (Ed.), *Natural Theories of Mind*, pp. 63–78. Oxford: Blackwell.

Malcolm, N. (1962). Wittgenstein's *Philosophical Investigations*. In V. C. Chappell (Ed), *The Philosophy of Mind*, pp. 74–100. Englewood Cliffs, NJ: Prentice-Hall.

Mead, G. H. (1934). *Mind, Self, and Society* (C. W. Morris, Ed.). Chicago, IL: University of Chicago Press.

Meltzoff, A. N. (2002). Elements of a developmental theory of imitation. In A. N. Meltzoff and W. Prinz (Eds), *The Imitative Mind: Development, Evolution, and Brain Bases*, pp. 19–41. Cambridge: Cambridge University Press.

Merleau-Ponty, M. (1964). The child's relations with others (W. Cobb, Trans.). In M. Merleau-Ponty, *The Primacy of Perception*, pp. 96–155. Evanston, IL: Northwestern University Press.

Ogden, C. K. and Richards, I. A. (1985). *The Meaning of Meaning*. London: Routledge. (Original work published 1923.)

Perner, J. (1990). *Understanding the Representational Mind*. Cambridge, MA: MIT/Bradford.

Piaget, J. (1972). *The Principles of Genetic Epistemology*. London: Routledge & Kegan Paul.

Premack, D. and Woodruff, G. (1978). Does the chimpanzee have a theory of mind? *Behavioral and Brain Sciences*, 4, 515–26.

Ricks, D. M. and Wing, L. (1975). Language, communication and the use of symbols in normal and autistic children. *Journal of Autism and Childhood Schizophrenia*, 5, 191–221.

Sartre, J. -P. (1956). *Being and Nothingness* (H. E. Barnes, Trans.). New York, NY: Washington Square

Scheerer, M., Rothmann, E., and Goldstein, K. (1945). A case of "idiot savant": An experimental study of personality organisation. *Psychological Monographs*, 58,(269), 1–63.

Scheler, M. (1954). *The Nature of Sympathy* (P. Heath, Trans.). London: Routledge & Kegan Paul.

Searle, J. R. (1969). *Speech Acts*. Cambridge: Cambridge University Press.

Sigman, M. D., Kasari, C., Kwon, J. H., and Yirmiya, N. (1992). Responses to the negative emotions of others by autistic, mentally retarded, and normal children. *Child Development*, 63, 796–807.

Sorce, J. F., Emde, R. N., Campos, J., and Klinnert, M. D. (1985). Maternal emotional signaling: Its effect on the visual cliff behavior of 1-year-olds. *Developmental Psychology*, 21, 195–200.

Strawson, P. F. (1959). *Individuals*. London: Methuen.

Taylor, G. (1985). *Pride, Shame and Guilt*. Oxford: Clarendon.

Tomasello, M. (1999). *The Cultural Origins of Human Cognition*. Cambridge, MA: Harvard University Press.

Vygotsky, L. S. (1962). *Thought and Language* (E. Hanfmann and G. Vaker, Trans.). Cambridge, MA: MIT Press.

Warnock, M. (1976). *Imagination*. London: Faber and Faber.

Weeks, S. J. and Hobson, R. P. (1987). The salience of facial expression for autistic children. *Journal of Child Psychology and Psychiatry*, 28, 137–52.

Werner, H. and Kaplan, B. (1984). *Symbol Formation*. Hillsdale, NJ: Lawrence Erlbaum Associates Inc. (Original work published 1963.)

Wimmer, H. and Perner, J. (1983). Beliefs about beliefs: Representation and constraining function of wrong beliefs in young children's understanding of deception. *Cognition*, 13, 103–28.

Wittgenstein, L. (1958). *Philosophical Investigations* (G. E. M. Anscombe, Trans.). Oxford: Blackwell.

Wittgenstein, L. (1980). *Remarks on the Philosophy of Psychology, Volumes 1 and 2* (G. H. von Wright and H. Nyman, Eds; C. G. Luckhardt and M. A. E. Aue, Trans.). Oxford: Blackwell.

CHAPTER 49

DEMENTIA IS DEAD, LONG LIVE AGEING: PHILOSOPHY AND PRACTICE IN CONNECTION WITH "DEMENTIA"

JULIAN C. HUGHES

INTRODUCTION

It could be supposed that the tussles between essentialists and nominalists, as depicted by Scadding (1996), are no longer as rife as they once were. The Essentialists are those who think that the name of a disease stands for some discrete entity. As Scadding put it:

> Essentialist ideas about disease are implicit in colloquial speech. Diseases are regarded as causes of illness. The doctor's skill consists in identifying the causal disease and then prescribing the appropriate treatment. (Scadding 1996, p. 595)

This is simplistic and has no place in science, according to Professor Scadding, because life is more complex. The obvious complexities might lead us to conclude that the temptation to essentialism is one that is easily resisted. Using distinctions derived from Karl Popper (1902–1994), Scadding continued his discussion by characterizing nominalists, on the other hand, as those who:

> held that a universal was a name for a class of objects or events; the purpose of definition was to state the features by which a member of the class could be recognised. (p. 595).

He went on to say:

> Nominalists recognise that diseases have no existence apart from that of patients with them, and that the causal implications of a diagnosis in current disease terminology are widely varied. (p. 595).

So are we all nominalists now? It quickly becomes obvious that we are not, certainly not when we look at the popular media. Take this headline: "Scientist's eureka moment that found a 'cure' for Alzheimer's," which appeared in the *Herald Scotland* newspaper (Hamill 2010). It is essentialist in the sense that it treats Alzheimer's disease as if it is one thing, for which there can potentially be a (single) "cure." As we shall see, what exactly "Alzheimer's disease" is needs to be considered critically, but it is certainly not a simple entity. In any event, the headline suggests that Alzheimer's disease is a single, concrete thing—as if there is some *thing* called Alzheimer's—and is, in this sense, essentialist in the way described by Scadding.

Actually, and unfortunately all too predictably, the headline was sensationalist, because the breakthrough (the "cure") was only in test tubes and mice and was not, in any case, demonstrated in mice with Alzheimer's disease! Instead, the research centered on an enzyme, protein phosphatase 2A (PP2A), which was switched on by a commonly used antidiabetic drug called metformin. Inducing PP2A activity in this way reduced the phosphorylation of a protein called tau. And the excessive phosphorylation of tau is thought to play an important part in the formation of neurofibrillary tangles in the brains of people with Alzheimer's disease. Neurofibrillary tangles are thought to be crucial in causing this disease. So metformin may help to reduce Alzheimer's disease. The science is impressive. At the end of their paper, here is what the scientists say:

> Our data therefore suggest a potential beneficial effect of long-term metformin treatment and raise the hope that metformin would have a neuroprotective and prophylactic effect in patients with the predisposition for [Alzheimer's disease]. (Kicksteina et al. 2010)

Now, the reason for going into the details of the science (at least to a degree) is because I shall later shed doubt on some of the concepts that underpin the claim that metformin might be a "cure" for Alzheimer's disease. One might note, in passing, that the initially excusable "hope," that metformin might be protective against Alzheimer's disease, seems less excusable if there are doubts that the findings will be replicated in mice with Alzheimer's (let alone in humans) and even less excusable in the face of doubts about the broader argument. To anticipate, the role of neurofibrillary tangles in Alzheimer's is itself not clear-cut. But I want, in any case, to consider the implications of the statement that metformin might help "in patients with the predisposition for [Alzheimer's disease]." The statement is predicated on its being useful and meaningful to talk of those who might be *predisposed* to Alzheimer's disease (presuming there is such an entity). It might be argued, however, that what we see is a predisposition to essentialism, not just in the popular press, but also in scientific journals. Not only might we have a cure for the thing called Alzheimer's disease, but also for those *patients* who are predisposed: "patients" implying that they are already sick because of the thing or things that constitute the predisposition to the thing called Alzheimer's disease!

In this chapter I shall, first, pursue arguments that tend against the idea that "dementia" or "Alzheimer's" pick out any essential thing. It becomes very clear that there is no entity that can be called "dementia." "Alzheimer's pathology" can be used as shorthand for the type of pathology that Aloïs Alzheimer (1864–1915) described just over one hundred years ago, which chiefly involved amyloid plaques and neurofibrillary tangles. But it also becomes obvious without too much work that it is neither sensible nor useful to speak of Alzheimer's disease in an unproblematic way, especially when it comes to research, because of the lack of precision concerning the boundaries of the notion of Alzheimer's disease.

Thus, I shall argue that dementia is dead (and Alzheimer's is problematic). Much of the discussion will focus on the importance of evaluative judgments in making diagnoses. This is shown very clearly when it comes to discussion of mild cognitive impairment (MCI), which is said to be a pre-dementia state. This is an example of advances in scientific knowledge leading to more complex value judgments; but there are other examples, such as the use of biomarkers to diagnose dementia.

As an alternative paradigm, I shall turn to ageing. There are reasons to believe that it makes more biological sense to think in terms of the ageing brain when it comes to neurodegenerative diseases of old age, rather than to try to split them into discrete entities. This, too, carries philosophical and practical commitments.

One of those commitments is that "dementia" is placed in a broader field. In the final section of the chapter I shall explore the nature of dementia as a feature of the world: dementia-in-the-world even. Ageing is not something that we do solely at the end of our lives. It starts shortly after conception. So we should celebrate ageing in the way that we should celebrate life. In this context, the death of "dementia" (with all of its stigmatizing baggage and illicit presuppositions) looks like an unqualified good. Instead we should look more broadly at dementia-in-the-world as a feature of our ageing lives. This should all become clearer as the discussion progresses.

The Death of Dementia

Dementia is not one thing. According to Berrios (1987), "The term 'dementia' and the concept of cognitive failure came together sometime during the eighteenth century." The core meaning of "dementia" has tended to include "cognitive failure, chronic behavioural dislocation and psychosocial incompetence" (Berrios 1987). Of course, clinicians and scientists working in the field know that dementia is not one thing. It is a syndromal or umbrella term, used to cover a number of conditions, which are more precisely defined by other diagnostic labels such as Alzheimer's disease, vascular dementia, dementia with Lewy bodies, and frontotemporal degeneration.[1] None the less, common parlance still carries the sense that there is a (single) thing being picked out by the word, which is not helped by the colloquial use of "dementia" as if it can be used interchangeably with "Alzheimer's disease." Another tendency has been for "dementia" solely to be associated with cognitive impairment; indeed the stereotypical image of the person with dementia involves poor memory. This has a number of consequences.

First, research has tended to focus, until relatively recently, on the cognitive aspects of dementia. This tendency has been rectified to a degree as people have acknowledged the equal importance of non-cognitive symptoms. There is now a significant research effort looking at the behavioral and psychological symptoms of dementia (BPSD) (Ballard et al. 2001). Secondly, there has been the tendency to regard cognitive function as the be-all and end-all. Post (1995) referred to our "hypercognitive" society, in which the forgetful person finds that he or she is denied a standing as a moral agent. Elsewhere he has written: "Because

---

[1] I am not intending to offer fuller descriptions of these conditions in this chapter, but would refer the reader to relevant chapters of Jacoby et al. (2008).

memory is a form of power, we can sometimes find in those who have lost such power the opportunity to mock and ignore, sending the message that their very existence rests on a mistake" (Post 2006, p. 224). This tendency would, therefore, feed into the associated tendency to stigmatize people with dementia. Thirdly, it has encouraged a biomedical view of "dementia," because cognitive function is something that can be easily measured (by memory tests and the like) and the loss of cognitive function has closely correlated with particular pathophysiological deficits (e.g., Perry et al. 1978), which has provided the impetus for pharmacological fixes. The (essentialist) idea that there will be a treatment for "dementia"—a magic bullet—has persisted.

The redirection of focus from cognitive to non-cognitive symptoms and signs has, at least, taken us back toward the historical core meaning of the term as "cognitive failure, chronic behavioral dislocation and psychosocial incompetence" (Berrios 1987), where attention has to be paid to a wider range of issues than purely cognitive function. Still, we might wish to note that the historical core meaning of "dementia" has been pejorative: failure, dislocation, and incompetence. And this brings us to an arresting insight. For it might have been thought that a quite unique aspect of "dementia," in the field of philosophy of psychiatry, was its organic basis. If "dementia" is to do with loss of memory, which is to do with the loss of cholinergic neurons in the brain, then it is easy enough to discuss it factually as if it were an organic disease, where evaluative decisions might have to be made in connection with, for instance, treatment, but not in connection with what (in essence) "dementia" actually *is*. But it turns out that value judgments attach to the core meaning of "dementia." It is by no means simply a matter of scoring above or below a cutoff on a memory test. "Dementia" affects the whole person, and judgments about dementia must, accordingly, be whole-person judgments.

For a number of reasons, therefore, "dementia" as a concept is problematic. A number of opinion pieces have now appeared in the literature questioning whether the term "dementia" should be retained. Trachtenberg and Trojanowski (2008) have questioned the ethical basis of such a diagnosis, which is after all insulting: the etymology of "dementia" suggests that the person is out of his or her mind, which seems akin to calling someone an "idiot"! Thus, just as words such as "imbecile" or "moron" have disappeared as diagnostic terms, so it should be with "dementia." Hachinski (2008), a leading researcher in the field, suggested that "dementia" "combines categorical misclassification with etiologic imprecision.... To achieve clarity of thought and unity of purpose, current thinking about these disorders must shift." Hence, we find that the Neurocognitive Disorders Work Group, who are considering revisions for the fifth edition of the *Diagnostic and Statistical Manual of Mental Disorders* (DSM-5), has proposed that the term "dementia" should be replaced by "major neurocognitive disorders" (American Psychiatric Association 2010). Elsewhere, I have suggested an alternative, namely, "acquired diffuse neurocognitive dysfunction" and I have considered the value judgments that emerge in connection with the notion of "dementia" (Hughes 2011). There are important quibbles concerning the exact words we should use to capture the syndromal (umbrella) diagnosis. For instance, it is important to catch both the cognitive element of dementia and the broader brain dysfunctions (suggested by "neuro-") in order to mark out these conditions from, on the one hand, other mental disorders such as schizophrenia and, on the other, physical disorders, such as multiple sclerosis, despite the possibility of sufferers of both such disorders showing evidence of acquired diffuse neurocognitive dysfunction at some stage. But these nosological technicalities need not detain us here. What is clear is that evaluative judgments surround the notion of "dementia," as might be expected given that this is a ubiquitous feature of psychiatric diagnoses (Sadler 2004). The importance of facts *and* values in medical practice, in particular in connection with psychiatry, should now, in the wake of the work of Fulford (1989, 2004), be a commonplace assumption. But the point has to be made and remade. Nowhere is this more evident than in connection with MCI and it is, in particular, the evaluative concerns around the notion of MCI that sound the death knell of "dementia."

To many working in the field of "dementia," this would seem to be a highly paradoxical claim. MCI is considered to be a pre-dementia state. It is a term that describes "a condition or conditions where subjects have recognizable degrees of objective cognitive impairment which fall short of current standardized definitions for either a dementia syndrome in general or for particular disorders" (O'Brien 2008). So, rather than MCI presaging the end of "dementia" in a conceptual sense, it is seen as the place to target treatment in order to end "dementia" by curing it! However, whether or not it will be possible one day to predict "dementia" in an accurate manner and to initiate curative treatment before it has yet begun, the notion of MCI does raise considerable conceptual issues.

Proponents of MCI see it as "a useful clinical entity that does serve a practical function and hopefully will lead to a better quality of life for aging persons" (Petersen 2006). As time has gone on the number of possible *entities* that MCI might be has increased. We now have early or late, amnestic or non-amnestic, single- or multiple-domain MCI. The reason for this proliferation of entities is precisely an attempt to refine the criteria so that MCI has better predictive value. But the evaluative problem, of central importance to the concept, is that not everyone with MCI will progress to full-blown "dementia." So there is a value judgment involved in deciding to tell someone they have a condition that may or may not be normal. MCI is certainly not, therefore, a value-free diagnosis. In a systematic review, the conversion rate from MCI to "dementia" was about 10% per year (Bruscoli and Lovestone 2004). Elsewhere, much higher conversion rates are reported, but this seems to depend on recruitment strategies and the strictness with which diagnostic criteria have been applied (O'Brien 2008). Even with rigorous selection and diagnosis, 20% of those with MCI are still well (that is, they do not have "dementia") six years later.

Even if we appreciate that MCI might be useful for some, a "diagnosis" of MCI is not entirely benign. It can cause stigma (including self-stigma), alienation, and anxiety (Corner and Bond 2006; Sabat 2006). There just is "an essential ambiguity" to the status of MCI, which concerns whether or not it is pathological (Thornton 2006). Furthermore, there is a variety of institutional and cultural factors that influence the clinical use of the "diagnosis" of MCI (Moreira et al. 2008). The concept of MCI seems to have been accepted by many clinicians and researchers in the field of "dementia," even if it remains a contested notion (Graham and Ritchie 2006a, 2006b). There are, however, skeptics who would contend that MCI is a manifestation of normal ageing and not a disease (Gaines and Whitehouse 2006; Whitehouse 2006).

And this is the conceptual rub. No one can say for sure that a person with MCI, by whatever classification, will definitely develop "dementia." In some cases there is clear pathology of another sort, such as depression. But in some, it will just have to be said that the objective evidence of cognitive impairment that they (or someone else) have noticed was nothing more than a variant of normal ageing. I shall say more about normal ageing later in this chapter, but for now it is important to note that the line between normality and a pre-dementia state cannot be identified for certain.

One of the problems with the proposed DSM-5 notion of "major neurocognitive disorders," which at least satisfies a type of descriptive criterion (because the dementias *are* neurocognitive disorders), is that it was linked to the joint introduction of a new term: "minor neurocognitive disorders," which has subsequently been changed to "mild neurocognitive disorders" (where the change to "mild" from "minor" is itself significant if it represents the effect of lobbying by the proponents of MCI). Mild neurocognitive disorders include the notion of MCI. But the problems associated with MCI are not circumvented by this new terminology. This is both because there will still be evaluative decisions required to judge between what amounts to a major and a mild neurocognitive disorder and because there is a pathological spectrum at a biological level. For instance, in a recent community study involving autopsies, 33% of the brains of 134 people with MCI had macroscopic infarcts (i.e., strokes, which in someone with dementia would support a diagnosis of vascular dementia), but 54% showed Alzheimer's pathology (i.e., the so-called plaques and tangles) and 19% had mixed pathologies (Schneider et al. 2009). Even in the purest type of MCI, amnestic MCI (which is tightly defined to have the greatest chance of conversion to Alzheimer's disease), the researchers found heterogeneous pathologies. The pathological messiness of MCI, which in any case is not meant to be a disease state, gestures at the likely lack of any *essential* pathological features to "dementia."

In what sense, then, is MCI the death knell of "dementia"? Well, first, I have already suggested that, to increase the certainty of conversion to "dementia," MCI needs to be subcategorized so that its features are closer to the type of "dementia" under consideration. In other words, MCI only really starts to work if it is acknowledged that there are different types of "dementia." MCI emphasizes that there is not just one thing called "dementia." Secondly, MCI shows the difficulties surrounding attempts to establish boundaries around conditions that appear more frequently in ageing. The lack of a clear boundary between normal ageing and MCI introduces the possibility of a biological spectrum. In which case, presupposing that the spectrum runs on from MCI into disease states, the idea that "dementia" itself refers to anything like a natural kind becomes more doubtful. It is clear, then, that if a natural kind is something (not depending on human construction) that has essential properties or features, "dementia" is unlikely to be such a thing. Accordingly, MCI ushers in the death of "dementia" as a natural kind or objective biological entity: it emphasizes the extent to which there is no one thing that is "dementia" and, moreover, it suggests "dementia" has no essential component to make it the thing that it is supposed to be. "Dementia" has no essential reference.

In terms of nosology, killing off "dementia" is a swift affair. Diagnosis usually tells us something about the pathology of the disease, about its manifestations, or about its treatment. Thus, for example, once we hear that someone has prostate cancer, we know the location of the problem and the histopathology; we also know something about its prognosis. If we hear that someone is manic, we can guess how they might be talking and behaving. If we hear that someone has tuberculosis, we know both the likely (although it is not the sole) cause, *Mycobacterium tuberculosis*, as well as the type of treatment that will help (e.g., the antibiotic rifampicin). But "dementia" tells us none of these things. The pathology may involve amyloid plaques and neurofibrillary tangles, or a stroke, or a meningioma. We do not know, just by hearing that someone has "dementia," what the prognosis is likely to be: it could be from weeks to years. We do not know whether the person will present with cognitive symptoms or with Parkinsonism. The treatment might involve a variety of drugs or it might involve the insertion of a ventriculo-peritoneal shunt for normal pressure hydrocephalus. "Dementia," as a nosological entity, therefore, is otiose and should be regarded as dead.

FACTS AND VALUES AND ALZHEIMER'S DISEASE

Having accepted that we need a better umbrella term than "dementia" to cover all the different forms of acquired diffuse neurocognitive dysfunction, we might yet think that the particular types of disease can be easily distinguished. After all, we have consensus statements or international guidelines for Alzheimer's disease, vascular dementia, Lewy body dementia, fronto-temporal dementia, and so on (see Jacoby et al. 2008 for details). Yet the complexities of life, which Scadding (1996) referred to, as epitomized by real patients are such that doubts can be raised even about these specific diagnoses. As usual, the doubts surround the boundaries and have the same thrust: we need to guard against the tendency toward essentialism.

But the debate is also about values. It has, after all, been recognized for some while that our empirical approach to the world cannot be value-neutral. Many years ago, Gunnar Myrdal (1898–1987) discussed the possibility of a purely factual analysis independent of any valuations and concluded:

> This assumption is naïve empiricism: the idea that if we observe, and continue to observe, reality without any preconceptions, the facts will somehow organize themselves into a system which is assumed to pre-exist. But without questions there are no answers. And the answers are preconceived in the formulation of the questions. The questions express our interests in the matter. The interests can never be purely scientific. They are choices, the products of our valuations. (Myrdal 1958, p. 51).

Thus, we can probe the values that surround Alzheimer's disease which reveal it to be problematic. This in itself is odd, given that "Alzheimer's" is a notion that has become almost colloquial, as if there is no doubt about its standing as a disease entity. But even the history of the term shows how our interests "can never be purely scientific." The first use of "Alzheimer's disease" occurred in the eighth edition of Emil Kraepelin's (1856–1926) *Handbook of Psychiatry*, which appeared in 1910, four years after Alzheimer had described the case of Auguste D. and three years after his first written presentation of her case (Maurer et al. 1997). Kraepelin's use of the term could be seen as a purely factual matter: his friend and associate had discovered a new disease, so his name should (correctly) be associated with it. There may, however, have been other issues: in establishing this as Alzheimer's disease, Kraepelin helped boost the standing of his own institution in Munich. There was, too, a broader scientific endeavor, which was to establish the organic basis of psychiatric disease. One of the charges against Kraepelin is that he played down the vascular changes identified by Alzheimer in Auguste D. in order to establish this as a pure new disease, but many cases of Alzheimer's disease also show vascular pathology. Viewing Alzheimer's disease almost solely in terms of amyloid plaques and neurofibrillary tangles and regarding this as unique, as opposed to being a condition linked to other similar cases, may have been the result, therefore, of particular social pressures and of a perspective driven by certain evaluative concerns, namely the need to find pure pathology in keeping with an essentialist attitude toward diseases. Even if the true historical account is more complicated than this, because pathologists in 1906 approached their work with a different set of concerns (Berrios 1990), the relevance of evaluative judgments is not in doubt.

In an important paper, Richards and Brayne (2010) ask "What do we mean by Alzheimer's disease?" They point to two challenges that face "the pathology-led model of Alzheimer's disease." First, plaques and tangles do not always lead to cognitive impairment. Secondly, the pathology is often heterogeneous, so that in nearly 46% of those with clinically diagnosed Alzheimer's disease there is mixed pathology, which often includes atherosclerotic changes of the sort seen by Alzheimer, but downplayed by Kraepelin. Richards and Brayne (2010) point out that there is no easy correlation between pathology and cognitive impairment, so that we cannot even identify a neat spectrum running from normality to disease. This picture is of difference: different life courses involving different exposure to different risk factors that lead to different mixtures of different pathologies. The true picture, therefore, is far removed from essentialism and recalls, instead, Ludwig Wittgenstein (1889–1951) saying that a motto for his book *Philosophical Investigations* might have been a line from *King Lear*: "I'll teach you differences" (Rhees 1981, p. 171). Instead, Richards and Brayne (2010) think it might make more sense to speak of an Alzheimer's *syndrome*. And they continue:

> If Alzheimer's disease is a diffuse clinical syndrome, there is unlikely to be a therapeutic silver bullet, notwithstanding the dominant research endeavour towards finding effective drug treatments. (p. 866)

The reason Alzheimer's needs to be understood as a syndrome and not a disease is because of its problematic edges; and the problem at the edges is to do with values. At the clinical level, value judgments have to be made concerning where normality ends and MCI turns into a disease. At the pathological level, Alzheimer's pathology is found in normal older people and in the types of acquired diffuse neurocognitive dysfunction (i.e., "dementia") other than Alzheimer's disease, whilst other types of pathology are also found in Alzheimer's disease (see Jacoby et al. 2008 for details). It might be retorted that there are scientifically deduced cutoffs, both in terms of cognitive tests and in terms of criteria for deciding on a pathological diagnosis. But these cutoff scores reflect (at some level) broader judgments that are not based on anything other than evaluations that this or that should, on the whole, be regarded as abnormal. For, indeed, no scale, whether clinical or pathological, can draw a line that does not have exceptions. Hence, for example, in the famous study of an order of American nuns, Snowdon (2003) concluded:

> Given nearly the same location, type, and amount of neuropathologic lesions, participants in our study show an incredible range of clinical manifestations, from no symptoms to severe symptoms. (p. 453)

It is partly for this reason that any research that claims to be leading to a cure of Alzheimer's disease, such as the work involving metformin with which I started, must be questioned. For if the aim is to eradicate neurofibrillary tangles, we should remember that "normal" people have neurofibrillary tangles too and, moreover, people with Alzheimer's also have amyloid plaques, Lewy bodies, atherosclerosis, and so on. Since we have not been able to define Alzheimer's in a precise way, a precise cure is precluded.

This lack of precision does not mean, of course, that nothing can be called abnormal, because in most cases the evaluative judgment will not be called into question. As Fulford suggests in his second ("squeaky wheel") principle of values-based medicine:

> We tend to notice values only when they are diverse or conflicting and hence are likely to be problematic. (Fulford 2004, p. 209)

Values diversity becomes noticeable in connection with neurocognitive disorders at the boundaries. One response, driven (perhaps) by a repressed hankering after essentialism, is to think that closer scientific scrutiny will lead to a degree of precision that will do away with the need for evaluative judgments. Thus, for instance, in recent years we find a paper putting forward new research diagnostic criteria for Alzheimer's disease (Dubois et al. 2007). The authors acknowledge problems with insufficient diagnostic specificity in connection with Alzheimer's disease and the difficulties surrounding MCI, including the lack of a clear boundary between MCI and Alzheimer's disease. Their solution is to offer new criteria according to which the cornerstone is the finding of an episodic memory deficit, which they estimate should pick up 86–94% of cases. In addition to this core criterion, there must also be at least one biological footprint of the disease in terms of either structural imaging, biomarkers detected in cerebrospinal fluid, molecular imaging, or a dominant genetic mutation within the person's immediate family (Dubois et al. 2007). The authors of this paper exercise a good deal of caution in pointing out that uncertainty still surrounds many of the criteria they suggest; but their expectation is that matters will be clarified with further empirical work. Interestingly, however, they reflect that:

> Although most of these questions will receive empirical answers in the future, this will not entirely resolve an issue that is also philosophical, around whether an approach primarily based on applied clinical judgment or one based on fully operational definitions will work better for the research diagnosis of [Alzheimer's disease]. At this point we favour the former approach of clinical judgment being applied to the determination of each criterion. (Dubois et al. 2007, p. 743)

This holds out the possibility that at some stage everything might be operationalized, but it is interesting that these authors, whose tendency and expertise are in the realm of biological psychiatry, should currently favor clinical judgment. This is surely a reflection of the reality that the judgments cannot be based on facts alone, but must still be evaluative. A key issue for philosophy of psychiatry is whether such judgments will ever be settled simply by the application of rules, criteria or algorithms. A focus on the person in context, rather than on physical processes running a law-like course, tends toward the conclusion that judgments will always be nuanced:

> A skilled practitioner is able to make judgements that aim to get situations right. In mental health care, this involves a complex inter-relation between factual, meaningful and evaluative aspects. Within each of these aspects, judgements will depend on the relations between different reasons pulling in different ways. Thus, the overall judgement is based on an appreciation of a complex whole, but this is not to say that the interaction of the factors that make up the whole can be predicted algorithmically. (Thornton 2007, p. 232)

In connection with the complexities of the ageing brain this attitude seems sensible. In their paper, Richards and Brayne (2010) similarly concluded that there might be benefits to looking at the complexity rather than trying to lump things together:

> No straightforward correspondence exists between higher mental function and the burden of lesions in the ageing brain. If this shifts the focus away from detailed diagnostic classification made on the basis of assumed clinical-pathological correlation and towards a global pragmatic approach to the needs of patients and carers, and to modifiable lifetime risk factors, then the apparent loss of scientific precision is a gain to clinical practice. (p. 866)

Long Live Ageing

So, if we accept that "dementia," as a concept, is dead and if we accept that "Alzheimer's disease" is (at least) problematic, what might we turn to in order to fill the conceptual and practical hole? It is important to recognize, of course, that the conceptual gap is also practical: in both the clinic and in the research laboratory there is a problem to be solved. People suffer from neurodegenerative diseases. Well, in a sense the problem is not to do with nomenclature, although how we name things will be important. We can think of these conditions using a variety of terms, e.g., under the umbrella of acquired diffuse neurocognitive dysfunction, or of major neurocognitive disorder, which might include reference to Alzheimer's syndrome or to one of its more precisely worked out components. But how do we conceptualize this whole area, given that there will inevitably be boundary issues involving evaluative and pragmatic judgments?

We certainly do not have to desert the realities of basic biology. The central issue is to do with categorizing the ageing brain, as Richards and Brayne (2010) suggest. In their book, *The Myth of Alzheimer's*, Peter Whitehouse and Daniel George (2008) similarly point to the notion of ageing as the key concept to be grasped and understood. This is how Whitehouse would explain matters to a patient:

> All people have brains that age over time, and all our brains age in different ways.... It's important that you know that ... you're not diseased, even though your memory loss may be more pronounced than others your age. (Whitehouse and George 2008, p. 10)

Instead, Whitehouse sees the problem as one of cognitive ageing and would rather focus attention on broader issues to do with overall quality of life:

> Quality of life can be improved ... by staying mentally and physically active and addressing the range of ecological factors that influence your cognitive health ... Having a sense of purpose in life and a sense of belonging to a family and community is also critical to individual well-being. (Whitehouse and George 2008, p. 147)

The problem is to do with ageing and the way in which, in particular, our brains age. And my suggestion is that recognition of this fact helps to locate our discussion in a better framework.

First, this instantly eradicates the difficult boundary between these conditions and normal ageing. There need be no dichotomy between normal and abnormal ageing, there is simply ageing and difference. For a host of complicated reasons, we all age differently. We all have different narratives, which can be—none the less—grouped or separated for different purposes.

Secondly, talk of ageing makes biological sense. It might well be that diseases of ageing (Alzheimer's, arthritis, most cancers, cardiovascular disorders, stroke disease, and so on), which are currently researched as if they are individual, discrete entities (perhaps with essences), are really manifestations of an underlying reality, namely that we age. As Kirkwood (2006) has suggested,

> Although there have been unquestionable benefits from the labeling of neurodegenerative conditions such as [Alzheimer's disease] as distinct clinical entities, not least the removal of some of the stigma previously associated with *senile dementia*, the biology of aging suggests that too rigid an approach to classification is of doubtful validity and may even get in the way of understanding what is really going on. The debate about MCI not only illustrates the problems with trying to classify what in truth may be unclassifiable, but also may help us to see more clearly the importance of focusing on underlying causes and their effects. (p. 81)

Thirdly, before it is suggested that this pathologizes or medicalizes ageing, we need to see that ageing is—in the way that "dementia" is not—a broadening concept. "Dementia" focuses down onto one aspect of ageing and then focuses us on a cognitive and neuropathological conception of that one aspect; whereas ageing itself suggests a host of biological, psychological, social and spiritual concerns. The possibility of difference (of alternative ways to experience life) was obviously Bavidge's concern when he wrote:

> The thought that human consciousness emerges, develops, and ages should remind us not to pathologize old age.... there are mixed costs and benefits attending all stages of life. It is only when these become dysfunctional that we should start treating them as pathological symptoms. We should think of old age as offering alternative rather than impaired ways of experiencing life. (Bavidge 2006, p. 49)

Fourthly, predicated on the mundane (but nevertheless fascinating) point that we start to age from soon after conception (Kirkwood 2006), it is reasonable to argue that ageing is not just about old age, it is also about living. Suddenly the perspective on neurodegenerative diseases opens up in terms of how we should think of them, biologically, psychologically, socially, ethically, and spiritually. Our approach has to be broad: housing will be a key issue, as will medication, but the possibility of aromatherapy is also not ruled out, nor are the beneficial effects of music and dance (Hughes 2011; Hughes et al. 2010). In fact, everything is ruled in. The broadening perspective of ageing, once this is seen as a proxy for living, changes the subject in ways that are creative and potentially therapeutic. And it should be no surprise that the turn toward ageing also represents a deepening of the questions that are being asked. For now the questions are not merely about the boundaries of our concepts and the value judgments that surround decisions about different diagnoses, but are about the nature of our lives and what we make of them in the face of the vicissitudes that will come our way. In short, what is at issue becomes the nature of our being as such.

DEMENTIA-IN-THE-WORLD EVEN?

That "dementia" raises issues of such fundamental significance should be no surprise. The nature of the conditions covered by the term threatens every aspect of our being as human beings—and noticeably our standing as beings of intellect. But every other aspect of our personhood or selfhood is also challenged by "dementia" in ways that raise questions both about our identities as the same individuals over time, as well as about the (qualitative) nature of our individuality (for further philosophical reflections on these points see Hughes et al. 2006).

If there are challenges, there are also possibilities. For instance, in recent years the importance of embodiment in connection with working with people with "dementia" has come to the fore, because this is, after all, a quintessential aspect of our standing as beings of this kind (Kontos 2004). The developments in this field draw, inter alia, on the notion derived from Maurice Merleau-Ponty (1908–1961) of the body-subject (Matthews 2002). This has direct application to "dementia," especially in the later stages of the condition when the person's only means of communication may be through gestures and movements, which may or may not convey specific meaning, but which can be viewed as meaningful in some broader sense (Dekkers 2010). There are profound links between our embodied ways of being-in-the-world and our standing as persons (Hughes 2001):

> For our being-in-the-world cannot really be separated, except in abstract thought, from our embodiment. We are, on this view, essentially biological beings: our personhood, our manner of being-in-the-world, is rooted in our biological character. (Matthews 2007, p. 103)

At the same time, however, the nature of our being-in-the-world also involves our subjectivity and our intersubjectivity. This notion of the world—that is, the human world as such—means that however we are, we are situated in an interdependent context. The tendency for "dementia" to focus our perspective narrowly is counteracted by the idea that, even in the grip of "dementia," we are "in-the-world": dementia-in-the-world even.

"Dementia," then, is always dementia-in-the-world (Hughes 2011). The intention is that we regard "dementia" differently. The idea is not that there are people in-the-world who "have dementia." Having dementia (or acquired diffuse neurocognitive disorder) is part of the broad experience of being-in-the-world humanly with all that this entails. To put the point in another way, we should not think of dementia as an entity, nor even should we think merely in terms of acquired diffuse neurocognitive dysfunction, we should think in terms of our standing as beings of this sort (in the world) who age. The challenge is ageing in the human world. Dementia is part of that challenge and needs to be conceptualized in this broad way.

Dementia-in-the-world is a way of being *in-the-world*, which is characteristically *being-with-others*. It is a culturally and historically situated manner of being-in-the-world. This (culturally and historically) embedded being is who I am, where the importance of my personal (cultural and historical) background is essential to any understanding of my narrative. Hence, to understand my current behavior—to see its meaning—may well involve a good deal of interpretation, as well as a good deal of experience (Widdershoven and Berghmans 2006). My being is physically embodied, so that biological investigations aimed at understanding my state and attempts to alleviate my suffering should be as thorough as possible. But my life is also personal, both in the sense that it is *my* history (and neither simply that of some body nor that of some statistical aberration), and in the sense that it is intimate and private. So, to alleviate my suffering, you need to take notice of the personal details of my life: my story is essential (Stokes 2008). In addition, my life will typically involve others: to understand me you have to understand the ways in which I am positioned or co-constructed as a self by those who know (and do not know) me (Sabat 2001; Sabat and Harré 1992).

In short, to understand what I am as a human being, you have to understand my world, where any human world must be both multifaceted and multilayered. In one sense, then, dementia-in-the-world implies that we can never do enough: everything lies open to further iterative enquiry, because meaningful understanding of another just is a hermeneutic process (Widdershoven and Widdershoven-Heerding 2003).

In another sense, however, there is something shared at a deeper, existential level by our being-in-the-world-with-others. According to Martin Heidegger (1889–1976) it is part of human nature to experience care (*Sorge*). This is a basic feature of our being-in-the-world, which is associated with the anxiety of simply existing. This is not the everyday meaning of "care," which refers to an emotional state. Instead it has to be understood as an existential state, one that is part of our being as human existents (Dasein). Dasein must also engage in a practical way with the things of the world. This response on the part of Dasein Heidegger termed "concern" (*Besorgen*). But at the most fundamental level of importance for the human existent was Heidegger's notion of "solicitude" (*Fürsorge*):

> But those entities towards which Dasein as Being-with comports itself … are themselves Dasein. These entities are not objects of concern, but rather of *solicitude*. (Heidegger 1927/1962, p. 157)

In the end, therefore, our engagement with dementia-in-the-world is a reflection of our engagement in our own lives with the existential concerns that are part of our own being-in-the-world. "Dementia" is part of ageing and ageing is part of life; but it is our life lived as human beings amongst others. And the critical issue for us at this existential level is that of solicitude. That is, once we see our existence (our ageing in the world) from a certain perspective, the suggestion from Heidegger is that we should experience engagement with others in a particular sort of way, which he captures by the notion of solicitude.

Conclusion

Scadding's (1996) characterization of nominalists, who claim that "diseases have no existence apart from that of patients with them," is highly pertinent. There is no essence to "dementia"; instead there are individual people with different experiences of life who are ageing in different ways. They require different sorts of help. The old paradigm, which treated the different forms of "dementia" as if they were entirely discrete entities, is no longer applicable. We see instead differences. But these differences will be, in the nature of things, as varied as there are ways of being-in-the-world. The person with "dementia" will need *care*ful treatment (biological, psychological, social, and spiritual); but he or she also requires solicitude: in the old (but still valid) jargon of psychotherapy, being-with rather than doing-to.

We arrived at the notion of dementia-in-the-world through attention to the evaluative judgments that surround the boundaries of our essentialist inclinations toward pathologically specified disease entities. As an alternative, we must engage with the world of ageing—our world—where values diversity has to be negotiated amidst the complexity of living our lives in different ways with others (Fulford 2004). This requires investigation and treatment of ageing brains. And, at a fundamental level—the level of being-in-the-world humanly—it also requires solicitude, with all that this might entail in terms of changes to our practical arrangements for and social attitudes toward our ageing lives.

Acknowledgments

I am very grateful to Professor Bill Fulford and to Dr Richard Gipps for full and useful comments on an earlier draft of this chapter, which have saved me from some errors; those that remain are my own.

References

American Psychiatric Association (2010). *American Psychiatric Association DSM-5 Development*. [Online] Available at: <http://www.dsm5.org> (accessed November 30, 2010).

Ballard, C., O'Brien, J., James, I., and Swann, A. (2001). *Dementia: Management of Behavioural and Psychological Symptoms*. Oxford: Oxford University Press.

Bavidge, M. (2006). Ageing and human nature. In J. C. Hughes, S. J. Louw, and S. R. Sabat (Eds), *Dementia: Mind, Meaning, and the Person*, pp. 41–53. Oxford: Oxford University Press.

Berrios, G. E. (1987). Dementia during the seventeenth and eighteenth centuries: a conceptual history. *Psychological Medicine*, *17*, 829–37.

Berrios, G. E. (1990). Alzheimer's disease: A conceptual history. *International Journal of Geriatric Psychiatry*, *5*, 355–65.

Bruscoli, M. and Lovestone, S. (2004). Is MCI really just early dementia? A systematic review of conversion studies. *International Psychogeriatrics*, *16*, 129–40.

Corner, L. and Bond, J. (2006). The impact of the label of mild cognitive impairment on the individual's sense of self. *Philosophy, Psychiatry, & Psychology*, *13*, 3–12.

Dekkers, W. (2010). Persons with severe dementia and the notion of bodily autonomy. In J. C. Hughes, M. Lloyd-Williams, and G. A. Sachs (Eds), *Supportive Care for the Person with Dementia*, pp. 253–61. Oxford: Oxford University Press.

Dubois, B., Feldman, H. H., Jacova, C., Dekosky, S. T., Barberger-Gateau, P., Cummings, J., *et al.* (2007). Research criteria for the diagnosis of Alzheimer's disease: revising the NINCDS–ADRDA criteria. *Lancet Neurology*, *6*, 734–46.

Fulford, K. W. M. (1989). *Moral Theory and Medical Practice*. Cambridge: Cambridge University Press.

Fulford, K. W. M. (2004). Facts/values. Ten principles of values-based medicine. In J. Radden (Ed.), *The Philosophy of Psychiatry: A Companion*, pp. 205–34. Oxford: Oxford University Press.

Gaines, A. D. and Whitehouse, P. J. (2006). Building a mystery: Alzheimer's disease, mild cognitive impairment, and beyond. *Philosophy, Psychiatry, & Psychology*, *13*, 61–74.

Graham, J. E. and Ritchie, K. (2006a). Mild cognitive impairment: ethical considerations for nosological flexibility in human kinds. *Philosophy, Psychiatry, & Psychology*, *13*, 31–43.

Graham, J. E. and Ritchie, K. (2006b). Reifying relevance in mild cognitive impairment: an appeal for care and caution. *Philosophy, Psychiatry, & Psychology*, *13*, 57–60.

Hachinski, V. (2008). Shifts in thinking about dementia. *Journal of the American Medical Association*, *300*, 2172–3.

Hamill, J. (2010). Scientist's eureka moment that found a 'cure' for Alzheimer's. *Herald Scotland*, November 23. Available at: <http://www.heraldscotland.com/news/health/scientist-s-eureka-moment-that-found-a-cure-for-alzheimer-s-1.1070170> (accessed November 23, 2010).

Heidegger, M. (1962). *Being and Time* (J. Macquarrie and E. Robinson, Trans.). Malden, MA: Blackwell. (Original work published 1927.)

Hughes, J. C. (2001). Views of the person with dementia. *Journal of Medical Ethics*, *27*, 86–91.

Hughes, J. C. (2011). *Thinking Through Dementia*. Oxford: Oxford University Press.

Hughes, J. C., Lloyd-Williams, M., and Sachs, G. A. (Eds) (2010). *Supportive Care for the Person with Dementia*. Oxford: Oxford University Press.

Hughes, J. C., Louw, S. J., and Sabat, S. R. (Eds) (2006). *Dementia: Mind, Meaning, and the Person*. Oxford: Oxford University Press.

Jacoby, R., Oppenheimer, C., Dening, T., and Thomas, A. (Eds) (2008). *Oxford Textbook of Old Age Psychiatry*. Oxford: Oxford University Press.

Kicksteina, E., Kraussa, S., Thornhilld, P., Rutschowe, D., Zellere, R., Sharkey, J., *et al.* (2010). Biguanide metformin acts on tau phosphorylation via mTOR/protein phosphatase 2A (PP2A) signaling. *Proceedings of the National Academy of Sciences of the United States of America*, *107*(50), 21830–5. Available at: <www.pnas.org/cgi/doi/10.1073/pnas.0912793107> (accessed November 23, 2010).

Kirkwood, T. B. L. (2006). Alzheimer's disease, mild cognitive impairment, and the biology of intrinsic aging. *Philosophy, Psychiatry, & Psychology*, *13*, 79–82.

Kontos, P. C. (2004). Ethnographic reflections on selfhood, embodiment and Alzheimer's disease. *Ageing and Society*, *24*, 829–49.

Matthews, E. (2002). *The Philosophy of Merleau-Ponty*. Chesham: Acumen.

Matthews, E. (2007). *Body-Subjects and Disordered Minds: Treating the Whole Person in Psychiatry*. Oxford: Oxford University Press.

Maurer, K., Volk S., and Gerbaldo, H. (1997). Auguste D and Alzheimer's disease. *Lancet*, *349*, 1546–9.

Moreira, T., Hughes, J. C., Kirkwood, T., May, C., McKeith I., and Bond, J. (2008). What explains variations in the clinical use of mild cognitive impairment (MCI) as a diagnostic category? *International Psychogeriatrics*, *20*, 697–709.

Myrdal, G. (1958). *Value in Social Theory: A Selection of Essays on Methodology* (P. Streeten, Ed.). London: Routledge & Keegan Paul.

O'Brien, J. (2008). Mild cognitive impairment. In R. Jacoby, C. Oppenheimer, T. Denning, and A. Thomas (Eds), *Oxford Textbook of Old Age Psychiatry*, pp. 407–15. Oxford: Oxford University Press.

Perry, E., Tomlinson, B., Blessed, G., Bergmann, K., Gibson, P., and Perry, R. (1978). Correlation of cholinergic abnormalities with senile plaques and mental test scores in senile dementia. *British Medical Journal*, *2*, 1457–9.

Petersen, R. C. (2006). Mild cognitive impairment is relevant. *Philosophy, Psychiatry, & Psychology*, *13*, 45–9.

Post, S. G. (1995). *The Moral Challenge of Alzheimer's Disease*. Baltimore, MD: Johns Hopkins University Press.

Post, S. G. (2006). *Respectare:* Moral respect for the lives of the deeply forgetful. In J. C. Hughes, S. J. Louw, and S. R. Sabat (Eds), *Dementia: Mind, Meaning, and the Person*, pp. 223–34. Oxford: Oxford University Press.

Rhees, R. (Ed.) (1981). *Ludwig Wittgenstein: Personal Recollections*. Oxford: Basil Blackwell.

Richards, M. and Brayne, C. (2010). What do we mean by Alzheimer's disease? *British Medical Journal*, *341*, 865–7.

Sabat, S. R. (2001). *The Experience of Alzheimer's Disease: Life Through a Tangled Veil*. Oxford: Blackwell.

Sabat, S. R. (2006). Mild cognitive impairment: What's in a name? *Philosophy, Psychiatry, & Psychology*, *13*, 13–20.

Sabat, S. R. and Harré, R. (1992). The construction and deconstruction of self in Alzheimer's disease. *Ageing and Society*, *12*, 443–61.

Sadler, J. Z. (2004). *Values and Psychiatric Diagnosis.* Oxford: Oxford University Press.

Scadding, J. G. (1996). Essentialism and nominalism in medicine: logic of diagnosis in disease terminology. *Lancet, 348,* 594–96.

Schneider, J. A., Arvanitakis, Z., Leurgans, S. E., and Bennett, D. A. (2009). The neuropathology of probable Alzheimer's disease and mild cognitive impairment. *Annals of Neurology, 66,* 200–8.

Snowdon, D. A. (2003). Healthy aging and dementia: findings from the Nun Study. *Annals of Internal Medicine, 139,* 450–4.

Stokes, G. (2008). *And Still the Music Plays: Stories of People with Dementia.* London: Hawker Publications.

Thornton, T. (2006). The ambiguities of mild cognitive impairment. *Philosophy, Psychiatry, & Psychology, 13,* 21–7.

Thornton, T. (2007). *Essential Philosophy of Psychiatry.* Oxford: Oxford University Press.

Trachtenberg, D. I. and Trojanowski, J. Q. (2008). Dementia: a word to be forgotten. *Archives of Neurology, 65,* 593–5.

Whitehouse, P. J. (2006). Demystifying the mystery of Alzheimer's as late, no longer mild cognitive impairment. *Philosophy, Psychiatry, & Psychology, 13,* 87–8.

Whitehouse, P. J. and George, D. (2008). *The Myth of Alzheimer's: What You Aren't Being Told About Today's Most Dreaded Diagnosis.* New York, NY: St. Martin's Press.

Widdershoven, G. A. M. and Berghmans, R. L. P. (2006). Meaning-making in dementia: a hermeneutic perspective. In J. C. Hughes, S. J. Louw, and S. R. Sabat (Eds), *Dementia: Mind, Meaning, and the Person,* pp. 179–91. Oxford: Oxford University Press.

Widdershoven, G. A. M. and Widdershoven-Heerding, I. (2003). Understanding dementia: A hermeneutic perspective. In K. W. M. Fulford, K. Morris, J. Z. Sadler, and G. Stanghellini (Eds), *Nature and Narrative: An Introduction to the New Philosophy of Psychiatry,* pp. 103–11. Oxford: Oxford University Press.

CHAPTER 50

···

WHAT IS ADDICTION?

···

WALTER SINNOTT-ARMSTRONG

AND HANNA PICKARD

Clinicians debate whether addiction is a disease (Heyman 2009; Hyman 2005; Leshner 1997; Pickard and Pearce, in press). Philosophers and lawyers argue about whether addicts are morally or legally responsible (Sinnott-Armstrong, in press). Scientists disagree about which drug users to include in experimental studies of addiction. People wonder whether their friends or they themselves are addicted—and what that means. None of these issues can be settled until we determine what addiction is. That is the task of this chapter.

THE CHALLENGE

It is not easy to define addiction. One problem is that addiction takes many forms. There is wide variation in who is addicted, what they are addicted to, and the precise form, health effects, and motivation for the addiction.

Paradigmatic addictive substances are illegal drugs, including heroin, cocaine, morphine, barbiturates, and amphetamines. People can also become addicted to legal drugs, including alcohol, nicotine, caffeine, and prescribed medications, such as benzodiazepines and hypnotics (including Z drugs, as they are commonly known). In addition, popular culture and expert opinion increasingly count forms of behavior as addictions: for instance, gambling, sex, work, food, shopping, and Internet surfing or gaming (cf. Ross 2008). Propensity and rate of drug use leading to addiction varies across population group and kind of substance. Substances also differ with respect to health risks: from lung cancer and sclerosis of the liver, to malnutrition and risk of mental illness. The existence and nature of withdrawal symptoms also vary across kind of substance and, no doubt, individual addict. Physical withdrawal from heroin is comparable to a bad flu. In contrast, cocaine withdrawal is more like depression, with loss of energy and interest. Alcohol withdrawal is the most severe, with risk of hallucinations, delirium tremens, and death.

There is also variation in who gets addicted. Addiction occurs across levels of socioeconomic status (SES), intelligence (IQ), and education. Still, rates of addiction are positively correlated with low SES, low IQ, adolescence and early adulthood, childhood abuse, stress, psychiatric disorders (in particular, personality disorders), and religion (unsurprisingly, Mormons don't get addicted as often as others).

In addition, the motivation for drug use varies. Müller and Schumann (2011) identify the following eight goals of non-addictive consumption: (1) improved social interaction, (2) facilitated sexual behavior, (3) improved cognitive performance, (4) coping with stress, (5) alleviating psychiatric symptoms, (6) novel perceptual and sensory experiences, (7) hedonia or euphoria, and (8) improved physical and sexual appearance. Many of these motivations may survive once consumption becomes addiction (Pickard 2011). Further, once addicted, people may use drugs to maintain normal functioning and avoid withdrawal, as when former heroin addicts take up methadone maintenance.

Such variation issues a challenge to define addiction. A definition needs to specify what is common and peculiar to all these cases that make them count as cases of addiction. We need a definition to know what addiction is.

Definitions

Just as there are various kinds of addiction, so too there are various kinds of definition. When a definition is required, especially in philosophy or science, we need to establish the kind needed (Sinnott-Armstrong and Fogelin 2009).

Dictionary definitions report common usage. However, common usage can be very loose and vague, so dictionary definitions are often useless or misleading in philosophy and science. Stipulative definitions are likely to be more precise, but, because they are stipulative, they too may be useless or misleading. When we ask what addiction is, we need a definition that is neither a dictionary definition nor a stipulative definition. Instead, we need what is called a precising (or sometimes theoretical) definition.

A precising definition picks out a relatively precise class of conditions that lies within the limits of common usage (and so is not arbitrarily stipulative) but does not reflect all the vagueness of common usage (and so is not a dictionary definition). The goal of precising definitions is to be useful, either theoretically or practically. This pragmatic element in precising definitions might seem unusual, but it is not. The purpose of the standard definition of water as H_2O is to simplify theories of chemical bonding. For this reason, the definition is neutral with respect to the exact isotopes of hydrogen and oxygen, for isotopes are not relevant to chemical bonding. Similarly, precising definitions of death may be chosen partly for their usefulness in medicine, or, alternatively, moral theories. Precising definitions cannot stray too far from common usage if they are not to mislead. Nor should they conflict with our best scientific or theoretical understanding of the subject matter if they are to be accurate. But they are judged in large part by their usefulness, relative to a particular purpose.

The question we must therefore ask is: Which purposes should a precising definition of addiction serve? The answer is: several. Clinicians need to decide whom to treat. They need a definition of addiction that is relevant to that aim. Health insurance companies need to decide for whom they are willing to pay for treatment. The goals of insurers are, of course, not always consonant with the goals of treatment. Law courts need to decide whether a defendant is criminally responsible and so should be held straightforwardly accountable before the law and potentially imprisoned, or whether they should be remanded to a treatment program. These courts will have different purposes than clinicians or insurers. Scientists who study addiction want a definition that allows them to collect data in ways that enable precise scientific generalizations and theories. Finally, individuals need to decide how to think and feel about friends and family members who abuse drugs. Personal relationships can be affected significantly according to whether or not a person is seen as addicted. The definitions resulting from these various purposes can inform one another. They can also potentially, at least to some degree, conflict. But the purposes are all legitimate in their particular context.

As a result, there may be multiple definitions of addiction, each appropriate to different purposes and contexts. Or, if there is a single definition, it will need to include a variable term like "significant" that gets filled in differently in different contexts. (That is the kind of definition that we will propose here.) Either way, it is important to keep this pragmatic issue in mind in assessing various proposed definitions of addiction.

Symptoms

The *Diagnostic and Statistical Manual of Mental Disorders, Fourth Edition, Text Revision* (DSM-IV-TR; American Psychiatric Association 2000) defines substance dependence (which is synonymous with addiction) thus:

> A maladaptive pattern of substance use, leading to clinically significant impairment or distress, as manifested by three (or more) of the following, occurring at any time within the same 12-month period:
>
> (1) tolerance
> (2) withdrawal
> (3) using more than was intended
> (4) persistent desire or unsuccessful efforts to control use
> (5) a great deal of time spent obtaining, using, or recovering
> (6) reduction in other important activities because of use
> (7) continued use despite knowledge of its causing a persistent or recurrent physical or psychological problem.

This definition was formulated by a committee of leading experts for use by practicing psychiatrists and clinicians.

This definition is useful for at least one clinical purpose. If a prospective patient has three or more of these symptoms, along with "clinically significant impairment or distress," that could be a reasonable basis for treating the individual for addiction. It could also justify inclusion of addiction as a condition that we expect health insurers to cover and public health providers, such as the UK National Health Service, to treat. After all, people with three or more of these symptoms, leading to clinically significant impairment or distress, need help, which psychiatrists and clinicians may be in a position to provide.

The difficulty is that the polythetic nature of this definition means that very different patterns of substance use and attendant problems will all count as addiction. This limits this definition's capacity to fulfill another core clinical purpose of diagnosis, namely, to establish prognosis and indicate treatment course. For instance, compare (a) a drug user who develops tolerance and withdrawal, who spends a great deal of time obtaining drugs and correspondingly reduces other important activities, and whose anxiety about ensuring a regular supply of drugs reaches clinically significant proportions, but who has no other symptoms—no overuse, no unsuccessful efforts to stop, no clear recognition of the connection between use and anxiety; with (b) a drug user who routinely uses more than intended, makes unsuccessful efforts to control use, and continues use despite knowledge of its causing persistent and recurrent physical and psychological problems which together lead to clinically significant impairment and distress, but who has no other symptoms—no increased tolerance, withdrawal, or reduction in other activities, and little time spent obtaining, using, or recovering.

From a clinical perspective, both patients should be treated. But appropriate treatment is symptom dependent. In the first case, treatment (depending on the drug of abuse) is likely to require medically supervised gradual reduction in use and management of withdrawal symptoms, medication and/or cognitive behavioral therapy for anxiety, and life skills coaching for developing replacement activities. In contrast, the treatment for the second case is unlikely to require medical supervision, as opposed to any number of therapeutic interventions designed to improve control, develop strategies for relapse prevention, increase self-esteem and self-worth, and identify and address any underlying reasons for use as well as the attendant physical and psychological problems. In short, because of the polythetic nature of the diagnostic criteria, the DSM-IV-TR does not offer a unified set of diagnostic criteria for addiction. This limits its capacity to establish prognosis and indicate treatment course. Of course, clinicians take case histories, and in that context they can tailor treatment to individual needs. Nonetheless, this disunity suggests that the definition could in principle be improved in order to better serve clinical practice.

It also means that the DSM-IV-TR definition of substance dependence cannot adequately serve scientists who study the neural bases or psychological mechanisms of addiction, or philosophers who are interested in whether addicts are appropriately held responsible for their drug-connected and drug-consequent behavior. There is likely to be too much variety among individual addicts diagnosed with substance dependence according to the DSM-IV-TR for science to discern a unified set of neural bases and psychological mechanisms, or for philosophers to construct any unified, general principles for responsibility ascriptions to addicts. For the purposes of scientists and philosophers, then, we also need a different definition.

Appetites

Philosophical definitions of addiction tend to be pithy. Foddy and Savulescu define it thus: "An addiction is a strong appetite" (2010, p. 35). Of course, we now need to know what an appetite is. They define an appetite as: "a disposition that generates desires that are urgent, oriented toward some rewarding behavior, periodically recurring, often in predictable circumstances, sated temporarily by their fulfillment, and generally provide pleasure" (Foddy and Savulescu 2010, p. 35). So much for pithiness. Note that this definition does not restrict addiction to substances: arguably, as mentioned earlier, the appetite could be for gambling, sex, work, food, shopping, or the Internet (cf. Foddy 2011).

From a scientific or philosophical point of view, this definition does have some advantage over that in DSM-IV-TR. It enables scientists to seek the neural bases and psychological mechanisms for such strong appetites, and philosophers to ask whether people are responsible for what they do as a result of such strong appetites.

Nonetheless, Foddy and Savulescu's definition is too narrow. To see why, it is useful to import the distinction between liking and wanting as developed by the theory of incentive sensitization (Robinson and Berridge 1993). We engage in some activities because we get pleasure or reward from them. In short, we like them. For example, many people like watching comedies, or eating ice-cream, or physical thrills. But we also engage in some activities because we are motivated to do them regardless of whether we expect to get any pleasure or reward from them. In short, we may want to do them, but not because we like to do them. These motivations may be various, but, in the case of addiction, the theory is that addictive wants are triggered by drug-related cues that have become associated through sustained, heavy use with consumption: they are perhaps not unlike the desires of a salt-deprived rat for salty water. The salty water does not taste good even to the rat: the rat does not like the water. But it nonetheless wants the water very much (Robinson and Berridge 1993).

Foddy and Savulescu's definition of appetite seem to combine liking with wanting. They mention "rewarding behavior" and "pleasure," so liking seems essential to addiction on their account. But then their phrase "a disposition that generates desires that are urgent" sounds more like the wants of a salt-deprived rat. Hence, they seem to require that addicts both (strongly) like and (strongly) want to use drugs.

This double requirement is a problem, because some extreme addicts report no longer liking the drugs that they nonetheless want. Perhaps that is why Foddy and Savulescu add "generally" before "provide pleasure" in their definition, since people in general do get pleasure from drugs. However, Foddy and Savulescu's definition is also too broad, because it fails to distinguish addiction from heavy use based on strong desire. One of us has a disposition that generates urgent desires to play golf, and those desires periodically recur in predictable circumstances: when the sun shines. The desired activity generally provides pleasure: playing golf is rewarding. And the desire can be sated temporarily: playing eighteen holes usually does it. According to Foddy and Savulescu's definition, this desire counts as a strong appetite to play golf and hence as an addiction to golf. However, although golf might be as good a candidate as any for a behavioral addiction, if there is any, this case is not an addiction to golf. The author in question has no difficulty quitting, when it rains or even when it shines (if there is a good reason not to play golf), and playing golf does not cause significant personal harm or risk of harm (unlike skiing). In these ways, the author's relationship to golf is substantially different from a heroin addict's relationship to his needle (for discussion of that relationship, see Pates and McBride 2005).

Thus, Foddy and Savulescu's definition hides important differences and does not capture the core of our common understanding of addiction, for it allows far too much to count. Foddy and Savulescu might be happy to include regular golfers as addicts, but a precising definition needs to distinguish a strong appetite for golf leading to "heavy golf use" from heroin addiction in order to capture common usage, let alone prove theoretically useful to scientists and philosophers.

CONTROL

What is the difference between heavy use and addiction? A natural answer is: control. The importance of control in understanding addiction is reflected in three of the diagnostic criteria of the DSM-IV-TR definition given earlier: (3) using more than was intended, (4) persistent desire or unsuccessful efforts to control use, and (7) continued use despite knowledge of resulting persistent or recurrent physical or psychological problems. It is equally present in common understanding and testimony. To take one famous example, Burroughs (1959, xxxix) says that "dope fiends" are "not in a position to act in any other way" and "cannot act other than they do." Indeed, the reason why the strong appetite for golf described earlier seems not to count as addiction is that the author can stop playing or can play less.

What exactly does it mean to say that addicts *cannot* stop taking drugs? At one end of the spectrum of possible interpretations lies the "cannot" of hard determinism. Hard determinists often claim that nobody can act in any way other than they do. Here "cannot" means something like: holding fixed the laws of nature and past history, only one future course of events can obtain.

This use of "cannot" does not violate any semantic rules, but it does not shed any light on addiction. It cannot distinguish addicts from non-addicts, since addicts are no more or less determined than anyone else. So, whatever it means to say that addicts lack the ability to stop taking drugs, it cannot mean that their behavior is determined by the laws of nature and past history.

At the opposite end of the spectrum, the term "cannot" is also used in statements like this: "I cannot go out tonight, because I have to work." This use of "cannot" does not deny that one has the physical and psychological ability to go out. All it denies is that one has good enough reason. The point is that it would be irrational or at least irresponsible to go out, given the greater importance of work. No doubt, some addicts might claim that they cannot quit using drugs because it would be irrational or irresponsible for them to quit (perhaps because their gang will kill them or their family if they stop using drugs). However, that is not what addicts normally mean when they claim to lack the ability to stop. They do not seem to mean that they have the physical and psychological ability but lack good enough reason to quit (but see Pickard 2011, 2012 for a dissenting view).

Then what does it mean to say that addicts lack the *ability* to stop or that they *cannot* stop taking drugs? Burroughs exaggerates when he claims that he cannot act "in any other way," but there is a grain of truth beneath his exaggeration. The truth is that his physical and psychological ability to control his use is reduced: he lacks the degree of control that we normally expect people to have over their behavior.

So, what is control? Two accounts are common. One focuses on wants and claims that an agent has control over a type of action if and only if:

1. If they want overall to perform that type of action, then usually they do it; and
2. If they want overall not to perform that type of action, then usually they don't do it.

On this account, golfers have control over playing golf if and only if they usually play golf when they want overall to play golf and usually do not play golf when they want overall not to play golf. The qualification "usually" is necessary because they might fail to play golf when they want to because the only golf course is closed or their car breaks down or they miss their starting time. Occasional lapses do not prove lack of control. Similarly, the qualification "overall" is necessary because desires can conflict. If a golfer decides not to play, even though he has some desire to play, because he has a stronger desire to go swimming, then the golfer still has control over whether he golfs or swims. First-order desires (to golf) can also conflict with second-order desires (not to desire to golf). Such conflict and ambivalence can produce significant uncertainty, confusion, oscillation, and, hence, unclarity about what an agent in fact wants overall or how they or we could ever come to know what they want overall. (Holton and Schute (2007) offer a similar account of control that is based on overall judgments rather than wants.)

Such want-based accounts of control contrast with reasons-responsiveness accounts (cf. Duggan and Gert 1979; Fischer and Ravizza, 1998). On this kind of account, an agent has control over a type of action if and only if:

1′. If they have a strong overall reason to perform that type of action, then usually they do it; and
2′. If they have a strong overall reason not to perform that type of action, then usually they don't do it.

On this account, golfers have control over playing golf if and only if they usually play golf when they have strong overall reason to play golf and usually do not play golf when they have strong overall reason not to play golf.

These accounts might seem very close, especially to internalists who assume that all reasons are based on desires (Williams 1979/1981). However, these accounts come apart in various cases that are relevant to addiction. First, if agents have no reason to fulfill some desires, then those agents can act on their desires without being responsive to reasons. For example, some heavy users claim that they want drugs in the sense of having a strong desire even though they no longer like them or get any pleasure from them (and also would not suffer withdrawal if they quit). If so, these users might have control over their drug use on the want-based account because they take drugs when they want to and cease when they want not to. However, such users would lack control on reasons-responsiveness accounts if they continue to use drugs because of their strong wants even when they know that they have little or no reason to use drugs and strong reason not to use drugs.

These accounts of control also come apart in another kind of situation: Imagine that a desire to take drugs causes a user to think only about drugs and then forget about or not notice conflicting considerations, such as detrimental effects on self or loved ones. This user would want not to take drugs if he paid attention to the reasons not to take drugs, but his desires for drugs prevent him from becoming aware of those conflicting considerations (at least at the time when he takes drugs), so he does not actually want not to take drugs. Then it can be true that he takes drugs when he wants and does not take drugs when he wants not to take drugs, so he has control on the want-based account. Nonetheless, he lacks control on the reasons-responsiveness account, because he does not respond to the reasons that he never notices or becomes aware of. (It still might be true that he would respond to reasons that he did notice, so he would have control on a third account that adds "they know" before "they have" in (1′) and (2′).)

It is not completely clear which of these accounts of control is most appropriate for a definition of addiction. Here we will usually talk in terms of what the agent wants overall, because it is a less philosophically technical and controversial notion than reasons, and one can have control over irrational or less-than-perfectly rational behavior. Nonetheless, fans of reasons-responsiveness may recast our discussion into their favored terms, if they want.

With this rough account of control in place, we can now see how various factors can remove or reduce control. Consider an analogy. Suppose that one wants overall (or has and recognizes a strong reason) to lift a heavy weight off the floor for a substantial period of time. If so, how could one fail to lift the weight for that time? Putting aside extreme situations, such as death, external restraint, or changes in the laws of nature, a number of more ordinary factors can affect one's agency. Most obviously, one might not be strong enough to lift that much weight, either because the weight is too heavy or because one is weakened by disease. In addition, one might get tired of holding up the weight. Or one's attention might lapse or, alternatively, one's attention may become fixed on the relief that would come from putting the weight down. Or one might not try hard enough or exert enough willpower, possibly because of some conflicting desire that persists despite one's overall desire to hold up the weight or because one's self-conception is decidedly not as a weight-lifter. These factors correspond to the kinds of factors that reduce control over drug use (for further discussion of some of these factors, see Pickard 2012; Pickard and Pearce, in press).

First, the desire to use drugs can become strong and habitual. Immoderate long-term drug use can affect neural mechanisms. Many drugs directly increase levels of synaptic dopamine, which, over time, may affect normal processes of associationist learning related to survival and the pursuit of rewards (for a review, see Hyman 2005). Once drug-related pathways are thus established, cues associated with the drug use cause addicts to be motivated to pursue the reward of drugs to an unusually strong extent. Moreover, there is increasing evidence that as drug use escalates, control devolves from the prefrontal cortex to the striatum, in line with a shift from action-outcome to stimulus-response learning (for a review, see Everitt and Robbins 2005). Drug use becomes increasingly habitual: more wanted than liked, more automatic than deliberately chosen. Acting against strong and habitual desire requires willpower: an active attempt to resist the pull of the drug (cf. Levy 2010).

Second, it takes effort and resolve to keep exercising willpower. Exercising willpower depletes its strength in the short term but can increase it in the long term, much like a muscle (Muraven and Baumeister 2000). The longer willpower is exercised, the more depleted resources may become. So, the need for addicts to persevere in resisting the desire to use drugs, especially in the face of strong associations and cues, may weaken their willpower, potentially to depletion. This is one reason why many clinical interventions require addicts to remove themselves from their habitual environment, or at least identify and as much as possible steer clear of drug-related triggers.

Third, attention and cognition affect the capacity for long-term control. In addition to affecting strength of desire and habit, drug associations and cues may cause intrusive, incessant, obsessional drug-related thinking. This in turn may make it very difficult for addicts to recall and attend to non-drug-related desires and values or to the positive consequences of abstinence and the negative consequences of use. This may produce a "judgment-shift" whereby, faced with immediate temptation, prior resolutions are abandoned on the ground that they do not express present desires and values. Addicts overestimate the benefits of using drugs (including the pleasure or relief they will get) and the costs of not using (including the likelihood and intensity of cravings and withdrawal pains); and underestimate the harms of using (including health effects) and the benefits of not using (including the value of other activities as well as friends). They also seem to discount the future in extreme ways: hyperbolically (Ainslie 2001). And some addicts fail to take in or use information about fictive losses—losses in what they would have gained if they had acted differently—that is relevant to rational choice (see Chiu et al. 2008 on smokers).

Fourth, an addict who resolves to stop using drugs will still experience some motivational conflict with the appetite that constitutes their addiction. Even if they want overall to stop using, the desire for drugs does not thereby disappear. This is why techniques such as motivational interviewing can be clinically helpful to motivate some addicts to change: the aim is to explore and resolve ambivalence, highlighting the positive consequences of abstinence and the negative consequences of use.

Moreover, abstinence for many addicts requires undergoing withdrawal symptoms, which may be physically unpleasant, or even life threatening in certain cases if they do not seek medical advice and management. In addition, for many addicts, drug use may provide relief from life's various miseries, especially strong negative emotions and other psychopathological symptoms (for discussion, see Pickard 2012; Pickard and Pearce, in press). Until alternative methods of coping have been learned or the underlying distress alleviated, the psychological cost of abstinence is high. There can also be positive consequences associated with addiction, such as the possibility of status, role, and community within an established drug culture and network, and the corresponding construction of a positive self-conception. Many addicts have lost family and friends due to their addiction, so they might have few social and employment opportunities outside of the drug culture and community. The costs of forsaking drugs is then potentially very high, unless and until alternative, comparable goods within a non-drug-using culture and community are on offer.

These factors, in combination, show how or why control can be reduced in addiction. Desires for drugs can be strong and habitual. Willpower can get depleted. Drug-related associations and cues can affect cognition and attention. Drug use may serve psychological, social, and economic functions that produce motivational conflicts and oscillations. For all these reasons, even if heavy users want overall (and recognize strong reasons) to abstain, they still might not usually abstain, and then their control is understandably diminished.

We can now add control to the definition of addiction: Addiction is a strong and habitual want that significantly reduces control. To say that the strong and habitual want causes the reduction in control is not to say that it is the sole cause. As detailed earlier, multiple factors, in combination, often contribute to diminished control. It is important to remember that the strong and habitual want is usually only part of what causes the reduction in control.

Notice that this definition applies equally to the majority of addicts who are ambivalent and, at least on occasion, try unsuccessfully to control their use, and also to those "willing addicts" who endorse their addiction and never try to control their use (Frankfurt 1971). What makes "willing addicts" willing is that they want overall to use drugs; so they do what they want overall to do when they use. Nonetheless, if ex hypothesis they became "unwilling" and no longer wanted to use (or if they came to recognize strong overall reasons not to use), then they would still use at least usually. This is what makes "willing addicts" addicts.

Notice also that control comes in degrees, depending on the range of situations in which the agent acts in accordance with wants or reasons. Thus, control can be reduced without being extinguished completely. For addiction, the reduction or loss must be significant.

This notion of significance cannot be captured in a purely descriptive statistical way. Any measure of standard deviation from the mean level of control in the general population could only be arbitrarily selected as defining significance. Instead of being purely mathematical, the notion of significance at stake is pragmatic. This should not be surprising given the essential pragmatic function of precising definitions (discussed earlier). Within legal contexts, both criminal and civil, degree of control is relevant to legal responsibility; in psychiatric contexts, degree of control is relevant to decisions about diagnosis and treatment; in family and friendship, degree of control may be relevant to the possibility of sustaining relationships despite harm perpetrated toward self and others. More generally, we suggest that it is appropriate to count heavy drug use as a case of addiction if the degree of control falls below the degree of control that captures what is at stake in making a judgment about addiction in that context. Hence the definition of addiction as a strong and habitual want that significantly reduces control must be understood as a precising definition. It is to be judged in large part by its usefulness, relative to a particular purpose, in yielding a verdict on what counts as addiction and who is an addict. No doubt, the verdict may shift from context to context, according to what is at stake. Nonetheless, the general principle on which these various verdicts are based is consistent across contexts: the question in each case is whether the reduction in control is significant in the context.

Harm

This definition of addiction still might seem to lack an essential element. Desire and loss of control are, after all, also often associated with romantic love. Head over heels in love, one can become single-minded, obsessed, and devoted at the expense of many other goods.

Nonetheless, love differs in at least one crucial way from drugs and behaviors that many count as addictions. Only in extreme and unusual circumstances is love genuinely dangerous. Addictions, in contrast, typically cause serious harm to self. This is reflected in the DSM-IV-TR definition, which requires distress or impairment for addiction. In other words, it is only when a condition normally causes harm that it counts as an addiction.

Is the reference to harm essential? A critic might object that some addictions can be harmless. For instance, consider the following cases. Sue has a strong desire for alcohol and would find it extremely difficult to stop or even reduce her drinking if she tried. Nonetheless, her drinking does not seem to affect her life adversely. She works for a company where her colleagues go out for several drinks every day after work. Drinking with them improves Sue's social and professional life in various ways. If she didn't drink with these colleagues, she would not be as professionally successful. Or consider Joe, who is a gambler. He, too, would struggle to stop or reduce the frequency and time spent gambling, so he lacks control over whether or not he gambles. Nonetheless, he successfully controls which games he plays and which bets he places. He plays games of skill, like poker, rather than games of pure chance, like slot machines. Joe is very good at gambling. He plays games that he can win, and he wins a lot. He ends up richer and happier than he would be if he did not gamble so much. Moreover, he probably would not gamble so much were he not addicted to gambling.

How should we diagnose Sue and Joe? There are three possibilities. One possibility is that Sue and Joe are not addicts because they are not harmed by their behavior. A second possibility is that Sue and Joe are addicts, but, because they are not harmed by their behavior, that shows that addictions are not all harmful. A third possibility is that Sue and Joe are addicts who are harmed by their conditions, despite their happiness and successes in business and gambling.

According to this third possibility, what distinguishes successful addicts, like Sue and Joe, from their counterparts, who are equally successful but not addicted to alcohol or gambling, is simply that Sue's and Joe's control is significantly reduced. Such diminution of control can arguably count as harmful in itself. One reason is that, in nearby possible worlds with only minor differences in circumstances, Sue's and Joe's behavior causes them substantial harm. If Sue's company is bought by teetotalers, then her inability to control her drinking could cost her her job. If Joe fell in love with a woman who disliked gambling, his inability to control his gambling could cost him his happiness. Diminished control thus brings a substantial risk of further harm if it avoids harm only in a very narrow environmental niche. This risk of harm can itself arguably count as a harm. If it is, then Sue and Joe do not present counterexamples to the claims that addictions cause harm.

On this third view, it is not necessary to add any clause about harm to the definition of addiction, because the loss of control will already ensure risk of harm at a minimum. Nonetheless, to be explicit, we will expand our precising definition to say that an addiction is a strong and habitual want that significantly reduces control and leads to significant harm. As before, to say that the want and reduction in control cause harm is not to say that they are the sole causes. Many factors typically contribute to the harms of addiction.

In this definition, harm includes death, pain, distress, and dysfunction, as well as substantial risk of these within a normal environment. Like control, harm comes in degrees, and disagreement may occur as to when the degree of harm or degree of risk of harm counts as significant. Some cases will be clear, as when drug use results in death. Other cases will be unclear, as when Sue's and Joe's reduced control creates or constitutes risk of unhappiness. In unclear cases, verdicts may depend on context and purpose. For instance, Joe's risk of harm may not be significant enough for psychiatric treatment to be compulsorily imposed as opposed to made available should he choose it, but it may be significant enough to the woman he counterfactually loves to cause her not to love him in return.

Many definitions leave scope for disagreement as to how and when they apply to individual cases. This caveat is especially true of precising definitions in general and of our precising definition of addiction in particular. Nonetheless, this definition can still provide a consistent principle for determining what counts as addiction across different contexts and cases.

One final advantage of this definition is that it does not apply to normal romantic love, which does not lead to significant harm. It thus captures the intuitions expressed in common usage of the term, which distinguishes addictions from other extreme forms of behavior in part on the basis of harm. Note that, interestingly, it might apply to the kind of love that sometimes ties an abused woman to her abusive partner. But this kind of love—if love indeed it is, as opposed to fear or coercion—is arguably pathological. In contrast to normal romantic love, it is not obviously wrong to see such love as a form of addiction. In this case, perhaps the exception proves the rule.

Conclusion

Addiction is a strong and habitual want that significantly reduces control and leads to significant harm. Control and harm come in degrees. Addicts have *some* control over their choices and actions, but they do not have *full or normal* control; and hence they have *less* control than non-addicts (including non-addicted drug users).

This point about degrees of control and harm might seem obvious and innocuous, but it undermines many traditional debates. There is a long-standing debate about whether or not addiction is a form of compulsion (see, e.g., Charland 2002; Foddy and Savulescu 2006; Leshner 1997; Levy 2010; Pickard 2012; Pickard and Pearce, in press). Those who deny that addiction is a form of compulsion and claim that addicts have control seem to require a lot for compulsion and only a little for control. Those who claim that addiction is a form of compulsion and claim that addicts lack control seem to require a lot for control and a little for compulsion. One way to resolve this debate is to recognize that it may be fruitless: the debate is arguably about whether this particular glass is half-full or half-empty, when obviously it is both. The point about control and harm coming in degrees allows us to move forward: addiction is a form of compulsion to the degree that an addict lacks control.

Another long-standing debate is over whether addiction is objective or subjective. This debate can also be resolved by recognizing that, even if degrees of control and harm exist independently of our purposes, our purposes can still determine where we should draw a line between significant and insignificant harms and losses of control and, hence, between addicts and non-addicts. Compare vision. Optometrists can determine whether a person's eyesight is 20–20, 20–30, 20–40, or 20–400; as well as whether a person is colorblind, nearsighted or far-sighted, or has less than usual night vision. Still, optometry by itself cannot define when visual acuity is sufficient to get a license to drive a car or a bus, to pilot a plane, to get disability benefits, or to serve in the military or the police. The lines between adequate and inadequate vision are drawn at different places for different practical purposes, depending on the likelihood and harms of different kinds of mistakes in different circumstances.

The same goes for lines between addicts and non-addicts. As we have emphasized, clinicians, insurers, courts of law, friends and family, and scientists have various purposes. Courts may draw the line relatively high in order to count fewer people as addicts and thereby hold more people responsible for crimes. Insurers also may wish to count as few as possible as addicts, so that they will have to pay for as few claims as possible. Private citizens, in contrast, might draw the line relatively low in order to count more of their friends as addicts so that they can find more ways of maintaining good relations and offering care and support when relationships flounder due to drug use. Clinicians may draw the line in the middle, with regard to who is most likely to benefit from treatment. And scientists might draw the line between addicts and non-addicts so as to discover the highest correlations with neural or psychological mechanisms or genetic or environmental factors.

This variation in where the line between addicts and non-addicts should be drawn may be confusing if the rationale behind it is not explicit. But there is nothing illegitimate about drawing the line at different places for different purposes (compare again visual acuity). We simply need to be explicit about what we are doing and avoid the temptation to ask and answer overly simplistic questions about whether or not a person is *really* an addict. Instead, we must ask about the degree of diminished control and harm they suffer and about whether or not, given the particular context and what is at stake, we are justified in counting a person an addict. Such questions are often very difficult to answer, especially in contexts where time is limited and practical consequences are real. Nonetheless, good practice in all contexts where questions of addiction arise—from the courts to the clinic, from the personal to the laboratory—demands that we recognize that control and harm come in degrees and that judgments about where to draw the line between addicts and non-addicts can be made only relative to particular contexts and purposes.

REFERENCES

Ainslie, G. (2001). *Breakdown of Will*. New York, NY: Cambridge University Press.

American Psychiatric Association. (2000). *Diagnostic and Statistical Manual of Mental Disorders, Fourth Edition, Text Revision*. Washington, DC: American Psychiatric Association.

Burroughs, W. S. (1959). *Naked Lunch*. New York, NY: Grove Weidenfeld.

Charland, L. (2002). Cynthia's dilemma: consenting to heroin prescription. *American Journal of Bioethics*, 2(2), 37–47.

Chiu, P. H., Lohrenz, T. M., and Montague, P. R. (2008). Smokers' brains compute, but ignore, a fictive error signal in a sequential investment task. *Nature Neuroscience*, 11(4), 514–20.

Duggan, T. and Gert, B. (1979). Free will as the ability to will. *Nous*, 13, 197–217.

Everitt, B. J. and Robbins, T. M. W. (2005). Neural systems of reinforcement for drug addiction: from actions to habits to compulsion. *Nature Neuroscience*, 8, 1481–9.

Fischer, J. M. and Ravizza, M. (1998). *Responsibility and Control: A Theory of Moral Responsibility*. Cambridge: Cambridge.

Foddy, B. (2011). Addicted to food, hungry for drugs. *Neuroethics*, 4(2), 79–89.

Foddy, B. and Savulescu, J. (2006). Addiction and autonomy: can addicted people consent to the prescription of their drug of addiction? *Bioethics*, 20(1), 1–15.

Foddy, B. and Savulescu, J. (2010). Relating addiction to disease, disability, autonomy, and the good life. *Philosophy, Psychiatry, & Psychology*, 17(1), 35–42.

Frankfurt, H. (1971). Freedom of the will and the concept of a person. *Journal of Philosophy*, 68, 5–20.

Gert, B. (2005). *Morality: Its Nature and Justification*. New York, NY: Oxford University Press.

Heyman, G. (2009). *Addiction: A Disorder of Choice*. Cambridge, MA: Harvard University Press.

Holton, R. and Schute, S. (2007). Self-control in the modern provocation defence. *Oxford Journal of Legal Studies*, 27(1), 49–73.

Hyman, S. (2005). Addiction: A disease of learning and memory. *American Journal of Psychiatry*, 162, 1414–22.

Leshner, A. I. (1997). Addiction is a brain disease, and it matters. *Science*, 278(5335), 45–7.

Levy, N. (2010). Addiction and compulsion. In T. O'Connor and C. Sandis (Eds), *A Companion to the Philosophy of Action*, pp. 267–73. Oxford: Blackwell.

Müller, C. and Schumann, G. (2011). Drugs as instruments—a new framework for nonaddictive psychoactive drug use. *Behavioral and Brain Sciences*, 34(6), 293–310.

Muraven, M. and Baumeister, R. F. (2000). Self-regulation and depletion of limited resources: Does self-control resemble a muscle? *Psychological Bulletin*, 126, 247–59.

Pates, R., McBride, A., and Arnold, K. (Eds) (2005). *Injecting Illicit Drugs*. Oxford: Blackwell.

Pickard, H. (2011). The instrumental rationality of addiction. *Behavioral and Brain Sciences*, *34*(6), 320–1.

Pickard, H. (2012). The purpose in chronic addiction. *American Journal of Bioethics Neuroscience*, *3*(2), 40–9.

Pickard, H. and Pearce, S. (in press). Addiction in context: Philosophical lessons from a personality disorder clinic. In N. Levy (Ed.), *Addiction and Self-Control*. New York, NY: Oxford University Press.

Robinson, T. E. and Berridge, K. C. (1993). The neural basis of drug craving: an incentive-sensitization theory of addiction. *Brain Research*, *18*(3), 247–91.

Ross, D., Sharp, C., Vuchinich, R. E., and Spurrett, D. (2008). *Midbrain Mutiny: The Picoeconomics and Neuroeconomics of Disordered Gambling*. Cambridge, MA: MIT Press.

Sinnott-Armstrong, W. (in press). Are addicts responsible? In N. Levy (Ed.), *Addiction and Self-Control*. New York, NY: Oxford University Press.

Sinnott-Armstrong, W. and Fogelin, R. (2010). *Understanding Arguments: An Introduction to Informal Logic, Eighth Edition*. Belmont, CA: Wadsworth.

Williams, B. (1979). Internal and external reasons. (Reprinted in Williams, B. (1981). *Moral Luck*, pp. 101–113. Cambridge: Cambridge University Press.)

CHAPTER 51

IDENTITY AND ADDICTION: WHAT ALCOHOLIC MEMOIRS TEACH

OWEN FLANAGAN

FOLLOW THE PRONOUNS

There is something it is like to be an alcoholic, first personally, to the alcoholic himself. There is something the alcoholic is like to his loved ones, something he is like to those he is, or aspires to be in "I–Thou" relationships with, his good friends, his children, parents, and spouse. And there is something the alcoholic, perhaps any alcoholic, is like in the eyes of third parties—from the perspective of the courts or the medical doctors or the social workers, psychologists, and psychiatrists who deal with him, who categorize, diagnose, prognosticate, and treat him.[1]

First personally, alcoholism, at least the variety I am interested in here, involves mental obsession and craving—as well as bewildering problems with dosing according to well-hatched, seemingly rational plans—"This time exactly two martinis before dinner and then only half a bottle of wine with dinner." To the various second persons—the "yous"—in

---

[1] I am not committed to the ultimate usefulness of the concept of "alcoholism." I am interested in the shape and contours and extent of the phenomenon whatever it is called. It may be that the word "alcoholism" should go. The advantage of using it here is that most of the memoirs I have read, possibly most that are written, are by individuals with a certain kind of severe drinking problem, which is called "alcoholism." Both recent versions of the *Diagnostic and Statistical Manual of Mental Disorders* (DSM-IV and the upcoming DSM-5) and National Institute on Alcohol Abuse and Alcoholism (NIAAA) speak of Alcohol Use Disorders (AUDs). These include: (a) alcohol abuse, a condition characterized by recurrent drinking resulting in failure to fulfill major role obligations at work, school, or home; persistent or recurrent alcohol-related interpersonal, social, or legal problems; and/or recurrent drinking in hazardous situations, and (b) alcohol dependence (also known as alcoholism), a condition characterized by impaired control over drinking, compulsive drinking, preoccupation with drinking, withdrawal symptoms, and/or tolerance to alcohol.

relationship with the alcoholic, he is undependable, preoccupied, irritable, delicate; a liar. From the impersonal third-person point of view of the judge, the doctor, or the mental health professional, the alcoholic ("he/she," "it," "they") is a danger to public safety, the man with high blood pressure/kidney damage/liver disease, or an individual with a malfunctioning brain.

Each perspective speaks a truth, part of the truth, about alcoholism. Paying attention to each perspective is "the natural method" (Flanagan 1992, 2011, in press) for understanding any psychobiosocial phenomenon, a social kind, not a natural kind, which has phenomenological, behavioral, social, cultural, genetic, and neurophysiological aspects or features. Each way of seeing, thinking, and speaking changes the other perspectives, a phenomenon Ian Hacking calls "looping" (1995). Looping works this way: An alcoholic who has primarily first-personal experience of his own control failures, hangovers, and blackouts, experiences himself, who he is, differently from the same type of drinker who is also perceived by loved ones, what I call second persons, as worrisome, unreliable, a "fuck up." First-personal recognition of a drinking problem often leads to wonder and worry, to a certain amount of private denial. Second-person disapproval, even ordinary loving concern, changes the phenomenon by encouraging the alcoholic to minimize, conceal, dissemble, and lie to others. This increases his maddening bewilderment and self-loathing, further energizing the now first- and second-personal cycle of minimizing, concealment, dissembling, and lying. Caroline Knapp in *Drinking: A Love Story*, writes about the eventual structure of intimate relationships: "Mostly we lie" then we drink "to drown the guilt and confusion … the slow erosion of integrity" (Knapp 1997, p. 196). This repetitive pattern enhances the self-pity and self-loathing. "I hated myself for living like this, but by that time I felt I'd lost control over the script" (p. 206).

And, finally, for the alcoholic, his loved ones, and third parties how he is experienced, seen, and understood will vary depending on whether the larger culture from the impersonal third-person point of view thinks drinking, or heavy drinking, is shameful or not, a taken-for-granted or rare part of everyday life, and whether it sees him, and people like him, as "ill," or "weak," some of each, or, as was once incredibly believed, suffering from an allergy (this gem still appears in the so-called "Big Book" of Alcoholics Anonymous (AA; 1939/2001)).

At the theoretical level, each perspective constrains the other. When eventually all three perspectives are brought into reflective equilibrium, we will have as good an understanding of the phenomenon, "alcoholism," alcohol abuse, alcohol dependency, as we can get. We are a very long way from such an understanding at present.

Here I focus on the subjective side of alcoholism, specifically about what memoirs of alcoholism teach about alcoholism, and argue that a common theme in many memoirs is that drinking, sometimes heavy drinking, a prerequisite of addiction, was modeled, endorsed, and eventually achieved in a way that involves deep identification.[2] Alcoholism

---

[2] I use the terminology of "deep identification" to indicate identification that is neither ephemeral nor long lasting but shallow (like certain fashion tastes), but rather identification that is woven into the fabric of a life, that cannot be discarded without feeling some sort of self-loss. The depth might involve, at one end of the spectrum, one's central commitments and projects—commitment to a drinking life as such—or, at the other end of "deep identification," it might involve the implication of the behavior in many things, even everything, one does, e.g., eating, socializing, love, sex, romance, writing.

often, possibly usually, involves participation in a lifestyle, not some sort of hijack, midbrain mutiny, compulsion, or take-over.

Some worry that if memoirs produce knowledge it is idiopathic, about a single individual, and thus not systematic. Memoirs, one might lament, are just "stories." Others worry that memoirs don't produce knowledge at all, not even idiopathic knowledge, because the memoirist is playing to an audience, and thus engaged in some form of spin. A memoir, on this view, falls more on the side of fiction than non-fiction. And then there are worries about self-serving biases, reliability of memory, and representativeness (Radden and Varga, Chapter 9, this volume).

Here, I set such legitimate worries about accuracy and systematic knowledge-production aside, and argue that alcoholic memoirs, even assuming that they suffer from objectivity problems such as the latter, nonetheless serve an important function, and not just whatever cathartic function they serve for the author. First, addiction memoirs, "hyper-narratives,"— think of the breathlessness, the relentlessness, the irrepressible, intricate texture of David Foster Wallace's *Infinite Jest* (1996), or Hubert Selby Jr.'s *Requiem for a Dream* (1978) or *Last Exit to Brooklyn* (1964), or Jeet Thayil's *Narcopolis* (2012)—capture in fast-paced form, function, and feel the fine-grained texture of an actual or possible addict's mind and life. Hyper-narratives remind us that the thin, "hypo-narrative," typological regimen of diagnostic manuals (Sadler 2005; Tekin 2011, in press), which characterizes substance abuse in terms of a small set of general criteria, can conceal the obvious fact that the alcoholic is a person, an individual, who relates to his drug of choice, what David Foster Wallace, calls "the Substance," in idiosyncratic ways, and for whom overcoming the addiction, and attaining an equilibrium without the Substance requires attention to the particular details of how alcohol (or some other Substance) is woven into the fabric of his life. Second, the alcoholic who attempts to speak truthfully about what being in the grip is like, even if he does not get it exactly right even about himself, deserves a say in determining what alcoholism is because alcoholism, is a complex psychobiosocial disorder with an irreducible first-person what-it-is-to-be like-ness. DSM-IV, and the soon-to-be-fully-unveiled DSM-5, speak truthfully, as far as we know, about the general contours of alcoholism and alcohol abuse given the data. But if one wants to know what it feels like to be an alcoholic, one is much better off reading, say, Charles Jackson's *Lost Weekend* (1944), the best description ever of the phenomenology of alcoholic craving, scheming, the multiple kinds of alcoholic forgetfulness, forgetfulness of what one said and did, of the alcoholic's self-degradation, self-loathing, of the abject awfulness of his predicament, the suicidal despair. Jackson, channeling his first-personal knowledge of alcoholism through his fictional protagonist, played by Ray Milland in the Academy Award-winning movie of the same name, writes of the alcoholic's "desperate need … that shook him on days such as these. His need to breathe was not more urgent" (Jackson 1944, p. 41). Many alcoholics will agree that this is what it can seem like to be in the grip, as fundamental, as ineliminable a need, as breathing. Breathing. *Spiritus.* That which indicates that there is still some life, or at least, at the limit, not-death.

The alcoholic is not normally positioned to speak authoritatively for those he affects (even though he might have been affected by alcoholics himself), nor is he normally positioned to know how his brain is functioning or malfunctioning. But, or so I say, the alcoholic has a certain authority when it comes to saying what it is like for him to have the particular relationship with alcohol that he has (Flanagan 2011, in press). He also has a certain responsibility to use this authority to effect what is ultimately a matter of consensual social epistemology, saying what we mean and ought to mean when we talk about this phenomenon that we call, possibly simplistically, "alcoholism."[3]

Memoirs of alcoholism provide a powerful epistemic base for discussing common and uncommon features of alcoholism, and for responsibly influencing the dialectic of first-, second-, and third-person determination of what alcoholism is, how it is described, and how it is best treated. Reading the powerful thick descriptions of what it is like to be an alcoholic by gifted writers is one locus of control that the community of alcoholics has, or, at least, can leverage over how they are understood, for *verstehen*-framing, for how their *dasein* is seen by themselves and others. My aim is to say some helpful things about alcoholism—again, perhaps, it is just a kind of alcoholism—at a medium level of grain that I see revealed in memoirs, to explore what some memoirs teach about some real patterns among alcoholics.

I have some experience with all three pronominal positions: I am an alcoholic, most everyone in my family of origin is dead or in recovery (or was when they died) from alcoholism; I have been the subject of legal, medical, and psychiatric evaluation for my alcoholism; and I know some about what mind science reveals about alcoholism.

One more pronominal point: I speak here mostly, but not exclusively, of "he's" and "him's." I am almost certain that despite whatever general, possibly even universal characteristics define "alcoholism," that there are many different ways of being alcoholic or, what may be different, being an alcoholic, different forms of life that constitute being alcoholic, possibly that partly constitute alcoholism, "the alcoholisms." The kind of life I am most familiar with, and relate to the best when I read memoirs, is that of a certain kind of male drinker, white, middle class, growing up in the second half of the twentieth century.

VARIETIES OF ALCOHOLIC MEMOIRS

There are four different kinds of alcoholic memoirs. One kind of memoir is advertised as the true story of the drinking life of the author, call these *true alcoholic memoirs*. Examples are: Augusten Burroughs, *Dry: A Memoir* (2003), Pete Hamill, *A Drinking Life: A Memoir* (1995), Caroline Knapp, *Drinking: A Love Story* (1997), and Jack London, *John Barleycorn: 'Alcoholic Memoirs'* (1913/2009).

Second, there are *fictional memoirs*. These are written by alcoholics (or other kinds of addicts), but use all the devices of fiction, including fictional protagonists to channel or express what the author knows about what it is like to be an alcoholic. Examples are: Charles Jackson, *The Lost Weekend* (1944/1996) and David Foster Wallace, *Infinite Jest* (1996).

A third kind of memoir of alcoholism is comprised of the forty-five personal stories in the fourth-edition Big Book of Alcoholics Anonymous (1939/2001). Call these *AA memoirs*.

---

[3] The authority here consists in the alcoholic saying how things "seem" to him about his experiences or about himself. It is psychological or phenomenal authority, not necessarily epistemic authority. He could be wrong about the way things really are, for example, what is going on in his brain, about how and why he became an alcoholic, and so on. Indeed, he can even be wrong about how things seem, for example, that he seems unable to control using or that his situation seems hopeless, and he might change his judgments about "seemings" in the dialectic of information sharing between his phenomenology and more generic psychological, behavioral, and neurobiological information sources. The "natural method" (Flanagan 1992) is committed to fallibilism of all data sources including the first-personal sources.

These short stories are memoirs that follow the AA script of sharing "experience, strength, and hope" in the form of a story of "what it was like, what happened, and what it is like now" by people who attribute their recovery to AA. Then there are book-length AA memoirs like Nan Robertson's, *Getting Better: Inside Alcoholics Anonymous* (1988) and Marya Hornbacher's *Sane: Mental Illness, Addiction, and the 12 Steps* (2010). AA memoirs are a brand, regimented by the AA conception of alcoholism as a "chronic, progressive, and fatal disease" that can be arrested, not cured; but only if the alcoholic seeks and abides the spiritual solution contained in the twelve steps (and twelve traditions) of AA.

Finally, some of the most vivid memoirs of alcoholism are ones in which the story of alcoholism is absent or recessive, easily unnoticed. Call these *recessive alcoholic memoirs*. For example, William Styron's *Darkness Visible* (1990), a memoir of his terrible depression, starts—both the book and the depression—when Styron stops drinking because he is an alcoholic. And two amazing memoirs of manic-depression, Kay Redfield Jameson's *An Unquiet Mind: A Memoir of Moods and Madness* (1995) and Marya Hornbacher's *Madness: A Bipolar Life* (2009) involve essentially stories of a common accompaniment of bipolar disorder, alcoholic drinking. I focus here primarily on what the first three kinds of memoirs teach: true alcoholic memoirs, fictional memoirs, and AA memoirs. *Recessive alcoholic memoirs* are a goldmine worthy of independent treatment, in large part because of evidence that alcoholism is closely associated with other psychiatric disorders (Pickard and Pearce, in press).

THERE ARE PLACES I REMEMBER

If *Caenorhabditis elegans*, the common transparent roundworm, 300 neurons worth of mental muscle, could write a memoir, it, co-winner of five Nobel Prizes, would tell you that it takes a fancy to the same addictive substances that people do *and* that it also likes the environments—whatever corresponds to a saloon or a meth-lab or a crack house for *C. elegans*—in which it was introduced to "the Substance," whatever it is. According to the authors, the "findings suggest that, like vertebrates, *C. elegans* display a conditioned preference for environments containing cues previously associated with drugs of abuse, and this response is dependent on dopamine neurotransmission" (Musselman et al. 2012).[4]

For roundworms, and much more so for rats and humans, there is normally a complex associative network, a wide ecology, one that transcends the boundaries of the organism, that is not only associated with the addiction, but that partly makes up the addiction. One consequence is that the contours and boundaries of addiction cannot, out of respect to the phenomenon, be specified only in terms of the haywire neurobiology of, say, the dopaminergic system. The evidence suggests that alcoholism involves a messed up psychobiology, for example, abnormal craving for alcohol and eventually a malfunctioning "off switch," such that once one starts drinking there is no telling when (days, weeks, years) one stops

---

[4] Interestingly, among the roundworms, "dopamine deficient mutants" do not easily become addicted. And when they do, their addiction does not easily generalize to the wider associative ecology. Among rats, the majority of rats like humans, on the order of 90%, are resistant to cocaine addiction even when the supply is unlimited (Ahmed 2012). All rats like cocaine, but most will pass on it if there are other, better goods, e.g., sugar water, available. Some, the real addicts, won't.

(Berridge and Robinson 2011; Di Chiara 2004; Koob and Le Moal 2006).[5] But alcoholism also involves social, cultural, and historical habits, modes of being, habits of heart and mind, and social communion that are often part of a person's "deep self."

Well, that is not quite right. One might argue plausibly that there is a variety of kinds of alcoholics or alcohol abusers or alcoholic dependent persons (A_1, A_2 ... A_n), taxonomized across multiple dimensions. One dimension would be the degree of obsessive thinking about alcohol and physical craving for alcohol. Another would be behavioral, the degree and reliability of the pattern whereby, if an individual drinks, he can't stop until he falls asleep or otherwise goes unconscious. Another dimension would relate to what kind of mood change is sought through alcohol—to calm one's nerves, quell fear, or to make one feel happier or, what is different, more gregarious. Finally, there is the degree to which the person endorses, embraces, values, and identifies with a certain drinking lifestyle.[6] The mother who drinks privately at home does not identify with her drinking life; the saloon cowboy does.[7]

This last point raises the prospect that there are persons who are addicted to alcohol, but who live nothing like what could be called an alcoholic lifestyle, where by "alcoholic life-style," I mean, in the present case, a way of living that involves both dependency *and* a famil-iar "male" life of social and gregarious drinking.[8] We might conceive that the "female" life of largely private medicinal drinking is a way some, mostly female, alcoholics drink, but that it is not an alcoholic lifestyle in the sense that it is endorsed or valued by the wider culture, and thus is not a way of being alcoholic that in virtue of the mechanism of "looping" is likely to

---

[5] "Broken off switch" is metaphorical. I cannot know from the subjective, first-person phenomenological pose, whether or how accurately the metaphor describes the underlying psychobiology. It may be that a better picture, also fitting how it seems, is that there comes a point where even when I form a conscious intention or resolution not to use, I use. This is compatible with my intention or resolution-forming equipment being broken, or that equipment working fine but the connection between that equipment and the system that "wants/needs the drink," being broken, or all that working and the switch itself being broken (for good philosophical work on forming intentions and keeping them, see Bratman (2007), Holton (2009), and Levy (2010); for interesting psychological work on willpower see Baumeister and Tierney (2011)).

[6] It is a practical question whether the person who "drinks like a fish," gets into trouble (with his own conscience, other people, the law) for this, but who is neither mentally obsessed, nor craves alcohol when he is not using, and could stop if he tried to stop, is on the chart as a bona fide alcoholic or borderline. In the Big Book, such an individual is described as a "certain kind of hard drinker," not a "real alcoholic." Some college students fit the bill. One tactic is to call such people "alcohol abusers," not alcoholics.

[7] Regarding female drinking patterns, there may be different places that women tend to drink relative to men, publically versus privately, and there may also be different psychological states that different genders, like different individuals, characteristically, use to go via drinking. Caroline Knapp (1998) identifies with the chapter in Nan Robertson's *Getting Better*, where Robertson speaks about her alcoholism. Knapp writes that Robertson's husband used to say "'When Nan gets bombed, she goes off into some little room in her mind, and pulls down the shade.' [T]hat line stuck with me for many years. It was quite unlike anything I'd ever imagined of alcohol I'd encountered in the past: the manly and tough drinker, or the smooth and elegant drinker. *She goes off into some little room in her mind and pulls down the shade*. Without stating so explicitly, that image has to do with the places alcohol can take you. It had to do with transportation, with the very real—and to alcoholics, enormously seductive—phenomenon of taking psychic flight, ingesting a simple substance and leaving your self behind" (Knapp 1998, p. 64).

[8] Many aspects of "male" drinking style are open to women, especially white, college-age women. But even in this case, there are different gender rules, really permissions, related to drinking, as well as to sex, and aggression while drinking.

involve what I call deep-self identification, a way of drinking alcoholically that the alcoholic himself, at least initially, endorses, admires, even relishes.[9]

Likewise, some pill addicts get addicted to pain-killers (opiates) after surgery without there being any complex form of social life that they are introduced to and in which their addiction develops. The medication does the job. They get hooked, and they do what they need to get it. That's all there is to it.[10] Because social drinking, especially among males, is widely endorsed, involves a host of well-known social scripts, and because alcoholism takes time to develop, it is uncommon for men to become addicted to alcohol in the narrow sense without also being alcoholic in some wider sense. But again there is the stereotype of a certain type of female alcoholic, who drinks alone, acquires a set of dispositions, habits, predictable feelings and cues, which constitute "her drinking life," her-way-of-being-a-drinker, as she develops the obsession, craving, and "off switch" problems.[11] Her script, like the script of the opiate addict, is familiar, but it is not socially endorsed as attractive. It is not something one is likely to value and endorse in its own right.

For anyone with an addiction, the individual needs to change, and renegotiate his or her relation to his or her drinking or drug life, if and when he or she decides to stop, heal, and eventually create a new and improved version of herself. This can be really hard because of the *C. elegans* effect. Alcohol, for the alcoholic, is not an external thing in the world that he can choose to take or leave. The world itself, the way he sees and does the world, the *lebenswelt*, the nature of *every* action he performs is partly constituted by some relation (conscious seeking at one end, conscious suppressing at the other end) his action has to ethanol.

I intend this thesis—that the alcoholic's world is different because every action is saturated in alcohol, in its relation to alcohol—to be understood literally and in a strong way. For the alcoholic, at least for a certain kind of alcoholic, if, as is standard in philosophy of action, an action is defined as (mental intention/motive + behavior), then there comes a time in which none (or very few) of his actions are not constituted by some mental relation, frequently conscious or semiconscious, he has to alcohol. The same behavior, say walking to work, is just walking to work for person A, and it is exercise for person B. The behavior is

---

[9] Hanna Pickard, a philosopher, who also works with addicts in the UK, and who emphasizes, as I do the "purpose(s)" of addiction (2012), writes helpfully (personal correspondence) that many of her lower socioeconomic status female patients (many/most of whom were abused and suffer from comorbid personality disorders) drink the way I describe a certain American male style of drinking, "they do it socially, with pride, and fight in pubs." This reinforces my point about both the varieties of alcoholism and variation in identification with lifestyles that involve heavy drinking.

[10] The pill addict who gets hooked in this way, accidently, we might say, without working at a lifestyle, is different from the addict who seeks to use drugs the way the elders around him do. These sorts of addicts do "deep-self identify" with their addiction. See footnote 18.

[11] When I reflect on the genealogy of my own alcoholism, I think it best to say this: At some point in my mid-twenties I developed a very strong desire/need to drink regularly. My "on switch" worked perfectly, too well. But, in retrospect, my "off switch" showed signs of working erratically, like an actual "on–off" switch that sometimes needs toggling to turn off—perhaps jiggling the toilet flush handle is a better analogy. The problem worsened, until I got to the point where it made sense to say the "off switch" is really broken. The point is that the broken "off switch" metaphor is compatible with the breaking being a continuous degradation of functioning rather than abrupt and all-or-none. One reason it may be hard to get the alcoholic-in-waiting, the borderline alcoholic, to see where he really does seem headed, is because, up until to the bitter end, with a lot of toggling and jiggling, he has normally/eventually/with effort/lots of jiggling, etc. succeeded in getting himself stopped when necessary.

the same, but the action is different, different constituitively, because the intention or motive differs. So it is for the alcoholic. There comes a time in the lives of most alcoholics when doing their job is performing the task the job requires, say selling automobiles, teaching a class, *and* planning the next drink. Alcoholism is that psychologically absorbing. Even if it is common for particular actions to be partly constituted by whatever penumbra surrounds them, the alcoholic penumbra is different. It shadows and thus clouds every action, every type of action he performs.

It follows that if the alcoholic has to change how he acts, there is a non-trivial sense in which he has to change *the* world. In some cases, the world that has to change is not only the world in which all his actions are now alcoholic—as they are for the prescription drug addict, the woman who only drinks alone, and for John Barleycorn—but one with which there is also "deep-self identification." I do not intend to say that all kinds of alcoholism involve "deep-self identification." The John Barleycorn case, as described by Jack London, does; but the life of the prescription drug addict or the women who drinks alcoholically in private perhaps do not. "Deep-self identification" marks cases where the alcoholic approves of, endorses, and values (or, at least, once did) how he is living as a drinker. In such cases, as in the others, the alcoholic's actions are all alcoholic for the reasons just given, and, in addition, he, or a former self, or some part of his current self, approves of, identifies with, how he is.

The Astounding Illusion

Identifying one's self as an alcoholic is helpful, possibly necessary, in order to stop using, in order to actually receive, hear, and absorb the horrifying message that total abstention is the only solution. The fantasy of every alcoholic is that there is a nearby possible world in which he discovers a decorous dosing regimen, and drinks like a perfect gentleman or lady. "The idea that somehow, someday he will control and enjoy drinking is the great obsession of every abnormal drinker. The persistence of this illusion is astounding. Many pursue it into the gates of insanity or death" (AA 1939/2004, p. 30). To crush this fantasy—"The delusion that we are like other people, or presently may be, has to be smashed" (AA 1939/2004, p. 30)—the alcoholic has to identify with the class of other souls who have crossed the line, whose "off switch" is malfunctioning. The community of people with malfunctioning or broken "off switches" have in common exactly one thing: their "off switch" is broken. Perhaps they have other things in common too, but the alcoholic is encouraged "to identify, not compare." At first, this is hard to do because the alcoholic is beyond merely "liking" alcohol, enjoying its effects—he wants it, needs it, craves it, has-to-have-it; and the last thing he can now imagine is that he must stop doing what he has overwhelming need and desire to do, namely, drink. Normally, by this stage, he also has lots of experience with attempting to moderate or stop, and zero reason for confidence that he can do so.

The program of Alcoholics Anonymous says this: You can "quickly diagnose yourself. Step over to the nearest barroom and try some controlled drinking. Try to drink and stop abruptly" (AA 1939/2004, p. 31). Jack London writes about his own descent from ordinary heavy drinker to something more: "A poor companion without a cocktail, I became a very good companion with one. I achieved a false exhilaration, drugged myself to merriment ... It was at this time

I became aware … I *wanted* it, and I was *conscious* that I wanted it … [O]nly in retrospect can I mark the almost imperceptible growth of my desire" (London 1913/2009, pp. 161–162). Eventually, London writes, "There was no time in my waking time, that I didn't want a drink" (p. 183). The alcoholic is "restless, irritable and discontent" if his required and planned fix is delayed. This mood lifts, or perhaps, the awfulness settles, with the first drink. The first drink leads normally to other drinks, and drunkenness. The next day he hates himself again. The cycle repeats. Caroline Knapp calls this the "The mathematics of self-transformation." "Discomfort + Drink = No Discomfort … the dynamic is simple: alcohol makes everything better until it makes everything worse, it does so with such easy perfection, lifting you, shifting you—just like that—into another self" (1998, p. 66).

Going to AA meetings is one way to hear stories about the common features, the obsessive thinking, the craving, the broken "off switch,"—the fairly universal inability "to try some controlled drinking"—as is reading the first 168 pages of the Big Book, which describe the common experience of having reason to stop drinking and the inability to do so, the failed negotiations with self and others, the obsession, and the craving. This is the part about which David Foster Wallace says, "Identifying, unless you've got a stake in Comparing, isn't very hard to do. Because … all the stories of decline and fall and surrender are basically alike, and like your own." The rest of the Big Book consists of 400 pages worth of short stories, AA memoirs. This makes sense because AA is a method of recovery that was discovered when two well-educated, white, male professionals, Bill W. and Dr Bob, both by then in desperate straits, found that sharing their stories, "as they relate to alcohol," worked to stop their drinking and then to help them stay stopped.

Many heavy drinkers can and do moderate when they have a good reason to do so, when, for example, the drinker's health or job or a relationship that matters is at stake (Vaillant 1995). Indeed, the Big Book distinguishes between "a certain kind of hard drinker" and the "real alcoholic," (AA 1939, p. 30), or perhaps it is a certain extreme kind of alcoholic, by way of this contrast: the first can stop when he has reason to do so; whereas, the "real" or "true alcoholic" can't stop when he has good reason to do so. His "off switch" really is broken. In the real deal, the need or desire to drink is not reasons-sensitive or reasons-responsive in the normal way.[12] The system, or perhaps it is a subsystem, ballistically yields drinking from the overpowering desire to drink, and is not cognitively penetrable in the normal ways by reason, from the person level. Because familiar modes of exercising will power, and making and keeping resolutions, don't work for such souls, unusual tactics of self-manipulation— tying oneself to the mast, Antabuse to make one sick if one takes a drink, and social support—rehab, retox, AA meetings—are often required to leverage the system to a new, often unfamiliar way of being.

Even if alcoholism is a spectrum disorder, there is a location on the spectrum, where all those who lie rightward, are legitimately described as "true alcoholic" or "alcoholic type-n,"

---

[12] The system is not completely reasons-insensitive, not completely cognitively impenetrable. Although it can be very hard, most alcoholics, like other kinds of addicts, can respond to powerful incentives: "Your children will be taken away unless you seek help." Baumeister and Tierney's (2011) work on willpower is relevant here. Willpower is conceived as a kind of mental muscle that weakens with exercise in the same way that one is unable to do more than a certain number of reps at a high weight on a weight machine. The alcoholic who has fought the desire to use all day long is vulnerable by, say cocktail hour, because he has been using his willpower all day long. The good news is that, just as with weight training, strength of will can increase over time, although possibly not soon enough.

where type-n is defined in terms of an inability to moderate, to control usage, to drink like a normal person. True alcoholics can stop drinking. It is hard. But many do.[13] What they cannot do is find a decorous dosing regimen, often not even for one day. The "off switch" is broken. If they drink one drink, even one sip, craving sets in, and then the drinks, not the person, so we say, starts drinking, and all bets are off. Once after seven years of sobriety (well, I was using benzos—a very very dry martini, I now think), but without seeking any social support in AA or elsewhere, I took a sip of champagne, and by the end of the week was drinking alcoholically, again. Craving, powerless, out-of-control. I kept drinking for ten more years. I wanted to die. The only thing between death and me was that if you are dead you can't use. I lived to use. I could not imagine being alive in my body and not using. It was as simple and as degrading as that. Then I got lucky. I found my way into (one more) rehab, got a program, and retired my *denier* (although my *fantasizer*—romantic meals, martinis, fine wine—still pops up from time to time).[14]

Every person who has crossed the line is like every other addict, "all the stories of decline and fall and surrender are basically alike, and like your own." So here the identification required for stopping the cycle is identifying with the community of other users, 'We admitted we were powerless over 'the Substance,' and making the humbling admission that, as far as this Substance goes, I am just a token of the type 'alcoholic.'" One needs to make the "terrible acknowledgement that some line has been undeniably crossed." This sort of identification is difficult because the *denier* wants to find the escape hatch, the reason that, why, and how I can use like a normal person. But I can't. For those who pass the AA diagnostic of failing when they step up to the bar and try some controlled drinking, complete abstention is the only solution.

How do the AA memoirs in the Big Book help? The simple answer is that the forty-five stories in the current edition, unlike the stories in the first edition, which were only about low bottom, seemingly incorrigible, middle-class, white male alcoholics, include stories

[13] Depending on how one carves the phenomenon, there is evidence that most alcoholics, at least, most alcoholic-dependent people, who stop, do so on their own. The National Institute on Alcohol Abuse and Alcoholism's 2001–2002 survey (NESARC 2006) of more than 43,000 adults using questions based on criteria in the DSM-IV (which as I write, look like they will be pretty much the same in DSM— "stop-using-Roman-numerals"—5) found that twenty years after the onset of alcohol dependence, about three-fourths of individuals are in full recovery. About 75% of persons of those who recover from alcohol dependence do so without seeking any kind of help. Only 13% ever receive specialty alcohol treatment. See also Vaillant (1995) for evidence of fairly large numbers of men, especially, who are, at least, problem-drinkers and who moderate or stop without causing too much first-, second-, or third-personal harm or drama. Pickard (2011) and Pickard and Pearce (in press) argue that the hard-nuts-to-crack, the ones who don't "mature out," are likely heavy drinkers who also have personality disorders.

[14] Caveat. Hanna Pickard helpfully asks about the way I speak in this paragraph. "Craving, powerless, out-of-control"; "After the first one, the drinks take the drinks." I myself wonder and worry (Flanagan (2011, in press) about narrative construction in terms of the *episteme* that is AA, and these ways of speaking are definitely "AA-speak," an AA authorized way of talking about alcoholism. A judicious gloss on "powerlessness" without the associated commitment to the disease model would be that the (many/ most) alcoholic has a hell of a time stopping and staying stopped. With regard to the idea that after the first drink, the drinks take the drinks, this is clearly metaphorical and best understood as a way of saying that the alcoholic, because he has such a hell of a time stopping and staying stopped, needs all-hands-on-deck (reason, willpower) to keep his resolve, and the minute he takes the first drink these, reason and willpower, are compromised, undermined, taken off-line. Failure to keep one's resolve produces self-loathing, which produces desire for the drug that diminishes it, and thus the cycle repeats.

about both men and women, of various of ethnicities (Amerindian, black, Hispanic), sexual preferences, socioeconomic statuses, and who came into "the program" at various stages in the progression, in a few cases before there was incontrovertible evidence that the "off switch" was permanently damaged, and sometimes before full-blown obsession, craving, and degradation set in. One point is that at least some members of AA who introduce themselves at meetings with the (almost) universal "I am Owen and I am alcoholic," might not be of the "true," or "real alcoholic" variety as defined in 1939, although most are already experiencing difficulty controlling drinking from the stories they tell.

These AA memoirs reveal some common themes: many alcoholics liked the effects of alcohol from early on, especially the effects of mitigating fear and anxiety and reducing social awkwardness.[15] But there is nothing in the AA memoirs (how could there be?) that is evidence that alcoholics are more sensitive in these ways than other people, or more socially awkward than average, only that the people who become alcoholics found that alcohol had these medicinal effects (Vaillant 1995, has found no personality traits that distinguish alcoholics from non-alcoholics). Until it didn't. Until it produced more and worse fear and anxiety than it ever originally soothed. Until it turned the once well-lubricated charmer and bon vivant into a boor, a loud and boisterous asshole, an arrogant prick, a pathetic old sot.

The main function, the raison d'etre, for including these memoirs in the Big Book, is to make it easier for people who drink too much (for their own and public safety), who crave alcohol, obsess about drinking, and have a broken "off switch," to relate, to see that there are others who are like them in their relation to alcohol, as well as in other salient, identity constitutive ways—young, African American, gay, rich, poor, "gone to the finest schools" or not, and so on.

One worry about AA memoirs is that they were all written by people who got sober in AA, who are true believers in AA, and who conceptualize their alcoholism and their recovery according to the *episteme* that is AA (Flanagan, in press). This is unproblematic if one is only concerned with helping souls who are trying to get sober *in* AA, since regimenting the alcoholic's self-understanding in terms of that particular therapeutic conception is known to work about as well as any other way of conceiving alcoholism, and such an individual is already antecedently inclined to buy into that way of thinking. He is, after all, in "the program," reading its literature, and so on. So no harm, no foul. And in any case, almost all the stories are heartfelt testimonials of hope that recovery from a desperate condition is possible.

DRINKING AND THE "DEEP SELF"

AA memoirs help alcoholics identify themselves as a token of the type, a key on that piano, one of the batch, which is important for smashing the illusion that one is unique and can be, possibly once again, a moderate social drinker. These memoirs, as well as the stories one hears at meetings, help the alcoholic stop drinking, and normally, with the help of others,

---

[15] Müller and Schumann (2011) provide a fairly comprehensive inventory of all the different perfectly understandable reasons ordinary people might be motivated to drink or take drugs, from social lubrication, to relief from anxiety, to novel psycho-physical experiences.

to keep the resolution and stay stopped. But many people get sober outside of AA. George Vaillant's (1995) gold standard longitudinal studies indicate that many "hard drinkers," moderate and modify their drinking in their thirties and fourties in the context of marriage, family, and work. And the 2001–2002 *NESARC* (2006) study on alcohol abuse and dependency in America indicates that as many as three-fourths of the Americans with something in the vicinity of a drinking problem learn to moderate or abstain without reaching a low bottom, joining AA, or going into rehab (there is some evidence that rehabilitation rates for people who go into rehab or AA, often both, are much lower than the rate for people with various kinds of drinking problems as analyzed by NESARC.) Some of these may have been "true alcoholics," alcoholic type-n. The point is that many of these people learned to moderate or stop drinking without AA. It may be that people who find their way into AA or rehab are unrepresentative of all the kinds of alcoholics. We do not know much about how the former problem drinkers who learned to moderate or abstain experienced their own drinking, as a problem or not, and whether it was easy or hard to stop drinking.

But we do know that there are many alcoholics who stopped drinking for good outside of AA. I have a brother who has been sober for thirty years without AA. And Pete Hamill is a well-known example of a memoirist who got and stayed sober outside of AA. Both my brother and Hamill were able to smash the "astounding illusion" of type-n alcoholism. In both cases, there was resolution to abstain rather than moderate. And there was a strong dose of cognitive behavioral self-therapy. My brother decided one cannot be an addict and a rock/ice climber, serious bike racer, competitive half-marathoner, and ultra-marathoner. Hamill, who had great talent as a writer and aspired to be an accomplished one, used a conscious trick: drinkers are forgetters, writers are rememberers. "I had forgotten material for twenty novels" (Hamill 1995, p. 261).

AA memoirs, as well as true alcoholic memoirs and fictional alcoholic memoirs—these latter are AA-independent (minimally they are not officially endorsed by AA)—also teach that there is a second, underestimated sense of identification beyond the "identify, don't compare," "I really am the sort of person who can't touch this stuff at all (one day at a time)," sort. This second sort of identification involves understanding that many addicts start using as part of a social and therapeutic lifestyle, and consciously identify with the drinking life, or better, identify with one of the several kinds of drinking life that are scripted by the culture *and* not proscribed, possibly endorsed. We—some of us, at any rate—liked, even loved the lifestyle. We endorsed it. This is why mere abstention is often not sufficient for healing the alcoholic. He needs to change the way he is in some deep way.[16] One consequence of recognizing this second sense of addictive identification is that the idea that addiction is a brain disease is undermined (Graham 2010, Chapter 32, this volume). Every culture ever known works to make habits of heart and mind identity-constitutive, sometimes for all members of a group ("I am an American"), sometimes for people of a certain age, ethnicity, gender. But whenever such identification is engendered, all systems (including the brains of the individuals acquiring these habits—Dewey says that "character is the interpenetration

---

[16] In AA, people will advise that the alcoholic needs to change "peoples, places, and things" that are triggers. But soon the alcoholic will hear that he has a "soul-sickness, that alcoholism is only a symptom, and that he really must change "everything" about himself. I think there is something seriously confused about this even internal to the program of AA. Drinking is the problem. The grain of truth here is that many alcoholics will have to change a lot about their identity, their identifications, in order to stop, stay stopped, and gain serenity.

of habits")—are functioning properly, the ways they are supposed to, not malfunctioning. If there is an aspect of heavy drinking, among a certain class of users, that is a neurobiological malfunction it is still only an aspect of the problem. And if it is a disease at all it is, as the kids in Leonard Bernstein's *West Side Story* plead to Officer Krumpke about their juvenile delinquency, "a social disease."

Paying attention to this second sense of identification, "deep-self identification," undermines the idea that the solution is just "putting the plug in the jug." It is not, because the alcoholic often drinks, even in the insane, excessive, dangerous way he does, as part of who he is. And thus something more is needed than just stopping. The point can be put provocatively in terms of what philosophers sometimes call the "deep self."[17] Some philosophers think that the addict does not identify with "the Substance." Harry Frankfurt (1971) thinks the heroin addict is unwilling and that her desire is "external," something she does not "identify" with; whereas Timothy Schroeder and Nomy Arpaly (1999) think that such cases are better described in the language of "alienation," which is mostly a quibble about what to call something that is genuinely unwanted, unwelcomed, an intrusion in one's being. I say that in some cases of addiction, specifically a certain kind of alcoholism, we need to understand that part of the grip comes precisely from the fact that the alcoholic identifies deeply and is not alienated from a certain lifestyle that includes alcoholic drinking.

Some but not all of the things that I do, some but not all of the ways I am, are endorsed by me. I value them. I identify with them. I work to cultivate them. Traits and ways of being that I have and disapprove of, try to get rid of, work to change or remove, are aspects of myself or parts of me that I do not identify with; in some cases I am estranged and alienated from these traits, dispositions, and characteristics. The more a trait, disposition, style or way of being is one that I value and identify with, the more it is part of "my deep self."

There is a scene in Woody Allen's classic *Annie Hall* in which children tell not what they want(ed) to be when they grow up, but what they actually become as adults. One boy is the president of a plumbing company, another sells Jewish prayer shawls, and a third boy says, "I used to be a heroin addict. Now I'm a methadone addict." This is funny for a variety of reasons, but one reason in the heroin–methadone case involves the absurdity of anyone, anywhere, having an overall aspiration that could yield, as a downgrade from "the ideal," being a junkie or an alcoholic under-the-bridge, unless it be a cruel joke on the boy who wished to be a Great Outdoorsman.

The boy who wished to be the President of the United States and becomes the president of the plumbing company, like the boy who wished to start a business like Macy's and now sells tallits (prayer shawls) in Borough Park, have a connection to an ideal that make sense because it connects practically and conceptually to a well-known, widely endorsed childhood fantasy, to a socially approved script. The last boy makes no sense.[18] There is no

---

[17] See Frankfurt (1971), Watson (1975), and Wolf (1987) for details of the "deep self" view. See footnote 2. I am using deep self identification to refer not only to a person's central and stable attitudes, commitments, projects, and traits but also to any social, cultural, and historical habits, modes of being, habits of heart and mind, and social communion that a person's life is attuned to and implicated in, intertwined with. A test: if a person reflectively thinks that he will not be himself without a certain habit of heart and mind, then it is a component of his deep self.

[18] A dear friend, a black man, now a minister, from East St. Louis, tells me that when his older cousins came home from Vietnam there was, in his hood, social endorsement of being a drug user, a prerequisite for being an addict. It was part of an acceptable script for being a manly man. See footnotes 9 and 10.

connection, none whatsoever, between what he hoped for his life, his aspirational identifica-tion, and what he is, what he has become. His life is a cruel joke. What happened?

It is commonly said, including by addicts, that addiction is akin to hijacking or alien abduction, or more mundanely, that it is akin to getting cancer. No one ever aspired to become an addict. People choose to drink or use recreationally—"socially," as we say—and then there is a hostile take-over by "the Substance," whatever it is. One book on the psycho-biology of addiction speaks of a "mid-brain mutiny" (Ross et al. 2008), making one think along the lines of small teams of reckless Somalian pirates on speed boats scaling the hulls of huge oil tankers in the straits of Hormuz, and managing to actually take over many millions of dollars' worth of sea vessel and its cargo. Now, suddenly, unbelievably, the ship is under the control of a rag tag team of inepts, who themselves have nothing to lose, unless and until something very creative is done, essentially until either a huge ransom is paid or there is a skillful shot through the hearts of the pirates by Navy snipers. Otherwise the ship and its cargo are doomed.

But is addiction really like that—a hostile takeover, a hijacking, an alien abduction? Or is alcoholism specifically like that? Or is the lifestyle of the well-lubricated drinker, the suc-cessful bon vivant, something many alcoholics identify with, want to be, think that can be, and be for good—before they begin to drink alcoholically, before the "off switch" breaks? Many philosophers think that addiction is a good example of cases where free will is lacking, and that it is lacking because the agent is alienated from her using self, dis-identifies with that self, denies that it is her deep self.

There is an important sense in which this picture is misleading. The philosopher Peg O'Connor (2012) writes:

> In the 'hijacked' view of addiction, the brain is the innocent victim of certain substances—alcohol, cocaine, nicotine or heroin, for example—as well as certain behaviors like eating, gambling or sexual activity. The drugs or the neurochemicals produced by the behaviors overpower and redirect the brain's normal responses, and thus take control of (hijack) it. For addicted people, that martini or cigarette is the weapon-wielding hijacker who is going to compel certain behaviors.

She goes on and explains that the hijack analogy breaks down at a certain point:

> A hijacker comes from outside and takes control by violent means. A hijacker takes a vehicle that is not his; hijacking is always a form of stealing and kidnapping. A hijacker always takes someone else's vehicle; you cannot hijack your own car. That is a type of nonsense or category mistake. Ludwig Wittgenstein offered that money passed from your left hand to your right is not a gift. The practical consequences of this action are not the same as those of a gift. Writing yourself a thank-you note would be absurd.
>
> The analogy of addiction and hijacking involves the same category mistake as the money switched from hand to hand.

Minimally, most alcoholics participate in the development of their alcoholism. They chose to drink. The martinis did not sneak up on them and pour themselves into their mouths or brains. Furthermore, many, not all, alcoholics, a subtype of the type "alcoholic," identify with a lifestyle that involves heavy drinking. Hardly anyone wishes or intends to become an alco-holic, a person with a broken "off switch," who finds his way to addiction. But many aspire to a drinking life. It is not uncommon for certain individuals, especially I think men, perhaps it is only white men of a certain social class or ethnicity—I am not sure nor do I intend to make any sweeping generalizations—to desire to enter into an originally mysterious life form that involves drinking essentially. AA memoirs, true alcoholic memoirs, and fictional memoirs, even many recessive alcoholic memoirs (William Styron, after all, is a writer and American writers in the second half of the twentieth century drink), all speak this truth.

Here are three reasons that would-be alcoholics seek and gain entry to a form of life that involves drinking, that is endorsed by the elders, and thus that involves "deep-self identification":

- Especially for men, heavy drinking is modeled in certain places and times as manly.
- Drinking is (was) modeled as a source of creativity.
- Alcohol is modeled as an anxiety reducer and social relaxant and is discovered to be helpful in being at home in one's body, in feeling safe.

Insofar as feeling at home among others and in one's own body, being a good exemplar of one's gender, and being creative are valued, aspirational goods, and insofar as alcohol is associated with these goods, then a drinking life is one the culture scripts and offers up as a good one. At least it did.

Deep Self and Manly Men

In *A Drinking Life* (1994), Pete Hamill vividly describes the association of drinking with being a man of a certain sort, a manly man, a working-class Irishman in Brooklyn during and after World War II. His father modeled the ways of the bar life. The neighborhood bar was a hopeful place, a place for conviviality. "This is where men go, I thought; this is what men do" (1994, p. 17). As an altar boy he discovers that wine is essential to the mysterious sacramental zone of life. Alcohol is involved in transubstantiation!

In Hamill's world there was no shaming of adult drunkenness. This matters. According to George Vaillant (1995), coming from a family or ethnic group that does not disapprove of adult drunkenness, especially one that jokes about/approves of adult drunkenness, makes the normal male social drinker highly vulnerable to alcoholism. Every birth, baptism, first communion, confirmation, beginning of war, end of war, death, and funeral constitutes a reason to drink. Every important ritual involved essentially male drinking. "And so the pattern had begun, the template was cut. There was a celebration and you got drunk. There was a victory and you got drunk. It didn't matter if other people saw you; they were doing the same thing. So if you were a man, there was nothing to hide. Part of being a man was to drink" (Hamill 1994, p. 57). In the films all the Brooklyn boys of the 1950s, men drank:

> In those westerns, in the gangster movies, in the war movies, and even the love movies, the men were always drinking. They shot each other in saloons and nightclubs. They got drunk on leave and got into wild, hilarious fights in waterfront bars. Some of the movie drunks were comical, some mean. With the exception of a few cowboys, even the heroes drank whiskey. They never got drunk. (Hamill 1994, p. 43)

Notice the model: Everyone, even the hero, drinks. But the hero "never got drunk." The model is to tow that line. "I didn't want to be a drunk. [A]nd yet drinking started to seem as natural to real life as breathing" (Hamill 1994, p. 107). Hamill, eventually in the throes of addiction, angry at himself and the world, now getting falling down drunk like his father, pub brawling like the ordinary grubby and rowdy ranch hand, still held to the "astounding illusion" that he could be an exceptional drinker, like the heroic upstanding Marshall who frequents the saloon, but is somehow above the fray, or like "Bogart in *Casablanca*, sitting at the bar in a pool of bitterness, drinking his whiskey. I would be like that. I would just drink, quietly and angrily and say nothing" (p. 114).

Over half a century earlier in one of the very first true alcoholic memoirs, *Jack Barleycorn* (1913/2009), Jack London tells us that, "Drink was the badge of manhood" (p. 28). The saloon was also the context, in some ways the only context, in the life of the docks of Oakland, in which men were social:

> A newsboy on the streets, a sailor, a miner, a wanderer in far lands, always where men came together to exchange ideas, to laugh and boast and care to exchange ideas, to laugh and boast and dare, to relax, to forget the dull toil of tiresome nights and days, always they came together over alcohol. The saloon was the place of congregation. Men gathered to it as primitive men gathered around the fire of the squatting-place or the fire at the mouth of the cave. (London 1913/2009, p. 3)

But then, years later after embracing the life of drink, identifying with it, wanting it, London finds himself in this degrading situation at the end of a long sea journey. The ship docks and he is filled with anticipation of being a cultural tourist in Japan, learning about the country, its people, seeing its temples and gardens. "We lay in Yokohama harbor for two weeks, and about all we saw of Japan was its drinking places where sailors congregated" (London 1913/2009, p. 97).

London wrote at a time when the common view was that "true chemical dipsomania" was exceedingly rare, which if it—"true dipsomania"—is defined as immediate addiction after first ingestion, is almost certainly true. He also thought that alcohol was a stimulant, which it is, or can be, phenomenologically-speaking, although it is not so classified pharmacologically, according to which it is a depressant. Here he channels the complex mental-behavioral habit formation involved in becoming an alcoholic:

> I am convinced that not one man in ten thousand, or in a hundred thousand, is a genuine chemical dipsomaniac. Drinking, as I deem it, is practically entirely a habit of mind. It is unlike tobacco, or cocaine, or morphine, or all the rest of the long list of drugs. The desire for alcohol is quite peculiarly mental in its origin. It is a matter of mental training and growth, and it is cultivated in social soil. Not one drinker in a million began drinking alone. All drinkers begin socially, and this drinking is accompanied by a thousand social connotations ... These social connotations are the stuff of which the drink habit is largely composed. The part that alcohol plays itself is inconsiderable, when compared to the part played by the social atmosphere in which it is drunk. (London 1913/2009, pp. 205–206)

Here, London dramatically overstates the lack of addictive properties of ethanol, but he is right to emphasize both the individual choices involved, and the "thousand social connotations that are the stuff of which the drink habit is largely composed." In this way he can be read as forcefully resisting the picture of the alcoholic as the victim of a mutiny or hijacking.

And he should know because he was sometimes a pirate himself—one time hilariously pirating a salmon boat already, as he learned in a bar, pirated by other adventurers.

Deep-Self Identification and
the Romantics of Drinking

Drinking, a necessary condition of becoming a drinker, possibly a heavy drinker, eventually even, although no one aspires to it, becoming an alcoholic, is presented in many cultural niches—perhaps it is even a dominant trope—as a site of adventure, love, romance, sex, possibility, creativity. These are things that matter to people, sites of identification. Augusten Burroughs's, *Dry*, a compelling memoir of a gay male alcoholic, working in the New York City advertising industry in the 1990s, reminds us that, in many way, just like Jack London's Oakland saloon culture for working class men, that bars in New York City (and many other American cities) were suddenly the public places gay men went for conviviality, sex, romance, possibly love, in the last decades of the twentieth century, and still into the first decades of the twenty-first century. "You'll never know who you'll meet or where you'll end up. It's like this fucking incredible vortex of possibility. Anything can happen at a bar" (Burroughs 2003, pp. 23–24).

And, of course, the bar, gay or otherwise, often proclaims its romantic qualities and possibilities. After Burroughs's first attempt at abstinence, he goes into a bar and sees what it offers:

> An expansive bar begins near the door and stretches back into blackness for what is probably miles … Behind the bar, colorful liquor bottles are lit from below like fine art. [T]hey look breathtakingly beautiful. Seeing them, I am filled with longing. It's not an ordinary craving. It's a romantic craving. Because I don't just drink alcohol. I actually love it. I turn away. (2003, p. 136)

Burroughs, many months beyond his last drink, knows what he wants, but this time his will works:

> *A Ketel One martini please, very dry with olives*, I want to say. "Um just a selzer with lime," I say instead. I might as well have ordered warm tap water or dirt. I feel that uncool. And suddenly, it's like I can feel how depressing alcoholism really is. Basements and prayers. It lacks the swank factor. (p. 137)

The bar, the place of "breathtaking beautiful" backlit bottles, "the fucking vortex of possibility," the repository of the alcohol he does not merely drink but "actually loves," is contrasted with the life of recovery that embodies all that is "uncool" and un-"swank."

Besides the glamour and conviviality and sexy elegance associated with certain kinds of drinking, there is also, in certain communities, the association of drinking with creativity.

In Charles Jackson's *Lost Weekend* (1944), the alcoholic protagonist at thirty-three, Jesus' age when he was crucified, wizened, a prematurely hollow shell, looks into the mirror of the bar and wonders whether the boy he once was, if he could have seen ahead, would have seen and then admired the pathetic sot of a grown man he has become. It is the inverse of the

Woody Allen methadone joke, told from the desperate pose of the alcoholic in his cups. He gives this deluded answer to his own question:

> Of *course* he would accept it! It was crystal clear, like a revelation (suddenly he was feeling brighter, more alert and clear mentally, than he ever had in his life). That kid, could he have seen this face, the man of today, certainly would have accepted it—he would have loved it! The idol of the boy had been Poe and Keats, Byron, Dowson, Chatterton, all the gifted miserable and reckless men who had burned themselves out in tragic brilliance early and with finality ... There was poetic justice in those disillusioned eyes and the boy would have known it and nodded in happy recognition. (Jackson 1944, pp. 15–16)

I get this. I knew in eighth grade that Poe was a genius and died an alcoholic death, as did Chatterton, of "days of wine and roses" fame." I knew that Dylan Thomas and James Joyce were great Celtic writers *and* alcoholic by my junior year in High School. And I was taught by my father that the bar at the Algonquin Hotel on 59 West 44th Street, two blocks from his office, was the place where Dorothy Parker and other brilliant writers and thinkers gathered to drink and share important ideas. Magic happened at the Algonquin Round Table. Drinking and creativity were linked indelibly, romantically linked, in my sixteen-year-old imagination. I took my future wife there on our first date. Kay Redfield Jamison's *Recessive Alcoholic Memoir, Touched with Fire: Manic-Depressive Illness and the Artistic Temperament* (1993), is a telling study of the linkage in cultural imagination of manic-depression and drinking, often alcoholic drinking.[19]

The TV series *Mad Men* makes much, in its first few seasons, of the profane version of what I took to be a sacred linkage between creativity and drink, when men-in-suits trying to pitch cigarettes, potato chips, and disposable diapers, drink heavily at the office to get inspiration for their ad campaigns. Augusten Burroughs describes the extension of this culture in the advertising industry into the 1990s. It's true. I had many multi-martini lunches in the 1980s and 1990s with friends in advertising, friends whose reward in the wee hours involved doing lines of coke in clubs. It was swank. There are many recent exemplars of a profane Hollywood version of the artist whose *dasein* is devoted to the performance of being a party animal with occasional stays in celebrity rehab. It is true, of course, that alcohol, like other drugs, alters one's thinking and breaks down certain inhibitions. But it is an odd and naïve thought that it has genuine aesthetic powers. I remind myself that Dylan Thomas was dead at thirty-nine, James Joyce at fifty-nine.

THE DEEP-SELF AND BEING
AT HOME IN ONE'S BODY

There are many ways that drinking, and all that is associated with it, can gain entry in the fabric of one's being, become part of one's deep-self, and become identity constitutive. When

---

[19] If Hanna Pickard's (2012) surmise that addiction is a chronic and relapsing condition only for users who also have psychiatric problems, then "recessive alcoholic memoirs" deserve much more attention than I give them here.

I was wanting to date again in middle age, after divorce and new-found sobriety, I spoke to my psychiatrist a lot about what I knew about dating. The answer was not much. What I had learned in high school was that if you were trying to get a date—at a party, for example—you drank. And if you were lucky enough to get a date, you drank. And if you intended to make out, you (and the girl) really better have had drinks. Beer, whiskey sours, 7&7's would all do. The important thing was that romance, sex, and drinking necessarily went together. My shrink and I decided that I, as a newly sober middle-aged man, needed to learn how to kiss a woman sober. Hum.

Peter Hamill explains the basic situation better than I can:

> Drinking was an integral part of sexuality, easing entrance to its dark and mysterious treasure chambers. Drinking was a sacramental binder of friendships. Drinking was the reward for work, the fuel of celebration, the consolation for death or defeat. Drinking gave me strength, confidence, ease, laughter; it made me believe that dreams really could come true. (1995, pp. 146–147)

It may be that in certain cultures—these are always far away in the South Pacific—entry into the zones of dating, love, sex, and romance are negotiated effortlessly. But that is not typical in America. Sex is fraught. After a sweet riff on the innocent unguarded friendships of late childhood, Augusten Burroughs writes humorously, "Then you get pubic hair and everything changes. Pubic hair signals the beginning of your demise" (2003, p. 91).

Liquor is good for allaying awkwardness; it is an excellent lubricant if you are planning to sin, and a perfect tonic for assuaging the guilt of having sinned. The lesson is not all that hard-to-learn. It works, and in some cases, the solution becomes engrained in the way one does the world in its most important and magical zones.

The general point is that love and sex are great goods. Most adults want to live in such a way that these goods have a central place in their lives. But, for some of us, at any rate, we acquire skill at love and sex and drinking at the same time in the same places with fellow drinkers. According to the *C. elegans* effect, this much is bound to make them associated in the mind of such souls. But the linkage can easily become constitutive. Drinking and sex, even love, are part of the same activity. Learning how to kiss a woman sober, as a middle-aged man, is a bit humiliating. The point is a general one. For an individual whose drinking life and love life involve deep-self identification, it can be necessary to decouple activities that are independent and best kept apart, but that are coupled deeply for historical reasons in one's person.

THE FEELING OF "SAFETY ITSELF"

Wittgenstein says that one of the deepest desires or longings we have as humans is to feel "absolute safety." Wittgenstein thought the desire or need was at the root of the human attraction to the transcendental. Perhaps there is a kind of ultimate safety in the divine's embrace, a safety there isn't, that there can't be, in my parents' abode. Being at ease with oneself and, what is different, with one's compatriots, is less than a feeling of absolute safety, a feeling that one is completely protected, completely immune to harm, to pain, to suffering. But it is closer to that feeling than the ordinary experience of everyday vulnerability.

Drinking, for some, seems to produce something in this vicinity, which explains part of its attraction.

It is commonplace to hear that drinking begins as a form of self-medication, even that alcoholism is self-medication. There is some truth in this. Alcoholism requires using alcohol, and for people who keep at it long enough to become addicted, they must like something about "the Substance." Normally this is an effect not, at least at first, the taste of "the Substance" itself.

Becoming an alcoholic or drug addict requires using—choosing to use—enough of "the Substance" over a long enough period of time for whatever mid-brain mutiny that amounts to the "off switch" being broken to occur—assuming, for argument's sake, it does occur. At that point in time, one feels as if one has lost normal cognitive control over drinking or using, and one's behavior indicates that this is so. Some people start to use because others do, because it is endorsed and expected in their community, among people like them. And the using eventually causes the "off switch" to malfunction. Others use because they like the feeling even if drinking or using are not accepted, endorsed, or encouraged in their community. They use to gain the feeling. They chase it. But the feelings they chase—the "it"—are multifarious in kind, dependent on the drug of choice and the person. For some the feeling chased is a positive ecstatic one; for others it is a state of negation, a feeling of not being scared.

It is mainly when using is for control—suppression, modification, and/or elimination—of negative hedonic states that the self-medication trope makes sense. Using this way is not uncommon. The very first time I drank at the age of thirteen—a half-glass of hard cider— the main feeling I had on the walk home was that I felt not scared. I would not have said before that walk that I felt fearful or unsafe. But that first drink of ethanol lifted a fear I did not know I had.

In *Drinking: A Love Story*, Caroline Knapp describes both the social endorsement and then eventually her first-personal discovery of the safety effects of drinking: "Growing up, I had an unsafe feeling. From early on, drinking provided the feel of a psychological safety net" (1998, p. 69). Even before she experienced the fear lifting when she herself used, she saw that something magical, also a quieting of fear or tension, occurred during cocktail hour. She writes this from the pose of a little girl, a sort of semi-participant observer in a familiar American middle-class ritual:

> I liked the ritual long before I started to drink myself. Without realizing it, I had learned to look forward to it. My parents were normally so quiet: they'd sit on the sofa, my mother knitting and my father staring out the window, and a tension would hang over the room like a fog, a preoccupied silence that always made me feel wary, as though something bad were about to happen. My mother would say something about her day—about how she' d ordered some new curtains say, or taken the dog to the vet—and even though my father didn't ignore her in any obvious way, you' d get the sense that he wasn't listening, that his thoughts were about six blocks down the street. Five minutes would pass like that, or ten. Then he' d drink his martini, perhaps pour the second one. He' d begin to loosen up, and within a few minutes it would feel as though all the molecules in the room had risen up and rearranged themselves, settling down into a more comfortable pattern. (1998, pp. 38–39)

Later Knapp describes a dinner out with her father, who had introduced her to "martinis, Spanish sherry and single-malt Scotch." Now she could engage, genuinely participate, in the ritual where the "molecules rise up and rearrange themselves." And she knew how to modify her own anxiety and awkwardness.

> I sat on my hands, I remember feeling that particularly acute brand of teenage awkwardness, unable to think of a word to say, and I remember a thick interminable silence. I also remember an empty feeling, a wariness, something I often felt in my father's presence—looking for some nod of encouragement or approval from him, hoping for something to fill the gap between us … [B]ut then the wine came, one glass and then a second glass. And somewhere during that second drink, the switch was flipped. The wine gave me a melting feeling, a warm light sensation in my head, and I felt like safety itself had arrived in that glass, poured out from the bottle and allowed to spill out between us … the discomfort was diminished, replaced by something that felt like a kind of love. (1998, pp. 39–40)

Learning to drink in the way Knapp did (and the way I did too) involves acquiring a habit, learning an activity, participating in a form of life, for the sake of producing effects that answer to deep psychological needs, such as feeling safe, secure, not scared, not anxious, not awkward. Simply removing the alcohol when it starts to produce terrible effects and—as it often does—loses its ability to bring the safe feeling (or for others, the happy feeling) it once produced, stops one problem. But there is still the matter of having tampered with a major source of the person's feeling safe in the world. Minimally, he or she will need to learn new habits or activities that can help achieve, insofar as possible, a similar sense of being safe, minimally of being OK with himself, with who he is and how he does his life (Pickard 2012; Pickard and Pearce, in press).

CONCLUSION

So, what do memoirs teach about what it is like to be alcoholic? One answer is that they reveal that for a certain kind of alcoholic, perhaps mainly the ones who write memoirs or have low bottoms, possibly both, that alcoholism is woven into the fabric of their everyday lives. Such people, in the grip, were not hijacked by alcohol, they entered into, often they were inculcated into a form of life, a way of being in which drinking alcohol served one or more identity constitutive functions. For these individuals drinking, drinking heavily, is part of the way they are. They identify with drinking. Drinking is part of who they are, in some deep way, or better perhaps, in several deep ways. One implication is that our descriptions of what alcoholism is, of the varieties of alcoholism, must, in order to respect the phenomenon, include a way of speaking about this kind of alcoholic, and this kind of alcoholism. There is no doubt that there are aspects of this kind of alcoholism that involve narrow features of the brain and the body, for example, which make alcohol produce pleasant as opposed to unpleasant or wanted versus unwanted feelings, and that eventually produce in some souls, but not all, obsession and craving, and malfunctioning on and off switches. But for the sorts of individuals who reveal themselves in the memoirs I've discussed, their alcoholism includes much more than brain states and oddly functioning on and off switches. Their personhood, their character, is constituted, in part, by a history of drinking, by a set of identifications and practices that involve alcohol, and that make these individuals who and what they are. Alcoholism, of this sort, at any rate, is a wide ecological phenomenon; it involves the deep-self.

The identity constitutive and wide ecological features of alcoholism are not facts that an individual with first-person expertise as an alcoholic discovers by introspection; but they are facts that reveal themselves, to him or her and to us, when a first person expert (perhaps only some) reflects on and then describes his or her alcoholic life.

Besides the implications for taxonomy, for description, and for explanation, the deep-self analysis has implications for treatment, minimally, for what is involved in recovering from alcoholism. One needs to be especially cautious here. For some disorders neither their complex developmental history, nor their current wide ecology, are relevant to their treatment. Cancers can be cured with interventions that require no knowledge of their history, and my four-and-a-half-decade-old bad tennis serve—despite being a well-engrained, relational, way-I-am, the way-I play-tennis—can be fixed by a good coach without my personal identity being involved or undermined in the fix. To the degree that alcoholic drinking is woven into the fabric of an individual's life the situation is different. No matter how much relief is brought to the self, and to second- and third-person parties who are in relation with the alcoholic, by his putting a "plug in the jug," the more drinking is part of who he is, the more identity-reconstituting and reconfiguring work remains to be done after he stops drinking. Sometimes, perhaps often, alcoholism is an absorbing, full-time way of being in the world. Undoing alcoholism as a form of life, and not more narrowly as just a drinking problem, involves fairly radical undoing and then redoing of oneself. It gives the alcoholic an opportunity that many people never have. But it, identity reconstitution, presents formidable challenges. It is not clear where or on whom the burden falls to do all the identity reconstituting work. Surely the alcoholic-in-recovery bears the mother lode of responsibility for it. But it is important for all the second and third parties to recognize that such work is part of the process of recovery and that stopping drinking means only that the alcoholic doesn't drink. It does not mean he is healed or no longer alcoholic. Many alcoholics say they are alcoholic, rather than "were" alcoholic, long after they have stopped drinking, possibly until they die. This is a good way of reminding oneself and others that alcoholism is commonly a matter of the way one is, not merely a matter of the way one drinks, or the way one's brain is or might be messed up. It is also a way of respecting the phenomenon and the person.

ACKNOWLEDGMENTS

I am grateful to Tyler Curtain, Richard Gipps, George Graham, Carl Kenney, Peg O'Connor, Hanna Pickard, Jennifer Radden, and Serife Tekin for extremely helpful comments.

REFERENCES

Ahmed, S. H. (2012). The science of making drug-addicted animals. *Neuroscience*, 211, 107–25.

Alcoholics Anonymous (2001). *Alcoholics Anonymous* [Big Book]. New York, NY: Alcoholics Anonymous World Services. (Original work published 1939.)

Arpaly, N. (2006). *Merit, Meaning, and Human Bondage: An Essay on Free Will*. Princeton, NJ: Princeton University Press.

Baumeister, R. F. and Tierney, J. (2011). *Willpower: Rediscovering the Greatest Human Strength*. New York, NY: Penguin Press.

Bayne T. and Levy N. (2006). The feeling of doing: Deconstructing the phenomenology of agency. In N. Sebanz and W. Prinz (Eds), *Disorders of Volition*, pp. 49–68. Cambridge, MA: MIT Press.

Berridge, K. C. and Robinson, T. E. (2011). Drug addiction as incentive sensitization. In J. Poland and G. Graham (Eds), *Addiction and Responsibility*, pp. 21–54. Cambridge, MA: MIT Press.

Bratman, M. (2007). *Structures of Agency: Essays*. Oxford: Oxford.

Burroughs, A. (2003). *Dry: A Memoir*. New York, NY: Picador.

Di Chiara, G., Bassareo, V., Fenu, S., De Luca, M. A., Spina, L., Cadoni, C., *et al.* (2004). Dopamine and drug addiction: the nucleus accumbens shell connection. *Neuropharmacology*, *47*(Suppl 1), 227–41.

Fingarette, H. (1988). *Heavy Drinking: The Myth of Alcoholism as a Disease*. Berkeley, CA: University of California.

Flanagan, O. (1992). *Consciousness Reconsidered*. Cambridge, MA: MIT Press.

Flanagan, O. (2011). What is it like to be an addict? In J. Poland and G. Graham (Eds), *Addiction and Responsibility*, pp. 269–92. Cambridge, MA: MIT Press.

Flanagan, O. (in press). Phenomenal authority: The epistemic authority of Alcoholics Anonymous. In Levy, N. (Ed.), *Addiction and Self-Control*. Oxford: Oxford.

Frankfurt, H. (1971). Freedom of the will and the concept of a person. *Journal of Philosophy*, *68*, 5–20.

Frankfurt, H. (1988). *What We Care About: Philosophical Essays*. New York, NY: Cambridge University Press.

Graham, G. (2010). *The Disordered Mind: An Introduction to Philosophy of Mind and Mental Illness*. New York, NY: Routledge.

Hacking, I. (1996). The looping effects of human kinds. In D. Sperber and A. J. Premack (Eds), *Causal Cognition*, pp. 351–83. Oxford: Oxford University Press.

Hamill, P. (1995). *A Drinking Life: A Memoir*. Boston, MA: Back Bay Books.

Heyman, G. M. (2009). *Addiction: A Disorder of Choice*. Cambridge, MA: Harvard University Press.

Holton, R. (2009). *Willing, Wanting, Waiting*. Oxford: Oxford University Press.

Hornbacher, M. (2008). *Madness: A Bipolar Life*. Boston, MA: Houghton-Mifflin.

Hornbacher, M. (2010). *Sane: Mental Illness, Addiction, and the 12 Steps*. Center City, MN: Hazeldon.

Jackson, C. (1944). *The Lost Weekend*. (Reissued 1996.) Syracuse, NY: Syracuse University Press.

Jamison, R. K. (1993). *Touched with Fire: Manic-Depressive Illness and the Artistic Temperament*. New York, NY: Free Press.

Jamison, K. R. (1995). *An Unquiet Mind: A Memoir of Moods and Madness*. New York, NY: Vintage.

Jellinek, E. M. (1946). Phases in the drinking history of alcoholics: Analysis of a survey conducted by the official organ of Alcoholics Anonymous. *Quarterly Journal of Studies on Alcohol*, *7*, 1–88.

Jellinek, E. M. (1960). *The Disease Concept of Alcoholism*. New Haven, CT: Hillhouse.

Knapp, C. (1997). *Drinking: A Love Story*. New York, NY: Dial Press.

Koob, G. F. and Le Moal, M. (2006). *Neurobiology of Addiction*. London: Elsevier.

Levy, N. (2010). Resisting 'weakness of the will.' *Philosophy and Phenomenological Research*, *LXXXII*(1), 134–55.

London, J. (1913). *John Barleycorn: 'Alcoholic Memoirs'*. (Reprinted 2009.) Oxford: Oxford University Press.

Loewenstein, G. (1996). Out of control: Visceral influences on behavior. *Organizational Behavior and Human Decision Processes*, *615*, 272–92.

Müller, C. P. and Schumann, G. (2011). Drugs as instruments—a new framework for nonaddictive psychoactive drug use. *Behavioral and Brain Sciences*, *34*(6), 293–310.

Musselman, H. N., Neal-Beliveau, B., Nass, R., and Engleman, E. A. (2012). Chemosensory cue conditioning with stimulants in a Caenorhabditis elegans animal model of addiction. *Behavioral Neuroscience*, *126*(3), 445–56.

National Epidemiologic Survey on Alcohol And Related Conditions (NESARC). (2006). *NESARC 2001–2002*. [Online.] Available at: <http://pubs.niaaa.nih.gov/publications/AA70/AA70.htm>.

O'Connor, P. (2011). The fallacy of 'the hijacked brain.' *New York Times*, June 11. Available at: <http://opinionator.blogs.nytimes.com/2012/06/10/the-hijacked-brain/>.

Pickard, H. (2012). The purpose in chronic addiction. *AJOB Neuroscience*, *3*(2), 40–9.

Pickard, H. and Pearce, S. (in press). Addiction in context: Philosophical lessons from a personality disorder clinic. In N. Levy (Ed.), *Addiction and Control*. Oxford: Oxford.

Robertson. N. (1988). *Getting Better: Inside Alcoholics Anonymous*. (Reprinted 2009.) Lincoln, NE: iUniverse.

Ross, D., Sharp, C., Vuchinich, R. E., and Spurrett, D. (2008). *Midbrain Mutiny: The Picoeconomics and Neuroeconomics of Disordered Gambling: Economic Theory and Cognitive Science*. Cambridge, MA: MIT Press.

Sadler, J. (2005). *Values and Psychiatric Diagnosis*. Oxford: Oxford University Press.

Schroeder, T. and Arpaly, N. (1999). Alienation and externality. *Canadian Journal of Philosophy*, *29*(3), 371–88.

Selby, H. Jr (1964). *Last Exit to Brooklyn*. New York, NY: Castle Books.

Selby, H. Jr (1978). *Requiem for a Dream*. New York, NY: Da Capo Press.

Solinas, M., Chauvet, C., Thiriet, N., El Rawas, R., and Jaber, M. (2008). Reversal of cocaine addiction by environmental enrichment. *Proceedings of the National Academy of Sciences of the United States of America*, *105*, 17145–50.

Styron, W. (1990). *Darkness Visible*. New York, NY: Vintage.

Tekin, S. (2011). Self-concept through the diagnostic looking glass: Narratives and mental disorder. *Philosophical Psychology*, *24*, 357–80.

Tekin, S. (in press). Self-insight in the time of mood disorders: After the diagnosis, treatment. *Philosophy, Psychiatry & Psychology*.

Thayil, J. (2012). *Narcopolis: A Novel*. New York, NY: Penguin.

Vaillant, G. E. (1995). *The Natural History of Alcoholism Revisited*. Cambridge: Harvard.

Wallace, R. J. (1994). *Responsibility and the Moral Sentiments*. Cambridge, MA: Harvard University Press.

Wallace, D. F. (1996). *Infinite Jest*. Boston, MA: Back Bay Books.

Wallace, R. J. (1999). Addiction as defect of the will: Some philosophical reflections. *Law and Philosophy*, *18*(6), 621–54.

Watson, G. (1975). Free agency. *Journal of Philosophy*, *72*(8), 205–20.

Watson, G. (1999). Disordered appetites. In J. Elster (Ed.), *Addiction: Entries and Exits*, pp. 3–28. New York, NY: Russell Sage Foundation.

Watson, G. (2004). *Agency and Answerability: Selected Essays*. Oxford. Oxford University Press.

Wolf, S. (1987). Sanity and the metaphysics of responsibility. In F. Schoeman (Ed.), *Responsibility, Character, and the Emotions: New Essays in Moral Psychology*, pp. 46–62. Cambridge: Cambridge University Press.

Yaffe, G. (2001). Recent work on addiction and responsible agency. *Philosophy & Public Affairs*, *30*, 178–221.

CHAPTER 52

PERSONALITY DISORDER AND VALIDITY: A HISTORY OF CONTROVERSY

PETER ZACHAR AND ROBERT F. KRUEGER

INTRODUCTION

There are very few, if any, constructs in psychiatry that are more conceptually encumbered than that of personality disorder. How so? Because personality disorder inherits not only all the problems associated with the concept of "personality," but also all the problems associated with the concept "psychiatric disorder." Personality alone encompasses biological-genetic, developmental, social-cultural, perceptual-cognitive, motivational-emotional, existential-phenomenological, and behavioral psychology. Most of the validity issues relevant to these areas are also relevant to personality and its disorders.

In this chapter we will review the historical development of the concepts of personality and personality disorder in psychology and psychiatry before turning to an exploration of several validity-related questions that intersect the interests of psychologists, psychiatrists, and philosophers. These include the role that values should play in the conceptualization of personality disorders, the nature of pathology in personality disorders, and the extent to which personality traits can or should be considered to be causal entities that carve nature at the joints.

FROM SELF TO PERSONALITY

Many modern definitions of personality emphasize that it is a pattern of organized psychological characteristics (e.g., traits, motivations, conflicts) that are stable across time and situations, that make individuals unique, and that determine thoughts, emotions, and behaviors.

> Personality is the dynamic organization within the individual of those psychophysical systems that determine his characteristic behavior and thought. (Allport, 1961, p. 28)

> Personality refers to an individual's characteristic patterns of thought, emotion and behavior, together with the psychological mechanisms—hidden or not—behind those patterns. (Funder 1997, p.1)

One philosophically interesting claim in these definitions is that personality plays a causal role in the generation of thoughts, feelings, and behaviors. This claim predated the modern construct of personality, emerging in reflections on the nature of the self. Although a construct called *the self* began to appear in late antiquity, the psychological self as a bearer of thoughts and emotions was introduced only during the seventeenth and eighteenth centuries (Berrios and Marková 2003).

In nineteenth-century France, the term personality (personnalité) came to be seen by psychologists as a naturalistic alternative to metaphysical and quasi-spiritual notions about the unity and simplicity of the self (Lombardo and Foschi 2003). The academic philosopher turned psychologist Théodule Ribot believed the psychopathology of altered consciousness showed that self (or "personality") was not a unity, and its components could be studied in a scientific way. At this time the concept of "dissociation" was introduced as a pathological counterpart to the empiricist's notion that the association of ideas is the normal process by which minds are formed. The concept of dissociation was further developed by the neurologist Pierre Janet and later given significant credence in the USA by William James (1890) in his highly influential text *The Principles of Psychology* (Taylor 2000).

The Bostonian psychiatrist Morton Prince's interest in what he called "multiple personality" was directly influenced by James' appropriation of French ideas. Articles on personality appeared regularly in *Journal of Abnormal Psychology* which was founded by Prince in 1906 (Barenbaum and Winter 2003).

During the first decade of the twentieth century, character and personality were used interchangeably, but the term "character" carried moral connotations that came to be seen as inappropriate in a clinical context. One advantage of the term personality in mental health settings was that it allowed psychiatrists to put issues of morality and immorality aside in favor of non-judgmental clinical conceptualizations. After its adoption by the medical community in the USA, personality came to be considered to be more appropriate than character as a topic of scientific study—it was a considered a natural psychological attribute like memory and perception (Danziger 1990; Nicholson 2003).

In 1921, Prince's journal was renamed *The Journal of Abnormal Psychology and Social Psychology* and the psychologist Floyd Allport became its co-editor. The very first issue of the renamed journal included an article titled "Personality traits: Their classification and measurement" by Allport and his younger brother Gordon. Psychological measurement in the Galtonian tradition had been an alternative to experimental work as an approach to scientific psychology for at least a decade, but beginning in the 1920s it became an increasingly respectable alternative.

The development of intelligence tests for use in educational settings represented psychology's original foray into "psychometrics." Danziger (1990) points out that it soon became clear that early intelligence tests had only a limited predictive value—even in educational settings. More importantly, many considered them less than helpful in the US military's efforts to assign draftees to positions in World War I; it would take additional efforts to arrive at modern, reliable and valid intelligence tests. After the war ended, it was suggested that personality traits might be more predictive of real world behaviors than IQ scores. The assessment of personality traits was quickly adapted to the paper-and-pencil methods for assessing IQ in large groups that had been developed during the war and a new tool/instrument was born—the personality inventory.

The American Psychological Association accepted ownership of Prince's journal in 1926, leading to a large expansion of scientific articles in comparison to the clinical case reports favored by Prince (Barenbaum and Winter 2003). By the late 1930s the study of personality had become a unified content area in psychology, as signified by the increased number of researchers who specialized in the study of personality, entire courses on personality being offered in university psychology departments, and the inclusion of a distinct chapter on personality in most introductory textbooks (Nicholson 2003).

This establishment of personality as a research specialty at this time is exemplified by the work of two men, namely, Gordon Allport (1937) and Henry Murray (1938). Many psychologists were involved in the development of personality as a specialization, but Allport and Murray, who both had the imprimatur of Harvard University, are often singled out.

Allport is associated with making the study of personality distinct from both clinical and social psychology. Although he followed the medical tradition by arguing for use of the secular term "personality" instead of "character," he also advocated the study of the normal rather than the abnormal personality. His work in the measurement of normal traits represents the beginning of the empirical tradition in the psychology of personality. Until relatively recently, this tradition was segregated from psychiatric classification.

In addition to his concern with normality and health, Allport also emphasized the whole person and the subjective self. Psychologists later termed this foray into the study of normality *humanism*. Trait theorists, with their roots in faculty psychology, have always been interested in the biological basis of traits. In contrast, the humanistic psychologists were primarily interested in exploring meaning and personal values. In the 1950s, humanistic psychology was embraced by the rapidly expanding specialties of clinical and counseling psychology (Rogers 1951). Like the academic personality researchers, the humanistic clinical psychologists also had limited interest in psychiatric classification and diagnosis.

Unlike Allport, Murray was not trained as a scientific psychologist and he was a hostile critic of conventional academic psychology (Nicholson 2003). Nor did his preference for case studies and case conferences endear him to the Harvard psychology department. Yet, Murray's Freud-inspired theory of needs became influential in clinical psychology, as did other psychodynamic models including those of Jung, Adler, Horney, and Fromm (Hall and Lindsey 1957). What became of this tradition will be briefly explored at the end of the next section.

To summarize this section, the construct of personality represents a secularization of "character" for use in a medical context. It is also an heir to philosophical theories of the subsistent self. As a research specialty in psychology, personality was "normalized" and considered to be qualitatively distinct from psychopathology. Two forms this normalization took was the psychometric measurement of traits and the humanistic concern for individual subjectivity and meaning.

PERSONALITY AND THE CONCEPT

OF DISORDER

The history of personality disorder begins with the origin of modern psychiatry in the nineteenth century. Our story commences with the French physician Benedict Morel's introduction of dementia praecox in the 1850s, which he tied to the notion of degeneration. According to Morel, degeneration was an irreversible physical and mental deterioration from a higher to a lower form. Morel also believed that degeneration represented a fall from grace in the theological sense (Gilman 1985) and referred to the signs of degeneration as *stigmata* (Carlson 1985). Morel believed that once the degenerative process got going in a family, the offspring became increasingly degenerate. Those initially affected were nervous and violent. Subsequent cohorts were more likely to be epileptic, hysterical, and hypochondriacal. As degeneration proceeded, family members became eccentric and unpredictable, with dementia praecox being one of the later, final manifestations of the decline (Carlson 1985).

It is common to consider dementia praecox (later renamed schizophrenia) and its associated psychotic symptoms (especially delusions) as the prototype of insanity. It is, however, also historically accurate to say that the hypothetical process of degeneration itself was for a time an equally important theoretical model of insanity, including within its scope the notion of the morbid personality.

As degeneration theory spread it came to refer to deviates of all stripes and colors, including sexual deviates, criminals, the mentally retarded, and so-called inferior races. The moral dimensions to these categories were readily identified as character flaws. Prominent figures in the study of "degenerates" in the 1870s include Valentin Magnan in France, Cesare Lombroso in Italy, Henry Maudsley in England, and Richard von Krafft-Ebbing in Austria (Carlson 1985; Pick 1989; Shorter 1997,).[1] Depending on the thinker, the presumed etiological factors included alcohol and drug use, masturbation, poisoning, harsh climates, harsh working conditions, poor diet, neglect, and parental turmoil.

Crucially important was the integration of the degeneration hypothesis with mid-nineteenth-century evolutionary theory, whereby degeneration became a natural rather than a theological concept. This process was facilitated by the 1844 publication of *Vestiges of the Natural History of Creation*, authored anonymously by Robert Chambers. It was Chambers, not Darwin, who introduced the larger British public to evolution and the naturalistic approach to history. Referring to the *Vestiges* as a "Victorian sensation," Secord (2000) reports that the book was widely read (and condemned) by all strata of society and the public scandal led Darwin to delay publication of his own evolutionary theory for fourteen years.

In the *Vestiges*, Chambers claimed that evolution could be both progressive and retrogressive (i.e., degenerate). This bidirectional notion can be traced back to the origin of evolutionary thinking in the speculative work of Buffon in the eighteenth century, but through *Vestiges*

---

[1] Carslon (1985) notes that the French thinker Abbé Raynal included emigrated white Americans in his examples of degeneration. Both Benjamin Franklin and Thomas Jefferson objected.

the degeneration hypotheses permeated British Society. For example, in the literature of this time Mr Hyde, Count Dracula, the half-human half-animal creatures of Dr Moreau, and the Morlocks from *The Time Machine* were all depictions of degenerates (Pick 1989).

An additional nineteenth-century development important to the construct of personality disorder was the extension of the term "insanity" to cases that did not involve what currently what might be called a disorganized psychosis. For example, in 1801 Pinel introduced the classification *manie sans délire*. Berrios (1993) notes that the meaning of these terms have changed so much that we cannot assimilate them to our current notions of mania and delusions, and that Pinel's new classification primarily referred to a deviation from a state of "total insanity" in which rationality was somewhat preserved. Depression without psychotic features and obsessions and compulsions would be included in this category. Esquirol's 1810 notion of *monomania* was an alternative conception of partial insanity. Monomania explained some kinds of abnormal behavior by positing a single, fixed delusion that had radiating effects throughout consciousness and behavior, but did not entail a comprehensive disorganization of mental faculties (Goldstein 1987). J. C. Prichard's 1835 concept of *moral insanity*, which Berrios (1993) claims bears no resemblance to the modern construct of psychopathy/antisocial personal disorder, also belongs in this tradition of classifying non-psychotic mental disorders.

The notions of degeneration, character, and partial insanity came together most explicitly in J. A. Koch's 1891 concept of *psychopathic inferiority*. Koch used personality traits such as trouble-maker, arrogant, morose, and touchy to describe these conditions, the more severe forms of which he considered to be the result of a process of degeneration (Berrios 1996; Schneider 1923/1950).

The work of Emil Kraepelin was a major influence on many aspects of psychiatric thinking both before and after the turn of the century. In *Lectures on Clinical Psychiatry*, Kraepelin (1904) described the morbid personality as a state of permanent psychopathic inferiority— a term he used for stable and unremitting conditions with a hereditary basis. Morbid (or "degenerate") personality specifically referred to a group of narcissistic, irresponsible, and disagreeable individuals:

> If such a personality is measured by the standard of a law-court, it is simply that of a criminal and a swindler. Yet the physician cannot escape from the conviction that the patient has a congenital incapacity for a regular course of life, stronger than all education, experience, and self-control (Kraepelin 1904, p. 302).

As Kraepelin notes, such patients would seem normal in a casual encounters or upon a first meeting. The morbidity could only be gleaned by looking at the pattern of a whole life.

At some point in the first decade of the twentieth century, the tide against degeneration began to turn in psychiatry. This was likely a combination of improved information about hereditary processes in psychiatry and elsewhere, and growing philosophical disagreements with the social and political claims of its most committed advocates. Kraepelin largely abandoned the hypothesis by 1918 (Carlson 1985).

By the time that Kurt Schneider wrote *Psychopathic Personalities* in 1923, degeneration theory, and with it the notion of morbid personality, were much less tenable. For Schneider (1923/1950), "psychopathic personality" was a general term for all personality disorders. He considered these to be clinical, not moral conditions. Schneider defined abnormal personality in an objective, statistical sense as *deviation from an average range*. What made an abnormal personality clinically-relevant (psychopathic) was whether it led to either personal suffering on the part of the patient or to the suffering of others. Schneider also stated that psychopathic personalities were conditions that lay outside the narrow confines the disease-oriented approach to medicine and were not literal illnesses.

One additional contribution to the historical development of the construct of personality disorder must be mentioned. Late in his career, Freud (1921/1960) proposed what has come to be known as his structural (id, ego, and superego) model of personality. The development of this theory by thinkers such as Reich (1949) and Hartmann (1958) became influential in the USA. In particular, clinical psychologists who specialized in diagnostic testing came to see their task as developing a model of the patient's personality (Rapaport et al. 1945; Shapiro, 1965). This applied not only to hysteria and paranoia, but also to depression and schizophrenia. The third edition of the *Diagnostic and Statistical Manual of Mental Disorders* (DSM-III; American Psychiatric Association 1980) in 1980 is often given credit for raising interest in personality disorders by separating their diagnosis from the diagnosis of other mental disorders,[2] but it is rarely noted that in doing so the DSM-III created a greater distinction between personality and other mental disorders than previously existed in the American approach to psychopathology.

Philosophical Issues and Validity

The philosophical issues relevant to the validity of personality disorders can be parsed in different and partially overlapping ways. Many of the issues discussed in the psychological and psychiatric literature do not map neatly onto the professional concerns of philosophers. For example, the technical issue of whether a personality construct is distributed in the population as a true class (a "classical category") or as a continuous dimension dominates the scientific literature, but barely registers on the philosopher's own conceptual radar.

The three validity issues we will explore are rooted in the history just reviewed and they also represent ongoing concerns in psychology and psychiatry. They were selected because they could benefit from sustained philosophical exploration, i.e., explicit philosophical work has an important role to play in the development of solutions/resolutions. Furthermore, these issues are readily registered on the radar of psychiatrists, psychologists, and philosophers.

Issue one: What role do values and considerations of character play in the conceptualization of personality disorders?

Consider this passage from Jonathan Franzen's novel *Freedom*:

> A game could be made of trying to get Patty to agree that somebody's behavior was "bad."
> When she was told that Seth and Merrie Paulsen were throwing a big Halloween party for their

---

[2] For example, "Axis I" would code for psychiatric disorders such as depression. "Axis II" would code for personality disorders and personality traits. "Axis III" would code for medical conditions such as type II diabetes.

twins and had deliberately invited every child on the block except Connie Monaghan, Patty would only say that this was very "weird." The next time she saw the Paulsens in the street, they explained that they had tried *all summer* to get Connie Monaghan's mother, Carol, to stop flicking cigarette butts from her bedroom window into their twin's little wading pool. "That is really weird," Patty agreed, shaking her head, "but you know it's not Connie's fault." The Paulsens, however, refused to be satisfied with "weird." They wanted *sociopathic*, they wanted *passive-aggressive*, they wanted *bad*. (Franzen 2010, pp. 5–6)[3]

As will be reviewed in more detail later in this chapter, many psychologists believe that the universal structure of human personality is best modeled in terms of five broad traits—called by some *The Big Five*. Interestingly, when psychologists attempt to model the structure of normal personality at levels higher than the Big Five, they find two superfactors that Digman (1997) terms Alpha (α) and Beta (β) and De Raad and Barelds (2008) call virtue and dynamism. Virtue is said to capture the moral aspects of character such as kindness, reliability, and decency. Dynamism encompasses features such as enthusiasm and energy. Such findings suggest that despite the historical attempt to naturalize the morally-laden notion of *character* by introducing the construct of *personality*, the moral aspects have not been eliminated.

Much the same is true in the realm of psychopathology. DeYoung (2010) has termed Alpha "stability" and Beta "plasticity," and has noted that the best markers of Alpha are descriptors with negative valence (e.g., "I get out of control"), whereas positively valenced descriptors correspond with Beta (e.g., "I express myself easily"). Simms, Yufik, and Gros (2010) have shown empirically that negative valence is a potent predictor of personality disorder, whereas positive valence is considerably less relevant. Essentially, personality disorder as conceptualized in the contemporary psychiatric literature pertains to the tendency to behave in a negatively valenced fashion. Character and virtue are therefore inextricably interwoven into the fabric of personality disorders.

It is in this light that one should consider a variety of positions on the "mad versus bad" problem with respect to personality disorders. John Sadler (2005) notes that modern societies have to be careful about medicalizing what they consider immoral behavior. He is particularly concerned about those conditions that most people would consider to represent violations of moral norms. For example, every single criterion for identifying conduct disorder such as cruelty and theft represents a violation of moral norms. This does not mean that conduct disorder is not a legitimate disorder, but the possibility that bad behavior has been inappropriately medicalized should not be dismissed.

In the domain of personality disorder, Louis Charland (2004, 2006) has argued that the Cluster B personality disorders such as borderline, narcissistic, and antisocial are morally bad groupings of behaviors that have been inappropriately medicalized. Charland argues that if all the morally-laden diagnostic criteria for these conditions were eliminated, there would be nothing left to diagnose. Furthermore successful treatment of these "disorders," he claims, would be more akin to moral conversion.

Such assertions have to be considered with some care. As we have seen, after the abandonment of the construct of the morbid personality, personality disorders have not been considered to be disease-like entities along the lines of schizophrenia. Their "medical" status resides on the border between the dysfunctional and the disliked. Furthermore, if any

---

[3] Excerpt from "Good Neighbors" from *Freedom* by Jonathan Franzen. Copyright © 2010 by Jonathan Franzen. Reprinted by permission of Farrar, Straus and Giroux, LLC.

particular personality pattern is considered to lie within the fuzzy boundaries of the medical (i.e., be dysfunctional), there is no reason for thinking that the relevant capacity failures cannot include moral capacities.

Zachar and Potter (2010) respond to Charland by claiming that, instead of seeing moral theory as a threat to the study and treatment of personality disorders, moral theory can appropriately inform psychiatric thinking about personality disorders. In particular they explore the conceptual resources of virtue theory.

According to Zachar and Potter the concept of flourishing in virtue theory has a much larger scope than those philosophical notions of "morality" that emphasize prescribing law-like rules for governing behavior. Virtue theorists, who emphasize the importance of thinking about what kind of persons we should be rather than thinking about what rules should govern our behavior, would not expect that notions of morality, goodness, health, and adaptivity can be completed segregated.

Zachar and Potter also argue that if one decides to conceptualize traits along the lines of virtue theory with pathology/vice existing at the poles and virtue/health being in between, one should not be too concrete about the evaluative implications of any position within that structure. The golden mean is not an arithmetic mean but a dynamic balance point that represents a "better" (not perfect) response given all one's competing obligations and goals. The adaptiveness of any trait should be evaluated in the context of the person's situation. It should also be evaluated in the context of other traits which can compensate for or exacerbate any negative impact on adaptiveness.

One does not have to agree with Charland regarding the "moral, not medical" nature of personality disorders to be concerned about medicalization. Carl Elliott (1996, 2003), for example, withholds final judgment about the pathological status of personality and related states of character, but remains concerned about the consequences of medicalizing common personality traits. Part of his concern, very interestingly, relates to people's ambivalent attitudes about medicalization. Contemporary society cannot seem to decide whether medicalization (e.g., conceptualizing debilitating shyness as social phobia) is a scientifically improved or a shallower way to think about traits.

The risk of over medicalization is greater when normal personality traits are included in the assessment and the scales are bipolar. Consider what has arguably become the dominant test for measuring normal personality, the *NEO-Personality Inventory* (NEO-PI-R and recently NEO-PI-3). Some NEO-PI-R advocates conceptualize traits as being structured like virtues, with the extreme ends of each dimension being considered pathological (Widiger and Mullins-Sweatt 2009). The problem with most bipolar personality dimensions such as those in NEO-PI-R is that they were not designed specifically to measure psychopathology (Krueger et al. 2011). For example, the NEO-PI-R has scales to measure varieties of "agreeableness" but not scales to specifically index the conceptual opposite of agreeableness, i.e., frankly hurtful and antagonistic interpersonal behavior.

One of the flaws of many early clinical tests, particularly projective instruments such as the Rorschach Inkblot Test, was that nearly everyone given the test in a clinical situation was judged to be pathological because the examiners were looking for psychopathology. This overpathologizing problem potentially applies to using the NEO-PI in a clinical context as well. For example, consider the *NEO Problems in Living Checklist* which is sold with the third edition of the test (NEO-PI-3). The *Checklist* provides pathological interpretations for the extreme end of every scale, including all thirty facet scales (i.e., the scales have a bipolar structure). An example is the agreeableness facet named "trust." High scores can potentially signal being gullible and naïve and low scores signal being paranoid and jealous. With bipolar dimensional models there is also a risk that moderately high scores can be dubbed "subthreshold," and be considered potentially pathological. The authors of the test, Costa and McCrae, are also concerned about over-medicalization and caution again using the *Checklist* in this "cookbook" way, noting that these are only possibilities that must be independently confirmed (Costa and McCrae 2010). A more direct way to attenuate inappropriate medicalization is to calibrate trait scales to measure psychopathology itself. This is the approach taken by tests such as the *Minnesota Multiphasic Personality Inventory* (MMPI).

Another import feature about the latest edition of the MMPI that addresses some of the concerns of Charland and Elliot is that the scales are unipolar not bipolar. When scales are unipolar, high scores can be considered pathological whereas low scores generally have no specific interpretation. Many people can take the MMPI and have no interpretable scores, i.e., they are not experiencing the kinds of clinical problems that are assessed by the test. It is an empirical question as to whether high and low scores can be interpreted, but the advantages of designing scales to be unipolar should not be dismissed. This does not completely solve the problem of over-medicalization. Unipolar scales interpreted in a context-free manner can be harmful as well, but relative to bipolar scales that assess normal personality, the risk of harm is reduced.

Issue two: What makes personality "pathological"

One of the problems that arose after personality disorder was separated from degeneration theory and the disease model was justifying its pathological status. As might be expected, a plurality of models are used to justify the attribution of "disorder" to personality. Some of these models require minimal inferences and tend to be less controversial. The more inferences required, the more debatable the model. Those models that view personality disorders as inherently pathological rather than clinically-relevant are the most debatable. We will review six models. Our listing of the models is based on a discussion by Zachar (2011) which itself was influenced by conceptual work on the relationship between personality disorders and other psychiatric disorders (Dolan-Sewell et al. 2001), and on the relationship between temperament, personality traits, and personality disorders (Clark 2005).

The *vulnerability model* claims that personality disorders are clinically-relevant conditions in the same way that conditions such as hypertension and hypercholesterolemia are clinically relevant. They are clinically relevant because they are risk factors for the development of less controversial disorders. For hypertension the increased risk is for cardiovascular and cerebrovascular disease. For personality disorders the increased risk includes depressive disorders, anxiety disorders, eating disorders, and psychosis (McGlashan et al. 2000; Oldham et al. 1995).

The *pathoplasticity model* claims that personality disorders are clinically relevant conditions because they affect the course and outcome of other psychiatric disorders. Not only are people with personality disorders more vulnerable to developing other psychiatric disorders, when they do develop them they tend to develop them earlier in life, have more severe symptoms, and worse outcome (Clark 2007).

The *spectrum model* claims that personality disorders represent milder expressions of the same genetic predispositions that underlie more serious disorders (Lenzenweger 2006;

Meehl 1962). An early version of this model favored by Kraepelin (1907) and Kretschmer (1925) held that personality disorders represent milder manifestations (formes frustes) of serious psychiatric disorders. Examples of personality disorders that have been hypothesized to exist on a spectrum include schizotypal, schizoid, and paranoid personality disorders (schizophrenic spectrum) cyclothymic personality disorder (bipolar spectrum) and depressive and anxious personality disorders (internalizing spectrum) (Kendler et al. 1993; Phillips et al. 1995; van Valkenburg et al. 2006).

The *decline in functioning model* is best represented by degeneration theory, i.e., personality disorder represents a developmental unexpected decline in functioning (or morbid change). As we have seen, the very idea of regression to a more primitive type (atavism) is no longer considered an empirical possibility. A residue of degeneration may be detected, however, in the concept of genetic anticipation—which occurs in trinucleotide repeat disorders such as Huntington's disease (Carpenter 1994). The more repeats, the earlier the onset of the disease, and in theory the number of repeats can increase over generational time. The risk that genetic anticipation could result in some eugenics-like social policies is always a possibility, although at this point finding empirical support justifying its application to personality disorders seems far-fetched.

Another possible formulation of the decline in functioning model would be personality change due to: (a) severe emotional trauma, (b) a previous psychiatric illness, or (c) a general medical condition such as a brain injury. In these cases the personality-relevant symptoms are the same kinds of symptoms that define DSM and ICD personality disorders. All these overlapping symptom clusters are potentially maladaptive, with a main difference being that some clusters of symptoms (such as seen in brain injury patients) can be explained with respect to an aberrant causal history where other clusters (the personality disorders diagnosed in the DSM) cannot. What counts as an aberrant causal history, however, is a vexing philosophical problem. Does sexual abuse count? If so why do not all victims of sexual abuse develop personality disorders? As George Graham (2010) might say—experiences of abuse do not always "gum up the works"—one has to consider not only causal events, but also the particular pattern of vulnerability and resiliency variables on which they act.

The *impairment-distress model* is favored by Kurt Schneider (1923/1950), proponents of the five-factor model (Widiger 2006), and the authors of the DSM-IV. In addition to statistical abnormality, advocates of this perspective argue that personality styles and traits can be considered disordered if they reliably lead to distress or impairment in social and occupational functioning. In some versions of this model, the impairment is partly explained with respect to inflexibility/dyscontrol (Widiger 2006).

The *capacity failure model* emphasizes the failure to develop one or more psychological capacities that contribute to normal functioning. Unlike the decline in functioning model where capacities are lost, according to this model they never develop. It is therefore expected that the problematic symptoms associated with a personality disorder will be evident from a young age, often by the teenage years. Personality disorders in this sense are not like acquired conditions such as tuberculosis or major depression. One could think of them as developmental disorders similar to autism, except that they tend to emerge in adolescence rather than childhood. This is more explicit in the DSM-IV, with conduct disorder considered as necessary to diagnose antisocial personality disorder, but it is presumed for all other personality disorders.

As is true with all models that specify the nature of the dysfunction, there must be some notion of what counts as normal functioning—which requires speculation. Two popular ways of conceptualizing "normal" are the natural function approach (Millikan 1984; Wakefield 1992) and the causal-role approach (Cummins 1983). Natural functions refer to functions that exist because they were produced by natural selection. The casual-role approach is ahistorical and more mechanistic. Function refers to the causal contribution that a specific capacity plays in the overall functioning of an organism.

Some recent research has begun to make some headway on the problem of modeling capacity failure. For example Roel Verheul and colleagues note that a high level of neuroticism is not itself a capacity failure. In order to move toward a more substantial notion of personality pathology, they present a list of sixteen normal capacities that are relevant with respect to personality disorders (Verheul et al. 2008). These capacities include emotional regulation, purposefulness, enduring relationships, responsible industry, and cooperation. They further propose that severe personality disorders are cases in which a large number of these fundamental capacities are compromised.

Based on this brief survey, we conclude that a plurality of models is needed for understanding the nature of personality pathology. No single model seems able to adequately justify the pathological status of personality disorders, and those that attempt to do so more directly require making theoretical inferences that goes beyond the evidence. More work on an adequate theory of pathology for personality is still required.

Issue three: Is personality a causal entity?

One aim of our selective historical review was to contextualize this third, very difficult issue. Psychologists who study personality from the standpoint of trait theory claim that the contention of Allport that normal and abnormal are qualitatively distinct has been empirically refuted—not only with respect to personality, but with respect other disorders such as depression and schizophrenia (Clark 2005; Livesley et al. 1998; Smith and Combs 2010). For example, the current best evidence indicates that the distinction between depressed mood and normal mood does not represent a carving of nature's joints, but a practically useful cut on an underlying continuum of mood similar to a distinction between short and tall (Watson 2005). Those who emphasize what psychologists call the *quantitative* (difference in degree) rather than the *qualitative* (difference in kind) distinction between normal and abnormal are termed dimensional model proponents.

Psychologists who advocate a dimensional approach are also inching toward making personality foundational to the conceptualization of psychopathology in general as did the Freudian ego psychologists mentioned previously, but they remain skeptical about the medical model approach of the psychodynamic tradition which emphasized case studies and the identification of personality types such as borderline, histrionic, and narcissistic. The new personality-oriented psychopathologists argue that the symptom space of personality pathology can be more comprehensively described by empirically-supported trait models (Trull and Durrett 2005; Widiger and Trull 2007).

Let us introduce the issue of the casual role of traits by briefly turning to philosophical history. In his *A Treatise of Human Nature* the empiricist philosopher David Hume argued that we have no experience of the existence of a self. All we have experiences of are organized bundles of sensations and perceptions. These bundles succeed each other in a systematic way and are more-or-less similar from one to the next (in our memory). What we call the self, says Hume, represents the reification of that similarity into a subsistent entity, but it is not a real causal entity.

Behavioral observations indicate that people who are anxious in many situations are also likely to be fearful, self-conscious, and emotionally overwhelmed—supporting an inference that they are high on the dimensional construct of neuroticism. According to an empiricist, the dispositional term neuroticism encodes information about probabilities. When it is doing its job, neuroticism is an inference ticket for knowing which behaviors are correlated with each other and for developing expectations about what patterns are more likely to occur in the future. For empiricists, the hypothetical construct of neuroticism is an instrument that we use to organize and navigate information about human behavior, but it is not a real entity in the head any more than the subsistent self was an entity in the head for Hume.

As we say in early this chapter, the conceptual heirs of the subsistent self in modern scientific psychology are personality and personality traits. In the science of psychometrics, personality traits are considered to be *latent variables*. Latent variables are mathematical abstractions that represent hidden causal structures that determine motives, perceptions, interests, and behaviors. Latent variable models lead contemporary trait theorists, in contrast to the instrumentalism of the empiricists, to adopt *scientific realism* about personality traits. As we will see in the following sections, trait realists believe that universal causal models for psychology are likely to be grounded in biology. From their perspective neurotic traits such as being fearful and self-conscious are only surface properties. Neuroticism proper, they believe, refers to an endogenous physiopsychological entity that exerts a causal influence—it produces the neurotic pattern of behavior.[4]

The received view: Traits as causal entities in the person (the FFM perspective)

What Whitehead (1926) named the fallacy of the perfect dictionary is the hypothesis that humans have considered all the fundamental ideas that are relevant to understanding experience and encoded them in language. The perfect dictionary hypothesis, however, remains the underlying assumption of the *lexical approach* to trait theory. For example, the lexical theorist Raymond Cattell (1943b, 1943a) claimed to have developed a representative sample of the population of personality traits, which he then submitted to statistical analysis to see if it could be reduced to a small number of general constructs with minimal loss of information. Cattell's (1945) original model had twelve dimensions.[5] Advocates of the received view claim that it slowly became clear that trait models containing numerous and specific personality variants could be collapsed into a more general five-dimension model (Fiske 1949;

[4] In contrast to the philosophical empiricist's emphasis on the particular, the contingent, and the probable, most contemporary trait theorists are seeking *universal*, *necessary*, and relatively *certain* knowledge of why things happen. Hence, they could be considered rationalists rather than empiricists.

[5] The twelve factors were derived from data gathered by observer ratings. When the factors were measured by test items and the data analyzed was based on self-report, four additional factors for a total of sixteen emerged.

Norman 1964; Tupes and Christal 1958). Different studies, they claim, independently discovered the same five dimensions, irrespective of whether the data were based on self-report or peer observations. Termed the "Big Five," these dimensions are called: (1) surgency (extroversion), (2) agreeableness, (3) conscientiousness, (4) neuroticism, and (5) intellect/openness to experience.

In the late 1980s, Paul Costa and Robert McCrae developed a personality test to measure the Big Five (called the *NEO Personality Inventory*, NEO-PI). Rather than seeking to discover personality factors, they set out in an a priori fashion to measure what had already been identified by the "inductive" methods of the lexical theorists. In adopting an explicitly scientific realist position regarding the nature of traits, Costa and McCrae have become the best-known representatives of the received view. This is exemplified in their introduction of the term "five-factor model" (FFM)—by which they mean a comprehensive scientific (explanatory) model of personality (McCrae and Costa 2008).

According to the FFM narrative, subsequent to the model's introduction, these traits were shown to be highly stable over a period of several years (McCrae and Costa 2003). FFM advocates also report that the model has been replicated across all cultures studied so far, suggesting that the traits are domain general personality factors (McCrae and Costa 2008). The stability and cross-cultural consistency of the traits has led to a judgment of *universality* (McCrae and Costa 1997). The additional discovery that personality traits have genetic bases has resulted in the assertion that these traits are grounded in nature not culture or experience (McCrae 2004).

A plurality of contrarian views

Independent discovery?

What responses do *contrarians* have with respect to the received view? One response is to dispute the FFM discovery narrative. In this narrative, the five-factor model is psychology's version of the discovery of the J/ψ particle in physics: *different research teams working independently with separate methodological strategies made the same discovery*. As happened in physics, this narrative is taken to justify adopting a realist view about the discovered entities.

In contrast, Block (1995) argues that rather than starting from scratch and finding the fixed world structure waiting to be discovered, the various psychological research programs ended up the same place, roughly, because they began in the same place, roughly. They were looking for a five-factor model based on clues from a shared set of previous findings. In designing the research, trait terms were also included and excluded with such an outcome in mind. What happened, according to Block, was not independent discovery, but planned replication.

Universality?

Here are McCrae and John (1989) addressing the question of *why* there are five factors:

> We believe it is simply an empirical fact, like the fact that there are seven continents on earth or eight American presidents from Virginia. Biologists recognize eight classes of vertebrates (mammals, birds, reptiles, amphibians, and four classes of fishes, one extinct), and the theory of evolution helps to explain the development of these classes. It does not, however, explain

why *eight* classes evolved, rather than four or eleven, and no one considers this a defect in the theory. There are, of course, reasons why human beings differ along each of the five personality dimensions—reasons to be found somewhere in evolution, neurobiology, socialization, or the existential human condition. But it is probably not meaningful or profitable to ask why there happen to be just five such dimensions. (p. 194)

A contrarian can dispute such scientific realism by questioning the universality assumption. Several thinkers point out that although the five-factor model has been found in other cultures, so have alternative models, including three-, six-, seven-, and eight- factor models (Almagor et al. 1995; Ashton and Lee 2001; Clark and Watson 1999; De Raad 2009; De Raad and Barelds 2008). Advocates of models with greater than five factors argue that meaningful aspects of personality (such as honesty and hedonism) are distinct factors (Ashton and Lee 2001). Along a similar line of reasoning, it has been argued that the FFM is blind to the trait of schizotypy/psychoticism (Harkness et al. 1995; Shedler and Westen 2004; Zachar 2008).

De Raad and Barelds note (2008) that different combinations of personality items tend to emerge depending whether the data being analyzed are verbs, nouns, trait adjectives, or some combination of all three. Almagor et al. (1995) also state that different dimensions emerge depending on whether evaluative terms are included or excluded. Finally, Simms et al. (2010) provide evidence that these evaluative dimensions contribute additional information, beyond the FFM, that is relevant to the prediction of personality disorder.

With respect to the current chapter the most important example of this complex relationship between the kind of data used (input) and the solution (output) is what happens when the data are psychiatric symptoms. One of the most consistent findings in the past fifteen years is that patterns of comorbidity among many mental disorders can be accounted for by two superordinate dimensions, internalizing (INT) and externalizing (EXT). Comorbidity refers to the tendency for putatively distinct mental disorders to co-occur more often than predicted by chance. INT and EXT were originally derived in the work of the psychologist Thomas Achenbach on the structure of psychiatric problems in children (1995) and have turned out to be fruitful in understanding disorder co-occurrence in adults (Krueger 1999; Krueger et al. 1998). Put simply, internalizing disorders involve experiencing *emotional dysregulation*—it is what depression and anxiety disorders have in common. Externalizing disorders involve acting out emotional dysregulation in ways that most societies deem illegal. It is what antisocial personality disorder (doing things that would be grounds for arrest) and illicit substance dependence have in common.

Eaton et al. (2010) argue that INT and EXT are stable, present across cultures, and genetically meaningful. These dimensions are not, however, derived from the FFM in a direct fashion. This is because the FFM is derived from everyday language for describing normal personality, whereas INT and EXT are derived from mental disorder definitions used by psychiatrists. From the FFM standpoint, INT and EXT are likely blends of personality factors and therefore heterogeneous—for example, both are correlated with neuroticism (Krueger and Markon 2006). Externalizing also shares variance with antagonism (low agreeableness) and negligence (low conscientiousness (Krueger et al. 2011). Within the domain from which they were derived (mental disorders), however, INT and EXT are single and coherent factors. Returning to the geographical analogy, this would be like discovering seven continents while surveying them on a ship, but only two while surveying them from an airplane.

One of the goals of the scientifically oriented psychopathologists is to propose explicit mathematical models of various "symptom spaces" and compare them with each other in terms of adequacy. One could call this a *neo-Galilean* approach—meaning the goal is to construct mathematical models that best account for the subject matter being studied. Models that have what Krueger calls *structural validity* (Krueger and Eaton 2010) should fit the data according to specific mathematical criteria of adequacy (termed "goodness of fit"). Although psychiatry has typically used a natural history approach along the lines of Sydenham and Darwin, these recent psychometric developments in mathematical modeling constitute a research tradition that is more similar to modeling approaches used in other sciences.

Interestingly, the Big Five tradition is more mathematically-based than is the FFM for two reasons. First, the "FFM" is typically not associated with a model that transcends operationalization, but rather, with a single instrument—the NEO-PI-R (Costa and McCrae 1992). Abstract models and their concrete measures are not the same thing. Models are partial representations of particular domains[6] (Giere, 1999), but as we have noted, some thinkers have interpreted the NEO-PI-R scales as being identical with the five factors. Second, an important feature the NEO-PI-R is its division of the five factors into subscales (facets). For example, anxiety, angry hostility, and depression are facets of the neuroticism factor. This hierarchy, however, was derived rationally, as opposed to being inductively found in the data as were the Big Five. It may even be that clinically useful facet scales are too specific to emerge in models that capitalize on partialing shared variance (Krueger et al. 2011). This makes facets more like countries than continents.

To conclude this section, while the successful replication of the five factor model across different samples is impressive, there is too much variability in various factor structures to say that there is one and only one universal and fixed structure of personality consisting of extraversion, conscientiousness, agreeableness, neuroticism, and openness. In scientific realist lingo the five-factor model is at best an approximation to a circumscribed reality.

Biological, therefore, carving nature at its unique joints?

Another important assumption of the received view is that if a trait can be shown to have a biological basis, then it is both scientifically valid and "real." A crucial area of research in this respect has been behavioral genetics. The workhorse of behavioral genetics has been the twin study, which involves comparing identical and fraternal twins to get a handle on genetic and environmental contributions to human individual differences (Plomin et al. 2008).

A large number of reliable personality constructs seem to have heritabilities around 0.50 (Krueger and Eaton 2010), meaning that half of the total variation in all personality traits can be traced to genotypic differences among persons. For example, basic aspects of emotional temperament such as neuroticism are heritable to essentially the same degree as individual differences in the tendency to resonate with art and literature (i.e., openness to experience).

Why there seems to be so little variance regarding the heritability of personality traits raises interesting methodological and conceptual questions. One possibility, pursued by Krueger et al. (2008) is that the 50% figure is an average, across a range of "micro-environments" in which the heritability might differ notably. More technically, genetic and environmental influences on a phenotype such as personality are *moderated* (changed by) other variables.

For example, Krueger et al. (2008) examined the extent to which genetic and environmental influences on personality vary as a function of the relationships between adolescents

---

[6] It is worth noting that mathematical models are partial representations of theories just as theories are partial representations of some substantive domain.

(seventeen-year-old twins) and their parents. They found that, averaging across parent–child relationships, the heritability of neuroticism was 50%, similar to other findings in the literature. However, this 50% figure averaged across a wide range of relational scenarios that had a notable impact on the genetic and environmental architecture of personality variation. In relationships where there was a high level of conflict, the heritability of neuroticism was considerably diminished, and the level of family environmental influence was as strong as the level of genetic influence. This suggests that "the environment" and "genes" may not have consistent direct effects on personality, but rather, that these forces are in dynamic interplay. In environments where family conflict existed, that environment was relevant to personality variation. One therefore has to be careful about generalizing heritability estimates from one sample to the next, and also about assuming that a high heritability estimate proves that the trait in question is carving nature at its systematic joints.

Latent variables as causal entities?

Other critics question the essentialist assumptions underlying the latent trait model (Cramer et al. 2010; Kendler et al. 2011). Analogous to the notion of a single factor called pure g that underlies all individual differences in academic ability, trait essentialists assume the existence of a quality of pure neuroticism which some people display more of than others. In McCrae and Costa's model, how much neuroticism someone has is fixed by biology.

According to psychometric theory, test items are fallible indicators that can triangulate on the latent trait. That is to say, when psychologists measure neuroticism using a scale composed of many items (e.g., life is a strain for me), everyone who scores very high or very low on the scale could be said to have or lack this quality. In theory, different items can possess higher or lower doses of the latent trait of neuroticism and should be worth more or less points. People who are average on the trait should get there by agreeing with the average and low dose items, and not agreeing with high dose items. There is also promising evidence that constructing scales of this type is an empirical possibility (Watson et al. 2007, 2008).

Following up on a point made by Grove and Vrieze (2010), however, one must also consider the possibility that as long as items are preselected to be unidimensional, such a "dose response" structure is itself preselected. If a theory is used to guide the selection of empirical data, then to what extent can the data be said to confirm the theory? This is a difficult question. At the very minimum, if data can be selected to cohere with a theoretical model (e.g., the latent variable model for neuroticism), then at least the theory resists falsification by being empirically adequate.

Throughout the history of science, the validity of new scientific instruments has been subject to debate, often because there is no independent way to assess what the instruments are indicating. When Galileo claimed that his telescope revealed four moons around Jupiter, it was not possible travel to Jupiter to see if he was correct. Similar concerns arose with the introduction of microscopes and particle accelerators—and more recently with factor analysis and its emphasis on latent variables, realistically interpreted.

Borsboom (2008) specifically questions the assumption that the results of factor analysis indicate the existence of latent variables as endogenous entities that cause the patterns of thought, emotions, and behaviors that are encoded in item responses. In an earlier article Borsboom and his colleagues argued that realist assumptions (as opposed to instrumentalist and constructivist assumptions) are inherent to the logic of latent variable models, but construing latent variables as real causal variables in persons is not among those assumptions

(Borsboom et al. 2003). According to Borsboom and colleagues, we cannot justifiably say that Woody Allen's obtaining of a high score on our neuroticism scale was the causal result of his possessing a high dose of the latent variable N. What we can justifiably say is that people whose position on N is similar to Woody Allen's tend to obtain high scores on the neuroticism scale. It is like saying that people who earn a high score on a college admissions tests tend to succeed in college but not like saying that a latent variable called college admissions aptitude caused Bill Clinton to do well in college.

In this view, once all the internal factors that lead Woody Allen to obtain a high score on the neuroticism scale are listed, we would not gain additional information by adding "Neuroticism" to the list. The latent variable of N is not an endogenous causal entity in the scientific realists sense, but an emergent population property that accounts for individual differences. This is similar to a point made in Meehl's (1954) exploration of clinical and statistical prediction: Statistics provide information about population probabilities.

How then are we to understand individuals? Borsboom argues that an alternative model would explain patterns (either personality or personality disorders) by means of direct causal relationships between emotions, thoughts, and behaviors. In this view, the symptoms (fallible indicators) are not the result of a hidden causal essence behind the pattern (the latent variables such as neuroticism and antagonism), but are directly causally related to each other. For example, the borderline personality symptom "affective lability" may causally influence the symptom of "identity instability," and an unstable identity may recursively help maintain a labile affective temperament. According to this kind of "network model," borderline personality is a name for a casual system rather than a manifestation of a latent structure in the head.

As Borsboom et al. (2003) note, however, these competing models are subject to empirical test. For these same reasons, Krueger et al. (2010) call causal network model theorists to task for not directly comparing network models to latent variable models, and suggest one reason that they do not do so is because the type of model they propose is not well suited to achieve goodness of fit because it admits too many variables. Essentially, network models are relatively lacking in parsimony because they posit numerous direct connections among specific and narrow symptoms, as opposed to positing more unifying theoretical principles to help account for numerous specific empirical observations. Some important virtues of more parsimonious latent variable models, Krueger et al. claim, is their heuristic value for generating progressive research program (in a Lakatosian sense) and their potential for organizing the domain in what Phillip Kitcher (2001) calls a "well-ordered" way.

To conclude this section, there is some reason to doubt every one of the claims that five factor model advocates make to justify their scientific realism about personality traits. The five factors were not simply discovered, they may not represent the fixed, universal structure of personality, they are biologically based but in a complex dynamic way, and it is not clear that latent variables must be conceptualized as endogenous causal entities.

Conclusions

The concept of personality disorder, from its very inception, has been infused with philosophical assumptions and controversies. We showed how personality became a secularized version of character in the medical community, and how the concept of personality disorder developed beyond is roots in degeneration theory and the disease model. The problems of the relationship between personality and issues of character and of what makes personality "pathological" still persist. The issue that is likely of most concern to conceptually minded scientific psychologists, that about the ontological and causal status of latent traits, are also the most philosophically difficult issues reviewed in this chapter. With respect to the problem of latent traits, the conceptual problems that are of concern to psychologists and psychiatrists are difficult for outsiders to grasp, as are the concerns of philosophers. We realize that this means that there may be no natural audience that is interested in solutions that integrate these various sets of concerns, but contend anyway that a variety of research programs in psychology and psychiatry could benefit from philosophical attention to these problems.

References

Achenbach, T. M. (1995). Empirically based assessment and taxonomy: Applications to clinical research. *Psychological Assessment*, 7, 261–74.

Allport, G. W. (1937). *Personality: A Psychological Interpretation*, Oxford, England, Henry Holt.

Allport, G. W. (1961). *Pattern and Growth in Personality*. New York, NY: Holt, Rinehart, and Winston.

Almagor, M., Tellegen, A., and Waller, N. G. (1995). The big seven model: A cross-cultural replication of the basic dimensions of natural language trait descriptions. *Journal of Personality and Social Psychology*, 69, 300–37.

American Psychiatric Association (1980). *Diagnostic and Statistical Manual of Mental Disorders, Third Edition*. Washington, DC: American Psychiatric Association.

Ashton, M. C. and Lee, K. (2001). A theoretical basis for the major dimensions of personality. *European Journal of Personality*, 15, 327–53.

Barenbaum, N. B. and Winter, D. G. (2003). Personality. In D. K. Freedheim (Ed.), *Handbook of Psychology: Volume 1 History of Psychology*. Hoboken, NJ: John Wiley and Sons.

Berrios, G. E. (1993). European views on personality disorders: A conceptual history. *Comprehensive Psychiatry*, 34, 14–30.

Berrios, G. E. (1996). *The History of Mental Symptoms*. Cambridge: Cambridge University Press.

Berrios, G. E. and Marková, I. S. (2003). The self and psychiatry: A conceptual history. In T. Kircher and A. David (Eds), *The Self in Neuroscience and Psychiatry*, pp. 9–39. Cambridge: Cambridge University Press.

Block, J. (1995). A contrarian view of the five-factor approach to personality description. *Psychological Bulletin*, 117, 185–215.

Borsboom, D. (2008). Psychometric perspectives on diagnostic systems. *Journal of Clinical Psychology*, 64, 1089–108.

Borsboom, D. G., Mellenbergh, G. J., and Van Heerden, J. (2003). The theoretical status of latent variables. *Psychological Review*, 110, 203–19.

Carlson, E. T. (1985). Medicine and degeneration: Theory and praxis. In J. E. Chamberlin and S. L. Gilman (Eds), *Degeneration: The Dark Side of Progress*, 121–44. New York, NY: Columbia University Press.

Carpenter, N. (1994). Genetic anticipation: Expanding tandem repeats. *Neurologic Clinics*, 12, 683–97.

Cattell, R. B. (1943a). The description of personality: Basic traits resolved into clusters. *Journal of Abnormal and Social Psychology, 38*, 476–506.

Cattell, R. B. (1943b). The description of personality: I. Foundations of trait measurement. *Psychological Review, 50*, 559–4.

Cattell, R. B. (1945). The description of personality: Principles and findings in a factor analysis. *American Journal of Psychology, 58*, 69–90.

Charland, L. C. (2004). Moral treatment and the personality disorders. In J. Radden (Ed.), *The Philosophy of Psychiatry: A Companion.* New York, NY: Oxford University Press.

Charland, L. C. (2006). Moral nature of the DSM-IV cluster B personality disorders. *Journal of Personality Disorders, 20*, 116–25.

Clark, L. A. (2005). Temperament as a unifying basis for personality and psychopathology. *Journal of Abnormal Psychology, 114*, 505–21.

Clark, L. A. (2007). Assessment and diagnosis of personality disorder: Perennial issues and an emerging reconceptualization. *Annual Review of Psychology, 58*, 227–57.

Clark, L. A. and Watson, D. (1999). Temperament: A new paradigm for trait psychology. In L. A. Pervin and O. P. John (Eds), *Handbook of Personality: Theory and Research* (2nd edn), pp. 399–23. New York, NY: Guilford Press.

Costa, P. T., Jr and McCrae, R. R. (2010). *NEO Problems in Living Checklist.* Lutz, FL: PAR.

Cramer, A. O., Waldrop, L. J., van der Mass, H. L., and Borsboom, D. (2010). Comorbidity: A network perspective. *Behavioral and Brain Sciences, 33*, 137–50.

Cummins, R. (1983). *The Nature of Psychological Explanation.* Cambridge, MA: The MIT Press.

Danziger, K. (1990). *Constructing the Subject.* New York, NY: Cambridge University Press.

De Raad, B. (2009). Structural models of personality. In P. J. Corr and G. Mathews (Eds), *The Cambridge Handbook of Personality Psychology*, pp. 323–46. New York, NY: Cambridge University Press.

De Raad, B. and Barelds, D. P. H. (2008). A new taxonomy of Dutch personality traits based on a comprehensive and unrestricted list of descriptors. *Journal of Personality and Social Psychology, 94*, 347–64.

Deyoung, C. G. (2010). Toward a theory of the Big Five. *Psychological Inquiry, 21*, 26–33.

Digman, J. M. (1997). Higher-order factors of the big five. *Journal of Personality and Social Psychology, 73*, 1246–56.

Dolan-Sewell, R. T., Krueger, R. F., and Shea, M. T. (2001). Co-occurrence with syndrome disorders. In W. J. Livesley (Ed.), *Handbook of Personality Disorders: Theory, Research, and Treatment*, pp. 84–104. New York, NY: Guilford Press.

Eaton, N. R., South, S. C., and Krueger, R. F. (2010). The meaning of comorbidity among common mental disorders. In T. Millon, R. F. Krueger, and E. Simonsen (Eds), *Contemporary Directions in Psychopathology*, pp. 223–41. New York, NY: Guilford.

Elliott, C. (1996). *The Rules of Insanity.* Albany, NY: State University Press of New York.

Elliott, C. (2003). *Better than Well.* New York, NY: Norton.

Fiske, D. W. (1949). Consistency of the factorial structures of personality ratings from different sources. *Journal of Abnormal and Social Psychology, 44*, 329–44.

Franzen, J. (2010). *Freedom.* New York, NY: Farar, Straus and Giroux.

Freud, S. (1960). *The Ego and the Id.* New York, W. W. Norton and Company. (Original work published 1921.)

Funder, D. C. (1997). *The Personality Puzzle.* New York, W. W. Norton and Company.

Giere, R. N. (1999). *Science without Laws.* Chicago, IL: University of Chicago Press.

Gilman, S. L. (1985). Sexology, psychoanalysis, and degeneration: From a theory of race to a race to theory. In J. E. Chamberlin and S. L. Gilman (Eds), *Degeneration: The Dark Side of Progress*, pp. 72–96. New York, NY: Columbia University Press.

Goldstein, J. (1987). *Console and Classify*. Cambridge: Cambridge University Press.

Graham, G. (2010). *The Disordered Mind*. London: Routledge.

Grove, W. M. and Vrieze, S. I. (2010). On the substative grounding and clinical utility of categories versus dimensions. In T. Millon, R. F. Krueger, and E. Simonsen (Eds), *Contemporary Directions in Psychopathology*, pp. 303–23. New York, NY: Guilford.

Hall, C. S. and Lindsey, G. (1957). *Theories of Personality*. New York, NY: Wiley.

Harkness, A. R., Mcnulty, J. L., and Ben-Porath, Y. S. (1995). The Personality Psychopathology Five (PSY-5): Constructs and MMPI-2 scales. *Psychological Assessment, 7*, 104–14.

Hartmann, H. (1958). *Ego Psychology and the Problem of Adapation*. New York, NY: International Universities Press.

James, W. (1890). *The Principles of Psychology*. New York, NY: Holt.

Kendler, K. S., Mcguire, M., Gruenberg, A. M., O'Hare, A., Spellman, M., and Walsh, D. (1993). The Roscommon Family Study: III Schizophrenia-related personality disorders in relatives. *Archives of General Psychiatry, 50*, 781–8.

Kendler, K. S., Zachar, P., and Craver, C. (2011). What kinds of things are psychiatric disorders. *Psychological Medicine, 41*, 1143–50.

Kitcher, P. (2001). *Science, Truth, and Democracy*. New York, NY: Oxford University Press.

Kraepelin, E. (1904). *Lectures on Clinical Psychiatry*. New York, NY: William Wood and Company.

Kraepelin, E. (1907). *Clinical Psychiatry*. New York, NY: Macmillan.

Kretschmer, E. (1925). *Physique and Character*. New York, NY: Harcourt Brace.

Krueger, R. F. (1999). The structure of common mental disorders. *Archives of General Psychiatry, 56*, 921–6.

Krueger, R. F., Caspi, A., Moffitt, T. E., and Silva, P. A. (1998). The structure and stability of common mental disorders (DSM-III-R): A longitudinal-epidemiological study. *Journal of Abnormal Psychology, 107*, 216–27.

Krueger, R. F. and Eaton, N. R. (2010). Personality traits and the classification of mental disorders: Toward a more complete integration in DSM–5 and an empirical model of psychopathology. *Personality Disorders: Theory, Research, and Treatment, 1*, 97–118.

Krueger, R. F., Eaton, N. R., Clark, L. A., Watson, D., Markon, K. E., Derringer, J., *et al.* (2011). Deriving an empirical structure of personality pathology for the DSM-5. *Journal of Personality Disorders, 25*, 170–91.

Krueger, R. F. and Markon, K. E. (2006). Reinterpreting comorbidity: A model-based approach to understanding and classifying psychopathology. *Annual Review of Clinical Psychology, 2*, 111–33.

Krueger, R. F., South, S. C., Johnson, W., and Iacono, W. (2008). The heritability of personality is not always 50%: Gene-environment interactions and correlations between personality and parenting. *Journal of Personality, 76*, 1485–522.

Krueger, R. F., Young, C. G., and Markon, K. E. (2010). Toward scientifically useful quantitative models of psychopathology: The importance of a comparative approach. *Behavioral and Brain Sciences, 33*, 163–4.

Lenzenweger, M. F. (2006). Schizotaxia, schizotypy, and schizophrenia: Paul E. Meehl's blueprint for the experimental psychopathology and genetics of schizophrenia. *Journal of Abnormal Psychology, 115*, 195–200.

Livesley, W. J., Jang, K. L., and Vernon, P. A. (1998). Phenotypic and genetic structure of traits delineating personality disorder. *Archives of General Psychiatry, 55*, 941–8.

Lombardo, G. P. and Foschi, R. (2003). The concept of personality in 19th century French 20th century American psychology. *History of Psychology, 6*, 123–42.

McCrae, R. R. (2004). Human nature and culture: A trait perspective. *Journal of Research in Personality*, 38, 3–14.

McCrae, R. R. and Costa, P. T., Jr (1997). Personality trait structure as a human universal. *American Psychologist*, 52, 509–16.

McCrae, R. R. and Costa, P. T., Jr (2003). *Personality in adulthood: A five-factor theory perspective.* New York, NY: Guilford.

McCrae, R. R. and Costa, P. T., Jr (2008). The five-factor theory of personality. In O. P. John, R. W., Robins, and L. A. Pervin (Eds), *Handbook of Personality*, pp. 159–81. New York, NY: Guilford.

McCrae, R. R. and John, O. P. (1989). An introduction to the five factor model and its implications. *Journal of Personality*, 60, 175–215.

Mcglashan, T. H., Grilo, C. M., Skodol, A. E., Gunderson, J. G., Shea, M. T., Morey, L. C., *et al.* (2000). The collaborative longitudinal personality disorders study: Baseline axis I/II and II/II diagnostic co-occurrence. *Acta Psychiatrica Scandinavica*, 102, 256–64.

Meehl, P. E. (1962). Schizotaxia, schizotypy, schizophrenia. *American Psychologist*, 17, 827–38.

Millikan, R. G. (1984). *Language, Thought, and Other Biological Categories.* Cambridge, MA: The MIT Press.

Murray, H. A. (1938). *Explorations in Personality.* New York, NY: Oxford University Press.

Nicholson, I. A. M. (2003). *Inventing Personality: Gordon Allport and the Science of Selfhood*, Washington, DC: American Psychological Association.

Norman, W. T. (1964). Toward an adequate taxonomy of personality attributes: Replicated factor structure in peer nomination personality ratings. *Journal of Abnormal and Social Psychology*, 66, 574–83.

Oldham, J. M., Skodol, A. E., Kellman, H. D., and Hyler, S. E. (1995). Comorbidity of axis I and axis II disorders. *The American Journal of Psychiatry*, 152, 571–8.

Phillips, K. A., Hirschfeld, R. M. A., Shea, M. T. and Gunderson, J. G. (1995). Depressive personality disorder. In W. J. Livesley (Ed.), *The DSM-IV Personality Disorders*. New York, NY: The Guilford Press.

Pick, D. (1989). *Faces of Degneration.* Cambridge: Cambridge University Press.

Plomin, R., Defries, J. C., McClearn, G. E., and McGuffin, P. (2008). *Behavioral Genetics.* New York, NY: Worth.

Rapaport, D., Gill, M. M., and Schafer, R. (1945). *Diagnostic Psychological Testing.* Chicago, IL: Yearbook Publishers.

Reich, W. (1949). *Character Analysis.* New York, NY: Farrar, Strauss, and Giroux.

Rogers, C. R. (1951). *Client Centered Therapy.* Boston, MA: Houghton Mifflin.

Sadler, J. Z. (2005). *Values and Psychiatric Diagnosis.* New York, NY: Oxford University Press.

Schneider, K. (1950). *Psychopathic Personalities.* London: Cassell. (Original work published 1923.)

Secord, J. A. (2000). *Victorian Sensation.* Chicago, IL: The University of Chicago Press.

Shapiro, D. (1965). *Neurotic Styles.* New York, NY: Basic Books.

Shedler, J. and Westen, D. (2004). Dimensions of personality pathology: An alternative to the five-factor model of personality. *American Journal of Psychiatry*, 161, 1743–54.

Shorter, E. (1997). *A History of Psychiatry.* New York, NY: John Wiley and Sons.

Simms, L. J., Yufik, T., and Gros, D. F. (2010). Incremental validity of positive and negative valance in predicting personality disorder. *Personality Disorders: Theory, Research and Treatment*, 1, 77–86.

Smith, G. T. and Combs, J. (2010). Issues of construct validity in psychiatric diagnosis. In Millon, T., Krueger, R. F., and Simonsen, E. (Eds), *Contemporary Directions in Psychopathology*, pp. 205–25. New York, NY: Guilford.

Taylor, E. (2000). Psychotherapeutics and the problematic origins of clinical psychology in America. *American Psychologist*, 55, 1029–33.

Trull, T. J. and Durrett, C. A. (2005). Categorical and dimensional models of personality disorder. *Annual Review of Clinical Psychology*, 1, 355–80.

Tupes, E. C. and Christal, R. C. (1958). *Stability of Personality Trait Rating Factors Obtained Under Diverse Conditions*. Lackland Air Force Base, TX: US Air Force.

Van Valkenburg, C., Kluznik, J. C., Speed, N., and Akiskal, H. S. (2006). Cyclothymia and labile personality: Is all folie circulaire? *Journal of Affective Disorders*, 96, 177–81.

Verheul, R., Andrea, H., Berghout, C. C., Dolan, C., Busschbach, J. J. V., van der Kroft, P. J. A., *et al.* (2008). Severity indices of personality problems (SIPP-118): Development, factor structure, reliability, and validity. *Psychological Assessment*, 20, 23–34.

Wakefield, J. C. (1992). The concept of mental disorder: On the boundary between biological facts and social values. *American Psychologist*, 47, 373–88.

Watson, D. (2005). Rethinking the mood and anxiety disorders: A quantitative hierarchical model for DSM-V. *Journal of Abnormal Psychology*, 114, 522–36.

Watson, R., Deary, I., and Austin, E. (2007). Are personality traits items reliably more or less 'difficult'? Mokken scaling of the NEO-FFI. *Personality and Individual Differences*, 43, 1460–9.

Watson, R., Roberts, B., Gow, A., and Deary, I. (2008). A hierarchy of items within Eysenck's EPI. *Personality and Individual Differences*, 45, 333–5.

Whitehead, A. N. (1926). *Science and the Modern World*. London: Cambridge University Press.

Widiger, T. A. (2006). Tough questions of morality, free will, and maladaptivity. *Journal of Personality Disorders*, 20, 181–3.

Widiger, T. A. and Mullins-Sweatt, S. N. (2009). Five-factor model of personality disorder: A proposal for *DSM-5*. *Annual Review of Clinical Psychology*, 5, 197–220.

Widiger, T. A. and Trull, T. J. (2007). Plate tectonics in the classification of personality disorder: Shifting to a dimensional model. *American Psychologist*, 62, 71–83.

Zachar, P. (2008). Real kinds but no true taxonomy: An essay in psychiatric systematics. In K. S. Kendler and J. Parnas, J. (Eds), *Philosophical Issues in Psychiatry: Explanation, Phenomenology, and Nosology*, pp. 327–67. Baltimore, MD: Johns Hopkins University Press.

Zachar, P. (2011). The clinical nature of personality disorders: Answering the neo-Szazian critique. *Philosophy, Psychiatry, & Psychology*, 18, 191–202.

Zachar, P. and Potter, N. N. (2010). Personality disorders: Moral or medical kinds – or both. *Philosophy, Psychiatry, & Psychology*, 17, 101–17.

CHAPTER 53

PERSONAL IDENTITY AND IDENTITY DISORDERS

STEPHEN R. L. CLARK

MULTIPLE PERSONALITY DISORDER/ DISSOCIATIVE IDENTITY DISORDER AND ITS ATTRACTIONS

The American Psychiatric Association's (2000) *Diagnostic and Statistical Manual of Mental Disorders, Fourth Edition, Text Revision* (DSM-IV-TR), provides the following criteria to diagnose Dissociative Identity Disorder (DID):

1. Two or more distinct identities or personality states are present, each with its own relatively enduring pattern of perceiving, relating to, and thinking about the environment and self.
2. At least two of these identities or personality states recurrently take control of the person's behavior.
3. The person has an inability to recall important personal information that is too extensive to be explained by ordinary forgetfulness.
4. The disturbance is not due to the direct physiological effects of a substance (such as blackouts or chaotic behavior during alcohol intoxication) or a general medical condition (such as complex partial seizures).

Accounts of the disorder suggest that those who provide, who are, the evidence for this disorder are usually in acute distress, but those who wish to believe in it find the idea almost exhilarating. At the least we *might* have been otherwise than we are, and those unrealized possibilities still hover at the back of our minds. Perhaps we could someday realize those other lives, without the pain of abandoning our present: we could at least "act out of character"—on the understanding that we wouldn't wholly lose our characters. More soberly, many of us would welcome a personality who positively enjoys collecting data, or preparing reports for the local administration, while leaving other personalities to enjoy themselves in their own way. At the same time, we remember that such divisions bring their own problems, and suspect that those who apparently succeed in dividing themselves up must have suffered serious trauma in the past, and be plagued by missed appointments and self-hatred in the present. Some of us believe that "multiple personality" reveals a truth about us all, that none of us is the simple, heroic self that we pretend. Others suspect that it is a wish to avoid responsibility that causes some of us to pretend not to be the selves that actually we are. Yet others hope that there is some better, stronger spirit resident within us, who might someday speak. It maybe some of us are merely fascinated and aghast.

Philosophers may be especially entranced, for a rather different reason. What is it that grounds our notion of identity, and particularly *personal* identity? Can the rules we tacitly employ to identify someone as "the same person" from one year to the next cope with thought experiments, about memory loss, personality change, split-brain experiments, *Star Trek* transporters, or bodily resurrection? "Real-life" cases where commonsensical identity is seriously challenged seem to provide more solid material on which to test our philosophical intuitions. This was Kathy Wilkes' argument in *Real Persons* (1984): the thought experiments are unhelpful, precisely because they are imaginary. The *real* cases show us more exactly what the problems are, and how we might deal with them. We can say anything we please about future or counterfactual possibilities. We cannot be so cavalier when confronted by the people therapists describe, but have some chance of discovering real solutions—ones that enable patients, therapists, judges, and the rest of us to cope. Maybe there really *could* be creatures whose bodies were animated by several distinct individuals. Maybe there could be intelligent creatures who reproduced like amoebas, or whose offspring had immediate access to all the memories of their lineage. Maybe there will one day be creatures inhabiting a merely virtual environment, complex computer programs which speak and think as if they were really us. Maybe there could even be creatures that existed discontinuously, emerging from the happy nothing to take up their fissured lives without having existed at all in the meantime. But all these things are fantasies: we here-now, it is commonsensical to think, are singular, bodily beings who exist continuously from birth (or more plausibly, conception) until death (or possibly, brain death). We may not be as simple or as simple-minded as we sometimes think, but our identities survive chronic amnesia, fugue, repentance and dissociation. The thing that I identically am is this living body here, however much I may have forgotten about its history, and however much I wish to disown that past.

But perhaps there are at least two challenges to be met. First of all, the stories of "multiple identities" cast doubt on the easy assumption that there is always one clearly defined person (one will and intellect) to be associated with each physical body—and thereby suggest that something more is involved in our own continued being than the merely bodily. Second, the very distinction between "thought experiments" and "real-life cases" may be subverted by the suspicion that personal identity, whether in the supposedly "normal" cases or the "pathological," is a function of the stories that we variously tell. Maybe both the victims and their therapists are following a script, whether they know it or not; maybe we all are.

WHAT PSYCHIATRISTS SAY

What are the cases now subsumed under the title "Dissociative Identity Disorder," and formerly as "Multiple Personality Disorder" (MPD)? The history of the diagnoses has been told by many, including Braude (1995), Crabtree (1997), Hacking (1995), and Spanos (1996). In brief, it begins in nineteenth-century France with cases of "double consciousness": individuals who either spontaneously, or under hypnosis, underwent a change of personality, forgetting their pasts and constructing new lives for themselves. Some of these cases could easily, in an earlier day, have been diagnosed instead as victims of demonic possession—and there continued to be some association with "spiritist" interpretations of the data even when the diagnosis spread to America. In such cases as that of "Miss Beauchamp" (Prince 1908), other features emerged. First, there might be more than two apparently separate personalities. Second, though the personality that was initially presented to the therapist claimed not to know about or remember the thoughts and actions of the "other," one or another such "other" ("alter," as it came to be called) professed to be continually conscious of the others' thoughts and actions, while insisting that these were not her own. Morton Prince, who was responsible for managing and publicizing the Beauchamp case, insisted that the "real Miss Beauchamp" could only emerge and take control of her life by the exorcism of the one alter, "Sally," who seemed to be aware of (and to dislike) all the others. In effect, he treated Sally as an invading demon, despite his claim that all the alters were fragmented parts of one original personality. The diagnosis ceased to be fashionable once Freudian interpretation became more popular: perhaps because the diagnosis of MPD was associated with the suggestion that such alters began as the response of imaginative children to serious abuse. If Freud was right in his later opinion,[1] most of the stories of abuse (which usually only emerged during therapy) were fables, and could not therefore identify the *cause* of such radical dissociation. The abuse and the multiple personalities were both confabulations. After a long gap Thigpen and Cleckley's study of *The Three Faces of Eve* (1957), modeled on the Beauchamp case, brought the diagnosis back into fashion.

In more recent years, it has been easier to believe in child abuse, and that the children hid this abuse even from themselves, by inventing someone else to endure it. Spanos (1996) has argued, with some justice, that there is little external evidence for the notion that we can so readily suppress childhood memories, or recall what happened before we were two or three years old, or that what is "retrieved" in the therapeutic conversation is veridical. Memories aren't stored unchangeably in some recess of our minds, but constantly reinvented and renarrated, often to the point of obvious fiction. Some accusations of abuse are justified, but almost certainly not all.

---

[1] See Freud (1935/1952, pp. 36–37). It is important to add that Freud did not deny that children were sometimes abused: he merely abandoned the idea that *everyone* who presented a problem must have been raped in their childhood.

It is also notable that the *number* of alters in each individual case has expanded beyond belief: where the nineteenth-century originals manifested only two or three, mutually unknown, personalities, later cases have shown four, twenty, or several hundred—helped along by the strategy of treating each and every changing mood or memory as the work of some significant other. "In systems where extreme splitting occurs, clients may report a host of personality fragments created to do specific tasks, such as cooking, cleaning the house, or going to school" (Hacking 1995, p. 19)—or does this only mean that—unsurprisingly—they don't think about cooking when they are heading off to school?

The number of cases has also grown: some therapists have never seen a plausible example of the disorder; a very few therapists treat all the ones that there are—and almost all therapists and patients are American. Perhaps the diagnosis is merely fashionable. Or perhaps the disorder itself is fashionable: that is, it is not merely a name devised by therapists for confused and unhappy clients, but an actual condition which therapist and patient conspire, consciously or not, to create. By this account, even Miss Beauchamp, in her several guises, was only describing her changing relations with Morton Prince (Spanos 1996, p. 226), and Prince—consciously or not—colluded with this story—as others have colluded with other fashionable frenzies. "The increases over time in the number of alters per MPD patient is reminiscent of the increases in the number of demon selves that were commonly manifested in demoniacs who were exposed to protracted series of exorcisms during periods of peak interest in demonic possession" (Spanos 1996, p. 232).

Or perhaps there is more going on than Spanos would admit. There are after all, *false* or at least unconvincing claims to be thus multiple. The case of Ken Bianchi, for example (see Spanos 1996, pp. 237–239), reads very clearly (*pace* Beahrs 1982, pp. 202–222) as the attempt of a clever serial killer to *pretend* that an alter, "Steve," was responsible for crimes that "Ken" did not remember. In other cases, the alters speak more plausibly in their different characters, and have less reason to attempt deceit (see, e.g., Oltmanns et al. (1991, pp. 54–72), and the personal testimony of such as Sizemore (1989) or Oxnam (2006)). The fact that only a few therapists, and those mostly American, can easily identify the disorder is not of itself evidence that they are deceived or deceiving. "The physical sciences abound with examples of phenomena that no one noticed until there was a theory to make one look" (Hacking 1995, p. 90).

So what is going on? Current diagnostic criteria require "the presence of two or more distinct identities or personality states that recurrently take control of the individual's behavior, accompanied by an inability to recall important personal information that is too extensive to be explained by ordinary forgetfulness" (DSM-IV-TR). According to the website of the International Society for the Study of Trauma and Dissociation (<http://www.isst-d.org/default.asp?contentID=76>):

> It is now recognized [*sic*] that these dissociated states are not fully-formed personalities, but rather represent a fragmented sense of identity. The amnesia typically associated with Dissociative Identity Disorder is asymmetrical, with different identity states remembering different aspects of autobiographical information. There is usually a host personality who identifies with the client's real name. Typically, the host personality is not aware of the presence of other alters. The different personalities may serve distinct roles in coping with problem areas. An average of 2 to 4 personalities/alters are present at diagnosis, with an average of 13 to 15 personalities emerging over the course of treatment. Environmental events usually trigger a sudden shifting from one personality to another.

This account is confused, or confusing. On the one hand, we are to suppose that there are "distinct personalities"; on the other, these only "represent a fragmented sense of identity." One personality is identified as "the host," although she is usually unaware of—and so does not contain or control—her alters. At times, multiples are described as weirdly unlike singletons like ourselves. At others, they seem only to be doing what any of us might do. This is how one (alleged) victim of the sort of ritual abuse that Spanos and others doubt has actually occurred (and who might seem likely to be an extreme example of the syndrome) describes the experience:

> To me, having multiple personalities does not feel like I have lots of people living inside my body. Rather I find myself thinking and talking to myself in different tones and accents. Some of the voices that talk in my mind sound like children. When I allow them to talk to other people they don't talk like children to impress anyone or be dramatic. I have to talk like that sometimes in order to express what I need to say. I can't say it in my adult voice.... Then there are the deep-raspy intent voices that say the earnest things you could imagine. When they talk, I feel hard inside, I feel cold and calculating. (Hacking 1995, p. 32; cited from Smith 1993, p. 25)

A cure for the disorder (if that is what it is) would then be simply to facilitate the inner conversation, in the recognition—already implicit in this self-description—that there is only one person involved: "It is a mistake to consider each personality totally separate, whole or autonomous. The other personalities might best be described as personality states, other selves or personality fragments" (Coons 1984, p. 53). And in that case there is no need to silence the different selves, as though self-reinforcing monologues are a sounder basis for our characters and actions than a conversation.

On the other hand, Chris Sizemore (the original "Eve" described by Thigpen and Cleckley) reports that "despite authorities' claims to the contrary, my former alters were not fragments of my birth personality. They were entities, whole in their own rights, who coexisted with my birth personality before I was born [*sic*]. They were not me, but they remain intrinsically related to what it means to be me" (1989, p. 211). Oxnam, a distinguished scholar diagnosed as a multiple late in his life agrees: "alters must be seen as real people. They have their own unique experiences, abilities, memories. Alters have enormous differences—in voices, demeanor, literacy levels, even heart rates. Most of all they have their own identities and feelings. Deny that 'realness' and MPD therapy won't work" (Oxnam 2006, p. 63: quoting his therapist Jeffery Smith). By renaming Multiple Personality Disorder as Dissociative Identity Disorder psychiatrists have sought to suggest that victims are only at one end of a continuum, and that alters are not truly distinct agents, who can be held severally responsible for their actions and their arguments. As Hacking observes "as dissociative identity disorder becomes the official diagnosis and practice ... opportunities for intentional action [by alters] may fade away" (Hacking 1995, p. 237). If my car is driven competently from A to B, while I—the supposed driver—daydream, must Someone Else have been driving? Could that other someone have decided to go somewhere else, or stopped for a secret meeting? If I—the present speaker—don't recall this episode, is there Another who could talk about it? A diagnosis of MPD requires a positive answer; a diagnosis of DID need not.

The stories told of and by multiples may not be fraudulent, nor merely fashionable, and yet still be, exactly, stories. On this account, the theory that abused children split apart so as to hide memories of the trauma in a secret self may perhaps be replaced by the notion that it is the *adult* patients who compose a story of past abuse, of hidden memories, and disparate personalities in order to cope with some *present* trauma. It may even be that there are many more multiples around than therapists suppose, and that most of them aren't traumatized at all (Beahrs 1982, p. 86): only the ones having difficulties ever approach a therapist, and mostly in America! In Midgley's words, "some of us have to hold a meeting every time we want to do something only slightly difficult, in order to find the self [that is, the personality] who is capable of undertaking it" (Midgley 1984, p. 123). Are all of us covert multiples?

The decision to speak of DID rather than the older MPD may also be a step on the way to abandoning the very notion of a discrete syndrome. The condition is ranked alongside other dissociative disorders, typically involving "depersonalization" (see Simeon and Abugel 2006), "derealization," amnesia, identity confusion, and identity alteration. Three other conditions are also identified within this group: dissociative amnesia, dissociative fugue, and depersonalization disorder. But all these are identified with one or more of the named characteristics, without any clear account of their etiology. It may be that "DID" cases only happen to have particular features which do not really amount even to symptoms, let alone a syndrome. It may be that neither the partial amnesia, nor even the existence of alters, are really the most significant features of such cases: all that we can identify are varying degrees of "depersonalization" (feeling that one's body, actions, status and feelings are not one's own) and identity confusion. "DID has three clinical criteria: identities, switching, and amnesia. Each criterion is required; all must be simultaneously co-present" (see Dell 2001, p. 15; Dell and O'Neill 2009)—but in the absence of any known underlying cause of the conjunction this may be as nominal a definition as, for example, speaking of red-haired, left-handed, male speakers of Esperanto as a class. Very probably there are such people (let's call them—arbitrarily—borogoves), but nothing else of interest can be said of them, nor is there any reason to distinguish them as a class from people with some other range of characters. Eating disorders, for example, are commonly associated with abusive voices that tell their victim that she doesn't deserve to eat, or even to exist (see, e.g., Schaefer and Rutledge 2004). One commentator adduces this as a reason to suspect that at least some anorexics may "have MPD":

> Frequently, MPD patients present themselves to the clinician with a variety of psychophysiological symptoms. Eating-disorder symptoms may be one of these, and may include the following: binge eating, self-induced vomiting, laxative abuse, excessive exercising, body image distortion, self-starvation, fluctuations in body weight, and nausea.... The pathological eating behavior [in some of these cases] was so severe that some patients matched DSM-III-R diagnostic criteria for an eating disorder. Clinicians dealing with eating disorders should be aware that some patients may represent a subgroup in whom the underlying cause for the eating disorder may be MPD. These patients seldom respond to conventional treatment modalities used in eating-disorders programs, and only when the underlying multiplicity is identified and treated by a trained clinician, will the patient's eating-disorder symptoms improve. (Torem 1990; see also Hacking 1995, p. 151)

This isn't implausible. Anorexics, in addition to housing an abusive voice, are also often alienated from their various *social* personae, and feel themselves to be insincere in almost all they do. But if "MPD" does not identify an underlying cause, but only a set of symptoms, it would be as easy to suggest that those patients who most clearly present themselves as multiples are suffering from a generic "dissociative disorder," contingently combined with other mental problems. Or rather, the proof will lie in Torem's final sentence: What is the most effective treatment for any of these conditions? "What are known as *externalizing conversations* can flush the presence and operations of anorexia/bulimia [the abusive voice] into the open" (Maisel et al. 2004, p. 81): in other words, demanding a response from the "disease entity" itself, the possessing demon or personality state, and so treating it as an agent with its own destructive purposes and customary techniques. And who is the "original" self: the alert, courteous and intelligent self that many anorexics display in public, or the anxious and self-hating self that cooperates with the disease? Or neither?

On the other hand, Hacking (1995, pp. 96–112) has argued, plausibly, that the actual arguments for believing in a "dissociative continuum," ranging from commonplace confusions all the way to seriously fissured multiples, are poor: it may still be true that there is a distinct, unusual syndrome, not closely related to less striking dissociations. The traumas that apparently prompt many patients to create their alters no more define the disorder (*pace* Allison 1998) than the precise mechanism of infection *defines* any other disease (as though catching the HIV virus from a dirty needle made it a different disease than catching it from unprotected sex, or from bushmeat). We don't yet know what the underlying mechanism is that permits this degree of dissociation (a term which merely puts a name to the condition). And the association with eating disorders may have a different moral. Crabtree (1997), without endorsing any strong belief in possession, reports that there are at least therapeutic advantages in accepting that hypothesis while dealing with multiples—and almost everyone involved in the care and management of anorexic patients (whether therapists, nurses, doctors, care-givers or the victims themselves) will end up speaking of "the disease" as exactly such an intrusive demon (see, e.g., Schaefer and Rutledge 2004). Maybe the "spiritist" interpretation is right after all.

In brief, the present psychotherapeutic evidence is inconclusive. These pathological cases don't offer any definite answer to the philosophical puzzles, or none that are any more compelling than the thought experiments of less informed philosophers. In fact, they seem to depend upon the philosophical puzzles: what is the difference between a "distinct personality" and a "personality state"? What is it to be or not to be an individual agent? Are there demons? Are these matters of fact, or matters for moral decision (see Box 53.1)?

The Metaphysics of Identity

Philosophical discussions of personal identity have usually begun from the assumption that any reasonable theory of what is involved in such identity must confirm common judgments: called upon to prove my own identity I produce my birth certificate, passport, driving license. If there are any doubts about the authenticity of these documents, I appeal to friends and family, to medical and dental records, perhaps to traces of DNA. Commonsensically, I am an identifiable physical organism, with a unique history, however little I remember of past years, and however changed, in disposition, beliefs and character from what I was. People do also, sometimes, speak as if I could be "a different person" (just in that my disposition, beliefs and character have changed), or observe that I am "a different person" at home and at work, in public display and in private (it would indeed be peculiar if I weren't). But such changes don't usually amount to much. Legally and morally I am the very same person as committed whatever follies I would now like to disown: the very fact that I would like to disown them, even forget them, is proof that they are mine! But there may be more extreme alterations: if I wake one morning in complete ignorance of any personal past, and must reconstruct a life on the basis of what I am told and what I can find to do, can I be held responsible for acts I can't remember, and understand as little as anyone else? It may still be true that I am the same creature as before, the same physical organism, precisely because the explanation for this schism is to be found in what this organism has suffered: the former creature has not simply been replaced. But I am not in every sense the same person. Conversely, many contemporary fantasies—and also, of course, more traditional beliefs about the resurrection of the dead—suggest that I might find myself awakened in a newly created body long after the destruction of the one that is typing these words: the same person, but not the same human creature (perhaps not human at all). Must such an awakened revenant decide instead that, notwithstanding clear similarities of character and apparent memory (as well as the universal agreement of friends and family), he is not after all the person that he momentarily supposes? Is it enough that, for all practical purposes, he is "just as good" a Stephen as the one that wakes "normally" tomorrow morning? Perhaps physical continuity is not all that matters, at least for some senses of "personal identity." Nor is the issue simply to do with memory: our memories are fluctuating, disorderly and partial at the best of times. According to Oxnam, "probably the biggest difference between 'normal multiplicity' and MPD is that most people recall what happens when they move through their array of personae. By contrast, MPD is characterized by rigid memory walls that prevent such recall until therapy begins to break down the barriers" (Oxnam 2006, p. 5). But this exaggerates the openness of our usual memory: most people probably *don't* recall very much of what they did in another guise (until they are forced to remember)! Not only don't I easily remember what the person I apparently am was doing several years ago, I often cannot recall what he was doing ten minutes ago, nor why I have gone to the kitchen. Granted that the diagnostic criteria for DID explicitly exclude such "normal forgetfulness," is there any clear criterion for what is "normal" or what is really required for unambiguous identity? Creatures who didn't thus forget what they were doing might reasonably think we were *all* multiples.

Maybe the revenant could count as me even if he *doesn't* seem to remember much of what I've done, but behaves as if he did. Maybe we are simply wrong to expect a singular, definite answer in all cases of presumed identity: being the same person or creature from one moment or one year to the next isn't after all an "all or nothing" affair, and there may be no "objective" answer to the question, any more than there is an objective answer to questions about the proper boundaries of a nation-state, or how long it has existed. The United Kingdom has its cumulative origin in successive Acts of Union (1707, 1800, 1927), but "England" has no such definite beginning, nor any clear spatial boundaries. Once such a nation-state exists, there is a powerful tendency to read it back into the past—as though first-century Gaul was really France-in-waiting. Just so, we *imagine* our past history as embryos and infants even though our *personal* being did not—so some suppose—begin till the times we can, with some effort, remember.

Are we entities any more distinct, stable or objective than nation-states or cities? René Descartes's conclusion—like Augustine's—was that he knew himself to exist in the very act of considering whether or not he did, and simultaneously knew that this existence wasn't the same as any physical presence. What certainly existed wasn't René Descartes, but a thinker, known in the act of thinking. It is perhaps unfair to reply, with Bertrand Russell, that all he could be sure of was that there was a thought, and not that there was a non-material substance which did the thinking. It is enough that there was thinking. But that thinking is at least not as active, and self-directed, as some Cartesians have supposed. Most of the thoughts that float across the sphere of my attention are disconnected, or loosely associated, fragments: try listening to your thoughts, or try to focus them. It is an important step in self-knowledge to be made to realize just how fluid and uncontrolled our ordinary thinking is.

> Whence came the soul, whither will it go, how long will it be our mate and comrade? Can we tell its essential nature? … Even now in this life, we are the ruled rather than the rulers, known rather than knowing…. Is my mind my own possession? That parent of false conjectures, that purveyor of delusion, the delirious, the fatuous, and in frenzy or senility proved to be the very negation of mind. (Philo, *On Cherubim*, 1929, vol. II, p. 77)

And again:

> It is a hard matter to bring to a standstill the soul's changing movements. Their irresistible stream is such that we could sooner stem the rush of a torrent, for thoughts after thoughts in countless numbers pour on like a huge breaker and drive and whirl and upset its whole being with their violence…. A man's thoughts are sometimes not due to himself but come without his will. (Philo, *De Mutatione Nominum*, 1929, vol. V, pp. 239–240)

What we cannot control is not our own: even my mind is not my own, or at any rate no more *mine* than are the involuntary motions of my body. In distinguishing myself from the body, as was customary long before Descartes, I also distinguish *myself* from my mind!

Multiplicity is the norm. So also is passivity. It may be exceptional for people to suppose that the thoughts they find themselves thinking are not really "theirs," that these have been put into their heads by Martians, demons or the government. Thinking that one's thoughts, or one's bodily movements, all belong to "someone else," or to no-one at all, is easily supposed a symptom of insanity or at any rate a failure to be properly engaged with one's own life (it is part of what "depersonalization" means). But maybe those who are thus diagnosed have simply noticed, and melodramatically described, what really is, for most of us, the case. They are "our" thoughts in that we are immediately aware of them (or rather there is an immediate awareness of them), but not ours, because we do not actually *think* them, in the sense that they would vanish if we chose to stop (see Stephens and Graham 1994).

> "Know Yourself" is said to those who because of their selves' multiplicity have the business of counting themselves up and learning that they do not know all the numbers and kinds of things they are, or do not know any one of them, nor what their ruling principle is, or by what they are themselves. (Plotinus 1966–1988, *Ennead* VI 7 (38), 41.22–26)

Those who seek to follow the Delphic instruction—so St Hesychios was to say—find themselves, as it were, gazing into a mirror and sighting the dark faces of the demons peering over their shoulders (Palmer et al. 1979, p. 123).

In brief, neither multiplicity nor passivity are new discoveries. Descartes left us with the impression that self-knowledge was our normal and necessary condition: the earlier tradition makes it clear that such knowledge is difficult, and "single-heartedness" a distant, luminous goal. The aim of meditation in many different traditions is to learn to distinguish oneself from the ordinary objects and the ordinary affects that afflict us, and to discover the one Good for which the self is made. "It is not one and the same Goodness that always acts the Faculties of a Wicked man; but as many several images and pictures of Goodness as a quick and working Fancy can represent to him; which so divide his affections, that he is no *One thing* within himself, but tossed hither and thither by the most independent Principels and Imaginations that may be" (so said the Cambridge Platonist, John Smith (1618–1652): Patrides 1969, p. 172).

How could it be otherwise? The unity and coherence of any merely material object, even of any living creature, is always a matter of degree. Some (e.g., slime moulds) find it useful to split up into their component cells, and only re-unite when they need to emigrate. We aren't the sort of creature that literally and physically divides itself, but we clearly do—and should—have different ways of behaving, feeling and thinking in different circumstances. We should also prefer an interior conversation to an interior monologue! Spiritist and materialist can here agree. As creatures with bodies, passions and parts, we are not wholly different in kind from cooperative colonies, and our mental life rides on biochemical exchanges whose complexity we cannot analyze. Very fortunately, we are not left to make conscious choices about everything that matters for the survival of these colonies: fortunately, since we would have no idea how to make them. Even our brains, it seems, are compounded of many modules. Some of these have a fairly precise physical location; others are distributed through our brains and spinal column. Recent philosophical attention (e.g., Parfit 1987) has tended to focus on "split-brain" experiments, in which each hemisphere of our brain appears to house or facilitate a distinct body of knowledge, capacity and desire (and some earlier accounts of MPD supposed that there were only two distinct personalities, one for each hemisphere). But the brain and body can be divided or hampered in many ways, and our mental and moral lives are altered accordingly. "I suspect," says Beahrs (1982, p. 9), "that our brains permit us to organize our mental life in at least as many ways as societies can be governed." Not all these modules or organs have any voice with which to express themselves, and any conversation with them (so to speak) will be indirect—but still possible. If we change our diet, our pattern of breathing, our physical exercises, our day-dreams or even our philosophy, there will be concomitant responses in our heart, lungs, liver, gonads and other glands. Some of them will amount to instructions ("Don't drink so much orange juice!" "Relax your shoulder muscles!"). Others may open up new aspects of our sensory world, or excite particular selves and strategies: porn, caffeine, alcohol and chocolate especially so. The Persians, so Herodotus tells us in his *Histories* (I.139), required that all serious decisions be taken twice: once drunk and once sober. They were possibly wise. After all, even the most sensible of us don't always know why we act or think as we do. Often, something other than our conscious selves seem to be directing us, something with its own reasons, motives and attitudes: something, in other words, that is itself a personal agent. Whether that agent is wiser than our conscious selves may be moot: it is at least rather different. Allowing it to speak, and to argue, may save us from its preemptive sabotage of what we consciously desire, and the sort of brutal exasperation "Sally" felt for "Miss Beauchamp."

Let us suppose then that our identity at any one time is fractious and easily fractured, and that our identity over time is not easily settled. The promises we feel bound to keep, the follies for which we feel responsible, reveal our own opinion about who and what we are—which may not always be the opinion others have: we won't be allowed to ignore our serious compacts on the plea that we don't any longer much like the self that made them. We teach our children who they are to think themselves by requiring them to acknowledge their mistakes, and praising them for their accomplishments—even if they don't at the time have much conception of their own continued being. Multiples, on this account, are seriously confused about what they are expected to acknowledge: they believe, it seems, that acts they don't understand or approve of can't really have been theirs, because those acts don't express their *present* selves, or what they want their selves to be. Because they were not theirs, they must have been someone else's—and the image of Another Self emerges from that error. But of course this is an error only by social agreement: in fact, we could suspect, even our ordinary Self is just such an artifact. We pretend to ourselves and others that there is Someone responsible for all the acts of our acknowledged past, Someone who must fulfill our present promises. We might instead decide that there is really no one, and that the various acts and words and feelings are, essentially, unowned.

By this last account, apparent singletons and multiples alike need to be disabused, disillusioned and enlightened by the Buddhist insight: that there is no self. In the *Questions of King Milinda* (which is Menander, ruling in the second century BC in north-west India) the Buddhist philosopher Nagasena explains to Menander that no complex entity is anything but a collection of parts: better still, such words as seem to name that complex entity are only convenient designations for what has no substantial being. "Nagasena" itself is "but a way of counting, term, appellation, convenient designation, mere name for the hair of the head, hair of the body.... brain of the head, form, sensation, perception, the predispositions and consciousness. But in the absolute sense there is no ego to be found" (Radhakrishnan and Moore 1957, pp. 281–284; see also Dennett 1991, pp. 210, 416).

But there is an alternative. The thoughts, feelings, and images that sweep across our consciousness, and that may briefly absorb us are not the same as the self, considered simply as that consciousness. Our error is to *identify* with the passing thoughts. Our release is to draw ourselves back from them, even from those with which we are most tempted to identify. Billy Milligan, whom the American courts—briefly—excused for rape and assault on the plea that he suffered from MPD, described the process whereby different personae moved out into control of their shared body as one of stepping into the light of a spotlight from the corners of a dark room (Crabtree 1997, p. 82, after Keyes 1981). One interpretation of the metaphor is that it is the light itself that is the self. At least that does to some extent match the implications of meditative practice in many traditions. If "the mind" is a complex of mental microbes (the earlier label, coined by Ritchie (1891, p. 22), for what have more recently been called "memes"), then we need another expression (say "the Self") for the light or space within which these complexes take shape. The Self is not identical with "that parent of false conjecture," or swarming congregation. Techniques for recognizing it differ: ranging from the "sudden enlightenment" of Ch'an Buddhism to the prayerful devotion of Christian monks or the rational inquiry of Platonists. One way of understanding Descartes' cogito itself (which is also Augustine's) is as a record of a real experience, the revelation of one's self as something more than its thoughts and visions (see Holscher 1986, pp. 126ff).

The point is not "merely philosophical." Philosophy here meets with psychotherapy. One way of coping with the apparent onset of MPD, or even with accusing voices, is to draw the victim's attention not to other thoughts or regions of the mind, but to the Self, the Centre. By redescribing what she is enduring, by not being trapped into allegiance to a particular thought-chain, she may become aware of her original selfhood (which is unlikely to be the personality or mind she had or displayed "before," let alone the one that strikes the therapist as most obviously "normal"). Conversely, the point is not "merely psychotherapeutic." One of the best proofs that we are right to identify with the self, the light, the center is that such willed identification may help to release patients from their real distress. But without some assurance that the theory itself is coherent that "proof" might be no better than pragmatic, and the theory just another fiction. I doubt that its truth can ever be entirely demonstrated. It is at least not disproved by modern or post-modern commentary, and is compatible with the stories told about DID/MPD, passivity and our ordinary lives. Without some sense of the Self, we shall be reduced to thinking ourselves mere aggregates of squabbling voices.

Our predecessors (and many of our contemporaries) would have agreed that our surface consciousness, the self we present to the world, is not the only power at work in us. They would also have agreed that we are always telling stories about our lives and about the world. But the point is to know when to tell *true* stories, and to know what stories are true. The pathological phenomena that are grouped together as dissociative disorders don't themselves determine our metaphysics: to that extent, they are no more use than the thought-experiments of philosophers, and the conclusions drawn by therapists are no more authoritative than the philosophers' intuitions. But their experience, and their clients', may nonetheless be amenable to a different reading than any preferred by present-day common sense.

Watching out for the Daimon

According to the currently fashionable judgment "DID clients are individual people who experience their minds as consisting of separate personalities that are able to function autonomously. Yet they are single persons" (Hacking 1995, p. 134; see also Gunnarsson 2009). But as Hacking also observes (1995, p. 19) "some clients … experience these parts as spiritual entities that are separate from themselves." And this latter judgment is truer to the accounts originally given by multiples and psychologists in the nineteenth and early twentieth centuries. MPD, as both Crabtree and Spanos have observed (though with opposite effect), is early associated with theories of possession. And it is Possession that is the commoner theory.

Bourguignon (1989) compares two accounts: one, by Lasky (1978) of a multiple, "Mrs G."; the other, by Pressel (1978), of a case of spirit possession in Brazil. The authors, a therapist and an anthropologist, have different methods, and different attitudes.

> Their reactions to the alternate personalities are correspondingly different. Lasky notes that, in spite of earlier hints of Candy's existence, he "had not lent credence" to Mrs. G.'s "second, separate personality." When Candy does appear, he is surprised and responds cautiously, telling her that he "would like to learn … which part of Mrs. G. she represented." This statement of disbelief in her existence infuriates Candy, who replies that "she did not *represent* anything, she was herself" (Lasky 1978, p. 370, italics in original). Candy insists that she is a separate person, sharing a body with Mrs. G., who essentially agrees. She, the core personality, tells Lasky that Candy "usually seemed to be someone else who knew her very well and seemed almost 'to sit on my shoulder, like a little bird'" (Lasky 1978, p. 364). This perception of Candy as separate and alien is confirmed when Mrs. G. says that though she may be embarrassed at Candy's actions, she does not feel any guilt for them. That is, she does not feel responsible for Candy's behavior. The therapist, however, does not entertain such a possibility. To him, Candy is a splitoff part of Mrs. G. herself, "resulting from a developmental defect of the ego" (Lasky 1978, p. 364). For comparison we turn not to Pressel's views on Margarida but to those of Joaõ and his fellow Umbandistas. They do not consider Margarida as a split-off part of Joaõ's own principal personality, but as a separate being. She is one of several spirits that "possess" him at intervals. In local parlance, he is her *cavalho* or "horse" whom she "mounts." She does so

by temporarily displacing his personality and taking over his body. What happens on these occasions is her responsibility, not his. Margarida is believed to be a "disincarnate" spirit, that is, the spirit of a deceased person (after Pressel 1977).... In other words, the alters of Mrs. G. and of Joaõ—who live in different cultural settings, and who seek help from different types of healers—have different ontological status: for the American psychotherapist, it is possible, although unusual, for persons to suffer from defective ego development, to use dissociation, or "splitting" rather than repression as a principal ego defense mechanism, and as a result to develop "multiple personalities." For Umbandistas, the world is peopled by disincarnate as well as incarnate spirits. Having unfinished business in the world, they seek out persons with mediumistic capacities (Bourguignon 1989, pp. 374–376).

The Brazilian rationale is matched by an Indian. For nine months in the year Hari Das is a manual labourer and prison guard. In the remaining three months he is the medium of a Hindu god: "you become the deity. You lose all fear. Even your voice changes. The god comes alive and takes over. You are just the vehicle, the medium. In the trance it is God who speaks, and all the acts are the acts of the god—feeling, thinking, speaking" (Dalrymple 2009: ch. 2). In both these cases, and many others, the possession (as it is perceived) is socially approved, and mostly confined to particular ritual circumstances. One interpretation, easier for Western common sense, is that this is a form of theatre, hardly different from the techniques used by actors to evoke (rather than invoke) a character. At best, it is an attempt to find a decent place in society for seriously damaged multiples. But this is not how it seems to the participants. There may be moments when a great actor does manage to incarnate a spirit. But the participants in such rituals do not consider themselves great actors, nor do they remember any details of what "they" do while possessed. Nor do they suppose merely that the gods are their own hidden selves, as though Hari Das's evocation of the god Vishnu were evoking only Hari Das's Vishnu. It is thought to be possible instead that someone else will take on the role, the god, when Hari Das has to retire. Nor do they seem to be damaged.

The robust metaphysical response to this would simply be to deny that there are or even could be non-corporeal entities of this sort. Even this claim might not finally settle the matter: viral infections don't only affect our *bodies*. Some of them affect our minds: temperament, desires and maybe even beliefs. Cat-lovers may have been infected with the same virus that, apparently, renders mice susceptible to feline charm! Only a few years ago stomach ulcers were routinely explained as a psychosomatic response to *stress*: the discovery that they are bacterial in origin, and cured by antibiotics, has relieved many victims, and embarrassed older doctors. It may be that future psychologists will also be embarrassed at the discovery of simple bacterial or viral causes of the mental disorders whose victims they now patronize—and also of the mental disorders that are now usually admired (egoism, ambition, anthropocentrism, scientism)! Or maybe there are no simple physical correlates of the infection or contagion: maybe instead we should consider these possessive spirits as "mental microbes." Common sense itself is compounded of mental microbes, voices advising us to purchase this or that, to swoon over celebrities and punish deviants. Perhaps they are more than fashions. Perhaps they are indeed devils. And maybe some are angels.

This conclusion, of course, is a deliberate challenge to the materialist metaphysic that, without much actual argument, now possesses most of the West.

Despite the many cases described as MPD or DID, and despite the efforts of many thoughtful therapists and victims, it is still not clear either that there is a genuine syndrome present in all or most or many of these cases, or that—on the contrary—there is a dissociative continuum, in which some unfortunates merely suffer a little more intensely and confusingly what all of us endure. Ralph Allison, a therapist notorious for his use of literal exorcism to displace what he has come to suspect are genuinely invasive spirits (whether of the deceased, or of more diabolical origin), also distinguishes firmly between MPD and the latterly more popular diagnosis DID:

> Dissociation is a life saving mental mechanism which very highly hypnotizable abused patients used to stay alive, by creating alter-personalities. Emotional Imagination is a ubiquitous ability which all but the demented can use to create Imaginary Companions, both internal and external. Dissociation is the separation of certain aspects of the personality into two or more parts, while imagination is the creation of new images and features which never existed before (Allison 1998, p.126).

Genuine victims of MPD, he suggests, were easily hypnotizable children traumatized before the age of seven, when their original personality retreated into the background and successive alters, both benign and malign, took center stage. DID, he suggests, has a different history: after the age of seven, the other personalities involved in the patient's life to console them for lesser traumas are imaginary companions. The former, MPD, are chiefly women; the latter, DID, chiefly men—and those men mostly found in jail. "The criminals used as "hit-men" Internalized Imaginary Companions (IIC's), not alter-personalities. They used Emotional Imagination instead of Dissociation" (Allison 1998, pp. 126ff). Allison builds the proposed etiology of the conditions into his definition, but he may also have sufficient reason to distinguish their overt symptoms.

He also draws attention to the phenomenon of the "inner self helper," a voice and character which distinguishes itself from the patient and seeks to assist her (Allison 1980, 1998; see Beahrs 1982, p.117). One odd story—this from a study of eating disorders—recounts how one abused girl prayed desperately for spiritual support, and promptly encountered a frog willing to sit on her hand. "It occurred to her that she could bring the spirit of the frog inside of her and carry this spirit with her, This arrangement seemed agreeable to the frog, and henceforth Margaret and her frog became inseparable" (Maisel et al. 2004, p. 231). From such encounters, we may suspect, cultural practices grow. They also draw attention to a traditional pattern. Not all the voices that seem to come from outside merely dispossess the "host." Nor are they all indifferent to the host's being and welfare. In older terms they may be "guardian angels," "*daimones*" rather than demons: at once superior in power and knowledge to the ordinary self, and also in some way serving as a "higher" self with whom the host must one day identify:

> If a man is able to follow the spirit (*daimon*) which is above him, he comes to be himself above, living that spirit's life, and giving the pre-eminence to that better part of himself to which he is being led; and after that spirit he rises to another, until he reaches the heights. For the soul is many things, and all things, both the things above and the things below down to the limits of all life, and we are each one of us an intelligible universe, making contact with this lower world by the powers of soul below, but with the intelligible world by its powers above. (Plotinus 1966–1988, *Ennead* III.4 [15], 3.18–24)

Here-now, we may find ourselves advised and even bullied by our *daimon*—as "Sally" bullied "Miss Beauchamp"—but if all goes well we shall find ourselves awakening to that "higher" self, and find yet another guiding star above us. This traditional account is at odds in one respect with the commonest modern hope: the dominant goal of therapy is usually "integration" (aka silencing the conversation), though there are occasional voices advising that it may be enough to achieve a reasonably stable and cooperative family of personalities (Haddock 2001, chapter 8). Even Prince, who decided to drive Sally away (for no better reason, it seems, than that he found her intolerably perky), imagined that she was merely retreating to "the unconscious," where she belonged, and where her talents and wit could be utilized by the newly dominant personality, "the real Miss Beauchamp." "After successful integration," so Ross (1996, pp. 226–227) reports, "MPD patients function much better than before, and can be released from the mental health system." But older traditions—as well as having a more critical attitude to normality—took the possible need for exorcism more seriously: the imagined ascent back up to heaven required us to strip off the characters we have accumulated here, including the "normal" one. The therapists who disapproved of Allison's exorcism of the more hostile and angry multiples in his charge (see Allison 2000) may not have thought him simply deluded (after all, it is not uncommon for therapists to play along with their clients' belief-sets and stage dramatic scenes in the hope of effecting a "cure"). The problem may have been rather that they didn't suppose that *any* element of the patient's soul should be so roughly removed (so Beahrs 1982, pp.129, 141–165). But surgery, however brutal, may occasionally be necessary. There are some selves, or would-be selves, that must be acknowledged only to be dismissed, just as there are some possible lifestyles that we shouldn't even discuss, some voices that we shouldn't lend any strength to: whether exorcism "works" is another matter.

The other crux, of course, is indeed that there may be disagreement about the *origin* of alters, especially those that Allison identifies as Imaginary Companions. The persona that is first presented to the world, and the therapist, is itself Imaginary: someone or something devised to deal with the outer world, usually by an abject conformity. Is it possible that the companions are *invoked*—as people around the world suppose that gods, demons and the departed dead may be invoked? Or are they "only imagined"? What is of more philosophical interest, perhaps, is whether there is any clear distinction between these options.

What is it, after all, to "imagine" something? Our predecessors would have found our belief in our own *creativity* odd. The sculptor locates the statue in the marble, and rubs or chips away at the stone till it emerges. The composer *hears* the music that he then writes down. Only what is really there already can truly and vividly be imagined. The image of some superior angel that we think we create for ourselves is actually that angel's presence to us. Conversely, the image we create for ourselves (we think) of a life less disciplined, less virtuous, is that very life's own struggle to emerge from the dark backward of our souls. Nor is there much reason to suppose that our own images are very different from anyone else's.

In conclusion, it is probably safe only to suggest that the data do confirm the existence of troubled persons, who believe themselves to be governed or beset by several personalities, often at odds with each other. There may be no single syndrome responsible for all the cases. Some patients are variously dissociated, depersonalized, and forgetful. Some seem to speak with many voices, including voices that vary from the diabolical to the briskly angelic. How precisely patients, therapists, and armchair theorists choose to describe the events will depend on their prior metaphysical commitments, and the only test of those commitments that the cases offer is whether or not a particular treatment seems to "work." But there will also always be disputes about what is to count as "working." Is it enough that people find friends and useful occupation? Or should we, like our philosophical forebears, hope for a higher calling?

Box 53.1 Extract from *Mirror Dance*

He wondered where Mark had gone.

People came, and tormented a nameless thing without boundaries, and went away again. He met them variously. His emerging aspects became personas, and eventually, he named them, as well as he could identify them. There was Gorge, and Grunt, and Howl, and another, quiet one that lurked on the fringes, waiting.

He let Gorge go out to handle the force-feedings, because Gorge was the only one who actually enjoyed them. Gorge, after all, would never have been permitted to do all that Ryoval's techs did. Grunt he sent forth when Ryoval came again with the hypospray of aphrodisiac. Grunt had also been responsible for the attack on Maree, the body-sculptured clone, he rather thought, though Grunt, when not all excited, was very shy and ashamed and didn't talk much.

Howl handled the rest. He began to suspect Howl had been obscurely responsible for delivering them all to Ryoval in the first place. Finally, he'd come to a place where he could be punished *enough. Never give aversion therapy to a masochist. The results are unpredictable.* So Howl deserved what Howl got. The elusive fourth one just waited, and said that someday, they would all love him best.

They did not always stay within their lines. Howl had a tendency to eavesdrop on Gorge's sessions, which came regularly while Howl's did not; and more than once Gorge turned up riding along with Grunt on his adventures, which then became exceptionally peculiar. Nobody joined Howl by choice.

Having named them all, he finally found Mark by process of elimination. Gorge and Grunt and Howl and the Other had sent Lord Mark deep inside, to sleep through it all. Poor, fragile Lord Mark, barely twelve weeks old.

Ryoval could not even see Lord Mark down in there. Could not reach him. Could not touch him. Gorge and Grunt and Howl and the Other were all very careful not to wake the baby. Tender and protective, they defended him. They were *equipped* to. An ugly, grotty, hard-bitten bunch, these psychic mercenaries of his. Unlovely. But they got the job done.

He began to hum little marching tunes to them, from time to time.

Reproduced from *Mirror Dance*, Lois McMaster, Chapter 26, © 1994, Lois McMaster Bujold. Originally published by Baen Books. Reproduced here with permission of the author.

Lois McMaster Bujold is best known for her engaging and psychologically acute space opera, usually focused on a disabled military genius in a far-future society conditioned to fear difference. This particular episode is concerned rather with her hero's clone brother, reared in still worse conditions as a potential assassin, and here captured and tortured. His broken personalities enable him to cope: at once distinct centres of consciousness and servants of the whole. Whether there really are such experiences remains uncertain: at least the story, and its more immediate and maybe-factual cognates provide metaphors for living.

ACKNOWLEDGMENTS

This chapter reworks some of the data, theories, arguments and ideas contained in Clark, S. R. L. (1996). Minds, Memes and Multiples. *Philosophy, Psychiatry & Psychology, 31*, 21–28; see also Clark, S. R. L. (1991). How many selves make me? In D. Cockburn (Ed.), Human Beings , pp. 213–33. Cambridge: Cambridge University Press; Clark, S. R. L. (1992); Descartes' debt to Augustine. In M. McGhee (Ed.), *Philosophy, Religion and the Spiritual Life*, pp. 73–88. Cambridge: Cambridge University Press; Clark, S. R. L. (1996). Commentary on Stephen Braude's "Multiple Personality and Moral Responsibility." *Philosophy, Psychiatry &*

Psychology, 3 , 55–8; Clark, S. R. L. (2003). Constructing persons: The psychopathology of identity. *Philosophy, Psychiatry, & Psychology, 10,* 157–60; Clark, S. R. L. (2009). Plotinus: Charms and countercharms. In A. O'Hear (Ed.), *Conceptions of Philosophy,* pp. 215–31. Cambridge: Cambridge University Press.

References

Allison, R. B. (1998). Multiple personality disorder, dissociative identity disorder, and internalized imaginary companions. *Hypnos, 25*(3), 125–33.

Allison, R. B. (1999). *Mind in Many Pieces: Revealing the Spiritual Side of Multiple Personality Disorder* (2nd edn). Los Osos, CA: Cie Publishing.

American Psychiatric Association (2000). *Diagnostic and Statistical Manual of Mental Disorders, Fourth Edition, Text Revision.* Washington, DC: American Psychiatric Association.

Beahrs, J. O. (1982). *Unity and Multiplicity: Multilevel Consciousness of Self in Hypnosis, Psychiatric Disorder and Mental Health.* New York, NY: Brunner/Mazel, Inc.

Bourguignon, E. (1989). Multiple personality, possession trance, and the psychic unity of mankind. *Ethos, 17,* 371–84.

Braude, S. R. (1995). *First Person Plural: Multiple Personality and the Philosophy of Mind* (2nd edn). London: Rowman and Littlefield.

Coons, P. (1984). The differential diagnosis of MP: A comprehensive review. *Psychiatric Clinics of North America, 7,* 51–7.

Crabtree, A. (1997). *Multiple Man: Explorations in Possession and Multiple Personality.* Toronto: Somerville House.

Dalrymple, W. (2009). *Nine Lives: In Search of the Sacred in Modern India.* London: Bloomsbury.

Dell, P. F. (2001). Why the diagnostic criteria for dissociative identity disorder should be changed. *Journal of Trauma and Dissociation, 2*(1), 7–37.

Dell, P. F. and O'Neil, J. A. (Eds) (2009). *Dissociation and the Dissociative Disorders: DSM-V and Beyond.* New York, NY: Routledge.

Dennett, D. C. (1991). *Consciousness Explained.* Boston, MA: Little Brown & Co.

Freud, S. (1952). *Autobiographical Study.* New York, NY: W. W. Norton & Co. (Original work published 1935.)

Gunnarsson, L. (2009). *Philosophy of Personal Identity and Multiple Personality.* London: Routledge.

Hacking, I. (1995). *Rewriting the Soul: Multiple Personality and the Sciences of Memory.* Princeton, NJ: Princeton University Press.

Haddock, D. B. (2001). *The Dissociative Identity Disorder Sourcebook.* New York, NY: McGraw Hill.

Holscher, L. (1986). *The Reality of the Mind: Augustine's Philosophical Arguments for the Human Soul As a Spiritual Substance.* London: Routledge & Kegan Paul.

Keyes, D. (1981). *The Minds of Billy Milligan.* New York, NY: Random House.

Lasky, R. (1978). The psychoanalytic treatment of a case of multiple personality. *Psychoanalytic Review, 65,* 355–80.

Maisel, R., Epston, D., and Borden, A. (2004). *Biting the Hand That Starves You: Inspiring Resistance to Anorexia/Bulimia.* New York, NY: W. W. Norton and Co.

Midgley, M. (1984). *Wickedness.* London: Routledge and Kegan Paul.

Oltmanns, T. F., Neale, J., and Davison, G. C. (1991). *Case Studies in Abnormal Psychology*. Hoboken, NJ: John Wiley and Sons.

Oxnam, R. B. (2006). *A Fractured Mind: My Life With Multiple Personality Disorder*. London: Fusion Press.

Palmer, G. E. H., Sherrard, P., and Ware, K. (Eds) (1979). *Philokalia*. London: Faber.

Parfit, D. (1987). *Reasons and Persons* (3rd edn). Oxford: Clarendon Press.

Patrides, C. A. (Ed.) (1969). *The Cambridge Platonists*. Cambridge: Cambridge University Press.

Philo of Alexandria (1929). *Collected Works* (F. H. Colson and G. H. Whitaker, Trans.). London: Heinemann, Loeb Classical Library.

Plotinus (1966–1988). *Enneads* (A. H. Armstrong, Trans.). London: Heinemann, Loeb Classical Library.

Pressel, E. (1977). Negative spirit possession in experienced Brazilian Umbanda spirit mediums. In V. Crapanzano and V. Garrison (Eds), *Case Studies in Spirit Possession*, pp. 333–64. Hoboken, NJ: John Wiley and Sons.

Prince, M. (1908). *The Dissociation of a Personality*. New York, NY: Longmans, Greene & Co.

Radhakrishnan, S. and Moore, C. (Eds) (1957). *Sourcebook of Indian Philosophy*. Princeton, NJ: Princeton University Press.

Ritchie, D. G. (1891). *Darwinism and Politics*. London: Swan Sonnenschein and Co.

Ross, C. A. (1990). Twelve cognitive errors about multiple personality disorder. *American Journal of Psychotherapy*, 44, 348–56.

Ross, C. A. (1996). *Dissociative Identity Disorder: Diagnosis, Clinical Features and Treatment of Multiple Personality* (2nd edn). Hoboken, NJ: John Wiley and Sons.

Schaefer, J. and Rutledge, T. (2004). *Life Without Ed: How One Woman Declared Independence from Her Eating Disorder and How You Can Too*. New York, NY: McGraw Hill.

Simeon, D. and Abugel, J. (2006). *Feeling Unreal: Depersonalization Disorder and the Loss of the Self*. New York, NY: Oxford University Press.

Sizemore, C. (1989). *A Mind of My Own*. New York, NY: William Morrow.

Smith, M. (1993). *Ritual Abuse: What it is, Why it Happens, How to Help*. San Francisco, CA: Harper.

Spanos, N. P. (1996). *Multiple Identities and False Memories: A Sociocognitive Perspective*. Washington, DC: American Psychological Association.

Stephens, G. L. and Graham, G. (1994). Self-consciousness, mental agency and the clinical psychopathology of thought-insertion. *Philosophy, Psychiatry & Psychology*, 1, 1–10.

Thigpen, C. and Cleckley H. M. (1957). *The Three Faces of Eve*. London: Secker and Warburg.

Torem, M. S. (1990). Covert multiple personality underlying eating disorders. *American Journal of Psychotherapy*, 44, 357–68.

Wilkes, K. (1984). *Real People*. Oxford: Clarendon Press.

SECTION VII

EXPLANATION AND UNDERSTANDING

CHAPTER 54

INTRODUCTION: EXPLANATION AND UNDERSTANDING

For much of its history, the pairing of explanation and understanding has been taken to express an opposition between natural science and human science or interpersonal understanding more broadly. Further, the opposition was taken to express the limits of both. The kind of insight offered by one was impossible to achieve by the other. This was Jaspers' view. Whilst psychiatry should contain both approaches, and whilst the very same events could be approached using either (he thought that every event could, in principle, be explained and, more surprisingly, all except primary delusions could also be understood), concentration on only one risked diminishing the insight.

Given that understanding is an implicit thread through much of the rest of this handbook, this section concerns not what cannot but rather what can be studied scientifically. On the assumption that psychiatry is based, in part at least, on natural science, what is the nature or the general shape of that science? Some of the chapters aim at getting right the nature of component parts of a scientific world view. What, for example, is the nature of causation and its connection, if any, to the existence of mechanisms? If psychiatry rests on a taxonomy of mental disorders, what kind of kinds does that involve? If they merit the title "natural kinds," what exactly are those? Should taxonomy aim at reliability and validity and are these in tension?

Others concern potentially fruitful scientific approaches. One chapter addresses not a priori arguments against the identity in principle of mind and brain but rather what concretely can be learnt about the mind from subpersonal brain mechanisms studied using contemporary imaging techniques. Another addresses how phenomenology—the philosophical approach with which Jaspers was familiar—can be combined with neurology to produce a unified discipline which augments both.

The overall moral of the section is that psychiatry can properly claim to contain—if not be restricted to—a scientific discipline but one which requires a twenty first century *philosophy* of science. The conception of science which dominated philosophy at the start of the twentieth century assumed that things were much simpler than they have proved to be. That conception was a poor fit for a discipline facing the empirical and conceptual challenges that psychiatry has taken on. Once, however, one realizes that there can be different kinds of (natural) kinds; that causal links need not be restricted to well-behaved levels of explanation but can cross levels (if, indeed, such talk of levels fits actual findings); that there are varieties of validity and reliability with opposing virtues etc. then one has a more appropriate understanding of the nature of science to shed light on psychiatric practice.

In Chapter 55, "Causation and Mechanisms in Psychiatry," John Campbell returns to a theme he has been developing in a number of recent papers on psychiatry and psychology. Taking the question of whether poverty causes mental illness as a first example, he argues against some assumptions that have been taken to constrain causation and then for a positive view. There is no need to assume that only particular kinds of cause can have particular kinds of effects belonging to the same "level of explanation." Second, although we find it natural and fruitful to look for them, there need be no mechanisms mediating cause and effect. But third, causation can be thought of in the light of potential interventions. In the example given, if intervening on poverty has effects on mental illness then poverty—possibly brutely—causes mental illness.

Rachel Cooper argues in Chapter 56, "Natural Kinds," that debate about whether mental disorders can be natural kinds has been distorted by assuming that such kinds have to be like the kinds picked out by the periodic table in chemistry. There are, however, different views of kinds in different natural sciences (e.g., kinds of rock in geology). In consequence, Cooper argues for a relaxed view: natural kinds are kinds picked out by the sciences. Such kinds, of whatever sort, can ground explanations and predictions. Thus, although kinds of mental disorder differ from the kinds recognized by sciences such as chemistry in various ways, they may yet be natural kinds.

The first challenge Dominic Murphy addresses in Chapter 57, "The Medical Model and the Philosophy of Science," is to characterize what the "medical model" might mean especially in the context of psychiatry. He distinguishes a minimalist from a stronger version. The former adopts appropriate empirical methods, such as epidemiology or evidence of dose–response relationships for drugs and is "recognizably medical in terms of the information it collects, the concepts it employs, and the practices it supports." But it "makes few, if any, commitments about what is really going on with the patient." By contrast, a stronger version adds to this a commitment that disease is a breakdown in normal functioning due to a pathogenic process unfolding in some bodily system. The chapter then explores how such a view of psychiatry as an instance of cognitive neuroscience concerned with the subpersonal causes of psychiatric signs and symptoms can address issues such as the proper level of explanation and/or the value-based nature of illness.

In Chapter 58, "Reliability, Validity, and the Mixed Blessings of Operationalism" Nick Haslam starts by providing a careful overview of the various concepts of reliability and validity and explores their interrelation. He then uses this to assess the benefits and the costs of the reliability inspired turn to operationalist diagnosis begun in DSM-III. Although nuanced, he argues that whilst it may have helped to explore the relationships between diagnoses and other relevant clinical phenomena, and also improved communication across theoretical and cultural divides, it may also have contributed to the proliferation of mental disorders, the resulting problem of comorbidity, and a distorted conception of some forms of psychopathology where its focus on observable features may have led to a systematic neglect of others.

Chapter 59, "Reduction and Reductionism in Psychiatry," examines the prospects of relating the phenomena described in psychiatry to lower-level, biological and chemical, theory. Kenneth Schaffner distinguishes between "sweeping reductionism," in which a powerful biological theory explains the whole of psychiatry en masse, with "creeping reductionism," in which particular psychiatric phenomena are given explanations in specific lower-levels terms. Using recent genetic and neuroscientific work on the symptoms of schizophrenia as an example, Schaffner argues that it illustrates patchy, creeping reductionism in which merely some aspects of schizophrenia are explained in lower-level terms. Nevertheless, even this modest picture is a form of reduction as it meets three key conditions: (1) the explainers are a partially decomposable microstructure in the organism/process of interest, (2) the explanandum is a higher-level macro property, and (3) bridge laws permit the relation of macrodescriptions to microdescriptions.

Chapter 60, "Diagnostic Prediction and Prognosis: Getting from Symptom to Treatment," by Michael Bishop and J. D. Trout, looks first at diagnosis and then prognosis and treatment. The first half provides an overview of the evidence concerning the effectiveness of a variety of approaches to diagnosis starting with subjective methods, semi-structured and structured clinical interviews, and statistical prediction rules (SPRs). It transpires that the last approach trumps all others: "when based on the same evidence, the predictions of well-constructed SPRs are at least as reliable, and are often more reliable, than the predictions of human experts." The second half of the chapter discusses assessment of the effectiveness of treatments including a discussion of what counts as a placebo control in the case of talking therapies.

In Chapter 61, "Clinical Judgment, Tacit Knowledge, and Recognition in Psychiatric Diagnosis," Tim Thornton takes Michael Polanyi's famous slogan that "we can know more than we can tell" and his discussion of knowledge of anatomy to assess the role of tacit knowledge in psychiatric diagnosis. Against a view of tacit knowledge as context-dependent and practical, he argues for its ineliminable role in diagnosis even in cases of very thorough phenomenological description.

Two chapters, in different ways, sketch the possibilities for particular scientific approaches to the study of mind. In Chapter 62, "Neural Mechanisms of Decision-Making and the Personal Level," Nicholas Shea argues that more general philosophical arguments concerning the relation between personal- and subpersonal-level descriptions (e.g., Davidsonian arguments that personal-level descriptions cannot be reduced to subpersonal-level descriptions) leave open the possibility that light can be shed on the nature of human experience through neural imaging work. He outlines one particular study of the neural basis of reward-guided decision-making in which imaging suggests that a particular psychological approach or model is realized in the imaged brain activity. Shea goes on to outline how such an approach might also shed light on addiction and schizophrenic delusions.

In Chapter 63, "Psychopathology and the Enactive Mind," Giovanna Colombetti sketches an account of recent enactivist approaches to the mind, which draws on the phenomenology of Merleau-Ponty but also neuroscience. Specifically, she outlines the interplay of three key themes in enactivism: the "neurophenomenological" integration of first- and third-person data concerning lived experience and physiological activity for the study of consciousness; its emphasis on the integration of cognition and emotion; and the direct bodily and affective nature of intersubjectivity.

The final chapter of the section (Chapter 64), Michael Lacewing's "Could Psychoanalysis be a Science?," addresses its titular question. Although the particular issues outlined concerning the characteristic forms of psychoanalytic theory and practice and the way evidence for it can be marshaled both on its own terms and in combination with other approaches are distinctive, the chapter also serves as a microcosm for the issues that face psychiatry more broadly when critics ask about its scientific status.

CHAPTER 55

CAUSATION AND MECHANISMS IN PSYCHIATRY

JOHN CAMPBELL

INTERVENTIONS

Causation is not simply a matter of correlation. You cannot straightforwardly draw conclusions about what causes what from data about what is correlated with what. Consider, for example, the case of poverty and mental illness. There has long been thought to be a correlation between the two. But on the face of it, there are a number of different causal hypotheses that could explain this correlation. Maybe there is some third factor that causes both poverty and mental illness. Or it could be that poverty causes mental illness. Perhaps some people have a genetic vulnerability to mental illness that is only exposed by the stresses of poverty. Or perhaps the direction of causation is the reverse. Perhaps mental illness causes poverty. The natural suggestion is that the question could be resolved by an experiment. But here, as often in psychiatry, it is at first difficult to imagine an experiment that is practically possible.

An unexpected insight into the problem appeared in the course of an eight-year longitudinal study of the development of psychiatric disorders. Beginning in 1993, 1420 children aged nine, eleven, and thirteen years old were recruited for the study, from eleven counties in western North Carolina. Three hundred and fifty of them were American Indian children, living on a reservation crossing two of those eleven counties. In 1996, a casino opened on the reservation, and from then on every tribal member received a percentage of the profits, paid every six months. So here we have a "natural experiment." The amount paid out was enough to lift many of the affected families out of poverty. It was thus possible to look at the correlation between being lifted out of poverty and the incidence of mental illness. Suppose poverty does not cause mental illness. Suppose that the correlation is because of some third factor, a common cause, or because mental illness causes poverty. Then there should be no significant difference between the incidence of mental illness in the group that has been lifted out of poverty and those that have not been lifted out of poverty. On the other hand, if there is a difference in the incidence of mental illness among those who have been lifted out of poverty and those who have not been lifted out of poverty, that must reflect a causal connection from poverty to mental illness. Costello et al. (2003) found that there was indeed a correlation between mental illness and being lifted out of poverty, confirming that poverty is a cause of mental illness.

This particular study illustrates many of the key points about causation in psychiatry. Most strikingly, it displays the ineliminable role of the notion of an "intervention" in explaining the distinction between cause and correlation. Mere observation of a correlation between poverty and mental illness, however sustained, will not of itself lay bare what pattern of causal connections is underpinning the correlation. To find what the causal connections are is a matter of finding what happens when some factor—such as the action of an experimenter, or the construction of a casino—comes from outside the system we are considering and acts on one of the variables in the system, such as income.

To be fully explicit about the picture of causation that scientists typically work with here, we have to be more explicit than scientists usually are about the notion of an "intervention" that we are using. Of course, there are many points at which you might take issue with the Costello et al. study, but the underlying picture of what it is for there to be a causal connection between two variables, such as poverty and mental illness, seems reasonably clear. The picture is that for X to be a cause of Y is for X and Y to be correlated under interventions on X. Equivalently, we might state the idea by saying that for X to be a cause of Y is for it to be the case that in some cases, were there to be an intervention on X, there would be a difference in the value of Y.

Of course, the idea of an "intervention" is itself a causal notion, so we are not here explaining causation in terms of something else. This "interventionist" analysis is nonetheless an articulation of the approach to causation routinely presupposed by experimental science in general, not just psychiatry. The idea is that a causal claim is equivalent to a statement about the result of an idealized experiment. To say that smoking causes cancer is not just to say that smoking and cancer are correlated. It is to say that were there to be an ideal experiment in which the level of smoking in a community was varied, there would, for some variations at any rate, be a difference in the level of cancer (cf. e.g., Woodward 2003). (Of course, variation between ninety-nine and one hundred cigarettes per day might not make any difference to cancer levels; but there will be some variations for which there is a difference in cancer level.)

Thinking of things in this way puts a lot of pressure on the notion of an "intervention." In a randomized controlled trial, for example, the point of the design is to ensure that the experimental intervention meets some stringent conditions. Suppose, for example, that we have a basic setup to test whether a particular drug causes recovery from illness. We "randomly" assign our subjects to one of two groups. One group receives the drug treatment and the other (the control group) does not. We look at the rates of recovery from illness in the two groups and if the group receiving the treatment has better recovery rates we conclude that the drug causes recovery from illness. The point of the "randomization" is to try to ensure that (a) there is no hidden common cause of receipt of the drug treatment and recovery from illness (otherwise, for example, it might happen that the patients who were most energetic in trying to ensure their recovery were both getting into the treatment group and recovering better, not because of their treatment but because of the various other strategies they independently used to achieve better health), and (b) that there is no "accidental" factor systematically differentiating the patients in the treatment group from those in the control group that might affect recovery. The Costello et al. study used a number of more sophisticated strategies to try to achieve that same effect of "randomization" in its cohorts. In practice, there is always a question about whether such conditions have been met in any particular trial. But if the experimental intervention does meet all the relevant conditions, then a causal conclusion is implied by the results.

The basic ideas I am setting out about the connection between intervention and causation were explicitly characterized by Pearl (2000), Spirtes et al. (1993), and, in some ways most fully, by Woodward (2003). Following Woodward and Hitchcock (2003), we could define the notion of an "intervention" in terms of the notion of an "intervention variable." Suppose we have a family of variables in terms of which we are trying to characterize the causal functioning of a system. For example, we might consider "poverty" and "mental illness" to be a fragment of a full family of variables specifying the causes of mental illness. Then an "intervention variable" will be something that comes from outside the system, seizes control of our candidate "cause" variable X, and makes a difference to it. (Thus, for example, the action of an experimenter in administering a drug, or the construction of a casino and its consequent impact on earnings.) The causal question is whether there is then a difference in the value of our candidate outcome variable Y. The intervention variable I will have to meet a number of conditions (Woodward and Hitchcock 2003):

1. I causes X.
2. I does not cause Y otherwise than by X.
3. I is not correlated with any Z causally relevant to Y otherwise than via X.
4. I suspends X from its usual causes.

If these conditions are met, then we can say that for X to be a cause of Y is for X to be correlated with Y under interventions on X. For this definition to work, there are further conditions that must be met by the family of variables that we are using to characterize the system. For example, we might set two conditions on the variables in the family: (1) that they should be "independent" of one another (that is, each variable should relate to an aspect of the system distinct from any other variable), and (2) the family should be "complete," in the sense that there is no variable not in our family that is a common cause of some pair of variables in the family. We need some conditions like these if we are going to be able to read off the existence of a causal connection from the existence of a correlation under interventions between two variables. In the absence of condition (1), a correlation under interventions might merely reflect the fact that the two variables are not distinct, rather than a causal connection. In the absence of condition (2), the existence of a correlation under interventions between X and Y may reflect the operation of a hidden common cause of X and Y, rather than a causal connection between X and Y. But once all these points are in place, it is open to us to characterize the relation between causation and intervention in terms of correlation under interventions.

This approach to causation is of great importance to psychiatry. The reason it matters is that in principle, variables of any type whatever can be used: the variables X and Y could be economic, biological, psychological, or anything else. This matters because, in psychiatry at the moment, there seems in practice to be no one privileged level of causal explanation. A contemporary, biologically oriented psychiatrist might feel strongly that, in principle, psychiatric causation must ultimately be understood in terms of the operation of brain systems. A psychiatrist from a psychodynamic tradition might feel strongly that ultimately, mental illness has to be understood in terms of psychological variables. The empirical evidence at the moment, however, simply indicates the operation of a wide range of factors at different levels all being implicated in the causation of disorders. A characteristic survey of the factors underlying alcohol use, for example, would include a range of social, psychological, and genetic factors (cf. Kendler 2012). An interventionist characterization of causation allows us to make sense of a picture on which causation can occur with a collection of any type of variables.

The interventionist picture of causation allows us to address a number of problems that arise quite sharply in connection with talk about causation in psychiatry. These include:

1. The idea of a "level" of causal explanation. There are many different kinds of vocabulary that we can use to describe human beings as causal systems. To take a single broad contrast, we can describe human beings in mentalistic terms, and we can describe them in terms of their biology. What is the best way to describe human beings in characterizing the causal functioning of psychiatric disorders?
2. The idea of a "mechanism" underlying a psychiatric disorder. Many researchers in psychiatry would describe themselves as attempting to find the mechanisms underlying one or another disorder, or set of symptoms. But what notion of "mechanism" is being used here? People sometimes talk about psychological or brain mechanisms. But what is meant by that?

I will discuss these ideas in turn.

LEVELS OF EXPLANATION

It is a natural idea that there are strong a priori constraints on what a causal explanation in psychiatry must look like. A striking formulation of the main point here was given by Christopher Frith (1992). Frith wrote:

> Certain causal explanations for schizophrenia symptoms are simply not admissible. For example, I think it is wrong to say, "thought disorder is caused by supersensitive dopamine receptors," or "hallucinations occur when the right hemisphere speaks to the left hemisphere via a faulty corpus callosum" …
>
> Consider statements of the type "alien thoughts are caused by inappropriate firing of dopamine neurons." Let us assume that it is true that there is an association between alien thoughts and abnormal dopamine neurons. Nevertheless, the explanation is clearly inadequate. It says nothing about the nature of hallucinations nor the processes that underlie them. It does not say anything about the role of dopamine neurons within the physiological domain. Some might argue that, empirically, these details are irrelevant, because it is sufficient and important to demonstrate an association. This approach is very dangerous. In clinical research it is usually only possible to demonstrate association as opposed to causation ….
>
> A better, but still unsatisfactory way of linking mind and brain might be to say that "random, unnatural firing" of neurons lead to the patient having abnormal mental experiences. This is a dualist position in which the mind and the brain send messages to each other. This explanation

is inadequate because it does not explain how the mind normally distinguishes between a natural and an unnatural mental experience. At the neural level there must be a mechanism that permits a distinction between unnatural firings and those that form a proper part of a larger scheme....

My approach will be to develop as complete as possible an explanation at the psychological level. In parallel with this there should eventually be a complete explanation at the physiological level. (Frith 1992, p. 27)

It is, I think, very difficult not to sympathize with the point Frith is making here. It is, however, not easy to find a proper place for his idea. On the analysis I proposed in the "Interventions" section, there is indeed a distinction to be drawn between correlation and causation. But that distinction is drawn in terms of what happens under interventions. For dopamine neurons to be causing alien thoughts is not a matter merely of there being a correlation between particular firing rates of dopamine neurons and the experience of alien thoughts. It requires that an intervention on dopamine neurons would be correlated with a difference in the experience of alien thoughts. While that is certainly difficult to organize in practice, it is by no means impossible. But Frith's point is that the appeal to dopamine neurons is "at the wrong level" to give us a causal explanation of alien thoughts. What does that mean?

On the face of it, Frith is appealing to an idea that was decisively criticized by David Hume: the idea that there are a priori connections between cause and effect variables, so that we can tell well enough in advance of empirical inquiry that a particular variable cannot be the cause of a particular outcome. Of course it is natural to suppose that the world must exhibit a certain "intelligibility" to us, and to suppose that an attempt to explain the phenomena we encounter is a matter of trying to show that despite their apparently arbitrary nature, there is an underlying structure that has an a priori intelligibility. That seems to have been one of the impulses behind the mechanistic philosophy of seventeenth-century physics. It seems also to be one of the impulses behind the idea one finds in contemporary philosophy, that all psychological causation must be an exercise of rationality. Arguably, the form that this idea takes in contemporary science is that there are "levels of explanation." The suggestion here is not that we can know a priori which specific variables are the causes of which specific outcomes. The idea is rather, as the earlier quotation from Frith suggests, that each variable occupies a particular "level" and that only variables from the same level can function as causes of an outcome. What "level" a variable occupies is an a priori matter. It's not, in general, a matter for empirical discovery whether a variable is psychological or physiological, for example. Hume's critique of the idea of such a priori connections between cause and effect is brief and trenchant:

Every effect is a distinct event from its cause. It could not, therefore, be discovered in the cause, and the first invention or conception of it, a priori, must be entirely arbitrary. And even after it is suggested, the conjunction of it with the cause must appear equally arbitrary ... A man must be very sagacious who could discover by reasoning that crystal is the effect of heat, and ice of cold, without being previously acquainted with the operation of those qualities. (Hume 1748/1975, part IV/I)

Hume's point seems devastating to the idea of a priori constraints on what can cause what. There is after all no reason to suppose that the world we inhabit has been constructed so as to be penetrable by human reason. In principle, anything can be a cause of anything else. To take Frith's example once more, how can it be ruled out that the irregular firing of dopamine neurons could be a cause of alien thoughts? What we have here might simply be one of those arbitrary cause–effect relationships on which our world is grounded. The relationship can be discovered empirically. We can find whether interventions on the firing of dopamine neurons are correlated with the occurrence of alien thoughts. But why should there be any more "intelligibility" to a causal relationship than that?

I think that it is always important to bear Hume's uncomfortable point in mind when dealing with talk about "levels of explanation"; I think that it is genuinely easy to use the talk of "levels" as a way of bringing back the comforting idea of an intelligible world. But there is much more to be said on Frith's behalf. First, we might remark that in understanding the operation of a complex system, it is usually helpful to distinguish a level at which one gives the "box-and-arrow" description of the functional organization of the system, from a level at which one describes how that functional structure is implemented. For example, we can distinguish between the wiring diagram for a complex piece of electrical equipment, such as an amplifier, and a direct description of the physical constitution of the various pieces of wire and so on constituting it. To explain a malfunction of the equipment by saying "what causes the volume to drop out is the copper wire W overheating" is not adequate, even if there is a correlation under interventions between the volume drop-out and wire W overheating. To understand what's going on here, we really do need the wiring diagram together with an explanation of which box wire W is implementing, together with some understanding of the purely physical implications of overheating in wire W. Furthermore, there is a philosophical position according to which a psychological description of a human being is merely a description of their functional structure (Levin 2010). On this view, describing the psychological causes of someone's actions is actually a matter of giving a box-and-arrow diagram of the way in which that person is functionally organized. Saying "alien thoughts occur because of irregular firing of dopamine neurons" is, on this view, strictly analogous to saying that "what causes the volume to drop out is copper wire W overheating." So you might argue that similarly, the explanation of alien thoughts in terms of dopamine neurons needs to filled out by a fuller box-and-arrow description of the subject's psychology and where the alien thoughts fit in, and an account of which box the dopamine neurons are implementing, together with a purely physiological description of the consequences of dopamine neuron firing rates.

Of course, even with all that said, it remains true that in our electronics example, the statement, "what causes volume to drop out is wire W overheating," will be strictly true, if volume drop-outs are correlated under interventions on the overheating of W. It's only that there is some broader kind of explanation and understanding that we have when the functional architecture of the system is made explicit by a wiring diagram and we understand how W fits in. Similarly, it may be strictly true that "alien thoughts are caused by the firing of dopamine neurons," even if a broader understanding is provided by a functional characterization of the psychological system that generates alien thoughts.

You might argue that Frith's comments are not merely an appeal to the contrast between a functionalist level of explanation and an implementational level. Rather, you might argue, he should be read as appealing the specific architecture of classical cognitive science. On Marr's classic formulation, there are characteristically three levels in psychological explanation (Marr 1982, pp. 24–27). These are:

1. The computational level, at which we specify which task the system under study is performing.

2. The level of the algorithm, at which we specify the computational procedures that are used to accomplish the task.

3. The level of implementation, at which we say which biological systems are realizing these computational algorithms.

It is natural to wonder whether psychiatry should not in the end be aiming at such an approach to causal explanation (cf. Huys et al. 2011), and you might regard Frith's comments as implicitly appealing to some such picture as this, on which an account of the causes of alien thoughts must ultimately be integrated into a Marr-style explanation of the functioning of the system that generates our thoughts. There are, however, some basic problems. First, there typically may be nothing identifiable as "the computational point" of the kind of system we are dealing with in psychiatry. If we describe the workings of a complex engine, an air-conditioning system, for example, there will be something that a particular component, such as a regulator, is doing in the system. But that need not be a computational point; the air conditioning system is not fundamentally a computer. Similarly, whatever it is that underlies the recognition of thoughts as one's own in humans, there is no a priori reason to suppose that it is a computational system. More generally, there is no a priori reason to suppose that the systems involved in the generation of psychiatric disorders are, in general, computational systems. Consider, for example, the way in which depression is generated. There may be computations involved. It may be that computations relating to one's own social standing, for example, are implicated in the slide from humiliation to depression. But that does not show that the system we are considering here is fundamentally computational. Compare: a regulator in an air-conditioning system may have a chip that compares the outside temperature to the temperature inside the building and computes from that the pressure at which air should be circulated. It does not follow that the air-conditioning system is fundamentally a computer. Similarly, there may be some adaptive point that depression serves, but it does not follow that it is a computational point. Secondly, there is no reason to suppose that in general, a system implicated in the generation of psychiatric symptoms will have just one specifiable point. Does thought have just one adaptive point? Does depression? The psychology of the individual is a holistic system that has developed in a complex environment with many different demands on the individual. It does seem possible, in the case of early vision, to single out just one thing that a system is for: edge-detection, for instance. In the case of highly interconnected personal-level psychology, it is very much harder to single out a specific system and assign it a single point. Thirdly, in the case of visual systems, we have a relatively firm grasp on the distinction between correct and incorrect functioning of a system. In the case of psychiatric symptoms, it is very much harder to understand when we have correct as opposed to incorrect functioning. Consider, for example, the way in which grief is generated by bereavement. Is that the correct functioning of a system? If similar symptoms are generated in you by social humiliation, is that the system functioning correctly? It seems evident that we do not have a firm grasp on these distinctions.

Summing up, it does not seem that in psychiatry it will always be possible to identify "the" computational task that a system ought to perform, relative to which we could describe the algorithms performing that task and the physiology realizing those algorithms. It is difficult to take classifications over straightforwardly to psychiatry from the study of other, more "modular" areas of the mind. More generally, even the picture of ordinary psychological terms as functionally defined is not obviously correct (cf. Levin 2010), and it does not seem that psychiatry as such should take on any general commitment to functionalism. In general, it seems best to work with the minimal interventionist picture of causation, as involving a family of variables correlated with an outcome under interventions on those variables.

Mechanisms

I began with the Costello et al. (2003) study of the impact of poverty on mental illness. Notice that although it confirms that poverty causes mental illness, the study itself says absolutely nothing about the mechanism by which poverty causes mental illness. This is a quite general feature of experimental investigations into the existence of causal connections. Suppose, for example, that we have a randomized controlled trial to determine whether a particular drug has any impact on recovery from some illness. Suppose the trial is well executed and does establish a causal connection. The mechanism by which the drug is affecting recovery is a further question. Nonetheless, researchers usually feel very strongly that there "must" be a mechanism linking cause and effect. The idea of causation without a mechanism would strike most people as baffling. This is another element in Frith's comment quoted earlier, the sense that, as he puts it, "there must be a mechanism" that is not described if we say merely that alien thoughts are caused by the irregular firing of dopamine neurons. It is, therefore, natural to wonder whether characterizing causality in term of correlation under interventions is not relatively superficial. Isn't the true nature of causation to be found in the analysis of mechanisms?

The trouble with that way of putting things is that there is no way of explaining what a "mechanism" is without appealing to the idea of an intervention. To say what is and what is not a working part of a mechanism you have to ask: what would happen if this component were otherwise? And the counterfactual question you are asking here is a question about what would happen under an intervention (cf. Craver 2007).

Furthermore, the notion of a "mechanism" in general is remarkably obscure. In the case of the hypothesis that poverty causes mental illness, Costello et al. did suggest a possible "mechanism" by which variation in income might be making a difference to mental health. Two of the mental health outcomes they measured related to opposition conduct and deviant behavior. Their suggestion was that relief from poverty affected the amount of time that was available for parental supervision of children, and that this in turn was affecting oppositional conduct and deviant behavior. In what sense is this a "mechanism"? The simplest description is that we now have some causal variables intermediate between poverty and mental health. Poverty causes them, and they cause mental illness. Is that all there is to finding a "mechanism," that we find some further causal variables? If so, then the demand for a "mechanism" is something that can never be put to rest. Given any two variables, one of which is a cause of the other, we can always ask for further causal variables to be found between them. We have no way so far of distinguishing the case in which we have found a mechanism and can stop, from the case in which we do not have a mechanism at all, only a causal connection.

I think that the demand for mechanisms once again stems for our desire to find causal connections penetrable by reason, a desire to find our world fundamentally intelligible by us. This is the demand for intelligibility that Hume criticized. Hume's point was that causal connections are fundamentally arbitrary, and that there can be no demand that human reason should find them "intelligible."

In the case of physical objects, the classical conception of "intelligible causation" was the transmission of motion by impulse. Suppose one billiard ball collides with another, and the second one moves off. Why did that happen? The classical picture was that this needs no explanation; there could be nothing more intelligible in terms of which you might explain this phenomenon. So all explanation of physical phenomena should take the form of showing it to be nothing more than complex mechanical phenomena involving, in the end, no more than the transmission of motion by impulse. Hence the great mechanist program of seventeenth-century science. The mechanist program was, of course, completely mistaken. In particle physics today we find nothing of the intrinsic intelligibility that people had hoped for: we find only Hume's arbitrary conjunctions, impenetrable to reason. Still, a legacy of that program survives in our present-day insistence that "there must be a mechanism" when we are looking at the causation of psychiatric phenomena. The suggestion is that in explaining how alien thoughts can be caused by dopamine neurons, or mental illness by poverty, we must find an underlying, presumably biological, level at which we do have "something like" contact phenomena.

In the case of human psychology, our prototype of intelligible causation, the analog of the transmission of motion by impulse, is rationality. We take it that when we have an explanation of behavior in terms that make it rationally comprehensible, we can stop there. For example, if we ask why people spend more in times of high inflation, we think we have given a satisfying explanation if we can say why spending more in such a situation would seem rational, given what people believe and want. In contrast, suppose we have people who move from (a) perception of a row of empty tables in a café, to (b) belief that the world is ending. Here we have the sense of a kind of spooky "action at a distance" that demands some kind of filling-in, to explain how we got from this perception to that belief.

Now a demand for "mechanisms" that is rooted in a pre-Humean demand that causal connections should be penetrable by reason does not seem defensible. Causal connections as such are fundamentally arbitrary associations under interventions with "distinct existences." Since cause and effect are distinct existences, the relation between them cannot be penetrable by reason. It's just a mistake to elevate into a priori truths our own tendencies to think comprehensible the transmission of motion by impulse, or rational psychological transmissions. This point is particularly important to bear in mind in psychiatry, where we frequently encounter psychological causation that does not appear to be rational.

To illustrate what I mean by letting go the demand for "mechanisms," consider a simple model. There are a number of predictors of major depression, both psychological and biological. Suppose that we give them a causal interpretation. Thus, suppose that, in line with the findings of Kendler et al. (2003), we take it that humiliation, particularly humiliation with a social twist, is a cause of major depression. Suppose too that, in line with a great deal of speculation, we assume that problems in serotonin transporter mechanisms are causes of major depression (cf. Lotrich and Pollok (2004) for a skeptical review, however). Now not everyone who is humiliated becomes depressed. Suppose we think of serotonin problems as related to one's resilience in the face of humiliation. Now we have two factors that have been identified as coordinate causes of depression. We might assume that this can be tested by using extensive longitudinal studies, in which there are "natural interventions" on humiliation or on serotonin. So we have a pair of variables of two different types, psychosocial and biological, that jointly generate depression. What is the "mechanism" by which these two variables jointly generate depression? It might be, of course, that we can give a reductive analysis of humiliation, as consisting in some particular biological condition. But suppose for the moment that this turns out not to be possible; suppose, for example, that insofar as we can find brain correlates of humiliation, they are massively multiple, non-uniform, scattered, and not always co-present. "Humiliation" is still a reasonably well-defined psychological variable. We simply may not be able to find some systemic "mechanism" by which humiliation and serotonin imbalances produce depression; certainly we have no a priori guarantee that there is such a thing. The idea that "there must be a mechanism" does not seem to be empirically grounded. It seems, rather, to be the expression of an a priori insistence that causal connections must somehow be penetrable by reason. As we have seen, that is a natural and persistent idea. But it seems to be wrong, as Hume pointed out. The correct empirical approach is simply to find which collections of variables are correlated under interventions with outcomes of psychiatric interest. Whether there is a single "level" or "mechanism" in terms of which everything can be understood is not a matter to be settled a priori. After all, what is the neural correlate of poverty?

Causal Grammars and Control Variables

There is another way of thinking about the idea that "there must be a mechanism." Philosophers have often distinguished between two levels at which one can characterize scientific theorizing:

1. The general pattern, or patterns, of explanation that one finds in a particular well-established domain of science, as opposed to
2. Particular explanations of particular phenomena in that domain (cf. Godfrey-Smith 2003).

So, for example, suppose we find a genetic predictor of vulnerability to a particular physical disease, such as cancer. At an early stage of the investigation, we might find that we are fairly confident that the genetic characteristic is a cause of cancer, but not understand the details of how it is bringing about cancer. When we say in this case that "there must be a mechanism" by which the genetic base brings about cancer, we need not be appealing to any a priori ideas about how causal explanation must go. We may rather be appealing to the existence of many detailed explanations of how genetic factors generate physical illnesses, and demanding something similar in this case.

This idea can be developed within the framework of the broadly interventionist account of causation I have sketched so far. All that we have as yet required of our cause variables is that intervention on them should make a difference to the values of our outcome variables. But there are further constraints we should put on the family of variables that we use to characterize the causal dynamics of a complex system. Most of the problems that are usually discussed under the heading of "levels of explanation" or "mechanisms" can be thought of in this way. What we have to leave behind is the idea that these matters should be addressed by a priori reflection. Correlatively, we will also leave behind the idea that there is some *contrast* between thinking of causation as a matter of what happens under interventions, and thinking of causation as a matter of what mechanisms there are linking one phenomenon to another. It's natural to think in terms of a contrast here: one thinks of the "mechanisms" as being the actual-world nuts and bolts, the rods and levers, that underpin the truth of counterfactuals about what would happen were there to be an intervention. As we have seen, the trouble is that we have no way of saying what is and what is not a working part of the machine without appealing to facts about what would happen under an intervention on that part. And in psychiatry in general, we have no idea what the "machine" in general might be. Of course the brain will play an important role in any future psychiatry; but so too will economic, social and psychological variables. Still, I think that we can find what is right in the idea of "mechanisms" of causation in psychiatry by looking at the considerations that should govern our choice of a family of variables to characterize the causal functioning of whatever system we are considering.

Joshua Tenenbaum and his colleagues have begun developing the idea of a "causal grammar," on analogy with a grammar for a language (cf. e.g., Tenenbaum and Griffiths 2007). The idea is that in any domain, there are principles governing the construction of a well-formed causal explanation. Consider, for example, some simple types of causal explanation of physical diseases. We can think of ourselves as having a family of variables divided into three classes:

1. Behaviors (understood broadly to include aspects of the environment one is in, e.g., working in a coal-mine).
2. Diseases
3. Symptoms of diseases.

We typically think in terms of patterns in which type-1 variables cause type-2 variables, which in turn cause type-3 variables. Of course, in any particular case disagreement is possible over just which behaviors are causing just which diseases, and over which diseases cause which symptoms. But these are disputes within the same general framework. In contrast, the idea that coughing, for example, causes one to work in a coal-mine, seems barely comprehensible. The idea is that this suggestion would violate a principle of "causal grammar." It's not that the suggestion is a priori absurd or incoherent, you can perfectly well imagine situations in which that is what happens. It's rather that this is a logical possibility not recognized in the kind of framework for theorizing about diseases that we ordinarily use. It is, as it were, "grammatically inadmissible." The correctness of a "causal grammar" is itself, of course, an empirical matter. It might turn out that our current framework for theorizing about diseases should be overturned. But that kind of paradigm shift, in Kuhn's term, is a much more radical change than merely moving to recognition that smoking, for instance, is one of the causes of cancer.

Of course, the simple description I gave earlier, of ways of thinking about the causes and effects of diseases, is far too simple even for this particular case. The constraints on what a medical researcher would think an adequate description of the causes and effects of a disease are far more various and subtle than my earlier description suggests. And the possibilities for the formal characterization of causal grammars are far richer than I have suggested (Griffiths and Tenenbaum 2007). But from our present synoptic perspective, these are matters of relative detail and complexity.

My proposal is that we should leave behind the picture of a "mechanism" as the collection of rods and levers that underpins the truth of counterfactuals about what would happen under an intervention. Instead, we should think of causal explanation as a matter of finding a family of variables interventions on which make a difference to the value of our outcome variable, governed by the causal grammar for that domain. The question now is what sense we can have of the right "causal grammar" for descriptions of causation in psychiatry.

Consider the following collection of variables proposed as causally implicated in alcohol dependence (from Kendler 2012): (1) latent genetic risk, (2) aldehyde dehydrogenase (ALDH; a group of enzymes implicated in alcohol oxidation) variants, (3) variants in the gamma-aminobutyric acid (GABA; a neurotransmitter) receptor system, (4) childhood sexual abuse, (5) frontal lobe dysfunction, (6) impulsivity, (7) peer deviance, (8) social norm expectations, (9) taxation. These are, plainly, variables of quite different types. Yet none of them seem to be redundant, given the others. Is there some privileged "level" or "mechanism" in terms of which all these causes of alcohol dependence should be understood? You might argue that after all, the brain is implicated in all of these causal connections, and that therefore, the "level" of the "mechanism" is the level of brain physiology. The problem with this line of argument is immediately evident. Consider the impact of taxation on alcohol dependence. Brains are implicated here. Does it follow that the causal impact of the cost of alcohol on incidence of alcohol dependence is best analyzed by brain imaging? The absurdity of supposing that the causation here has to be understood in terms of brain mechanisms is particularly evident, but a similar point will evidently apply to many of the other causal factors listed earlier.

Still, this list of causes of alcohol dependence may seem unsatisfyingly haphazard. We have the various symptoms of alcohol dependence and the various causes above. Mustn't there be some "core" or bottleneck in the disorder, through which those various causes are funneled to generate the symptoms? The trouble is that there is no evidence for such a bottleneck. There might be one, but there is no evidence for it.

The problem is that we do not have a family of satisfying, well-established explanations of particular psychiatric disorders that could provide patterns for the explanation of further disorders. Rather, the case of alcohol dependence discussed seems to be the general case in psychiatry at the moment. We can find collections of factors that have been established to be predictive of a particular disorder. Often, we can go further and make the claim that interventions on those factors would make a difference to whether the patient contracts the disorder. And that is all there is to our understanding of psychiatric disorders. We have no further patterns of complete, satisfying explanation of a disorder to which to appeal in explaining what a complete explanation of, for example, alcohol dependence might look like. If you look, for example, at the earlier list of causes of alcohol dependence, then you may feel impelled to say, "but there must be a mechanism" by which these factors severally and jointly generate alcohol dependence. By this you mean that there must be filled-out explanation of a familiar sort that would include these variables as elements, and show their role in a bigger picture. That's what you have in mind when you say, for example, that "there must be a mechanism" by which smoking causes cancer. The trouble is that in the case of psychiatry, as opposed to physical illness, there are no "filled-out explanations of a familiar sort" to which to appeal as explaining what one means when one says "mechanism." You literally do not know what you are talking about.

There is a more conservative way in which we could try to structure our investigations into the causes of psychiatric disorders. We have to look for variables interventions on which are correlated with differences in our outcome variables. There will be many families of variables that do that. Each candidate family of cause variables for our outcomes will have to consist of variables that are independent of one another, in the sense mentioned earlier, of relating to "distinct existences" in Hume's phrase. And we will want it to be complete, in the sense that there is no common cause of any two variables in the family that is not itself in the family. But there are going to be further conditions that can make one family of variables a better candidate than another for being a way of describing the causal functioning of the system.

A start is provided by Austin Bradford Hill's criteria for causation (Hill 1965). Hill gave a number of criteria, let me select just three: size, specificity, and dose–response relationships. Suppose we are considering whether smoking is a cause of cancer. The first point is that the size of the correlation between the two is a factor in assessing the evidence for a causal relationship. If smoking increases the risk of cancer by a factor of 200, that is a stronger case for a causal relationship than if the increase in risk is a factor of 1.2. The second point is that the case for having correctly identified a causal relationship, such as the relationship between smoking and cancer, is stronger if the cause variable, smoking, predicts a change in the value specifically of the outcome variable, cancer, rather than, for instance, a more general tendency to ill health. The last point is that the case for a causal link between smoking and cancer is strengthened by the existence of a dose-response relationship between the two: the greater the number of cigarettes smoked, the greater the risk of cancer.

These kinds of criteria for causation are evidently of great practical importance. But it has always been difficult to see what place, if any, they have in an analysis of causation itself. For on the face of it, there could in principle be causal connections even though these conditions were not met. What I want to suggest is that they can be read as providing criteria for variable choice. Given two families of variables that we can use to characterize the causes of a particular outcome, we can decide between them by choosing the family of variables that provides the best "control panel" for our outcome, in the sense of providing the variables intervention on which results in big, specific and systematic (dose–response) changes in our outcome variable. These are comparative rather than absolute criteria. It could be that our best "control panel" for a psychiatric outcome will, in absolute terms, seem to provide variables that do not have particularly strong, specific or systematic impacts on the outcome. But it will nonetheless be the candidate family of cause variables that has the best score by these criteria.

We could in principle construct a set of fine-grained biological variables that, cell-by-cell, gives a complete picture of the condition of a brain. Alternatively, we could in principle construct a set of psychological variables that gives a complete picture of someone's psychology. These two sets of variables would not be independent of one another. The physical and the psychological variables are not describing "distinct existences" in Hume's sense. So we could not simply take the union of the two sets of variables to give us the causes of psychiatric disorders. They are competing candidates for the characterization of the causes of disorders. They are likely to have different problems. The set of fine-grained biological variables is unlikely to hold variables that have specific or systematic relationships to the outcomes of interest in psychiatry. There is no one cell, for example, whose firing-rate will have a strong, specific and systematic correlation with major depression. The set of psychological predicates is likely to do better on that score, but is unlikely to be complete, in the sense that it will need supplementation by biological variables (e.g., recall the possibility that serotonin levels constitute the difference between those who are resilient in the face of humiliation and those who contract depression). Fortunately, our choice of a set of variables to characterize the causes of disorders is not confined to the purely biological or the purely psychological. The situation illustrated by the collection of causes for alcohol dependence listed earlier is typical of the current situation in psychiatry: a motley collection of variables of quite different types. Such a motley list may in the end prove to be the best "control panel" possible for a given disorder: that is, the collection of variables interventions on which are best correlated with strong, specific, and systematic changes in the disorder itself. For the moment, at any rate, that seems to be the situation with the analysis of causation in psychiatry. It is natural to feel that one must go beyond that, to find "the mechanisms" on which these causal relations depend. But my point has been, not that this feeling is wrong, but that there is no saying what it means.

References

Costello, E. J., Compton, S. N., Keeler, G., and Angold, A. (2003). Relationships between poverty and psychopathology: A natural experiment. *Journal of the American Medical Association*, *290*(15), 2023–9.

Craver, C. (2007). *Explaining the Brain*. Oxford: Oxford University Press.

Frith, C. (1992). *The Cognitive Neuropsychology of Schizophrenia*. Hillsdale, NJ: Lawrence Erlbaum Associates.

Godfrey-Smith, P. (2003). *Theory and Reality: An Introduction to the Philosophy of Science*. Chicago, IL: University of Chicago Press.

Griffiths, T. L. and Tenenbaum, J. B. (2007). Two proposals for causal grammars. In A. Gopnik and L. Schulz (Eds), *Causal Learning*, pp. 323–45. Oxford: Oxford University Press.

Hill, A. B. (1965). The environment and disease: Association or causation? *Proceedings of the Royal Society of Medicine*, *58*, 295–300.

Hume, D. (1975). *An Enquiry Concerning Human Understanding*. Oxford: Clarendon Press. (Original work published 1748.)

Huys, Q. J. M., Moutoussis, M., and Williams, J. (2011). Are computational models of any use to psychiatry? *Neural Networks*, *24*, 544–51.

Kendler, K. S. (2012). Levels of explanation in psychiatric and substance use disorders: Implications for the development of an etiologically based nosology. *Molecular Psychiatry*, *17*, 11–21.

Kendler, K. S., Hettema, J. M., Butera, F., Gardner, C. O., and Prescott, C. A. (2003). Life event dimensions of loss, humiliation, entrapment, and danger in the prediction of onsets of major depression and generalized anxiety. *Archives of General Psychiatry*, *60*, 789–96.

Levin, J. (2010). Functionalism. In E. N. Zalta (Ed.), *The Stanford Encyclopedia of Philosophy* (Summer 2010 Edition). [Online.] Available at: <http://plato.stanford.edu/archives/sum2010/entries/functionalism/>.

Lotrich, F. E. and Pollok, B. G. (2004). Meta-analysis of serotonin transporter polymorphisms and affective disorders. *Psychiatric Genetics*, *14*, 121–9.

Marr, D. (1982). *Vision*. San Francisco, CA: W. H. Freeman.

Pearl, J. (2000). *Causation*. Cambridge: Cambridge University Press.

Spirtes, P., Glymour, C., and Scheines, R. (1993). *Causation, Prediction and Search*. New York, NY: Springer-Verlag.

Tenenbaum, J. B., Griffiths, T. L., and Niyogi, S. (2007). Intuitive theories as grammars for causal inference. In A. Gopnik and L. Schulz (Eds), *Causal Learning*, pp. 301–22. Oxford: Oxford University Press.

Woodward, J. (2003). *Making Things Happen: A Theory of Causal Explanation*. Oxford: Oxford University Press.

Woodward, J. and Hitchcock, C. (2003). Explanatory generalizations, part 1: A counterfactual account. *Nous*, 37, 1–24.

CHAPTER 56

....

NATURAL KINDS

....

RACHEL COOPER

What are natural kinds? Are mental disorders natural kinds? Why does it matter? Let's start with rough and ready answers, and then assess complications later.

Paradigmatically, natural kinds are the kinds of thing or stuff that are classified by the natural sciences. The periodic table provides perhaps the best example of the potential importance of natural kinds for science. The periodic table provides a classificatory basis for chemistry that enables different types of stuff to be classified, and via this classification, for them to be understood and controlled. Thus, once I have determined that a particular chemical sample is lead, say, I know how it will behave and how to treat it if I wish to use it in various ways. Classification grounds explanations and predictions, and enables us to control a domain. If mental disorders are natural kinds, perhaps we can hope that one day psychiatric classification will ground psychiatric theory and practice in a way that approaches the successes of the periodic table in grounding chemistry.

In the philosophy of psychiatry, debates over whether mental disorders can be natural kinds emerge because kinds of mental disorder are manifestly different from chemical kinds in various ways. While chemical kinds are precise, psychiatric kinds are fuzzy. While chemical kinds are objective, the identification of psychiatric kinds is value-laden. Psychiatric classification involves classifying people, and unlike chemical elements, people can respond to being classified in various ways. Later in this chapter I will go through these differences, one-by-one, and argue that despite them, mental disorders may be natural kinds.

Thus we have our rough and ready answers: natural kinds are kinds picked out by the sciences. Identifying natural kinds is worthwhile because such kinds can ground explanations and predictions and enable us to gain control over a domain. Although kinds of mental disorder differ from the kinds recognized by sciences such as chemistry in various ways, they may yet be natural kinds (though this will not be shown until later in this chapter). Now for the complications.

What are Natural Kinds?
Three Traditions Distinguished

In this chapter we will focus on natural kinds understood as the kinds that are picked out by scientific classifications. However, the literature on natural kinds can be hard to navigate as different authors mean different things when they talk of natural kinds and are interested in different sorts of problem. Other authors have also noted the heterogeneity of natural kind concepts and suggested various classifications (Haslam 2002a; Murphy 2006; Zachar, in press). I suggest that we can usefully divide the literature into three traditions:

First, and I think most importantly for the philosophy of psychiatry, there is the tradition on which we will focus, call it the "kinds-in-science" tradition (e.g., Dupré 1993, 2001, 2006). This tradition is impressed by the power of classification in science and is interested in those kinds that facilitate such successful classifications. Paradigmatic examples of natural kinds are taken to be chemical kinds and biological species. When writers in this tradition seek to understand natural kinds they seek to understand kinds like these, and how they can be employed in scientific practice.

Second, there is an Aristotelian tradition. In the Aristotelian tradition, talk of natural kinds is taken to be of importance not only for explaining the behavior of members of a kind (as in the kinds-in-science tradition) but also for making sense of problems concerned with identity, development, and change (Ayers 1981; Brody 1973; Megone 1998). For Aristotelians, the character of an individual depends on what kind of thing it is, and the ways in which individuals can change while yet retaining their identity thus depends on the natural kind to which they belong. Thus a caterpillar changing into a butterfly continues to be the same individual, because such changes are part of the natural development of individuals of that type, while a caterpillar that is eaten by a bird ceases to be. Aristotelians take biological kinds to be key examples of natural kinds. Within the philosophy of psychiatry, Chris Megone employs Aristotelian traditions of natural kinds in making sense of mental disorder (1998, 2000). Megone argues that humans are essentially rational animals and that mental disorders can be understood as states that inhibit human flourishing. Aristotelian approaches might also be used to make sense of some of the problems that mental disorders can raise for questions relating to the identity of persons. In some dissociative conditions, for example, we may wonder whether identity is destroyed or fragments. Insofar as the Aristotelian tradition makes use of natural kind talk in understanding the development and destruction of individuals it might prove useful for exploring such issues. To date, and as far as I am aware, however, such work has yet to be undertaken.

Third amongst our traditions of natural kinds, there are New Essentialists (e.g., Ellis 2001, 2002). New Essentialists are principally interested in essences. An "essence" or "essential property" is a property that all members of a kind share that determines their nature. In the case of chemical elements, for example, the essence would plausibly be the atomic number. While Aristotelians also talk of essences they can be distinguished from New Essentialists as their very different metaphysical stance leads them to nominate very different candidates for "essences." Aristotelians will suggest that "being a rational animal" might be the essential property of humans. New Essentialists think of essences as being the properties fundamental physics and chemistry find explanatory. New Essentialists have principally been interested in the metaphysical implications of a kind having such an essential property; for example, some have argued that natural laws are necessary. They have restricted their interest to those kinds, such as fundamental particles and chemical elements, which plausibly do have essences in their sense. Insofar as other kinds, such as biological species, fail to have such essences, thinkers working in this tradition simply lose interest in them. This tradition is of the least interest for the philosophy of psychiatry as it is highly unlikely that kinds of mental disorder will have essential properties in the same sort of way as chemical elements.

These three traditions use the term "natural kind" slightly differently and are concerned with slightly different issues. Within the philosophy of psychiatry, confusions between them have resulted in much misunderstanding. Misunderstanding between those adopting a kinds-in-science approach (according to which natural kinds may or may not have essences) and essentialist approaches (on which natural kinds must have essences by definition) has resulted in much discussion failing to get beyond the stage where one author takes the plausible absence of essences to show that mental disorders cannot be natural kinds (e.g., Haslam 2002b; Zachar 2000), while another argues that mental disorders can be considered natural kinds on some non-essentialist account of natural kinds (e.g., Cooper 2005). In order to avoid such misunderstandings, when talking about kinds it is best to be explicit about what one has in mind, and also to bear in mind that there are various different usages in circulation.

RETURNING TO THE KINDS-IN-SCIENCE TRADITION: HOW DOES IDENTIFYING NATURAL KINDS PLAY A ROLE IN SCIENCE?

How does identifying natural kinds play a role in science? If we limit ourselves to thinking about kinds such as the chemical elements, the answer to this question may at first seem clear. Why is it we can expect all samples of some element to behave similarly? Because, all samples of an element share an "essential property"; they all have the same atomic number, and this ensures that they will have the same chemical properties. In theoretically important respects, all samples of a particular element are interchangeable.

Turn to biological species, however, and we will soon see that thinking in terms of essential properties will not quite do. Classifying biological individuals into different species has proved highly successful as a classificatory strategy; members of a species can be expected to behave in similar ways. However, plausibly it is not the case that all members of a species share some essential property. Within a species, diversity is the rule at both the genetic and phenotypic level. As John Dupré (1981, 1993) has powerfully argued there are simply no essential properties to be found.[1]

Within the kinds-in-science tradition on which we are focusing, several accounts of kinds have been developed with the aim of explaining how it is that kinds like biological species can successfully ground explanations and inductive inferences even though members of the species do not share some essential property. Insofar as any kinds of mental disorder might be expected to be rather like other biological kinds these accounts are of particular interest for the philosophy of psychiatry.

John Dupré has offered an account that he calls promiscuous realism (1981, 1993). He asks us to consider the entities of some domain mapped into a multidimensional space where the different dimensions map onto different properties (as in cluster analysis). Entities that are similar to each other will form clusters in such a space. Dupré suggests that kinds such as biological species can be identified with some such clusters. Of course, in the multidimensional space, not only biological species, but also multitudes of other clusters may be identified—some will correspond to classifications at levels higher or lower than species, for example, families, and varieties, will also be identifiable. The key claim for Dupré is that the world is such that some individuals are objectively similar to each other.[2] They share similar properties and will thus behave alike. In my 2005 *Classifying Madness*, I argue that a Dupré-style account can fruitfully be applied to kinds of mental disorder.

In another cluster-type account, Richard Boyd has argued that we might usefully think of biological species as being "homeostatic property clusters" (1988, 1991). Like Dupré, Boyd argues that members of a species share a cluster of properties, but in addition Boyd emphasizes that this is for a reason. Homeostatic mechanisms ensure that members of the kind will continue to be alike—in the case of biological species these mechanisms include gene flow between members of the species, and environmental pressures that mean that those organisms which survive must all be capable of surviving in the same environmental niche. The difference between Dupré's account and Boyd's is that Boyd requires homeostatic mechanisms to "glue together" a property cluster, whereas Dupré requires no glue. In the philosophy of psychiatry, Dominic Murphy suggests that Boyd's account of natural kinds might accommodate certain mental disorders (Murphy 2006, pp. 338–341).

---

[1] Dupré argues that there are no necessary and sufficient criteria for species membership. It will not do to say that members of a species can interbreed. Not only is such a criterion inapplicable to asexual species, but it also runs into problems dealing with sterile organisms, hybrid organisms, etc. It will not do to rely on criteria of ancestry. While it is true that rabbits have rabbit ancestors and hares have hare ancestors, this is not enough to distinguish rabbits from hares, as some other criterion will be required to distinguish the ancestor rabbits from the ancestor hares. Nor can measures of genetic or phenotypic similarity be used to pick out co-members of a species. Some species are more heterogeneous than others, so there is no level of difference that is necessary and sufficient to mark species boundaries.

[2] The claim that some pairs of entities are objectively more similar to each other than other pairs is common to all accounts of natural kinds. To illustrate, two twin tigers would be said to be more similar to each other than some other pairs of entities, for example, a tiger and a balloon. Such similarities are seen as objective features of the world. The tiger twins share more properties than do the tiger and the balloon. Such claims are compatible with many metaphysical accounts of properties, but not with all of them. In particular, there are certain nominalist positions on which the idea that some pairs of entities are more similar than others makes no sense (for example, Goodman 1972). Discussing the details of the various accounts of properties is far beyond the scope of this chapter. Interested readers might consult Mellor and Oliver (1997), or Armstrong (1989).

A further account of biological kinds has been produced by Ruth Millikan (1999). She emphasizes the role of copying mechanisms that make it the case that biological kinds are fundamentally historical kinds, with the similarity of organisms of a species ensured by the fact that copying mechanisms make offspring like their parents. Turning to mental disorders, copying mechanisms may also play a role in explaining why cases of a kind are alike. Ian Hacking has developed a number of case studies of epidemic mental disorders where unconscious copying mechanisms result in similar cases occurring (Hacking 1995a, 2010). Marion Godman (2011) is currently developing the idea that certain kinds of mental disorder can best be understood as historical kinds.

Plausibly different accounts might work best for different mental disorders. Millikan-style copying, for example, will clearly have a greater role to play in some mental disorders than others. There is still work to be done figuring out exactly which account of kinds will work best for which kinds of mental disorder.

Reasons why Natural Kinds of Mental Disorder Might Seem Problematic

A number of writers have suggested that kinds of mental disorder cannot be natural kinds. In this section I examine their arguments.

On gaps

It is frequently assumed that natural kinds should be discrete—that is, when the members of any two natural kinds are plotted in a multidimensional space, there should be a gap between them (DeSousa 1984, p. 565; Haslam 2002b; Mill 1973, p. 123; Reznek 1987, p. 42; Samuels 2009). I suggest, however, that gaps, where they occur, are not important. The important thing about natural kinds is that members of a natural kind are all objectively similar to each other. The basic idea is that the causal structure of the world is such that certain entities are to a large extent interchangeable, in the sense that their similar properties mean that they can be expected to behave in much the same fashion. Thus, once I have learnt how to grow one radish seed, I will be able to grow any radish seed, because they really are all much the same—the similar causal natures of the seeds mean that they will need the same sorts of environmental conditions to flourish. When it comes to grounding predictions and explanations and enabling us to control the world, it's the similarities between members of a kind that do all the work. Some kinds are gappy (e.g., chemical elements, as atomic numbers only come in integer numbers) and some kinds vary along dimensions (e.g., alloys), but this difference doesn't much matter. Alloys provide nice examples of continuously varying kinds that can yet ground explanations and predictions. If I know the makeup of a sample of alloy I can predict its properties just as accurately as if I know the identity of a sample of pure metal. For this reason I suggest that we should consider kinds that vary along dimensions to also be natural kinds. Given that such dimensional kinds can do all the important work of traditional discrete natural kinds there is no benefit in restricting the term "natural kind" to discrete kinds.

Turning to consider mental disorders, discussion by those who argue that mental disorders might in some cases be better represented by a dimensional, as opposed to a categorical, classification system has revolved around two sorts of case. First, there are cases where one type of disorder seems to merge into another—thus, for example, depressive disorders might run into anxiety disorders. Second, there are cases where a disorder fades into the normal range. Once again depression provides an example, as there seems to be no natural dividing line between normal unhappiness and mild depression. In both cases, I suggest, that the really important question is whether cases that are classified together genuinely share properties. Whether there are any sharp boundaries that can be drawn between the kind "depression" and other kinds is then a distinct, and less important, question.

On values

On many accounts, a condition is only a disorder if it is a bad thing (Cooper 2002; Flew 1973; Fulford 1989; Reznek 1987; Wakefield 1992). Given that disorders are defined partly in value terms, but that natural kinds need to be defined with regard to natural properties, it may thus look like types of disorder cannot be natural kinds (as an example of someone who takes this line of argument see Peter Zachar (2000b)).

We can respond to this worry by thinking through an analogy. Weeds are unwanted plants, and so whether a particular plant is considered a weed or a flower can vary with the tastes of the gardener. The umbrella category "weed" is defined in terms of values and is not a natural kind. However, the different species of weed, such as dandelion and dock, are still natural kinds. Although whether a particular plant counts as a weed depends on values, the fact that it is a dandelion, or a dock, depends solely on its natural properties. Similarly, while the category "mental disorder" is value-laden and does not form a natural kind, conditions that are commonly disorders—schizophrenia, depression, and so on—may still be natural kinds. To complete the analogy, let's imagine that some particular process underpins cases of schizophrenia. Let's suppose that such a process occurs within some individual, but in that person the process does no harm—they hear voices but are not harmed by their condition. In such a case, I suggest we could say that the individual has schizophrenia, but not a disorder. While schizophrenia is frequently a kind of disorder, in cases where it does no harm, it might simply be considered a kind of difference. In the same way, while dandelions are generally weeds, the dandelions in my wild flower garden are not weeds, though they are still dandelions. I conclude that types of condition that are usually mental disorders might be natural kinds even though the umbrella category "disorder" is not a natural kind.

My reasoning here would imply that someone could have schizophrenia and yet not be mentally ill. Some would take terms such as "schizophrenia" to be themselves value-laden and would say that someone biologically and psychologically of the "schizophrenic-type," but who is not harmed by their condition, does not have schizophrenia. I suspect that current concepts of "schizophrenia" are insufficiently defined for it to be clear whether the term is itself value-laden, or whether it is a purely descriptive term that falls under a value-laden umbrella category (as the "weed" analogy would suggest). Building on work by Joseph Laporte (2004), I think it likely that the extension of such terms will become more precise in the future as the relevant linguistic communities reach a consensus on how such terms should be used.

In his book *Natural Kinds and Conceptual Change* (2004), Laporte uses case studies to examine controversies that have emerged in the history of science because the extension of terms is sometimes not as precise as emerging circumstances require. For example, he considers how the scientific community reacted to the discovery that samples of jade fall into two chemically distinct kinds. Laporte argues that prior to the discovery it was indeterminate whether "jade" referred to all samples of a particular chemical structure or to all samples with particular superficial characteristics. Following the discovery that samples of "jade" fall into two chemical varieties it was necessary for the fuzziness of the extension to be clarified and it was eventually decided that "jade" would apply to both varieties.

I suggest that the discovery that some voice-hearers are not harmed by their condition brings out indeterminacies in the extension of "schizophrenia" in a way analogous to that in which the chemical discoveries brought out indeterminacies in the extension of "jade." Whether one should think of terms like "schizophrenia" as value-laden or, as the weed analogy suggests, as a purely descriptive term that falls under a value-laden umbrella term will ultimately be a matter for decision by the relevant linguistic communities (primarily mental health professionals, researchers, and service users). The factors to be weighed in making such a decision will be complex. Still, the weed analogy shows that it would be possible to precisify terms like "schizophrenia" and "depression" in such a way that they became confirmed as natural kind terms.

On cultural shaping

The "natural" in "natural kind" should be read as in "natural law" as opposed to "present in the garden of Eden." Some natural kinds are man-made; plutonium is an example. Still, there might be thought to be something problematic about the extent to which kinds of mental disorder are shaped by culture. Plausibly, mental disorders have varied greatly across cultures and history. This may lead one to doubt that natural kinds of disorder can be picked out. Maybe the disorders that are found in one context are simply different to those that are found in another? Depending on the sorts of cultural shaping that occur, different responses to this worry are appropriate.

Superficial variation

As an example of superficial variation consider how the content of delusions varies with time and place. In Europe, in the early modern period, there were people who believed themselves to be made of glass or earthenware (Speak 1990). Nowadays deluded people have different fears. Such variation is easy to understand. It's commonly the case that the superficial properties of members of natural kinds vary with environmental conditions. For example, apple trees can be grown tall or flat against walls depending on how they are pruned. Variation at a superficial level is fully compatible with types of mental disorder being natural kinds.

Deeper cultural molding

More profound types of cultural molding may also occur. In *Creating Mental Illness* (2002), Allan Horwitz makes a convincing case that "most nonpsychotic symptoms stem from general underlying vulnerabilities that may assume many different overt forms, depending on the cultural context in which they arise … Cultural processes, not the unfolding of natural disease, structure the overt manifestation of symptoms into recognizable entities" (p. 108). Horwitz argues that whether a vulnerable and distressed person manifests a disorder characterized by depression, or anxiety, or somatization, or some other symptom, depends on their cultural context. If Horwitz is right, then not only "superficial" properties shift with cultural setting.

In thinking through such cases of "deep molding," considering some of the kinds that occur in other natural historical sciences can be illuminating. Specifically, let us consider the different sorts of igneous rocks that are recognized by geologists. These rocks are all formed from magma. All the different igneous rocks are made from the same basic stuff, but their characteristics vary depending on the conditions under which they were formed. The size of the crystals in the rock depends on the rate of cooling, for example. Igneous rocks are classified according to their chemical composition and their history (both of which can vary continuously). Classifications of rock are complex. Still, the different kinds of rock can be considered natural kinds. Samples of a kind of rock are objectively similar to each other and distinguishing rock kinds is useful for grounding explanations and inductive inferences.

If Horwitz is right and different anxiety-depression type disorders are formed into distinct entities by cultural context, then we can think of such disorders as being kinds analogous to the different kinds of rock distinguished by geologists. Admittedly such historical natural kinds may only occur under certain conditions (in *Mad Travelers* (1998) Ian Hacking shows this is the case for fugue, for example). Still, though such disorders may occur for a limited time or in limited places, within those constraints the kinds operate like normal natural kinds. Historical natural kinds—such as kinds of rock, and culturally formed type of mental disorder, can usefully be considered natural kinds, I suggest, because the kinds can support explanations and inductive inferences and feature in law-like generalizations. The individuals that fall into such kinds are "repeatables" in the sense that any two specimens of basalt, or any two cases of fugue, can be expected to have much in common.

At this point some may worry that in suggesting that even some culturally formed mental disorders can be considered natural kinds, I have come a very long way from what many have meant when they talk of natural kinds. My kinds need not have essential properties, can vary along continua, and can be historically contingent, in that they may only arise under certain historical conditions. The reason I think it's reasonable to call such kinds natural kinds is that they are up to the job of grounding explanations and predictions. To take an example, anorexia may plausibly be a culturally formed mental disorder, and yet is the sort of kind that can help ground psychiatric science. We can know that anorexia is hard to treat, anorexia is very dangerous, many women with anorexia will cease menstruation, and so on.

Interaction

Over the last few decades, Ian Hacking's work has stressed the importance of the fact that humans respond to being classified in ways that other classified entities do not (1986, 1988, 1992, 1995a, 1995b). A child who is told they are stupid may stop trying at school and fall behind yet further; a diagnosis of "problem drinking" may come to motivate abstinence; a whole class of people may respond to a classification with new forms of resistance, as in "fat pride." Such interactions between classifications and behavior mean that "human kinds"— the kinds classified by the human sciences—become moving targets. No sooner has a kind been picked out than behaviors shift and classifications have to be revised.

One of Hacking's best developed examples of such "looping effects" concerns multiple personality disorder (1995a). When cases of multiple personality disorder were first reported, a person with multiple personality disorder would typically possess just two or three clearly distinct personalities. Over time, however, the symptoms of people with multiple personality disorders shifted. Hacking makes a convincing case that the shift in symptoms was in part caused by changing prototypes of the disorder being made available in the media. The media tended to report more florid cases, and over time people with multiple personality disorders started to present with more and more personalities, and as their numbers increased, these personalities became more diverse and also more fragmentary. Note that Hacking's claim is not that patients intentionally copy the symptoms of publicized cases. Rather the mechanism is more subtle and subconscious, but still the consequence is that a distressed individual will most likely manifest distress in ways that are culturally recognized.

At certain points in his work, Hacking has claimed that interaction between kinds and their classification, as seen in the case of multiple personality disorder, marks an important distinction between natural kinds and human kinds, such that human kinds cannot be natural kinds. Previously, I have argued that Hacking is wrong on this point (Cooper 2004). The gist of my argument is this: It is true, as Hacking has claimed, that human kinds shift in response to classificatory practices, and this requires classifications to be updated. However, this is not sufficient to show that human kinds cannot be natural kinds. Other types of natural kind also shift in response to pressures that only affect kinds of their particular type. For example, types of domestic animal and plant shift as a result of selective breeding and only types of domestic animal and plant can be selectively bred (Boyd 1991). It is of course important to note that particular types of kind are vulnerable to shifting under different types of pressures, but there is no reason to think that these differences mark any fundamental metaphysical distinctions.

Hacking also proposed a supplementary argument, which used Elizabeth Anscombe's claim that intentional actions are intentional under a description to argue that the new descriptions formulated by the human sciences made new types of action logically possible (Anscombe 1957; Hacking 1986, 1995a). I have argued that this argument is based on a misinterpretation of Anscombe's work (Cooper 2004). Her claim that intentional actions are only intentional under-a-description should be interpreted as being equivalent to the claim that an intentional actions is only intentional qua some aspect (an example she gives is one where a bird intends to land on the twig qua a way to get the seed, but not qua a way to land in the bird trap) (Anscombe 1971). This translation of Anscombe's claim makes it clear that formulating new descriptions does not make new actions logically possible.

In his most recent work, Hacking has himself shifted away from talking of natural and human kinds on the basis that talk of "natural kinds" has become so laden with metaphysical baggage that the term in now best avoided (2007). This is a claim with which I am sympathetic, although the approach suggested in this chapter is that rather than jettisoning the terminology one should be explicit about what one has in mind when talking about natural kinds.

Functionally defined kinds

A number of writers have argued that psychological kinds cannot be natural kinds because they are functionally defined (McGinn 1991). Functionalists about the mind claim that mental states are characterized by their causal role. That is, the nature of a mental state is fixed by the types of stimuli that typically produce it, its causal relations with other mental states, and the types of behavior that it typically produces. Thus, for example, fear is a state that is characteristically produced by stimuli like charging bulls, snarling dogs and aggressive gun men, interacts with other mental states, such as the belief that help can be summoned, and leads to behavior like screaming for help and running away. Functionalism implies that mental states can be multiply realized. Any state that fits the right causal role counts as a mental state, no matter what its physical realization. Thus, while my fear of dogs is realized by some neural state, your fear might be realized by some quite different brain state, and a robot's fear would be realized by electronics. Given that cases of the same psychological kind (e.g., fears) can be physically unalike, these kinds look very unlike prototypical natural kinds, where the similar behavior of members of the kind occurs because the members are physically similar.

This problem can be dealt with in at least two ways. First, and most simply, we can note that the claim that mental states are theoretically multiply realizable is compatible with all human mental states being realized in much the same way (Kim 1993, pp. 305–335). In robots and Martians fears may be realized by all sorts of different systems, but in humans all fears may be linked to some particular anatomy. This means that human psychological states of a kind may all be physically alike.

Second, we can note that even when the kinds of some domain are functionally defined when they are working properly, the kinds of breakdown that occur need not be functionally defined. Consider electronic components, for example. These are functionally defined— anything that behaves like a capacitor is a capacitor, and capacitors can be made of different materials. Still, the ways in which capacitors can break down depend on the physical stuff that different types of capacitor are made of; for instance, some are brittle while others are not. Insofar as we might think of mental disorders as arising when normal mental functioning breaks down it is consistent to think that, even if normal mental states are functionally defined, abnormal ones might not be. For example, I might be a functionalist about normal beliefs and desires, and yet also think that human mental states are vulnerable to certain types of disruption that are characteristically caused by drinking too much alcohol. In the same sort of way that only brittle capacitors are vulnerable to breaking by smashing, only thinkers with a certain biology will be vulnerable to certain sorts of mental disruption. Being a functionalist about normal mental states is thus compatible with thinking that kinds of mental disorder may be natural kinds.

Admittedly, being a functionalist about normal mental states is also compatible with thinking that mental disorders are functionally-defined. In order to motivate this position, though, some further reason for thinking that mental disorders are functionally-defined would need to be provided. David Papineau (1994) presents an argument for thinking that any disorders that can be characterized as stemming from dysfunctional patterns of learnt behavior and thinking will be functionally defined. However, the scope of Papineau's argument is limited, as many mental disorders cannot plausibly be seen to have their origins in faulty learning.

ON FINDING NATURAL KINDS

OF MENTAL DISORDER

When seeking natural kinds the aim is to find categories that map the causal structure of the domain being classified. How might natural kinds of disorder best be identified? The distinction between the context of discovery and the context of justification has fallen from favor in recent philosophy of science, but appealing to something like it is here useful. The basic thought is as follows: The key task is to group cases together in such a way that co-members of a category really are importantly similar to each other. Co-members of a category should share properties that mean they can be expected to behave in similar ways. Depending on one's account of kinds, one might also require that these similarities can be explained by the existence of homeostatic mechanisms or via copying. How such a classification is achieved doesn't matter.

Within current psychiatry, research traditions seek to construct classifications in various ways. Most dominant is the approach associated with the *Diagnostic and Statistical Manual of Mental Disorders* (DSM), but there are also competing traditions that propose that classifications might be developed using the methods of numerical taxonomy, or propose radical overhauls to classification on the basis of some theory or other.

Though they may not describe their aim in these terms, I take it that research programs such as that associated with the DSM aim at discovering natural kinds of mental disorder. A basic assumption of the DSM project is that discovering kinds of mental disorder will be important for grounding psychiatric theory. Furthermore, the procedures for revising the DSM assume that fixing the boundaries between kinds will be informed by empirical evidence. In seeking natural kinds of disorder, the DSM has tended to rely on tradition which is then revised as more and more empirical data is found. The sorts of evidence appealed to when the DSM is revised (rates of comorbidity, family studies, drug response, differences in age of onset, etc.) can reasonably be hoped to enable us to map the causal structure of the domain of mental disorders. One might have concerns about the ways in which non-scientific factors might affect the process of DSM revision. Plausibly the classification has been affected by lobbying that is politically or financially motivated (Cooper 2005; Kutchins and Kirk 1997). Since the days of the DSM-III, however, the processes for revising the DSM have become less open to distortion. For example, committees are now expected to publish details of the literature on which they have based their decisions (in the DSM-IV *Sourcebooks* (Widiger et al. 1994, 1996, 1997), and online for the DSM-5) and those serving on the committees responsible for revisions are expected to limit their financial links with the pharmaceutical industry (see, e.g., guidelines of committee membership; American Psychiatric Association 2010). One might still worry that, insofar as the default position is that disorders remain between successive editions of the DSM, problematic categories inherited from DSM-III will remain. Still, the basic approach of the DSM-system to seeking natural kinds—start with a classification system and revise it as new evidence suggests—is a reasonable way to seek to achieve a classification of natural kinds, at least so long as one assumes that the traditional classification system from which the DSM has tried to progress via incremental stages is on roughly the right tracks. One worry is that if the initial classification was thoroughly misguided then the DSM process of revision, which allows revisions only when an advance over the existing classification can be proven, may not allow the classification system to ever reach an optimal state. Rather the classification could get stuck at a suboptimal point, in the same way in which evolving organisms can get stuck at local maxima in fitness space.

Worries such as this lead those who do think that the starting point for the DSM is likely unsatisfactory to suggest full-scale overhaul. Some theorists have suggested classifications based on some overarching theory—maybe, evolutionary theory (Murphy 2006) or developmental approaches. Insofar as such classifications depend on the theoretical approach used to develop them they can only be expected to be as good as the theory behind them. Alternative approaches to classification involve the use of statistical methods to find kinds of disorder from raw data. On occasion, the proponents of "numerical taxonomy" have claimed that their approach is purely empirical and generates theory-free classification systems (e.g., Sokal and Sneath 1963). The claim that the techniques of numerical taxonomy are theory-free is misguided. Before the techniques of numerical taxonomy can be applied one must decide which properties will be entered into the analysis, and decide which of the various statistical techniques to apply. One's theories will shape decisions at both these levels (Cooper 2005, chapter 3). Still, though they are not theory-free, the techniques of numerical taxonomy offer one approach to seeking natural kinds of disorder.

What if the categories developed by different classificatory approaches fail to correspond to each other? For example, what if a classification that is developed on the basis of treatment response fails to correspond to that developed by geneticists, which in turn fails to correspond to that used by those taking a developmental perspective? We can note that such a situation also occurs in other sciences. Within biology, for example, Dupré has convincingly argued that the species concepts that are required in different areas of biological research fail to correspond to each other (Dupré 2001). While ecologists find it most useful to classify species on the basis of current characteristics, evolutionary theorists find it better to classify on the basis of ancestry. Dupré suggests that in such a situation different scientific subdisciplines should be free to classify as they find most useful. On Dupré's metaphysical picture, the world is a complex place. Many categories can usefully be picked out for different scientific purposes, and so there are multiple sets of natural kinds that different subdisciplines might find it useful to classify.

WHICH DISORDERS AREN'T NATURAL KINDS

In this chapter we have come a long way from the traditional idea that natural kinds will be eternal, discrete, and possess essential properties. I have argued that a looser notion of natural kinds is sufficient to give us kinds that can do the important work of grounding inductions, explanations, and predictions. We can say that natural kinds are groups of entities that are genuinely importantly similar to each other (and where, depending on one's account, theses similarities might be explained by the existence of homeostatic mechanisms or via copying). If we take this approach, are there any kinds of mental disorder that will fail to be natural kinds?

Finding natural kinds of mental disorder can still be expected to be difficult, and some current categories of mental disorder will fail to be natural kinds because they fail to group together cases that are similar to each other in any causally important respect. Most obviously, ragbag categories included in the DSM for completeness, such as Psychosis NOS, will fail to be natural kinds for this sort of reason. It may also turn out that some prima facia more respectable diagnoses fail to pick out natural kinds of disorder because they lump together heterogeneous cases. For example, if schizophrenia turns out to be an umbrella term for a number of conditions with differing underlying causal structures then schizophrenia would fail to be a natural kind.

IMPLICATIONS OF MENTAL DISORDERS BEING NATURAL KINDS

If types of mental disorder are natural kinds, what are the implications? Occasionally, it is claimed that if types of people fall into kinds then there are ethical or political implications. In *The Disorder of Things*, Dupré claims that when types of people are considered to form distinct natural kinds "it is inevitable that any systematic differences that are found will be taken to be explained, or explicable, in terms of the intrinsic differences between members of the two kinds" (1993, p. 253). This leads "to the legitimation of conservative politics and to the discouragement of proposals for significant social change" (1993, p. 256). Here, I think Dupré is simply mistaken. Take an example of human natural kinds—men and women—and consider some of the systematic differences between them. On average, women give birth to more children and are paid less than men. Here we have no problems recognizing that some but not all of the differences are due to intrinsic differences, and that some but not all of the differences might be ameliorated by progressive social policies. Believing in human natural kinds is compatible with holding any range of political views.

One implication that I think is important is that if types of mental disorder are natural kinds then this means that there may be grounds for optimism that one day successful therapies will be developed that will enable the mass treatment of disorders. If mental disorders are natural kinds, then this means that one case of a kind can be expected to behave like other cases of that kind. All cases of a kind will be alike in important respects. This means that a treatment that works for one of the kind can be expected to work for all. As a consequence, if mental disorders are natural kinds, then we can hope that "black-box" therapies may one day be available. A black-box technology is one that a consumer can simply buy off-the-shelf (so named because they are typically sold in a black box) (Mackenzie 1993). Black-box technologies may originally have been hard to develop, but have now been perfected so that they can be produced on an industrial scale, and delivered in a form that can be used reliably by people who don't understand how they work. Lasers offer an example. Originally getting lasers to work was very difficult, but now they can be bought off-the-shelf. Successful drug therapies would provide the most straightforward example of black-box therapies. Developing drugs is, of course, difficult. However, once the right chemical has been found, drug treatments can ideally be refined to the stage where they can be produced on an industrial scale and taken with reliable effect by people with little understanding. Think of paracetamol, or the contraceptive pill.

It will only be possible to develop black-box therapies for mental disorders if the disorders are natural kinds. The therapies can only be developed to work reliably insofar as the problems of those in the treatment group are all fundamentally similar. Note that although drug therapies offer the clearest promise of black-boxability, other forms of therapy might also be black-boxable. Suppose it turns out that depression can reliably be cured if a person plays football for half an hour a day, and spends an hour talking to others. Such a therapy would be black-boxable in my sense, as it is the sort of therapy that can be packaged such that it can be reliably reproduced by unskilled therapists (or reliably used for self-treatment). Ultimately the reason why it matters whether mental disorders are natural kinds is that if it is possible to classify mental disorders in such a way that cases that are importantly theoretically similar are classified together, then it may be possible to develop treatments that can successfully treat all cases of a kind.

Conclusions

In this chapter we have examined accounts of natural kinds, and asked whether types of mental disorder might be natural kinds and why it matters. We started by noting that different theorists define "natural kind" in different ways and are interested in different problems. One of the key claims of this chapter is that the variety of uses of the term "natural kind" means that it is important to be explicit exactly what one means when talking about natural kinds and to be clear what points are at issue. I have suggested that if we are interested in natural kinds insofar as they support explanations, inductions, and predictions then the key question for the philosophy of psychiatry is whether it will be possible to classify mental disorders in a way that maps the causal structure of the domain of mental disorders. The aim is to classify cases together when they are similar to each other in causally important ways and to classify them apart when there are no such similarities. Depending on the models of mental disorder that turn out to be correct, the similarities between cases of mental disorder that are important might be similarities with regard to neurotransmitter levels, or genetic abnormalities, or developmental history, or patterns of learnt responses, or whatever, or some combination of such similarities.

We examined various objections to mental disorders being natural kinds (in this weak sense) and showed how they could be overcome. I argued that classifications that distinguish natural kinds of mental disorder might be created in a variety of ways. We saw that the implications of there being kinds of mental disorder are important and yet ethically and politically limited. If there are natural kinds of mental disorder then we can hope that a treatment that successfully treats one-of-a-kind might also treat others-of-that-kind. Ultimately this is why searching for natural kinds of mental disorder is worthwhile.

References

American Psychiatric Association (2010). *Board of Trustee Principles*. [Online.] Available at: <http://www.dsm5.org/about/Pages/BoardofTrusteePrinciples.aspx>.
Anscombe, E. (1957). *Intention*. Oxford: Basil Blackwell.

Anscombe, E. (1971). Under a description. (Reprinted in Anscombe, E. (1981). *Metaphysics and the Philosophy of Mind*. Oxford: Basil Blackwell.)

Armstrong, D. (1989). *Universals: An Opinionated Introduction*. Boulder, CO: Westview Press.

Ayers, M. (1981). Locke versus Aristotle on natural kinds. *Journal of Philosophy*, 78, 247–72.

Brody, B. (1973). Why settle for anything less than good old-fashioned Aristotelian essentialism. *Nous*, 7, 351–65.

Boyd, R. (1988). How to be a moral realist. In G. Sayre-McCord (Ed.), *Essays on Moral Realism*, pp. 181–228. Ithaca, NY: Cornell University Press.

Boyd, R. (1991). Realism, anti-foundationalism and the enthusiasm for natural kinds. *Philosophical Studies*, 61, 127–48.

Cooper, R. (2002). Disease. *Studies in History and Philosophy of Biological and Biomedical Sciences*. 33, 263–82.

Cooper, R. (2004). Why Hacking is wrong about human kinds. *British Journal for the Philosophy of Science*, 55, 73–85.

Cooper, R. (2005). *Classifying Madness*. Dordrecht: Springer.

De Sousa, R. (1984). The natural shiftiness of natural kinds. *Canadian Journal of Philosophy*, 14, 561–80.

Dupré, J. (1981). Natural kinds and biological taxa. *The Philosophical Review*, XC, 66–90.

Dupré, J. (1993). *The Disorder of Things*. Cambridge, MA: Harvard University Press.

Dupré, J. (2001). In defence of classification. *Studies in History and Philosophy of Biological and Biomedical Sciences*, 32, 203–19.

Dupré, J. (2006). Scientific classification. *Theory Culture Society*, 23, 30–2.

Ellis, B. (2001). *Scientific Essentialism*. Cambridge: Cambridge University Press.

Ellis, B. (2002). *The Philosophy of Nature*. Chesham: Acumen.

Flew, A. (1973). *Crime or Disease?* London: The Macmillan Press.

Fulford, K. W. M. (1989). *Moral Theory and Medical Practice*. Cambridge: Cambridge University Press.

Godman, M. (2011). Grounding natural kinds in the "special sciences." PhD thesis submitted to King's College London.

Goodman, N. (1972). Seven strictures on similarity. In *Problems and Projects*, pp. 437–47. Indianapolis, IN: Bobbs-Merrill.

Hacking, I. (1986). Making up people. In T. Heller, M. Sosna and D. Wellbery (Eds), *Reconstructing Individualism*, pp. 222–36. Stanford, CA: Stanford University Press.

Hacking, I. (1988). The sociology of knowledge about child abuse. *Nous*, 22, 53–63.

Hacking, I. (1992). World-making by kind-making: Child abuse for example. In M. Douglas and D. Hull (Eds), *How Classification Works*, pp. 180–238. Edinburgh: Edinburgh University Press.

Hacking, I. (1995a). *Rewriting the Soul*. Princeton, NJ: Princeton University Press.

Hacking, I. (1995b). The looping effects of human kinds. In D. Sperber and A. Premark (Eds), *Causal Cognition*, pp. 351–94. Oxford: Clarendon Press.

Hacking, I. (1998). *Mad Travelers*. Charlottesville, VA: University of Virginia Press.

Hacking, I. (2007). Natural kinds: Rosy dawn scholastic twilight. *Royal Institute of Philosophy Supplement*, 61, 203–39.

Hacking, I. (2010). Pathological withdrawal of refugee children seeking asylum in Sweden. *Studies in History and Philosophy of Biological and Biomedical Sciences*, 41, 309–17.

Haslam, N. (2002a). Kinds of kinds: A conceptual taxonomy of psychiatric categories. *Philosophy, Psychiatry, & Psychology*, 9, 203–17.

Haslam, N. (2002b). Natural kinds, practical kinds, and psychiatric categories. *Psycholoquy*, *13*. Available at: <http://psychprints.ecs.stonon.ac.uk/>.

Horwitz, A. (2002). *Creating Mental Illness*. Chicago, IL: University of Chicago Press.

Kim, J. (1993). *Supervenience and Mind*. Cambridge: Cambridge University Press.

Kutchins, H. and Kirk, S. (1997). *Making Us Crazy*. New York, NY: The Free Press.

Laporte, J. (2004). *Natural Kinds and Conceptual Change*. Cambridge: Cambridge University Press.

MacKenzie, D. (1993). *Inventing Accuracy: A Historical Sociology of Nuclear Missile Guidance*. Cambridge, MA: MIT Press.

McGinn, C. (1991). Mental states, natural kinds and psychophysical laws. In *The Problem of Consciousness*, pp. 126–52. Oxford: Basil Blackwell.

Megone, C. (1998). Aristotle's function argument and the concept of mental illness. *Philosophy, Psychiatry, & Psychology*, *5*, 187–201.

Megone, C. (2000). Mental illness, human function and values. *Philosophy, Psychiatry & Psychology*, *7*, 45–65.

Mellor, D. H. and Oliver, A. (1997). *Properties*. Oxford: Oxford University Press.

Mill, J. S. (1973). *Collected Works of John Stuart Mill* (J. Robson, Ed.). London: Routledge.

Millikan, R. G. (1999). Historical kinds and the "special science." *Philosophical Studies*, *95*, 45–65.

Murphy, D. (2006). *Psychiatry in the Scientific Image*. Cambridge, MA: MIT Press.

Papineau, D. (1994). Mental disorder, illness and biological dysfunction. In A. Griffiths (Ed.), *Philosophy, Psychology & Psychiatry*. *Royal Institute of Philosophy Supplement 37*, pp. 73–82. Cambridge: Cambridge University Press.

Reznek, L. (1987). *The Nature of Disease*. London: Routledge & Kegan Paul.

Samuels, R. (2009). Delusion as a natural kind. In M. Broome and L. Bortolotti (Eds), *Psychiatry as Cognitive Neuroscience*, pp. 49–79. Oxford: Oxford University Press.

Sokal, R. and Sneath, P. (1963). *Principles of Numerical Taxonomy*. San Francisco, CA: W. H. Freeman and Company.

Speak, G. (1990). An odd kind of melancholy: Reflections in the glass delusion in Europe (1440–1680). *History of Psychiatry*, *1*, 191–206.

Wakefield, J. (1992). The concept of mental disorder—on the boundary between biological facts and social value. *American Psychologist*, *47*, 373–88.

Widiger, T. A., Frances, A. J., Pincus, H. A., First, M. B., Ross, R. R., and Davis, W. W. (Eds) (1994). *DSM-IV Sourcebook Volume 1*. Washington, DC: American Psychiatric Association.

Widiger, T. A., Frances, A. J., Pincus, H. A., First, M. B., Ross, R. R., and Davis, W. W. (Eds) (1996). *DSM-IV Sourcebook Volume 2*. Washington, DC: American Psychiatric Association.

Widiger, T. A., Frances, A. J., Pincus, H. A., First, M. B., Ross, R. R., and Davis, W. W. (Eds) (1997). *DSM-IV Sourcebook Volume 3*. Washington, DC: American Psychiatric Association.

Zachar, P. (2000a). Psychiatric disorders are not natural kinds. *Philosophy, Psychiatry, & Psychology*. *7*,167–182.

Zachar, P. (2000b). *Psychological Concepts and Biological Psychiatry: A Philosophical Analysis*. Amsterdam: John Benjamins.

Zachar, P. (in press). Beyond natural kinds: Toward a "relevant" "scientific" taxonomy in psychiatry. In. H. Kincaid and J. Sullivan (Eds), *Mental Illness and Natural kinds*. Cambridge, MA: The MIT Press.

CHAPTER 57

···

THE MEDICAL MODEL
AND THE PHILOSOPHY
OF SCIENCE

···

DOMINIC MURPHY

INTRODUCTION

In this chapter I will sketch an account of psychiatric explanation with roots in contemporary philosophy of science and suggest that it is a natural fit with what I will call the strong interpretation of the medical model in psychiatry. I will start by distinguishing between strong and minimal ways to understand the medical model before I move on to talk about explanation. The basic idea of this chapter is that the logic of the medical model, together with recent developments in the sciences of the brain, suggests that psychiatry should be seen as a kind of cognitive neuroscience. The second part of the chapter discusses some issues in applying mechanistic explanatory models to mental disorders. Recent philosophical work on explanation in the cognitive neurosciences has seen it as *mechanistic* explanation. A mechanistic explanation shows how components of a system interact to give rise to the phenomenon to be explained.

THE MEDICAL MODEL

What is the medical model?

Defining the medical model in a satisfactory way is difficult. A recent paper (Shah and Mountain 2007, p. 375) offered this: "the 'medical model' is a process whereby, informed by the best available evidence, doctors advise on, coordinate or deliver interventions for health improvement. It can be summarily stated as 'does it work?'" As a piece of rhetoric this is likely to be unpersuasive, since few convinced opponents of the medical model are likely to think, "Well then, I must not be interested in the best available evidence, or perhaps I don't consider health improvements to be the aim of my work." The more grievous problem with this definition is that it is so broad as to be uninformative. Contrast it with another broad definition of what is supposed to be a rival psychiatric orientation, the biopsychosocial model. Ghaemi (2010, pp. 62–63) dissects a recent discussion of the biopsychosocial approach that presents it as having six "central aspects." Taken together these add up to the claim that the biopsychosocial model integrates a variety of perspectives and makes the patient's circumstances central to the provision of clinical care along several dimensions. Ghaemi argues that none of these differentiate the biopsychosocial approach from several other traditions in psychiatry.

Very general definitions that elide differences between research programs may capture an important fact about clinical procedure, viz., that many clinicians operate with a rough and flexible set of assumptions and rules of thumb that can be shared across whatever they take their theoretical orientations to be. However, if you are a philosopher of science trying to understand and evaluate research programs and traditions of inquiry, you like the issues that divide them to be nice and stark. To understand how different research programs make their different channels of inquiry through the world and succeed (or do not) in telling us how the world works, we need to be able to find a set of claims that let us tell them apart, while at the same time allowing for changes in traditions over time and not cutting things so finely that coherent shared assumptions dissolve into myriad individual practices.

If we constrain Shah and Mountain's definition by limiting what counts as evidence for diagnosis and outcome, though, it arguably does capture a broadly held commitment to what we might call a minimal interpretation of the medical model. A minimalist interpretation offers a general commitment to empirical methods, such as epidemiological information or information about dose–response relationships for particular drugs. It could also include information about risk factors such as genes or family environments, and see disorders as syndromes—sets of signs and symptoms that occur together and have a predictable history. These bodies of information are all recognizably medical, and permit the gathering of further information about diagnosis, prognosis and treatment (Bishop and Trout, Chapter 60, this volume). The minimal interpretation is therefore recognizably medical in terms of the information it collects, the concepts it employs, and the practices it supports, but it makes few, if any, commitments about what is really going on with the patient. What is characteristic of what I'll call the strong version of the medical model is a set of commitments about the nature of mental illness that treat it as a disease and suggest a set of further philosophical commitments about explanation which I will explore in subsequent sections.

The strong interpretation of the medical model

A minimal interpretation about the medical model, then, makes no commitments about the underlying physical structure of mental illness. But the strong interpretation does. It says that what psychiatrists describe as "mental illnesses" are diseases that are causally explained by their underlying pathophysiology. It is committed to specific causal hypotheses in terms of abnormalities in underlying neurobiological systems, which are responsible for the observed patterns of signs and symptoms. An example of the view is Nancy Andreasen's (2001, pp. 172–176) argument that an explanation of mental illness will ultimately cite destructive processes in brain systems, just as bodily diseases are explained by such processes in other organs. The process can mediate the effects of cultural forces or other environmental risk factors. Nor does the cause of disorder have to completely destroy a brain system: it may be enough to put the system into a stable but chronically dysregulated state. The way to understand the scientific part of the two-stage view, then, is that there are, in psychiatry, phenomena that fit the conception of disease as a destructive process realized in bodily organs that predominates in biomedicine generally.

Many skeptics see this stress on pathophysiology as an invitation to reductionism, leading to a search for molecular or genetic mechanisms that misses much of what is important about mental illness. But strong reductionistic programs (Kandel 2005) reflect a metaphysical taste for a privileged level in nature rather than the logic of medicine. The basic commitment of the medical model is this: a disease is a breakdown or suboptimal deviation in normal functioning due to a pathogenic process unfolding in some bodily system. Breakdowns need to be understood in the light of the normal case.

What might a competitor to the medical model look like? Well, many approaches to mental illness might share some aspects of the minimal medical model, such as the use of statistically sophisticated epidemiological information. However, there are a number of ways to reject core properties of the medical model as I present it. One could reject the very notion of mental diseases. One way to do this would be to, as some psychoanalysts did, dispute the very idea that there is a distinction between the mentally healthy and the mentally ill. Without going so far, one might nonetheless think that mental disorders are just not enough like diseases more generally to make the assumptions of the medical model very useful (Arpaly 2005). Another way to reject a key assumption of the medical model would be to accept that the normal causal explanations of the life sciences apply to organic brain conditions but deny their usefulness for explaining abnormalities in human experience. The medical model assumes that we can talk about some brains as dysfunctional and others as falling within normal or neurotypical ranges of functioning, and that the explanation of the abnormalities can be carried out using the vocabulary of some favored science of the brain. It does not require us to limit ourselves to biochemical explanations, but it does assume that causal explanations are possible using the resources of, for example, as I shall suggest, cognitive neuroscience. If you think that no such causal explanations can do much to increase our understanding of human minds, you are likely to find the medical model unpersuasive. Rejecting the medical model does not commit you to rejecting materialism about human beings, but it does commit you to rejecting a fundamentally mechanistic view about what people are like.

Brains

Biological systems normally contribute to the overall functioning of an organism, which we can think of as a wider set of systems that maintain themselves in equilibrium. A collection of integrated systems adds up to an organism, which, though dependent on the environment and relating to it in myriad ways, does not fit into it as a component of a wider system in the way that an organ fits in to a physiological system. The physiological systems all help to maintain in being an organism that strives to survive and reproduce. It was Claude Bernard (1865/1927) who argued that the major systems in the human body seek to maintain homeostasis—in his favorite example, by regulating the chemistry of the blood. Organisms can only explore and transform the external environment if they have sufficient internal stability. On this view the answer to the question "What are the major physiological systems for?" is "To keep the internal environment stable." Bernard missed the other important dimension—behavior evolved not just to maintain the organism in being but also to enable it to reproduce, and that involves a number of bodily changes of state. Nevertheless, the basic idea is sound: organisms are a hierarchy of biological systems that make contributions to the systems that contain them, all the way up to the level of the organism.

Suppose we think of diseases as departures from normal functioning, as the strong medical model does. Then understanding disease means understanding the normal function of bodily systems, and in psychiatry that typically means the systems that make up the brain. Mental diseases are instances of the brain not doing what it should, so we need to understand normal function and pathological function in terms that make that perspicuous—we ask what the system has evolved to contribute to the overall system that it partly constitutes, and how it is failing to do that. As Thagard (2008, p. 340) puts it clearly:

> The circulatory system consists of a set of components—the heart, veins, arteries, and blood—that interact to provide nutrients to the rest of the body. This mechanism is susceptible to many kinds of breakdown, such as defects in the heart valves, blockage in the arteries due to plaque and blood clots, and abnormal growth of blood cells. These breakdowns can arise because of many kinds of interacting causal factors, from internal ones such as defective genes to external ones such as infectious agents.
>
> Similarly, the explanation of mental diseases requires specification of the normal functioning of the brain and other relevant organs, along with precise description of the different kinds of breakdown that can impede mental functioning.

The specification of the system and the specification of the ways it can break down need to mention whatever concepts are necessary for understanding. The components of the brain are systems that govern the cognitive, sensory, and motor capacities of the person. It is normal in the neurosciences these days to view these systems as processing information. Cognitive scientists now employ computational models based on conceptions of information processing developed in the middle of the twentieth century, but the basic idea of the central nervous system as a computational system dates back to the late nineteenth century, and the development of ideas that biological relations among parts of the nervous system can be modeled mathematically as dynamic transformations of the weights assigned to energy levels in and between cells, so that the output of a neuron is a function of the inputs to it. Furthermore, some of the energy flowing through the system was modeled as sensory information ultimately derived from the environment, and specific states of at least sensory systems could be correlated with external states of affairs. This conception of the nervous system informs Freud's early thinking about the mind, and was common among his teachers. Much of it survives today in recognizable form as connectionism (Glymour 1992).

So a tradition within neuroscience since the nineteenth century understands the brain as an information-processing organ—in which, for example, learning is a process that adjusts connections between cells. We should distinguish this wider tradition from more recent claims which are characteristic of cognitive psychology, viz., that thought is manipulation of symbols: physical entities with semantic and syntactic properties. In my 2006 book (Murphy 2006) I followed a wing of the strongly medical psychiatric community in urging that psychiatry should adopt the methods of contemporary cognitive neuroscience, as they descend from the information processing tradition, in order to carry forward the research program contained in the ideas of the medical model, in which classification and causal explanation will be ultimately founded on the neurophysiological organization of the mind. This approach is only one way to apply the medical model, and makes a bet that cognitive neuroscience is able to account for psychological phenomena by treating them as computational processes (though not necessarily symbolic process, rather than connectionist ones). Skeptics about computational approaches to cognition can adopt other neuroscientific applications of the medical model. The worry is that those rival approaches lack the resources to deal with cognitive processes.

The medical model, conjoined to the tradition of information-processing physiology, asserts that the explanation of these personal-level problems lies in the failure of subpersonal systems to function in their normal way. It is individual subjects, not parts of their brain, who are psychotic. But the explanation of why somebody is psychotic will cite problems with subpersonal mechanisms like the executive system in dorsolateral prefrontal cortex and its relations—perhaps, a failure of inhibition—with cognitive systems that have evolved to subserve thought that are less tethered to reality (Gerrans, in press). An explanation in terms of the physiology of cognition does not rule out a broader range of upstream factors as sources of the functional disruption. Following Kraepelin, we can distinguish etiology and pathology. An explanation of why Jane undergoes a psychotic episode could make reference to her recent trauma, or a failure to negotiate certain developmental challenges and a reliance on very destructive defense mechanisms (such as massive splitting and projection). To fit in with the logic of the medical model in its strong guise, however, such processes would need to have, among their effects, a realization of a destructive or dysfunctional disease process in the brain. The ensuing neuropathology is just what the disease amounts to, on the strong interpretation of the medical model. That does not mean that the pathology must always arise in the same way, but if mental disorder is brain disease then there must be in every case a neuropathology—an abnormal state of a subpersonal system—that realizes the disease.

These subpersonal systems are cognitive systems involved in the regulation of social behavior. There is no reason to suppose that they must be explained reductively, if that means employing only the concepts of low-level molecular neuroscience or genetics. They should be explained using whatever concepts are necessary to explain them, and nothing in the logic of the medical model rules that out. In another sense, though, the medical model does offer reductive explanations, in that it assumes that the mind decomposes into components and shows how the components work in concert to produce abnormal behavior. Normal behavior is produced by the components of the mind working together as they should. (Interpreting that "should" is a hard problem in the philosophy of psychiatry, as we will see in a moment. But in some guise it is a problem for every concept of mental disorder.)

Kincaid (2008, p. 375) has argued that it is unreasonable to see the understanding of the normal function of biological systems as part of the medical model. We can investigate depression (his example) based on "partial and unsystematic" understanding of its causes, as we do with organs in medicine more generally. But Kincaid identifies the possession of background theory with having a "complete wiring diagram of the organism from fertilization to maturity" (p. 377). Furthermore, he sees the search for such wiring diagrams as reflecting a view of science as a search for laws of nature and natural kinds. But these commitments do not seem to hang together quite so tightly: a background theory of what a system does can be quite vague, but without some understanding of a system's typical function it is difficult to see how we could reach the conclusion that there was something wrong with it.

Functions and norms

A theory of normal function could comprise a number of partial wiring diagrams arrived at by piecemeal investigation, and it does not have to be driven by a desire for explanation in terms of kinds participating in laws. I shall suggest shortly that mechanistic explanations appear to fit the medical model better than explanations in terms of laws. We do not need, despite Kincaid's worries, a complete theory of how biological systems work in order to conduct fruitful research. The issue is whether, at a minimum, there needs to be some rough theoretical frameworks and shared empirical claims within which abnormalities can be identified and outcomes assessed. We should expect these theories to be informed by developing work on psychopathology and to influence that work in their turn, as both inquiries mature.

This point stands even if you think that determinations of mental disorder are sensitive, in the first place, to judgments about norm violation rather than abnormal function. Suppose it is true that we make judgments about whether someone is ill, in the first place, just by making assumptions about them based on their behavior's violating certain norms. The mentally ill, as a class, may have nothing in common beyond the fact that their behavior strikes us as deviant. It still might be the case that each type of deviance is associated with an objective non-typical or dysfunctional cognitive or neurological cause. Cooper (2007 and Chapter 56 this volume) and Murphy (2006) have drawn an analogy between the concept of mental disorder and that of weed. Weeds are not a scientifically relevant category of entities. We can perhaps say that a weed is a fast-growing species that negatively impacts on economically valuable crops, usually through competition for nutrients, sunlight, and space. What fixes the extension of "weed" (and similar concepts like "vermin" or "precious metal") is a set of contingent human interests that can change over time.

There is nothing inherently dysfunctional about a weed; weeds are just species that we don't like because of certain interests that we have. So "weed" is not a technical term in ecology and the science of weeds is just the science of plants and animals, put to special use. "Weed" rarely appears within publications in reputable ecological journals, but nonetheless there is real, explanatory mind-independent knowledge to be had about each sort of "weed." Suppose that determining that a condition is a disorder is like determining that a plant is a weed. The diagnosis is determined by value judgments we have already made. The proponent of the medical model can still say that the underlying condition is a genuine cognitive and/or biological disorder. Of course, further inquiry might lead us to reject the initial judgment altogether. The science might suggest that there is nothing neurologically abnormal going on at all, which would support claims that we are not dealing with a real mental illness. But just as there is a genuine biological story to be told about how weeds attack crops, there could be a genuine neuropsychological account of abnormalities of the subpersonal systems that produce the signs and symptoms that folk psychology or social norms interpret as indicators of mental illness. The fact that a kind is constituted by human interests does not mean that the members of the kind cannot be understood scientifically in ways that explain why they attract that particular kind of human interest. A sociological account can explain why people are seen as deviant. The further question is why they are seen as mentally ill, rather than deviant in some other way. Boyer (2011) argues that what he calls the *intuitive detection* of mental disorder involves judging that a particular type of behavior is so different from what the culture expects that it appears to be evidence that some mental systems are dysfunctional. If true, Boyer's theory explains what sociological theories unsupplemented by psychology struggle to account for, which is why some deviant behaviors seem pathological rather than attractive, eccentric, criminal, or immoral. But even if a mixture of culture and cognition explains why we make judgments of pathology, it can still be the case that, as the medical model bets, there is real, explanatory mind-independent knowledge to be about underlying dysfunctions in each sort of genuine mental illness. Or it could be that the science is entirely directed by the value judgments, so that what we think of as a dysfunction is, metaphysically speaking, no such thing. It could merely be a brain state we don't like, because of the behavior it gives rise to. The medical model bets that we can distinguish dysfunctional brains from merely unpopular ones. We need an account of natural function and dysfunction to do that, which is a hard demand to meet (Roe and Murphy 2011), but notice that an account of biological dysfunction is a medical problem, not a peculiarly psychiatric one. The medical model in psychiatry inherits the philosophical problems of medicine as well as the promise of it.

Graham (2010, pp. 53–58) offers a different criticism of the medical model, which turns on the (plainly correct) observation that most mental disorders are the product of several different causes rather than one, or in his terms, a set of propensities rather than a "single main cause" (p. 55) as in bodily diseases like malaria. However, this objection can be met if we distinguish between the realization of a disease and its more proximate causes. Many diseases have a number of different possible causes that interact with genetic propensities; lung cancer is not just caused by smoking, for example, but also by inhaling various pollutants such as asbestos or coal dust. What the different causes have in common is their subsequent destructive effect on the respiratory system via the replication of abnormal cells of various sorts. We lack a comparably detailed story for mental disorders, but the logic would be same. The proponent of the strong medical model bets that the different causes of a mental disorder will tend to render a set of subpersonal systems abnormal in the same way across the affected population, even if the details of the cases vary according to accidents of biography. It is not in dispute that the subjective intentional life of the patient makes a difference to how mental illness is experienced and manifested in different people. The medical model's fundamental contention is that all these people, despite the varieties in their presentations, have something in common at the subpersonal level: their neuropsychological systems are disrupted in ways that we make sense of using the explanatory resources of the neurosciences, including cognitive or intentional concepts.

Are mental disorders natural kinds?

Kincaid and Graham both charge, on slightly different grounds, that the conception of mental illness as akin to physical disease I outline here is committed to the idea that mental illnesses are natural kinds. Insofar as the medical model borrows much of its basic intellectual structure from a wider set of ideas about the nature of disease, there is clearly something to this charge; so are mental illnesses natural kinds, according to the medical model? Several theorists have recently argued that Richard Boyd's homeostatic property-cluster theory (HPC) (Boyd 1990, 1991) provides us with the right way to think about the kindhood of mental disorders (Beebee and Sabbarton-Leary 2010; Kendler et al. 2011; Parnas et al. 2010; Samuels 2009). On the HPC view a kind is defined by a set of properties that vary somewhat among its members, although causal mechanisms make it the case that the properties are more or less jointly instantiated. When inductive reasoning works, thinks Boyd, it works because we have latched onto underlying causal mechanisms that bring about the clustering. Successful inductions track the observable manifestations of the causal mechanisms responsible for the characteristics of the kind. The mechanisms, we might say, leave an identifiable causal signature in the world.

The HPC account seems to suit mental disorders. They often vary across cases, with characteristic symptoms sometimes absent even when the patient presents a typical cluster of signs and symptoms. So it is understandable that theorists who are sympathetic to the medical model in psychiatry should be drawn to the homeostatic property cluster idea. The existing *Diagnostic and Statistical Manual of Mental Disorders* (DSM) nosology (American Psychiatric Association 2000) comprises what Kendler et al. (2011) call practical kinds. Practical kinds strive to classify patients in ways that meet goals that fit a minimal interpretation of the medical model, such as prediction, discovery of risk factors, or direction of treatment. These are pragmatic goals, and DSM diagnoses should not be assumed to be natural kinds, which would demand a causal classification based around underlying mechanisms, just as the strong version of the medical model assumes.

In sum: The strong version of the medical model goes beyond a general commitment to data gathering and treatments according to medical standards, and sees mental illness as causally depending on abnormal or dysfunctional processes in subpersonal systems. There are many ways of understanding these systems, which are dealt with by sciences concerned with, intuitively, many different levels of explanation from the cognitive to the molecular. Recent philosophy of science has a lot to say about how to explain phenomena like these. Let's turn now to explanation.

Explanation

Mechanisms

Mental illnesses are complicated phenomena; they are mixtures of behavioral, psychological, and physical signs and symptoms which appear to depend on many different causes. The same condition in different people also varies in length and severity. Most cases of depression, for example, remit after about four months, but a small minority of people suffer for years. Major depressive episodes are associated with several kinds of pathophysiology, but none of these are present in all depressive subjects, and no one of them is specific to depression. The monoamine depletion hypothesis, for example, contends that the underlying pathophysiology is a shortage of the neurotransmitters serotonin, norepinephrine, or dopamine. It has led to the mass-marketing of drugs but remains unconfirmed despite decades of effort. Twin studies, and observation of afflicted families, do indicate genetic risk factors for depression. Optimistic judgments that the gene for depression has been found, however, have always been premature. A form of the serotonin transporter gene *5-HTT* is involved in emotional regulation and response to threat (Hariri and Holmes 2006) and the gene appears to be involved in building the receptors for the neurotransmitters mentioned by the monoamine hypothesis. But although the gene may affect some people in ways that increases their chances of depression, it is not the gene for depression. As Kendler et al. showed on the basis of extensive twin studies (2006, p. 115), major depression is a classic "multifactorial disorder." A range of factors affect your chances of contracting major depression. Genes certainly make a difference, but so do factors like the extent of the child abuse you suffered, the state of your marriage, and your history of substance abuse, as well as stressful environmental events like unemployment or bereavement. The association between these stressful life events and major depression is, say Kendler and Prescott (2006, p. 281), at least partly causal, which raises the question of causal explanation.

For example, suppose we want to understand the mechanism by which neurotransmitters are released (Craver 2007, pp. 4–6). This involves finding answers to questions such as: Why does depolarization of an axon terminal lead to neurotransmitter release, and why are neurotransmitters released in quanta? The answers involve pointing out various entities, including various intracellular molecules, and showing how their properties allow them to act. The entities interact with each other to give rise to the phenomena that we want to explain. An explanation with these features is mechanistic. In recent years philosophers have stressed the way in which explanation in many sciences, above all the biological and cognitive, depends on finding mechanisms (Bechtel and Richardson 1993; Craver 2007; Schaffner 1993; Tabery 2009). Rather than seeing explanation as a search for laws, we seek the parts within a system of which the structure and activities explain the phenomena produced by the system. Philosophers disagree over exactly how to characterize mechanisms, but it is agreed that mechanisms: (a) comprise component parts that (b) do things. Strife arises over how to understand the activities of the parts. Are they also primitive constituents of a mechanism or just activities of the constituent components (Tabery 2004)? But it is generally agreed that a mechanistic explanation shows how the parts and their interactions give rise to the phenomenon we want to explain.

Central to Craver's account of mechanistic explanation is the display of relations of causal relevance between phenomena at different levels of explanation (Craver 2002). Causal relevance is defined in terms of manipulability and intervention. Events at one level are causally relevant insofar as they make a difference at another level. Causal relevance depends on realization. Levels of explanation, on this account, are actually descriptions of the same processes at different levels of resolution. A delusion can be understood in personal terms as a psychotic episode in the life of an individual that depends on relations between different psychological processes in different brain systems. These in their turn involve cells whose operations can be studied in terms of the systems that constitute them, and so on down to the molecular level. On this account, explanation in neuroscience, as in biology more generally, involves describing mechanism(s) at each level in ways that make apparent the relationships between causally relevant variables at different levels (Woodward 2010). Showing the causal relations between levels lets us integrate models of phenomena drawn from different areas of neuroscience. Clinical data, imaging studies, and other high-level psychological information ultimately need to be systematically related to models of low-level phenomena such as the effects of neurotransmitter activity.

Presented in this way the basics of mechanistic explanation involve a perspective on levels of explanation that should look familiar to philosophers and cognitive scientists. It is reminiscent of Marr's (1982, pp. 24–25) distinction between three levels of explanation in cognitive science. The highest specifies the computational task accomplished by the system of interest. It tells us what the goal of the system is, specified in terms of what it computes. The middle level describes the actual representations and algorithms that carry out the goal. The lowest level tells us how brain tissue or other material substrates, such as the parts of a machine, can implement the algorithm. Should we, then, follow this picture and conceive of psychiatry as a science of many-level processes?

Levels

Marr's three levels are different representations of the same process, which he called the construction of a three-dimensional representation of the world from two-dimensional data. This understanding of levels fits Craver's (2007) picture of mechanistic explanation outlined earlier, with its stress on causal relevance. Causal relevance tells you how it is that something happening at one level makes a difference at another level: it is because the lower-level system is a part of the higher-level system. The worry is that this account will fail to do justice to the fact that in psychiatry distinct causal processes mesh together phenomena that are not nested like Russian dolls in this way.

Data from large-scale twin studies provide evidence that three main causal routes to major depression exist (Kendler and Prescott 2006, pp. 333–338). Different causal histories of depression depend on the interaction of genes with psychological characteristics like neuroticism and low self-esteem, as well as other mental illnesses. Kendler and Prescott's model also incorporates accidents of biography, such as the early loss of a parent, sexual abuse in childhood, divorce, and insufficient social support. They also report (2006, p. 159) that episodes of "humiliation in a public setting" are powerful predictors of major depression. There is no straightforward pathway from gene to depression, but rather a complicated network of (probably non-linear) relations among variables that mediate between genes and phenotypic outcomes. The mechanistic approach aims to integrate these different variables, but it seems that it can only do so if the causes of depression can be represented as taking place in one system that is describable at different levels, because the mechanistic approach aims at showing how systems are nested within each other at different levels. The topmost level of the hierarchy is the brain as a whole, and the explanation can certainly integrate processes occurring in different brain areas—in that sense the brain can be treated as a whole system.

But since the causes of many mental illnesses include a mix of genes and environmental factors we need to think about how environmental factors can be understood within the mechanistic program. These are different kinds of processes, not different levels at which one process can be represented by the theorist. If we were dealing, like Marr, with one process describable in different ways, then we could anticipate an integrative account in which higher-level variables get mapped on to lower-level ones. But even though it is hard enough to imagine a molecular or neurological reduction of a psychological construct like humiliation it is even harder to imagine a reductive analysis of sociocultural factors like unemployment or childhood sexual abuse. They have brain effects, but the brain effects vary across classes of individuals in ways that depend on other environmental and genetic contexts (see Kendler and Prescott (2006) for a comprehensive review.)

Appealing to levels of explanation is unobjectionable if it just involves a reminder that we need to relate variables of many sorts. But it is not clear that we have any principled grounds for sorting phenomena into levels, especially once we move beyond the organism: Are unemployment and bereavement processes at different levels? Marr did have a principled basis for distinguishing levels. He imagined them as descriptions of the same process (the construction of a three-dimensional image from two-dimensional retinal impacts) couched in the vocabularies of different sciences. But when we move outside the skull and begin introducing environmental factors and other kinds of cause, the Marrian picture looks less plausible.

One way to deal with this problem is to assume that we can ignore the outside world because information about it is represented in the brain. Adolphs (2010), for example, assumes that social neuroscience begins with the transduction of social information, so that social factors are relevant only insofar as the system represents them. If that is right as a general strategy, then all we have to worry about is how the brain represents social information and the relations of the systems that do the representing to other systems that regulate behavior. Then the mechanistic program can carry on unamended. Methodological solipsism of this type will work as an explanatory strategy if we want to preserve the mechanistic understanding of the biological hierarchy in an enduring system. It will uncover proximate mechanisms and the causal relevance relations between them. It will not help us to isolate the relevant environmental factors and understand their effect on the organism (because we have to know what they are first to make the solipsistic strategy work).

A different option preserves much of the mechanistic approach but takes a different view of causal relevance and a more relaxed view of levels. Campbell (2008) argues for an interventionist approach to causation. This is the view that when we say X is a cause of Y we are saying that intervening on X is a way of intervening on Y (Pearl 2009; Woodward 2003; Woodward and Hitchcock 2003): manipulating one variable makes a difference to another. This is not a reductive analysis of causation, since it makes use of causal ideas—it just states that questions about whether X causes Y are questions about what would happen to Y if we did something to change X. Kendler and Campbell (2009) have argued that an interventionist model provides a rigorous way of articulating the idea that any combination of variables might characterize the causes of a disorder, whilst at the same time providing a clear test of what variables are actually involved, thus avoiding a simple-minded holism that just says that lots of things are relevant. Kendler and Campbell advance a picture of psychiatric explanation that looks for control variables that make a difference to behavior, such as humiliation or genetic factors. But they do not expect to fit all the variables into a natural hierarchy in which events at one level are reductions of events at a higher level. On this picture, environmental processes are part of the overall explanatory system in their own right, not just qua representations in the hierarchy of brain systems. We can continue to look for mechanistic stories at many levels of explanation in the brain, but we do not have to face the worry of reducing environmental factors. On Kendler and Campbell's story, unemployment is a genuine cause of depression insofar as it makes a systematic difference to depressed patients, even if there is no explaining unemployment in terms of a mechanism. It is a genuine cause of depression in virtue of its difference-making properties.

Those difference-making properties cross levels. Depression counts as a cause of something neurological in its own right, and not just insofar as it is mediated by mechanisms that realize it. That is, cause and effect are related across levels. Kendler and Campbell contend (2009, p. 997) that interventionism "permits the clear separation of causal effects from the mechanistic instantiations of those effects," thus directly confuting the approach favored by Craver and Bechtel (2007, p. 554) who argue that it stretches the concept of causation to breaking point to admit interlevel causes: they say that "to accept interlevel relationships as causal violates many of the central ideas associated with the concept of causation." Craver and Bechtel argue that we explain effects in terms of interlocking parts, and the relation across levels, they affirm, is one of constitution, not causation; causation can only be intralevel. Events at a level cause subsequent phenomena at that level, which realize higher-level phenomena. Interlevel causation, on this view, amounts to something causing itself, because different levels are different ways of talking about the same thing. Causal relevance is the relation borne by phenomena at one level to the lower-level phenomena they depend on, but causal relevance is not causation. The dispute here turns in part, then, on philosophical views about the nature of causation. Campbell (2008) argues on broadly Humean grounds that that we simply cannot tell in advance of inquiry what causal relations obtain in nature. We simply have to take our causal relations where we find them, including interlevel ones.

Appealing to levels of explanation in psychiatry, then, can either be a reminder that we need to relate variables of many sorts in explaining the causes of disorder. Or it can represent a commitment to seeing psychiatric explanation in terms of a biological hierarchy, with systems built up out of other systems. The debate over how to understand mechanisms and processes at different levels is partly an empirical one and partly bound up with philosophical views on reduction, explanation, and causation. I will suggest later that proponents of the medical model might adopt an interventionist account of causation which permits causal relations across levels. This approach allows for causal factors that are environmental or sociological, as well as factors internal to the organism that permit a fully mechanistic explanation. I think this causes no trouble for the medical model. The strong interpretation of the medical model can say that a disease is a destructive process realized in the human brain but caused by many interweaving factors. In that sense, it is a mistake to say that a disease is caused by a brain process. It just is a brain process, but the process itself admits of many causes.

I will move on to discuss a further problem. As well as great diversity in causal factors, psychiatry also confronts the problem of diverse symptoms; many mental illnesses take a different form in different people. Although two people might both be diagnosed with major depression, they need share few symptoms. Both are very likely to feel miserable and lose interest in activities they normally enjoy. However, one might lose weight, sleep less, and becomes physically agitated while the other sleeps more and becomes lethargic and tormented by feelings of guilt and thought of suicide. The philosophical problem arises from the confrontation between the great variation in clinical reality and the need to simplify in order to render that reality scientifically tractable. In summary form, the problem is: What are we trying to explain when we explain a mental illness? Is it a diverse set of real-world phenomena, or some simplified representation of those phenomena? In the latter case, we do not explain the phenomena directly, but we construct a model of the phenomena of interest, show how causal and explanatory relations work in the model, and then point to resemblances between the simplified model and the more complicated actual phenomena.

Disorders as statistical networks

One way to start thinking about what we have to explain in psychiatry is to borrow Thagard's (1999, p. 114–115) account of diseases as networks of "statistically based causal relations" discovered using epidemiological and experimental methods. This fits the picture that Kendler and Prescott present for depression quite neatly (although their models are designed to incorporate both causal relations and mere correlations). Thagard's causal-statistical networks, like Kendler and Prescott's path models, provide "a kind of narrative explanation of why a person becomes sick" (p. 115). They incorporate information about the typical course of a disease as it unfolds over time, including information about typical risk factors for the disease—such as the finding that heavy use of aspirin increases acid secretion which makes a duodenal ulcer more likely. The causal network does not specify how each causal factor produces its effects, though. It is really a descriptive model that lets us ask the question: What facts make it true that people get sick in these ways?

In effect we have a set of exception-prone generalizations about the pathways a disorder takes: people in this situation are likely to become depressed unless such and such intervenes. And when they are depressed they will probably have the following experiences, unless they have these other ones. Thagard's idea of a narrative is helpful here; path models represent typical stories about characteristic ways of getting sick that isolate control variables. But a narrative by itself might not explain anything; if it is explanatory, it is because earlier events mentioned in the narrative pick out the causes of later events.

Cooper (2007) presents a way of thinking about psychiatric explanation that fits the idea that diagnosis gives us tools to construct a narrative of the patient's current state and future prospects. She argues that at least some mental illnesses are natural kinds, and *natural history explanations* work by "invoking natural kinds" (2007, p. 47). Once we know what kind an object belongs to, we can explain and predict its behavior based on its kind membership. We can explain that a substance has expanded upon being heated because it's a bit of metal, and metals expand when heated. And, it is hoped, we can explain why Laura hears voices by appealing to the fact that she has schizophrenia. And our confidence that she is schizophrenic warrants predictions about her future.

We often find ourselves with narratives that tell us how someone gets sick, and it might be that a useful narrative is one which isolates the temporally prior variables and lets us see how later phenomena depend on them. One way to think about this is that a good narrative is one that talks about a natural kind of the HPC type we mentioned earlier. If we have a natural kind, with some causal structure underpinning it, the systematic dependence of later states on earlier ones is easy to grasp: they depend on the causal mechanisms that give rise to the properties of the condition, and variation in patient histories is only to be expected, as HPC kinds do not have uniform observable properties, but clusters that manifest a typical causal signature.

From histories to causes

Cooper argues that a natural history explanation needs to cite natural kinds to be helpful. But the explanations do not need to mention the actual causal mechanisms responsible for the behavior of the members of the kind. We can know that a disease will unfold in a predictable way even if we are ignorant of its underlying pathophysiology. The history of psychiatry offers a number of instances in which pharmacology has led to the recognition of new kinds even in the absence of detailed causal knowledge. For example, Cade's (1949) discovery that lithium greatly inhibited the startle reflex and other forms of anxiety in guinea pigs was useful even without good information about their underlying cognitive neurobiology, since it led him to predict that whatever was going on might also apply in humans, thereby suggesting a shared causal pathway raising the possibility that some forms of anxiety constitute a distinct kind. A similar example was the discovery in the early 1060s that imipramine, introduced as an antidepressant, benefited patients who had been diagnosed with anxiety disorder in a specific way. Imipramine reduced the incidence of acute bursts of anxiety in these patients, suggesting the existence of a distinct kind of anxiety condition— what we would now call panic disorder—that had been hitherto unrecognized as distinct from chronic anxiety.

Invoking kinds give us power over the world, by making it easier to predict, control, or mitigate the outcomes we care about. One philosophical question we can ask, of course, is whether science wants anything more. If you think science just aims for empirical adequacy, then it may seem that sorting patients into kinds is enough, provided that we can understand the course of the disease.

In particular, natural history explanations fit a conception of diseases as syndromes unfolding over time that is enshrined in both DSM-IV-TR and the minimal construal of the medical model. It does not deny that there are causal processes, but sees mental illnesses as collections of signs and symptoms with characteristic histories. They doubtless depend on physical processes but are not defined or classified in physical terms. This picture of disease naturally goes along with the employment of natural history explanations, since they too invoke natural kinds without worrying about the mechanisms that explain the behavior of members of the kind. It's enough to be able to identify kind membership, thereby giving us a degree of explanatory and predictive control.

Natural history explanations fit Thagard's disease network nicely; if a disease network provides a narrative account of why people get ill, and predicts some outcomes, we can see it as a graphical representation of the historical pathway typical of a kind. Much epidemiological work in psychiatry fits the pattern here; we try to isolate the causal factors that define a disease history that is met with regularly. These histories display relations between variables that show how later phenomena, like the symptoms of depression or substance abuse, depend on earlier phenomena, like the genes you were born with, or the parental abuse you endured.

Unlike some of the more homespun examples, the natural histories uncovered by systematic longitudinal research can be quite surprising and genuinely explanatory. But (as Cooper and Thagard both suggest) they leave us with a lot to do if we want to provide mechanistic explanations of key factors.

Causal explanatory strategies

The natural history approach tracks the operation of hitherto unknown causes by sorting patients into kinds with a presumed common nature, based on the natural history of their conditions, or on other grounds such as differential responses to drugs. If they license reliable inductive inferences, we assume, as on the Boydian picture, that we are tracking hidden causal factors that the observable syndrome depends on.

Cooper suggests (2007, p. 174, n. 2) that natural history explanations provide us with what Murphy (2006) calls causal discrimination, as opposed to causal understanding. We can know two kinds are causally different even if we don't why they are different, because the details of the underlying causal structure evade us. Different types of plant may need to be put in the ground at different times, or in different seasons, in order to maximize crop yield, for instance, and we may be able to predict accurately that different patients will respond to different drugs even if the basis for these differences remain unknown. But we assume that these differences rest on an underlying causal structure. In psychiatry, differential diagnosis follows a similar logic, but skeptics wonder if the degree of variation makes the predictions too unreliable for this approach to really work.

Our complete explanatory job is to explain the observed causal-statistical network by identifying the mechanisms inside the organism and the external factors that affect them, either by developing a model of the natural hierarchy or by developing models of control variables. The problem, of course, is the sheer variety of the phenomena, which does not give us the degree of epistemic security we get when we sort phenomena into kinds in other sciences. One way to make this variety tractable, suggested by the natural history approach, is to look for some stable phenomena that do not vary. These are not likely to be found at the level of diagnoses, because in many cases two people with the same diagnosis will exhibit different behaviors and other symptoms depending on their personal lives, cultural background, other mental illnesses, and so on. There is too much variety at the level of diagnosis. So we must search for smaller units of explanation.

We can think of this first approach as zooming-in on one small portion of the overall network, looking for a unit that has enough stability across histories to allow for an explanation in which there are cause–effect regularities; if the underlying causal structure is too diverse, look for causal units that stably replicate across patients, explain them, and then put these well-understood parts together to explain individuals. Another advantage of this approach is that it promises to treat patients as individuals rather than clumping together into kinds that they only approximately fit.

This zoom-in approach is exemplified by Bentall (2003) and Spaulding et al. (2003). They both look for the smallest unit of reliable explanation or manipulation. Spaulding et al. argue from a clinical perspective for seeing patients as collections of "problems," with the problems in each case drawn from a repertoire of clinically significant phenomena that different patients exemplify in different ways. For Spaulding et al., the relevant sciences for identifying problems span many levels of analysis from the intracellular to the sociocultural. Their examples of relevant explanatory factors include low levels of cortisol and learning deficits (pp. 127–130). Their multilevel approach fits with the medical model as I have presented it, although they tend to think in terms not just of pathological phenomena but also of problems in living. In that sense their picture incorporates elements of the medical model within a broader, clinically focused outlook.

Bentall argues that diagnoses like depression or schizophrenia have proved helpless in the face of all the variation that patients exhibit. There is no such thing as schizophrenia because schizophrenia is not a natural kind. He thinks "we should abandon psychiatric diagnoses altogether and instead try to understand and explain the actual experiences and behaviors of psychotic people" which he terms *complaints* (2003, p. 141). The same argument might apply to other psychiatric categories. There are no mental disorders as traditionally under-stood, but a diverse range of psychotic phenomena that combine in different ways in differ-ent people. I call this approach zooming-in, because it aims for finer detail than traditionally recognized diagnoses.

For example, Bentall (2003, chapter 15) objects to the old model of inferring thought disorder on the basis of disordered speech. He sees disordered speech as a failure of com-munication, which is especially likely when subjects are emotionally aroused. In Bentall's tentative model, initial deficits in working memory caused by emotional arousal interact with other deficits in semantic memory, theory of mind, and introspective monitoring. The result is a failure to communicate and a lack of self-awareness of one's failure to communi-cate (which distinguishes psychotic patients from normal subjects in the grip of powerful emotions who are struggling to get their ideas across). This is a stable phenomenon, in the sense that we can give the same causal story in all cases of thought disorder, thus giving us a robust account that transfers across patients. A general theory of schizophrenia would have too many qualifications and varieties to transfer in this way.

Bentall thinks that the disease model of mental illness should be abandoned and replaced by one centered on complaints, but his approach is at home in my cognitive neuropsychi-atric interpretation of the strong medical model in nearly every way, since one of his com-plaints is effectively a mini-disease which permits the application of the mechanistic account I sketched earlier. Complaints are disorders of psychological systems that can be studied in isolation.

Approaches like this exist in philosophy of science accounts that seek to render tracta-ble some complex biological phenomena. Mitchell (2003) proposes an "integrative plural-ism" which tries to isolate individual causes and model them individually, seeing how each makes a causal contribution on its own. Theorists then put together a collection of models of individual phenomena and try to integrate them by applying multiple models as seems nec-essary to explain a particular case. Mitchell's approach zooms-in in its search for decompos-ing, but she envisages isolating causes that can recombine—such as genes or interpersonal difficulties—rather than searching for explanations of particular clinical phenomena like thought disorder (see also Tabery 2009). This is similar to the way Spaulding et al. (2003) seek the development and integration of causal models in the service of developing a com-prehensive clinical understanding of people and their problems.

This approach looks for stable, replicable units of psychiatric explanation. Bentall favors cognitive psychological explanations of his putative complaints, but his emphasis on phe-nomena produced by psychological systems is an invitation to the mechanistic account of explanation that we saw earlier. He explains psychological phenomena as the effects of subpersonal systems that are themselves composed of further systems describable at lower levels. Bentall concentrates on components of presently recognized diagnoses rather than the diagnoses themselves, which he rejects (at least in psychosis) But we should distinguish the claim that depression or schizophrenia should be abolished from the claim that tracing phenomena down to subpersonal systems will bring about some diagnostic revision in our current categories, which every proponent of the medical model should countenance. The medical model foresees a nosology built on causal explanation. The current DSM nosology has quite different foundations, and so revision of the current nosology looks very likely.

Existing conditions are pragmatic constructions, not genuine causally based catego-ries. Causal explanation may well upset many existing assumptions. We should expect the diagnostic landscape to change if the program of tracing abnormalities in subpersonal sys-tems is carried out; hitherto unsuspected ruptures in our categories may result from the rec-ognition that patients who look alike in fact suffer from conditions that depend on different underlying abnormalities. Equally, of course, increased knowledge of the brain may lead us to see what we now take to be different syndromes as manifestations of the same problem. These are all live empirical possibilities, and it may be that Bentall's complaints do turn out to be the right grain of diagnosis for the medical model. But there are also reasons to think they might not.

Zooming-in and zooming-out

Is zooming-in the way to apply the medical model? We will always want to develop explana-tions of particular phenomena, such as thought disorder. What is distinctive about Bentall's approach is his denial that useful psychiatric kinds exist at a broader level. There is always the chance that some finer causal discrimination will uncover an even more stable structure. Zooming-in faces the problem of knowing when to stop. There will always be some variation at the level of the complaint. Theory-building can handle this problem by finding a grain of description that permits useful modeling. The objection is not that science will be paralyzed by endless subdivision, but that zooming-in should not be thought of as an alternative to idealization. Any search for commonalities across patients will involve some degree of ide-alization. The rival approach, zooming-out, is another form of idealization, but zooms out to think in terms of idealized patients, rather than idealized problems.

Zooming-out begins by accepting that mental illness almost always depends on complex interactions between diverse lower-level phenomena and tries to deal with this variety by treating disease networks as idealizations that are more or less similar to actual histories. The serious problem that zooming-in faces is that Bentall's complaints are not strongly independent of one another—the presence of some of them do seem probabilistically to imply the presence of others, which suggests that underlying mechanisms are responsi-ble for clustering observable properties together, as Boyd's HPC account of natural kinds suggests.

In Murphy (2006) I argued that the variety of phenomena within many psychiatric diag-noses forces us to explain psychiatric phenomena not by looking for stable regularities but by constructing exemplars. An exemplar is an imaginary patient who has the ideal textbook form of a disorder. This might be something Thagard's (1999) disease network, and the nar-rative it provides. An exemplar applies to one disorder, so our imaginary patient has only that disorder, and the textbook needs to be thought of as a statement of the final theory, not any current work in psychiatry. Like zooming-in, the approach assumes that commonalities across patients will be revealed by inquiry. The idea is to model all the causes that contribute to a natural history so as to explore how they work together in different contexts to produce the various outcomes of interest, and then understand patients as idiosyncratic instances of the exemplar. When we explain a disease, we construct an exemplar and model it. But the causal structure that explains the exemplar resembles real world patients to varying degrees. So when we talk about individuals we explain their symptoms by identifying processes in the patient and showing how they resemble some part of the model. And because it is instru-mental concerns that drive our search for explanations in psychiatry, as in medicine more generally, the clinically significant relations between disease, model, and patient are likely to be highly context specific; they will be determined in part by whether they offer opportunities for successful therapeutic interventions, which depend not just on how the world is arranged, but also on what our resources and opportunities are.

The exemplar lets us identify *robust processes* (Sterelny 2003, pp. 131–132, 207–208) that are repeatable or systematic in various ways, rather than the actual processes that occur as a disorder unfolds in one person. But we do not stop there: the ultimate goal is causal understanding of a disease. We build a model to represent the pathogenic process that accounts for the observed phenomena in the exemplar. To explain an actual history in a patient is to show how the processes unfolding in the patient resemble those that are assumed to occur in the exemplar. Exemplars provide an idealized form of the disorder that aims to identify the factors that remain constant despite all the individual variation. Not every patient instantiates every feature of an exemplar, and so not every part of a model will apply to a given patient. Once we understand the resemblance relations that exist between parts of the model and the exemplar, we can try to manipulate the model so as to change or forestall selected outcomes in the real world.

Ghaemi (2003, chapter 12) offers a different defense of zooming-out. He argues that current DSM diagnoses function as ideal types in Weber's sense. An ideal type is an analytic construction that isolates the crucial features of some social phenomenon (like "capitalism" or "bureaucracy") and ignores the inessential or local. An ideal type of capitalism, for example, would isolate all those features that make capitalism distinctive and are analytically important for social science, even though the ensuing picture may not correspond accurately to capitalism as actually manifested in any society. One way to understand Weber's idea is just as a forerunner of modeling, in which essential variables are isolated and inessential ones put aside (Engerman 2000, pp. 257–258). That makes Weber's approach a forerunner of contemporary model-based approaches to science, and the exemplar idea outlined earlier would be an application of the ideal type to psychiatry.

Ghaemi, though, locates the ideal type in a different tradition, that of hermeneutic understanding most closely associated in psychiatry with the phenomenological tradition. This approach looks for meaningful psychological connections between phenomena and is contrasted with causal, scientific explanation. However, this seems to reflect an impoverished view of both explanation and of the resources available for the explanation of mental states. Your reasons might play a distinctive role in justifying your actions, in getting me to understand your point of view, and in making sense of your actions relative to a broader depiction of your nature, but there seem obvious cases in which reasons, and other meaningful states like beliefs, do causally explain actions. My belief that owning a dog will make you happy, together with my desire to cheer you up, causally explains why I buy you a puppy. Most philosophers now are happy to think of reasons as causes. On my approach, the correct way to think about reasons is that they are representations in the brain (although these may not correspond exactly to states of mind recognized by everyday psychology).

Jaspers (1963, p. 304) argued that the "rules of causality" take the form of inductively derived scientific laws that subsume particular cases. It may well be true that there are no general laws in psychology governing connections between states of mind and behaviors. But there is no reason to accept, with Jaspers, the idea that explanations in science are statements that must cite laws. Explanations in the cognitive and biological sciences are usually not law governed, but mechanistic; they explain a phenomenon in terms of interacting causal processes. Meaningful mental states can explain behavior in the absence of general laws, although that is not the only way in which we use them to interpret the behavior of others.

Conclusion

I have suggested that the medical model can be given a strong interpretation as a branch of cognitive neuroscience concerned with the subpersonal causes of psychiatric signs and symptoms. I further argued that some version of mechanistic explanation looks like the appropriate philosophical program for such an account of psychiatry to follow, although many details remain unresolved—how should we think of levels of explanation in psychiatry or address causal relations across levels? Indeed, it is not clear what we should try to explain—idealized diagnoses or phenomena of more modest scope. The medical model is not a proven success, but it is a set of ideas with excellent scientific and philosophical pedigrees, and it provides ample opportunities for both philosophical and empirical theorists to explore.

References

Adolphs, R. (2010). Conceptual challenges and directions for social neuroscience. *Neuron*, 65, 752–67.

American Psychiatric Association (2000). *Diagnostic and Statistical Manual of Mental Disorders, Fourth Edition, Text Revision*. Washington DC: American Psychiatric Association.

Andreasen, N. C. (2001). *Brave New Brain*. New York, NY: Oxford University Press.

Arpaly, N. (2005). How it is not "just like diabetes": Mental disorders and the moral psychologist. *Philosophical Issues*, 15(1), 282–98.

Bechtel, W. and Richardson, R. C. (1993). *Discovering Complexity: Decomposition and Localization as Strategies in Scientific Research*. Princeton, NJ: Princeton University Press.

Beebee, H. and Sabbarton-Leary, N. (2010). Are psychiatric kinds "real"? *European Journal of Analytic Philosophy*, 6(1), 11–27.

Bentall, R. (2003). *Madness Explained*. London: Penguin.

Bernard, C. (1927). *Introduction to the Study of Experimental Medicine*. New York, NY: Macmillan. (Original work published 1865.)

Boyd, R. (1990). What realism implies and what it does not. *Dialectica*, 43, 5–29.

Boyd, R. (1991). Realism, antifoundationalism, and the enthusiasm for natural kinds. *Philosophical Studies*, 61, 127–48.

Boyer, P. (2011). Intuitive expectations and the detection of mental disorder: A cognitive background to folk psychiatries. *Philosophical Psychology*, 24, 95–118.

Cade, J. (1949). Lithium salts in the treatment of psychotic excitement. *Medical Journal of Australia*, 2(36), 349–52.

Campbell, J. (2008). Causation in psychiatry. In K. Kendler and J. Parnas (Eds), *Philosophical Issues in Psychiatry*, pp. 196–216. Baltimore, MD: Johns Hopkins University Press.

Cooper, R. (2007). *Psychiatry and Philosophy of Science*. Stocksfield: Acumen Publishing.

Craver, C. (2002). Interlevel experiments and multilevel mechanisms in the neuroscience of memory. *Philosophy of Science*, 69(S3), 83–97.

Craver, C. F. (2007). *Explaining the Brain*. New York, NY: Oxford University Press.

Craver, C. F. and Bechtel, W. (2007). Top-down causation without top-down causes. *Biology and Philosophy, 22*, 547–63.

Engerman, S. L. (2000). Max Weber as economist and economic historian. In S. Turner (Ed.), *The Cambridge Companion to Weber*, pp. 256–71. Cambridge: Cambridge University Press.

Gerrans, P. (in press). *The Measure of Madness. Philosophy and Cognitive Neuropsychiatry*. Cambridge, MA: MIT Press.

Ghaemi, S. N. (2003). *The Concepts of Psychiatry*. Baltimore, MD: Johns Hopkins University Press.

Ghaemi, S. N. (2010). *The Rise and Fall of the Biopsychosocial Model*. Baltimore, MD: Johns Hopkins University Press.

Glymour, C. (1992). Freud's androids. In J. Neu (Ed.), *The Cambridge Companion to Freud*, pp. 44–85. Cambridge: Cambridge University Press.

Graham, G. (2010). *The Disordered Mind*. New York, NY: Routledge.

Hariri, A. R. and Holmes, A. (2006). Genetics of emotional regulation: the role of the serotonin transporter in neural function. *Trends in Cognitive Science, 10*(4), 182–91.

Jaspers, K. (1963). *General Psychopathology* (J. Hoenig and M. W. Hamilton, Trans. from the German 7th edn). Manchester: Manchester University Press.

Kandel, E. R. (2005). *Psychiatry, Psychoanalysis, and the New Biology of Mind*. Arlington, VA: APA Publishing.

Kendler, K. and Campbell, J. (2009). Interventionist causal models in psychiatry: Repositioning the mind-body problem. *Psychological Medicine, 39*, 881–7.

Kendler, K. S., Gardner, C. O., and Prescott, C. A. (2006). Towards a comprehensive developmental model for depression in men. *American Journal of Psychiatry, 163*, 115–24.

Kendler, K. S. and Prescott, C. A. (2006). *Genes, Environment, and Psychopathology: Understanding the Causes of Psychiatric and Substance Use Disorders*. New York, NY: The Guilford Press.

Kendler, K. S., Zachar, P., and Craver, C. (2011). What kinds of things are psychiatric disorders? *Psychological Medicine, 41*, 1143–50.

Kincaid, H. (2008). Do we need theory to study disease? Lessons from cancer research and their implications for mental illness. *Perspectives in Biology and Medicine, 51*, 367–78.

Marr, D. (1982). *Vision*. San Francisco, CA: W. H. Freeman.

Mitchell, S. (2003). *Biological Complexity and Integrative Pluralism*. Cambridge: Cambridge University Press.

Murphy, D. (2006). *Psychiatry in the Scientific Image*. Cambridge, MA: MIT Press.

Parnas, J., Nordgaard, J., and Varga, S. (2010). The concept of psychosis: A clinical and theoretical analysis. *Clinical Neuropsychiatry, 7*, 32–7.

Pearl, J. (2009). *Causality* (2nd edn). Cambridge: Cambridge University Press.

Roe, K. and Murphy, D. (2011). Function, dysfunction, adaptation? In P. Adriaens and A. Block (Eds), *Maladapted Minds*, pp. 216–37. Oxford: Oxford University Press.

Samuels, R. (2009). Delusion as a natural kind. In M. Broome and L. Bortolotti (Eds), *Psychiatry as Cognitive Neuroscience: Philosophical Perspectives*, pp. 49–80. Oxford: Oxford University Press.

Schaffner, K. (1993). *Discovery and Explanation in Psychology and Medicine*. Chicago, IL: University of Chicago Press.

Shah, P. and Mountain, D. (2007). The medical model is dead: Long live the medical model. *British Journal of Psychiatry, 191*, 375–7.

Spaulding, W., Sullivan, M., and Poland, J. (2003). *Treatment and Rehabilitation of Severe Mental Illness*. New York, NY: Guilford Press.

Sterelny, K. (2003). *The Evolution of Agency and Other Essays*. Cambridge: Cambridge University Press.

Tabery, J. (2004). Synthesizing activities and interactions in the concept of a mechanism. *Philosophy of Science, 71*, 1–15.

Tabery, J. (2009). Difference mechanisms: explaining variation with mechanisms. *Biology and Philosophy, 24*, 645–64.

Thagard, P. (1999). *How Scientists Explain Disease*. Princeton, NJ: Princeton University Press.

Thagard, P. (2008). Mental illness from the perspective of theoretical neuroscience. *Perspectives in Biology and Medicine, 51*, 335–52.

Woodward, J. (2010). Causation in biology: Stability, specificity, and the choice of levels of explanation. *Biology and Philosophy, 25*, 287–318.

CHAPTER 58

....

RELIABILITY, VALIDITY, AND THE MIXED BLESSINGS OF OPERATIONALISM

....

NICK HASLAM

Psychiatric diagnosis can be seen in many ways—as a vital basis for treatment planning or a sinister means of pigeonholing the deviant, a clinical art or a mechanical chore—but it is fundamentally an exercise in assessment. Accordingly, if we wish to evaluate it we must pay attention to reliability and validity, the two key goals of psychological assessment. Diagnostic instruments and practices should be both reliable and valid, and efforts to revise them should be guided by these desiderata. Such efforts are not straightforward, as reliability and validity are complex concepts and pursuing them can produce unwanted side effects. Indeed, some of the controversial historical changes in psychiatric diagnosis can be understood as outcomes of a misguided attempt to pursue one at the expense of the other.

I begin this chapter by examining the multiple senses of reliability and validity in the psychometric literature and then explore the nature of their relationship. Following these technical preliminaries I turn to the question of operationalism in psychiatric diagnosis, focusing in particular on the revolutionary changes inaugurated by the third edition of the *Diagnostic and Statistical Manual of Mental Disorders* (DSM-III; American Psychiatric Association (APA) 1980). The mixed blessings of this radical overhaul of diagnostic practice are then critically examined.

On the one hand, by privileging reliability and striving to be atheoretical the DSM-III and subsequent editions arguably impoverish the description of mental disorders by screening off phenomenology and psychodynamics. Their operational approach may also contribute to distorted understandings of some forms of psychopathology, the proliferation of disorders, and the misrepresentation of dimensional phenomena as categories. On the other hand, by avoiding theory-saturated and highly inferential concepts these diagnostic systems arguably reduce diagnostic disagreement, promote clinical communication, and stabilize the meaning of diagnostic entities. Whether these advantages outweigh the disadvantages is a major point of disagreement within the field.

I argue that some of the criticism of operational diagnosis is based on a misconception of what it aims to do. Rather than being full *definitions* of mental disorders, operational diagnostic criteria are better understood as identification procedures that are intrinsically partial, indirect, and simplified. Understood in this limited way, they should not be expected to do justice to the richness of clinical phenomena or to reflect the ontological status of what they identify. Instead they should be evaluated primarily on pragmatic grounds: Do they serve useful communicative and epistemic functions by enabling clinicians and researchers to agree on what they treat and study (reliability), and do they help to predict things that matter about psychopathology, including those that might advance our theoretical understanding of it (validity)?

RELIABILITY

The reliability of an assessment procedure or instrument represents its trustworthiness and freedom from measurement error. Reliable tools yield knowledge that is robust, replicable, and consistent. Several species of reliability are recognized. The forms of trustworthiness that each embodies are diverse, relating to the consistency among the elements of an assessment instrument, between users of the instrument, and between different times when the instrument is used to assess the same people. Reliability therefore refers to internal, interpersonal, and intertemporal consistency.

Internal consistency is a form of reliability that refers to the degree of empirical coherence among the elements of an assessment tool, such as the items of a personality inventory. It is usually measured as a function of the correlations among these elements, so that tools whose elements all intercorrelate strongly have high internal consistency whereas those whose items correlate weakly, not at all, or negatively have low consistency. Grounding this sense of reliability is the idea that if the elements of an assessment tool fail to covary in a consistent manner then they cannot be assessing the same phenomenon. Measurement error in this sense refers to the failure of the elements of an instrument to cohere systematically, as they should if they tap a single underlying phenomenon.

Whereas internal consistency refers to consistency among multiple elements of an assessment instrument, *interrater reliability* refers to consistency among multiple users of the instrument. An instrument is reliable in this sense if different assessors draw similar conclusions about the same person being assessed, such as by arriving at the same psychiatric diagnosis, and instruments that fail to yield substantial agreement lack reliability. Once again, the rationale for this form of reliability is straightforward. If two mental health professionals administering the same diagnostic interview to a single patient tend to disagree on the patient's diagnosis then that interview is not a trustworthy source of diagnostic knowledge. Whatever the source of that disagreement—whether it reflects differences intrinsic to the assessors, to differences in their implementation of the assessment, or to differences in the inferences they draw from its findings—it raises fundamental doubts about the replicability of the information that the assessment instrument generates. The findings of an assessment tool that is unreliable in this sense depend excessively on who deploys it rather than what it aims to measure.

Reliability also has a temporal dimension. An assessment device that has *re-test reliability* yields consistent information about its targets across time. If a psychological test provides very divergent scores for the same person assessed at two times then the test lacks reliability in this sense. An important qualification of this statement is that re-test reliability should only be high for attributes that should in theory be stable over time, such as personality traits or psychiatric diagnoses, and would not be expected for measures of transient states such as moods. If the to-be-assessed attribute is understood to be enduring, then any assessment that delivers fluctuating findings about individuals over time suffers from measurement error and hence unreliability.

Validity

The validity of a psychological test concerns the extent to which inferences drawn from the test are empirically well-founded. Like reliability, validity has a number of recognized forms or facets. The concept is fundamentally triple-barreled, with psychometric theorists distinguishing *content, criterion-related*, and *construct* validities. A valid instrument assesses the content of what it is intended to assess, is empirically related to suitable external criteria, and is associated with other instruments in a way that accords with the theoretical understanding of the construct it is intended to measure. Needless to say these three barrels do not always run parallel, and are to some degree independent of one another. An assessment tool may measure something other than what its developers believe but still predict external criteria successfully, or it may map accurately onto its intended construct but be predictively useless. For these and other reasons it is important to distinguish these kinds of validity.

As noted earlier, a test's *content validity* refers to the adequacy of its coverage of the content of what it aims to measure. As Cronbach and Meehl (1955, p. 282) argue, it "is established by showing that the test items are a sample of a universe in which the investigator is interested." A test of a particular mental disorder, for example, should contain items that refer to its primary clinical or other associated features, and if the test systematically fails to sample part of the universe of relevant features—like a test of arithmetic ability that contained no subtraction items—it can be said to lack content validity.

Criterion-related validity is not a matter of the "internal" properties of a test—whether it covers its measurement domain appropriately—but represents the degree to which a test enables successful prediction of variables that are external to it. In practice, validity of this sort is demonstrated by empirical associations between an assessment instrument and criteria located in the future (e.g., treatment response, recidivism, suicide; known as predictive validity), in the present (e.g., correlations with other contemporary clinical phenomena; known as concurrent validity), or even in the past (e.g., associations with the prior course of illness or factors of possible etiological relevance such as early life experiences).

In many cases psychological and psychiatric attributes or processes have no single obvious criterion for external validation, and their internal validity cannot be directly established. In these cases a third kind of validation, dubbed *construct validity*, is required (Cronbach and Meehl 1955). The construct validity of a psychological test represents its embedding in a web of empirical relationships with other constructs—a "nomological net"—that help to fix and clarify its meaning. Construct validation involves demonstrating that the test assesses a hypothetical process, state, or structure, and so requires that the test be associated with other phenomena that the hypothetical entity should be associated with, and not be associated with phenomena with which that entity should not be associated. For example, a test of schizotypal personality should correlate with measures of magical thinking and social anxiety but not with measures of depression and compulsiveness.

These three forms of validity help to organize a classic discussion of diagnostic validity by Robins and Guze (1970; see Cloninger 1989), who proposed five phases of validation. Their first, the precise clinical description of a disorder, refers to content validity and their second, fourth, and fifth phases—validation through correlating the disorder with laboratory findings, examining its future course with follow-up studies, and observing its associations across generations in family studies—involve criterion-related validity. Robins and Guze's third phase, in which the disorder is delimited from others, can be seen as a process of construct validation that clarifies distinctions between the hypothetical clinical entity and similar alternatives.

The key issue for our current purposes is that neither validity nor reliability is a monolithic concept, and that the distinct forms do not strongly imply one another. An instrument may have strong criterion-related validity, enabling useful predictions about non-test predictive criteria, but nevertheless lack content and construct validity. Equally, a psychological test might have strong internal consistency but weak re-test reliability. For these reasons it is questionable to make unqualified claims about assessment instruments simply "having" reliability and validity.

Reliability–Validity Relations

The reliability and validity of assessment procedures are conceptually distinct and they are empirically established by different means. They are nevertheless related, in that reliability is a necessary but not sufficient condition for validity. In short, reliability constrains or imposes a ceiling on validity. For instance, an assessment tool that utterly lacks reliability—whether because its elements do not cohere, different assessors obtain inconsistent findings, or its findings are temporally unstable—cannot demonstrate criterion-related validity by predicting phenomena outside the test itself. Just as a thermometer whose readings fluctuate randomly or are different for different readers cannot robustly predict heat-related phenomena such as sweating and freezing, so a psychological test cannot predict important clinical phenomena to the extent that its measurements are inconsistent. Translating this point into statistical terms, if a variable is assessed with measurement error then any "true" correlation that it has with another variable will be diluted in proportion to that error.

Validity imposes no comparable constraint on reliability. Although an unreliable test cannot be valid, it is entirely possible for an invalid test to be reliable. People can generate reliable estimates of the brightness of ambient light, but if this is intended as a means of assessing ambient temperature it lacks validity. This asymmetrical relationship between reliability and validity means that the former is in some respects more fundamental. Consequently, it is not unreasonable for developers of assessment methods, such as psychological tests or diagnostic interviews, to pay special attention to reliability and concentrate their efforts on enhancing it. Although doing so does not guarantee validity, it is a validational necessity. As we shall see, this preferential attention to reliability over validity has left a controversial legacy in the study of psychiatric diagnosis and classification.

The fact that reliability may be a prerequisite for validity might seem to imply a positive or at worst a null relationship between these properties: increased reliability should enable increased validity even if it does not guarantee it. However an inverse relationship is possible in some situations, so that the pursuit of reliability comes at the cost of validity. Arguably such a price has been paid in the historical changes in psychiatric diagnosis to which we now turn.

Reliability and Validity in Psychiatric Diagnosis

Issues of diagnostic reliability, validity, and their relationship arose most forcefully in response to the DSM-III in 1980. This manual presented a radical overhaul of psychiatric nosology that, because it has served as a kind of pivot-point in the field, continuing to guide subsequent DSM editions, is not merely of historical interest. Although the history of its development is somewhat contentious, several key points about their precursors are not in serious question. First, the preceding edition of the manual, the DSM-II (1968), bore a strong theoretical imprint of the psychodynamic approach that dominated the field at the time. Psychodynamic terminology permeated the text, most notoriously the concept of "neurosis." In the case of hysterical neurosis, for example, the manual indicated that "Symptoms characteristically begin and end suddenly in emotionally charged situations and are symbolic of the underlying conflicts" (APA 1968, p. 39). Second, the DSM-II contained 182 diagnostic categories which were described in often impressionistic ways without clear-cut diagnostic algorithms. Third, studies of diagnostic agreement between clinicians (i.e., interrater reliability) using the DSM-II yielded rather modest results, implying that agreement was rarely good and was sometimes little better than chance. Partly in consequence of the apparent looseness and unreliability of the diagnostic status quo, several influential researchers working in the 1970s developed stricter sets of diagnostic criteria for selected psychiatric conditions, notably the so-called Feighner criteria (Feighner et al. 1972) and the Research Diagnostic Criteria (Spitzer et al. 1978).

The DSM-III initiated several fundamental changes to psychiatric classification. More than one hundred new diagnostic categories were added and the diagnostic manual itself swelled to almost four times the earlier edition's page count. Terminology with a psychodynamic origin or connotation was purged, as was material related to etiology, in favor of avowedly "atheoretical," descriptive, and behavioral language. One casualty was the concept of "neurosis," an idea judged to carry too much psychoanalytic freight. Individual mental disorders were no longer described in DSM-II's holistic manner, in which each condition was summarized in a single paragraph that gave little explicit guidance on how diagnostic judgments should be rendered. Instead, DSM-III provided detailed enumerations of diagnostic criteria that each addressed a relatively narrow kind of observable behavior and invited a binary present/absent decision. These itemized criterion sets were accompanied by explicit instructions for making diagnostic decisions, which involved necessary features, exclusion criteria, and quantitative requirements such as minimum symptom durations and thresholds for polythetic symptom lists (i.e., the number of criteria that must be met for a diagnosis to be made). By this means diagnostic decision-making became governed by explicit rules for combining criteria, replacing the holistic pattern-matching process that DSM-II entailed. With DSM-III the diagnostic process also became increasingly dominated by structured diagnostic interviews, which aimed to standardize diagnostic practice by providing uniform question wording.

To illustrate, the DSM-II contained a disorder called "obsessive-compulsive neurosis," and described it with a brief syndrome portrait in the form of a verbal slab.

> This disorder is characterized by the persistent intrusion of unwanted thoughts, urges, or actions that the patient is unable to stop. The thoughts may consist of single words or ideas, ruminations, or trains of thought often perceived by the patient as nonsensical. The actions vary from simple movements to complex rituals such as repeated handwashing. Anxiety and distress are often present either if the patient is prevented from completing his compulsive ritual or if he is concerned about being unable to control it himself. (APA 1968, p. 40)

The DSM-III, in contrast, changed the disorder's name to "obsessive-compulsive disorder" and described it with a long list of clinical features including variants of many that had been laid out in the previous edition but also extending to demographic features and differential diagnosis. Explicit rules required patients to meet a set of criteria for obsessions or compulsions, and also criteria for clinically significant distress or impairment.

These many diagnostic alterations can be understood narrowly as an attempt to secure diagnostic reliability and broadly as an imposition of an operationalist philosophy of science. The technical goal of enhancing reliability, usually understood in the interrater sense, was the dominant expressed rationale among the DSM-III's developers. Criticizing the extent of diagnostic disagreement under DSM-II, Robert Spitzer and colleagues endeavored to minimize it as far as possible, and almost all new features of the DSM-III can be viewed in this light. Provision of specific diagnostic criteria should improve reliability by simplifying the cognitive task of the diagnostician. Expressing these criteria in standardized interview questions should reduce variation between diagnosticians in the manner and method of information gathering. Making criteria refer to observable behaviors rather than inferred psychological dynamics should enable intersubjective agreement. Eliminating theory-saturated concepts from diagnostic decision-making should discourage unreliable depth-psychological inferences. Formulae for combining diagnostic criteria into diagnostic decisions should remove opportunities for judges to integrate their diagnostic impressions in idiosyncratic ways. By improving diagnostic reliability by these means, the developers of the DSM-III aimed to provide a more solid foundation for psychiatric research, which requires a robust and replicable method of identifying clinical groups, and also for psychiatric practice, where enhanced diagnosis might improve treatment planning and efficacy.

Although the DSM-III's wholesale changes to diagnostic practice can be viewed in this way simply as a pragmatic attempt to increase reliability, it can also be seen as the product of a distinct logical empiricist philosophy of science and measurement, usually referred to as *operationalism*. Based on Bridgeman's work on the philosophy of physics and developed in relation to psychiatric taxonomy by Hempel (1965), the operationalist approach to scientific classification maintains that concepts should be identified by explicit operations or procedures that precisely define the concepts' meaning. These "operations" could be interpreted liberally for psychiatry as clinical observations, but it was crucial that they were reliable in the sense of having "intersubjective uniformity," which we would recognize as interrater reliability. Indeed, influential psychiatric thinkers such as Kendell (1975), who drew approvingly on Hempel's work, gave special attention to the need for reliability and the concrete and "objective" diagnostic features that enable it.

Hempel's approach to psychiatric classification supposes that diagnostic entities should be described by observable properties that define their necessary and sufficient conditions, namely empirically established features that people who merit the diagnosis must have and that only they have (Schwartz and Wiggins 1986). The aim of this exercise is to generate sets of features that afford clear, precise, and scientifically well-founded meanings for diagnostic entities, as well as rigorous procedures for determining when these features apply to individuals. According to Hempel, these diagnostic descriptions should also be incorporated into systematic theories and laws about the mental disorders in question, including their etiology. Psychiatry tends to lack systematic etiological theories of this sort, as Hempel recognized, but should aspire to develop them. The institution of operational definitions of real diagnostic entities was an important step toward their development.

Hempel's advocacy of operationalism for psychiatric diagnosis was later taken up by an influential group of research psychiatrists who developed what came to be known as the neo-Kraepelinian approach to diagnosis. The key tenets of their approach, echoing those of Emil Kraepelin's descriptive psychopathology of the early twentieth century, include the desirability of explicitly codified and scientifically supported operational diagnosis. However they extend well beyond such technical matters to a broad commitment to a biomedical view of the field (Klerman 1978). The neo-Kraepelinians considered psychiatry to be a branch of medicine that dealt with discrete mental illnesses that categorically distinguished the sick from the normal, and they believed that psychiatry should emphasize biological etiologies. Their nosological preferences gave shape to the DSM-III (Compton and Guze 1995).

Criticisms of DSM-III and Operational Diagnosis

The DSM-III attracted criticism from many fronts, many more sociohistorical than philosophical, but for our purposes those that relate to reliability and validity are of greatest concern. I will focus on four criticisms that are especially pertinent. Although these are framed as criticisms of DSM-III in particular, and were first expressed in reference to it, they have continuing relevance to later editions (DSM-III-R, DSM-IV, DSM-IV-TR), which have substantially retained the original's approach.

1. *Did the DSM-III succeed in its stated goal of increasing interrater reliability?* The simplest reliability-related criticism of the DSM-III's operationalist approach is that diagnostic agreement failed to improve substantially in its wake. Kirk and Kutchins (1994), for example, argue that published studies of diagnostic agreement show little

or no improvement from DSM-II to DSM-III, even under research conditions, such as extensive training of diagnostic interviewers, which should maximize interrater reliability. It is difficult to challenge the view that the DSM-III's improvements to reliability were oversold and frequently modest and incremental rather than large and revolutionary. By implication, the limited success of DSM-III's operational approach in enhancing reliability, one of its primary motivations, either represents the intrinsic misguidedness of that approach or the inadequacy of its implementation.

2. *Did the operational nature of DSM-III diagnostic criteria omit more suitable clinical features?* Some critics argue that by focusing diagnostic criteria on clinical features that are directly observable and, in theory at least, "atheoretical," the DSM-III provides impoverished descriptions of its disorders. In psychometric language, the system's emphasis on (interrater) reliability comes at a cost of (internal) validity. Criticisms of this sort tend to come from writers with psychodynamic or phenomenological commitments (e.g., Parnas and Zahavi 2002). Their common thread is that by omitting psychodynamics or experiential subtleties the DSM-III's diagnostic criteria do not accurately characterize core features of particular disorders, and may not validly pick out true cases of the disorder. A psychoanalytically-oriented critic might argue that the use of projection as a defense mechanism is a core aspect of paranoid personality, and that any diagnostic criterion set that omits it, whether on grounds of theoretical agnosticism or the unobservability of unconscious defenses, will thereby lack content validity. A phenomenologist might make similar claims about the omission of aspects of self-awareness from diagnostic criteria for schizophrenia.

3. *Did the DSM-III's operational approach lead to a distortion of certain diagnoses?* A related criticism is that an exclusive reliance on observable, behavioral features for diagnosis may lead not only to error in the specification of a mental disorder, but to a systematic distortion. It can be argued that by tilting diagnostic decision-making toward such features the DSM-III may have invalidly narrowed some of its disorders. This criticism has been expressed in relation to antisocial personality disorder (ASPD), which came into being as a replacement for psychopathy in DSM-III. Psychopathy has two underlying components, one related to antisocial and delinquent behavior and the other an interpersonal style marked by callousness, lack of empathy, and other emotional and social-cognitive deficits. The latter component is less directly observable and thus more difficult to capture in behavior-focused criteria. As a result, the DSM-III ASPD criteria arguably overemphasize antisocial conduct and thus fail to capture adequately the broader clinical pattern, as well as overdiagnosing people with histories of offending (Ogloff, 2006).

4. *Did the proliferation of recognized mental disorders in DSM-III represent an invalid form of nosological "splitting"?* DSM-III's striving for reliability can also be held at least partly responsible for the sharp increase in the number of disorders over the previous edition. Whereas most critiques of the DSM-III's emphasis on reliability have focused on diagnostic agreement (interrater reliability), this claim addresses internal consistency instead. It argues that by placing emphasis on homogeneous clusters of observable features, the DSM-III over-differentiates psychopathology, preferring classificatory "splitting" over integrative "lumping." Striving for internal consistency can promote splitting because larger, looser, and therefore more inclusive sets of features can usually be subdivide into smaller, more highly correlated subsets.

The potential over-differentiation may endanger validity to the degree that commonalities among "split" clinical entities may be overlooked. Some writers have argued that the DSM-III's operational stance may systematically overlook these commonalities by omitting diagnostic features that are not directly observable and require a degree of inference. Two behaviorally-defined syndromes that are superficially distinct might share an underlying mechanism or process that supplies a valid link between them. The demise of the concept of "neurosis" illustrates the point. DSM-II employed this overarching term to link disorders in which anxiety "may be felt and expressed directly, or it may be controlled unconsciously and automatically by conversion, displacement and various other psychological mechanisms" (APA 1968, p. 40). By disallowing reference to inferred (e.g., conversion and displacement) rather than directly observable processes, the DSM-III classifies these conditions separately rather than unifying them under the neurotic umbrella. Which classificatory decision is the more valid is an open question.

DSM-III's apparent reliability-driven tendency to over-differentiate disorders may have implications beyond validity. In a further irony, the splitting of psychiatric conditions that is promoted by an emphasis on internal reliability can weaken interrater reliability. Any increase in the number of disorders in a psychiatric classification adds to the number of ways in which diagnosticians can disagree, and differential diagnosis is made especially difficult when two similar disorders are distinguished within the psychopathological space that was previously occupied by a single condition. The proliferation of similar diagnoses that may have a common underlying pathological process—which Parnas et al. (2008, p. 580) refer to as an "atomization of psychopathology"—also adds to the problem of "comorbidity," the tendency for patients to receive multiple diagnoses. This kind of spurious comorbidity due to splitting not only misrepresents the patient's difficulties but also creating difficulties for clinicians in the prioritizing of treatment.

Whether or not all of these criticisms of DSM-III's operational approach to diagnosis have merit, they demonstrate the complexities involved in the pursuit of reliability. Although it is true in theory that certain forms of reliability enable validity, they may also impair validity and even weaken other forms of reliability. The DSM-III's pursuit of interrater reliability has arguably reduced the content validity of its disorder descriptions by omitting certain types of clinical features, such as those that are linked to particular theoretical positions or that are inferentially demanding. Its pursuit of internal consistency, coupled with the emphasis on observable behavior in its diagnostic criteria, may have over-differentiated psychopathology (i.e., "splitting") so that some disorders are invalidly narrow. The resulting proliferation of diagnoses may have come at a cost of interrater reliability (i.e., diagnostic agreement).

ADVANTAGES OF OPERATIONAL DIAGNOSIS

Arguments of this sort suggest that the reliability-driven turn to operational diagnosis, begun with DSM-III and continuing in later editions, has come at a considerable cost. If the quest for reliability can endanger rather than merely enable validity then the rationale for the descriptive, atheoretical, behavioral, and rigidly proceduralized approach to diagnosis that DSM-III embodies is seriously undermined. However, there are also good reasons why de-emphasizing reliability in future diagnostic systems might be problematic.

Critics who advocate against the DSM raise a variety of objections. Some of these are not directly related to issues of psychometric reliability and validity, such as the DSM's supposed lack of a coherent concept of mental disorder, its malign influence on psychiatric practice and education, the role of particular political or industrial interests in formulating it, or its contamination by various kinds of bias. I will set these aside and focus on objections relevant to the topic of this chapter. These objections tend to focus on issues of validity rather than reliability.

As we have seen, some writers invoke content validity by objecting to the exclusion of phenomenological or psychodynamic dimensions in the characterization of particular disorders. Some take issue with the apparent arbitrariness of diagnostic cutpoints, such as duration criteria or thresholds for polythetic symptom lists. Some argue that certain disorders are over-inclusive, their boundaries invalidly broad so that people who are not disordered receive diagnoses. Similarly, some critics argue that by drawing diagnostic boundaries at all, the DSM rests on an invalid assumption that mental disorders are discrete categories. This supposed ontological error, which is often traced back to the neo-Kraepelinian assumption that mental disorders are biomedical disease entities, is sometimes held responsible for the tendency for people to reify and essentialize mental disorders. I address some of the weaknesses of these criticisms of operational diagnosis in the next section.

Problems with the inclusion of theory-based diagnostic features

Although these criticisms may have merit in pointing to forms of invalidity within the dominant approach to psychiatric classification and diagnosis, some of them underestimate the problems that unreliability can cause. For example, the operationalist approach adopted by DSM-III's developers may indeed have led to a systematic neglect of certain kinds of phenomena in the characterization of mental disorders, such as forms of subjectivity, defense mechanisms, or intrapsychic conflicts. This neglect may have been justified on the grounds that diagnostic criteria should be "generally atheoretical." At least some of these phenomena may have valid and even strong linkages to particular disorders, and in this sense their omission would amount to a lack of content validity in their diagnostic criteria (i.e., the sampling of clinical features from the universe of the disorder would be biased). Nevertheless, if phenomenological and psychodynamic attributes and processes cannot be judged reliably by diagnosticians then their validity as signs of a disorder is psychometrically worthless. If there is a phenomenological sign X that experts have reason to believe is strongly associated with disorder Y, but which is so subtle or slippery that even trained clinicians cannot agree when it is present, then including the sign as a diagnostic feature will reduce the Y's reliability to the detriment of its criterion-related validity.

Phenomenological writers seem to recognize that their desire to increase the content validity (as they see it) of mental disorders by including aspects of subjectivity in diagnosis may lead to a reduction in reliability. As Mishara (1994, p. 147) observes, "phenomenology cannot compete with empirical approaches in producing reliable results." However, this recognition does not seem to appreciate the costs involved in any such loss of reliability. Interrater reliability may not guarantee validity, as we have seen, but anything that reduces reliability will correspondingly reduce the capacity for psychiatric diagnoses to predict external criteria. Criterion-related validity matters both for practical clinical reasons—e.g., the capacity of diagnostic decisions to predict treatment response—and for the scientific development of the field. Interrater disagreement constrains the capacity of researchers to find new relationships between mental disorders and other phenomena, such as etiological factors, epidemiological correlates, and so on. Any alteration to diagnostic practice that aims to improve content validity by including new clinical features but has the side effect of impairing interrater reliability can therefore have detrimental consequences.

There is some precedent for this sort of detrimental effect in psychometrics. Projective tests, such as the famous Rorschach inkblots, have been promoted by psychodynamic clinicians as having validity in part because they assess deep aspects of the personality that self-report inventories cannot reach. They are therefore claimed to have content validity for assessing personality dynamics. However, these instruments have been plagued by weak interrater reliability, even when efforts have been made to standardize their administration, scoring, and interpretation. Partly as a result, in head-to-head comparisons with self-report inventories they tend to have poorer criterion-related validity (Wood et al. 2003). Opposition to the use of projective tests can therefore be justified either by opposition to the psychodynamic theoretical commitment of the tests—much as the DSM excludes theory-identified content from its diagnostic criteria—but also, and perhaps more legitimately, by recognition of the empirical deficiencies in criterion-related validity of these tests.

My claim here is not that phenomenological or psychodynamic aspects of clinical presentations are invariably or intrinsically lacking in interrater reliability or in criterion-related validity. Rather, I argue that as these aspects tend to be less amenable to reliable judgments than observable behavior, diagnostic criteria that rely on the latter can be expected to have less criterion-related validity, even if the former might add to content validity. A sensible middle way forward would be to relax the requirement that all diagnostic criteria should be atheoretical and behavioral, but insist that all clinical features considered for inclusion as criteria demonstrate acceptable levels of interrater reliability. Chronic use of a defense mechanism or aberrant forms of subjectivity might be considered as diagnostic criteria if they contribute to content validity, but only if they also show psychometric credentials of interrater agreement (see Vaillant 1985).

The need for a shared understanding of psychopathology

Another consideration that critics of operational diagnosis tend to neglect, including champions of theory-linked diagnostic features, is the need for any diagnostic system to serve as a shared medium of communication. Classifications such as the DSM must be useable by multiple constituencies that vary in their theoretical commitments and in their social contexts. Ideally any diagnostic system will be acceptable to clinicians with diverse theoretical orientations and will be used in comparable ways, picking out comparable clinical groups, in different countries and cultures. This consistency of endorsement and application is far from assured—a diagnostic system that adopts any explicit theoretical approach will be unacceptable to clinicians who do not share it, and there has been evidence of striking cross-cultural differences in diagnostic practices. A pre-DSM-III example revealed much more liberal application of the schizophrenia diagnosis in the USA compared to the UK in the late 1960s (Kendell et al. 1971), one study finding that American psychiatrists viewing a videotaped diagnostic interview were thirty-three times more likely to diagnose the patient with schizophrenia than British psychiatrists viewing the same videotape, who in their turn were eighteen times more likely than their American colleagues to diagnose hysterical personality. For all their possible failings, and despite the impossibility of any classification being truly "atheoretical," diagnostic systems that strive to avoid theory-specific concepts and that lay out clear-cut operational diagnostic criteria have the best chance of being widely usable and of carrying similar meanings across different national and cultural contexts.

On pragmatic grounds, therefore, operational diagnosis of the sort embodied by DSM-III and later editions has several advantages. Its relative theoretical agnosticism and procedural strictness should increase the utility of diagnostic classifications and the confidence that groups of patients identified as having a disorder in different locations are comparable. These implications are important for clinical and scientific communication. Practitioners and researchers need a common nomenclature and a common set of understandings of mental disorder, even if they appreciate that these shared understandings are partial and theoretically unsatisfying. As Allen Frances, architect of the DSM-IV, has remarked (2010, p. 6), "the DSM is necessarily more about forging a common language than in finding a truth." As languages go it is also deliberately basic. An operational diagnostic system should be seen not as a lingua franca that captures all the richness of clinical phenomena in a universally acceptable way, but as a simplified pidgin that clinicians of different orientations can use to transact their shared business, while speaking their preferred first language—phenomenology, psychoanalysis, cognitivism—within their tribes. A lingua franca is unachievable and a Babel of diagnostic languages is unworkable, so for all its crudeness a pidgin may be the best option.

Categories or dimensions?

Many of the criticisms of operationalism as embodied in recent editions of the DSM are directed at categorical diagnosis. The DSM produces binary diagnostic decisions—disorder or no disorder—on the basis of explicit criteria. This commitment to categorical diagnosis has been criticized on multiple validity-related grounds, including arbitrariness in the criteria used to make these decisions and excessively liberal criteria leading to overdiagnosis. More fundamentally, many critics have argued that psychopathology may not be composed of bounded categories, and that the DSM is invalid in making categorical diagnoses unless evidence of discrete categories is found (Kendell and Jablensky 2003). Instead, it is argued that most mental disorders do not conform to the neo-Kraepelinian assumption of discrete disease entities or psychiatric natural kinds (Haslam 2000; Zachar 2000), and that the differences between normality and abnormality, and between different forms of abnormality, are matters of degree. A dimensional view of psychopathology is therefore seen as more valid than the categorical view enshrined in DSM (Helzer et al. 2008; Widiger and Samuel 2005).

The scientific evidence on these matters is becoming increasingly clear. With respect to the underlying structure of psychopathology, a recent quantitative review of 177 taxometric research studies (Haslam et al, 2012) found that most psychopathological variation is latently continuous (dimensional) rather than categorical. Psychiatric nature may have few joints to carve. This finding directly contradicts the neo-Kraepelinian assumption that mental disorders are discrete disease entities. Furthermore, a large meta-analysis by Markon et al. (2011) found that dimensional measures of psychopathology tended to have greater reliability (15%) and much greater criterion-related validity (37%) than categorical measures, an advantage that held for all major classes of mental disorders.

Research findings such as these challenge categorical diagnosis, indicating that diagnosing disorders as dichotomously present or absent misrepresents their underlying structure and impairs reliability and validity. Whether the operationalist approach to diagnosis is directly responsible for these failings is questionable, however. The classification systems that preceded DSM-III also rendered categorical diagnoses, and merely did so through a more flexible and less formalized decision process. Moreover, unlike its predecessors the DSM-III and subsequent editions explicitly disavow the idea that making categorical diagnoses implies an ontological commitment to mental disorders being discrete categories. The DSM-IV, for example, makes "no assumption that each category of mental disorder is a completely discrete entity with absolute boundaries dividing it from other disorders or from no mental disorder" (APA 1994, p. xxii). In this fashion, the way in which mental disorders are represented in the diagnostic manual and identified in clinical practice is detached from their latent structure, which is screened off as the kind of etiology- and theory-related matter that the DSM's descriptive approach forswears. Although the DSM-III emerged from a neo-Kraepelinian matrix that was aligned with a biomedical disease model of mental disorders, its operationalism can be at least partially removed from that matrix. An operational approach to psychiatric diagnosis need not rest on the belief that mental disorders are discrete disease entities.

Instead of resting on a biomedical disease model, psychiatric classifications can justify categorical diagnosis on pragmatic grounds. Categorical diagnosis simplifies clinical communication and treatment planning, even if it does not correspond to the underlying (dimensional) nature of the psychopathology to which it refers. In a similar fashion, obesity and hypertension tend to be diagnosed categorically on the basis of semi-arbitrary body mass index (BMI) and blood pressure thresholds, despite an appreciation that each falls on a seamless continuum. Thus, scientific findings that mental disorders tend not to be latent categories do not directly challenge the DSM's use of categorical diagnoses, if these diagnoses are properly understood as pragmatic simplifications, like diagnosing someone as overweight if their BMI exceeds thirty. Findings that categorical diagnosis carries a validity penalty are more problematic, but they are again not specific to recent versions of the DSM or directly linked to its operationalism. Earlier versions of the DSM also rendered categorical diagnoses, and dimensions can also be assessed operationally.

This discussion raises an important point. Many of the criticisms of operationalism in psychiatry implicitly challenge it on the grounds that operational diagnoses are deficient as definitions of mental disorders. These definitions supposedly provide impoverished descriptions of mental disorders and misrepresent their underlying nature. However, operational diagnostic criteria should not be seen as constituting full definitions but only as partial, indirect and contingent specifications. As Hempel (1965, p.143) noted, sometimes a measuring instrument only provides "a *partial definition*, or better, *a partial criterion of application*, for the term under consideration (or for the corresponding concept)." Malmgren (1993, p.58) illustrates such an indirect and contingent identification procedure:

> By "blackbird" is meant that kind of bird, the males of which you can often hear singing loudly and beautifully from treetops in Göteborg on early March evenings.

We would not mistake this statement for a full definition of "blackbird," let alone an account of the category's ontological status or causation, but it is akin to the observation-based identification rules that make up the DSM.

CONCLUSIONS

Psychiatric diagnosis remains a contentious topic, and as it involves assessment these contentions will often implicate reliability and validity. In this chapter I have tried to show that these properties are complex and interrelated. The advent of the operationalist approach to diagnosis has had implications for reliability and validity, and a balanced appraisal must acknowledge that these implications are ambivalent. Operational diagnosis has probably had a positive impact on diagnostic agreement (interrater reliability), which would be expected to bolster empirical relationships between diagnoses and other clinically and scientifically relevant phenomena (criterion-related validity). It has also probably had a beneficial impact on the communicative value of psychiatric diagnoses across theoretical and cultural divides and the confidence that research findings obtained in different locations can refer to comparable patient groups. These are significant achievements and should not be ignored or trivialized by critics, whose contrary proposals may set them back.

At the same time, operational diagnosis may have contributed to the proliferation of mental disorders, the resulting problem of runaway comorbidity, and a distorted conception of some forms of psychopathology where its focus on observable features may have led to a systematic neglect of others. It may also have led to an impoverished understanding of descriptive psychopathology among people in the mental health field—and their educators—who mistake DSM diagnostic criteria for full definitions of mental disorders. This mistake is a critical and common one; it loads DSM descriptions with more meaning than they can bear, and then criticizes them when they collapse under the weight of unreasonable expectations. Operational diagnoses are delimited identification procedures, not comprehensive clinical formulations. They should be evaluated primarily on the pragmatic grounds of whether they identify meaningful clinical groupings, provide a common ground of working concepts for clinicians and researchers, and allow them to make helpful inferences and discoveries about patients. Whether recent systems for psychiatric diagnosis meet these criteria is a separate question.

REFERENCES

American Psychiatric Association (1968). *Diagnostic and Statistical Manual of Mental Disorders, Second Edition*. Washington, DC: American Psychiatric Association.

American Psychiatric Association (1980). *Diagnostic and Statistical Manual of Mental Disorders, Third Edition*. Washington, DC: American Psychiatric Association.

American Psychiatric Association (1994). *Diagnostic and Statistical Manual of Mental Disorders, Fourth Edition*. Washington, DC: American Psychiatric Association.

Cloninger, C. R. (1989). Establishment of diagnostic validity in psychiatric illness: Robins and Guze's method revisited. In L. N. Robins and J. E. Barrett (Eds), *The Validity of Psychiatric Diagnosis*, pp. 9–18. New York, NY: Raven Press.

Compton, W. M. and Guze, S. B. (1995). The neo-Kraepelinian revolution in psychiatric diagnosis. *European Archives of Psychiatry and Clinical Neurosciences*, 245, 196–201.

Cronbach, L. J. and Meehl, P. E. (1955). Construct validity in psychological tests. *Psychological Bulletin*, 52, 281–302.

Feighner, J., Robin, E., Guze, S., Woodruff, R., Winokur, G., and Munoz, R. (1972). Diagnostic criteria for use in psychiatric research. *Archives of General Psychiatry*, 26, 57–63.

Frances, A. (2010). DSM in philosophyland: Curiouser and curioser. *Bulletin of the Association for the Advancement of Philosophy and Psychiatry*, 17, 3–7.

Haslam, N. (2000). Psychiatric categories as natural kinds: Essentialist thinking about mental disorders. *Social Research*, 67, 1031–58.

Haslam, N., Holland, E., and Kuppens, P. (2012). Categories versus dimensions in personality and psychopathology: A quantitative review of taxometric research. *Psychological Medicine*, 42, 903–20.

Helzer, J. E., Kraemer, H. C., and Krueger, R. F. (Eds) (2008). *Dimensional Approaches in Diagnostic Classification: Refining the Research Agenda for DSM-V*. Washington, DC: American Psychiatric Association.

Hempel, C. G. (1965). Fundamentals of taxonomy. In *Aspects of Scientific Explanation and Other Essays in the Philosophy of Science*, pp. 137–54. New York, NY: Free Press.

Kendell, R. E. (1975). *The Role of Diagnosis in Psychiatry*. Oxford: Blackwell.

Kendell, R. E., Cooper, J. E., Gourlay, A. J., Copeland, J. R., Sharpe, L., and Gurland, B. J. (1971). Diagnostic criteria of American and British psychiatrists. *Archives of General Psychiatry*, 25, 123–30.

Kendell, R. E. and Jablensky, A. (2003). Distinguishing between the validity and utility of psychiatric diagnoses. *American Journal of Psychiatry*, 160, 4–12.

Kirk, S. A. and Kutchins, H. (1994). The myth of the reliability of DSM. *Journal of Mind and Behavior*, 15, 71–86.

Klerman, G. L. (1978). The evolution of a scientific nosology. In J. C. Shershow (Ed.), *Schizophrenia: Science and Practice*, pp. 99–121. Cambridge, MA: Harvard University Press.

Malmgren, H. (1993). Psychiatric classification and empiricist theories of meaning. *Acta Psychiatrica Scandinavica*, 88, 48–64.

Markon, K. E., Chmielewski, M., and Miller, C. J. (2011). The reliability and validity of discrete and continuous measures of psychopathology: A quantitative review. *Psychological Bulletin*, 137, 856–79.

Mishara, A. L. (1994). A phenomenological critique of commonsensical assumptions in DSM-III-R: The avoidance of the patient's subjectivity. In J. Z. Sadler, O. P. Wiggins, and M. A. Schwartz (Eds), *Philosophical Perspectives on Psychiatric Diagnostic Classification*, pp. 129–47. Baltimore, MD: Johns Hopkins University Press.

Ogloff, J. R. (2006). Psychopathy/antisocial personality disorder conundrum. *Australian and New Zealand Journal of Psychiatry*, 40, 519–28.

Parnas, J., Sass, L. A., and Zahavi, D. (2008). Recent developments in philosophy of psychopathology. *Current Opinion in Psychiatry*, 21, 578–84.

Parnas, J. and Zahavi, D. (2002). The role of phenomenology in psychiatric diagnosis and classification. In M. Maj, W. Gaebel, J. J. López-Ibor and N. Sartorius (Eds), *Psychiatric Diagnosis and Classification*, pp. 137–62. New York, NY: John Wiley.

Robins, E. and Guze, S. B. (1970). Establishment of diagnostic validity in psychiatric illness: Its application to schizophrenia. *American Journal of Psychiatry*, 126, 107–11.

Schwartz, M. A. and Wiggins, O. P. (1986). Logical empiricism and psychiatric classification. *Comprehensive Psychiatry*, 27, 101–14.

Spitzer, R., Endicott, J., and Robins, E. (1978). Research diagnostic criteria: Rationale and reliability. *Archives of General Psychiatry*, 35, 773–82.

Spitzer, R. L. and Fleiss, J. L. (1974). A reanalysis of the reliability of psychiatric diagnosis. *British Journal of Psychiatry*, 125, 341–7.

Vaillant, G. E. (1985). An empirically derived classification of adaptive mechanisms and its usefulness as a potential diagnostic axis. *Acta Psychiatrica Scandinavica*, 71(Suppl 319), 171–80.

Widiger, T. A. and Samuel, D. B. (2005). Diagnostic categories or dimensions? A question for the Diagnostic and Statistical Manual of Mental Disorders—Fifth Edition. *Journal of Abnormal Psychology*, 114, 494–504.

Wood, J. M., Nezworski, M. T., Lilienfeld, S. O., and Garb, H. N. (2003). *What's Wrong with the Rorschach?: Science Confronts the Controversial Inkblot Test*. San Francisco, CA: Jossey-Bass.

Zachar, P. (2000). Psychiatric disorders are not natural kinds. *Philosophy, Psychiatry, & Psychology*, 7, 167–82.

CHAPTER 59

....

REDUCTION AND
REDUCTIONISM IN
PSYCHIATRY

....

KENNETH F. SCHAFFNER

A number of scientists and philosophers have argued that biology, and even more so psychology and psychiatry, involve phenomena, types of concepts, and forms of explanation which are *distinct* from those employed in the physical sciences. The reductionistic alternative is to view these phenomena, concepts, and modes of explanation as only prima facie distinct and ultimately definable in terms of (or fully explainable and perhaps replaceable by) concepts and modes of explanation drawn only from the physical and chemical sciences, and in the case of psychology, only from the biological sciences in addition to physics and chemistry. The issue of reduction (and reductionism) in both biology and the sciences of the mind provokes vigorous debate. Reduction to a number of scientists often has the connotation that biological and or psychological entities, as implied by the earlier statement, are "nothing but" aggregates of physicochemical entities. This can be termed "*ontological* reductionism" of a strong form. A closely related but more *methodological* position is that sound scientific generalizations are available only at the level of physics and chemistry, or in *molecular* biology.[1] In philosophy of science, a major extended debate about the concept of reduction has also revolved around what has been termed *intertheoretic* reduction. Essentially intertheoretic reduction is the *explanation* of a *theory* initially formulated in one branch of science by a theory from another discipline.

Reductionistic and antireductionist themes have their counterparts in psychiatry, where the focus is, as will be developed in the following pages, on the reduction of *mental or psychiatric disorders*. The discussion also often overlaps with the related topic of the *etiology* of psychiatric disorders. A major feature of many psychiatric disorders found in the third edition of the *Diagnostic and Statistical Manual of Mental Disorders* (DSM-III) through DSM-IV-TR, the tenth revision of the International Classification of Diseases (ICD-10) "Mental Disorders" chapter, and thus far in the developing DSM-5, is their prima facie lack

---

[1] These distinctions are developed in more detail and with reference to examples and to the literature in Schaffner (1993, chapter 9).

of any organic basis and etiology. DSM-IV-TR notes that "the etiological basis for most psychiatric conditions remains elusive" (American Psychiatric Association 2000, p. 2). Further, reflecting the atheoretical stance of the volume with respect to etiology, psychosis of a psychiatric type is to be ruled out if an organic or medical condition may have caused the condition (p. 14). This is a reasonable position if its intent is to exclude similar appearing but quite distinct disorders such as amphetamine psychosis. In the past two decades, however, a number of researchers have begun important investigations into etiological and molecular aspects of the functional psychoses, including schizophrenia and bipolar affective disorder.

These inquiries, in the case of schizophrenia, include both the elaboration of complex reductionistic models of the disorder(s), molecular etiologies, as well as attempts to determine genetic markers and an imaging basis for the disorder. Neurobiological models of schizophrenia developed by Lewis and by Harrison and Weinberger, to be discussed later in this chapter, can be construed as ways to bring molecular neurobiology to bear on psychiatric disorders both providing reductions as well as advancing research into the disorder's etiology. These neurobiological models can supplement molecular genetic studies that attempt to identify the gene (or far more likely *genes*) that are partially causative of the disorder (see section "Schizophrenia as a possible paradigm of a reducible mental disorder"). Neurobiological models, genetic studies, and neuroimaging approaches can also synergistically intercalate with a developmental approach to schizophrenia (see, e.g., Lewis and Levitt 2002) and potentially provide cellular and biochemical markers for the disorder, leading to improvements in diagnosis and treatment. In the light of such developments, more attention needs to be given to the possibility of important organic etiological features in disorders such as schizophrenia. However, molecular approaches to mental disorders such as schizophrenia are quite complex and partial—complications that I believe will require some preliminary philosophical clarifications prior to considering some representative ongoing reductionistic advances in psychiatry.

Kinds of Reduction

One distinction that needs to be introduced at the outset is between two kinds of reductionism. The first is what I call "sweeping reductionism," where we have a sort of "Theory of Everything" and there is *nothing but* those basic elements—for example, a very powerful biological theory that explains all of psychology and psychiatry. The second kind is "creeping reductionism," where bit by bit we get fragmentary explanations using interlevel mechanisms. In neuroscience, this might involve calcium ions, neurotransmitter dopamine molecules, genes, neuronal cell activity, and neural circuits, among other things, and of the sort we will encountered in the schizophrenia examples later on. Sweeping reductionism, I think, is probably non-existent except as a metaphysical claim. There is, however, some scientific bite in trying to do something like this in terms, say, of reducing thermodynamics to statistical mechanics or reducing optics to electrodynamics, but even these sweeping reductions tend to fail somewhat at the margins. In any event, I do not think that sweeping reductionism really has much in the way of cash value in the biological and psychological sciences. It is a scientific dream for some, and for others, a scientific nightmare.

Creeping reductionism, on the other hand, can be thought of as involving partial reductions—reductions that work on a patch of science. Creeping reductionism is what, for example, neuroscientists do when they make models and propose mechanisms. Creeping reductions do not typically commit to a nothing-but approach as part of an explanatory process. Rather, they seem to tolerate a kind of pragmatic and pluralistic parallelism akin to partial emergence, working at several levels of aggregation and discourse at once. And creeping reductions are consistent with a co-evolutionary approach that works on many levels simultaneously, with cross-fertilization. I will return to this notion of creeping reduction using psychiatric exemplars further in the sections "Schizophrenia as a possible paradigm of a reducible mental disorder" and "A partial reduction model in philosophy of science."

Disorders as Overlapping Models

Before we can discuss the specifics of reduction in psychiatry, we need to introduce a few general comments about *what* exactly is being reduced. The issue of how to define a "mental disorder" generally, and to a first approximation anyway, independent of any issues of reduction or etiology, has been one of the most vexing for both psychiatrists and philosophers of psychiatry. Other entries in this handbook will address the more general issues and examples that cluster around this issue, including naturalistic approaches (e.g., Kingma, Chapter 25) as well as non-naturalistic analyses (e.g., Bolton, Chapter 28; Fulford and van Staden, Chapter 26). Specific proposals in the psychiatric diagnostic manuals of both the American Psychiatric Association in the DSMs and the *International Classification of Disorders*, "Mental Disorders" chapter, including proposed definitions and supporting analyses are discussed in Sections V, on Descriptive Psychopathology and VI, on Assessment and Diagnostic Categories. The present article is not able to address these more far-ranging issues, but confines itself to a brief discussion of some logical and epistemological features of psychiatric disorders.

I will begin by briefly defending a view of a mental disorder as a family of over-lapping prototypical multilevel models. This defense is based on some of my previous work on the role of theory in biology and medicine (Schaffner 1980, 1986, 1993), but a very similar view was then further and independently developed in the psychiatric literature in the late 1990s. Within psychiatry proper, this prototype approach is consistent with Bleuler's classic description of schizophrenia, as well as with emerging indications of an underlying genetic heterogeneity of schizophrenia(s). The prototype approach to mental disorders was argued for and underwent a test implementation in the work of Mezzich (Cantor et al. 1980), was subsequently commented on favorably by (Frances et al. 1990), and then further developed by (Lilienfeld and Marino 1995, 1999). This view of a psychiatric disorder also has implications for reductionistic (and molecular genetic and biological) methodology, in the sense that it allows for a more dimensional and less categorical approach to disorder reduction. In the following sections "Schizophrenia as a possible paradigm of a reducible mental disorder" and "A partial reduction model in philosophy of science" I will examine what it means for a disorder to be reduced (or to be in the process of reduction) to a molecularly associated/definable entity or entities (Schaffner 1993, 2006, 2013). Finally in the concluding section, I will consider briefly the ramifications that this analysis has for more precise disorder definition(s), etiology, diagnosis, and therapy, as well as some implications for DSM-5 (and for later DSMs and ICD iterations), as well as for the emerging Research Diagnostic Criteria (RDoC) initiative of the National Institute of Mental Health.

What might be called the standard approach to contemporary psychiatry can be found in the DSM-IV-TR volume and in ICD-10 "Mental Disorders" chapter, and in related treatment texts that describe a variety of ways to address the collection of "mental disorders" found in the diagnosis texts. This suggests that to the first approximation, issues of reduction in psychiatry would be directed at providing biological and even physical-chemical characterizations of those disorders as well as physical-chemical-biological explanations of them. There are some changes in disorder definition projected for DSM-5, and thus also for ICD-11, but these are not expected to be major departures, even though dimensional approaches will figure more in these new developments. Such disorders are in the main presented as categories, and later in this chapter we will look at the category of schizophrenia as a representative example, but the categories do not present necessary and sufficient conditions for the application (diagnosis) of the category in any given patient. Since there can be many specific cases that satisfy the conditions for a diagnosis of a disorder, they are better thought of as "polytypic" (or "polythetic") categories, or in my view, a collection of prototypes related by similarity.

There are other models that can capture such variation and relation by similarity, which will be remarked on further, but for various reasons I believe that an overlapping prototype approach has the strongest case. From my perspective, what we encounter in biology, and I would argue eventually in psychiatry as we proceed reductively, are families of models or mechanisms with, in any given subdiscipline, a few prototypes. These prototypes are typically interlevel: in biology they *intermingle* ions, molecules, cells, cell–cell circuits, and organs, in the same causal/temporal process. In psychiatry the currently intermingled levels are primarily behavioral data obtained from patients' acquaintances and patients' subjective reports, intercalated in research contexts with genetic and neurobiological/imaging information. In both biology and psychiatry prototype models are related to each other by dimensional similarity, and there are many interforms. These partially overlapping interforms are often referred as a "spectrum" in psychiatry, as in "autistic spectrum" and "schizophrenia spectrum." The prototypes functioning as markers or signposts in spectra in this view are in effect *narrow classes*—ones which do allow for law-like/probabilistically causal predictions, and explanations—including in some cases for individuals. Extensive variation among the models and mechanisms in biology is a natural consequence of the result of how evolution operates: by replicating entities with many small variations, and assembling odds and ends—thus what Jacob called "tinkering" (Jacob 1977). And this kind of evolutionary variation is also currently evident in recent genetic studies of schizophrenia, about which more later.

A prototype approach has other independent arguments in its support in addition to consistency with the way that relationships among biomolecular models seem to behave. Psychologists, beginning with the pioneering work of Rosch in 1975, have argued that prototype representations are closer to the way that humans think naturally than are other more logically strict approaches to concepts (Rosch 1975a, 1975b). For additional comments on Rosch's approach as well as two alternatives, see Machery (2009, chapter 4).

Let me conclude this section by drawing together some of the themes and relating them to our general chapter topic of reduction. Generally acknowledging a prototype approach in psychiatry allows a dimensional approach to be integrated naturally into the received view of psychiatric disorders. Since I have argued that a prototype approach is also encountered extensively in the biological sciences, including molecular biology and neuroscience, this may facilitate the cross connections needed to accomplish the patchy reductions we find in the relation between psychiatry and molecular biological neuroscience.

Schizophrenia as a Possible Paradigm of a Reducible Mental Disorder

I now want to turn to some general issues associated with the molecular explanation of a specific and representative mental disorder, schizophrenia. I will begin by summarizing some diagnostic features of schizophrenia that are likely to appear in DSM-5 in 2013. Then I shall turn to some recent work in the molecular genetics of schizophrenia. Both of these subsections will serve as a backdrop to one more detailed example and a second account that will be sketched in outline that utilize in part the genetic advances, but also go beyond them to introduce the neurological circuits and molecular biological pathways that lead to schizophrenic symptoms. Those two exemplars will function as the specifics from which we can generalize a more philosophical account of reduction in psychiatry, albeit a partial reduction.

A summary of the features of schizophrenia that are targets for reduction

Here we will consider what may be the main features of schizophrenia. DSM-IV-TR's account of the disorder would possibly do, but I would rather try to anticipate what is likely to appear in mid-2013 as DSM-5's account of schizophrenia. If the preliminary postings on the DSM-5 website (<http://www.dsm5.org>) hold, there will be very few major changes from the DSM-IV-TR account. The symptoms listed in the next paragraph have some temporal qualifications attached to them, which I will summarize after the diagnostic definition is presented.

There are five what are termed "Criterion A" or active-phase symptoms of schizophrenia:

1. Delusions
2. Hallucinations
3. Disorganized speech
4. Grossly abnormal psychomotor behavior, including catatonia
5. Negative symptoms, e.g., diminished emotional expression or avolition.

These five core symptoms require that two or more of them be present for a significant amount of time during a one-month period (excepting successful treatment), and one of these symptoms must come from the first three listed—traditionally termed "positive symptoms." The disorder in some form needs to be persistent for a six-month period, and there is a requirement that there be a significant decrease in various aspects of personal functioning.

(The diagnosis also includes several exclusionary conditions, such as the symptoms not being caused by an abused drug or by a different medical condition.)

The picture of schizophrenia presented here is essentially that of a fully developed form of schizophrenia. Extensive research on the disorder indicates that it is part of a "schizophrenic spectrum," including a variety of less severe syndromes, such as schizotypal personality disorder. Also, related research strongly suggests that schizophrenia is a developmental disorder, typically manifesting itself after puberty, but not after forty years of age (Lewis and Lieberman 2000). Schizophrenia frequently begins with a somewhat ill-defined "prodrome," on which there has been considerable and continuing investigation as well as controversy. For more discussion on this topic see Schaffner and McGorry (2001).

In the past decade, a number of investigators of schizophrenia have argued that a set of *cognitive* symptoms are more fundamental than these five classical "Criterion A" symptoms. In point of fact, the two reductionistic models summarized in the "Two neuroscience models of schizophrenia" subsection, focus in on these cognitive symptoms. The rationale for that focus is presented in that subsection, but toward the end of the subsection some concerns expressed by the DSM-5 schizophrenia task group concerning the current diagnostic *specificity* of the cognitive symptoms will be noted. These cognitive symptoms, which include deficits in working memory, can also be construed as endophenotypes or intermediate phenotypes that may provide a stronger signal of genetic variation on the clinical syndrome. (For a now classical article on the notion of endophenotypes, see Gottesman and Gould 2003.)

What remains to be done in the next two subsections is first to illustrate what a partial reduction of a psychiatric disorder looks like in some detail in practice, and then to explore what type of reduction analysis this fits, there drawing on the philosophical literature on reduction.

Advances in schizophrenia genetics in the first decade of the twenty-first century

After a period in the years roughly from 2002 through 2007 when the picture regarding schizophrenia genes seemed to be clearing, the situation has since 2008 become considerably more complex. During that five-year 2000s period, the discovery of two strong candidates as risk genes, and of several others as quite probable genetic liability factors, fueled optimism that we had "turned the corner" as regards molecular psychiatric genetics (Kendler 2004b). These and a small number of additional genes related to schizophrenia replicated to some extent, but their support now seems somewhat weaker, though these assessments could still change as active research in schizophrenia genetics continues. In several cases *chromosomal* abnormalities that point to specific genes, such as *DISC1*, have also been associated with schizophrenia.

Beginning in 2007, single nucleotide polymorphism (SNP) results from genome-wide analyses began to be available. Though we are all about 99+% alike genetically, with approximately three billion nucleotides constituting our DNA, this allows millions of potential variants. One type of variant is a SNP, which is a site in the DNA where different chromosomes differ in the base they have, e.g., a T has a C substitute. Each of the two possibilities is called an allele. The difference may not mean much regarding trait or disease, but these

SNPs can be used as markers along the entire DNA sequence (whence the whole genome or genome-wide language), and can be associated via a case–control type of design with differences between normals and individuals with a disorder, whence the A in what are called GWA studies, and sometimes just GWAS. GWAS was dependent on the availability of the HapMap initially completed (first phase) in 2005.

The HapMap project is a multi-institutional project identifying millions of common SNPs across various individuals and ethnic groups. Because of the cost of full genome sequencing (still the holy grail in a sense), the HapMap project proposed a shortcut. The HapMap project focuses only on *common* SNPs, those where each allele occurs in at least 1% of the population. With the development of microarrays (gene chips), this technology could be applied to scan for common SNPs in the hundreds of thousands of SNPs, even millions, very quickly. This is done by having up to millions of complementary sequences printed as the tiny dots of complementary DNA on a gene chip. The chip can then be processed in a laser scanner and automatically interpreted to reveal the SNP patterns in diseased/disordered individuals versus controls. Because of the multiple tests, the P-value for significance is set very low, at less than 5×10^{-8}.

These GWAS results identify loci, but not necessarily genes—though it is suspected relevant genes are close by (or may be identical with) the loci. Psychiatric geneticists have seen "a flood of such data" from GWAS, including a large consortium study of schizophrenia published in September 2011 in *Nature Genetics* (Ripke et al. 2011). Many of these newer studies also involve CNVs (copy number variations) as well as SNP studies. But the results to date do not seem to be any more productive of consistent replications, nor of odds ratios (Ors) greater than 1.2. (A gene or SNP with an OR of 1.2 roughly translates into an increase in risk of 20%, so from one in a hundred for population-wide schizophrenia risk to one in eighty.) Nor have GWAS yet illuminated the molecular pathways, though they show some promise of accomplishing that. More on this point later.

Including those with relatively weak support, the current literature which includes GWAS findings suggests that the number of schizophrenia susceptibility genes number over 100. Other analyses that initially cast their net even more widely (and are more tolerant of very weak evidence) have suggested that the genes may number in the thousands (see Ayalew et al. 2012). Discoveries continue at a rapid pace, and reporting on them can overwhelm even the databases tracking gene discoveries for psychiatric researchers. (For a reasonable current list (updated at the end of 2011) of schizophrenia susceptibility genes, see <http://www.szgene.org/>.)

In this chapter, I will only briefly discuss one of the frequently favored susceptibility genes related to schizophrenia, namely the neuregulin-1 gene. I picked this gene in part because of its role in the second reductionistic model covered later in this chapter. Neuregulin, however, has an effect size that is quite small, only about 1.2 in terms of ORs. In contrast, Mendelian disorder genes, such as the Huntington's chorea gene, have effect sizes about 100 times as strong (Kendler 2005).

Neuregulin-1

The *NRG1* gene was found on chromosome 8p21–22 by Stefansson et al. (2002) using the deCODE Icelandic population database (and also data from a mouse model). A whole-genome scan provided suggestive evidence for the 8p12–21 region, and a follow-up study using higher resolution techniques focused in on two large risk haplotypes. Application of an early application of the SNP strategy then disclosed a core haplotype with a highly significant association with schizophrenia and which contained the *NRG1* gene (Stefansson et al. 2003). This gene produces a molecule affecting neuronal growth and development, as well as glutamate and other neurotransmitters, and also glial cells (see Moises et al. 2002). The NRG1 protein isoforms may additionally affect myelin in the brain. Neuregulin is believed to be regulated by a post-synaptic cell receptor known as ErbB3/4. The *NRG1* effect is small, accounting for approximately 10% of the schizophrenia risk in the Icelandic population, but the association has also been confirmed in a Welsh study and one Chinese populations, though not in another Chinese population (Hong et al. 2004) nor in the Irish high-density study (Thiselton et al. 2004). Again, the effect size is tiny in comparison with Mendelian genes, being less than 1.2 in terms of ODs, and there is extensive population heterogeneity (Gong et al. 2009). The *NRG1* gene, the *ERB4* gene, and its pathway, however, figures prominently in our second model of schizophrenia, as recently summarized in Law et al. (2012). More will be said about *NRG1* later in connection with our reduction examples.

Two neuroscience models of schizophrenia

There have been a number of largely speculative attempts to propound a theory of brain activity at the chemical level which might account for the behavior and cognitive aspects of schizophrenia. This subsection begins by providing an overview of what we might call the "Lewis Model of Schizophrenia." The model is situated within a broader context of evolving concepts of schizophrenia, including the additional attention since the late 1990s to cognitive dimensions of the disorder, for example, disturbances in memory. As noted earlier, a number of investigators see these deficits as a "core domain" of schizophrenia, perhaps underlying a number of aspects of the disorder, though they are not as dramatic as the traditional hallucinations and delusions. An important aspect of the Lewis model is that it provides mechanisms and pathways that terminate in effects on human brain gamma frequency oscillations, now believed to be one of the key underlying factors in brain function and dysfunction, such as schizophrenia. The Lewis model fits into the increased attention to the neurotransmitters glutamate and gamma-aminobutyric acid (GABA), which are as relevant to schizophrenia today as was dopamine originally (Kendler and Schaffner 2011). The Lewis approach also intercalates with an overlapping model developed by Harrison and Weinberger, our second model, which is also more explicitly back grounded by the role of the *NRG1* gene mentioned earlier, including its downstream pathways. Though this section focuses on the Lewis model, at its close some of the significant features of the Harrison–Weinberger model will also be noted.

The attention to gamma oscillations, as perhaps a key factor in schizophrenia, is quite recent. A useful recent review article summarizes some of this work as follows:

> There has been a fascinating convergence of evidence in recent years implicating the disturbances of neural synchrony in the gamma frequency band (30–100 Hz) as a major pathophysiologic feature of schizophrenia. Evidence suggests that reduced glutamatergic neurotransmission via the N-methyl-D-aspartate (NMDA) receptors that are localized to inhibitory interneurons, perhaps especially the fast-spiking cells that contain the calcium-binding protein parvalbumin (PV), may contribute to gamma band synchrony

deficits, which may underlie the failure of the brain to integrate information and hence the manifestations of many symptoms and deficits of schizophrenia. (Woo et al. 2010, p. 173)

This review article adds further that gamma oscillation disturbances might affect important developmental aspects of the schizophrenia pathophysiology, as well as introduce "excito-toxic or oxidative injury to downstream pyramidal neurons, leading to further loss of synapses and dendritic branchings," both in prodromal and early phases of the disorder.

The extent to which gamma oscillation pathologies can be identified with standard schizophrenia symptoms is still under discussion and requires further research in psychiatry. This review article just cited, however, does provide a number of references that support these connections, stating that "gamma abnormalities have been found to be associated with various symptom domains of schizophrenia, such as hallucinations, thought disorder, disorganization, and psychomotor poverty'." (For references see Woo et al. 2010, p. 3.) As noted earlier, the Lewis model is one of the more detailed models that account for gamma oscillation disturbances in schizophrenia.

Lewis, who along with most of his research collaborators is at the University of Pittsburgh, was profiled in a recent issue of *Nature*. There, the current director of the National Institute of Mental Health, Thomas Insel, MD, wrote of the Lewis investigations into schizophrenia that the model "provides something this field really needed: a framework for linking observations at the molecular, cellular and systems levels. We haven't had a story that crossed those levels of explanation before. And his story, whether it pans out in all its details or not, is invaluable for doing that" (Dobbs 2010). In addition to levels integration, the Lewis model also has had some preliminary practical results, and has led to some phase II clinical trials conducted with novel compounds predicted to improve cognitive dysfunction in schizophrenia.

The Lewis model argues for the importance of cognitive dimensions of schizophrenia, noting that "cognitive deficits are present and progressive years before the onset of psychosis, and the degree of cognitive impairment is the best predictor of long-term functional outcome" (Lewis et al. 2012).

In one of the Lewis group's most recent reviews, they write:

> Deficits in cognitive control, a core disturbance of schizophrenia, appear to emerge from impaired prefrontal gamma oscillations. Cortical gamma oscillations require strong inhibitory inputs to pyramidal neurons from the parvalbumin basket cell (PVBC) class of GABAergic neurons. (Gonzalez-Burgos and Lewis 2012)).

The central element in the Lewis model, then, is the circuit that involves these inputs from the parvalbumin (PV) basket cells to the brain's pyramidal neurons using the GABA neurotransmitter, though pyramidal cells themselves use the neurotransmitter glutamate. (There are actually two types of basket cells that we need not discuss in this simplified account, and there is also another type of cell, chandelier cells, which assist in the regulation of the oscillatory activity of the pyramidal neurons as noted briefly later.) In addition, there are two important input regulating receptor types for glutamate, one is termed the NMDAR (N-methyl-D-aspartate receptor) introduced briefly above in the discussion of gamma oscillations, these being under the influence of several type(s) of schizophrenia susceptibility genes including *NRG1*. There is also an additional glutamate receptor type, abbreviated as AMPAR (a-amino-3-hydroxy-5-methyl-4-isoxazolepropionic acid receptor),

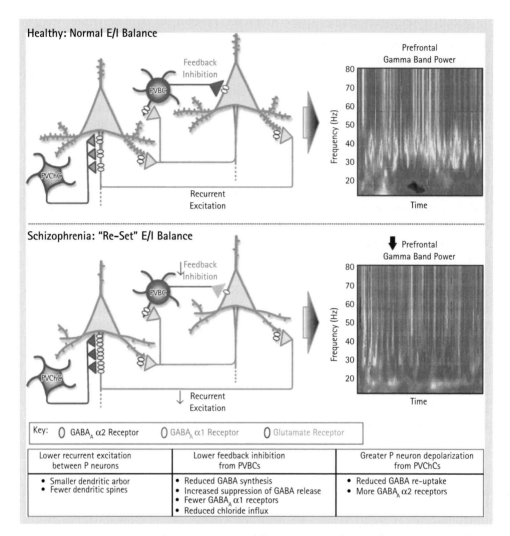

FIGURE 59.1 Connectivity between pyramidal neurons and parvalbumin-positive basket (PVBC) and chandelier (PVChC) cells in dorsolateral prefrontal cortex (DLPFC) layer 3. See text for explanation. Reprinted from *Trends in Neurosciences*, 35(1), David A. Lewis, Allison A. Curley, Jill R. Glausier, and David W. Volk, Cortical parvalbumin interneurons and cognitive dysfunction in schizophrenia, pp. 57–67, Copyright (2012), with permission from Elsevier.

which mediates fast synaptic neurotransmission. (The NMDAR is the main molecular mechanism controlling memory function, but a balance between both types of receptors may explain some features of pyramidal cell oscillation regulation. For details on this see Gonzalez-Burgos and Lewis (2012) and Lewis et al. (2012); also see Fig. 59.1.)

The Lewis model has evolved in the past three years from the form originally presented in Lewis and Sweet (2009) to one that now focuses more on the basket cell interactive role with pyramidal cells—see Lewis et al. (2012). This is an evolution that has largely been driven by additional empirical findings over these past three years. The current form of the model is most easily presented in the form of a published figure that contrasts the process lead-ing to gamma oscillations in normal cells versus schizophrenia affected cells (see Fig. 59.1). The figure shows several alterations in disordered cells. First, the key pyramidal cells mak-ing up 75% of the dorsolateral prefrontal cortex (DLPFC) engage in recurrent excitations regulated by feedback inhibition by the basket cells to produce stable gamma oscillations. However, the pyramidal cells are smaller in schizophrenia, and also have fewer dendritic spines due to the disorder. (Dendritic spines—tiny buttons found on the dendrites—both act to facilitate synaptic strength and assist in the transmission of electrical signals to the neuron's cell body.) The affected pyramidal cells thus cannot output as strong a signal to the regulating PV basket cells, which also may be downregulated by less effective NMDARs on those cells. This decreased signal induces a compensatory response in the basket cells, in the form of decreased inhibition via less (or less active) glutamate enzyme, itself control-led by the *GAD67* gene (thus there is an equivalent increased excitation by the basket cells). Recent evidence that the chandelier cells are excitatory suggests that they too are part of a (still insufficient) compensatory response. This net under-compensation results in a gamma oscillation output that is still suboptimal in comparison with healthy pyramidal cortex cells, yielding symptoms of disordered cognitive control.

A considerably oversimplified summary of the Lewis model might be:

> Pyramidal cell signal strength ↓(via smaller cells and decreased dendritic spines in SZ) plus NMDAR ↓→ PV basket cell activity ↓ (as feedback compensation) → pyramidal cell oscillation activity still insufficiently increased = schizophrenic symptoms (the types of symptoms varying depending on the circuits involved, thus memory in some areas and decreased tone sensitivity in the auditory region).

This model as described thus far does not examine in any detail what may be causing the decrease in NMDAR activity, which may be an important factor in schizophrenia, beyond an effect on the basket cells. An examination of NMDAR activity related to the Lewis model remains somewhat equivocal, with a recent article suggesting that "additional research is required to determine the particular cell type(s) that mediate dysfunctional NMDAR sig-naling in the illness" (Gonzalez-Burgos and Lewis 2012). Various additional hypotheses have been developed, one which identifies the *NRG1* malfunction and another more recent proposal by the Lewis group that cites dysbindin gene effects (Gonzalez-Burgos and Lewis 2012). The former (NRG1) hypothesis is the most developed in the literature, having been extensively researched by Harrison's group at Oxford, also working with Weinberger and his colleagues at the NIH (Weinberger is now Director at the Lieber Institute for Brain Development in Baltimore, Maryland.) An overview of the multiple pathways by which NRG1 may affect schizophrenia can be found in my Schaffner (2008a), and more recent hypotheses related to NMDA and long-term potentiation (including effects on pyramidal cells in the hippocampus) are developed in Deakin et al. (2011), Nicodemus et al. (2010), and Pitcher et al. (2011). A recent communication from the Harrison and Weinberger groups, based in part on animal model studies (mice and rats) as well as human lymphocytes and brain tissue, proposes "a genetically regulated, pharmacologically targetable, risk path-way associated with schizophrenia and with [NRG1 and] ErbB4 genetic variation involving increased expression of a PI3K-linked ErbB4 receptor (CYT-1) and the phosphoinositide 3-kinase subunit, p110δ (PIK3CD)")." (Law et al. 2012, p. 1).

Close inspection of the Lewis model publications, as well as alternative approaches such as the Harrison–Weinberger pathway just cited, indicate that there are a number of questions that remain to be answered about the details of the cells and circuits affecting schizophrenia. Furthermore, a focus on the cognitive deficits of schizophrenia emphasized by the Lewis model must not be interpreted as arguing for a major *clinical* diagnostic focus on these features; cognitive deficits will continue to be but an aspect of schizophrenia symptoms.

In point of fact, the DSM-5 "Psychotic Disorders" workgroup studying those disorders listed in a proposed category named "Schizophrenia Spectrum and Other Psychotic Disorders" has included cognition in their eight features or domains of schizophrenia. These eight domains are: Hallucinations, Delusions, Disorganized Speech, Abnormal Psychomotor Behavior, Negative Symptoms (Restricted Emotional Expression or Avolition), Impaired Cognition, Depression, and Mania. Each of these eight is recommended to be assessed on a quasi-dimensional scale of 0 (not present) to 4 (present and severe. Impaired cognition was not, however, included in the five (Criterion A) major diagnostic features of the disorder because the workgroup believed that cognitive impairment lacked the necessary *specificity*, being present in a number of other psychiatric disorders as well. They wrote that a "wealth of data suggest that this separation [from other disorders] is not sufficient to justify inclusion of cognition as a Criterion A symptom of schizophrenia (see: <http://www.dsm5.org/>).

The Lewis model and the overlapping Harrison–Weinberger model appear largely directed at capturing fully developed schizophrenia. There are other nascent models that aim at representing brain circuits that may be responsible for prodromal aspects of the disorder, but studies of these alternative circuits is in the early stages of research. One aspect of the prodrome that is of particular philosophical interest relates to early and subtle changes in the concept of the "self," and its property of "ipseity," or selfhood. For accounts of how changes in ipseity can be studied as well as references to brain circuits that may be responsible for these early changes in mental processing in developing schizophrenia see Nelson et al. (2009) and Parnas et al. (2005).

In spite of these diagnostic limitations, including, as noted earlier, incomplete knowledge of the details of the cells and (probably multiple) circuits affecting schizophrenia, we can abstract from these reductionistic models (with a focus on the Lewis model) what a reductionistic account of a representative psychiatric disorder involves.

A PARTIAL REDUCTION MODEL IN
PHILOSOPHY OF SCIENCE

As noted in the first section, there have been two contrasting approaches to reduction that I described as *sweeping* and *creeping*. A more formal variant of the sweeping type of reduction found in the philosophy of science has been the Nagel account of theory reduction, wherein large domains of a scientific subject are reduced by a theory developed in a quite distinct scientific subject area. Examples in the reduction literature include thermodynamics' reduction by statistical mechanics and optics' reduction by electrodynamics. (For references to this literature and an extended optics example see Schaffner, 2013). In an earlier essay on reduction in psychiatry with applications to schizophrenia (Schaffner 1994), I sketched a slightly modified version of that sweeping approach, which some refer to as the "Nagel–Schaffner model" (Dizadji-Bahmani 2010). But in subsequent years, I have come to believe that a "creeping" or partial reduction approach is more applicable in psychiatry. I continue to hold, however, that in physics something like a Nagelian type of theory reduction is largely applicable; again see Schaffner (2012) for details. Let me briefly sketch some of the reasons for this shift of position.

It turns out, after a general careful review of putative reduction examples in the history of science that ultimately all attempts at theory reductions in science are "incomplete," "partial," or "patchwork" in character. The nature and degree of the incompleteness varies with the type of science, however, and in physics, because of its "Euclidean" form of theories, virtually "systematic" or "sweeping" Nagelian-type reductions seem possible. It was the prospect of these sweeping reductions that motivated the original Nagel model of reduction and its application to the now canonical thermodynamics and statistical mechanics example. However, for classical Nagelian-type reductions to work well, the branches of science that enters into a reduction relation need to be axiomatizable in a fairly straightforward manner, that is, by using an integrated small number (three to six) of core scientific laws. Also connections between the reduced and reducing fields need to be straightforward and relatively simple, though the connections may well be far from obvious. (These connections are frequently referred to as "bridge laws," though I think other expressions such as "reduction functions" or even better "connectability assumptions" carry less philosophical baggage. This issue of "connectability" has generated a very large and often contentious literature in the philosophy of science; see Schaffner (2012) for references.)

Even in physics, though reductive expositions can give the *appearance* of a complete systematic reduction, closer inspection reveals this systematicity fails at the margins (Schaffner 2012). Further, in more complex sciences such as molecular genetics and neuroscience, both of these stringent conditions, simple axiomatizablity and simple connectability, fail in significant ways, though that they do fail, or would fail, was not necessarily obvious at the beginning of the Watson–Crick era of comparatively uncomplicated molecular biology. Furthermore, in psychology and psychiatry where *conscious experience* figures prominently, connectability will ultimately need to involve the thorny and contentious issue of what are termed "neural correlates of consciousness" (NCC) (Koch 2004). Some philosophers and scientists believe will these "correlates" will ultimately need to be *identities* (of mind entities and properties with brain entities and properties), and not just correlates of them. And this issue will also likely generate variants of what is termed in the philosophy of mind area "the hard problem" (Chalmers 1996).

In summary, more than sixty years of explorations and refinements of alternative reduction possibilities strongly support a more "creeping" form of reductions particularly in the biological sciences and the neurosciences. But this view, however, does not impugn the importance of such partial reductions. Such partial reductions amount to potentially Nobel-prize winning accomplishments in unifying and deepening significant though "local" areas of scientific investigation.

The background and locus of partial reductions in biology and the neurosciences

The models depicted in Fig. 59.1 from the Lewis et al. (2012) paper discussed in detail in the earlier section "Two neuroscience models of schizophrenia" are what I like to call *preferred causal model systems* (PCMSs) for the specific scientific article in which they appear. The model (or in this case two contrasting models representing healthy and schizophrenically disordered brains) is what accomplishes the partial reduction—more on this in the next few pages. The model is simplified and idealized, and uses causal language such as "provide recurrent excitation," "increased depolarization," and "resulting in." The *PCMS* is clearly interlevel, showing cells, parts of cells (dendrites), receptors, as well as connections among them (circuits) ultimately resulting in differing prefrontal cortex gamma band oscillations. I find that it is best to approach such models keeping in mind the scientific field(s) on which they are based, and the specific alternative explanations (model sketches in a sense) that a scientific article proposing the preferred model provides as contrasts within the field(s). Here, the fields on which the model draws are generally molecular genetics and especially neuroscience. Scattered throughout the article are occasional alternative but possible causal pathways or contrasting alternatives which are evaluated as not as good an explanation as those provided in the preferred model system. (One example in the Lewis article is the previous role of the chandelier cells, now modified in this article. Another alternative is noted in the second to last paragraph at the end of the article where what is explicitly termed an "alternative model" involving NMDA receptor hypofunction resulting in a GAD67 deficit in the PV neurons is noted, but mainly rejected.)

I will not say more about how fields and alternative explanations are characterized here, but interested readers can see Schaffner (2006) for additional details, albeit with somewhat different terminology. I should note here that the notion of a "pathway" appears to be especially prominent in models in the biomedical sciences, and here including psychiatry. Pathways appear to be more general than any specific mechanism that may be part of a pathway, but like "mechanisms," they are also typically interlevel in character. On this point, compare Schaffner (2011, p. 153) and Machamer (2000) on the issue of whether "mechanism language"—a prominent development since the later 1990s in philosophy of science—will suffice; also see comments in the concluding section of this chapter.

The preparation(s) or specific *experimental system(s)* investigated in the clinic and/or laboratory (this may include several data runs of the "same" experimental system) is identified in its relevant aspects with the (more abstract) preferred causal model system. In this Lewis article, which is partly a review article, several such data sources or experimental systems are noted, ranging from human patients with cognitive deficits due to schizophrenia, to stem cells derived from patients, to results based on mice and rat studies, some of which involve using hippocampal or brain slices. At the abstract or "philosophical" level, the reductive explanation proceeds by identifying the laboratory or clinical experimental system with the theoretical system—the PCMS—and exhibiting the event or process to be explained (in philosophy this is called the *explanandum*) as the causal consequence of the system's behavior. The *explanans* (or set of explaining elements) here uses molecular neuroscience and is mainly comparative rather than involving strict quantitative derivational reasoning, in the sense that in this chapter two qualitatively different end states—the prefrontal gamma band power—are compared and contrasted. The theoretical system (the PCMS) utilizes generalizations of varying scope, some from basic biochemistry involving the balance of chloride ions. Often these generalizations appeal to similarity analyses among like systems, especially different animal models and humans, to achieve the scope, as well as make the investigation of interest and relevance to other neuroscientists and psychiatrists. For those concerned with philosophical rigor, the preferred model system and its relations to model-theoretic explanation can be made more philosophically precise (and technical), along the lines suggested in other publications, including Schaffner (2006).

The discussion sections of scientific papers are the usual place where larger issues are raised, and where extrapolations are frequently found and future research proposed. In this Lewis paper, which is partly a review article and thus is not structured in the usual way that more specific scientific and medical papers are, with materials and methods, results, and a discussion section, the extrapolations and more general and future-looking comments are found at the end of the paper. In the Lewis paper, these comments are partly cautionary, noting that the current model is based on a "limited portion of cortical circuitry," as well as a proposal that additional studies involving connectivity patterns in the DLPFC, better methods to assess compensation, and further animal models are needed.

This explanation is both reductive and non-reductive

The Lewis example is typical of molecular neuroscience psychiatric explanations of behavior, including cognitive aspects. Behavior is an organismic property, and in the example the explanation appeals to entities that are *parts* of the organism, including molecularly characterized genes and molecular interactions such as receptor bindings and G-protein coupled receptor mechanisms—thus this is generally characterized as a *reductive* explanation. But it represents *partial* reduction—what I termed reduction of the *creeping* sort—and it differs from *sweeping* or comprehensive reductive explanations because of several important features.

1. The model does not explain *all* cases of schizophrenia; and different though somewhat related models can address other features of the disorder, e.g., prodromal features of schizophrenia.
2. Some of the key entities, such as the signal producing the gamma oscillations have not yet been fully identified.
3. The causal account utilizes what might be termed "middle-level" entities, such as neuronal cells, in addition to molecular entities. Further work that is even more reductionistic can address ion channels in the neurons, but this research is yet to come. (I discuss some of this ion channel work in connection with worm touch sensitivity in Schaffner (under review)).
4. It is not a quantitative model that derives behavioral and cognitive properties from a small set of axioms or even from rigorous general equations of state, but is causally qualitative and only roughly comparative.
5. Interventions to set up, manipulate, and test the model are at higher aggregative levels than the molecular, such as the traditional diagnosis of patients afflicted with schizophrenia and the use of brain slices.

The explanation does meet three conditions that seem reasonable for a reductive explanation, namely:

1. The explainers (here the preferred model system shown in Fig. 59.1) are a partially decomposable microstructure in the organism/process of interest.

2. The explanandum (the cognitive deficits) is a grosser (macro) typically aggregate property or end state.
3. Connectability assumptions (CAs), sometimes called bridge laws or reduction functions, are involved, which permit the relation of macrodescriptions to microdescriptions. Sometimes these CAs are causal sequences as depicted in the model figure where the output of the neurons under one set of conditions causes strong gamma band power, but in critical cases the CAs are provisional identities (such as weak gamma oscillations = cognitive deficits) which later may be expanded, perhaps to identities underlying neural correlates of consciousness (Koch 2004).

Though etiological and reductive, the preferred model system explanation is not "ruthlessly reductive," to use Bickle's phrase (Bickle 2003), even though a classical organismic biologist would most likely term it strongly reductionistic in contrast to their favored non-reductive or even antireductionist cellular or organismic points of view. It is a *partial* reduction.

SUMMARY AND CONCLUSION

In the past fifty years, a reductionistic approach in the biomedical sciences and in psychology has become far less imperialistic and considerably more fragmented and tentative. At present, the best fit of a model of reduction, and a research strategy related to such a model, is a partial or creeping one. Whether these more fragmented and multilevel model explanations can be "integrated" in some appropriate way(s), or whether they will remain stubbornly "pluralistic," and possibly even inconsistent is an answer for the future (but compare Dupré 1993; Kendler 2004a; Mitchell 2003, 2008, 2009). The vagaries regarding reductionistic approaches to schizophrenia encountered in the results of thousands of research papers in molecular psychiatry and the related fields of genetics and neuroscience might be represented pictorially in what has been termed a "watershed model" (Fig. 59.2).

The watershed model was originally introduced by Cannon and colleagues (Cannon 2010; Cannon and Keller 2006). In my slightly modified version of their figure, I have inserted a prodromic feature of schizophrenia ("Ipseity") following proposals by Nelson et al. (2009) and Parnas et al. (2005) to represent the effect of an alternative disordered neural circuit in this system. Cognitive Function Z, which could be Lewis types of memory deficits, is another circuit effect. The clinical syndrome at the base (or mouth of the river with subtly differing subcurrents in the outflow) is expanded to depict the kinds of overlapping disorders described earlier. Overall the tributaries and river system represent probabilistic causal pathways leading to clinical syndromes, and in any individual patient case, a truncated river system with pruned off tributaries would be the case, since not all instances of schizophrenia will be affected by all possible causes. In fact, if the rare variants hypothesis for schizophrenia holds (McClellan and King 2010; Visscher et al. 2012), there could be thousands of differing watershed models, only a small number of which would have strong overlaps with each other.

The accounts sketched in this chapter are consistent with the emerging analysis of schizophrenia likely to be presented in DSM-5 (and thus probably ICD-11), though go deeper

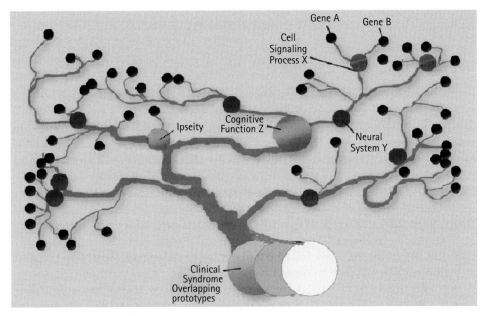

FIGURE 59.2 Modified from Cannon and Keller (2006) and Cannon (2010). A prodromic feature of schizophrenia ("Ipseity") is introduced (following Nelson et al. 2009; Parnas et al. 2005) to represent the effect of an alternative disordered neural circuit in this system. Cognitive Function Z, which could be Lewis-related memory deficits, is another circuit effect. The clinical syndrome at the base (or mouth of the river where there are subtly differing subcurrents in the outflow) is expanded to depict the kinds of overlapping disorders described in the "Disorders as overlapping models" section. Overall the tributaries and river system represent probabilistic causal pathways leading to clinical syndromes. See text for additional details. Republished with permission of Annual Reviews, Inc., from Annual review of clinical psychology, Cannon TD and Keller MC, 2, pp. 267-90, Figure 1 © 2005, Annual Reviews, Inc., permission conveyed through Copyright Clearance Center, Inc.

to speculate about possible etiological and reductionistic underpinnings. By emphasizing multilevel analyses in the partial reductions, the accounts should also resonate well with the developing National Institutes of Mental Health Research Diagnostic Criteria. (On this initiative and its "matrix" of newer psychiatric domains/constructs and units or levels of analysis, see <http://www.nimh.nih.gov/research-funding/rdoc/index.shtml>.) Where the account in this chapter may add to the RDoC matrix's units of analysis is in its suggestion that the concept of *pathways* can causally integrate (or at least significantly interrelate) etiology and pathology across several levels of analysis (for further discussion of this point, see Schaffner 2008a, 2008b) including clinical aspects of psychiatric disorders. It is evident, however, from a review of the psychiatric literature in 2012 that molecular psychiatry, in spite of its enormous strides in the past fifty years (Shorter 1998), is still in the early stages of identifying etiological features of psychiatric disorders. This should not be surprising, since the brain, the seat of the psyche, is the most complex of the human biological organs.

REFERENCES

American Psychiatric Association (2000). *Diagnostic and Statistical Manual of Mental Disorders, Fourth Edition, Text Revision*. Washington, DC: American Psychiatric Association.

Ayalew, M., Le-Niculescu, H., Levey, D. F., Jain, N., Changala, B., Patel, S. D., *et al.* (2012). Convergent functional genomics of schizophrenia: From comprehensive understanding to genetic risk prediction. *Molecular Psychiatry*, 17(9), 887–905.

Bickle, J. (2003). *Philosophy and Neuroscience: A Ruthlessly Reductive Account*. Dordrecht: Kluwer.

Cannon, T. D. (2010). Candidate gene studies in the GWAS era: the MET proto-oncogene, neurocognition, and schizophrenia. *American Journal of Psychiatry*, 167(4), 369–72.

Cannon, T. D. and Keller, M. C. (2006). Endophenotypes in the genetic analyses of mental disorders. *Annual Review of Clinical Psychology*, 2, 267–90.

Cantor, N., Smith, E. E., French, R. S., and Mezzich, J. (1980). Psychiatric diagnosis as prototype categorization. *Journal of Abnormal Psychology*, 89(2), 181–93.

Chalmers, D. J. (1996). *The Conscious Mind: In Search of a Fundamental Theory* (Philosophy of Mind Series). New York, NY: Oxford University Press.

Deakin, I. H., Nissen, W., Law, A. J., Lane, T., Kanso, R., Schwab, M. H., *et al.* (2011). Transgenic overexpression of the type I isoform of Neuregulin 1 affects working memory and hippocampal oscillations but not long-term potentiation. *Cerebral Cortex*, 22(7), 1520–9.

Dizadji-Bahmani, F., Frigg, R., and Hartmann, S. (2010). Who's afraid of Nagelian reduction? *Erkenntis*, 73, 393–412.

Dobbs, D. (2010). Schizophrenia: The making of a troubled mind. *Nature*, 468(7321), 154–6.

Dupré, J. (1993). *The Disorder of Things: Metaphysical Foundations of the Disunity of Science*. Cambridge, MA: Harvard University Press.

Frances, A., Pincus, H. A., Widiger, T. A., Davis, W. W., and First, M. B.(1990). DSM-IV: Work in progress. *American Journal of Psychiatry*, 147(11), 1439–48.

Gong, Y. G., Wu, C. N., Xing, Q. H., Zhao, X. Z., Zhu, J., and He, L.(2009). A two-method meta-analysis of Neuregulin 1(NRG1) association and heterogeneity in schizophrenia. *Schizophrenia Research*, 111(1–3), 109–14.

Gonzalez-Burgos, G. and Lewis, D. A. (2012). NMDA receptor hypofunction, parvalbumin-positive neurons and cortical gamma oscillations in schizophrenia. *Schizophrenia Bulletin*, 38(5), 950–7.

Gottesman, I. I. and Gould, T. D. (2003). The endophenotype concept in psychiatry: etymology and strategic intentions. *American Journal of Psychiatry*, 160(4), 636–45.

Hong, C. J., Huo, S. J., Liao, D. L., Lee, K., Wu, J. Y., and Tsai, S. J. (2004). Case-control and family-based association studies between the neuregulin 1 (Arg38Gln) polymorphism and schizophrenia. *Neuroscience Letters*, 366(2), 158–61.

Jacob, F. (1977). Evolution and tinkering. *Science*, 196(4295), 1161–6.

Kendler, K. S. (2004a). Psychiatric genetics: A methodologic critique. *American Journal of Psychiatry*, 162(1), 3–11.

Kendler, K. S. (2004b). Schizophrenia genetics and dysbindin: a corner turned? *American Journal of Psychiatry*, 161(9), 1533–6.

Kendler, K. S. (2005). "A gene for…": the nature of gene action in psychiatric disorders. *American Journal of Psychiatry*, 162(7), 1243–52.

Kendler, K. S. and Schaffner, K. F. (2011). The dopamine hypothesis of schizophrenia: An historical and philosophical analysis. *Philosophy, Psychiatry, & Psychology*, 18(1), 41–63.

Koch, C. (2004). *The Quest for Consciousness: A Neurobiological Approach*. Denver, CO: Roberts and Co.

Law, A. J., Wang, Y., Sei, Y., O'Donnell, P., Piantadosi, P., Papaleo, F., *et al.* (2012). Neuregulin 1-ErbB4-PI3K signaling in schizophrenia and phosphoinositide 3-kinase-p110delta inhibition as a potential therapeutic strategy. *Proceedings of the National Academy of Sciences of the United States of America, 109*(30), 12165–70.

Lewis, D. A. and Lieberman, J. A. (2000). Catching up on schizophrenia: Natural history and neurobiology. *Neuron, 28*(2), 325–34.

Lewis, D. A. and Levitt, P. (2002). Schizophrenia as a disorder of neurodevelopment. *Annual Review of Neuroscience, 25*, 409–32.

Lewis, D. A. and Sweet, R. A. (2009). Schizophrenia from a neural circuitry perspective: Advancing toward rational pharmacological therapies. *Journal of Clinical Investigations, 119*(4), 706–16.

Lewis, D. A., Curley, A. A., Glausier, J. R., and Volk, D. W. (2012). Cortical parvalbumin interneurons and cognitive dysfunction in schizophrenia. *Trends in Neurosciences, 35*(1), 57–67.

Lilienfeld, S. O. and Marino, L. (1995). Mental disorder as a Roschian concept: A critique of Wakefield's "harmful dysfunction" analysis. *Journal of Abnormal Psychology, 104*(3), 411–20.

Lilienfeld, S. O. and Marino, L. (1999). Essentialism revisited: Evolutionary theory and the concept of mental disorder. *Journal of Abnormal Psychology, 108*(3), 400–11.

Machamer, P., Darden, L., and Craver C. (2000). Thinking about mechanisms. *Philosophy of Science, 67*, 1–25.

Machery, E. (2009). *Doing Without Concepts*. Oxford: Oxford University Press.

McClellan, J. and King, M. C. (2010). Genomic analysis of mental illness: a changing landscape. *Journal of the American Medical Association, 303*(24), 2523–4.

Mitchell, S. D. (2003). *Biological complexity and integrative pluralism* (Cambridge Studies in Philosophy and Biology). Cambridge: Cambridge University Press.

Mitchell, S. D. (2008). Explaining complex behavior. In K. S. Kendler and J. Parnas (Eds), *Philosophical Issues in Psychiatry*, pp. 19–38. Baltimore, MD: Johns Hopkins University Press.

Mitchell, S. D. (2009). *Unsimple Truths: Complexity, Science and Policy*. Chicago, IL: University of Chicago Press.

Moises, H. W., Zoega, T., and Gottesman, I. I. (2002). The glial growth factors deficiency and synaptic destabilization hypothesis of schizophrenia. *BMC Psychiatry, 2*(1), 8.

Nelson, B., Fornito, A., Harrison, B. J., Yücel, M., Sass, L. A., Yung, A. R., *et al.* (2009). A disturbed sense of self in the psychosis prodrome: linking phenomenology and neurobiology. *Neuroscience and Biobehavioral Reviews, 33*(6), 807–17.

Nicodemus, K. K., Law, A. J., Radulescu, E., Luna, A., Kolachana, B., Vakkalanka, R., *et al.* (2010). Biological validation of increased schizophrenia risk with NRG1, ERBB4, and AKT1 epistasis via functional neuroimaging in healthy controls. *Archives of General Psychiatry, 67*(10), 991–1001.

Parnas, J., Møller, P., Kircher, T., Thalbitzer, J., Jansson, L., Handest, P., *et al.* (2005). EASE: Examination of anomalous self-experience. *Psychopathology, 38*(5), 236–58.

Pitcher, G. M., Kalia, L. V., Ng, D., Goodfellow, N. M., Yee, K. T., Lambe, E. K., *et al.* (2011). Schizophrenia susceptibility pathway neuregulin 1-ErbB4 suppresses Src upregulation of NMDA receptors. *Nature Medicine, 17*(4), 470–8.

Ripke, S., Sanders, A. R., Kendler, K. S., Levinson, D. F., Sklar, P., Holmans, P. A., *et al.* (2011). Genome-wide association study identifies five new schizophrenia loci. *Nature Genetics, 43*(10), 969–76.

Rosch, E. and Mervis C. B. (1975a). Family resemblances: Studies in the internal structure of categories. *Cognitive Psychology, 7*(4), 573–605.

Rosch, E. (1975b). Cognitive representation of semantic categories. *Journal of Experimental Psychology*, *104*, 192–233.

Schaffner, K. F. (1980). Theory structure in the biomedical sciences. *Journal of Medicine and Philosophy*, *5*, 57–97.

Schaffner, K. F. (1986). Exemplar reasoning about biological models and diseases: a relation between the philosophy of medicine and philosophy of science. *Journal of Medicine and Philosophy*, *11*(1), 63–80.

Schaffner, K. F. (1993). *Discovery and Explanation in Biology and Medicine*. Chicago, IL: University of Chicago Press.

Schaffner, K. F. (1994). Psychiatry and molecular biology: Reductionistic approaches to schizophrenia. In J. Sadler, O. Wiggins, and M. Schwartz (Eds), *Philosophical Perspectives on Psychiatric Diagnostic Classification*, pp. 279–94. Baltimore, MD: Johns Hopkins University Press.

Schaffner, K. F. (2006). Reduction: The Cheshire cat problem and a return to roots. *Synthese*, *151*(3), 377–402.

Schaffner, K. F. (2008a). Etiological models in psychiatry: Reductive and nonreductive. In K. S. Kendler, J. Parnas (Eds), *Philosophical Issues in Psychiatry*, pp. 48–90. Baltimore, MD: Johns Hopkins University Press.

Schaffner, K. F. (2008b). Theories, models, and equations in biology: The heuristic search for emergent simplifications in neurobiology. *Philosophy of Science*, *75*, 1008–21.

Schaffner, K. F. (2011). Reduction in biology and medicine. In F. Gifford (Ed.), *Philosophy of Medicine*, pp. 137–57. Amsterdam: Elsevier.

Schaffner, K. F. (2012). Ernest Nagel and reduction. *Journal of Philosophy*, *109*, 534–565.

Schaffner, K. F. (under review). *Behaving: What's Genetic and What's Not, and Why Should We Care?* Oxford: Oxford University Press.

Schaffner, K. F. and McGorry, P. D. (2001). Preventing severe mental illnesses—new prospects and ethical challenges. *Schizophrenia Research*, *51*(1), 3–15.

Shorter, E. (1998). *A History of Psychiatry: From the Era of the Asylum to the Age of Prozac*. New York, NY: John Wiley.

Stefansson, H., Sarginson, J., Kong, A., Yates, P., Steinthorsdottir, V., Gudfinnsson, E., et al. (2003). Association of neuregulin 1 with schizophrenia confirmed in a Scottish population. *American Journal of Human Genetics*, *72*(1), 83–7.

Stefansson, H., Sigurdsson, E., Steinthorsdottir, V., Bjornsdottir, S., Sigmundsson, T., Ghosh, S., et al. (2002). Neuregulin 1 and susceptibility to schizophrenia. *American Journal of Human Genetics*, *71*(4), 877–92.

Thiselton, D. L., Webb, B. T., Neale, B. M., Ribble, R. C., O'Neill, F. A., Walsh, D., et al. (2004). No evidence for linkage or association of neuregulin-1 (NRG1) with disease in the Irish study of high-density schizophrenia families (ISHDSF). *Molecular Psychiatry*, *9*(8), 777–83.

Visscher, P. M., Goddard, M. E., Derks, E. M., and Wray, N. R. (2012). Evidence-based psychiatric genetics, AKA the false dichotomy between common and rare variant hypotheses. *Molecular Psychiatry*, *17*(5), 474–85.

Woo, T. U., Spencer, K., and McCarley, R. W. (2010). Gamma oscillation deficits and the onset and early progression of schizophrenia. *Harvard Review of Psychiatry*, *18*(3), 173–89.

CHAPTER 60

....

DIAGNOSTIC PREDICTION AND PROGNOSIS: GETTING FROM SYMPTOM TO TREATMENT

....

MICHAEL A. BISHOP AND J. D. TROUT

Psychiatrists diagnose people with psychiatric conditions, and on that basis, psychiatrists make prognoses (i.e., predictions about how that condition is likely to turn out given a treatment). Psychiatric diagnosis and prognosis is fraught with important philosophical and conceptual problems. We can divide these into three categories:

1. *Metaphysical issues*: Is there such a thing as mental illness? What makes something a psychiatric condition? (Hacking 1995; Murphy 2006)
2. *Epistemological issues*: When are there good grounds for making a psychiatric diagnosis? What evidence justifies the belief that a course of treatment is effective? (Dawes 1994; Murphy 2006) Are our diagnostic categories the right ones? Are some psychiatric diagnoses self-fulfilling? (Szasz 1974)
3. *Moral issues*: What are a therapist's moral obligations to her patient? What is a just distribution of scarce psychiatric resources given the many people with psychiatric conditions whose suffering could be alleviated with treatment? (Dawes 1994)

As we cannot adequately cover all these issues here and our assigned topic is *diagnostic prediction and prognosis*, we propose to focus primarily on the epistemological issues that arise in contemporary psychiatric practice. And on occasion, we will note moral problems that arise along the way. This focus inevitably takes for granted the legitimacy of many of the psychiatric categories set forth in the *Diagnostic and Statistical Manual of Mental Disorders* (DSM). Needless to say, this is a tendentious assumption. Two pragmatic considerations justify the assumption. First, the philosophical issues we will discuss would still arise within many different views about the nature of mental illness. Second, the DSM categories are widely used and accepted in psychiatric practice, and so no other assumption about the nature of psychiatric conditions would be as useful for our purposes.

DIAGNOSIS

When an individual exhibits signs that suggest a potential medical condition, the first order of business is to arrive at a diagnosis. The literature on medical and psychiatric diagnosis typically distinguishes between "clinical" and "actuarial" techniques. The former involves a clinician using her experience to combine data in an informal, subjective manner; the latter involves a purely mechanical, reproducible procedure that can be programmed into a computer (Grove et al. 2000; Meehl 1954). But the clinical-actuarial distinction is by no means a clear one. A list of nine families of potential diagnostic methods follows, ordered very loosely in terms of how "structured" or "automated" they are—in terms of how much freedom the individual clinician has in carrying out the diagnostic method:

1. Gestalt: The clinician comes to an intuitive diagnosis on the basis of an interview, perhaps a cursory interview.
2. Projective techniques: The clinician presents the individual with an ambiguous stimulus (an inkblot or an open-ended instruction such as drawing a person or selecting a photograph), to which the individual can give a variety of responses. The response is assumed to represent a projection of the individual's personality and underlying disorder if there is one. As Meehl (1945) has noted, projective techniques can be more or less structured depending on the ambiguity of the stimulus presented, the variety of potential answers, and the rules for interpreting the response.
3. Experience: The clinician justifies her diagnosis entirely on the basis of her own past clinical experience with similar cases.
4. Subjective differential diagnosis: The clinician begins with a list of potential diagnoses and attempts to eliminate all but one item on the list. For example, some disorders involve delusions (e.g., delusional disorder and some schizophrenias). If the clinician can establish that a person does not suffer from delusions, these can be marked off the list.
5. Semi-Structured Interview: The clinician begins with a predetermined, ordered set of questions or themes that are to be addressed in the interview; but these are merely guides that leave considerable freedom to pursue (or not) issues in detail and in whatever order seems natural.
6. Structured Interview: The clinician begins with a prearranged menu of questions or surveys that she presents in a prearranged order, and a differential diagnosis is arrived at given the clinician's interpretation of the individuals' answers to those questions.
7. LEAD: LEAD is an acronym that stands for (a) "Longitudinal evaluation of symptomology," (b) "Evaluation by expert consensus," and (c) "All Data from multiple sources" (Spitzer 1983). A LEAD diagnosis is arrived at by expert diagnosticians reaching a consensus after they have considered a wide variety of longitudinal evidence about a patient.
8. Computer-aided structured interview: This works just like a structured interview except the clinician inputs her interpretation of the individuals' answers into the computer, and the computer delivers the differential diagnosis. (The computer might

also generate a set of potential diagnoses, perhaps ranked in terms of likelihood, and perhaps including suggestions about further screening procedures.)

9. Statistical Prediction Rule: The individual takes a paper-and-pencil or computerized test and a diagnosis is delivered by a purely mechanical algorithm that can be programmed into a computer.

One might quibble about this ordering but the first four methods seem clearly "clinical" and only the last one is entirely automated. So any lessons to draw from the diagnostic literature is unlikely to be framed starkly in terms of "clinical versus actuarial" diagnosis, but in terms of how much structure is externally imposed upon the individual clinician—or alternatively, how much freedom the individual clinician has in coming to a diagnostic judgment. Of course, one might venture that the expert clinician doesn't require the external regimentation imposed by more structured diagnostic techniques because the clinician has internalized that structure in acquiring her expertise. As we shall see, however, this proposition has not stood up well under empirical test.

In order to test the accuracy of a diagnostic method, we need a way to evaluate the accuracy of its diagnoses. The LEAD diagnosis is often taken to be the gold standard: a team of experts who consider all the best evidence about an individual over an extended period of time and who come to a consensus. Although we will follow convention on this point, we should note in passing that there is some room to be skeptical of LEAD. For example, how consistent are LEAD diagnoses across different teams of clinicians? There is evidence that group decision-making, even among experts, can go awry in various ways (Kerr et al. 1975; MacCoun and Kerr 1988; Stoner 1968). As far as we know, the reliability of LEAD has not been evaluated. Putting aside this concern, a practical worry about LEAD is that it is expensive. One way to understand the diagnosis literature in psychiatry is as a search for quicker, easier and cheaper diagnostic methods that approach the accuracy of LEAD.

The vicissitudes of subjective methods

A psychiatric diagnosis typically begins with a clinical interview. Prior to the introduction of formal training in DSM diagnosis in the 1970s and 1980s, subjective psychiatric diagnosis appears to have been a haphazard affair. In a stunning study, Cooper et al. (1972) found that in ten New York area hospitals the ratio of schizophrenia to manic depressive diagnoses was 12:1, whereas in ten London area hospitals the ratio was 1:1. All of these diagnoses were arrived at as a result of clinicians conducting standardized interviews. But when an international group of psychiatrists reviewed these diagnoses and applied "uniform diagnostic criteria ... the diagnostic distributions of patients entering a hospital in New York and London are to all purposes identical" (p. 2).

Even after the introduction of widespread training in standardized methods, subjective clinical diagnosis was still problematic. Lipton and Simon (1985) returned to one of the original New York hospitals from the Cooper study and carefully reevaluated a random sample of 131 patient diagnoses. The findings were shocking. Clinicians were not following the standardized procedures that were presumably part of their training: "Documentation of DSM-III criteria for assigned chart diagnoses was not present in 80% of the 131 charts reviewed." More substantively, they found many misdiagnoses. They confirmed "only sixteen out of eighteen-nine chart diagnoses of schizophrenia. Conversely, the raters assigned presumptive diagnoses of affective disorder to fifty patients, while only fifteen had received that diagnosis in their charts" (Lipton and Simon 1985, p. 370).

A serious problem with the overdiagnosis of schizophrenia is that such diagnoses are seldom reconsidered. This was dramatically demonstrated in the controversial Rosenhan study (1973) in which eight healthy people (three women and five men) gained admission to twelve different hospitals claiming (falsely) to have experienced auditory hallucinations. These "pseudopatients" falsified their names and vocations, but once admitted to the hospital, they were instructed to act normally and describe the events of their lives as they actually were. The pseudopatients had a strong desire to be discharged and so were "motivated not only to behave sanely, but to be paragons of cooperation" (Rosenhan 1973, p. 252). The nursing reports confirmed this—they "uniformly indicate that the patients were 'friendly,' 'cooperative,' and 'exhibited no abnormal indications'" (p. 252). In every case but one, the pseudopatient was admitted with a diagnosis of schizophrenia, and once labeled, "the pseudopatient was stuck with that label" (p. 252). It is no surprise that a person complaining of hallucinations would be admitted to a psychiatric hospital. What is surprising is that after an extended stay—an average of nineteen days and a maximum of fifty-two days—sanity was not detected by the hospital staff. Ironically, it was detected by many of the other patients:

> During the first three hospitalizations, when accurate counts were kept, 35 of a total of 118 patients on the admissions ward voiced their suspicions, some vigorously. "You're not crazy. You're a journalist, or a professor (referring to the continual note-taking). You're checking up on the hospital." (p. 252)

The clinicians' interpretation of the pseudopatients' histories were typically shaped by the diagnosis of schizophrenia. One person's changing relationships with his parents, which might go otherwise unnoticed, was interpreted as "ambivalence in close relationships" which is typical among schizophrenics. When the pseudopatients' note-taking was commented upon, it was interpreted as compulsive behavior or a manifestation of a poor memory.

In the Rosenhan study, the pseudopatients did not take any medication they were given. But the medication for schizophrenia is likely to contribute to the stickiness of the diagnosis. Lipton and Simon note that "once written, the diagnosis of schizophrenia became irrevocable and apparently was never reconsidered. The probability of such reconsideration was further lessened by the effects of the inevitable neuroleptics, prescribed in doses sufficient to 'quiet' the 'disturbing' symptoms" (Rosenhan 1985, p. 371).

If psychiatric diagnoses tend to be sticky, then it is particularly important that preliminary diagnoses be as careful as possible. In 1978, Pope and Lipinsky estimated that at minimum 100,000 patients in the USA with affective disorders were misdiagnosed as having schizophrenia. As a result, these patients were receiving inappropriate medication. Given the plausible assumption that some of these patients would have recovered with appropriate medication, it is not melodramatic to say that this scale of systematic misdiagnosis is tragic. To avoid this result, appropriate diagnostic techniques should put a very high premium on avoiding false positives (e.g., diagnosing non-schizophrenics as having schizophrenia).

We have so far considered the history of unaided DSM diagnoses. But what about prospective techniques, such as the Rorschach Inkblot Test and the Thematic Apperception Test (or TAT, in which the individual is asked to tell a story about a picture depicting an ambiguous social situation)? A 1995 study found that five of the ten instruments most commonly used by clinical psychologists were prospective techniques. Eighty-two percent of clinical psychologists sometimes administered the Rorschach test and 43% administered it frequently or always (Watkins et al. 1995). But in general, the accuracy of prospective techniques is unimpressive. A literature review found that just a few of the indexes derived from the TAT and the Rorschach test were accurate: "the substantial majority of Rorschach and TAT indexes are not empirically supported" (Lilienfeld et al. 2000, p. 27). What's more, projective techniques fail to provide much "incremental validity"—they do very little to improve accuracy over standard diagnostic techniques (Lilienfeld et al. 2000, p. 38).

The case against subjective methods does not end with their lack of accuracy. There is also evidence that subjective methods are tinged with racist, sexist, and class bias. Some clinical judgments about women, African Americans, and people of lower social classes tend to be both harsher and less accurate. Garb (1997) reviews this literature and concludes that, while in many cases bias does not appear to exist:

> misdiagnoses of schizophrenia occur more often for Black and Hispanic patients than for White patients when the patients have psychotic affective disorders. Another well-replicated finding is that diagnoses of antisocial personality disorder are more likely to be made for males than females while diagnoses of histrionic personality disorder are more likely to be made for females than males, even when males and females are described by the same case histories. Another important finding is that referrals for psychotherapy were more often made for middle-class clients than for lower-class clients … [A]ntipsychotic medications were more often prescribed for black patients than for other patients even when the Black patients were not more psychotic, and affective symptoms in severely mentally ill patients were more often untreated when patients were Black or Hispanic compared to when they were White. (pp. 113–114)

It is difficult to escape the judgment that when tested against well-confirmed diagnoses, highly subjective diagnostic techniques have an appalling track record.

This is a harsh verdict, but it does not apply only to psychiatric diagnosis. When medical diagnoses are tested against autopsies, the results are also abysmal. In a massive study of 2479 autopsies performed at 248 institutions, almost 40% "revealed at last one major unexpected finding … that contributed to the patient's death" (Zarbo et al. 1999, p. 194). Autopsy studies reveal surprisingly high rates of undiagnosed cancers. A study conducted at the Mayo Clinic found that among the 768 autopsied patients with a malignant tumor, 17% "harbored a malignancy unknown during the patient's life" (Avgerinos and Björnsson 2001, p. 776). In a hospital serving a largely indigent population, 44% of autopsied patients with malignant tumors had gone undiagnosed (Burton et al. 1998, p. 1246). A study with similar results was published by H. Gideon Wells—in 1923! Given this background, it would be stunning if subjective psychiatric techniques were highly accurate. The hard fact is that diagnosing disease, whether cancer or schizophrenia, is a very difficult business.

Semistructured clinical interviews

One might reasonably wonder whether the psychiatric misdiagnoses described in the previous section are the result of a lack of effective training. This is particularly plausible given the finding that 80% of the charts Lipton and Simon reviewed did not document the DSM criteria that would justify a diagnosis (Lipton and Simon 1985, p. 370). In part to overcome this sort of problem, clinicians are often trained to conduct a semistructured interview: "structured" insofar as it consists of a predetermined, ordered set of questions or themes that are to be addressed in the interview, and "semi" insofar as it is a guide that leaves considerable freedom for the interview to pursue (and presumably to not pursue) issues in detail and in whatever order seems natural. A well-known example of a semi-structured interview is the "Mental Status Examination" (MSE). It begins immediately, with the clinician noting the individual's appearance (grooming, hygiene, eye contact, appropriate dress, posture); topics raised include identifying information (age, sex, marital status, etc.), the individual's chief complaint ("What brings you here today?"), the history of that complaint (e.g., its onset, severity, timing, and potential causes such as drug or alcohol use), medical and psychiatric history (e.g., medications, past hospitalizations or past suicide attempts, family history), family and social history (e.g., schooling, military history, housing status, children, siblings, legal problems, hobbies), and so forth (Daniel and Gurczynski 2009).

Many studies have evaluated the MSE against confirmed diagnoses. In one study, experienced clinicians evaluated 200 diagnoses made by fifteen trainees who knew their diagnoses would be assessed (Skodol et al. 1984). The experts disagreed with seventy-three of the 200 Axis I diagnoses (diagnoses of clinical disorders such as depression and anxiety disorders) and twenty-two of the 200 Axis II diagnoses (diagnoses of personality disorders such as paranoia and schizophrenia). Of these errors, 78% of the Axis I errors and 59% of the Axis II errors were the result of a "failure to apply [DSM] criteria or conventions correctly" (Skodol et al. 1984, p. 253). While these results are bracing, it is important to note that most of the trainees' errors were fairly subtle:

> [I]n only 9 percent of [the Axis I] cases was the change from one DSM-III diagnostic class to another. According to the standards of most reliability studies, only these 18 cases would be instances of disagreements. Therefore, the majority of the changes were in the finer, more subtle discriminations between categories within a diagnostic class or between subtypes of a particular diagnostic category. (Skodol et al. 1984, p. 254)

Psychiatric diagnosis is a complex affair and "neither didactic training nor limited clinical experience with DSM-III can be expected to result in mastery of its intricacies" (Skodol et al. 1984, p. 254).[1]

We have explored the danger of false positives (diagnosing someone with a condition they don't have); but there is also the danger of false negatives (failing to diagnose someone with a condition they have). As a matter of fact there is evidence that, in the USA, these dangers have gone hand in hand: historically, people with affective disorders have often been diagnosed with schizophrenia instead. A potential explanation for this phenomenon is that clinicians, despite training, have misconceptions about affective disorders, and perhaps DSM disorders more generally. Rubinson et al. (1988) presents some disturbing anecdotal reports of clinicians misdiagnosing major depression (MD):

> [O]ne experienced clinician eliminated the diagnosis of MD for a middle-aged woman because she was able to laugh at a joke and because her mood improved briefly when her sister visited. Thus, lack of mood reactivity, a criterion item only for melancholia, was thought to be necessary for the broader diagnosis of MD as well.

---

[1] For more on the complexities of psychiatric diagnosis using DSM categories, see Murphy (2006, esp. chapter 2).

In another case, a trainee diagnosed borderline personality disorder in a clinging, phobic, tearful, 59-year-old man who had no marked vegetative signs [e.g., a sleep disorder, or a loss of appetite, libido] as part of his presenting picture. Psychotherapy was recommended. The patient was seen by another clinician and rediagnosed as having a major depressive episode despite the absence of significant vegetative signs. The patient responded to phenelzine (Nardil) with complete remission of his depressive syndrome and marked improvement in long-standing maladaptive interpersonal behavior (pp. 480–481).

To determine whether these sorts of misconceptions about major depression are common-place, Rubinson sent a fifteen-item true–false questionnaire to working clinicians to test their knowledge of major depression. The error rates for particular questions varied from 13% to 48%. For example, 48% of the clinicians surveyed believed that "at least one veg-etative sign" is essential for a diagnosis of MD. But this is not true. A vegetative sign is not essential for a diagnosis of MD. Forty-one percent believed that "The dysphoric mood found in major depression is of a 'distinct quality' from that seen in less severe depression, such as dysthymic disorder" (Rubinson et al. 1988, p. 481). But again, this is not true. The possibil-ity raised by this study is that clinicians are not properly diagnosing patients with atypical symptoms of MD. A clinician who sees a patient without vegetative signs might mistakenly dismiss MD as a potential diagnosis.

Structured and computer-aided structured interviews

Unstructured clinical interviews have a difficult history. And even semi-structured inter-views are problematic. The problem with these diagnostic tools is the potential for incon-sistent application. Researchers are well aware of this problem. "Although clinicians use [an unstructured interview technique] with unquestioning faith, researchers mostly avoid using it as an exclusive diagnostic method in clinical trials" (Miller et al. 2001, p. 256). To reduce inconsistency, diagnostic tools with more structure—and fewer opportunities for subjective judgment and hence inconsistent application—have been developed. A structured inter-view sets forth a predetermined, ordered set of questions; answers are coded by the clinician (which can involve quite subjective judgment) and the result is delivered by some formal rule. The result might come in the form of a diagnosis, a set of working diagnoses, or pos-sible further tests that might be administered. Given the level of automation in structured interviews, it is not surprising that computer programs have been developed to aid clini-cal interviews. Computer programs that aid in psychiatric diagnosis go back to DIAGNO developed in the 1960s (Spitzer and Endicott 1968). More recent programs include SCAN (Wing et al. 1990) and CADI (Miller et al. 2001).

Miller et al. (2001) compared three diagnostic methods: (a) the TDA (Traditional Diagnostic Assessment), an unstructured interview; (b) the SCID (Structured Clinical Interview for DSM), a paper-and-pencil structured interview; and (c) the CADI (Computer Assisted Diagnostic Interview), a computer-assisted structured interview. It should be noted that Miller gave the TDA an advantage: it was conducted by clinicians with at least twenty years' experience and who were faculty at a university affiliated with the hospital, while the SCID and the CADI were conducted by Miller and four trained hospital residents or fel-lows. The methods were administered to fifty-six psychiatric inpatients, and their accuracy was judged by the LEAD method (i.e., expert consensus after long-term evaluation of all the evidence). The results were dramatic: both structured interviews agreed with the LEAD diagnoses 85.7% of the time; the TDA, despite the expertise of the clinicians, agreed with the LEAD diagnoses only 53.8% of the time (Miller et al. 2001, p. 261).

What explains this dramatic difference in accuracy? Structured interviews force clinicians to ask all the relevant questions. Miller et al. (2001) noted that while the structured interviews evaluated all the Key Criteria ("those criteria … that must be evaluated before the linked diagnosis can be ruled in or ruled out" (p. 257)), the clinicians conducting the unstructured interviews on average evaluated only 53% of Key Criteria (p. 260). As a result, they failed "to search for all possible diagnoses and increasing the likelihood of missing the [LEAD] Consensus Diagnosis" (p. 262). For example, clinicians using the unstructured interviews significantly underdiagnosed schizoaffective disorder, "a diagnosis that requires the clinician to evaluate 11 Key Criteria" (p. 262). Structured interviews don't allow clinicians to cut corners once they're confident they have the right diagnosis.

Statistical prediction rules

Actuarial diagnoses, or statistical prediction rules (SPRs), combine evidence in a purely mechanical manner to deliver a diagnosis. SPRs require no clinical expertise to apply. One simply needs to plug the right quantities into a formula and properly solve that formula. SPRs can be programmed into a computer. In 1954, Paul Meehl wrote a "disturbing little book" in which he reported on twenty studies in which experts and actuarial models made their predictions on the basis of the same evidence. Since 1954, almost every non-ambiguous study that has compared the reliability of clinical and actuarial predictions has supported Meehl's conclusion (Grove and Meehl 1996). So robust is this finding that we have called it The Golden Rule of Predictive Modeling: when based on the same evidence, the predictions of well-constructed SPRs are at least as reliable, and are often more reliable, than the predictions of human experts. Even when experts are given the results of the SPR, they still do not outperform the formula (Goldberg 1968; Leli and Filskov 1984). Upon reviewing this evidence, Paul Meehl said:

> There is no controversy in social science which shows such a large body of qualitatively diverse studies coming out so uniformly in the same direction as this one. When you are pushing [scores of] investigations [140 in 1991], predicting everything from the outcomes of football games to the diagnosis of liver disease and when you can hardly come up with a half dozen studies showing even a weak tendency in favor of the clinician, it is time to draw a practical conclusion." (1986, pp. 372–373)

How can the Golden Rule be consistent with the fact that LEAD is the "gold standard" for psychiatric diagnoses? After all, if LEAD and a SPR disagree about a patient's diagnosis, then the SPR must be wrong. There is no inconsistency here. Remember that SPRs are by nature rigid: they take into account only certain lines of evidence and they combine those lines of evidence in a specific way. The Golden Rule says that SPRs defeat clinicians when both are restricted to only the evidence used by the SPR. But LEAD diagnoses take into account "All Data," including the results of SPRs.

A well-constructed SPR gives very accurate answers to very specific questions. SPRs are accurate but inflexible predictors. Consider perhaps the best known psychiatric SPR, Goldberg's Rule (Goldberg 1968). It diagnoses psychiatric patients as neurotic or psychotic on the basis of the scores of a well-known personality test, the Minnesota Multiphasic Personality Inventory (or MMPI). It answers a very specific question: Given only a patient's MMPI results, is that patient neurotic or psychotic? Goldberg's Rule is more accurate than experienced clinicians in answering this precise question. But it is impossible to use the Goldberg Rule by itself to make a diagnosis. That's because, as Graham notes, "the index is useful only when the clinician is relatively sure that the person being considered is either psychotic or neurotic." In fact, when the rule is applied to people without a psychiatric disorder or with a personality disorder, the Goldberg Rule judges most of them to be psychotic (Graham 1993, p. 225).

So one cannot properly apply the Goldberg Rule without having used some other diagnostic tools. But even when applied to an appropriate population, it would be irresponsible to use the Goldberg Rule to make a final diagnosis. Remember, Goldberg himself took his rule to have an accuracy rate of about 70% (Goldberg 1968). What's more, the psychiatric categories "neurotic" and "psychotic" are quite general. Clinicians need to make finer diagnoses. And so clinicians need to consider other lines of evidence which might well outweigh the MMPI evidence. A team of experts who arrive at a consensus after evaluating all the evidence about a patient over a long period of time, including the results of all the SPRs, will be more reliable than the Goldberg Rule.

This general lesson seems to apply to other SPRs. For example, a recent SPR predicts minor psychiatric morbidity on the basis of a standard assessment questionnaire (Wilkinson and Markus 1989). It is more accurate than clinicians at this specific task. But like the Goldberg Rule, this SPR answers a specific question about a coarse-grained diagnostic category ("minor psychiatric morbidity") on the basis of a single line of evidence. When it comes to psychiatric diagnosis, SPRs seem suited to make preliminary, coarse-grained diagnoses that do not stand alone but must be supplemented with more robust and powerful diagnostic techniques.

Why aren't there more useful SPRs for psychiatric diagnosis? After all, many SPRs are useful for other kinds of prediction; there are useful SPRs that predict criminal violence and recidivism, academic performance, credit-worthiness and the quality of the vintage of a red wine (Bishop and Trout 2005, pp. 13–14). So why not in clinical practice? We suggest a possibility: The paucity of SPRs in clinical practice is perhaps due to the dominance of the DSM as a standard of psychiatric classification. SPRs are powerful tools for predicting phenomena for which there are no clear and established diagnostic criteria. There is no manual that tells us that a prisoner will recidivate if he meets four of seven identifiable criteria. If there were, we wouldn't need a SPR; we could just run through the criteria and figure out if a person met four of them. The DSM identifies sets of symptoms that are sufficient for diagnosing psychiatric disorders. The criteria that must be met for a clinician to make a diagnosis of major depressive disorder are clear and established. To determine whether a patient meets these identifiable criteria is not a job for a SPR. But it's also not a job for an unaided clinician. It is a job for a trained clinician using a structured interview, which forces the clinician to explore all relevant DSM categories and criteria.

Prognosis and Treatment

Once a diagnosis is made, a range of treatment options, possible actions to take in response to the condition, will be considered. Treatment options will typically include no treatment (i.e., doing nothing), a single treatment (e.g., psychotherapy), or a range of different treatments (e.g., psychotherapy and drug therapy). A prognosis is a prediction about the future course or outcome of a condition given a treatment option. In what follows, we will not attempt to report or make judgments about what are the best treatments for particular disorders. Our purpose is to discuss some of the major practical, epistemological, and moral issues that arise for prognosis in psychiatry. We will endeavor to cite as examples some—but by no means all—studies that deserve to be taken seriously as we write this in early 2011.

Controlled experiments: The basics

A prognosis is justified by competently performed controlled experiments. Controlled experiments come in many varieties (e.g., randomized, prospective, retrospective). The reason controlled experiments are crucial can be made clear with a somewhat simplified example. A medical intervention is supposed to make a patient better; in other words, a treatment (e.g., a drug or a course of therapy) is supposed to *make a positive difference* to the patient. Let's distinguish two sorts of evidence we might possess about a treatment, T:

   A. The outcomes of many applications of treatment T.
   B. The outcomes of many applications of a placebo treatment.

Let's say that if one only has (A), one's evidence concerning treatment T is uncontrolled. One knows only what happens when T is applied. There are serious problems with attempting to draw conclusions about the effectiveness of T solely on the basis of uncontrolled evidence.

1. Researcher bias: If the clinician has a strong belief that T is an effective treatment—and if she is committed to using it, she often will—the clinician's interpretations of patient outcomes might be more positive than those of a neutral observer.
2. Attrition effects: Even if a clinician is scrupulously objective in assessing outcomes, his evidence is likely to make T appear more effective than it really is because of attrition: Patients for whom T is not effective are more likely to stop seeing the clinician than are patients for whom T is effective. So the clinician's evidence ends up being biased: it consists of an unduly large percentage of patients for whom T is effective.
3. Placebo effects: Even if an objective assessment shows that patients improved after receiving T, this might have been the result of a placebo effect: The improvement is the result of patients believing they are being treated rather than the specific ameliorative effects of the treatment.
4. Regression effects: Even if an objective assessment shows that patients improved after receiving T, this might have been the result of regression: Many disorders have symptoms that can vary in severity over time. If patients are more inclined to seek

out a clinician when symptoms are particularly severe, improvement might be the result of regression rather than the treatment.

5. Spontaneous improvement: Even if an objective assessment shows that patients improved after receiving T, some conditions improve on their own without any intervention; and so improvement might have been the result of the normal course of the patient's condition rather than the treatment.

Each of these factors might seem like a "mere possibility" that, like the specter of skepticism, can be waived off and ignored in real-life situations. But as we shall see, there is plenty of evidence that some of these factors are operative in common psychiatric situations (esp., placebo effects and spontaneous improvement). The other factors are commonly cited as justifying standard methodological practices in science (e.g., researcher bias and double-blind experiments). There is also an ethical issue in play: Suppose a researcher has uncontrolled evidence that patients seem to improve after T is employed, but the researcher has no evidence either way about whether any of the earlier listed undermining factors explain the improvement. Is it morally acceptable to proceed on the assumption that the improvement is the result of the T rather than one of the undermining factors *when there are widely accepted and readily available ways to control for such factors*? The way to rule out these confounding factors is to have a control. To properly assess T, we need to know what *difference* T makes to patient outcomes. And so we need to know what patient outcomes are when (A) treatment T is applied and when (B) a placebo, and not treatment T, is applied to relevantly similar cases.

Methodological issues

We have made the case for assessing psychiatric treatments with controlled experiments and we have raised some of the epistemological dangers that arise from relying on uncontrolled investigations. But there are methodological and ethical issues that arise that are unique—or at least particularly troubling—when trying to assess talk therapy. We want to address three of those issues.

What is the proper way to measure the "effectiveness" of a therapy?

In order to test the "effectiveness" of a treatment, we must address the question of what it is for a treatment to be effective. What counts as success in therapy? What is its proper goal? Without some general idea of what the goal of therapy is, it is folly to try to figure out which treatments help us to approach or achieve that goal. No doubt there are many different therapists who have many different views about what it is for therapy to be effective; likewise, different patients will want different things from therapy. But in most of the studies we will consider, the effectiveness of therapy is assessed by using standard and widely accepted psychological measures of depression, anxiety, well-being, etc. Most people would agree that such goals are important. Many people who seek out therapy are suffering and have difficulties functioning in the world. The studies we will discuss below advance strong evidence that therapy effectively alleviates people's suffering and helps them function more smoothly in the world. This is no mean feat.

One might reasonably wonder whether there is something more that therapy should be aiming for beyond the amelioration of psychic distress and dysfunction. This point is often made with a medical analogy: Surely therapy is supposed to do more than "merely treat symptoms." It should also aim to cure or resolve the "underlying causes" of a person's psychic distress. So what is the underlying cause that therapy should address? Some therapists contend that the goal of therapy is the acquisition of insights into one's unconscious processes; others insist that therapy must help one to act with full autonomy; still others will argue that successful therapy will help one find personal meaning in life; and other therapists have yet other ideas about what therapy must do to be effective. The symptom-underlying cause analogy is surely true: there is *some* underlying cause of a patient's psychological distress or dysfunction. These perspectives about the underlying causes of psychological distress that therapy should address are typically motivated by a rich theory of personality and the nature of mental illness. The open question is whether we have good evidence for thinking that any of these views is accurately describing the nature of the underlying cause of mental illness. While we cannot hope to address this large question here, there are some moral and epistemological standards one needs to meet in order to justify putting into practice a goal for therapeutic treatment.

In thinking clearly about implementing therapeutic goals in an epistemologically and ethically responsible way, it is important to recognize that therapy is scarce and valuable resource—in some cases, it is a life-saving resource. Any such resource raises issues of distributive justice: How is this scarce resource to be fairly distributed? Many important questions of distributive justice center on large-scale policy issues about the structure of a society's health care system. But some vital issues are of a narrower scale. For example, policies governing how therapists are licensed are essential to determining the supply of this important resource (Dawes 1994). Another factor that helps determine how many people will benefit from therapy is how the appropriate goals for therapy are set. Other things being equal, the more difficult the goals of therapy are to attain, the fewer people in need will receive therapeutic treatment. This does *not* imply that the goals of therapy should be extremely modest. Instead, it implies that certain moral and epistemological standards need to be met in order to implement a therapeutic goal—in order to spend valuable resources pursuing that goal with patients. To be morally justified in implementing a therapeutic goal, one must have good evidence that pursuing and achieving that goal brings significant benefits. And in order to have good evidence for this, the goal must be measurable.

In a society without any scarcity of resources, the inefficient use of resources would raise no issues of justice. But in our imperfect world in which many people who could benefit from therapy don't have access to it, there is a moral obligation to use scarce therapeutic resources efficiently (although this is, obviously, not the only requirement justice demands). One cannot justify expending valuable resources in pursuit of therapeutic goals when we have no evidence that this pursuit brings a significant benefit. We are not defending a general "triage" model of therapy in which resources must *always* be used to maximize expected efficiency. (There are mental health triage practices used for making emergency room decisions. But a general triage model would be much more radical—it would require that *every* therapeutic intervention, not just emergency room decisions, be justified by whether it is the most efficient distribution of resources. While we don't defend a general triage model, a general discussion that explored the promise and pitfalls of a general triage model would be enlightening.) Our contention is more modest: Given scarce resources, a therapeutic goal can be morally justified only if there is good evidence that pursuit of that goal tends to bring about reasonably significant benefits to their patients. How "significant"? This question cannot be answered in the abstract, outside of a particular context. But opportunity costs set the right context for answering this question: What benefits were foregone in pursuit of that goal? We do not contend that the benefits of pursuing a goal must always outweigh the opportunity costs of pursuing that goal—that would be the general triage model. But the benefits of pursuing that goal must be significant in relation to the foregone benefits of using those resources to deliver therapy to someone whose psychological disorder has gone untreated.

Given this general framework for thinking about therapeutic goals, it is clear that the goals of alleviating psychological suffering and distress and thereby helping people to function more effectively in the world pretty clearly satisfy the moral standard. These goals can be reasonably measured. And as we shall see, there is lots of evidence that therapy produces these sorts of benefits.

The medical analogy sometimes used to describe this situation—the reduction of pain, distress and dysfunction address "symptoms" but not the "underlying disease"—can be misleading in two ways. And we think it is crucial to avoid these misunderstandings. First, the medical analogy can be used (implicitly or explicitly) to deprecate therapeutic goals such as the amelioration of suffering, distress and dysfunction as relieving "mere symptoms." Even if this is true, the amelioration of debilitating or life-threatening symptoms without curing the underlying disease is often a very good thing. Human immunodeficiency virus (HIV) cannot be cured. But the development of antiretroviral drugs that relieve the symptoms of HIV is one of the most important and beneficial medical advances of the past twenty-five years. Indeed, many people might someday be able to take advantage of a cure for HIV precisely because antiretroviral drugs allowed them to survive its symptoms. The analogous point might hold true in the case of talk therapy as well. If there is some underlying disease that remains after therapy has reduced its symptoms, the amelioration of the symptoms can give a patient the opportunity to address the disease more effectively. The point to emphasize is that regardless of one's theoretical perspective, it is a mistake to deprecate therapeutic goals such as the amelioration of suffering, distress and dysfunction. And it is a mistake to underestimate the importance of studies that show the effectiveness of talk therapy in achieving these goals.

The second reason to be careful with the medical (disease-symptom) analogy is that there is no consensus on the nature of the "disease" to be addressed by talk therapy and it is an open question whether we have good evidence that some theory accurately describes it. Perhaps it's true that psychological disorders occur when people are stymied in their "self-becoming," or there are problems with the "quality or richness of their inner life," or they are incapable of "living authentically." It is difficult to assess claims about these matters because it is often unclear how to accurately measure these psychological properties of self-becoming, the quality or richness of a person's inner life, or the extent to which they are living authentically. Even if we cannot yet measure these properties directly, we can perhaps measure them indirectly in terms of their symptoms. Consider the following hypothesis:

> If psychological property C is causing measurable symptoms S (e.g., psychological suffering, distress or dysfunction), then a course of treatment that effectively brings about a reduction in the severity of the cause, C, will more effectively ameliorate the symptoms, S, than other courses of treatment.

The idea here is one that follows naturally from the disease-symptom medical analogy: Understanding how a disease works helps us effectively treat the disease and its symptoms. If pursuing the therapeutic goal of improving C does not lead to the amelioration of its symptoms, then this is evidence that either (a) this method of pursuing the goal of improving C is ineffective or (b) C is not the cause of symptoms. If this hypothesis is reasonable, then we must count as relevant studies that measure how effective certain treatments are at relieving "symptoms" such as psychological suffering, distress or dysfunction. They are one line of evidence for determining whether a therapeutic goal that is more ambitious than "merely" addressing symptoms actually succeeds in doing more than "merely" addressing symptoms.

One might reply to this line of thought by insisting that the sort of deep self-improvement that comes with therapy does not manifest itself in the alleviation of measurable symptoms. We can distinguish two different claims here. The weaker objection is that developing measures of complex psychological properties is a technically difficult business that can take years, and as a result the instruments for measuring the benefits of some form of therapy have not yet been developed. The stronger objection is that the benefits of therapy in principle cannot be measured. Against the stronger objection, one needn't be a falsificationist to have serious doubts about the epistemic integrity of a theory with no measurable consequences. But even the weaker objection, while epistemologically respectable, betrays a moral failure. As we have noted, given that many people who could benefit from therapy do not have access to it, there is a moral standard that a proposed therapeutic goal must meet. Pursuit of that goal should be reasonably expected to bring about a significant benefit. Otherwise, it is difficult to see how to justify expending resources in pursuit of that goal rather than in alleviating the suffering of people who do not have access to mental health care.

What is a placebo for talk therapy?

When it comes to testing the effectiveness of a drug, what counts as a placebo seems pretty straightforward: something that looks and is delivered like the drug but that has no ingredients that causally influence the condition being treated. (A placebo can't be entirely inefficacious—even a sugar pill will have *some* effects on the body.) Some have raised concerns about whether it makes sense to extend the placebo concept to talk therapy. Irving Kirsch, for example, has argued that it is conceptually impossible for there to be placebos in psychotherapy. The argument is that "to control for the psychologically produced effects of a particular treatment … it is important that the placebo have the same psychological properties as the treatment it is replacing" (Kirsch 2005, p. 796). But of course, this is impossible in the case of psychotherapy. To have "the same psychological properties" as the psychotherapy being tested, the placebo would have to *be* the psychotherapy being tested.

This is an odd argument. A placebo is not best understood as something that has the same psychological properties as the treatment being tested. Otherwise there could be no placebos for psychoactive drugs. Indeed, Kirsch himself has published a meta-analysis evaluating the effectiveness of antidepressants by pitting them against placebos (Kirsch et al. 2002). And presumably the placebos used did not have the same psychological properties as the antidepressants—otherwise they would have to *be* the antidepressants.

For our purposes, it is perhaps wise not to get too caught up in trying to define *placebo*. The idea of crucial importance for our purposes is that of a controlled experiment. What is central for our purposes is that a particular treatment regime—whether it involves drugs or talk—can make a *difference* to a person. This difference can be good, bad or indifferent. There is a lot of evidence we will cite later in this chapter that shows that psychotherapy can make a positive difference in the lives of people who are in considerable psychological distress. But some interventions might be systematically more effective than others. So let's suppose there is a family of therapeutic interventions that is motivated by a particular theory about the nature of mental illness in general or of a specific illness. We want to know what difference this particular therapeutic intervention makes to patients. So we compare that intervention to a cheap, easy intervention that is not motivated by any very sophisticated view about the nature of mental illness. Examples of such cheap, easy-to-do treatments include attention control training, "systematic ventilation" (in which patients talk about common childhood memories, e.g., one's first day at school), or general discussions that do not offer specific problem-solving strategies. Whether we call these interventions "placebos" or "interventions that should be less effective than any respectable therapy" does not matter. What matters is that such a study can tell us what *difference* the sophisticated intervention makes. If the interventions derived from a particular theoretical perspective systematically fail to be more effective than what are essentially "bull sessions" at relieving symptoms of psychological distress and dysfunction, this is prima facie evidence that there is something wrong with that theoretical perspective. But the failure is more than just epistemological. One cannot morally justify expending scarce and valuable resources on therapies that produce no measurable benefit when those resources could be used to relieve genuine suffering. We see no legitimate conceptual or epistemological grounds on which to question the importance of placebos in testing the effectiveness of talk therapy. There is, however, an important moral issue that we must address.

Are placebos morally justified?

In controlled studies of the effectiveness of any psychiatric intervention, the control group is either active (members of the group are given an alternative treatment or a placebo treatment) or passive (members are given no treatment at all). Serious ethical questions arise for studies that use placebo or passive control groups, as they involve intentionally withholding potentially effective treatment for people who might be in significant distress. There are a number of ways to dampen the negative moral impact of controlled studies. For example, wait-list studies involve passive controls in which the no-treatment group receives treatment after the study is concluded. Passive control group studies, however, raise worries about placebo effects: If the intervention was effective, was that the result of the specific intervention or was it the result of factors that appear in cheap interventions (e.g., bull sessions) not specifically designed to be effective for the disorder in question? Moral concerns about the placebo group can be allayed somewhat by the fact that placebo interventions are surprisingly effective compared to no-treatment groups. These concerns can be allayed further if the placebo group is given the therapeutic treatment at the conclusion of the study. Another potential justification for using control groups, whether active or passive, is the potential long-term benefits that come with possibly discovering effective treatments for mental disorders. Perhaps the best way to avoid moral concerns that come with controlled studies is to do a comparative study instead—a study in which a new therapy is tested against what is taken to be the best currently available treatment. Comparative studies, however, come with standard pitfalls associated with studies that lack a true control. What's more, given the possibility that the intervention under test will not be as effective as the best available treatment raises moral concerns. Some moral concerns associated with controlled studies can also be allayed by informing patients about the nature of the study and requesting their consent prior to their participation in the study.

For many disorders, therapy is more effective than no-treatment controls

There is a robust consensus among leading psychologists of the importance of empirically validating treatments with controlled studies: "A major shift in training is nearing completion in university-based clinical psychology programs, as advocates of traditional psychotherapies retire and have in large part passed the torch to younger, more empirically informed colleagues" (Westen and Morrison 2001, p. 875). But the empirical validation of psychiatric therapies is rife with problems. For one, different studies can have inconsistent results. This situation can be improved, at least somewhat, with careful meta-analyses. A meta-analysis is a study that takes a set of similar studies (e.g., similarly designed studies that address the same specific issue) and uses statistical techniques to systematically combine their results. This process is far superior to a narrative review, which simply describes inconsistent studies—or worse, ignores studies with which the reviewer disagrees. A competently done meta-analysis can provide strong evidence for a prognosis. But as we shall see, meta-analyses are not a panacea.

To appreciate the problems with psychiatric prognosis, it will be useful to focus on a relatively narrow range of the empirical literature. We will focus on the effects of therapy on depression and generalized anxiety disorder (GAD). This focus is not entirely arbitrary. The empirical literature on therapy is fairly large and these are two common psychiatric disorders. Nearly twenty-one million people over the age of eighteen in the USA suffer from a mood disorder,[2] and about forty million are afflicted with some kind of anxiety disorder.[3] These two conditions often co-occur, but even with the overlap more than one-seventh of the US population suffers from one or both of these disorders. Among anxiety disorders, GAD "is the most common anxiety disorder in primary care" (Ballenger et al. 2001, p. 55). Before continuing, however, we want to emphasize that our goal here is to not to recommend treatments for these conditions but to address moral and epistemological issues that arise in testing and confirming psychiatric prognoses.

Outcome studies compare a treatment group to a control group (no treatment, placebo, or another treatment). The effect size of the treatment under study is typically understood as follows:

> Effect sizes were computed as the mean of the [treatment] group ... minus the mean of the [control] group, divided by the standard deviation of the [control] group. Conceptually, the effect sizes reflect the distance the average ... therapy client was from the average [control] client, expressed in standard deviation units. (Dobson 1989, p. 415)

---

[2] See <http://www.nimh.nih.gov/health/publications/the-numbers-count-mental-disorders-in-america/index.shtml#Mood>.

[3] See <http://www.nimh.nih.gov/health/publications/the-numbers-count-mental-disorders-in-america/index.shtml#Anxiety>.

In a well-known meta-analysis, Smith and Glass (1977) compiled 375 controlled studies that evaluated ten different psychotherapy practices. They found reasonably large effect sizes for fear-anxiety reduction and for self-esteem (at 0.97 and 0.90, respectively), although effect sizes for other outcomes (adjustment, achievement) were more modest (p. 756). Smith and Glass conclude that "the typical therapy client is better off than 75% of untreated individuals" (p. 752). A follow-up improved upon the methods of the original study but nonetheless confirmed its results:

> When studies without adequate controls are omitted from analysis, the magnitude of effectiveness of psychotherapy remains moderately high.... Likewise, when groups that received therapy were directly compared with groups administered placebo treatment, therapy emerges as superior. (Landman and Dawes 1982, p. 511)

Dawes later admitted that he conducted this follow-up study because he was originally skeptical of the finding that therapy was effective: "I had become a 'reformed sinner'—someone who had originally been ready to ascribe the apparent effectiveness of psychotherapy to methodological flaws in the studies supporting it but who had now become a 'true believer'" (Dawes 1994, p. 54).

Let's focus on the outcome literature for therapy on GAD. GAD is diagnosed for people who exhibit excessive anxiety or worry over the course of at least six months that is difficult to control, and is associated with at least three of the following six symptoms: restlessness, fatigue, difficulty concentrating, irritability, muscle tension, and sleep disturbance. GAD is chronic, disabling and prevalent—it "is the most common anxiety disorder in primary care" and it is often associated with a range of other conditions, including depression (Ballenger, et al. 2001, p. 55).

What do we know about how to treat GAD? The spontaneous remission rate is 20–25% (Ballenger et al. 2001, p. 53). So almost a quarter of patients will get better regardless of their treatment, assuming that the treatment doesn't actually make them worse! Here again is a reason to be wary of uncontrolled experience. Clinicians who don't realize they get a 20–25% success rate for free might overestimate the effectiveness of their treatment for GAD. So let's turn to controlled studies. One fascinating clinical study assessed a cognitive behavioral treatment for GAD. Cognitive behavioral treatments begin with the principle that distorted attitudes are at the root of a person's psychological disturbances. Therapy involves teaching the patient to employ certain problem-solving strategies aimed at correcting the distorted attitudes. Ladoucer et al. embrace a model of GAD that takes it to be the result of four distorted attitudes: (a) an intolerance of uncertainty in everyday life, (b) the erroneous belief that worrying helps prevent or mitigate negative outcomes, (c) a non-productive reaction to problems (fear, lack of confidence), and (d) cognitive avoidance (2000, p. 958). The therapy was evaluated with a wait-list control study. The treatment group showed significant improvement in anxiety, worry, and depression; the control group did not. "Further, for all 26 participants, mean post-treatment scores are well within the nonclinical range on all measures" and the benefits were still significant a year later (Ladoucer et al. 2000, p. 962).

At this point, we can raise a general worry about many outcome studies: they often choose their participants very carefully. This is not an especially serious worry in the Ladoucer study. Of the forty-two potential participants interviewed, they excluded five "because they did not have GAD" and four more "because GAD was not their most severe disorder" (Ladoucer et al. 2000, p. 958). But as a general point, the lessons drawn from a study that sets very stringent entry criteria, even if it is otherwise methodologically pristine, might not generalize to the sorts of patients a clinician sees. "One of the most contentious issues in evidence-based practice is the extent to which results from randomized controlled trials can be generalized to routine clinical practice" (Stewart and Chambless 2009, p. 602). One meta-analysis, for example, found that:

> In the average study [reviewed] … two thirds of patients who present for treatment with symptoms of the disorder are excluded, and the more patients excluded and the more stringent the exclusion criteria, the more successful the treatment. For clinicians who cannot pick and choose their patients, the applicability of these findings to clinical practice is largely unknown. (Westen and Morrison 2001, p. 884)

This validity worry can be met with a meta-analysis that confirms the effectiveness of cognitive behavioral therapy (CBT) for anxiety disorders generally—not just in the laboratory but in clinical practice:

> Patients treated with CBT in clinically representative studies improved significantly and substantially from pretest when they completed treatment. Moreover, CBT for anxiety disorders produced significant pretest-posttest reductions in depression symptoms with large effects across panic disorder, PTSD [post-traumatic stress disorder], GAD, and OCD [obsessive-compulsive disorder], and a medium effect for social anxiety disorder. (Stewart and Chambless 2009, p. 601)

The study also found that training made a difference: "our results indicate that when therapists are not trained, do not use manuals, and are not monitored to ensure they are carrying out the intended treatment, outcome effect sizes decrease" (Stewart and Chambless 2009, p. 601). But the "training" referred to here is quite specific—for CBT to be effective, the practitioner must be trained in the proper use of the techniques of CBT. In fact, one study suggests that standardized treatment plans are more effective than therapist-generated treatment plans in treating anxiety disorders (Schulte et al. 1992). This lesson harkens back to our discussion of psychiatric diagnosis: therapists will typically do better for their patients if they follow empirically validated guidelines rather than improvise.

At this point, control concerns arise for both the clinical study and the meta-analysis. The Ladouceur study used a passive (wait-list) control group. Passive control group studies raise placebo effect objections: To what extent are the benefits of the treatment really the result of placebo effects? As for the meta-analysis, it synthesized the results of fifty-six different studies testing the effectiveness of CBT on adult anxiety disorders—in particular on panic, social anxiety, obsessive-compulsive, generalized anxiety, and post-traumatic stress disorders. Most of the studies did not include a control group. The measure for improvement in these studies was pretest–posttest (i.e., the difference in anxiety measures before and after treatment). While these uncontrolled studies showed significant pretest–posttest improvement, it's difficult to know how much of this improvement is the result of the therapy. Recall, again, the 20–25% spontaneous remission rate. Six of the studies included in the meta-analysis did include a control group, and in these studies, the effect size was 1.29, which "is comparable with a 78% improvement rate for [cognitive behavioral therapy] patients versus a 22% improvement rate for patients in the control conditions" (Stewart and Chambless 2009, p. 600). It is not clear, however, whether these control groups were active or passive; and as we have seen, passive control groups raise placebo effect worries.

Outcome studies for depression come to very similar conclusions. One meta-analysis found that the average (mean) effect size for cognitive therapy was over 2 when the control subjects received no treatment! In other words, "the average cognitive therapy client did better than 98% of the control subjects" on a standard measure of depression. However, all ten of the controlled studies compiled in this meta-analysis used passive controls, "either a no-treatment or a wait-list control" (Dobson 1989, p. 415). So again, we face the issue of placebo effects.

For many disorders, therapy works quickly

The problem of placebo effects becomes particularly acute because some evidence suggests that for many psychological problems relief often comes quickly—in some cases, suspiciously so. Kopta et al. (1994) estimate that a surprising percentage of people "would have improved after making an initial contact with the clinic but before attending the first session." For example, 40% of people who overeat showed significant improvement between the time they made contact with the clinic and the time they first saw a therapist, as did 24% of lonely people, 20% of people who are scared for no reason, and 50% of people with temper outbursts (Kopta et al. 1994, pp. 1011–1013). Another line of evidence suggests that therapy has a "ceiling effect"—after the initial boost, therapy doesn't bring much improvement. Dobson's meta-analysis, which showed a dramatic effect size for cognitive therapy in the treatment of depression, also concluded: "it appears that cognitive therapy has its effect independent of the length of therapy. Because the average length of therapy in the studies was only 14.9 weeks … it appears that cognitive therapy may have a relatively rapid effect on changing depressive self-report" (Dobson 1989, p. 417). In their meta-analysis showing the effectiveness of many different types of therapy on many different psychological disorders, Smith and Glass (1977) found essentially no correlation (−0.02) between outcomes and hours spent in therapy (p. 758).

Given these findings, it is reasonable to wonder whether the benefits of psychotherapy are the result of placebo effects, i.e., "non-specific factors" (e.g., the patient's establishing a relationship with a therapist, or expecting to receive an effective treatment, or feeling understood)—factors that are common to therapy in general but not to any specific therapeutic practice. To test this suspicion, we need to focus on studies that evaluate psychotherapy against placebo treatments—treatments that do not include specific techniques that are thought to be useful in treating the disorder in question.

The weight of the evidence to date suggests that therapy is more effective than placebo treatments. In a meta-analysis of studies that controlled for patients' expectations (i.e., patients had the same expectations for benefits in both the therapy and placebo groups), therapy was more effective than placebo treatments. And placebo treatments were more effective than passive (no-treatment) controls. "[E]ven when differences in subjects' expectations for improvement are controlled, the effects of psychological treatment remain roughly twice that of nonspecific factors" (Barker, et al. 1988, p. 590). Another meta-analysis came to the same conclusion: "The descending order of therapeutic effectiveness appears to be therapy, placebo, and [no-treatment] control conditions" (Grissom 1996, p. 980).

Why does therapy work?

Why is therapy more effective than placebo treatments? Intuitive answers abound: the experience and training of the therapist, the duration of the therapy, whether it was group or individual therapy, the diagnosis of the clients. It appears that none of these measures is strongly correlated with patient outcomes (Smith and Glass 1977, p. 758). What is the practical conclusion to draw from the failure of Smith and Glass to find a ready explanation for the effectiveness of therapy? We would counsel against two extreme reactions. The first is to assume that any kind of therapy is just as good as any other kind of therapy, no matter what the problem. First, the Smith and Glass study did not show that all treatments are equally effective for every psychological disorder. It showed that in the studies they compiled, therapy is effective but no type of psychotherapy was more effective than any other across the board. That is perfectly consistent with some specific treatment being particularly effective with some specific disorder. But to arrive at this sort of specific conclusion, we need good evidence in the form of controlled studies. This brings us to the second sort of reaction we would counsel against: Uncritical reliance on our intuitions or on the uncontrolled experience of a clinician. Consider the following claims:

- Some particular kind or school of therapy is the most effective for a wide range of disorders.
- Long-term therapy is better than short-term therapy.
- A highly paid, well-educated, experienced therapist will have better patient outcomes than a less-expensive lay counselor.

We submit that such claims, when justified solely on the basis of intuition or the uncontrolled experience of a clinician, should be viewed with skepticism. That's not to say they're always false, of course. As Robyn Dawes (1994) has emphasized, "Recovery is a base rate phenomenon. That is, in predicting the likelihood that a particular individual will recover, we can do little better than by predicting from the overall rate of recovery; we have no insight into exactly why some people get better while others don't" (p. 38). But claims about the effectiveness of a treatment, when backed up only by experience or intuition rather than controlled studies, are epistemically guilty until proven innocent.

The question of what the evidence supports is crucial, but it is not the only important normative issue raised by this literature. Note that the judgments we are naturally inclined to support tend to favor the more expensive treatment options. The opportunity costs of a medical system that allocates resources in a massively inefficient manner, particularly when many people suffering from psychological disorders go without treatment, raises obvious questions of justice and morality.

Long-term benefits

There is another problem we wish to touch on with respect to the empirical verification of prognoses and the validation of treatments. Given the quick benefits that come with therapy, we might worry about whether these benefits are ephemeral. The reason this is a worry is that there are very few controlled studies that test the long-term effects of therapy. And this is because the control group for such a study would have to receive no treatment or a pseudo-treatment for years. A meta-analysis of controlled studies done in the 1990s on the effects of therapy on depression, GAD, and panic disorder noted that "One of the most striking things about" the studies "is the sheer lack of data on follow-up at 12 months or longer." Measures of long-term effect sizes are extremely rare "primarily reflecting the ethical problem of keeping patients treatment free for such an extended period" (Westen and Morrison 2001, p. 881). On the basis of very few long-term studies, they conclude:

> The average patient in these studies who receives an active treatment is substantially better off than the average control patient at the end of treatment … The limited data available suggest, however, that the majority of patients do not show sustained improvement over 1 to 2 years, particularly for generalized affect states (depression and GAD). (Westen and Morrison 2001, p. 884)

CONCLUSION

The study of psychiatric diagnosis for the past fifty years has shown a steady trend in favor of more structured diagnostic techniques. In general, structured methods of diagnosis have been shown to be more accurate than methods that give clinicians considerable room for improvisation. Prognosis is a different story. While we can reasonably generalize that some forms of psychotherapy or some drug therapies tend to work well for people with specific disorders, individuals with the same DSM diagnoses respond differently to the same treatment. And so prognosis is inherently probabilistic—we have very little understanding of how to match a particular individual with a particular treatment. We are now in our fourth decade of research that employs meta-analyses to verify prognoses, and conclusions come laden with qualifications and uncertainties of scope. For example, for those with GAD, the evidence suggests one is likely to be better off with therapy. But one review notes that "there is no predictor to identify those patients who require long-term pharmacotherapy for anxiety disorders" (Thuile et al. 2008, p. 84).

We have explored some of the difficulties with empirically confirming prognoses. There are others we have not addressed. For example, someone wishing to conduct a meta-analysis on a well-studied disorder has hundreds, perhaps thousands, of potential clinical studies to choose from. As we have noted, meta-analyses employ exclusion criteria to rule out certain studies deemed irrelevant to the research question at hand, or in some way methodologically deficient. So it is possible that a pair of meta-analyses could come to conflicting conclusions on the same research question because they employ different exclusion criteria. The problem of biased exclusion criteria besets this literature (Westen and Morrison 2001). Long-term clinical studies will lose patients—especially control condition patients—which can compromise their scientific integrity (Weston and Morrison 2001). And if psychological disorders often co-occur (e.g., GAD and depression), it might not always be clear which disorder an effective treatment is ameliorating (Ballenger et al. 2001, p. 55; Barbee et al. 2003). With all these potential pitfalls, it is not surprising that clashes are vibrant in the empirical literature on psychiatric prognosis.

The best we can do today is to recognize that despite the difficulties inherent in the empirical validation of psychiatric treatments, responsible prognoses—and hence treatment decisions—must be based on competent empirical research. We still have much to learn about treating psychiatric disorders. New research is bound to point us in new and better directions. A hopeful vision of research that gives us a finer-grained understanding of how to treat psychiatric disorders is expressed by a recent meta-analysis of research on GAD: "In future research, large-scale multicenter studies should examine more subtle differences between treatments, including differences in the patients who benefit most from each form of therapy" (Leichsenring et al. 2009, p. 85). These imperatives for cooperation and for clear, multi-institutional research standards point beyond studies of GAD. Good science deserves our best efforts, as does every person who suffers with a psychological disorder.

REFERENCES

Avgerinos, D. V. and Björnsson, J. (2001). Malignant neoplasms: discordance between clinical diagnoses and autopsy findings in 3,118 cases. *Acta Pathologica Microbiologica et Immunologica Scandinavica, 109*(11), 774–80.

Ballenger, J. C., Davidson, J. R., Lecrubier, Y., Nutt, D. J., Borkovec, T. D., Rickels, K., *et al.* (2001). Consensus statement on generalized anxiety disorder from the International Consensus Group on Depression and Anxiety. *Journal of Clinical Psychiatry, 62*(suppl 11), 53–8.

Barbee, J. G., Billings, C. K., Bologna, N. B., and Townsend, M. H. (2003). A follow-up study of DSM-III-R generalized anxiety disorder with syndromal and subsyndromal major depression. *Journal of Affective Disorders, 73*(3), 229–36.

Barker, S. L., Funk, S. C., and Houston, B. K. (1988). Psychological treatment versus nonspecific factors: a meta-analysis of conditions the engender comparable expectations for improvement. *Clinical Psychology Review, 8*(6), 579–94.

Bishop, M. and Trout, J. D. (2005). *Epistemology and the Psychology of Human Judgment.* New York, NY: Oxford University Press.

Burton, E. C., Troxclair, D. A., and Newman, W. P. (1998). Autopsy diagnoses of malignant neoplasms: how often are clinical diagnoses incorrect? *Journal of the American Medical Association, 280*(14), 1245–8.

Cooper, J. E., Kendall, R. E., Gurland, B. J., Sharpe, L., Copeland, J. R. M., and Simon, R. (1972). *Psychiatric Diagnosis in New York and London; A Comparative Study of Mental Hospital Admissions* (Maudsley Monographs, no. 20). London: Oxford University Press.

Daniel, M. and Gurczynski, J. (2009). Mental status examination. In D. L. Segal and M. Hersen (Eds), *Diagnostic Interviewing* (4th edn), pp. 61–88. New York, NY: Springer.

Dawes, R. (1994). *House of Cards: Psychology and Psychotherapy Built on Myth.* New York, NY: Free Press.

Dobson, K. S. (1989). A meta-analysis of the efficacy of cognitive therapy for depression. *Journal of Consulting and Clinical Psychology, 57*(3), 414–19.

Garb, H. N. (1997). Race bias, social class bias, and gender bias in clinical judgment. *Clinical Psychology: Science and Practice*, 4(2), 99–120.

Goldberg, L. R. (1968). Simple models or simple processes? Some research on clinical judgments. *American Psychologist*, 23(7), 483–96.

Graham, J. R. (1993). *MMPI-2: Assessing Personality and Psychopathology* (2nd edn). New York, NY: Oxford University Press.

Grissom, R. J. (1996). The magical number.7 ±.2: meta-meta-analysis of the probability of superior outcome in comparisons involving therapy, placebo, and control. *Journal of Consulting and Clinical Psychology*, 64(5), 973–82.

Grove, W. M. and Meehl, P. E. (1996). Comparative efficiency of informal (subjective, impressionistic) and formal (mechanical, algorithmic) prediction procedures: the clinical-statistical controversy. *Psychology, Public Policy, and Law*, 2(2), 293–323.

Grove, W. M., Zald, D. H., Lebow, B. S., Snitz, B. E., and Nelson, C. (2000). Clinical versus mechanical prediction: a meta-analysis. *Psychological Assessment*, 12(1), 19–30.

Hacking, I. (1995). *Rewriting the Soul*. Princeton, NJ: Princeton University Press.

Kerr, N. L., Davis, J. H., Meek, D., and Rissman, A. K. (1975). Group position as a function of member attitudes: Choice shift effects from the perspective of social decision scheme theory. *Journal of Personality and Social Psychology*, 35, 574–93.

Kirsch, I. (2005). Placebo psychotherapy: Synonym or oxymoron. *Journal of Clinical Psychology*, 61(7), 791–803.

Kirsch, I., Moore, T. J., Scoboria, A., and Nicholls, S. S. (2002). The emperor's new drugs: An analysis of antidepressant medication data submitted to the FDA. *Prevention and Treatment*, 5(1), Art. 23.

Kopta, S. M., Howard, K., Lowry, J. L., and Beutler, L. E. (1994). Patterns of symptomatic recovery in psychotherapy. *Journal of Consulting and Clinical Psychology*, 62(5), 1009–16.

Ladouceur, R., Dugas, M. J., Freeston, M. H., Léger, E., Gagnon, F., and Thibodeau, N. (2000). Efficacy of a cognitive-behavioral treatment for generalized anxiety disorder evaluation in a controlled clinical trial. *Journal of Consulting and Clinical Psychology*, 68(6), 957–64.

Landman, J. T. and Dawes, R. M. (1982). Psychotherapy outcome: Smith and Glass' conclusions stand up under scrutiny. *American Psychologist*, 37(5), 504–16.

Leichsenring, F., Salzer, S., Jaeger, U., Kächele, H., Kreische, R., Leweke, F., *et al.* (2009). Short-term psychodynamic psychotherapy and cognitive-behavioral therapy in generalized anxiety disorder: A randomized controlled trial. *American Journal of Psychiatry*, 166(8), 875–81.

Leli, D. A. and Filskov, S. B. (1984). Clinical detection of intellectual deterioration associated with brain damage. *Journal of Clinical Psychology*, 40(6), 1435–41.

Lilienfeld, S. O., Wood, J. M., and Garb, H. N. (2000). The scientific status of projective techniques. *Psychological Science in the Public Interest*, 1(2), 27–66.

Lipton, A. A. and Simon, F. S. (1985). Psychiatric diagnosis in a state hospital: Manhattan State revisited. *Hospital and Community Psychiatry*, 36(4), 368–73.

MacCoun, R. J. and Kerr, N. L. (1988). Asymmetric influence in mock jury deliberation: Jurors' bias for leniency. *Journal of Personality and Social Psychology*, 54, 21–33.

Meehl, P. E. (1945). The dynamics of "structured" personality tests. *Journal of Clinical Psychology*, 1(4), 296–303.

Meehl, P. E. (1954). *Clinical versus Statistical Prediction: A Theoretical Analysis and a Review of the Evidence*. Minneapolis, MN: University of Minnesota Press.

Meehl, P. E. (1986). Causes and effects of my disturbing little book. *Journal of Personality Assessment*, 50, 370–5.

Miller, P. R., Dasher, R., Collins, R., Griffiths, P., and Brown, F. (2001). Inpatient diagnostic assessments: 1. Accuracy of structured vs. unstructured views. *Psychiatry Research*, *105*(3), 255–64.

Murphy, D. (2006). *Psychiatry in the Scientific Image*. Cambridge, MA: MIT Press.

Pope, H. G. and Lipinski, J. F. (1978). A reassessment of the specificity of 'schizophrenic' symptoms in light of the current research. *Archives of General Psychiatry*, *35*(7), 811–28.

Rosenhan, D. L. (1973). On being sane in insane places. *Science*, *179*(4070), 250–8.

Rubinson, E., Asnis, G. M., and Harkavy Friedman, J. M. (1988). Knowledge of the diagnostic criteria for major depression: a survey of mental health professionals. *Journal of Nervous and Mental Disease*, *176*(8), 480–4.

Schulte, D., Künzel, R., Pepping, G., and Schulte-Bahrenberg, T. (1992). Tailor-made versus standardized therapy of phobic patients. *Advances in Behaviour Research and Therapy*, *14*(2), 67–92.

Skodol, A. E., Williams, J. B. W., Spitzer, R. L., Gibbon, M., and Kass, F. (1984). Identifying common errors in the use of DSM-III through diagnostic supervision. *Hospital and Community Psychiatry*, *35*(3), 251–5.

Smith, M. L. and Glass, G. V. (1977). Meta-analysis of psychotherapy outcome studies. *American Psychologist*, *32*(9), 752–60.

Spitzer, R. L. (1983). Psychiatric diagnosis: are clinicians still necessary? *Comprehensive Psychiatry*, *24*(5), 399–411.

Spitzer, R. L. and Endicott, J. (1968). DIAGNO: a computer program for psychiatric diagnosis utilizing the differential diagnostic procedure. *Archives of General Psychiatry*, *18*(6), 746–56.

Stewart, R. E. and Chambless, D. L. (2009). Cognitive-behavioral therapy for adult anxiety disorders in clinical practice: a meta-analysis of effectiveness studies. *Journal of Consulting and Clinical Psychology*, *77*(4), 595–606.

Stoner, J. A. F. (1968). Risky and cautious shifts in group decisions: The influence of widely held values. *Journal of Experimental Social Psychology*, *4*, 442–59.

Szasz, T. (1974). *The Myth of Mental Illness*. New York, NY: Harper.

Thuile, J., Even, C., and Rouillion, F. (2008). Long-term outcome of anxiety disorders: a review of double-blind studies. *Current Opinion in Psychiatry*, *22*, 84–9.

Watkins, C. E., Campbell, V. L., Nieberding, R., and Hallmark, R. (1995). Contemporary practice of psychological assessment by clinical psychologists. *Professional Psychology: Research and Practice*, *26*(1), 54–60.

Wells, H. G. (1923). Relation of clinical to necropsy diagnosis in cancer and value of existing cancer statistics. *Journal of the American Medical Association*, *80*(11), 737–40.

Westen, D. and Morrison, K. (2001). A multidimensional meta-analysis of treatments for depression, panic, and generalized anxiety disorder: an empirical examination of the status of empirically supported therapies. *Journal of Consulting and Clinical Psychology*, *69*(6), 875–99.

Wilkinson, G. and Markus, A. C. (1989). Validation of a computerized assessment (PROQSY) of minor psychological morbidity by Relative Operating Characteristic analysis using a single GP's assessments as criterion measures. *Psychological Medicine*, *19*(1), 225–31.

Wing, J. K., Babor, T., Brugha, T., Burke, J., Cooper, J. E., Giel, R., *et al.* (1990). SCAN: Schedules for Clinical Assessment in Neuropsychiatry. *Archives of General Psychiatry*, *47*(6), 589–93.

Zarbo, R. J., Baker, P. B., and Howanitz, P. J. (1999). The autopsy as a performance measurement tool—diagnostic discrepancies and unresolved clinical questions: a College of American Pathologists Q-Probes study of 2479 autopsies from 248 institutions. *Archives of Pathology and Laboratory Medicine*, *123*(3), 191–8.

CHAPTER 61

CLINICAL JUDGMENT, TACIT KNOWLEDGE, AND RECOGNITION IN PSYCHIATRIC DIAGNOSIS

TIM THORNTON

INTRODUCTION

In this chapter, I will examine the role of clinical judgment in the recognition of psychiatric symptoms via the idea that this involves an ineliminable tacit dimension. I will do this by examining three authors (Polanyi, Ryle, and Wittgenstein) who offer support for the existence of some form of tacit knowledge. But I will place them in the context, in this section, of the dominant criteriological approach to psychiatric diagnosis and, in the final section, one reaction against it.

One reason for doubting, or playing down, a role for tacit knowledge in psychiatric diagnosis is the influence of operationalism in a quest for reliability for the last fifty years or so. There were two main factors which explain this.

Firstly, on its foundation in 1945, the World Health Organization (WHO) set about establishing an International Classification of Diseases (ICD). Whilst the chapters of the classification dealing with physical illnesses were well received, the psychiatric section was not widely adopted and so the British psychiatrist Erwin Stengel was asked to propose a basis for a more acceptable classification. Stengel chaired a session at an American Psychological Association conference of 1959 at which the philosopher Carl Hempel spoke. As a result of Hempel's paper (and an intervention by the UK psychiatrist Sir Aubrey Lewis) Stengel proposed that attempts at a classification based on theories of the causes of mental disorder should be given up (because such theories were premature), and suggested that it should instead rely on what could be directly observed, that is, symptoms.

In fact, Hempel's paper provided only *partial* support for the moral that was actually drawn for psychiatry. He argued that:

> Broadly speaking, the vocabulary of science has two basic functions: first, to permit an adequate description of the things and events that are the objects of scientific investigation; second, to permit the establishment of general laws or theories by means of which particular events may be explained and predicted and thus scientifically understood; for to understand a phenomenon scientifically is to show that it occurs in accordance with general laws or theoretical principles. (Hempel 1994, p. 317)

These two requirements—that terms employed in classifications should have clear, public criteria of application and should lend themselves to the formulation of general laws—correspond to the aims of *reliability* and *validity* respectively. But it was the former that was adopted by psychiatry as the key aim at the time. With respect to it, Hempel claims that:

> Science aims at knowledge that is *objective* in the sense of being intersubjectively certifiable, independently of individual opinion or preference, on the basis of data obtainable by suitable experiments or observations. This requires that the terms used in formulating scientific statements have clearly specified meanings and be understood in the same sense by all those who use them. (Hempel 1994, p. 318)

He commends the use of operational definitions (following Bridgman's (1927) book *The Logic of Modern Physics*), although he emphasizes that in psychiatry the kind of measurement operations in terms of which concepts would be defined would have to be construed loosely. This view has been influential up to the present WHO psychiatric taxonomy in ICD-10.

The second reason for the emphasis on reliability and hence operationalism was a parallel influence from within American psychiatry that shaped the writing of the third edition of the *Diagnostic and Statistical Manual of Mental Disorders* (DSM-III; American Psychiatric Association 1980). Whilst DSM-I and DSM-II had drawn heavily on psychoanalytic theoretical terms, the committee charged with drawing up DSM-III drew on the work of a group of psychiatrists from Washington University of St Louis. Responding in part to research that had revealed significant differences in diagnostic practices between different psychiatrists, the "St Louis group," led by John Feighner, published operationalized criteria for psychiatric diagnosis. The DSM-III Task Force replaced reference to Freudian etiological theory with more observational criteria. The Task Force leader, Robert Spitzer, later reported: "With its intellectual roots in St Louis instead of Vienna, and with its intellectual inspiration drawn from Kraepelin, not Freud, the task force was viewed from the outset as unsympathetic to the interests of those whose theory and practice derived from the psychoanalytic tradition" (Bayer and Spitzer 1985, p. 188 quoted in Shorter 1997, pp. 301–302).

This stress on operationalism has had an effect on the way that criteriological diagnosis is codified in DSM and ICD manuals. Syndromes are described and characterized in terms of disjunctions and conjunctions of symptoms. The symptoms are described in ways influenced by operationalism and with as little etiological theory as possible. (That they are neither strictly operationally defined nor strictly etiologically theory-free is not relevant here.) Thus one can think of such a manual as providing guidance for, or a justification of, a diagnosis offered by saying that a subject is suffering from a specific syndrome. Presented with an individual, the diagnosis of a specific syndrome is said to be justified because he or she has enough of the relevant symptoms which can be, as closely as possible, "read off" from their presentation. Such an approach to psychiatric diagnosis plays down the role of individual judgment or tacit knowledge amongst clinicians.

POLANYI ON TACIT KNOWLEDGE

Whilst the influence of operationalism deployed in the service of reliability aims to remove or reduce the presence of judgment and thus an uncodified tacit element in psychiatric diagnosis, there is a tradition in the history and philosophy of science (dating from about the same time) which stresses an ineliminable role for tacit knowledge in science. In this section, I will examine arguments offered by the chemist turned philosopher of science Michael Polanyi.

But first, what does Polanyi mean by "tacit" knowing or knowledge? (Polanyi himself talks of tacit *knowing* rather than knowledge. I will, nevertheless, use "knowledge" whilst talking about his views but will return to emphasize the practical dimension to what is tacit.) In this chapter, I will follow two clues. The first comes from the start of his book *The Tacit Dimension*:

> I shall reconsider human knowledge by starting from the fact that *we can know more than we can tell*. (Polanyi 1967b, p. 4)

The second clue comes from *Personal Knowledge* in which he says:

> I regard knowing as an active comprehension of things known, an action that requires skill. (Polanyi 1958, p. vii)

These passages suggest two features tacit knowledge might have: that it is not, or perhaps cannot be made, explicit and that it is connected to action, the practical knowledge of a skilled agent. I will start with the first claim and, in later sections, return to the second. The first (that we can know more than we can tell) continues:

> This fact seems obvious enough; but it is not easy to say exactly what it means. Take an example. We know a person's face, and can recognize it among a thousand, indeed among a million. Yet we usually cannot tell how we recognize a face we know. So most of this knowledge cannot be put into words. (Polanyi 1967b, p. 4)

The suggestion is that tacit knowledge is *tacit* because it is "more than we can tell." We cannot *tell how* we know things that we know tacitly. But what argument does he give for this? What are the limits on what can be said still leaving something that can be known?

In *Personal Knowledge*, Polanyi's strategy is to examine how what can be said or, more broadly, *articulated* both leaves room for, and depends on, something outside what can be articulated. There are two key arguments of relevance to this chapter. One depends on limits on the kind of representation available to summarize *explicit* knowledge in science, thus indicating a space for tacit knowledge. The other depends on an analysis of what is involved in recognition (an argument which promises to impact on diagnostic judgment), which also connects to Polanyi's views of how linguistic representation in general is possible. I will suggest that this latter argument is the fundamental argument but start with the former.

To examine the limits of scientific representation, Polanyi considers the understanding that a skilled surgeon has of the spatial configuration and orientation of organs in the body. He argues that this cannot be captured in a representation:

> The major difficulty in the understanding, and hence in the teaching of anatomy, arises in respect to the intricate three-dimensional network of organs closely packed inside the body, of which no diagram can give an adequate representation. Even dissection, which lays bare a region and its organs by removing the parts overlaying it, does not demonstrate more than one aspect of that region. It is left to the imagination to reconstruct from such experience the three-dimensional picture of the exposed area as it existed in the unopened body, and to explore mentally its connections with adjoining unexposed areas around it and below it.
>
> The kind of topographic knowledge which an experienced surgeon possesses of the regions on which he operates is therefore ineffable knowledge. (Polanyi 1962, p. 89)

The claim here is that three-dimensional spatial knowledge is ineffable, or tacit, because it cannot be captured in a representation. Polanyi goes on to argue that even if all human bodies were identical and even if there were a map comprising cross sections based on "a thousand thin slices" of the body, that in itself would not articulate the knowledge of a trained surgeon. Someone knowing merely the former "would know a set of data which fully determine the spatial arrangement of the organs in the body; yet he would not know that spatial arrangement itself" (p. 89). An additional act of interpretation or imagination is needed. But because that act cannot itself be encoded in a representation, according to Polanyi, it remains tacit.

This argument is a little surprising. Polanyi concedes that the set of cross-sectional representations, presumably alongside some further information about their inter-relations such as their order and distance apart, "fully determine(s) the spatial arrangement of the organs" and yet denies that this amounts to an articulation of the three-dimensional understanding.

Without the further information about the relations between the set of maps, the maps alone would not be an articulation of the skilled surgeon's knowledge. But then neither would they fully represent the arrangement of bodily organs. With the addition of that further information, however, why would this not count as an articulation of the surgeon's knowledge? If so, it would be explicit, rather than merely tacit, knowledge.

A further possible clue to Polanyi's thinking runs thus:

> The difficulty lies here entirely in the subsequent integration of the particulars and the inadequacy of articulation consists altogether in the fact that the latter process is left without formal guidance. The degree of intelligence required from the student to perform the act of insight which ultimately conveys to him the knowledge of the topography, offers here a measure of the limitations of the articulation representing this topography. (Polanyi 1962, p. 90)

But there remains something strange about this line of thought. If the *integration* of the partial representations, such as the set of cross sections, were left without formal guidance then it would be clear why the partial representations could not articulate the surgeon's knowledge. But neither would they *determine* the arrangement of organs as Polanyi has previously asserted.

The difficulty with interpreting this argument is that of balancing the claim that spatial configuration is both determined by what can be represented but remains ineffable and thus tacit rather than explicit. I think that the clue to its interpretation is to realize that whether a symbol logically determines anything always, according to Polanyi, depends on a tacit element. This is supported by a different argument:

> I may ride a bicycle and say nothing, or pick out my macintosh among twenty others and say nothing. Though I cannot say clearly how I ride a bicycle nor how I recognise my macintosh

(for I don't know it clearly), yet this will not prevent me from saying that I know how to ride a bicycle and how to recognise my macintosh. For I know that I know how to do such things, though I know the particulars of what I know only in an instrumental manner and am focally quite ignorant of them. (Polanyi 1962, p. 88)

Polanyi suggests that the skill involved in the example of recognizing a macintosh is akin to the practical skill of cycle riding. In both cases, the "knowledge-how" depends on something which is not explicit: the details of the act of bike riding or raincoat recognition. Whilst one can recognize one's own macintosh, in the example, one is ignorant, in some sense, of how. Thus how one does this is tacit.

If this argument were successful it would be of general significance because it would also apply to the recognitional skill which underpins classification such as diagnosis in psychiatry but also linguistic labeling generally. Indeed, Polanyi makes this connection explicitly.

[I]n all applications of a formalism to experience there is an indeterminacy involved, which must be resolved by the observer on the ground of unspecified criteria. Now we may say further that the process of applying language to things is also necessarily unformalized: that it is inarticulate. Denotation, then, is an art, and whatever we say about things assumes our endorsement of our own skill in practising this art. (Polanyi 1962, p. 81)

This connection between denotation and tacit recognitional skills appears to be the fundamental argument for the importance of tacit knowledge for explicit scientific accounts. Polanyi summarizes the connection thus:

If, as it would seem, the meaning of all our utterances is determined to an important extent by a skilful act of our own—the act of knowing—then the acceptance of any of our own utterances as true involves our approval of our own skill. To affirm anything implies, then, to this extent an appraisal of our own art of knowing, and the establishment of truth becomes decisively dependent on a set of personal criteria of our own which cannot be formally defined ... [E]verywhere it is the inarticulate which has the last word, unspoken and yet decisive. (Polanyi 1962, p. 70–71)

Note that the argument for the claim about the art of denotation being tacit seems to rest on an appeal to the apparently clearer case of the recognition of particulars—such as a particular macintosh—which, he argues, depends on features of which one is focally ignorant. There is a difference between the two cases. The example he gives concerns recognition of a particular macintosh as one's own among a pile of them. It is not the judgment that the object is a macintosh, but the recognition (re-cognition) of *that* particular macintosh. But nothing will turn on that difference in what follows and so I will ignore it.

To justify his claim about denotation he needs to defend the general claim that explicit recognition of something as an instance of a type, such as "macintosh," is based on the implicit recognition of subsidiary properties of which one is focally ignorant. In other words, to recognize a feature (F, say) one must (a) always recognize it in virtue of something else (subsidiary features G, H, and I, for example) of which (b) one is focally ignorant. But it is not clear that either part of this claim is true.

To consider the claim, it will help to make clearer what Polanyi means by focal attention and subsidiary awareness. Elsewhere he uses the sample of pointing to something using a finger:

There is a fundamental difference between the way we attend to the pointing finger and its object. We attend to the finger by *following its direction* in order to look at the object. The object *is then at the focus of our attention*, whereas the finger *is not seen* focally, *but as a pointer* to the object. This directive, or vectorial way of attending to the pointing finger, I shall call our *subsidiary awareness of the finger*. (Polanyi 1967a, p. 301)

In attending from the finger to the object, the object is the focus of attention whilst the finger, though seen, is not attended to. Note, however, that the finger is not invisible. It could itself be the object of focal attention were it attended to. This suggests that the first part of the general claim that Polanyi needs itself faces an objection based on a regress. The recognition of an instance of a type or kind depends on subsidiary awareness of something else which could have been the object of focal awareness and thus would have depended on subsidiary awareness of something else.

This is a potential rather than a vicious regress. (It is not that in order to have subsidiary awareness of something one must already or actually have had focal awareness of it or anything else. Combined with Polanyi's general claim, that thought would have generated a vicious regress.) Nevertheless, even the potential regress suggests something implausible about Polanyi's general claim. It does not seem reasonable to think that it is always the case that recognition of the instantiation of a kind depends on subsidiary awareness of something else. Take the case of the recognition that something is an instance of redness. Surely the recognition that x is red turns on a matter of focal awareness of its color, not subsidiary awareness of anything else?

Polanyi seems to assume that the question of how one recognizes something to be of an instance of a particular kind always has an informative answer (and to cover cases where it is not obvious what this is, the second move he makes is to assume that it is tacit). But whilst it sometimes may have an informative answer, there is no reason to think that it always has. In the next section I will return to this point. This line of thought puts the first part of Polanyi's claim—that to recognize a feature (F, say) one must (a) always recognize it in virtue of something else (subsidiary features G, H, and I, for example)—under pressure. What of the second aspect: that one must be focally ignorant of the subsidiary features?

Even in cases where one recognizes a particular as an F in virtue of its subsidiary properties G, H, I, *and cannot give an independent account of those properties*, it is not clear that one need be focally ignorant of them. It may be, instead, that the awareness one has of G, H, I is manifested in the recognition of something as an F or a particular F. One might say, I recognize that this is a macintosh (or even my macintosh) because of how it looks *here* with the interplay of sleeve, shoulder and color even if one could not recognize a separated sleeve, shoulder, or paint color sample as of the same type. Whilst it seems plausible that one might not be able to say in context-independent terms just what it is about the sleeve that distinguishes a macintosh from any other kind of raincoat (one may, for example, lack the vocabulary of fashion or tailoring) that need not imply that one is focally ignorant of, or not attending to, just those features that make a difference. Recognition may depend on context-dependent or demonstrative elements, such as recognizing shapes or colors for which one has no prior name. But if anything, that suggests one has to be focally aware, not focally ignorant, of them.

In summary, two claims seem to support Polanyi's case. First, one is sometimes focally unaware of features that underpin one's recognitional abilities. Second, one cannot always say in general terms on what features one's recognition depends. But these do not support the general claim that (focal) recognition of one feature always depends on merely subsidiary awareness of something else. And if not, then Polanyi has not offered a general reason to hold that recognition is a *tacit* skill.

The Tacit Element in Recognition

I argued in the "Polanyi on tacit knowledge" section that Polanyi's argument for the role of a tacit element in science turns on an argument that it is fundamental in recognition, including the recognition which underpins the "art of denotation." Polanyi suggests that tacit knowledge is that which falls outside linguistic articulation or representation. But such representation *presupposes* recognitional know-how rather than the other way round. So the know-how that constitutes recognition is not itself articulated but rather tacit.

I argued, however, that Polanyi's argument for the role of tacit knowledge in recognition is not successful because he has to assume that to recognize a feature (F, say) one must (a) always recognize it in virtue of something else (subsidiary features G, H and I, eg.) of which (b) one is focally ignorant. But neither point—(a) or (b)—is compelling. There are, however, two other arguments which were both framed at about the same time as Polanyi's and which seem to suggest limits both to what can be put into words (which resistance Polanyi takes to indicate tacit-status) and the importance of a practical dimension underlying linguistic competence, picking up Polanyi's second clue. These are Gilbert Ryle's argument that knowledge-how is a concept logically prior to the concept of knowledge-that and Ludwig Wittgenstein's regress argument concerning understanding a rule. I will now explore the extent to which these support Polanyi's emphasis on a tacit dimension.

Ryle's argument takes the form of a regress:

> If a deed, to be intelligent, has to be guided by the consideration of a regulative proposition, the gap between that consideration and the practical application of the regulation has to be bridged by some go-between process which cannot by the pre-supposed definition itself be an exercise of intelligence and cannot, by definition, be the resultant deed. This go-between application-process has somehow to marry observance of a contemplated maxim with the enforcement of behaviour. So it has to unite in itself the allegedly incompatible properties of being kith to theory and kin to practice, else it could not be the applying of the one in the other. For, unlike theory, it must be able to influence action, and, unlike impulses, it must be amenable to regulative propositions. Consistency requires, therefore, that this schizophrenic broker must again be subdivided into one bit which contemplates but does not execute, one which executes but does not contemplate and a third which reconciles these irreconcilables. And so on for ever. (Ryle 1945, p. 2)

There has been a recent flurry of literature on the precise nature of this argument and thus whether it is successful (e.g., Noë 2005; Stanley and Williamson 2001; for detailed assessment see Gascoigne and Thornton 2013). But it seems to involve something like the following regress:

Suppose all know-how can be articulated (put into words) as a piece of knowledge-that: grasping some proposition that p. Grasping the proposition that p is itself something one can do successfully or unsuccessfully, so it is also a piece of know-how. So, on the theory in question, it will involve grasping another proposition, call this q. But grasping the proposition that q is itself something one can do successfully or unsuccessfully, so it is also a piece of know-how. So, on the theory in question, it will involve grasping another proposition, call this r ... etc.

If the first step of the reductio is designed to "articulate" or represent a piece of otherwise merely tacit knowledge at the heart of recognition, it will lead to a regress. Ryle himself suggests that it can be used to undermine what he calls an "intellectualist legend" which attempts to explain practical knowing-how though a deeper, theoretical form of knowing-that based on grasping a proposition. His counter argument is that, since grasping a proposition can be done well or badly, the only way to avoid the vicious regress is to grant that intelligence can accrue to, and be manifested in, practical knowledge directly, without further theoretical explanation or underpinning. Knowing-how is more basic than knowing-that.

What is the relationship between Ryle's argument and Polanyi's views of tacit knowledge? On the one hand, it offers some nuanced support. Polanyi's claim that we know more than we can tell is one of his two main clues to tacit knowing, the second being the connection between knowing and personal skill (of which more below). Given that Ryle argues that knowing-how cannot be explained through knowing-that or grasp of a proposition—both paradigmatic of what can be put into words—if, following Polanyi's second clue, tacit knowledge is equated with practical knowledge then Ryle's argument suggests limits to the way or purpose of putting it into words. It cannot be *explained*, at least, in knowing-that terms.

But, on the other hand, the idea that practical knowledge can express intelligence directly—without needing to inherit it from grasp of a proposition—suggests the following thought which runs counter to Polanyi's claim that we know more than we can tell. (And thus it puts Polanyi's two clues in tension.) Consider the following piece of practical knowledge: the ability to recognize a raincoat as a macintosh and thus denote it "macintosh." Why is the denoting of raincoats as "macintoshes" not what articulating or expressing this piece of recognitional knowledge amounts to, thus discharging any tacit element? In this particular example, because it involves linguistic denotation, why is that not putting all the relevant knowledge in play *into words* (calling *this* coat a "macintosh," for example)? Why assume, as Polanyi does, that there is always a further, though tacit, answer as to how one recognizes that something is an instance of a general kind?

These questions flag a possibility that Polanyi neglects: that recognitional knowledge might both be fully expressible (and thus, intuitively, not tacit in the sense of silent) nor grounded in further tacit elements understood in the same way. But at the same time, Ryle does provide support for the fundamental importance of the practical dimension. Might that be used to justify a conception of tacit knowledge as "personal knowledge"—"an active comprehension of things known, an action that requires skill"—in Polanyi's phrase but independently of his own arguments?

I will address that question by looking at a related regress argument which dates from about the same time: Ludwig Wittgenstein's discussion of rule following. Wittgenstein considers what is grasped by someone who has grasped a mathematical rule or series which he approaches via the idea of teaching the +2 series:

> Now we get the pupil to continue a series (say + 2) beyond 1000—and he writes 1000, 1004, 1008, 1012.
>
> We say to him: "Look what you've done!"—He doesn't understand. We say: "You were meant to add *two*: look how you began the series!"—He answers: "Yes, isn't it right? I thought that was how I was *meant* to do it."—Or suppose he pointed to the series and said: "But I went on in the same way."—It would now be no use to say: "But can't you see ... ?"—and repeat the

old examples and explanations.—In such a case we might say, perhaps: It comes natural to this person to understand our order with our explanations as we should understand the order: "Add 2 up to 1000, 4 up to 2000, 6 up to 3000 and so on." (Wittgenstein 1953, section 185)

In passages such as these, Wittgenstein seems to stress the infinite possibilities of divergence and thus the infinite possibilities of a breakdown of communication. Given his concurrent criticisms, in surrounding passages of the *Philosophical Investigations*, of appeal to physiological mechanisms, mental talismans and platonic structures, objective features of the structure of reality and independent of us, to explain our grasp of going on in the correct way, it can seem the most fragile contingency that communication is possible (cf. Lear 1982). The problem is the apparent mismatch between, on the one hand, the idea of infinite range of rules and, on the other, the scanty resources for teaching them.

> Whence comes the idea that the beginning of a series is a visible section of rails invisibly laid to infinity? Well, we might imagine rails instead of a rule. And infinitely long rails correspond to unlimited applications of a rule. (Wittgenstein 1953, section 218)

But since teaching rules is possible only either by paraphrase, which merely postpones the problem of explaining the paraphrase, or by finite examples, which seem to underdetermine the rule which governs a potentially unlimited number of cases, grasp of a rule seems to need some further helping hand.

This line of thought suggests, albeit mistakenly, a role for tacit knowledge. The thought runs: since everything that can be said still allows for the kind of misunderstanding exemplified by Wittgenstein's hypothetical deviant pupil, the grasp of a rule that a normal pupil acquires must be based on something unsaid and implicit. It must depend on a tacit element. This seems to support Polanyi's slogan that we know more than we can tell. It can also seem to fit Wittgenstein's own conclusion:

> What this shews is that there is a way of grasping a rule which is *not* an *interpretation*, but which is exhibited in what we call "obeying the rule" and "going against it" in actual cases. (Wittgenstein 1953, section 202)

The problem with this thought is that it accepts what Wittgenstein opposes: an uncritical view of the metaphor of rules as rails "invisibly laid to infinity" fundamentally distinct from our capacity to articulate them. This is a platonic view of the underpinnings of our concepts which somehow latch onto the independent structure and is one of Wittgenstein's targets.

The platonic picture is reinforced by one response to the cases of deviant pupils. They show, according to this response, both that any finite set of examples underdetermines a correct understanding of the rule but also that such correct understanding must involve grasp of a structure which is independent of human judgment. Since no actual human enumeration of the pattern seems enough to determine it, it must be super-human. Hence the metaphor of rails laid to infinity. But whereas real rails can bend and break, the rails in the metaphor cannot. They are supernatural. With that picture of the way rules determine correct moves in place, there is a substantial role for tacit knowledge to bridge the gap between what can be made explicit in the sublunary realm and the ideal platonic standard.

This picture is wrong for two reasons, however. The first objection is that it undermines the possibility of communication. If understanding depends on a combination of something which can be expressed but which stops short of a rule and an inexpressible tacit element which fills the gap, how can the right tacit element be communicated in any particular case? The hybrid account cannot escape the problem that the deviant pupil seems to raise. The deviant pupil might fill in the gap with the wrong tacit element since nothing that can be expressed is enough to guide the selection of tacit element.

The second objection is that it is unnecessary. Whilst Wittgenstein rejects philosophical explanations (via mental mechanisms or platonic structures) of our grasp of rules (by pointing out they could not determine what they are supposed to), he does not promote a kind of skeptical gap between what can be manifested and what must be understood for communication, a gap that has thus to be filled by a tacit element. To the contrary, he undermines the idea that there is any such gap in the first place. For example, he argues that there is a conceptual connection between what a teacher can express and what a student can grasp in the examples which manifest the teacher's meaning:

> "But do you really explain to the other person what you yourself understand? Don't you get him to *guess* the essential thing? You give him examples,—but he has to guess their drift, to guess your intention."—Every explanation which I can give myself I give to him too.—"He guesses what I intend" would mean: various interpretations of my explanation come to his mind, and he lights on one of them. So in this case he could ask; and I could and should answer him. (Wittgenstein 1953, section 210)
>
> "But this initial segment of a series obviously admitted of various interpretations (e.g. by means of algebraic expressions) and so you must first have chosen *one* such interpretation."–Not at all. A doubt was possible in certain circumstances. But that is not to say that I did doubt, or even could doubt. (Wittgenstein 1953, section 213)

Recognizing that understanding can be expressed in examples, for those with eyes to see at least, undermines the idea that there is a gap between sublunary explanations and rules understood as platonic structures and thus a need, there, for tacit knowledge to bridge that gap. A finite series of examples, or a particular verbal explanation, or even a signpost, can express the very rule in question without the need for an underlying tacit interpretation. Thus there is no support in Wittgenstein's discussion of understanding for Polanyi's slogan that we know more than we can tell. What we know, we can express and in the case of denotation, put into words.

Wittgenstein's discussion also suggests a response to Polanyi's assumption that the focal recognition of one thing depends on tacit or subsidiary awareness of something else. If the role of the subsidiary elements serves as the tacit grounds for an understanding of what is focally recognized, if they provide a kind of interpretation of it, then Wittgenstein's discussion undermines that picture. The account of understanding as depending on a combination of an explicit and a tacit element cannot be generally true. This, thus, undermines the motivation for Polanyi's arguments in the previous section. Polanyi does not provide a reason to think that recognitional judgment is tacit nor to think that acts of denotation do not fully manifest one's recognitional know-how.

But whilst Ryle's and, especially, Wittgenstein's regress arguments do not support a connection between tacit knowledge and inexpressibility, they do suggest an important link between the practical groundings of knowledge and a more modest construal of the slogan that we know more than we can tell.

Consider a rule which can be partly codified in an informal statement such as that the digits always follow the pattern: "0, 2, 4, 6, 8, 0, etc." or more fully codified in an explicit mathematical formula or principle. Someone who understands such a rule may understand a general principle or perhaps a set of related principles using some of them to explain others. They may thus be able to articulate what they understand the rule to be in general and context-independent terms. Nevertheless, even with such a codifiable rule, understanding it cannot be independent of understanding its instances. One needs to know, in Wittgenstein's phrase, how to go on.

Wittgenstein gives an example of someone who grasps a series either with, or without, having a formula in mind:

> It is clear that we should not say B had the right to say the words "Now I know how to go on," just because he thought of the formula—unless experience shewed that there was a connexion between thinking of the formula—saying it, writing it down—and actually continuing the series …
>
>   We can also imagine the case where nothing at all occurred in B's mind except that he suddenly said "Now I know how to go on"—perhaps with a feeling of relief; and that he did in fact go on working out the series without using the formula. And in this case too we should say—in certain circumstances—that he did know how to go on. (Wittgenstein 1953, section 179)

The passage makes a connection between understanding and an ability to take part in a practice explicit. But there is also something implicit in this example. It involves *particular* cases. Whatever the general criteria there may be for understanding a rule, such as restating or summarizing it in general terms, such understanding also requires grasp that *this particular* number, for example, is the next number in the sequence. One needs to know how to recognize or proffer a particular number which—whatever its size, color, and font—counts as an instance of the rule because it is an instance of the next number, for example, 8.

This is the connection that lies at the heart of the rule following considerations. Understanding a general rule involves the ability to recognize particular cases. The regress argument targets attempts to explain this connection in non-practical terms. It undermines putative explanations of the practical ability to recognize new cases as instances of a general rule in other terms such as by invoking subpersonal mechanisms or supernatural and platonic structures. But as the example of the deviant pupil shows, when one abstracts away from our actual shared abilities and responses, it is impossible to recover what is understood when one understands a rule. Nothing impersonal can capture the way a subject can see, in the examples given, a general rule and then recognize new instances as going on in the same way. Thus both Ryle and Wittgenstein share an emphasis on what I called Polanyi's second clue: the practical groundings of knowledge.

But the regress arguments also suggest a qualified version of the first clue, especially as it applies both to recognition and more explicitly practical knowledge. The point is not that such knowledge cannot be expressed but that it cannot be expressed in context-independent terms. Practical knowledge requires context-dependent sensitivity. This suggests a way to draw on Polanyi's suggestions, if not his explicit arguments, for tacit knowledge. Tacit knowledge is best thought of as context-dependent practical knowledge or "personal knowledge" in Polanyi's phrase. Further, if the regress argument is correct, it lies at the heart of explicit knowledge that can be articulated or codified in context-independent terms.

So understood, it also seems relevant to psychiatric diagnosis. In particular, it is relevant to the dominance of the criteriological approach to diagnosis and its attempt to underpin reliability. The moral of the regress argument is that there are limits to the extent to which this can be achieved since codification rests on a bed of practical skills.

TACIT KNOWLEDGE, CLINICAL JUDGMENT
RECOGNITION, AND PSYCHIATRIC SYMPTOMS

I began by outlining the importance of reliability and thus the stress on operational-ism for psychiatric taxonomy and diagnosis. For the last half-century, syndromes have been defined in terms of conjunctions and disjunctions of symptoms which have them-selves been described in terms as free of etiology as practical. (For some conditions, such as post-traumatic stress disorder, that would be impossible.) Thus the diagnosis of a spe-cific syndrome is justified in a particular subject if he or she has enough of the relevant symptoms.

This approach is aimed at closing the potential gap between syndrome and subject and thus increasing inter-rater reliability among clinicians. Because of the way both ICD and DSM base syndromes on a combination of conjunction and disjunction of symptoms, it is possible that a syndrome so defined may apply to two individuals with little, or even no, overlap of symptoms. But these differences are codified rather than left to an overall uncodi-fied clinical judgment. Further, the heritage of operationalism suggests a hope that indi-vidual symptoms can be tied to subjects through a kind of measuring operation.

There remains, however, a potential gap between the textbook or diagnostic manual artic-ulation of a symptom and a presenting individual. The concepts of specific symptoms are, despite their specificity, general concepts that can be instantiated in an unlimited number of actual or potential cases. So how can one judge that a general concept applies to a specific individual case or individual person? How can one recognize that the individual exemplifies a type?

One can attempt to bridge this apparent gap in purely general and impersonal terms so as to codify psychiatric expertise. Textbooks of psychiatry can describe, rather than merely list, symptoms. But whatever descriptive account they give of symptoms, there will always be a distinction of kind between their general descriptions and concepts (which potentially apply to any number of individuals) and any particular presenting individual who may or may not exemplify or instance them. Determining that they do instance or exemplify such general concepts calls for clinical judgment.

The regress arguments from the previous section suggests that there are limits to the extent to which operational definitions or criteriological approaches to diagnosis can, in a quest for reliability, exclude the exercise of skilled individual judgment. It is thus worth not-ing that there has been something of an antioperationalist backlash within psychiatry.

Criticizing the ability of the DSM criteria to capture the nature of schizophrenia, Mario Maj, for example, argues that:

> One could argue that we have come to a critical point in which it is difficult to discern whether the operational approach is disclosing the intrinsic weakness of the concept of schizophrenia (showing that the schizophrenic syndrome does not have a character and can be defined only by exclusion) or whether the case of schizophrenia is bringing to light the intrinsic limitations of the operational approach (showing that this approach is unable to convey the clinical flavour of such a complex syndrome). In other terms, there may be, beyond the individual phenomena, a "psychological whole" (Jaspers 1963) in schizophrenia, that the operational approach fails to

grasp, or such a psychological whole may simply be an illusion, that the operational approach unveils. (Maj 1998, pp. 459–60)

In fact, Maj favors the former hypothesis. He argues that the DSM criteria fail to account for aspects of a proper grasp of schizophrenia: for example, the intuitive ranking of symptoms (which have equal footing in the DSM account). He suggests that there is, nevertheless, no particular danger in the use of DSM criteria by skilled, expert clinicians for whom it serves merely as a reminder of a more complex prior understanding. But there is problem in its use to encode the diagnosis for those without such an additional underlying understanding:

> If the few words composing the DSM-IV definition will probably evoke, in the mind of expert clinicians, the complex picture that they have learnt to recognise along the years, the same cannot be expected for students and residents. (Maj 1998, p. 460)

Maj's criticism that the DSM criteria do not capture a proper, expert understanding of the diagnosis of schizophrenia raises the question of how or why that could be the case. If the criticism is right, is it that the wrong criteria have been used: either the wrong symptoms and/or the wrong rules of combination? Or is there something more fundamentally wrong with the criteriological approach as applied to psychiatry? Josef Parnas suggests the latter. In a paper describing pre-operational approaches to taxonomy and diagnosis as a "disappearing heritage" he comments on an underlying difference in attitude towards signs and symptoms of schizophrenia.

> When the pre-DSM-III psychopathologists emphasized this or that feature as being very characteristic of schizophrenia, they did not use the concept of a symptom/sign as it is being used today in the operational approach. This latter approach envisages the symptoms and signs as being (ideally) third person data, namely as reified (thing-like), mutually independent (atomic) entities, devoid of meaning and therefore appropriate for context-independent definitions and unproblematic assessments. It is as if the symptom/sign and its causal substrate were assumed to exhibit the same descriptive nature: both are spatio-temporally delimited objects, ie, things. In this paradigm, the symptoms and signs have no intrinsic sense or meaning. They are almost entirely referring, ie, pointing to the underlying abnormalities of anatomo-physiological substrate. This scheme of "symptoms = causal referents" is automatically activated in the mind of a physician confronting a medical somatic illness. Yet the psychiatrist, who confronts his "psychiatric object," finds himself in a situation without analogue in the somatic medicine. The psychiatrist does not confront a leg, an abdomen, not a thing, but a person, ie, broadly speaking, another embodied consciousness. What the patient manifests is not isolated symptoms/ signs with referring functions but rather certain wholes of mutually implicative, interpenetrating experiences, feelings, beliefs, expressions, and actions, all permeated by biographical detail. (Parnas 2011, p. 1126)

The claim here is that the criteriological approach has the wrong model of psychiatric symptoms and signs in two respects. Just as smoke can mean fire or tree rings the age of a tree, the criteriological approach takes signs to be free standing items which causally indicate underlying states. (Smoke is distinct from, but can be caused by, fire and so in a particular context smoke can factively mean fire.) Furthermore, these relations are independent of one another: they are atomic. By contrast, Parnas suggests, psychiatric signs and symptoms are both essentially meaning-laden and also mutually interdependent wholes. It is the latter claim which plays the more important role in his criticism.

One argument for their interdependence is that it is only in particular contexts that symptoms are reliable. Thus, for example, mumbling speech is comparatively widespread (Parnas estimates 5% of the population) but in—and only in—the context of other features such as "mannerist allure, inappropriate affect, and vagueness of thought, it acquires a psychopathological significance" (Parnas 2011, p. 1126). So the effectiveness of the sign is context dependent. In some contexts it is indicative and in others not. But Parnas goes further by suggesting a more than merely additive view. Grasp of psychiatric symptoms is likened to seeing the figure of the duck-rabbit first as a rabbit and then suddenly as a duck: seeing the signs and symptoms under an overall aspect or Gestalt:

> A Gestalt is a salient unity or organization of phenomenal aspects. This unity emerges from the relations between component features (part-whole relations) but cannot be reduced to their simple aggregate (whole is more than the sum of its parts) ... A Gestalt instantiates a certain generality of type (eg, this patient is typical of a category X), but this typicality is always modified, because it is necessarily embodied in a particular, concrete individual, thus deforming the ideal clarity of type (universal and particular). (Parnas 2011, p. 1126)

So the model of diagnosis is one in which the skilled clinician grasps the right diagnosis as a whole in which different aspects can be seen as abstractions from that whole rather than as its basic building blocks. Such a view would accommodate Maj's suggestion that criteriological elements serve as reminders for already skilled clinicians. They do—on this view—in the sense that after the fact, such articulations of the overall picture are possible, as a musical note may be divided into its pitch, tone, and duration whilst it cannot be built up from those as independent building blocks. But that does not imply that the expert judgment of the whole could be built up from the individual criteria understood in isolation.

I think that this is also the clue to understanding the nature of Parnas and his colleagues' recent EASE project: the Examination of Anomalous Self-Experience. Prima facie, this might seem to be merely a more detailed version of a criteriological approach with a more thorough description of symptoms in a forlorn attempt to eliminate the need for clinical judgment in bridging the gap between general description and particular presenting individual. It is, after all, described by them thus:

> The Examination of Anomalous Self-Experience (EASE) is a symptom checklist for semi-structured, phenomenological exploration of *experiential* or *subjective* anomalies that may be considered as disorders of basic or "minimal" self-awareness. (Parnas et al. 2005, p. 236)

But despite this, the EASE approach stresses the need for flexible conversational relations between clinician and patient or client, rather than a structured interview, and the development of practical recognitional skills:

> The interviewer must possess good prior interviewing skills, detailed knowledge of psychopathology in general and of the schizophrenia spectrum conditions in particular, and he should pass an EASE 3-day training course, comprising (1) a 1-day theoretical seminar, (2)

a number of supervised interviews and (3) provisional assessment of reliability. (Parnas et al. 2005, p. 239)

In other words, the reliability of the method is underpinned by shared practical judgments as well as theoretical knowledge and fits Parnas' stress on a Gestalt or holistic view of the nature of diagnosis rather than a criteriological view.

To what extent, then, does the kind of diagnostic judgment outlined by Parnas depend on tacit knowledge? If one adopts the view of tacit knowledge as context-dependent practical knowledge there are two reasons to think so. First, and negatively, is the claim that the expertise involved cannot be codified in context-independent terms, as the DSM and ICD criteria require. But second, recognizing a diagnostic whole as a kind of Gestalt, seen with its own internal organization, is an example of the same kind of judgment involved in recognizing a new case as an instance of a grasped, prior rule or concept: an essentially context-sensitive judgment.

The operational approach attempts to codify psychiatric expertise and thus play down a role for a tacit dimension in clinical expertise. But philosophical analysis suggests that this project could never be completed. There is no alternative to a practical judgment, of "how to go on," in Wittgenstein's phrase. Maj's criticisms of the operational criteria for schizophrenia and Parnas' opposing view of the nature of diagnosis more generally suggest an alternative view of how diagnostic reliability might be achieved. This alternative accepts that diagnostic judgment cannot be so codified and takes it instead to be an exercise of skilled recognitional clinical judgment, a form of *tacit knowledge* under the most plausible understanding of that phrase.

REFERENCES

American Psychiatric Association (1980). *Diagnostic and Statistical Manual of Mental Disorders, Third Edition*. Washington, DC: American Psychiatric Association.

Bayer, R. and Spitzer, R. L. (1985). Neurosis, psychodynamics and DSM-III. *Archives of General Psychiatry, 42*, 187–96.

Bridgman, P. W. (1927). *The Logic of Modern Physics*. New York, NY: Macmillan.

Gascoigne, N. and Thornton, T. (2013). *Tacit Knowledge*. Durham, UK: Acumen.

Hempel, C. G. (1994). Fundamentals of taxonomy. In J. S. Sadler, O. P. Wiggins, and M. A. Schwartz (Eds), *Philosophical Perspectives on Psychiatric Diagnostic Classification*, pp. 315–31. Baltimore, MD: Johns Hopkins University Press.

Lear, J. (1982). Leaving the world alone. *Journal of Philosophy, 79*, 382–403.

Maj, M. (1998). Critique of the DSM-IV operational diagnostic criteria for schizophrenia. *British Journal of Psychiatry, 172*, 458–60.

Noë, A. (2005). Against intellectualism. *Analysis, 65*, 278–90.

Parnas, J. (2011). A disappearing heritage: The clinical core of schizophrenia. *Schizophrenia Bulletin, 37*, 1121–30.

Parnas, J., Møller, P., Kircher, T., Thalbitzer, J., Jansson, L., Handest, P., *et al.* (2005). EASE: Examination of anomalous self-experience. *Psychopathology, 38*, 236–58.

Polanyi, M. (1962). *Personal Knowledge*. Chicago, IL: University of Chicago Press.

Polanyi, M. (1967a). Sense-giving and sense-reading. *Philosophy*, 42, 301–25.

Polanyi, M. (1967b). *The Tacit Dimension*. Chicago, IL: University of Chicago Press.

Ryle, G. (1945). Knowing how and knowing that. *Proceedings of the Aristotelian Society*, 46, 1–16.

Ryle, G. (1949). *The Concept of Mind*. London: Hutchinson.

Shorter, E. (1997). *A History of Psychiatry*. New York, NY: John Wiley and Sons.

Stanley, J. and Williamson, T. (2001). Knowing how. *Journal of Philosophy*, 97, 411–44.

Wittgenstein, L. (1953). *Philosophical Investigations*. Oxford: Blackwell.

CHAPTER 62

NEURAL MECHANISMS OF DECISION-MAKING AND THE PERSONAL LEVEL

NICHOLAS SHEA

INTRODUCTION

How is study of the brain relevant to understanding the mind? A venerable body of opinion says that it isn't. Many in psychiatry and psychology, as well as in philosophy, still hold that it is a mistake to study the brain if you are trying to understand the mind. It would be like trying to figure out what an abacus does by plotting the physical dynamics of beads on wires. That might give you a reasonable grip on the trajectories of the beads but would entirely lose sight of the calculations being performed. Very few are explicit dualists, of course, but many think that because a straightforward reduction of the mental to the neural is untenable, we should study mental phenomena in isolation from goings on in the brain.

This chapter examines some of the obstacles to relying on neural information in understanding the mind. A major objection is formulated in terms of the distinction between personal and subpersonal properties ("Personal and subpersonal" section), objecting in particular to the idea of subpersonal representations ("Subpersonal representation" section). Multiple realizability presents a separate challenge ("The challenge from multiple realizability" section). The section entitled "Representational models and brain mechanisms" argues that the well-worked-out body of research on reward-guided decision-making has overcome those challenges. The "Applications" section shows how that work can be used to explain some real practical cases: interindividual differences in decision-making, choice behavior in addiction, and positive symptoms in schizophrenia.

An overarching theme is that this philosophical account suggests a particular perspective on patients, as people, that is relevant to the clinical situation. Neural evidence can explain the personal-level phenomenon of voluntary decision-making not because it shows how patients are being caused to act by their brain—the "brain made me do it" approach to the problem, which treats patients like mechanisms—but because it allows us to see why these personal-level processes should unfold in unusual ways.

PERSONAL AND SUBPERSONAL

Cognitive neuroscience purports to explain behavior by reference to recognizably psychological properties: perceiving a state of affairs, representing an outcome, valuing a reward. But it attributes those properties to parts of the brain. That presupposes that the mind can be unified with neuroscience relatively straightforwardly.

The unification is achieved via the idea of internal representations. A paradigmatic example of a representation is a written sentence, for example, "Snow is white." The sentence is a collection of marks on the page that also has semantic properties: it concerns some other things in the world (snow, whiteness) and can be true or false, depending on how the world is. Indeed, giving the conditions under which a written sentence is true does a lot to capture its meaning. The internal representations postulated by psychology and cognitive neuroscience share these features of paradigmatic representations. They are physical particulars, proper parts of people (wholly or substantially in the brain), that have semantic properties. These internal physical particulars enter into causal processes, and the way those processes unfold depends upon their physical properties. However, the system's dispositions to move between these physical particulars can be set up so as to be faithful to their semantic properties. That is the crucial insight behind the success of computers, and it is a critical assumption of information-processing psychology: intelligent behavior is a result of information processing over internal representations, which are internal particulars with semantic properties.

Cognitive neuroscience often goes further. Not only are there representations in the brain that are as physically real as words on the page, but a person may instantiate mental properties (e.g., perceiving a tomato or desiring orange juice) in virtue of having appropriate internal representations in the brain (neural representations of, e.g., features of the tomato or the subjective value of orange juice). The idea is that, when neural representations play the right functional role in the rest of the neural architecture, then they can be the basis on which a whole person has mental properties like perceiving and desiring.

A standard objection opposes the first move: the very idea of neural representations. Properties of people (and their brains and bodies) can be divided into those at the *personal level*[1] and those at the *subpersonal level* (Dennett 1969). The commonsense understanding of the mind, *folk psychology*, is at the personal level. Personal-level properties are those which are familiar from everyday descriptions of people and their mental lives: perceptual states like seeing, hearing and tasting; cognitive states like believing, desiring and remembering; emotional states and moods; feelings like being in pain; and so on. Explanations at the personal level rationalize actions in terms of mental states.

Even if the distinction cannot in the end be rigidly delineated, two characteristic features of the mind do allow us to pick out paradigmatic instances of personal-level properties. The first is consciousness. Conscious experiences are at the personal level, as are mental states

---

[1] I follow the convention of using italics when introducing a term by using, rather than mentioning it.

that can be brought to consciousness. For example, episodic memories are at the personal level, even when not being experienced occurrently, since they can come to be consciously experienced. So are unattended features of the visual field that can draw our attention and become conscious. The second characteristic feature is having contents that are suitable for explaining and justifying why a person acts as she does. It is not just a brute causal fact that perceiving chocolate makes a person reach out and take it. Combined with the near-universal desire for chocolate, the perceptual experience rationalizes the action.

By contrast, properties at the subpersonal level are not conscious and may not be suitable for rationalizing explanations. At the subpersonal level we can observe that a person's chocolate-seeking behavior correlates with (and is perhaps caused by) the firing of neurons in the orbitofrontal cortex, and that as the person eats more chocolate, the firing of those neurons attenuates and their chocolate-seeking behavior reduces. But the fact that a particular neuron in orbitofrontal cortex, call it neuron 42375, fires does not rationalize any of the actions it causes. We can describe various properties of neuron 42375: its neural type (e.g., pyramidal cell), anatomical location, network connections, and firing rate. But none of these throws any rational light on the action of eating a chocolate. Even if the person's reaching out to take the chocolate is caused in part by neuron 42375, neither its firing pattern, nor any other of its purely neural properties, rationalizes the action. Nor is neuron 42375 conscious. No one thinks that the activity of a single neuron is sufficient for consciousness, even if, integrated in the appropriate neural networks, this neuron were the basis for the neural difference between desiring chocolate and being satiated. So the firing pattern of neuron 42375 is a subpersonal property of the agent.

According to one influential view, explanations that deal in personal-level properties are of a distinctive kind, importantly different from the kinds of explanations offered in science, which deals in nomological generalizations about how the world happens to work (Hornsby 1997). John McDowell argues that it is a mistake to mix together properties from the two explanatory schemes:

> Concepts of the propositional attitudes have their proper home in explanations of a special sort: explanations in which things are made intelligible by being revealed to be, or to approximate to being, as they rationally ought to be. This is to be contrasted with a style of explanation in which one makes things intelligible by representing their coming into being as a particular instance of how things generally tend to happen. (McDowell 1985, p. 389)

Others think that there is no deep difference between personal- and subpersonal-level properties and that many acceptable explanations appeal to both (Rey 2001), in particular that it can be appropriate to explain a personal-level property like an action in subpersonal terms. Whether that is legitimate is one of the topics for this chapter. However, even those who refuse to dichotomize can still accept a rough-and-ready distinction, with the conscious, contentful states appealed to by folk psychology being paradigmatic of the personal level.

The personal–subpersonal distinction forms the basis of an attack of the very idea of subpersonal representation. The idea of representing is found at the personal level. If it thereby belongs to a different explanatory scheme, inapplicable to things like neural structures (which are not persons), then it would be a mistake to invoke the idea of neural representation at all. The acceptability of the idea of subpersonal representation therefore depends in part on how deep the divide is between the personal and subpersonal level. Those who rely on subpersonal representations need not subscribe to the view that they are of the same kind as personal-level representations like beliefs and desires. But they do have to assert the existence of a subpersonal variety of representation and reject the view that the personal–subpersonal distinction marks an insuperable explanatory divide.

This is not the place to mount a philosophical argument for the interaction between personal and subpersonal levels (see Davies 2000). However, its plausibility partly turns on whether there are actual cases where subpersonal-level facts furnish useful generalizations about personal-level phenomena. The aim of this chapter is to offer some worked examples of interaction between personal- and subpersonal-level properties.

Subpersonal Representation

Making space for subpersonal representation

Some have argued that scientific psychology can talk "as if" subpersonal physical particulars are representations, provided the representational talk is ultimately discharged in favor of unproblematic subpersonal-level properties (Hornsby 2000). However, scientists are not restricted to choosing between using the personal-level notion of representation metaphorically or not using it at all. Psychology and cognitive neuroscience can define and work with their own technical terms, including a subpersonal concept of representation (Davies 2000). Their use of subpersonal representation need not inherit all the properties of personal-level varieties of representation (beliefs, desires, perceptions, etc.); in particular the normativity and consciousness. Their commitment to the existence of subpersonal mental representations is unproblematic provided the notion of internal representation introduced earlier—that of subpersonal particulars interacting causally in virtue of physical properties in ways that respect associated semantic properties like their correctness or satisfaction conditions—does not introduce properties that are part of an explanatorily isolated realm.

Cognitive neuroscientists work out what a bit of the brain is representing by seeing how its response profile connects to the behavior of the organism and to features of the outside world. For example, some patterns of neural firing are said to represent the probability of reward (Yang and Shadlen 2007). They are thought to have that content because their firing rate correlates with the probability that choosing a particular stimulus will lead to a reward, in the context of evidence that the neural firing is causally important for the choice behavior. So the key question is whether there is a subpersonal variety of representation that comports with cognitive neuroscientific practice of this kind. Given scientists' use, various straightforwardly causal properties seem appropriate to characterizing these internal states, like carrying correlational information, and having various natural functions (Davies 2005).

The project of giving a fully-satisfying account of the contents that figure in subpersonal information-processing psychology remains an open philosophical question, and an important one. But there is no reason to doubt that the scientists' concept or concepts of subpersonal representation can be explicated without appeal to problematic properties like normativity and consciousness. As it is used in subpersonal contexts, representation is tied closely to other clearly subpersonal properties like correlation, natural information, isomorphism, natural teleology, and so on; not to people, their social relations, and associated norms. That is so whether or not subpersonal representation turns out to be reducible to other natural properties. A broadly reductive approach to subpersonal representation remains promising, although it is far from fully worked-out. But even if a reduction is not available, subpersonal representation may still be a perfectly acceptable physical property, on a par with other non-reducible properties in special sciences like biology, chemistry, and geology. It can be integrated with other scientific properties though generalizations and *ceteris paribus* laws without being reducible to them.

Either way, there is nothing constitutively normative about subpersonal representation. That is to say, it is not constitutive of an information processing state having the content it does that certain norms apply to that state. The difference between a correct and an incorrect representation is just another descriptive distinction. Norms may apply to that distinction, as they do to many other descriptive distinctions (e.g., whether a person is cycling on a road or on the footpath). For example, if a piece of information processing in the brain relies on a subpersonal representation in calculating how to satisfy your desires, it turns out to be false, and things go badly for you as a result, then we might indeed say there was something wrong, normatively, with the subpersonal representation. But the normativity is not built into the property of subpersonally-representing. In this domain correct versus incorrect is a descriptive distinction to which norms may attach. Even if personal-level representations were constitutively normative (which remains open to controversy), subpersonal representations do not share that feature. What they do share with personal-level representations is that something like correctness conditions or satisfaction conditions play a role in explaining behavior.

Interaction of subpersonal representations with the personal level

Having made space for subpersonal representations, whether reductive or non-reductive, the question arises as to their relation to personal-level representations like beliefs, desires, perceptions, and so on. On the most optimistic view personal-level representation will reduce to one or another variety of subpersonal representation. At the moment that looks unlikely. Even without reduction, however, there are many ways of integrating personal-level representation with the subpersonal that would not create an unbridgeable divide. The nature of personal-level representation may lie in its constitutive connections with other personal-level properties: various normative connections between representations *inter se*, or between states and actions, may be constitutive of their identity. But the personal and subpersonal levels may interact, for example where empirical findings at the subpersonal level show that a given personal-level conception does not correspond to a property that humans actually instantiate (Davies 2000). There may also be non-strict generalizations (admitting of exceptions or *ceteris paribus* clauses) or other explanatory relations connecting personal-level representations with subpersonal information processing.

Those who argue that personal-level properties fall on the far side of an unbridgeable gulf need to do more than to appeal to non-reducibility or anomalousness of the mental (in the sense of Davidson 1970), since anomalous monism is compatible with there being robust *ceteris paribus* laws linking the mental and the physical (Shea 2003). They need to show that the personal level resists any kind of explanatory integration with the subpersonal. The force of those arguments depends in part on the success of the cognitive neuroscientific enterprise. If scientific psychology discovers lots of robust generalizations linking the personal and subpersonal, then premises about the explanatorily hermetic status of personal-level properties start to look rather less secure.

The examples later in this chapter show that cognitive neuroscience has indeed had some success in integrating phenomena across the personal–subpersonal divide. Alive to the distinction, we can assess these examples without being beguiled by the familiarity of personal-level talk, aware of the possibility that personal-level properties could be being smuggled in and predicated of parts of the brain in inappropriate ways. Humans have a tendency to over-attribute intentionality, for example when we see intentions at work in floods and storms (Bloom 2004). So we should be careful that representation talk in cognitive neuroscience is not metaphorical or merely instrumental (eliminable "as if" talk), or straightforwardly false.

A second merit of marking the distinction is that it forces us to accept that different representational properties are in play. At the very least there is personal-level representation on the one hand and subpersonal representation on the other; more likely, there are several varieties of each. For the reasons discussed earlier, subpersonal representational content is likely to be rather different in kind than personal-level representational content. We don't have to subscribe to the thesis that brains and persons fall under incommensurable schemes of explanation to think that, as a matter of empirical fact, the firing of a single neuron just cannot have belief-type content. Most neuroscientists are extremely cautious about their claims, but there are still plenty of papers that overreach, especially amongst those that are picked up outside the field. So it is as well to be alive to inappropriate deployment of personal-level concepts.

Even if the personal–subpersonal distinction is not a huge gulf that undermines the very idea of subpersonal representation, as some claim, paying attention to the distinction does alert us to the important difference between attributing content to some aspect of neural activity as part of an information processing account of the performance of a task, on the one hand, and uncovering the constitutive basis of personal-level phenomena like believing, desiring, and perceiving, on the other.

The Challenge from Multiple Realizability

A second reason for caution about cognitive neuroscientific practice derives from a mainstream part of naturalistic philosophy of mind. The philosophical orthodoxy of the last forty years has been that mental states are multiply realizable in real physical systems, and are likely to be multiply realized in the brains of actual people. The prospect of finding a neural property shared by all and only those organisms that are in pain, say, which was the hope of the central state materialists of the 1950s and 1960s, has been displaced. However, cognitive neuroscience seems to have ignored the philosophical lesson about multiple realization and dived straight in to look for information processing mechanisms in the brain that are shared by many or all human subjects. What is the status of those findings, and of the philosophical motivations that they seem to contradict?

Standard practice in cognitive psychology is to proceed in a way that is independent of knowledge of brain mechanisms. From observing subjects' patterns of behavior in experimental settings, especially reaction times and patterns of error, but also dissociations between abilities in pathological cases, they build up a picture of how information is being processed so as to drive behavior. In principle these information-processing steps could be realized differently in different people's brains, and could even be realized differently in a given person's brain on different occasions.

The information processing account divides the mechanism leading to behavior into a series of boxes, each of which performs its own step or computation and then communicates the results to other stages of processing. The stages of processing are functionally defined. What makes it the case that a particular part of the brain is performing a particular part of the information processing is the functional role of that part of the brain. And those functional roles can be re-assigned dynamically. Analogously, a standard personal computer stores many representations in random access memory (RAM). There is no systematic correlation between different parts of a RAM chip and different kinds of stored information (hence "random"). Indeed, there is no strict mapping between the pieces of information appreciated by the user and the information stored at particular locations. The words that appear serially in a sentence on the screen need not be stored serially in RAM locations. So the computer analogy supports the idea that there may be only a very loose connection between stages of the true information processing account of the system's operation and the neural areas that are involved.

Before the rise of cognitive neuroscience, the practice of psychology tended to respect this assumption. Neuroscience might study the wiring of the brain and some of its basic mechanisms, like the synaptic plasticity involved in long-term potentiation and long-term depression, but the psychological level of description was taken to be relatively autonomous from these details, and multiply realized in them. With the rise of spatially-detailed brain imaging techniques like functional magnetic resonance imaging (fMRI) and positron emission tomography (PET) that assumption has been displaced by the assumption that some psychological functions are relatively consistently realized. Cognitive neuroscientists now look for repeatable, generalizable events in the brain that correspond directly to particular stages of the information processing story.

For example, it is now well established that there are fairly stable mappings between some basic psychological functions and particular brain areas. That is particularly true of functions that are proximal to input and output: the processing of basic perceptual features, and the motor programs that drive action sequences. Many of these commonalities apply, not only to all normal humans, but also to other primates. For example, the perception of movement depends upon visual area V5/MT and it is now very plausible that neural firing in this area is the basis of the content difference between different perceived directions of motion in both monkeys and humans (Rees et al. 2000). Similar results have been established for many other contents of perception. There is also a mapping between motor cortex and effectors that is generalizable across individuals. Such broad-level generalizations leave space for a lot of variable realization at the level of neural firing. In very simple brains like in the sea slug or nematode it is possible to re-identify individual neurons across individuals, with particular neurons being dedicated to the same range of functions in all members of the species (White et al. 1986). Nothing like that is true in primate cortex. The distributed patterns of neural firing that are the basis of representing a particular perceptual content vary between individuals.

Multiple realizability leaves it open that the same psychological state could be realized in different ways in the same individuals at different times. Here, too, neural evidence suggests that, even if mental properties are multiply realizable, actual variation in their realization is less disparate than it might be. FMRI data can be analyzed by powerful pattern classifiers to identify the detailed spatial patterns that are associated with different contents. For example, pattern classifiers can learn the distributed pattern of voxel activation in early visual areas that is characteristic of the orientation of edges being viewed (Kamitani and Tong 2005). At higher levels, pattern classifiers have been trained to predict, with reasonable accuracy, whether a subject intends to add or subtract a pair of numbers that are yet to be presented (Haynes et al. 2007). Although there are very many neurons in each voxel, these results show that representing the same content on different occasions has a relatively consistent effect on the local distribution of oxygenated hemoglobin, which is in turn coupled to local differences in firing rates (Mukamel et al. 2005). So these results demonstrate the relative intrapersonal stability of the distributed patterns of neural activation responsible for perceiving particular contents. They show that there can be a tight correspondence between a subject's instantiating a psychological property and what is going on in their brain. This suggests that there are cases where the mind-brain relation is intimate enough that neural data can be illuminating about personal-level phenomena. The relation appears to lie within the family of options in the metaphysics of mind that make neural data a good basis for inferences about personal-level phenomena.

There are three broad options in this family. The first is identity theory: that each psychological property is identical to some non-psychologically-specifiable, non-functionalist, property of a person's body and brain. The relevant non-psychological properties are likely to be complex, and the identities are likely to concern fine-grained properties—the state of feeling a sharp stabbing pain in the top right hand corner of the left big toe, rather than the more general property of feeling pain. The second option is functionalism: that psychological properties are constituted by causal relations to physically-specifiable inputs, outputs, and other functionally-specifiable states. However, as we've seen earlier, even if such functional properties are multiply realizable, there is enough commonality of realization that we are able to make reasonable inferences about a person's psychological state from observations of physical properties of the brain, at least for some states. The third option is some form of mere token physicalism, albeit one where there are quite robust *ceteris paribus* generalizations linking the psychological and the physical.

According to some philosophical views, for example a property dualism that takes the neural properties to be merely nomologically connected to mental properties, the deliverances of cognitive neuroscience are at best merely evidence of what mental state a person is in. However, according to all three of the physicalist views just mentioned, cognitive neuroscience is delivering more than mere evidence. The configuration of the person's brain is part of what makes it the case that they are in that psychological state: because the brain state is identical to, realizes, or provides the supervenience base for being in the psychological state.

It is tempting to view the neural evidence in quite a different way: that it concerns a brain state that causes me, the person, to be in a given personal-level psychological state. In non-specialist discussions of neuroscientific results, it is often said that the neural state is a cause of the mental state—that neuroscientists are discovering ways in which brains make people do things. However, if that is assumed to be true in all cases, it betrays an intuitive dualism about the mental. Although it is unsurprising that commonsense views subscribe to a kind of dualism about the mind, the philosophical arguments in favor of the physicalist positions listed earlier should lead us, on reflection, to reject this aspect of commonsense. Often the brain state is not just a regular cause, and therefore evidence of the person's psychological state. It is part of the constitutive basis of their psychological state. In this way neuroscience can deliver evidence of what makes it the case that a person instantiates various personal-level psychological properties.

Although not intended as a rigorous argument, the last two sections do indicate how philosophical concerns about the idea that neural properties have a role to play in explaining personal-level phenomena may be overcome. The next section turns to a worked-out example.

REPRESENTATIONAL MODELS AND BRAIN MECHANISMS

One of the best cases of convergence between a psychological information processing theory and an account of what is going on in the brain is offered by work on the neural basis of reward-guided decision-making. Subjects are asked to make a series of choices, for example, choosing between pairs of stimuli. Neither stimulus delivers a sure-fire reward, but there is a certain probability that each will be rewarded when chosen (e.g., 70% for A, 30% for B). Those probabilities may change during the experiment. Subjects are typically asked to make a series of rapid choices and typically have little awareness of why they choose as they do. Nevertheless, they often perform much better than chance, sometimes nearly optimally.

Mathematical models have been developed showing what the optimal choices are, given a certain string of choices and feedback. For example, if option A has mostly been rewarded in recent trials, it makes sense to distribute a high proportion of your choices to option A; but not exclusively so, otherwise you will miss out on finding out when the reward contingencies switch and B becomes the higher-value option.

Experiments measure the neural activity occurring in people and other animals when they perform these tasks. There turns out to be a surprising convergence between the way some of the mathematical models suggest that optimal actions ought to be calculated and the quantities that seem to be processed in parts of the brain in subjects carrying out such tasks.

There are many ways that a subject could decide what to do next, given a history of reward. For example, she could try to work out the causal structure of the system with which she is interacting. Or she could even try to second-guess the intentions of the experimenter. A simpler approach is to use an algorithm that keeps a running estimate of how much reward is delivered, on average, by each option. Reinforcement learning models take that approach. They use the feedback about the magnitude of reward received from taking an option in order to update a representation of the expected value of each option available in the situation.

A subclass of reinforcement learning models that have proven to be particularly successful are those that employ temporal difference learning (Sutton and Barto 1998). The temporal difference approach overcomes the problem that the reward received from an action may not be immediate. Some actions may be useful because they take the agent one step further toward being able to take an action that receives a payoff. The system keeps track of expected long-run rewards, but generates predictions about the reward expected at a time by taking the difference between long run rewards across that time step: $V_t - V_{t+1}$. In actor-critic models using temporal difference learning, an "actor" selects an action as a function of the relative long-run values of the available options. The critic generates a prediction about the amount of reward that should be delivered at the current time step, given that choice, and compares the prediction with the feedback actually received. It subtracts the expected reward from the reward actually received to generate a prediction error δ_t.

Prediction error at t = reward received at t – reward expected at t:

$$\delta_t = r_t - (V_t - V_{t+1})$$

The prediction error is used to update reward expectations to be closer to that actually experienced. The rate at which expected values are revised up or down in the direction of the most recent feedback is fixed by the learning rate α. The new expected value is the old expected value plus a fraction α of the prediction error δ_t.

The key finding in this literature is that something very like the prediction error signal posited by temporal difference models is found in the brain of subjects performing the task. So in single unit recording in macaques, dopamine neurons in ventral tegmental area (VTA) and substantia nigra pars compacta have been shown to have the response profile expected of a prediction error signal (Bayer and Glimcher 2005; Schultz 1998; Schultz et al. 1997). When an action that has not previously been rewarded leads to a reward, the neurons fire. As that action continues to be rewarded, their firing decreases, in line with the increasing expectation of a reward for that action that would be observed if the subject was updating its expectations based on reinforcement learning from the history of reward. Instead, it is now the predictive stimulus that elicits a prediction error signal. The predictive stimulus indicates a change of state, since it signals that a reward will be coming, so changes the agent's expectations about the long-run value of the current state. When the reward predicted by the stimulus is subsequently delivered on cue, it elicits no response, because it is fully predicted. In a further manipulation a predictive cue that has been learned is presented and the expected reward is omitted. In that case reduced firing is observed at the time of expected reward, consistent with the negative prediction error postulated by the temporal difference learning model.

Similar results are obtained in humans by looking at fMRI data about activity in the brain. FMRI measures the flow of oxygenated blood in parts of the brain (the "BOLD" signal), which reflects neural firing rates. Subjects are asked to perform the kind of probabilistic reward-based task described earlier. Parameters in the temporal difference model, principally the learning rate α, can then be estimated by fitting the model to subjects' choice behavior. The goodness of fit of the temporal difference model can also be assessed from examining the subject's behavior, and compared to rival models. Once parameters have been set, the model itself makes predictions about the prediction error that the agent should be generating on each trial, if it is calculating the quantities posited by the model. Trial-by-trial estimates of the prediction errors that the subject should calculate are then compared to the trial-by-trial variation in the BOLD signal in order to identify neural areas in which the BOLD signal covaries with prediction error (if there are any). This method consistently finds a reward prediction error signal in the VTA (D'Ardenne et al. 2008), and in areas in the ventral striatum to which dopamine neurons in the VTA project (Haruno and Kawato 2006; McClure et al. 2003; O'Doherty et al. 2003).

This impressive body of work is sometimes interpreted as showing directly that the brain implements the temporal difference learning algorithm in an actor-critic architecture, but that is too quick. The ubiquitous problem with imaging methods that the brain activity being recorded may just be a side effect of, rather than the constitutive basis of, the information processing which gives rise to the behavior in question has been partly addressed by obtaining converging evidence from a variety of sources (neurophysiology, fMRI, electroencephalography, transcranial magnetic stimulation, etc.). A more important problem concerns the validity of model-based analysis of fMRI data (Corrado et al. 2009).

It is likely that a whole family of algorithmic models would show a reasonable match to the empirical data (Mars et al. 2010). It is hard to differentiate the particular temporal difference learning model that is used to account for trial-by-trial variations in neural activity from other reinforcement learning models in which prediction error signals play a role. So we should reach a more tentative conclusion: that representations of expected values and reward prediction errors posited by temporal difference learning accounts, *or some closely-related quantities*, are being processed in the brain and probably have a causal role in generating choice behavior. To put this another way, we can conclude that the temporal difference learning model captures something important about the target phenomenon—the neural information processing underpinning reward-guided decision-making—but that the exact relation between model (temporal difference algorithm) and target (neural information processing) remains unclear at this stage. The philosopher of science Peter Godfrey-Smith has argued that it is a distinct advantage of model-based science in general that the relation between model and target can remain loose and unspecified as the enquiry proceeds (Godfrey-Smith 2006).

Even with this caveat, the cognitive neuroscience of reward-guided decision-making offers a worked-out example of our understanding of the mind–brain relation where relations between the psychological and neural levels turn out to be more tractable than some philosophical arguments suggest they might be. If psychological properties are functional kinds, it turns out in this domain that there is less multiple realization, both within and between subjects, than there might have been. Non-reductive physicalism remains a viable option as well, because there is no suggestion here of there being exceptionless laws linking the psychological with the neural. But the kind of radical anomalousness of the mental that some have expected is not observed in this field of activity.

What does this work say about whether there is an unbridgeable divide between personal and subpersonal levels? A deflationary answer is to argue that all of the data is subpersonal. Although conscious awareness has not been studied extensively in these paradigms, it does not seem that subjects are consciously aware of their reward expectations, of the reasons they choose as they do, or of the reasons that they revise their choice behavior after feedback (Pessiglione et al. 2008). But it is unsatisfactory to assimilate the whole pattern of behavior to the subpersonal level. The subjects are fully conscious normal adults, behaving as they do in the experiment because they have understood and are following instructions. In almost all experiments the stimuli are also consciously perceived. Subjects are motivated by the cash rewards available in the experiment and their behavior shows sensitivity to the structure of those rewards. It is hard to deny that they are acting voluntarily when they select one stimulus over another or push one button rather than another. Even if the psychological processes leading up to the behavior are forever unavailable to consciousness, therefore subpersonal, the thing to be explained—the subject's behavior—is a voluntary action at the personal level. So the temporal difference model together with its brain basis provides a putative subpersonal-level information-processing explanation of a personal-level phenomenon.

Although it is far from clear that this scheme of explanation will extend to cover all thought and action, it does offer a template for the relation between the personal and subpersonal levels that shows that they are not always separate and incommensurate schemes of description. When a subject makes a choice, neural data will allow us to differentiate between several alternative explanations of why they decide as they do. Perhaps a large prediction error was generated on the last trial and they have changed their valuations as a result, leading them to choose differently. Or it could be that there have been no prediction errors over a series of trials and the subject is continuing to choose as she was before. A third possibility is that the subject has changed choice, not because of a prediction error, but because this is one of the occasions when their stochastic decision rule has selected a low-value option. These are competing explanations of why the subject acts as she does on each occasion.

Neural evidence allows us to differentiate between these options, and hence explain something about why the subject acted as she did. The subpersonal processes behind these action choices are not like an external cause that compels the agent to behave one way rather than another. On the contrary, they are the very mechanisms that allow the agent's choices to reflect her overall plans (to comply with the experimental instructions) and desires (to take home as much money as possible from the experiment). They allow the agent's behavior to be responsive to incentives and feedback. So there is good reason for thinking that these mechanisms are part of what makes it the case that the agent's behavior is voluntary.

Two features of this framework are important for what follows. First is the existence of robust explanatory connections between personal-level phenomena (voluntary actions) and subpersonal mechanisms in which they are implemented. Second is the observation that the subpersonal properties are not acting as causes external to the agent, compelling her actions or moving her around like a mechanism. The connection is much more intimate than that (although consistent with several different approaches to the metaphysics of mind, as discussed earlier). If the subpersonal mechanisms captured by reinforcement learning models of reward-guided decision-making are part of what makes it the case that agents take voluntary decisions as they do, then malfunctions of those mechanisms can help explain how the personal-level mental life of patients goes awry in some of the cases studied by psychiatry. The model here is not of powerless agents being compelled by external forces outside of their control. Instead, the picture is of personal-level processes operating in an anomalous way because of systematic and explicable malfunctions in the way they unfold.

APPLICATIONS

Variability in learning from experience

In this section we will see three examples of the way the kind of work discussed earlier can explain interindividual variations and pathologies in voluntary action.

The first example deals with how swiftly we update our expectations in the light of unexpected feedback. When a piece of feedback fails to match expectations, a reward prediction error is generated. How much should expectations then be adjusted? The reward prediction error only reflects how far the expectation was awry. In a very static environment it would make sense to discount this information and rely instead on a long history of experience suggesting that the choice is generally rewarding and that this particular skipped reward is just a fluke. In a very changeable environment, on the other hand, an unexpectedly absent reward is much more likely to carry useful information, indicating that the probabilities of different actions being rewarded have changed, in which case it makes sense for reward expectations to be updated, so as better to reflect the new reward contingencies.

This difference has been probed in an experiment that manipulated the variability of the environment experienced by subjects in a pared down reward-based scenario (Behrens et al. 2007). During periods of stability the contingencies between stimuli and outcomes varied little and any failure to match expectations was more likely to be due to chance than to a change in the reward contingencies. During other periods in the experiment the reward contingencies changed rapidly, so reward prediction errors were much more likely to reflect the fact that the reward contingencies really had changed. Fitting a model of a Bayesian optimal learner to the behavioral data suggested that subjects altered their setting for the learning rate parameter (corresponding to α in the model discussed earlier) depending upon whether they were in a volatile or stable phase of the task. Neural activity in the anterior cingulate cortex (ACC) in subjects performing the task correlated with the estimates of volatility derived from the optimality model, suggesting that subjects were keeping track of the volatility of the environment and using it to weight the value of the information carried by a prediction error signal, thereby altering the rate at which they learnt from prediction errors.

Most interestingly for our purposes, the study found that variations in the size of this ACC signal across subjects predicted variations in their learning rates. Some subjects altered their estimates of expected value more than others when feedback failed to match expectations. If it is true that a learning rate is represented in the brain in a way that is reflected in ACC activity, and is sensitive to the volatility of the environment, then the variations in that represented value reflected in the BOLD signal generated by the ACC can explain why some subjects are more sensitive to unexpected feedback than others.

One criticism of reliance on brain imaging to explain behavior is that the brain data adds nothing to an observed difference in behavior. If subjects behave differently in two different experimental conditions, then we should expect there to be some differences in brain activation that reflect the contrast between those two types of behavior. Claiming that such differential brain activity explains the behavioral difference is indeed a bit thin because, taken alone, it doesn't tell us anything more about computations or psychological processes. We knew there would be some neural differences between two conditions and we find that there are. However, the explanatory framework described earlier goes much further. It explains changes in behavior (choosing one action rather than another) in terms of a series of computations carried out in the brain, including calculations of the reward prediction error. And it explains interindividual differences in behavior in terms of differences in another quantity, the learning rate, which is involved in the computations that constitute the making of a choice. So the neuroimaging data is not just telling us that there is some neural difference between conditions (which happens to be reflected in activity in the ACC). It gives us a window into the calculations being performed within the subject in the process of choosing an action. The evidence then allows us to explain subjects' behavior in terms of the mental representations which are being processed; and differences in behavior in terms of differences in the values being represented.

These representations are "hidden variables," which help choose between competing hypotheses consistent with the same range of behavioral data. They do not simply reflect a direct contrast between subjects or conditions. Instead, the brain imaging data is allowing us to choose between different hypotheses about the multistage internal computational processes that lead to behavior. It is precisely because such processes do not correlate with simple experimental parameters (stimulus type, behavior type, feedback type, etc.) that model-based brain imaging is so useful as an independent source of data about such internal processing.

In a separate series of experiments, Krugel et al. discovered that some interindividual differences in how quickly subjects adapt to changed reward contingencies can be explained by genetic differences in a gene involved in dopamine metabolism (recall that dopamine mediates the transmission of the prediction error signals discussed earlier) (Krugel et al. 2009). That is a second kind of case where features of the brain mechanisms that instantiate various calculations leading to behavior can be identified in a way that is relatively independent of the patterns of behavior. And this in turn means that such data can form part of an explanation of why subjects are behaving as they are.

So here we have a personal-level phenomenon—voluntary actions that are sensitive to rewards—an aspect of which is susceptible to subpersonal explanation. When people differ in how much they react to unexpected outcomes, this can be explained both by variations in how heavily they weigh feedback information computationally (reflected in the neural signal from ACC) and in genetic variations in the underlying mechanisms. Neither of these is an external cause of the agent's behavior. They are more likely to be constituents of the mechanisms that instantiate or realize their behavior.[2] So they give us an explanatory window onto the question of why individual subjects are the kind of (personal-level) decision-makers that they are.

The observation that genetic differences and differences in neural activation may predict and explain interindividual differences in personal-level phenomena like voluntary action may well be unsurprising. It is, however, more controversial when this framework is applied to pathologies in personal-level phenomena. Two examples are discussed next.

---

[2] In a similar vein, structural differences in white matter tracts between subjects can explain interindividual variability in behavior (Buch et al. 2010).

Addiction

The well-confirmed framework above for explaining reward-guided decision-making can also play a role in explaining pathological behavior. With the framework in place it should be immediately clear that errors in the prediction error signal could lead to radically false representations of expected value and thereby motivate behavior that is decoupled from actual rewards. Neurons originating in the VTA/substantia nigra signal prediction errors by releasing dopamine at their terminals in the striatum and medial prefrontal cortex. This dopamine release in turns drives the short-term plasticity by which representations of expected value are modified. A straightforward consequence is that any direct interference with the neuropharmacology of dopamine will stop this mechanism operating as it should.

That prediction is widely confirmed by data from rats, other primates, and humans. To take just one case, there is good evidence that at least some forms of drug addiction occur because of the abnormal action on the dopamine system. Cocaine acts directly in the brain to block dopamine reuptake in the postsynaptic terminal, thereby increasing the concentration of extracellular dopamine (Koob and Bloom 1988), and other addictive drugs have similar effects on dopamine concentration in synapses particularly in the ventral striatum (Johnson and North 1992). Recall that when the prediction error system operates normally, a large prediction error is generated when an unexpected reward is delivered. But as the same stimulus leads repeatedly to reward, the rewards become predicted and the prediction error signal declines. It seems that the direct pharmacological action of cocaine has the effect of perpetuating the production of a misplaced prediction error signal. That effectively tells the circuit calculating expected value that the experienced value of the action just performed was higher than expected so that the expected value for the next occasion should be revised upward. The result is that the represented expected value continues to increase even though the feedback is not experienced as hedonically pleasurable and is not increasingly intrinsically rewarding (Berridge and Robinson 1998; Wyvell and Berridge 2000). There is not yet consensus on the details of this explanation, but it is widely thought that the direct action of cocaine on the dopamine-mediated system for reward-guided decision-making is part of the reason that some addicts continue to be motivated to get their drug even when the feedback they experience as a result of taking the drug stops being hedonically positive (Hyman 2005).

There are two ways to understand this pathology. On one understanding, because of these effects of the drug on the brain, the addict is behaving in a way that is beyond her control. It is as if she were being compelled by an external force. Her drug-seeking behavior is being driven by a system that is external to her "self," or will or her capacity for voluntary self-control. The alternative picture sees the drug as acting on and altering the mechanisms that constitute personal-level voluntary behavior. If so, it's not that the addict's personal-level psychology is losing a battle with a strong external cause; it's rather that the constitution of the addict's personal-level psychology has been changed, via a non-standard route.

The fact that addicts' drug-taking behavior is sensitive to incentives is sometimes taken to be evidence addicts are ordinary decision-makers who prioritize the pleasure of taking their drug over other priorities (Foddy and Savulescu 2010). But the earlier model shows how a mechanism that implements decision-making can go wrong in ways that leave agents still showing sensitivity to incentives, but having represented pathologically high expected values for some outcomes. The fact that addicts' drug-taking behavior is still sensitive to rewards is some evidence against the first picture described earlier, which treats the addict's behavior as coming from outside of and overpowering the personal-level phenomena of voluntary action guidance. So it gives us reason to prefer the second picture according to which the drug has interfered directly with the mechanisms that generate representations of value that are partly constitutive of the personal-level phenomenon of acting voluntarily.

Which picture is correct has implications for clinical engagement with people suffering from a drug addiction. The balance of evidence to date seems to favor the second picture according to which at least some drug addictions are due to a pathology of the personal-level phenomenon of voluntary behavior. That would have the advantage from the clinical perspective of encouraging clinicians to engage with addicts as rational agents, rather than as mechanisms being pushed around by forces beyond their control (Pearce and Pickard 2010). The person with a drug addiction really is strongly motivated to take their drug, and that motivation feeds into the mechanisms of voluntary action control in many of the ordinary ways, allowing for complicated reasoning and forward planning. But they are suffering because the usual mechanisms that keep expected values aligned with feedback have been interfered with. Their motivational system is being driven by artificially-inflated expected values, induced by the persistence of a prediction error signal long after the experienced reward associated with drug taking is fully predicted, or has even abated entirely. Furthermore, this direct action of the drug on the brain also seems to block the normal routes by which our higher order desires—our conscious decisions about what to want or value—act on our first-order desires or motivations (Holton 2009).

In this way the dopamine system gives us a useful subpersonal explanation of the personal-level phenomenon of abnormal voluntary action. Exactly how that explanation will go, and what it means for treatment, will depend upon the details of the story, which are still being worked out. But the outlines of the account so far suggest that this is another case where a subpersonal-level understanding of the mechanisms that constitute a personal-level phenomenon will help us to explain and intervene on the personal-level problem. Rather than the subpersonal being a disempowering external cause—"my brain made me do it"—the subpersonal is coming in as part of what makes it the case that the patient is as she is: that the way that she chooses voluntarily works as it does. This body of work suggests that it would be wrong to treat those suffering from drug addiction as automata deprived of the capacity for rational agency. But nor are they just ordinary people with selfishly hedonistic values. The cognitive neuroscience gives us good reason to think that the values that go into their rational decision-making are produced in a non-standard, pathological way.

Delusions in schizophrenia

It is worth giving a final brief example, because of its tight connection with prediction errors and the dopamine system. A prominent theory of the positive symptoms of schizophrenia (e.g., hearing voices, loss of sense of agency) traces them to "dysconnection": abnormal regulation of N-methyl-D-aspartate-receptor-mediated synaptic plasticity by neuromodulators including dopamine (Stephan et al. 2009). The idea is that there is an underlying pathology in the way representations of the world are updated by error signals, caused by abnormal dopamine neurotransmission (Fletcher and Frith 2009).

To illustrate the approach, consider the phenomenon of hearing voices. A difference between inner dialogue and hearing the speech of others is that inner speech is predictable in a fine-grained way from the agent's occurrent beliefs and other mental states, in a way that the speech of others is not. The hypothesis is that there is a subpersonal mechanism that keeps track of this distinction in order to tell whether a voice is one's own or the voice of another. Now consider what happens if there is a problem with dopamine neuromodulation so that a false prediction error signal[3] is generated when the patient is engaging in inner speech. The speech which should generate no prediction error (matching prediction) falsely generates a large prediction error, indicating non-match, which is taken to indicate that the voice is the speech of another.

This way of explaining positive symptoms of schizophrenia is still controversial (Gallagher 2004). But the hypothesis is nevertheless interesting for our purposes because of what it illustrates about the potential relation between personal-level phenomena (the experienced life of a person suffering from schizophrenia) and subpersonal mechanisms. If the very mechanisms that are involved in weighing evidence and drawing conclusions in a roughly Bayesian-rational way are impaired, then the phenomenon itself becomes an interesting mix of the personal and subpersonal. The positive symptoms of schizophrenia are part of the experienced conscious life of the patient, and thereby belong to the personal level. But the kinds of rational connections that are the other paradigmatic feature of the personal level may have broken down very systematically. (Two-factor accounts of delusions are designed to do justice to that fact (Davies et al. 2001).) So here we have a subpersonal explanation of why the personal-level phenomenon should fail to exhibit all the signs of being at the personal level.

If a patient's experience of hearing voices can be explained by a pathology in the subpersonal mechanisms that constitute the normal capacity for responding to evidence in rational ways, then we again have a subpersonal factor that is more than just an external cause of the personal-level phenomenon. It is part of the constitutive basis of that phenomenon. But because it is operating abnormally, the nature of the personal-level phenomenon itself changes.

If all of that is right, it suggests that a very particular mindset may be called for in the clinical encounter. The appropriate mindset would recognize that what we have to deal with is not just a case of the patient being pushed around and compelled by some external cause. Nor would it be right to treat the patient as a mere mechanism. Rather, to engage with the problem is to engage with the person. But the dysconnection hypothesis suggests that the person himself is different. The clinician will have to be alive to the fact that a very central feature of interactions between persons—the way we evaluate and weigh evidence—may be impaired. The patient's personhood or capacity for agency may be altered in respects that normally underpin fluid interpersonal interactions. Of course, that will be no kind of news to the experienced clinician. What is worth remarking, though, is that appealing to subpersonal properties to explain the personal-level pathology in no way detracts from the need to treat the patient as a person, not a mechanism: a person whose psychological processes depart in a central way from the paradigm of the personal level, albeit in constrained and predictable ways.

---

[3] Or, on some views, a false estimate of the precision or confidence to be attached to the prediction error signal, and hence how strongly it should be weighted in subsequent processing.

CONCLUSION

Although there is not scope here to mount a full-scale rebuttal of the claim that there is an unbridgeable personal–subpersonal divide, the discussion shows that there are respectable philosophical positions according to which neural data can help explain personal-level phenomena. The cognitive neuroscience of reward-guided decision-making offers a well-worked-out example where there is sufficiently little variable realization that neurally based generalizations are tractable, and where there are indeed robust explanatory connections between the personal and the subpersonal. To illustrate the point we saw how subpersonal neural properties can explain particular phenomena: interindividual variability in weighing the value of new evidence about rewards, motivation in drug addiction, and delusions in schizophrenia. None of this requires us to treat people as mechanisms that are being pushed around by their brains. The framework strongly suggests instead that the neural properties appealed to in these explanations are part of what makes it the case that people are voluntary decision-makers, guided by their goals and sensitive to feedback. If so, this philosophical approach to issues in the metaphysics of mind is in sympathy with a clinical approach that treats patients as people rather than mere mechanisms.

ACKNOWLEDGMENTS

The author would like to thank Martin Davies and Neil Levy for discussion of the issues canvassed in the chapter; and Tim Bayne and Richard Gipps for comments on an earlier draft. The support of the John Fell OUP Research Fund, the Oxford Martin School, and the Wellcome Trust (grant 086041 to the Oxford Centre for Neuroethics) is gratefully acknowledged.

REFERENCES

Bayer, H. M., and Glimcher, P. W. (2005). Midbrain dopamine neurons encode a quantitative reward prediction error signal. *Neuron, 47*(1), 129–41.

Behrens, T. E. J., Woolrich, M. W., Walton, M. E., and Rushworth, M. F. S. (2007). Learning the value of information in an uncertain world. *Nature Neuroscience, 10*(9), 1214–21.

Berridge, K. C. and Robinson, T. E. (1998). What is the role of dopamine in reward: hedonic impact, reward learning, or incentive salience? *Brain Research Review, 28*(3), 309–69.

Bloom, P. (2004). *Descartes' Baby: How the Science of Child Development Explains What Makes Us Human.* New York, NY: Basic Books.

Buch, E. R., Mars, R. B., Boorman, E. D., and Rushworth, M. F. S. (2010). A network centered on ventral premotor cortex exerts both facilitatory and inhibitory control over primary motor cortex during action reprogramming. *Journal of Neuroscience, 30*(4), 1395–401.

Corrado, G. S., Sugrue, L. P., Brown, J. R., and Newsome, W. T. (2009). The trouble with choice: studying decision variables in the brain. In P. W. Glimcher, C. F. Camerer, E. Fehr, and R. A. Poldrack (Eds), *Neuroeconomics: Decision Making and the Brain,* pp. 463–80. Amsterdam: Elsevier.

D'Ardenne, K., McClure, S. M., Nystrom, L. E., and Cohen, J. D. (2008). BOLD responses reflecting dopaminergic signals in the human ventral tegmental area. *Science, 319*(5867), 1264–7.

Davidson, D. (1970). Mental events. In L. Foster and J. W. Swanson (Eds), *Experience and Theory*, pp. 79–101. Amherst, MA: University of Massachusetts Press.

Davies, M. (2000). Interaction without reduction: The relationship between personal and sub-personal levels of description. *Mind & Society, 2*(1), 87–105.

Davies, M. (2005). Cognitive science. In F. Jackson and M. Smith (Eds), *The Oxford Handbook of Contemporary Philosophy*, pp. 358–94. Oxford: Oxford University Press.

Davies, M., Breen, N., Coltheart, M., and Langdon, R. (2001). Monothematic delusions: Towards a two-factor account. *Philosophy, Psychiatry, & Psychology, 8*(2), 133–58.

Dennett, D. C. (1969). *Content and Consciousness*. London: Routledge.

Fletcher, P. C., and Frith, C. D. (2009). Perceiving is believing: A Bayesian approach to explaining the positive symptoms of schizophrenia. *Nature Reviews Neuroscience, 10*(1), 48–58.

Foddy, B., and Savulescu, J. (2010). A liberal account of addiction. *Philosophy, Psychiatry, & Psychology, 17*(1), 1–22.

Gallagher, S. (2004). Neurocognitive models of schizophrenia: A neurophenomenological critique. *Psychopathology, 37*(1), 8–19.

Godfrey-Smith, P. (2006). The strategy of model-based science. *Biology and Philosophy, 21*, 725–40.

Haruno, M. and Kawato, M. (2006). Different neural correlates of reward expectation and reward expectation error in the putamen and caudate nucleus during stimulus-action-reward association learning. *Journal of Neurophysiology, 95*(2), 948–59.

Haynes, J. D., Sakai, K., Rees, G., Gilbert, S., Frith, C., and Passingham, R. E. (2007). Reading hidden intentions in the human brain. *Current Biology, 17*(4), 323–8.

Holton, R. (2009). *Willing, Wanting, Waiting*. Oxford: Oxford University Press.

Hornsby, J. (1997). *Simple Mindedness: A Defence of Naïve Naturalism in the Philosophy of Mind*. Cambridge, MA: Harvard University Press.

Hornsby, J. (2000). Personal and sub-personal: A defence of Dennett's early distinction. *Philosophical Explorations, 3*, 6–24.

Hyman, S. E. (2005). Addiction: A disease of learning and memory. *American Journal of Psychiatry, 162*, 1414–22.

Johnson, S. W. and North, R. A. (1992). Opioids excite dopamine neurons by hyperpolarization of local interneurons. *Journal of Neuroscience, 12*(2), 483–8.

Kamitani, Y. and Tong, F. (2005). Decoding the visual and subjective contents of the human brain. *Nature Neuroscience, 8*(5), 679–85.

Koob, G. F., and Bloom, F. E. (1988). Cellular and molecular mechanisms of drug dependence. *Science, 242*, 715–23.

Krugel, L. K., Biele, G., Mohr, P. N. C., Li, S. C., and Heekeren, H. R. (2009). Genetic variation in dopaminergic neuromodulation influences the ability to rapidly and flexibly adapt decisions. *Proceedings of the National Academy of Sciences of the United States of America, 106*(42), 17951–6.

Mars, R. B., Shea, N. J., Kolling, N., and Rushworth, M. F. S. (2010). Model-based analyses: Promises, pitfalls, and example applications to the study of cognitive control. *Quarterly Journal of Experimental Psychology, 65*(2), 252–67.

McClure, S. M., Berns, G. S., and Montague, P. R. (2003). Temporal prediction errors in a passive learning task activate human striatum. *Neuron, 38*(2), 339–46.

McDowell, J. (1985). Functionalism and anomalous monism. In E. LePore and B. P. McLaughlin (Eds), *Actions and Events: Perspectives on the Philosophy of Donald Davidson*, pp. 387–98. Oxford: Blackwell.

Mukamel, R., Gelbard, H., Arieli, A., Hasson, U., Fried, I., and Malach, R. (2005). Coupling between neuronal firing, field potentials, and FMRI in human auditory cortex. *Science*, *309*(5736), 951–4.

O'Doherty, J. P., Dayan, P., Friston, K., Critchley, H., and Dolan, R. J. (2003). Temporal difference models and reward-related learning in the human brain. *Neuron*, *38*(2), 329–37.

Pearce, S. and Pickard, H. (2010). Finding the will to recover: philosophical perspectives on agency and the sick role. *Journal of Medical Ethics*, *36*(12), 831–3.

Pessiglione, M., Petrovic, P., Daunizeau, J., Palminteri, S., Dolan, R. J., and Frith, C. D. (2008). Subliminal instrumental conditioning demonstrated in the human brain. *Neuron*, *59*(4), 561–7.

Rees, G., Friston, K., and Koch, C. (2000). A direct quantitative relationship between the functional properties of human and macaque V5. *Nature Neuroscience*, *3*(7), 716–23.

Rey, G. (2001). Physicalism and psychology: Towards a substantive philosophy of mind. In C. Gillet and B. Loewer (Eds), *Physicalism and Its Discontents*, pp. 99–128. Cambridge: Cambridge University Press.

Schultz, W. (1998). Predictive reward signal of dopamine neurons. *Journal of Neurophysiology*, *8*(1), 1–27.

Schultz, W., Dayan, P., and Montague, P. R. (1997). A neural substrate of prediction and reward. *Science*, *275*(5306), 1593–9.

Shea, N. (2003). Does externalism entail the anomalism of the mental? *The Philosophical Quarterly*, *53*(211), 201–13.

Stephan, K. E., Friston, K. J., and Frith, C. D. (2009). Dysconnection in schizophrenia: from abnormal synaptic plasticity to failures of self-monitoring. *Schizophrenia Bulletin*, *35*(3), 509–27.

Sutton, R. S. and Barto, A. G. (1998). *Reinforcement Learning: An Introduction*. Cambridge, MA: MIT Press.

White, J. G., Southgate, E., Thomson, J. N., and Brenner, S. (1986). The structure of the nervous system of the nematode Caenorhabditis elegans. *Philosophical Transactions of the Royal Society of London. B, Biological Sciences*, *314*(1165), 1–340.

Wyvell, C. L. and Berridge, K. C. (2000). Intra-accumbens amphetamine increases the conditioned incentive salience of sucrose reward: enhancement of reward "wanting" without enhanced "liking" or response reinforcement. *Journal of Neuroscience*, *20*(21), 8122–30.

Yang, T. and Shadlen, M. N. (2007). Probabilistic reasoning by neurons. *Nature*, *447*(7148), 1075–80.

CHAPTER 63

....

PSYCHOPATHOLOGY AND THE ENACTIVE MIND

....

GIOVANNA COLOMBETTI

THE ENACTIVE APPROACH

....

The term "enaction" was originally introduced in philosophy of mind and cognitive science by Varela et al.'s *The Embodied Mind* to characterize a conception of mind and cognition profoundly different from the computational-representational one of mainstream cognitivism:

> We propose ... the term *enactive* to emphasize the growing conviction that cognition is not the representation of a pregiven world by a pregiven mind but is rather the enactment of a world and a mind on the basis of a history of the variety of actions that a being in the world performs. (Varela et al. 1991, p. 9)

The terms "history," "actions," "world," and "perform" underscore main features of the enactive mind, namely its *dynamical*, *embodied*, and *situated* character. Cognition is not "inside" the brain, representing information about the world, computing it according to internal rules, and eventually telling the body how to act; cognition is rather enacted or brought forth, over time, by the whole organism (not just its brain) situated in the world.

This view was not new, and Varela and colleagues indeed explicitly presented their work as a continuation of Merleau-Ponty's *The Structure of Behavior* (1942/1963) and *Phenomenology of Perception* (1945/1962). Merleau-Ponty had already defended the thesis of the thoroughly embodied and situated nature of the mind on the basis of phenomenological and empirical considerations, and had himself been influenced by Husserl and Gestalt psychologists (just to mention his most proximate sources). Varela et al. importantly brought these ideas into Anglo-American cognitive science, joining the efforts of authors such as Dreyfus (1972), who had already drawn on continental philosophy to criticize the possibility of symbolic artificial intelligence.

Since the publication of *The Embodied Mind*, the embodied, situated, and active character of cognition has been emphasized in particular by defenders of the view that perception and action are intimately tied together, indeed that they are mutually constitutive rather than mediated by an internal representational system (Hurley 1998; Noë 2004; O'Regan and Noë 2001). At the same time, supporters of the dynamical systems approach in cognitive science (Kelso 1995; Port and van Gelder 1995; Thelen and Smith 1994; Thelen et al. 2001) and situated robotics (Brooks 1991; Matarić 2002) have also underscored the temporal, embodied, and highly context-dependent character of various cognitive and motor abilities, fuelling the philosophical debate on the mind–body relationship and, more specifically, on the representational nature of the mind (cf. Clark 1997; Wheeler 2005).

It would be restrictive, however, to reduce the enactive approach to the view that cognition, and perception in particular, is active, embodied, and situated. Enactivism is a complex approach to the conceptualization and study of the mind that draws also on, for example, large-scale accounts of brain activity, philosophical and biological theories on the nature of living systems, the relationship of life to mind, and the nature of consciousness. All these threads have been woven together by Thompson (2007) in what can be considered the ultimate synthesis of the enactive approach, and more are already being spun (see the recent collection by Stewart et al. 2010).

For present purposes, I will pull out only those threads that are relevant to the main goal of this chapter, which is to illustrate points of convergence between enactivism and psychopathology, and to suggest possible ways to integrate them more explicitly. The threads I have chosen are the following:

1. Enactivism's insistence on the importance of developing rigorous first-person methods for the study of consciousness, and for the "neurophenomenological" integration of first- and third-person data, namely data about lived experience and data about physiological activity.
2. Enactivism's emphasis on the affective nature of cognition.
3. Enactivism's emphasis on the direct bodily and affective nature of intersubjectivity.

Let us now take a closer look at each of these points.

Neurophenomenology

Varela et al. (1991) already argued that cognitive science, in order to be a science of the mind, ought to pay serious attention to the study of consciousness. In particular, they emphasized the need to have a well-developed *first-person method* for such a study, which led them to discuss the very old and established Buddhist discipline of "mindfulness meditation." The latter consists in the cultivation of self-awareness by way of practices aimed at making one increasingly "present" to one's own mind, namely increasingly awake to the contents of one's own consciousness and to the "habits" of one's own mind.

This emphasis on the need for a systematic and disciplined observation of lived experience subsequently led Varela (1996) to elaborate his specific proposal for a *neurophenomenological* method that could integrate data about experience (first-person data) and data about brain activity (third-person data). According to Varela, the former are necessary to make sense of the latter; vice versa, the latter should be used to refine the former. From a philosophical standpoint, neurophenomenology can be seen as a method for "naturalizing phenomenology," that is, for making experience amenable to natural scientific enquiry.

Importantly neurophenomenology does not call for the *reduction* of the experiential level to the physiological one; it does not attempt, for example, to *translate* first-person data into third-person ones (for this approach, see Roy et al. 1999). Quite the opposite, it calls for the inclusion of first-person data *as such* in the natural-scientific enterprise of understanding how the organism enacts consciousness.

A few experiments have now been conducted under the neurophenomenological agenda.[1] In a much-cited study, Lutz et al. (2002) trained subjects to report precisely on their experience of coming to see a three-dimensional image from a "magic eye picture" (a two-dimensional random dot pattern with binocular disparities). This training allowed both subjects and experimenters to identify categories of experience (feeling "ready" to see the image, feeling completely "unready," and feeling in a middle state of "fragmented readiness") that were subsequently used to make sense of patterns of brain activity recorded while subjects looked at the dot patterns. Lutz et al. (2002) indeed were able to identify distinctive patterns of electroencephalographic (EEG) activity corresponding to the experiential states of readiness, unreadiness, and fragmented readiness respectively.

The fact that subjects were *trained* to observe and report on their experience is particularly significant, and characterizes this study as neuro-*phenomenological*. Importantly, training occurred via a mixture of "first-person" and "second-person" methods, namely via self-observation but also in interaction with an interviewer, whose role was to guide subjects to pay attention to different aspects of their experience. Furthermore, the interviewer asked "open questions" that did not constrain the range of answers the subjects could give.

It may be objected that there is nothing special or different about neurophenomenology compared to the more familiar cognitive-neuroscientific approach. After all, neurophenomenologists also appear to be looking for the neural correlates of consciousness; moreover, neurophenomenology is entirely brain-oriented and as such appears to be at odds with Varela's own embodied-enactive predicaments. There are, however, at least two important differences between neurophenomenology and cognitive neuroscience. First, neurophenomenology believes that it is not only possible but necessary to develop first-person methods to obtain reliable first-person data. Cognitive neuroscience on its part tries to minimize reliance on self-reports, which it generally sees as biased and untrustworthy, and takes behavior to be a more objective measure of cognitive activity. Whereas neurophenomenologists collect first-person data at the *beginning* of a study and use them as an "organizing analytical principle" (Gallagher 2003, p. 86), cognitive neuroscientists collect self-reports, if at all, only at the *end* of a study and mainly for control purposes. Second, neurophenomenology does not regard brain activity as *sufficient* for experience; it regards it as just *one part* of the broader organismic processes that underpin, or better enact, consciousness.[2]

Admittedly only a few neurophenomenological studies have been conducted so far, and the extent to which it is possible to map the structure and dynamics of lived experience onto the one of neural and perhaps even non-neural bodily activity remains an open question. For present purposes however, what matters is the *shift of attitude* toward lived experience that is entailed by neurophenomenology compared to mainstream cognitive neuroscience,

---

[1] For a comprehensive discussion of the neurophenomenological approach, including a summary of relevant experimental work, see Thompson et al. (2005).

[2] See Colombetti (in press) for a less brain-centered "neuro-physio-phenomenology" that aims at integrating data about experience with data about brain and non-neural bodily processes.

in particular the idea that the neuroscientific study of consciousness must include asking subjects what they feel without constraining their answers, and using their answers to shed light on the structure of specific experiences as well as the physiological activity supposedly enacting them.

Sense-making and the affective nature of cognition

In the enactive approach, cognition and affectivity are not regarded as two distinct psychological faculties. Rather, cognition *is* inherently affective. To see how, we need to look briefly at the notion of *sense-making* as it appears in Varela's later writings and subsequent elaborations of the enactive approach. This in turn requires a detour into the enactive conception of life and of its relationship to cognition. The whole story is quite complex and difficult to recount without introducing technicalities, but for present purposes it will suffice just to highlight some of its main points (for the details, see Thompson 2007, especially chapters 3, 5, and 6).

At the very roots of the enactive approach is the claim that all living systems are cognitive systems (Maturana and Varela 1980). Specifically, they are cognitive in virtue of their *autonomous* and *adaptive* nature. An autonomous system is defined as one whose constituent processes "(i) recursively depend on each other for their generation and their realization as a network, (ii) constitute the system as a unity in whatever domain they exist, and (iii) determine a domain of possible interactions with the environment" (Thompson 2007, p. 44). The paradigmatic autonomous system is the living cell. Multicellular metazoan systems, nervous systems, insect colonies, etc., however, are also autonomous, even if they do not have a material boundary; they are all importantly "operationally closed" systems, constituted by processes whose results remain within the system itself. Adaptivity on its part refers to the capacity of living systems to monitor and regulate themselves with respect to their conditions of viability, and to improve their situation when needed (Di Paolo 2005).

According to the enactive approach, the autonomous and adaptive nature of living systems makes them into *sense-making* systems, that is, systems that have a *perspective* or *point of view* from which they establish their own world of meaning—their *Umwelt*, to use Von Uexküll's (1934/2010) term.[3] As Weber and Varela (2002, pp. 117–118) succinctly put it: "[b]y defining itself and thereby creating the domains of self and world, the organism creates a perspective which changes the world from a neutral place to an *Umwelt* that always means something in relation to the organism." The *Umwelt* is thus not a world "outside" the living system in which the latter grows and moves, and into which it occasionally bumps; rather the living system enacts or performs its *Umwelt*, very much like one "lays down a path in walking" (to use Varela's analogy). Importantly, according to the enactive approach, the process of establishing a world of significance in this way is the basic "mark of the cognitive."

This characterization of cognition entails affectivity, in the broad sense that the living organism is never indifferent to its existence and environment. As Weber and Varela (2002) remark in several passages, the perspective or point of view of the sense-making living

---

[3] "*Umwelt*" literally means "world around" and is usually translated as "environment." The German term, however, is used here to refer specifically to the environment from the perspective of the living system.

system is *concerned*; the living system "is interested" and "cares" about its own continuation, so to speak.[4] This concern is the correlate of another important property of living systems, namely their inherent *purposefulness*: the constituent processes of a living system conspire to maintain its identity against a variety of perturbations; in other words the living system strives, as a function of its organization, to maintain itself and its conditions of viability. Finally, the very notion of an *Umwelt* is also affective in a broad sense: the *Umwelt*, as enacted by the organism, represents what is *relevant* or *salient* for the organism, what *matters* to it.[5]

From an enactive perspective then, it is not really possible to distinguish cognition from affectivity without providing a somewhat distorted notion of cognition. The separation of cognition and affectivity is an abstraction, the imposition of a distinction onto what is fundamentally a simultaneously cognitive-affective phenomenon.

A critical aspect of this view is that it is the *whole* organism, not just the brain, that makes sense of the world. This approach differs considerably from the one of mainstream affective science, according to which the faculty responsible for evaluating the world in relation to the subject's needs and concerns, the "appraisal," is typically characterized as a "non-bodily" cognitive process. The widespread assumption is that the appraisal is a cognitive process realized by some part of the brain, which evaluates various aspects of a situation and brings about a series of responses in body, behavior, feeling, etc.[6] Even when the cognitive appraisal is viewed as a component of emotion (e.g., Scherer 2009), it is still conceptualized as an intellectual or "brainy" event distinct from the rest of the organism. From an enactive perspective, on the other hand, the process of evaluating the world in relation to one's needs and concerns is enacted by the whole organism in virtue of its organization (for arguments, see Colombetti 2007, 2010; Colombetti and Thompson 2008).

Participatory sense-making

Another recent thread developed within the enactive approach regards the social dimension of cognition. In this context, De Jaegher and Di Paolo (2007) have proposed the notion of *participatory sense-making*, which extends the enactive notion of sense-making introduced earlier to the domain of "being together." They particularly emphasize that accounts of social cognition should not overlook the concrete face-to-face (or rather, we should say, body-to-body) interactions that pervade our daily living together, namely what Trevarthen (1979) originally dubbed "primary intersubjectivity," i.e., a set of embodied and affective skills involved in non-conceptual and pragmatic understanding of others. These interactions, they point out, typically enact or bring forth a specific form of *shared meaning* that cannot be reduced to each participant's own sense-making. The interaction, we can say, imposes a kind of second-order constraint over the participants, and develops a "life of its own" characterized by its own specific style of unfolding; in other words, the interaction develops its own form of autonomy. De Jaegher and Di Paolo (2007) particularly emphasize the character

---

[4] Weber and Varela (2002) draw largely on Jonas (1966/2001). See Thompson (2007) for a more detailed account of the relationship between enactivism and Jonas's conception of life.

[5] For a more detailed discussion of the affective nature of sense-making, see Colombetti (in press).

[6] Details vary from one theory of appraisal to the other (see Scherer et al. 2001 for an overview of the field).

of "coordination" of concrete social encounters, namely the sustained, non-accidental coupling between participants. The notion of coupling at play here is borrowed from dynamical systems theory; in simple terms, it refers to a process of continuous reciprocal influences between systems (organisms included), such that they can be considered one single system. The classic example is the one of two pendulums hanging from the same wall that end up oscillating at the same frequency (in virtue of the vibrations that each pendulum transmits to the wall), but the phenomenon is widespread in physical and biological systems.

We know that human intersubjectivity in particular is characterized by phenomena of spontaneous mimicking, mirroring, and affect attunement. The perception of facial expressions of emotions induces in the perceiver distinct facial reactions that mimic at least parts of the perceived expression (e.g., Dimberg et al. 2000). Neural mirror systems exist for both perception and emotion expression. The perception of another's specific goal-oriented action activates one's own neural motor system for that action; the perception of another's expression of disgust activates neural areas that are also active when one experiences disgust oneself (see Rizzolatti and Sinigaglia 2008 for an overview of the relevant findings). Furthermore, caregivers "attune themselves" to children by reproducing cross-modally the dynamic features of their affective states, such as intensity, timing, and shape (Stern 1985).

The enactive approach emphasizes that these modes of bodily and affective coupling are pervasive and continuous with "higher-order" phenomena of social cognition, such as cognitive empathy and enculturation (both discussed in Thompson 2007, chapter 13; see also Gallagher 2001). Even if during one's lifetime one will develop different modes of interacting with others, bodily and affective coupling is not transcended as the organism grows older. Other organisms are part of the environment in which we are situated, and interactions with them are a constitutive part of the process of enacting a world of significance.

Also, unlike mainstream positions in the so-called theory of mind debate, the enactive approach emphasizes the immediate and direct "understanding of the other" that characterizes concrete encounters. The idea is that in order to understand the other's actions or expressions, we need neither to recur to a "theory" (as in the so-called "theory theory"), nor to "simulate" the other's state in ourselves (as posited by the "simulation theory"). We do not infer the other's intentions and emotions via some intermediate mental operation, but we "directly" see the other's mind in her bodily attitude. Again, this point is borrowed from phenomenology, specifically from accounts of intersubjectivity and empathy developed by Stein, Scheler, and others (for references and discussion, see, e.g., Zahavi 2007).

CONNECTIONS WITH PSYCHOPATHOLOGY

Enactivist ideas so far have not been applied to develop worked-out theories and methods in psychopathology (for some initial discussions, see Drayson 2009; Fuchs 2009). There are, however, various points of contact between enactivism and current trends in psychopathology—most notably in *phenomenological psychopathology*. The latter emphasizes that lived experience ought to be taken seriously, without reducing it to neural activity and/or behavior. Phenomenological accounts of mental illness also underscore its bodily and situated character, as well as the profound transformations in the sense of reality and "being there" that it involves. The cognition-affect dichotomy has also begun to falter under these more existential accounts of mental disorders that emphasize changes in "feelings of being," rather than (or at least in addition to) "false beliefs." The enactive approach sits well also with pluralistic approaches to treatment which employ bodily practices to modify the organism's dynamics and its modes of relating to the world, including other people. I will now look at these points of contact in more detail and, when appropriate, develop them further into suggestions on how to elaborate a more explicitly "enactive psychopathology."

Toward a "neurophenomenological psychopathology"

We have seen that phenomenology, understood as the systematic analysis of the structures of experience, is central to the enactive approach; it is necessary for the scientific study of the mind, and in particular for progressing our understanding of how consciousness and physical processes are related. Not only is lived experience a fundamental aspect of mentality, but in order to study it, it is necessary to describe and analyze it as accurately as possible, and to develop appropriate tools and methods for this purpose.

Phenomenology as a descriptive and analytical tool has also been advocated in psychopathology since Jaspers (1913/1997). Jaspers advocated phenomenology as a method for providing concrete descriptions of patients' mental states, for analyzing their interrelations, and for identifying, differentiating and labeling them appropriately. He particularly valued patients' self-observation as a primary source of data, and open-mindedness on the part of the psychopathologist. The latter should neither be too impressed by specific claims on the part of the patient, nor restricted by theoretical presuppositions. Individual cases should be carefully scrutinized, with the aim of recognizing recurrent similar patterns within and across patients.[7]

Since Jaspers, phenomenology has made its way into psychopathology in a variety of ways, with the works of Binswanger, Minkowski, Straus, Buytendijk, and others (see Spiegelberg 1972 for a historical overview). Recent arguments for a role of the phenomenological method in psychopathology, and specific examples of the application of phenomenological categories to the understanding of mental disorders, can be found for instance in Fuchs (2005), Gallagher (2005), Mullen (2007), Parnas and Zahavi (2002), Ratcliffe (2008), Sass (1992), Sass et al. (2011), and Stanghellini (2004) (the list is not exhaustive). These works all resist and oppose the widespread reductionist attitude of much current psychiatry, which is interested in patients' lived experience primarily for the purpose of merely "spotting" symptoms already provided by the diagnostic manuals; once key symptoms are identified, experience is quickly left aside to examine "more objective" behavioral and neural data, and to identify appropriate pharmacological treatments.

This method is particularly limiting given that the diagnostic manuals provide very succinct snapshots of experience, intentionally leaving aside alleged irrelevant and distracting details. The result is a rather mechanical process in which there is little room for the

---

[7] Jaspers' phenomenological approach departs in various respects from Husserl's, in particular from the latter's quest for "essences," and more could be said about the relation between these two approaches. For the purposes of this chapter, however, I simply intend to point out the importance that both enactivists and some philosophers and psychiatrists grant to the development of methods for the exploration of consciousness.

identification of features of experience that have not been previously recognized as symptomatic. As Mullen (2007, p.114) complains, "[w]e now have generations of mental health professionals, many of whom have learned all the right questions. They may in the process, however, have lost the capacity to listen or to see what may challenge or otherwise discomfort the established diagnostic process."

By contrast, phenomenological psychopathology takes lived experience to be an essential aspect of mental illness that deserves full attention and that ought to be examined in detail. It uses existing phenomenological concepts and analyses (e.g., of self-awareness, temporal experience, background attunements), or develops new ones, in order to provide detailed and precise accounts of the experience of a variety of mental disorders. The results often challenge received views. Ratcliffe (2008), for example, uses his category of *existential feeling* to criticize accounts of delusions that only emphasize distortions of "beliefs." According to Ratcliffe, delusions involve fundamental changes in "how one finds oneself in the world" in terms of existential background orientations—as when we say that one feels "at home in the world," or alone, estranged, connected, in tune, etc. These ways of feeling are not directed at specific objects or events, but are backdrop orientations against which other experiences take place, and which also determine the kind of experiences one has or is likely to have. Like Heidegger's (1927/1962) moods, Ratcliffe's existential feelings are not merely contingent colorations of consciousness, but fundamental ways of being attuned to the world. They cannot be reduced to propositional attitudes, i.e., mental states such as beliefs that take propositions as objects ("I believe that this body is not mine," "I believe that someone is putting thoughts in my head"). Hence disorders such as Capgras' delusion, for example, where subjects report believing that other people (usually relevant others such as partners, relatives or close friends) are in fact impostors pretending to be them, cannot be reduced to mere false beliefs but encompass a deeper change in existential feeling, namely in how reality as a whole and oneself in it are experienced.

Valuing lived experience in psychopathology is not just an exercise in phenomenological analysis per se, but has relevant diagnostic and therapeutic implications. Classifications of mental disorders are notoriously fuzzy and fluid. More dramatically, they are, as Hacking (e.g., 1999, p.103) puts it, *interactive kinds*, they "can influence what is classified" and can be modified or replaced because they interact with what is classified. Interactive kinds induce "classificatory looping effects": the thing classified changes its behavior as a consequence of being so classified, which in turn requires a change in the original classification, and so on. These looping effects, as Hacking (1999) illustrates, are revealed in the history of the classification of psychopathologies such as mental retardation, childhood autism, and schizophrenia, as well as multiple personality disorder (Hacking 1995), and the now extinguished *fugue* (Hacking 1998). This history shows that psychopathologies are "moving targets"— their descriptions and classifications vary over time, and with them the behavior and experience of the people classified, which in turn induces new descriptions and classifications, etc. Hence both the way a mental disorder manifests itself in behavior and experience, and the diagnostic categories used to identify it, are subject to fluctuations and variations; looking up a pre-given fixed list of symptoms may thus become inadequate, or even a hindrance, to a comprehensive understanding of a specific condition.

The phenomenological approach in psychopathology is better suited than mainstream psychiatry to track these looping effects, because it aims to engage repeatedly with the patient to identify salient features of his life and experience, and to do so without imposing theoretical pre-conceptions and schemata. Mullen (2007, pp. 117–118) lists five stages that, in his view, ought to characterize a thoroughly phenomenological method in psychopathology. The first consists in facilitating spontaneous accounts of experience and behavior, without being guided by assumptions about what counts as pathological, reasonable, symptomatic, plausible, etc. A structured investigation may also be used that focuses on experiential categories such as experience of time, distance, direction, reality, causation, sense of control and agency, etc. This process should be repeated in the course of therapy, not just confined to preliminary stages. The second stage consists in "augmenting" self-accounts with artistic, literary, and philosophical works that also provide descriptions and analyses of experience with which the patient resonates. Third, the therapist should be empathetic and try to grasp the qualities of the patient's lived experience, as well as help him or her find words for it. This use of empathy should remain modest, and avoid imposition of pre-established theoretical frameworks and evaluations. In the fourth stage a summative description of the patient's experience and behavior is derived. Some ordering and systematization is applied at this point. In the final stage phenomenological categories are brought in to produce a provisional classification which may be modified after subsequent observation of experience and behavior.

This approach has a lot in common with neurophenomenology. Both methods reject a merely behavioristic and/or neurophysiological stance; they take lived experience seriously and do not attempt to reduce it to something else. Both methods strive to minimize theoretical preconceptions about the nature of experience; they encourage spontaneous reports, as well as an empathetic relationship between therapist and patient (or experimenter/interviewer and subject) to provide rich descriptions of lived experience and to reveal structures and invariants that might otherwise remain unnoticed, or that are not part of standard descriptions of symptoms. Also, importantly, both approaches share a conception of experience that is far from fixed or static, but rather moving, fluctuating and developing, subject to endogenous (neural, biological) as well as contextual (immediate environment, other people, near past or future events) and broader social-symbolic influences. In neurophenomenology, as we have seen, this conception of experience as dynamical and open implies that first-person data can, and should, be changed and stabilized with first- and second-person methods, as well as refined by third-person data. In phenomenological psychopathology, the same conception implies that a subject's experience needs to be repeatedly engaged with and explored in the therapeutic context, rather than limiting this investigation to the initial stages of the diagnosis. Neither approach assumes that no invariant whatsoever can be identified in experience; rather, both imply that part of the process of understanding lived experience involves exploring its flexibility and openness, and the way it responds to intervention.

Now, phenomenological psychopathology and neurophenomenology so far have been separate fields of inquiry, but it is possible to envisage a "neurophenomenological psychopathology" that extends the neurophenomenological method to the study of mental disorders. Such an approach would provide a bridge between biological and phenomenological strands within psychiatry, often considered incommensurable paradigms. Within such an integrated approach, lived experience would be explored systematically to identify relevant categories; the latter would then be used to organize and interpret data about neurophysiological activity; these data in turn could be used to identify finer-grained dimensions of experience.[8]

Gallagher's (2005) account of schizophrenia can be seen as a step in this direction. He draws on Husserl's analysis of time-consciousness to provide a phenomenological account of experiences of thought insertion and loss of sense of agency typical of the condition. In particular, he argues that schizophrenia may involve a disruption in the protentional dimension of time-consciousness, namely in the orientation toward what-is-to-come-next that, according to Husserl, characterizes all experiences of the present moment. According to Gallagher, ordinarily our sense of agency—the pre-reflective sense that I am the one generating my thoughts and actions—is always protentionally oriented toward what is to happen next. If that weren't the case, I would be constantly surprised by my thoughts and actions, as if they had just appeared, unexpectedly, in my experience and behavior; I would still have a sense of them as *my* thoughts and actions (sense of ownership would be retained), as in the case of ordinary unbidden memories, but I would not experience them as part of my agency. Gallagher proposes that this is just what happens in schizophrenia: the "protentional mechanism" is disrupted, and with it the sense that one is the intentional future-oriented source of one's thoughts and actions. The latter thus appear "inserted" by an outside source or force.

What makes Gallagher's discussion a step toward a neurophenomenological psychopathology is that he also compares his account with evidence from neuroscience, in particular with a study by Frith and Done (1988) showing that for 80% of schizophrenic subjects with positive symptoms, the EEG response to tones generated by the subjects themselves by pressing a button was similar in amplitude to the response generated to randomly occurring tones. Previous evidence had shown that in non-schizophrenic subjects, random tones generate a relatively larger response than self-generated ones. Gallagher thus suggests that Frith and Done's result confirms the view that schizophrenics fail to experience their own actions as self-generated, and rather experience them as surprising, as if they were generated from an outside source. These considerations could be used to design a neurophenomenological study that recorded neural activity as subjects reported their experiences "online," to see whether specific experiences of loss of sense of agency are indeed correlated with distinctive patterns of neural activity.

Another relevant approach here is Petitmengin et al.'s (2006) work on epilepsy. They employed a phenomenological method to explore in detail the nature of preictical symptoms (the experiences that usually precede an epileptic seizure). Specifically, they were able to distinguish between the experiences occurring during the "aura" (also known as simple

---

[8] One may note here that not *all* aspects of lived experience can be usefully linked to neurophysiological activity, and vice versa; there may be features of the structure of experience that are not amenable to being illuminated by third-person data. Take for example the notion of the "depth" of affective experience discussed by Ratcliffe (2010), which refers to the degree of specificity of the intentional object of an experience. On this account, the sadness for, say, the loss of one's favorite teddy bear is shallower than the sadness for one's inability to engage less than superficially with other people, which is in turn shallower than the sadness for the status of human rights in the world. These forms of sadness differ in existential import, and I agree that finding out that they corresponded to, say, different degrees of neural synchrony, would not be particularly interesting from a phenomenological-existential point of view. From the perspective of someone who is interested in how experience and physical processes are linked, however, it *would* be interesting to find out that the degree of specificity of the intentional object of an emotion corresponded reliably to different patterns of brain activity.

partial seizure), which is sudden and relatively brief (it lasts a few seconds or minutes), and the "prodromes," which are more progressive and can last up to a day. Unlike the aura, the prodromes have not been much investigated, and are not usually recognized and discussed in the clinical context.

The methodology that Petitmengin and colleagues employed to identify these differences in experience corresponds in many respects to the one recommended by Mullen (2007). They used a log form to ask hospitalized epileptic patients to reflect every morning on their state of fatigue, stress, and emotional condition in general, as well as on particular bodily, visual, and auditory sensations. Another log form with similar questions had to be filled in by the patients after each seizure; this form also asked patients to focus on the quality of their experience immediately before the seizure, to remember what they were doing then, at which moment they had started to feel specific sensations, how long did they last, and more. Similar questions were asked in another log form that patients had to fill after a "mini-crisis," namely a preictal episode that did not lead to a full seizure. These forms importantly alternated questionnaires in which subjects had to rate their current condition on a numerical scale, with more open questions in which subjects were asked to report and describe it in their own words.

Semistructured interviews were also used. In the first stage of the interview, patients were asked to recall a specific preictal experience, and to relive it by remembering in as much detail as possible the images, sensations, sounds, etc. associated with it. In the second stage, patients were asked to "slow down" the recollection of their experience, to attend to, thematize or make explicit aspects of it that had so far remained implicit or unnoticed. In the third stage, the interviewer helped the patients put their experience into words. At the end of the process the investigators extracted the "microstructure" of each personal experience (the precise sequence of sensations, feelings, etc. that constitute it) and detected regularities across experiences.

From a clinical perspective, this phenomenological work is in itself already very valuable. Epileptic patients are often only vaguely aware of how their experience changes in the hours preceding a seizure, yet they can learn to become more sensitive to these changes. This ability is particularly important for therapeutic purposes, because once subjects are able to "catch" preictal symptoms in time, they can also learn to engage in activities that delay or even prevent the onset of a seizure.

Petitmengin and colleagues' approach however is not "only" phenomenological but, like Gallagher's account of schizophrenia, attempts to bridge data about experience with data about neural activity. They compared the results of their phenomenological analysis with those of EEG measurements of the neural concomitants of preictal and ictal episodes. It had already been shown (e.g., Le Van Quyen et al. 2003) that about five minutes before the onset of a seizure, a decrease in synchronization or "phase-scattering" characterizes brain activity around the epileptogenic focus; these brain areas also tend to become relatively isolated compared to the interconnectivity characterizing the interictal phase (the phase between seizures free from ictal and preictal symptoms). Petitmengin et al. (2007) suggest that these phase-scattering may be characteristic of prodromes, as opposed to the neural synchrony that characterizes the ictal phase (including the aura). This suggestion, as they acknowledge, still has to be verified as no study has been conducted yet on the "real-time" correlation between the microdynamics of experience and those of brain activity. Such a study would count as thoroughly neurophenomenological.

In addition, a thoroughly neurophenomenological study of epilepsy could use data about neural activity to refine first-person data. Specifically EEG data could be used as *biofeedback* to help epileptic subjects become more sensitive to changes in their experience. Biofeedback as a technique involves continuously measuring some dimension of a subject's biological activity, and showing the measurement to the subject in real time, as it is taking place. In biofeedback therapy, subjects use the real time signal to monitor and regulate their awareness. Attempts to use EEG biofeedback to treat epilepsy go back to the 1970s (see, e.g., Cott et al. 1979); other dimensions of bodily feedback have been used since then to treat various conditions, such as migraine, muscle contraction, rheumatoid arthritis, and anxiety, including cardiophobia (Birbaumer and Kimmell 1979). Recent studies have shown that it is relatively easy to train subjects to regulate their emotion experience by using "real-time fMRI [functional magnetic resonance imaging]" (deCharms 2008). Johnston et al. (2010) targeted brain areas known to activate significantly during unpleasant emotions, and showed subjects various positive, neutral, and negative pictures (that is, pictures known to elicit pleasant, indifferent, and unpleasant emotion experiences respectively). Subjects received feedback about activity in these areas by looking at the picture of a thermometer whose temperature reflected increases in fMRI amplitude signal, and were instructed to regulate activity in the target brain regions by relying on the feedback. Interestingly, subjects were able to regulate activity in the target areas already from the first run.

Some mental disorders, starting with affective disorders, could be similarly approached by a neuroimaging-enhanced phenomenological method: subjects could become increasingly sensitive to changes in their awareness (like unpleasant or aversive feelings in response to specific stimuli that may initiate, for example, obsessive rumination) via the integrated use of self-exploration, second-person methods, and biofeedback, and eventually learn to divert or even prevent unwholesome experiences. It is notable that recent approaches to depression have started to integrate cognitive behavioral therapy, which is based on the analysis of thoughts and behavior, with "mindfulness" therapy (derived from Buddhist mindfulness practices) that requires clients to cultivate a heightened awareness of their experience, not only of recurrent patterns of thoughts, but also of a variety of bodily sensations and feelings (see Segal et al. 2001). This approach could be used to explore specific features or forms of the experience of depression, inform findings about neurophysiological (neural, but also bodily) processes, and also use the latter to refine understanding of the experience of depression.

To recapitulate, in this section I have illustrated one line of convergence between the enactive approach and psychopathology, notably the primacy that both neurophenomenology (which is an offshoot of the enactive approach) and phenomenological psychopathology attribute to lived experience and to the development of rigorous methods for its investigation. In addition, I have suggested that the neurophenomenological method may be fruitfully applied to the study of mental disorders to provide a bridge between the more mainstream biological approach in psychiatry, and phenomenological psychopathology.

Mental disorders as disorders of embodiment and situatedness

In spite of neurophenomenology's focus on the brain, as we have seen the enactive approach rejects the view that the mind is in the brain. Rather, it maintains that mind and experience are enacted or brought forth by the whole organism embedded in its environment.

Analogous views can be found in psychopathology (and, again, especially in phenomeno-logical psychopathology), in accounts of mental illness that emphasize its embodied and situated character versus the tendency to see it merely or primarily as a disorder of the brain. According to Fuchs (2009), for example, mental illness needs to be understood in the broader context of the embodied and situated nature of the person, namely as a disorder that straddles brain, body, and world. As he points out, even when it is possible to identify neural impairments accompanying specific mental disorders, the neurobiological charac-terization of the disorder does not do justice to the patient's condition. Of course this claim does not entail that neurochemical imbalances do not contribute to disorders of experience and behavior, or that a neurophenomenological approach could not reveal important neu-ral characteristics of such disorders. The point is rather that the causal factors relevant to mental disorders extend well beyond the skull, and consist of a broader complex system of reciprocal influences crisscrossing brain, body and world.

Fuchs himself suggests looking at schizophrenia "as a circular process, implying neu-ropsychological and biochemical dysfunction on the one hand and psychosocial alienation on the other" (Fuchs 2009, p. 230). In his account, biological imbalances contribute to with-drawal from the world in the prodromal phases of the condition; withdrawal subsequently leads to disruption of attunement to the world and other people, which feeds back onto the subject's condition and eventually leads to psychotic crises and appearance of delusions. Similar considerations apply to depression, which according to Fuchs (2001, 2009) consists in a complete breakdown of the continuous engagement and "synchronization" (his term) that characterize our everyday interactions with one another, as well as our relation to the environment more broadly. This breakdown results from an initial failure to cope with a major change, namely from a failure to re-synchronize with an altered world. The individual then retreats from the world by reducing her interactions with it, including other people. Social desynchronization eventually leads to "biological desynchronization," manifested physiologically in disturbances of neuroendocrine processes, temperature, sleep–wake and menstrual cycles, among other things. These organismic processes augment psychosocial desynchronization: the depressed person stops being in time, does not participate in joint decision-making, and at the level of concrete encounters a tendency toward stasis disrupts coordination with others in terms of bodily attunement (turn-taking, mutual expressivity, and gestuality).

With respect to autism, Peter Hobson (e.g., 2009) similarly argues that it is misleading to reduce it to the impairment of a specific cognitive skill within a brain module, such as the capacity to "read" other people's minds. In his view autism is best understood as primarily a disorder of one's affective engagement with others in face-to-face encounters, including the capacity directly to see feeling in facial expressions, to share feelings with others, and to understand what the other's emotions are directed toward. An impaired ability to read other minds, Hobson suggests, is the *result* rather than the cause of the autistic child's interper-sonal difficulties. Disruptions in the capacity to participate in bodily social-affective "forms of life" (to use Wittgenstein's term, as Hobson does) prevent the development of the capacity to share the other's experience and to take the other's perspective.

The embodied and situated nature of mental disorders is also apparent in accounts of the lived experience of mental illness. Existing accounts in phenomenological psychopathol-ogy underscore alterations in the experience of one's body and world, including other peo-ple. In the experience of depression, for example, one's own body comes to the foreground of awareness inducing a disproportionate absorption into one's bodily feelings and pain (Fuchs 2005, 2009). In social interactions, this self-absorption prevents depressives to enter into bodily and affective (gestural, expressive) resonance with others. Schizophrenia also comes with disorders of bodily self-awareness. Schizophrenics often have difficulties locating themselves ("Am I here or there? Am I here or behind?"; see Parnas and Sass 2001, p. 106) and their bodily parts feel disconnected. As some put it, schizophrenia specifically involves a disorder of *ipseity* or pre-reflective bodily self-awareness, namely of the ordinarily tacit awareness we have of our body as ours and as the agent of our actions (e.g., Parnas and Sass 2001; Sass 2004). It is argued in particular that schizophrenia involves bodily *hyper-reflexivity*, namely an automatic "popping into awareness" of bodily sensations that would ordinarily stay in the background. At the same time, this condition comes with several disorders in the experience of other people: the boundaries between oneself and others are experienced as blurred, and the generation and control of one's own actions and thoughts are often attributed to others; at the level of concrete interaction, schizophrenics appear to lack pre-reflective and pragmatic or commonsensical understanding of other's affectivity and intentionality (hence Stanghellini and Ballerini's 2004 term "schizophrenic autism"). In addition, the physical world appears alien and strange, flat and disproportionally detailed; objects and utensils do not afford the actions they normally do, and aspects or events in the world lose their salience. As Sass (2004) puts it, schizophrenia involves an experience of "unworlding."

Now, one could remark that none of these considerations refute the claim that any mental illness *really is* a neurochemical impairment, and that disruptions in bodily activity, situatedness, and experience are either causes or effects of such an impairment, but not events *constitutive* of the illness. Indeed most cognitive neuroscientists are ready to acknowledge that body and environment affect the brain, and vice versa, while they still think of the mind as somehow primarily dependent on, and/or even located in, the brain.

From an enactive perspective, however, to see the non-neural body and the environment as merely contingently related to one's mental life, including mental illness, is to misconstrue the relationship between the mind and the physical world. The brain does not sit in the organism as a central processing system, representing information about the world that comes to it through bodily sensory channels, and causing the body to act according to specific instructions. Rather the brain is physically entangled with the rest of the organism via a very complex network of continuous reciprocal exchanges of energy and matter (see Cosmelli and Thompson 2010 for a detailed account of the various dimensions of brain-body coupling). From a biological point of view, the brain is an organ able to perform its functions only when embedded in the context of an autonomous living being; living beings at the same time emerge from and are sustained throughout by the environment to which they are coupled. Thus the idea that one can isolate the nervous system from the network of causal interrelations in which it is so deeply embedded to designate it as the seat or source of mentality is a chimera. To construe mental illness as "merely" a neural impairment is equally misleading, the result of the same neurocentric prejudice.

Because of its emphasis on the embodied and situated nature of the mind, when it comes to treatment an enactive perspective calls for a pluralistic approach that does not exclude the use of drugs, but also favors "alternative" therapies such as bodily and interactive practices. Various such practices already exist—see, for example, Gutstein's (2009) Relationship

Development Intervention (RDI) approach to treating autism, which includes exercises of bodily coordination and turn-taking to restore affective resonance with others; music therapy, such as improvised music-making, is also used to engage autistic children in dialogical interactions and coordination with others (e.g., Wigram and Elefant 2009); and in Röhricht et al.'s (2009) bodywork treatment for chronic schizophrenia subjects are asked to engage in a variety of tasks involving their body, from dance movement therapy to Neo-Reichian body psychotherapy and sensory awareness. It follows from the preceding paragraph, however, that, from an enactive perspective, these practices are not mere indirect ways to act distally on the alleged primary source of mental illness, i.e., the brain; rather they act directly on concrete constitutive parts of the disorder. Irrespective of whether or not these practices end up affecting neural activity, they should be seen as directly manipulating the disorder itself.

Cognitive-affective shifts in mental disorders

Finally let us briefly consider the convergence between the enactive view that cognition is inherently affective, and current views in psychopathology. There is a close relationship between the enactive view that living systems are sense-making systems that enact their *Umwelt*, and the notion of existential feelings discussed by Ratcliffe (2008) and introduced earlier. The latter, as we saw, consist in feelings of how one "finds oneself in the world." They are thus world-oriented experiences, however at the same time they are *bodily* feelings—not in the sense that they take the body as an intentional object, but in the sense that they are bodily experiences of the world, experiences of the world-through-the-body. Likewise the enactive notion of sense-making implies that the world one finds oneself in (one's *Umwelt*) is always correlated to one's bodily structure and experience.

According to Ratcliffe (2008), disorders such as schizophrenia, depression, Capgras' syndrome, etc. involve radical shifts in existential feeling—as shown, for example, by changes in how one's own body is experienced, and correlatively by changes in how the world appears to the subject. From an enactive perspective, psychiatric disorders are to be understood as shifts in sense-making, resulting in an extraordinary and therefore often disconcerting *Umwelt*. Importantly, for both approaches these shifts are cognitive *and* affective at the same time. They are cognitive in the sense that they involve changes in perception, imagination, and understanding of others, which take different forms depending on the disorder in question. However, these cognitive changes are not appropriately characterized merely in terms of changes in one's propositional beliefs. Rather they involve deeper changes in what strikes one as salient; in what demands attention and affords interaction, and what does not anymore; in the awareness of one's possibilities of sensorimotor and affective relations to the world. These changes thus also encompass, crucially, the sphere of personal salience and affectivity, which thus cannot really be disentangled from their cognitive dimension.

Both notions of sense-making and existential feelings cut across the widespread conceptual divide between feelings, body, and intentionality/cognition. This divide is deeply entrenched in the analytic tradition of philosophy of mind and emotion, in which feelings are typically characterized as "mere feelings," that is, non-intentional conscious states dislocated from any meaningful action and interaction with the world. The same tradition typically sees bodily phenomena (behavior, expression, physiological changes, and bodily sensations) as mere effects of cognitive processes (such as judgments) that do not participate in the activity of making sense of the world. As we have seen, from an enactive perspective bodily processes are, rather, constitutive of the process of perceiving and interpreting the world, both experientially and subpersonally, and the distinction between cognition and affectivity is rejected accordingly. Existential feelings similarly cut across the distinction between cognition and affect, intentionality and bodily feelings. In existential feeling, the feeling body is constitutive of one's sense of reality; the latter is not provided by a disembodied faculty of cognition, but is given to the subject via the world-feeling body. To appeal to these notions to account for mental illness implies, then, acknowledging the complex holistic shift that this brings with it. Mental illness amounts neither only to disruptions of cognitive-propositional skills, nor only to alterations of affectivity and mood. Rather it involves a more radical and deeper cognitive-affective shift in how one makes sense of one's world including oneself in it.

CONCLUSION

In sum then, there are various common threads between the enactive approach, and current trends and practices in psychopathology. These common threads depend mainly on the fact that both the enactive approach and psychopathology have "phenomenological connections"; as such, they both value lived experience, emphasize the bodily and situated character of the mind, and the fact that what is constructed as salient depends constitutively on the organism's structure, interests, and goals.

To be aware of these commonalities is important to generate further ideas and methods. We have seen, for example, that an enactive neurophenomenological approach could be explicitly adopted to explore whether and how experience and neurophysiological processes correlate in mental disorders; also, emphasizing the complexity of the mutual relations of brain, body, and world, as enactivism does, can provide reasons within psychopathology as to why mental illness should not be reduced to neurochemical impairments, and as to why alternative forms of treatment such as bodily practices should be considered equivalent to drug-based therapy. These are only some initial ideas. Given the current thriving intellectual atmosphere surrounding both enactivism and psychopathology, I believe that more convergences are likely to be identified and developed into more precise research programs in the near future.

ACKNOWLEDGMENTS

Thanks to Adam Zeman for his comments on an early draft of this chapter, and to Richard Gipps for his thoughtful review and advice. This work has been funded by the European Research Council under the European Community's Seventh Framework Programme (FP7/2007–2013), ERC grant agreement nr. 240891.

REFERENCES

Birbaumer, N. and Kimmell, H. D. (Eds) (1979). *Biofeedback and Self-Regulation*. Hillsdale, NJ: Lawrence Erlbaum.

Brooks, R. (1991). Intelligence without representations. *Artificial Intelligence, 47*, 139–59.

Clark, A. (1997). *Being There: Putting Mind, Brain and Body Together Again*. Cambridge, MA: MIT Press.

Colombetti, G. (2007). Enactive appraisal. *Phenomenology and the Cognitive Sciences, 6*, 527–46.

Colombetti, G. (2010). Enaction, sense-making and emotion. In J. Stewart, O. Gapenne, and E. A. Di Paolo (Eds), *Enaction: Toward a New Paradigm for Cognitive Science*, pp. 145–164. Cambridge, MA: MIT Press.

Colombetti, G. (in press). *The Feeling Body: Affective Science Meets the Enactive Mind*. Cambridge MA: MIT Press.

Colombetti, G. and Thompson, E. (2008). The feeling body: Towards an enactive approach to emotion. In W. F. Overton, U. Müller, and J. L. Newman (Eds), *Developmental Perspectives on Embodiment and Consciousness*, pp. 45–68. Hillsdale, NJ: Lawrence Erlbaum.

Cosmelli, D. and Thompson, E. (2010). Embodiment or envatment? Reflections on the bodily bases of consciousness. In J. Stewart, O. Gapenne, and E. A. Di Paolo (Eds), *Enaction: Toward a New Paradigm for Cognitive Science*, pp. 361–86. Cambridge, MA: MIT Press.

Cott, A., Pavloski, R., and Black, A. (1979). The role of sensorimotor rhythm feedback in the biofeedback treatment of epilepsy: A preliminary report. In N. Birbaumer and H. D. Kimmell (Eds), *Biofeedback and Self-Regulation*, pp. 405–12. Hillsdale, NJ: Lawrence Erlbaum.

DeCharms, C. R. (2008). Applications of real time fMRI. *Nature Neuroscience Reviews, 9*, 720–9.

De Jaegher, H. and Di Paolo, E. A. (2007). Participatory sense-making: An enactive approach to social cognition. *Phenomenology and the Cognitive Sciences, 6*, 485–507.

Dimberg, U., Thunberg, M., and Elmehed, K. (2000). Unconscious facial reactions to emotional facial expressions. *Psychological Science, 11*, 86–9.

Di Paolo, E. A. (2005). Autopoiesis, adaptivity, teleology, agency. *Phenomenology and the Cognitive Sciences, 4*, 429–52.

Drayson, Z. (2009). Embodied cognitive science and its implications for psychopathology. *Philosophy, Psychiatry, & Psychology, 16*, 329–40.

Dreyfus, H. L. (1972). *What Computers Can't Do: A Critique of Artificial Reason*. New York, NY: Harper and Row.

Frith, C. D. and Done, D. J. (1988). Towards a neuropsychology of schizophrenia. *British Journal of Psychiatry, 153*, 437–43.

Fuchs, T. (2001). Melancholia as a desynchronization: Towards a psychopathology of interpersonal time. *Psychopathology, 34*, 179–86.

Fuchs, T. (2005). Corporealized and disembodied minds: A phenomenological view of the body in melancholia and schizophrenia. *Philosophy, Psychiatry & Psychology, 12*, 95–107.

Fuchs, T. (2009). Embodied cognitive neuropsychiatry and its consequences for psychiatry. *Poiesis & Praxis, 6*, 219–33.

Gallagher, S. (2001). The practice of mind: Theory, simulation or primary interaction? *Journal of Consciousness Studies, 8*, 83–108.

Gallagher, S. (2003). Phenomenology and experimental design: Toward a phenomenologically enlightened experimental science. *Journal of Consciousness Studies, 10*, 85–99.

Gallagher, S. (2005). *How the Body Shapes the Mind*. New York, NY: Oxford University Press.

Gutstein, S. E. (2009). *The RDI Book: Forging New Pathways for Autism, Asperger's and PDD with the Relationship Development Intervention Program*. Houston, TX: Connections Center.

Hacking, I. (1995). *Rewriting the Soul: Multiple Personality and the Sciences of Memory*. Princeton, NJ: Princeton University Press.

Hacking, I. (1998). *Mad Travellers: Reflections on the Reality of Transient Mental Illnesses*. Cambridge, MA: Harvard University Press.

Hacking, I. (1999). *The Social Construction of What?* Cambridge, MA: Harvard University Press.

Heidegger, M. (1962). *Being and Time* (J. Macquarrie and E. Robinson, Trans.). Oxford: Blackwell. (Original work published 1927.)

Hobson, R. P. (2009). Wittgenstein and the developmental psychopathology of autism. *New Ideas in Psychology*, 27, 243–57.

Hurley, S. (1998). *Consciousness in Action*. Cambridge, MA: Harvard University Press

Jaspers, K. (1997). *General Psychopathology* (J. Hönig and M. W. Hamilton, Trans.). Baltimore, MD: Johns Hopkins University Press. (Original work published 1913.)

Johnston, S. J., Boehm, S. G., Healy, D., Goebel, R., and Linden, D. E. J. (2010). Neurofeedback: A promising tool for the self-regulation of emotion networks. *NeuroImage*, 49, 1066–72.

Jonas, H. (2001). *The Phenomenon of Life: Toward a Philosophical Biology*. Evanston, IL: Northwestern University Press. (Original work published 1966.)

Kelso, J. A. S. (1995). *Dynamic Patterns*. Cambridge, MA: MIT Press.

Le Van Quyen, M., Navarro, V., Martinerie, J., Baulac, M., and Varela, F. J. (2003). Toward a neurodynamical understanding of ictogenesis. *Epilepsia*, 44, 30–43.

Lutz, A., Lachaux, J. -P., Martinerie, J., and Varela, F. J. (2002). Guiding the study of brain dynamics by using first-person data: Synchrony patterns correlate with ongoing conscious states during a simple visual task. *Proceedings of the National Academy of Sciences of the United States of America*, 99, 1586–91.

Matarić, M. J. (2002). Situated robotics. In L. Nadell (Ed.), *Encyclopedia of Cognitive Science*. London: Nature Publishers Group/Macmillan Reference Ltd.

Maturana, H. R. and Varela, F. J. (1980). *Autopoiesis and Cognition: The Realization of the Living* (Boston Studies in the Philosophy of Science, vol. 42). Dordrecht: D. Reidel.

Merleau-Ponty, M. (1963). *The Structure of Behavior* (A. Fisher, Trans.). Pittsburgh, PA: Duquesne University Press. (Original work published 1942.)

Merleau-Ponty, M. (1962). *Phenomenology of Perception* (C. Smith, Trans.). London: Routledge & Kegan Paul. (Original work published 1945.)

Mullen, P. E. (2007). A modest proposal for another phenomenological approach to psychopathology. *Schizophrenia Bulletin*, 33, 113–21.

Noë, A. (2004). *Action in Perception*. Cambridge, MA: MIT Press.

O'Regan, K. J. and Noë, A. (2001). A sensorimotor account of vision and visual consciousness. *Behavioral and Brain Sciences*, 24, 883–917.

Parnas, J. and Sass, L. A. (2001). Self, solipsism, and schizophrenic delusions. *Philosophy, Psychiatry & Psychology*, 8, 101–20.

Parnas, J. and Zahavi, D. (2002). The role of phenomenology in psychiatric classification and diagnosis. In M. Maj, W. Gaebel, J. J. Lopez-Ibor, and N. Sartorius (Eds), *Psychiatric Diagnosis and Classification*, pp. 137–162 (World Psychiatric Association Series). Chichester: John Wiley and Sons.

Petitmengin, C., Navarro, V., and Baulac, M. (2006). Seizure anticipation: Are neuro-phenomenological approaches able to detect preictal symptoms? *Epilepsy and Behavior*, 9, 298–306.

Petitmengin, C., Navarro, V., and Le Van Quyen, M. (2007). Anticipating seizure: Pre-reflective experience at the center of neuro-phenomenology. *Consciousness and Cognition*, 16, 746–64.

Port, R. F. and van Gelder, T. (Eds) (1995). *Mind as Motion*. Cambridge, MA: MIT Press.

Ratcliffe, M. (2008). *Feelings of Being: Phenomenology, Psychiatry and the Sense of Reality*. Oxford: Oxford University Press.

Ratcliffe, M. (2010). The phenomenology of mood and the meaning of life. In P. Goldie (Ed.), *Oxford Handbook of Philosophy of Emotion*, pp. 349–72. Oxford: Oxford University Press.

Rizzolatti, G. and Sinigaglia, G. (2008). *Mirrors in the Brain* (F. Anderson, Trans.). Oxford: Oxford University Press.

Röhricht, F., Papadopoulos, N., Suzuki, I., and Priebe, S. (2009). Ego-pathology, body experience, and body psychotherapy in chronic schizophrenia. *Psychology and Psychotherapy: Theory, Research and Practice*, 82, 19–30.

Roy, J. -M., Petitot, J., Pachoud, B., and Varela, F.J. (1999). Beyond the gap: An introduction to naturalizing phenomenology. In J. -M. Roy, J. Petitot, B. Pachoud, and F. J. Varela (Eds), *Naturalizing Phenomenology: Issues in Contemporary Phenomenology and Cognitive Science*, pp. 1–80. Stanford, CA: Stanford University Press.

Sass, L. A. (1992). *Madness and Modernism: Insanity in the Light of Modern Art, Literature, and Thought*. New York, NY: Basic Books.

Sass, L. A. (2004). Affectivity in schizophrenia: A phenomenological view. *Journal of Consciousness Studies*, 11, 127–47.

Sass, L. A., Parnas, J., and Zahavi, D. (2011). Phenomenological psychopathology and schizophrenia: Contemporary approaches and misunderstandings. *Philosophy, Psychiatry, & Psychology*, 18, 1–23.

Scherer, K. (2009). The dynamic architecture of emotion: Evidence for the component process model. *Cognition and Emotion*, 23, 1307–51.

Segal, Z. S., Williams M. G., and Teasdale, J. D. (2001). *Mindfulness-based Cognitive Therapy for Depression: A New Approach to Preventing Relapse*. New York, NY: Guilford.

Spiegelberg, H. (1972). *Phenomenology in Psychology and Psychiatry: A Historical Introduction*. Evanston, IL: Northwestern University Press.

Stanghellini, G. (2004). *Disembodied Spirits and Deanimated Bodies: The Psychopathology of Common Sense*. Oxford: Oxford University Press.

Stanghellini, G. and Ballerini, M. (2004). Autism: Disembodied existence. *Philosophy, Psychiatry, & Psychology*, 11, 259–68.

Stern, D. N. (1985). *The Interpersonal World of the Infant: A View from Psychoanalysis and Devlopmental Psychology*. London: Karnac.

Stewart, J., Gapenne, O., and Di Paolo, E.A. (Eds) (2010). *Enaction: A New Paradigm for Cognitive Science*. Cambridge, MA: MIT Press.

Thelen, E., Schöner, G., Scheier, C., and Smith, L.B. (2001). The dynamics of embodiment: A field theory of infant perseverative reaching. *Behavioral and Brain Sciences*, 24, 1–86.

Thelen, E. and Smith, L.B. (1994). *A Dynamic Systems Approach to the Development of Cognition and Action*. Cambridge, MA: MIT Press.

Thompson, E. (2007). *Mind in Life: Biology, Phenomenology, and the Sciences of Mind*. Cambridge MA: Harvard University Press.

Thompson, E., Lutz, A., and Cosmelli, D. (2005). Neurophenomenology: An introduction for neurophilosophy. In A. Brook and K. Akins (Eds), *Cognition and the Brain: the Philosophy and Neuroscience Movement*, pp. 40–97. New York, NY: Cambridge University Press.

Trevarthen, C. (1979). Communication and cooperation in early infancy: A description of primary intersubjectivity. In M. Bullowa (Ed.), *Before Speech: The Beginning of Interpersonal Communication*, pp. 321–47. Cambridge: Cambridge University Press.

Varela, F. J. (1996). Neurophenomenology: A methodological remedy for the hard problem. *Journal of Consciousness Studies*, 3, 330–50.

Varela, F. J., Thompson, E., and Rosch, E. (1991). *The Embodied Mind: Cognitive Science and Human Experience*. Cambridge, MA: MIT Press.

Von Uexküll, J. J. (2010). *Foray into the Worlds of Animals and Human*. (D. Sagan, Trans.). Minneapolis: University of Minnesota Press.

Weber, A. and Varela, F.J. (2002). Life after Kant: Natural purposes and the autopoietic foundations of biological individuality. *Phenomenology and the Cognitive Sciences*, 1, 97–125.

Wheeler, M. (2005). *Reconstructing the Cognitive World: The Next Step*. Cambridge, MA: MIT Press.

Wigram, T. and Elefant, C. (2009). Therapeutic dialogues in music: Nurturing musicality of communication in children with autistic spectrum disorder and Rett syndrome. In S. Malloch, and C. Trevarthen (Eds), *Communicative Musicality: Exploring the Basis of Human Companionship*, pp. 423–45. Oxford: Oxford University Press.

Zahavi, D. (2007). Expression and empathy. In D. D. Hutto and M. Ratcliffe (Eds), *Folk-Psychology Reassessed*, pp. 25–40. Dordrecht: Springer.

....

CHAPTER 64

COULD PSYCHOANALYSIS BE A SCIENCE?

....

MICHAEL LACEWING

Could psychoanalysis be a science? There are three ways of reading this question, which will structure our discussion:

1. Is psychoanalysis the kind of investigation or activity that could, logically speaking, be "scientific"? If we can defend a positive answer here, then it makes sense to ask:
2. Is psychoanalysis, in the form in which it has traditionally been practiced, and continues to be practiced, a science? If there are good reasons to doubt its credentials, then we might ask:
3. Is psychoanalysis able to become a science? This is a question about what is needed for the necessary transformation.

I shall argue that psychoanalysis can be a science in the first section, but that the historical debate raised important challenges to its methodology, viz., confirmation bias (§2.1), suggestion (§2.2), and unsupportable causal inference (§2.3). I argue that recent developments (§3.1–3.2) meet these challenges, and conclude with some reflections on the interdisciplinary nature of psychoanalysis (§3.3).

COULD PSYCHOANALYSIS (LOGICALLY) BE A SCIENCE?

....

This is a question about what psychoanalysis is and what counts as science, a question about our concepts of "psychoanalysis" and "science." Psychoanalysis involves both the clinical encounter and the production of psychoanalytic theory. It is a mistake to restrict the meaning of "psychoanalysis" to the interaction between analyst and analysand (§1.3), though this remains central to psychoanalysis. Psychoanalytic theory is a theory of the nature and functioning of the human mind, especially in relation to motives. Much of its evidential base rests in the clinical data—neurotic symptoms, dreams, present thoughts and emotions—but psychoanalysis has always gone beyond clinical data to appeal to data from other fields of enquiry (§3.3). Psychoanalysts have been active in producing some of this data, e.g., in child development or psychiatry, and in integrating the results into new psychoanalytic theory. It is the generation of psychoanalytic knowledge that is of central interest here, and so our immediate question is "Are the form of psychoanalytic knowledge and the method of its generation of a kind that could (logically) qualify as scientific?"

On the meaning of "science," I shall proceed pragmatically. I assume we have a rough conception that enables us to identify paradigmatic examples, and I shall argue by comparing psychoanalysis with "established" sciences, especially social psychology (§1.2) and the social sciences more broadly (§2.2).

1.1 But first, could psychoanalysis be a natural science? The most plausible defense of an affirmative answer rests on Freud's "economic" model of human psychology. The aim of his *Project for a Scientific Psychology* (1895) was "to discover what form the theory of psychical functioning will take if a quantitative line of approach, a kind of economics of nervous force, is introduced into it" (p. 296). Freud intended "to furnish a psychology that shall be a natural science" seeking to understand human psychology in terms of a "conception of neuronal excitation as quantity in a state of flow" (p. 296), governed by biological principles of homeostasis. The model he applied, popular at the time, was that of the reflex; energy in requires energy out, to prevent energy from building up dangerously within the system, which Freud argued is experienced as pain. And so neurons and the nervous system as a whole have a tendency to divest themselves of energy.

If the economic model were the core of psychoanalysis, there would be reason to consider it a natural science. But there would also be good reason to reject it. First, many of the claims of the economic model have been superseded by neuroscience. The nervous system does not operate on a reflex model, and does not tend to divest itself of energy. Neurons generate their own energy metabolically, rather than receiving it from outside stimulation, which therefore modulates, rather than creates, nervous system activity. Sensory surfaces are not conductors, but transducers, of external energy, converting it into electrochemical impulses of negligible energy but with varying frequency—and so the nervous system cannot be swamped by energy from outside, nor can energy be trapped in it. The energy within the system is not conducted—it is not a quantity in a state of flow—but is transmitted by propagation. Finally, the quantity of energy involved bears no correlation to the psychological state of the person; the nervous system uses information, not energy, to structure its activities (see Hobson 1988, esp. pp. 284–286; Holt 1965). Second, and perhaps most central to our enquiry, given this last claim, the clinical methods of psychoanalytic enquiry are inappropriate for generating knowledge of neural functioning.

Fortunately, psychoanalysis survives the demise of the economic theory. Freud repeatedly drew upon the economic model in his later psychological theorizing, e.g., he modeled psychic conflict as involving forces, understood associative links in content as involving energy pathways, talked of psychological ideas and experiences as cathecting neural networks, and analyzed psychic phenomena such as condensation and displacement in terms of transpositions of energy. This all needs to be reformulated just in terms of psychological content and processes. Freud sometimes approaches clinical questions in economic terms, e.g., narcissism (1914a), mourning (1917), and masochism (1924), and to the extent that psychoanalytic theories of these phenomena rest implicitly or explicitly on a mistaken conception of human beings as closed systems of fixed amounts of undissipated libido, the theories must be rethought. The theory of instincts, "our mythology" as Freud put it (1933, p. 94), must be translated into psychological terms, abandoned, or radically amended in the light of recent biological and neuropsychological investigations. All this can be or has been done.

These remarks leave open the possibility that psychoanalysis abuts neuroscience as a discipline, and there may be fruitful exchange (it may even be that neuroscience formulates a workable version of an "energy" concept). But psychoanalysis does not qualify as a natural science in its own right. This does not rule out the possibility that it may qualify as a social science, and it is to this question we now turn.

1.2 According to the "hermeneutic interpretation" of psychoanalysis, psychoanalysis is, at its heart, a process of self-reflection, self-interpretation and self-formation. This process can be transformative by opening up new ways of understanding ourselves and the meanings of our behavior, providing insights into previously unrecognized motives. The theoretical framework of psychoanalysis must therefore be an interpretation of this process in general terms (Habermas 1972). The roots of this view lie in a grand tradition, developed most famously by Dilthey (but also Brentano and Husserl), that holds that understanding the behavior of human beings, in particular the meaning of such behavior, is fundamentally distinct from scientific enquiry. On certain stronger interpretations of this view, no enquiries into this subject and so no social "sciences"—which include branches of psychology on any reasonable interpretation (social, educational, and personality psychology at least)—are sciences. Weaker interpretations accept the social sciences as such, but distinguish them from the natural sciences. On this view, psychoanalysis cannot be a natural science, but it could be a social science. But some hold the view that while there can be genuine social sciences, psychoanalysis is not among them, because of the individual nature of its subject matter as described.

There are a number of grounds on which we can contest this conclusion. First, some of the reasons put forward for thinking that neither the social sciences in general, nor psychoanalysis in particular, qualify as sciences rest on a narrow understanding of science, e.g., that science employs strict, universal laws or that all sciences are reducible to physics. While these are interesting philosophical debates, they fail to demarcate between recognized sciences and recognized non-sciences in the present. There are clearly branches of *natural* science, let alone social science, which no one knows how to reduce to physics and which do not employ strict, universal laws, but whose explanations of phenomena recognize the considerable role of historical contingency, e.g., paleontology and evolutionary biology. (This is not to say that there are *no* covering laws in these disciplines, but that scientific research and explanation carries on well enough without them in many typical cases.)

Second, a considerable portion of the strength of the original argument for the hermeneutic interpretation rested on a distinction between motives and causes (e.g., Ricoeur 1970, pp. 358–363, who approvingly cites Flew 1949; Peters 1950; Taylor 1964; Toulmin 1948): If motives are not causes, then explanations in terms of motives, such as those given in psychoanalysis, are not causal explanations; as scientific explanations are causal, psychoanalysis is not a science. Not only is the explanatory form different, to think of motives as causes is to reify them, and so to postulate metaphysically dubious entities. And the relation of causes to effects is always underwritten by (deterministic) laws, but there are no laws of this kind in psychology.

Two points challenge the inference. First, it is generally agreed that the original debate of the 1950s and 1960s was confused and worked with restricted conceptions of "cause" and "causal explanation" which have since been superseded. It is now clear that there is conceptual room for a range of causalist views that avoid the original objections (see O'Connor and Sandis 2010, part II).[1] And the way the debate has developed does not support the original claims about explanations in terms of motives. In large part as a response to Davidson's classic (1963) paper, the debate has focused on whether *reasons* are causes, or again, whether explanations of action in terms of reasons are causal explanations. But not all we wish to understand about an action is the reason for which the agent acted (there is also timing, manner, symbolic meaning, etc.), not all behavior is action, and not all motives are rational— by which I mean not just that people act irrationally because they take factors to be reasons when they are not; rather, not all motives involve the apprehension of reasons. We cannot reduce explaining the meaning of human behavior to an account of the reasons for which people act. To slam the door in anger does not typically involve taking anything as a reason for slamming the door (including the satisfaction one may gain from doing so), but my anger motivates my slamming the door, and saying that I was angry makes my slamming the door intelligible. Or, as a different example of meaning without rationality (though an example of imagination, not action), consider the expression of desires in dreams. Sticking uncontroversially to "transparent" dreams, such as dreaming of drinking when thirsty, the desire makes sense of and motivates the dream, but provides no reason for it (though it would rationalize the waking action of getting a drink). Goldie (2000, pp. 127ff.) provides a more complex example that combines emotional expression with imagination: scratching the eyes out of a photo of one's rival in love. Now, unconscious motives—of the sort discussed by psychoanalysis, but also those identified by social psychology, discussed later—do not always work through the provision of reasons for acting as the agent does. Even if we grant the view that *reasons* are not causes (or that reason-citing explanations are not causal explanations), this does not help the hermeneutic interpretation, since it does not support the claim that explanations citing motives are not causal explanations, at least when the motives do not give the agent's reasons.[2]

Second, the original argument entails that no branch of psychology seeking to investigate motives—or more generally, the meaning of human behavior—can qualify as a science. In response, we can argue that social psychology is rightly recognized as a science, given its methodology, the growth of agreed results, and its integration with other branches of psychology. We should not make its status as a science dependent upon the resolution of the philosophical debate over the precise relation between motives and causes. Scientific work

[1] For example, causalists need not maintain that motives are themselves *causes* of actions. They could instead hold that it is agents, not their beliefs, desires, or other psychological states, who bring about actions. They may claim that an agent acted as she did in virtue of certain motives, with this statement being understood as a causal explanation. Causal explanation, in turn, can be understood broadly as providing relevant information about the causal history of an occurrence, rather than citing the cause specifically, in a form amenable to universal law.

[2] For example, see Dancy (2000, pp. 167, 173–174), where he indicates that his book-length argument against considering reasons to be causes does nothing to rule out non-rational psychological explanations being causal. This includes not only non-rational motives, but also cases in which the motive cited, e.g., an emotional disposition or character trait, explains why the agent acted on the reasons they did.

with motives is, therefore, possible. That psychoanalysis offers explanations of behavior in terms of motives cannot, therefore, establish that it cannot be a science.

It is an important (and well-established) finding of social psychology that our behavior can be shaped by motives and meanings we are unaware of, and this can be investigated by recognized scientific methods. For example, subjects were asked to memorize word-pairs, and later given a word association task. Those who memorized "ocean-moon," when asked to name a detergent, were significantly more likely to say "Tide" (Nisbett and Wilson 1977, p. 243), but did not cite the relevant word-pair as motivating their answer. Likewise, many subliminal perception experiments work through the semantic content of the priming stimulus. Of course, the stimulus provides no *reason* for the response, but as already noted, we cannot restrict the project of self-understanding to rational explanation. Nevertheless, the hermeneut may object that this is the wrong sort of "meaning," the right sort having to do with "making sense" of our behavior.[3] This form of investigation doesn't do that, even if it explains it in some other way. It is therefore irrelevant to our discussion of whether psychoanalysis, which does attempt to make sense of our behavior, can qualify as scientific.

It is true that social psychology does not (often) concern itself with what the behavior and motive *mean to the individual*, while this is precisely what psychoanalysis does concern itself with (§1.3). But the line of argument just given is mistaken. First, we make sense—give the meaning—of behavior in ways that are broader than accounting for the meaning of the behavior to the individual; second, the influences on our behavior investigated by social psychology interact with the subjective meanings focused upon by the hermeneutic interpretation. The example just given provides a case in point. The semantic content of the stimulus is what makes sense of the response—the sense lies in the connection in content. The words mean something to the subject, and this meaning is part of the explanation offered on the basis of scientific enquiry; the same results cannot be expected with subjects who do not speak English or have not encountered a detergent named "Tide." (That the stimulus operates non-consciously is, of course, no objection. The hermeneutic interpretation of psychoanalysis must accept that the project of self-understanding allows both non-rational and also non-conscious motivation.[4])

Another example illustrates the close connection between social psychological explanations and the meaning of behavior to the individual. Consider Maier's (1931) classic

---

[3] We can identify four types of "meaning" that may be relevant to explaining human behavior. First, our psychology cannot be understood independently of intentionality and intentional content. Second, this content is, to a substantial degree, structured by language and the semantic meanings it makes available. Third, our mental states, with their intentional content and phenomenal character, are subjectively meaningful in a variety of ways. For example, they are cognitively meaningful as the means through which we conceptualize, think of and understand the world, and they are conatively meaningful both as preferences and evaluations directed toward the world, and as states toward which we take up (further) evaluative attitudes. Finally, we are rational creatures, and the (cognitive, conative, evaluative and semantic) meanings we make are governed by and answerable to rational discourse. The objection being considered is that the explanation appeals only to semantic meaning (type 2), but it is subjective meaning (type 3) that is relevant to the hermeneutic view.

[4] Whether or not the subject is conscious of the factors cited by the explanation undoubtedly alters the precise nature of the story to be told, as well as how we respond to and evaluate the behavior, e.g., in terms of whether we hold someone responsible for what they do. But this does not imply that explanations citing non-conscious factors do not "make sense" of the behavior.

experiment on problem solving. Two cords were hung from the ceiling, placed so that subjects could not, while holding one cord, reach the other. The room contained a variety of objects, e.g., poles, clamps, extension cords. Individual subjects were asked to tie the two cords together. Subjects easily discovered three solutions, after each of which they were asked to find a further solution. Many struggled at this point for several minutes, when Maier then casually started one cord swinging. Within a minute, subjects tied a weight to one cord, swung it like a pendulum, and thus brought it close enough to the second cord to tie the two together. Maier asked the subjects how they had come across the idea of the pendulum. None of them reported his action, but said it just occurred to them; the influence, therefore, was subliminal. Does Maier's action of swinging a cord provide an explanation of the subjects' doing so (less than a minute later) which "makes sense" of their behavior or not? I would argue it does. If the subjects had reported that they had seen Maier swing the cord, and this suggested the solution to them, and they had then enacted this solution, the explanation would, of course, make sense in the right way. That we are more influenced by situational factors than we can normally consciously report is an established finding of social psychology (Nisbett and Ross 1980). Yet many of these factors, if noted and considered consciously, can operate as reasons, interacting with our standing motives in rational and consciously recognizable ways.

Furthermore, the results of social psychological experiments can question the influence of the reasons we believe we act upon, and so present a challenge to explanations that *would* make sense if they were true. For example, two groups of students were asked to predict how much shock they would be willing to experience in an experiment on the effects of intense electric shock. One group were reassured that the shocks would cause no permanent damage, the other group was not. When asked if the reassurance had made a difference to their predictions, the first group replied that it had increased the level of shock predicted, i.e., the reassurance acted as one factor (among others) they had considered in predicting how much shock they were willing to take. The second group were asked, counterfactually, if such reassurance would have made a difference, and they reported that it would. However, there was no overall difference between the levels of shock predicted in the two groups (Nisbett and Wilson 1977, p. 246). So the reassurance appears not to make the difference the students claim it did. Understanding their predictions as a form of action, we can say that the students' actions were not influenced by a factor that they took themselves to be acting upon.

Given these considerations, we cannot rule out the investigations of social psychology as irrelevant to our attempts to make sense of ourselves, nor can we declare that the project of investigating the meaning of human behavior cannot qualify as a science.

1.3 There is yet a sense of "self-understanding," central to the psychoanalytic project, that contrasts with the type of investigation of motives described earlier. So even if the argument successfully defends the possibility of a science of motives, it does not establish whether psychoanalysis could qualify. This search for self-understanding is what cannot become a science, argues the hermeneut. This statement contains some truth: understanding individuals (oneself or others) is not a science, not least because every individual is unique in the contents and connections of their mental states. Researchers cannot make judgments evidenced in the usual experimental way regarding why an individual acts as they do on any given occasion, nor are laboratory control studies much use to someone trying to understand an individual in this way (such studies may suggest hypotheses, but cannot establish which is correct). But we would be wrong to think either that individual self-interpretation is all there is to psychoanalysis, or that nothing scientific can be done which can helpfully inform self-interpretation.

Psychoanalysis is not only about understanding individuals, with all the idiosyncratic contingencies of their mental content and history. It is also the construction of a general psychological theory, based on information about the *generic* processes and obstacles present in self-interpretation. Claims about transference, the many patterns of psychic defense, resistance, the understanding of dreams, unconscious emotions, the symbolic content of motives, and the influence of the past are part of this psychological theory. This theoretical apparatus, and the concepts it employs, can be used to generate explanations and predictions regarding human behavior. Clinical practice requires such a more general theoretical backdrop, and so any psychoanalytic approach to understanding ourselves must take some stance on these theoretical claims. These general claims (especially those concerning the clinical process) are often *assumed* by the hermeneutic interpretation—but they have been disputed by other psychological theories. Now, first, whether this psychodynamic picture of the mind is true or not makes a difference to how we should approach and understand the task of self-interpretation. For example, Timothy Wilson (2002), while acknowledging the immense contribution of Freud to psychology, argues that the results of social psychology indicate that we should turn *outward*, to our manifest behavior and situational influences, in order to understand ourselves, not inward, to our dispositions and their symbolic content. Second, general psychoanalytic claims can be supported or revised on the basis of extra-clinical results (e.g., Holt 2002; Masling and Bornstein 1983–1998; Solms and Turnbull 2002; Westen 1998, 1999) and the statistical analysis of clinical data (both across individuals and using "within-subject" designs, e.g., Dahl 1972; Gill 1982; Gill and Hoffman 1982; Kächele et al. 2008; Luborsky 1977, 2001); and there is a place for scientifically respectable case studies, even ones that involve no quantitative methods (Kazdin 1981).

We should conclude that even if the enterprise of understanding an individual's motives, and the meaning of their behavior to them, is not a science, psychoanalysis is not logically barred from being a science. It is committed to producing a general theory of psychic functioning, especially regarding motives, and this general theory informs the process of self-understanding emphasized by the hermeneutic interpretation. Having argued that psychoanalysis can be a science, we may now ask if it is one.

COULD PSYCHOANALYSIS (AS IT IS) BE A SCIENCE?

If psychoanalysis could logically be a science, does it instantiate one? The issue here is whether the form of psychoanalytic knowledge and the method of its generation qualify as scientific. Psychoanalysis presents us with a general theory of motivation, character, interpersonal relations and (aspects of) mental functioning, comparable to other such theories in empirical psychology. The form of this knowledge is scientific, so I shall focus on the question of method. A method can fail to be scientific if it cannot deliver the objectivity and rigor of science, or if it appeals to an evidential base that systematically fails to justify the inferences that are drawn from it. I shall therefore discuss three specific objections of this sort.

For the purposes of this section, I shall assume that the traditional methodology of psychoanalysis, viz. inferring its theoretical claims from clinical data presented as case studies, is its only method. This assumption is *narrow and out-of-date* in ways that will become apparent in §3.1 but it is useful for understanding the debate as it has been conducted.

2.1 Popper argued that scientific claims must be falsifiable—very roughly, they can (in principle) be tested against experience in such a way that it is possible for undermining evidence to come to light—and science proceeds by attempting to refute hypotheses. Those claims not refuted, despite vigorous testing, are (provisionally) held to be true. Popper (1963, pp. 34–38, 1983, chapter 2; see also 1995, pp. 87–89) argued that psychoanalytic claims are immunized against such testing, and so psychoanalysis is not a science.[5]

Popper begins by arguing that psychoanalysis proceeds by seeking out verifications of its theories, rather than falsifications (1995, p. 87; see also 1963, p. 38 footnote). Clinical data are "interpreted in accordance with established psychoanalytic theory," but genuine evidential support only comes from testing claims in ways that may demonstrate the claims are false. In effect, Popper diagnoses a type of confirmation bias, which involves the selective gathering, weighing, or interpretation of evidence that supports one's existing beliefs or favored hypothesis while neglecting or discounting evidence that tells against one's view.[6] Judged by standard psychoanalytic case study reports and key theoretical texts, many psychoanalysts have undoubtedly manifested confirmation bias in their handling and reporting of data.

Popper then argues that the logic of psychoanalysis is such that it cannot correct its confirmation bias, for two reasons. First, analysts' theories may influence the clinical data in such a way as to produce confirming evidence. Disconfirming evidence, therefore, doesn't emerge. We shall return to this issue of suggestion later. Second, psychoanalysis cannot countenance refuting evidence: not only do psychoanalytic concepts such as "ambivalence" make it "difficult, if not impossible" to agree on when a psychoanalytic interpretation has been falsified, but the theory attempts to explain "practically everything" about human behavior (Popper 1963, p. 34), allowing no conceivable event to refute it: "we can say, prior to any observation, that every conceivable observation will be interpretable in the light of psychoanalytic theory" (1995, p. 87).

Popper provides very little argument or evidence for this second claim, and it is unpersuasive. Freud claimed that "the theory of psychoanalysis is an attempt to account for two striking and unexpected facts of observation which emerge whenever an attempt is made to trace the symptoms of a neurotic back to their sources in his past life: the facts of transference and of resistance" (Freud 1914b, p. 16). If there were no evidence of either resistance or transference, the most important indicators of dynamic unconscious processes at work in the clinical setting, psychoanalysis would probably be placed beyond rescue. It is not *inconceivable*

---

[5] Popper's view of science has fallen into disfavor. It is generally agreed that scientific theories (as opposed to specific hypotheses) are not refuted by single observations or sets of observations, but rather, as Lakatos (1978) argued, through a widening gap between the facts that need to be explained and the explanations offered by the theory, a gap that brings the research program of the theory to a halt. Making adjustments to a theory and to the "auxiliary hypotheses" that link the theory to specific empirical predictions, in order to preserve the truth of the theory, is part of normal scientific procedure. However, Popper's objection to psychoanalysis, as I interpret it, can stand on its own.

[6] See Nickerson (1998) for a review.

that there should be no such evidence (though we may have to suppose much about human behavior to be different). For example, as evidence against resistance, we could observe that people are equally disposed to consciously recall and recognize motives that caused them psychic pain as those that did not, that situations that arouse feelings of helplessness or anxiety do not tend to increase rates of forgetting or other symptoms (see §3.1). Or again, against transference, we might observe that in their relation to their analyst, subjects remain calm, objective, and friendly over a span of months or years. Of course, highlighting psychoanalysts' *refusal* to countenance evidence against the theory shows only the presence of confirmation bias, not the impossibility of its correction. Such refusal is not universal: Grünbaum (1984, pp. 104–126) argues that there is significant evidence showing not only that central psychoanalytic claims are falsifiable, but that Freud (at least) gave up a good number as false on good grounds.

Rejecting Popper's claim does not show, however, that psychoanalysis, as traditionally practiced, can correct for confirmation bias. The charge is, therefore, important and remains unanswered, and I will return to it in §3.2.

2.2 The problem of suggestion has been a perennial challenge to the scientific rigor of psychoanalysis and the evidential soundness of its claims. The challenge is that some of the mental states of the analysand as evidenced in the clinical data are, in fact, brought about through the "suggestive" influence of the analyst. The clinical data is therefore not good evidence of the true structure and contents of the analysand's mind, and so not a secure basis for theorizing about the human mind. This was certainly the thought that Fliess presented to Freud (Freud 1954, pp. 334–337).

Hypnotic suggestion operates by explicit and forceful communication intended to alter a patient's mind by bypassing their conscious awareness of the idea communicated. Suggestion in psychoanalysis, if present, is unintended, subtle, and unconscious. It is best understood as a variety of "experimenter expectancy effect." Experimenter effects are influences that the experimenter has on the subjects of an experiment which are not the effects under investigation.[7] It has been shown that a variety of factors, from the experimenter's age to their need for social approval, can make a difference to how subjects respond in experiments (Rosenthal and Rosnow 2009, p. 327). Most relevant to the issue of suggestion, however, are expectancy effects: what the experimenter expects to happen, his or her favored hypothesis, subtly affects how subjects respond in favor of that expectation. The effects can be found in everyday life as well, e.g., in education:

> All of the teachers of an elementary school were told that a newly devised computer program was able to predict the intellectual development potential of children in their classroom. At the very beginning of the school year, a handful of children's names were selected completely at random and given to their teachers, who were told that those children would bloom intellectually in the academic year just begun. At the end of the school year those children whose names had been placed arbitrarily on the list of bloomers did, in fact, show greater intellectual gains than did the children in the control group. (Rosenthal 2000, p. 294)

---

[7] The leading researcher on experimenter effects for the last fifty years has been Robert Rosenthal, and his early work from the 1960s has not been surpassed or overthrown (see Rosenthal 1997; Rosenthal 2000; Rosenthal and Rubin 1978), such that Oxford University Press reissued his three major works in 2009 (Rosenthal and Rosnow 2009).

The theoretically-based expectations of the analyst thus might alter the clinical data so as to create "evidence" that supports those very expectations. The most prominent vehicles for suggestion are the analyst's interpretations and the reinforcing of certain types of patient communication (through vocalizations, displays of interest, etc.), with the authority of the analyst facilitating the patient's susceptibility to comply with the analyst's expectations (Erwin 1996, p. 96; Fisher and Greenberg 1977, p. 363).

It is generally recognized that the theories and values of the researcher are more likely to affect data in the social sciences, in part due to the nature of the interaction between researcher and subjects involving the need to interpret the meaning behavior has for the subject. But there are two reasons to think psychoanalysis faces a distinct challenge. First, experimenters produce greater expectancy effects when they appear professional, business-like but friendly, competent, and expressive in communication, and work in a "personal" space (Rosenthal 1976, chapter 15). On these criteria, psychoanalysts look set to produce the greatest expectancy effects of all, even setting aside traditional concerns about positive transference. Second, more generally, psychoanalysis does not avail itself of several established means for reducing biases, of which experimenter expectancy effects are one form. In a recent *Handbook of Applied Social Research Methods*, the researcher is encouraged to:

a. engage in intensive, long-term participant involvement, to enable more complete data and time to formulate alternative hypotheses;
b. collect "rich," i.e., detailed and varied, data;
c. secure "respondent validation," systematically soliciting feedback from participants on the conclusions drawn;
d. search for discrepant evidence;
e. "triangulate" conclusions, e.g., by drawing on diverse methods of collecting data, by looking at different sources of data, by reviewing findings using different researchers, and by interpreting the data in the light of different theories;
f. employ "quasi-statistics," i.e., using simple numerical results that can be easily extracted from the qualitative data;[8]
g. use comparisons with other groups (the role usually played by control groups in quantitative studies) or other studies. (Maxwell 2009, pp. 244–245)[9]

Psychoanalysis clearly fares well in relation to (a)–(c)—analyses last years, the data is highly detailed and covers many topics, and the analysand is constantly supplying feedback on the hypotheses presented by the analyst. (d) relates to confirmation bias, already remarked upon as a challenge.[10] The last three recommendations develop that challenge to the traditional psychoanalytic case study methodology. Some triangulation is achieved by the diversity of

---

[8] The term "quasi-statistics" comes from Becker (1970). Qualitative data often has an implicit quantitative element, e.g., in claims that something is "frequent" or "typical." Employing quasi-statistics seeks to make such quantitative elements more explicit, and enables researchers to assess, e.g., the number of discrepant cases, the percentage of sources they come from, and the amount of evidence relevant to a particular claim.

[9] Similar points are made in other handbooks on method, e.g., Patton (2000, chapter 9)—from which I have taken the helpful expansion on different types of triangulation. Patton also comments on the importance of training, which I discuss in §3.2.

[10] It is important to distinguish between suggestion and confirmation bias. Suggestion *changes* the clinical data in support of the theory; confirmation bias *misinterprets* the data in support of the theory.

individuals and their concerns, but there is no variety of method in gathering the evidence, and rarely are a variety of analysts with different theoretical perspectives asked to review the conclusions inferred from the data. The data is not recorded or presented in ways that facilitate statistical analyses. And comparisons of the kind that could prove corrective, e.g., with interpretations of similar phenomena in other psychoanalytic or non-psychoanalytic schools, are rarely drawn (see §3.2). Here, then, is an argument for thinking that psychoanalysis is not, as traditionally practiced, a science, because its method does not reduce bias sufficiently.

However, another means by which bias is overcome lies in corroboration. It is often not possible to tell, from the results of a single researcher, the degree to which expectancy effect has influenced the result. Replication by different experimenters (presumably with different expectations) is necessary. Rosenthal notes, "If all of a sample of experimenters obtain similar data we will not err very often if we assume that … no effects whatever associated with the experimenter have occurred" (Rosenthal and Rosnow 2009, p. 567). The methodology of a science necessarily involves the activity of a scientific community, and secure results are widely agreed upon, having been tested and confirmed by the results of many researchers.

We can appeal to corroboration, and on this basis reply to the charge of suggestion, for a limited, but central, range of claims in psychoanalytic theory.[11] Rubinstein (1976) famously argued that psychoanalysis is best seen as a "purely clinical" science (see also Klein 1976), and Wallerstein (1990, 2005) develops the case. He defines the clinical theory as the theory of transference and resistance, conflict and compromise, noting Freud's famous definition of psychoanalysis as "Any line of investigation which recognizes these two facts [of transference and resistance] and takes them as the starting point of its work" (1914b, p. 16). Wallerstein argues that the clinical theory is substantially held in common between the many psychoanalytic schools in mutual disagreement over metapsychology and etiological claims.[12] While Wallerstein's views have caused controversy, this has focused almost entirely on his claims about the relation of metapsychology to clinical data. Few commentators have taken issue over the consilience regarding clinical theory, and those that have focus more on the theory of clinical technique than the psychodynamic model of the mind and its clinical manifestations (see Abrams et al. 1989). Over the existence and nature of unconscious defenses against psychic conflict, and the implication of both such conflict and defense in the etiology of neurosis and a range of psychological traits, there is little disagreement (Rosenblatt 1989, pp. 90–91).

This is not a final answer to the problem of suggestion. Expectancy effects are put to rest more soundly when we get corroboration by different schools, and insofar as psychoanalysis can be considered a single school of thought in psychology, we must seek corroboration by

[11] For a more extensive defense of this claim, see Lacewing (2013).

[12] There is a common conception that the metapsychological and etiological disagreements are sustained by, and evidence of, the operation of suggestion, such that analysands tend "to bring up precisely the kind of phenomenological data which confirm the theories and interpretation of their analysts" (Marmor 1962, p. 289). The common conception is unsupported, however: confirmation bias could produce the same result. Hence it may *appear* that analysands produce data of the kind that supports the theoretical views of their analysts, but this appearance is in fact a product of the selection and presentation of the data by the analyst. Wallerstein (1990, p. 11) argues similarly that the data of different schools are comparable, but they are explained through different general theoretical frameworks, and this is possible because the theories are not tightly linked to the data.

non-psychoanalytic theories. This makes a general point about the nature of science—*no school of thought should stand in isolation from its rivals.* But where corroborative results within a school are established by a defensible methodology, its explanations enter as equal competitors, not to be dismissed from the outset as "unscientific." We have not yet secured this result for psychoanalysis, for the absence of the correctives in the social sciences—triangulation, quasi-statistics, and comparisons—and the threat of confirmation bias remain as reasons to think that, in its traditional form, psychoanalysis is not properly a science. We will turn to the issue of current and future developments in §3.

2.3 Our third methodological challenge comes from Adolf Grünbaum, who argues that the method of inferring the causes of clinical data from the clinical data is flawed (1984, chapter 3, 2004).[13] Causal inferences must be justified by use of Mill's canons (Mill 1904): to establish that X is the cause of Y, we must show that Xs make a difference to the occurrence of Ys by comparing (classes of) cases, either comparing the incidence of Ys in cases in which X occurs with ones in which it does not, and/or by comparing cases in which Y occurs to see whether X occurred or not. An example: to establish whether smoking causes lung cancer, we must compare the incidence of lung cancer in smokers and non-smokers; and/or we must examine cases of lung cancer to see whether the person smoked or not. If there is a higher probability that a smoker will have lung cancer than a non-smoker, and/or a higher probability that someone with lung cancer is a smoker than non-smoker, we may infer that smoking causes lung cancer. The clinical data, however, cannot furnish this kind of evidence. Take the central claim that neurosis results from repression (or better, from chronic psychic conflict together with the failure of psychic defense). Nothing in the clinical data alone could establish that the difference between neurosis and its absence is psychic conflict, because it does not record whether, in the general population, there are people who are not neurotic but nevertheless suffer from psychic conflict.

On the face of it, psychoanalysis proceeds by supposing that the interpretation of free associations can discover the psychological states that are the unconscious causes of the clinical data via connections in intentional content. In everyday life, Hopkins (1988) argues, we interpret voluntary behavior by placing it in relation to a motive or set of motives, which we take to have caused the behavior. The motive both explains and causes the behavior in virtue of its intentional content, while the behavior "inherits" its content from its cause. Most of the time, we must rely on background information and a range of behavior, e.g., to understand that someone is seeking revenge, we need to know more than that they deliberately seek to harm someone. We revise our interpretations, and so our causal inferences, as further evidence emerges, in line with the virtues of inference to the best explanation (accuracy, scope, coherence, simplicity, and plausibility). If this is what we, and psychoanalysts, are doing, Grünbaum argues, then we commit a fallacy of "thematic affinity": connections in intentional content or meaning between mental states, or between these and behavior, are no indication, on their own, of a causal connection. At the very least, we must draw upon background knowledge that rests on

---

[13] For this objection to apply, motives (and other mental states) must be causes of the behavior they bring about, i.e., the hermeneutic interpretation is false. I shall assume, with Grünbaum, that this is so. If the hermeneutic interpretation is correct, however, the general issue of how we justify our interpretations of the meaning of behavior still arises, and the discussion that follows may be understood in that light. For a more detailed discussion of Grünbaum's objection, see Lacewing (2012).

Mill's canons and establishes that certain types of mental state are the causes of certain types of behavior.

Grünbaum's conclusion, it will emerge, is defensible for a range of causal inferences in psychoanalysis, in particular those pertaining to the existence of metapsychological structures and the childhood causes of adult mental illness. But the general claim regarding thematic affinity is false. There is a logical or conceptual connection between the intentional content of a desire and the range of behavior it *typically* causes. What makes a mental state a desire, rather than some other type of state, is precisely the pattern of its causal and normative relations to behavior and other mental states. What gives a desire the content it has is also determined (in part) by such relations. The desire to get a drink is a *desire* and a desire *to get a drink* in virtue of its typical causes and effects. Hence to understand a desire is already to understand it in thematic affinity with the behavior it typically causes. This conceptual analysis entails that relations of intentional content are prima facie evidence of causal connections, and so Mill's canons are not necessary in the generation of background knowledge regarding the kinds of causal relations in which desires typically participate. Grünbaum is therefore wrong to think that appeal to thematic affinity is always fallacious.[14]

Nevertheless, experimental work, most famously by Nisbett and Wilson (1977) and Nisbett and Ross (1980), presents overwhelming evidence that people are poor at correctly identifying (all) the causes of their behavior, and prone to inventing false rationalizations. (Some examples were given in §1.2.) Instead, our inferences are guided by "judgments about the extent to which a particular stimulus is a plausible cause of a given response" (1977, p. 231). Wilson (2002) revisits and revises the argument in terms of a distinction between conscious and unconscious processes. Many processes, occurring as part of the "adaptive unconscious" mind, influence our preferences, decisions, and behavior, and in ways we would not think "plausible." As a result, our inferences from behavior to motives are accurate only when actual causal factors are plausible, and no plausible-but-irrelevant factors are present.[15] However, Nisbett and Ross (1980, p. 211) are clear that such everyday inferences do well enough most of the time, at least for voluntary behavior with a conscious motive. Furthermore, there is good reason to believe that typical mistakes in causal inference identified by Nisbett et al. are more common in situations that encourage casual or automatic responses, while thoughtfulness, motivation to understand, and social intelligence increase

---

[14] Two points. First, the conclusion can be made stronger: we *cannot* use Mill's canons to generate the background knowledge, because we cannot *conceptualize* or think coherently about the desire to get a drink without already thinking of the typical causes of getting a drink. For instance, it is incoherent to ask if the desire to get a drink might, in fact, typically cause people not to seek drink, but to seek sleep instead—for if, *per impossibile*, this were the case, we would no longer be talking about the desire for a drink. If X is, in part, constituted by its causal relations to Y, we cannot investigate whether X causes Y in the way Mill describes. Second, it should of course be acknowledged that behavior that *typically* manifests one motive may, in particular cases, be caused by another. Inference to the best explanation is not infallible, and we must be sensitive to patterns in behavior that would indicate this. But in particular cases, Mill's canons do even worse. Mill's canons establish relations between *types* of cause and their effects. For example, neither a statistical analysis of other occasions on which a singer has sung the national anthem, nor a statistical analysis of the various motives for which people generally tend to sing the national anthem, will alone provide an answer to why this singer sings it now (e.g., to impress her audience of patriots). Hopkins' method of interpretation, by contrast, is applicable to the particular case, even as it deploys general background knowledge.

[15] A further condition I do not discuss here is "availability" (see Nisbett and Wilson 1977, p. 251).

accuracy (Fletcher 1995, pp. 73–79; Gawronski 2004).[16] Hopkins' method is robust within limits.

But can the *everyday* method of inferring motives from behavior on the basis of intentional content be extended to become the basis for new *psychoanalytic* theories of unconscious motives? The three conditions that improve accuracy of inference are well-satisfied by psychoanalysts working in the clinical setting. As a result, such inferences may be rather more reliable than everyday ones. Nevertheless, I suspect the answer is "only so far," and this is why Grünbaum's challenge to psychoanalytic methodology is defensible. We should distinguish inferences from clinical data to:

   a. the present motives of the analysand in behaving as he does
   b. complex mental processes, such as defence mechanisms
   c. psychological structures, such as the superego or Klein's two "positions," and
   d. etiological accounts of the origins of any of (a) to (c).

Our everyday method of interpretation moves from current patterns of behavior to current motives (broadly construed). The forms of inference in (a) and (b) can be defended as an extension of this form of reasoning. With this information also comes information about psychic conflict. It is a central claim of psychoanalysis that such conflict is at the heart of neurosis, and the method of interpretation is capable of linking clinical data and such conflict in a way that can justify such a claim. (It is also on these claims that we argued there is corroboration.) However, our everyday method of interpretation has little (reliable) to say about inferences of types (c) and (d), and we need a further argument to think that metapsychological and etiological theories could be established in this way, without recourse to any data generated through the use of Mill's canons. There are too many factors of potential causal relevance to the formation of long-term dispositions, and many relevant non-psychoanalytic sources of evidence regarding the structure of the mind. Hence its traditional clinical methodology, if employed in isolation, does not enable psychoanalysis to provide scientifically respectable answers in these areas.

2.4 To finish our discussion of whether psychoanalysis is a science, it is worth switching perspectives. Rather than seeking to meet objections, is there an independent argument for a positive answer? One such argument can be made by appealing to the clinical results of psychoanalysis. Grünbaum (controversially) purports to find evidence of the following argument, defending Freud's central clinical claim that neurosis results from repression, in Freud's writings:

> (1) only the psychoanalytic method of interpretation and treatment can yield or mediate to the patient correct insight into the unconscious pathogens of his psychoneurosis, and (2) the analysand's correct insight into the etiology of his affliction and into the unconscious

---

[16] This evidence undermines the widespread view, first put forward by Ross (1977), that we suffer from a misleading theory about human behavior called the "fundamental attribution error": we assume that behavior is primarily the result of our "enduring and consistent dispositions" (Nisbett and Ross 1980, p. 31) rather than a response to the particular characteristics of the situation in which we act. We don't hold a faulty *theory* of human behavior, but we are, in *practice*, often too quick to attribute behavior to the agent's dispositions.

dynamics of his character is, in turn, *causally necessary* for the therapeutic conquest of his neurosis. (1984, pp. 139–140)

If these two claims are true, and if psychoanalysis is therapeutically successful, then this success validates the etiological hypotheses of psychoanalytic theory. The interpretations of the analyst must "tally" with the real causes of the analysand's neurosis, or cure will not follow (hence Grünbaum calls this the "Tally Argument"). However, the empirical support for (2) has been unforthcoming—"outcome studies" show that non-psychoanalytic therapies can be successful and there is even spontaneous remission. The argument fails.

In fact, recent evidence suggests caution about this conclusion. Certainly, there is no evidence to support that psychoanalytic therapy is *necessary* for "cure," but medical science does not work with necessary causes, only claims of relative causal efficacy. First, compared with spontaneous remission (no treatment), recent studies (e.g., Fonagy, et al. 2005; Leichsenring 2005; Milrod et al. 2007; Westen and Bradley 2005) show that psychotherapy (in general, not psychoanalysis specifically) has a considerable positive effect, with 80% of those treated ending up better than no-treatment controls. This effect size is as large as many medications for physical complaints, and greater than almost all treatments in cardiology, geriatric medicine, asthma, flu vaccination, and cataract surgery. Second, when it comes to comparing rival psychological therapies, some evidence is just now beginning to emerge that psychoanalysis is superior (see Shedler 2010 for a review). Why now?

First, most outcome studies compare rival psychotherapies with *short-term* psychoanalytic psychotherapy (up to six months), while some recent studies (de Maat et al. 2009; Knekt et al. 2008, 2011; Leichsenring 2011; Leichsenring and Rabung 2008) indicate that the benefits of psychodynamic psychotherapy become much more pronounced after six months' treatment, and that long-term psychodynamic psychotherapy *is* more successful in the long run, at least for chronic distress, mood, anxiety, and personality disorders. Second, outcome studies need something clear to measure, and it is less expensive to measure it over a short period of time, and so very few studies have measured what it is that psychoanalysis *now* would claim to be uniquely best at achieving, e.g., improving the patient's ability to tolerate a wider range of emotional experiences and be more emotionally "alive," to have a more satisfying sex life, to understand themselves and others in more nuanced ways, to live with greater freedom and flexibility. The empirical work is yet to be done on establishing whether there is an appropriate interpretation of "therapeutic success" according to which psychoanalysis uniquely delivers such success. However, such evidence would not demonstrate that it is veridical insight into the *origins* of the analysand's psychic structures of defense that is responsible for the therapeutic success, so etiological claims would still not be evidentially supported.

2.5 Our discussion has given us reason to believe that, as it is traditionally practiced, psychoanalysis is not a science. It faces challenges of confirmation bias, the absence of three standard correctives in the social sciences (triangulation, quasi-statistics, and comparisons), the absence of corroboration and the difficulty of defending its method of drawing inferences. The clinical theory does best, rebutting the last two objections at least, but this result could be greatly strengthened by finding solutions to the other issues. Given this assessment, it makes sense to ask:

COULD PSYCHOANALYSIS BE(COME) A SCIENCE?

There is a time lag in the our discussion "Could psychoanalysis (as it is) be a science?," and a narrowed focus on psychoanalysis as "traditionally practiced." The discussion ignores important developments of the last thirty years (with roots that extend throughout the history of psychoanalysis). A letter by Mary Target to the *New Scientist*, October 27, 2010, responding to an ill-informed article on the scientific status of psychoanalysis by Mario Bunge, states "The 54 signatories to this letter include distinguished researchers in psychoanalysis in the science faculties of leading world universities, who have acquired major public grants and have published papers in high-impact, peer-reviewed scientific journals." On this evidence, psychoanalysis is becoming accepted as a science. Two recent developments in psychoanalytic research are primarily responsible for this: an expansion of the methodology used to analyze the clinical data, and an interdisciplinary approach that utilizes findings from across psychology, including neuroscience. A third development, I shall argue, is additionally necessary, relating to the training and education of psychoanalysts. I consider the methodological issues first, and then comment briefly on training, before finishing with a comment on the interdisciplinary "turn."

3.1 The traditional clinical methodology of psychoanalytic theory involves defending claims on the basis of case studies. It does not utilize a variety of (statistical and non-statistical) forms of analysis of larger data sets. But the clinical data per se does not prevent deploying other methodologies,[17] and these may provide robust solutions to the objections considered in §§2.1-2.3. Robert Holt argues that

> [a] good deal can be done to test nonetiological hypotheses with the undeniably rich data of psychoanalyses, but only if they are fully recorded ... the data carefully if minimally censored to prevent recognition, and made available to all qualified researchers. Then at last we will have public and replicable data; then the researcher can be someone other than the therapist, and therefore truly disinterested and uncontaminated. (1985, p. 296)

Early examples of this kind of work include Dahl (1972), Luborsky (1977), and Gill (1982; and Gill and Hoffman 1982). Since then many such papers have appeared, testing hypotheses across clinical cases using statistical and quasi-statistical methods. Expanding clinical methodology in a different way, Kächele et al. (2008) have developed the single case study and significantly improved the rigor and objectivity of inferences drawn from it. They present the case study in eighty pages, followed by a 130-page analysis, with the evidence base of 517 audiotaped sessions made available to other researchers. A number of databases

---

[17] There is an ongoing debate over whether recording clinical sessions may influence the data; and whether more data is available to the analyst "live" than any recording can capture. It may be true that a fine level of detail and accuracy regarding the individual patient is lost, but there is good reason to think, from the work that has already been done, that enough remains—and remains the same—for general hypotheses to be tested.

of clinical material now exist, open to scrutiny and collectively running to tens of thousands of hours.

The introduction of these empirical methods of data analysis meets the three outstanding conditions on reducing bias left over from §2.2. Researchers can "triangulate" their conclusions, using a variety of methods, including "quasi-statistical" analyses and the comparison of findings across groups, either control groups or those used in other studies. An example: Luborsky (2001) seeks to identify the preconditions for recurrent symptoms, such as momentary forgetting, in psychotherapy. He examines the recurrence of seven symptoms manifested across seven audio-recorded analyses. The occurrence of symptoms is sampled in the context of the preceding thirty to fifty words and the preceding 300 to 400 words. These contexts are examined for psychological conditions they have in common. Twelve differentiating qualities were identified across the cases, and these were then rated for significance and intercorrelation, and five identified as most significant (viz., hopelessness, lack of control, anxiety, feeling blocked, and helplessness). A control group of contexts in which the symptoms were not manifest, chosen by arbitrary principles, was compared. Independent judges and a variety of scoring systems were deployed in generating the results. The five psychological conditions for symptom onset were then compared with a range of classical psychoanalytic theories, with "the most impressive conclusion" being the high match between the five conditions and those predicted by the theories (2001, p. 1148).

Similarly, the earlier appeal to corroboration, as a response to the challenge of suggestion, is strengthened if the corroboration remains once we deploy the new methodologies.

> With enough recorded treatments from a sufficient variety of analysts of all schools, it should be possible to find out just how far their patients' dreams, fantasies, childhood memories, etc. do systematically differ, and to what extent hypotheses of Freud's clinical theory hold, regardless of the nature of the treatment. If positive findings occur disproportionately more often in classical psychoanalyses ... that would imply that they are a consequence of suggestion. (Holt 1985, p. 295)

The absence of such positive findings is prima facie evidence of the absence of suggestion. Furthermore, from their interpretations of unconscious wishes and phantasies, psychoanalysts can make predictions regarding analysands' behavior (not specific acts, but classes of behavior, e.g., relation to authority figures) and postdictions regarding childhood events. Holt (1985, p. 301) notes that "Because so many thousands of us [psychoanalysts] have successfully made predictions and postdictions about particular cases informally ... the impression naturally arises that psychoanalytic theory has been thoroughly validated in clinical use." But he rightly argues that a stronger case rests on the new methodologies: "Predictions and postdictions must be regularly recorded, and then all relevant evidence recorded too, finally being judged blind, with control data, for relevance to the prediction (or postdiction)."

These developments do not take us beyond or outside psychoanalysis. The clinical data, and so the interaction between analyst and analysand, remain central, as the new methodologies are applied to clinical data. Only if psychoanalysis is mistakenly separated from the development of the psychoanalytic theory of the mind, e.g., by being identified exclusively with the attempt at facilitating individual self-interpretation, can the objection be made that these methods are no part of "psychoanalysis."

These methods do not solve the challenges facing the metapsychological and etiological theories noted in §2.3 and §2.4.[18] Here, psychoanalysis needs to turn toward interdisciplinary collaboration, on which I comment in §3.3.[19] But if we can meet the challenge of confirmation bias, these methods are sufficient to secure the clinical theory of psychoanalysis as scientific.

3.2 As noted in §2.2, one corrective to confirmation bias is to seek disconfirming evidence. Lord et al. (1984) and Hirt and Markman (1995) show that subjects who consider an *alternative explanation* of the evidence to the one they favor correct their confirmation bias. This simple strategy is more effective than attempting to be "fair and unbiased." It forces subjects to seek out evidence that distinguishes between rival explanations, which in turn leads to a better, more objective assessment of the evidence available. Thus, to avoid confirmation bias, the psychoanalyst needs to demonstrate that their preferred explanation is not merely "an" explanation, but better than alternatives. That is, psychoanalysis must explicitly adopt inference to the best explanation as its method, which is not merely a corrective to confirmation bias, but a key component of scientific method generally (Lipton 2004).

There are at least two "environments" in which psychoanalytic explanations compete. The first, "near" environment is the range of alternative psychoanalytic theories. What is necessary in developing theoretical psychoanalytic claims is an account that demonstrates one set of inferences is superior to those made by rival schools. The second, more "distant" environment comprises the range of non-psychoanalytic theories concerned with or impacting upon the data from which psychoanalytic inferences are drawn (e.g., alternative theories of dreaming and neurosis). To assess an inference as the best explanation, we need knowledge of the alternatives, and many of these may be generated outside the consulting room.

It may be that many of the phenomena that psychoanalysis seeks to explain simply do not have satisfactory alternative explanations, and that the unifying power of psychoanalytic explanation continues to provide reason to accept it. However, we can only know this to be true, if it is true, *if we know what these alternatives are*, and what the evidence is that supports them. Both factors change constantly—what was the best explanation may cease to be so, either because new evidence contra-indicates it or because a new, more powerful explanation is generated. The "environment of competition" can change, and has, of course, changed dramatically since Freud's initial proposals regarding the origin of neurosis 120 years ago.

[18] The disagreements between psychoanalytic schools regarding etiology and metapsychology are evidence either that everyone outside one's favored viewpoint is incompetent in drawing conclusions from clinical data or that clinical data doesn't determine the correct metapsychological theory. I prefer the second, more humble conclusion. It is noteworthy that as psychoanalysis has developed, so greater emphasis has come to be placed on working in the transference in the present, and less emphasis has been given to a reconstruction of the origin of neurosis. The usual reason offered for this shift is that the clinical data cannot reliably support historical reconstructions, but can give insight into present conflict.

[19] Of particular relevance to the etiological and developmental theories of psychoanalysis are the results of attachment theory (Ainsworth et al. 1978; Main and Goldwyn 1985; Cassidy and Shaver 1999; on the connections with psychoanalysis, see, e.g., Eagle 1997; Fonagy 2001; Fonagy and Target 2003, chapter 10; Holmes 2000).

Historically, psychoanalysts have not been good at practicing inference to the best explanation as described, failing to compare their claims to alternative theories. In this vein, a former editor of the *International Journal of Psychoanalysis* remarks that "by and large our standards of observation, of clarifying the distinction between observation and conceptualisation, and our standards of discussing and debating our observations are extraordinarily low; and they have received far too little attention" (Tuckett 1994, p. 865). In principle, at least, this issue can be resolved in the education and training of psychoanalysts. Such training would need to encourage psychoanalysts to test and compare explanations and theories, which in turn requires both that an atmosphere of intellectual enquiry and rigorous questioning is engendered and that trainees are provided with an education that covers a range of theories. Otto Kernberg (2000, 2006, 2007, 2010) complains that both are missing, and advocates a series of significant reforms to psychoanalytic training and education. He argues that many psychoanalytic training institutes fail to teach research skills and actively oppose original thought, and they ignore both the contributions of other schools of psychoanalysis and relevant information in non-psychoanalytic disciplines. The future development of psychoanalysis depends upon the integration of new knowledge from bordering disciplines.

A further reason to accept this last suggestion is that, to have confidence that a particular inference from clinical data is correct, we need to ensure that it does not directly conflict with well-established data elsewhere. It may be that a hypothesis has implications, e.g., relating to childhood development or mental processes, which are undermined by non-clinical data. On the other hand, non-clinical investigations may provide corroboration for an explanation first arrived at from clinical data, either in its existing form or in a modified form. This interaction between clinical and non-clinical data refines the explanation that is finally justified as "best." (This relation of psychoanalytic theory to non-clinical data should not, of course, be seen as a one-way street. Other psychological explanations and theories are just as beholden to well-established psychoanalytic clinical claims.) Working explicitly with inference to the best explanation as described can meet the objection from confirmation bias well enough to confirm the credentials of psychoanalysis as a science.[20]

3.3 It is well-known that Freud drew upon non-clinical sources in constructing psychoanalytic theory, most famously the work in neurology on which the economic model was based. But the full extent of his borrowings, laid out in Kitcher (1992), is rarely appreciated. From neurophysiology, Freud took ideas of neurons, psychic energy, and the reflex model of the mind; from psychology, associationism and the division of the mind into functional units; from psychiatry, the theory that neurotic behavior could be product of unconscious ideas, theories regarding the sexual origin of neurosis, and from his (and others') studies in aphasia, the claim that the idea of a thing and the idea of a word for a thing are separate (a claim that forms part of his theory of repression); from sexology, he took notions of infantile sexuality, stages of sexual development, and component instincts; and further borrowings are made from philology and sociology. From anthropology, he adopted an approach to understanding the mind by tracing lines of development from primitive ancestors, which can be

---

[20] Confirmation bias still occurs in scientific enquiry. For example, if a scientist hypothesizes that two events are causally related, this increases the chance that they will find supportive evidence and decreases the chance that they will find disconfirming evidence (Nisbett and Ross 1980, p. 97). Nickerson (1998, p. 194) suggests that it is the operation of science as an institution or community that neutralizes confirmation bias as far as it does.

detected not only in ancient cultures but in children and "primitive" people in the present. The same historical approach was taken from evolutionary biology and the theory of reca- pitulationism, which claims that ontogeny repeats phylogeny, i.e., the development of the individual organism passes through the stages of its evolutionary ancestors. Freud applies this form of explanation most famously to his theory that mental illness originates in earlier stages of psychosexual development.

These remarks show that engaging in interdisciplinary collaboration does not lead psy- choanalysis away from its roots, but returns it to them. More importantly, however, they show that in accepting any of Freud's claims that were influenced by or rested upon his bor- rowings from non-clinical sources, psychoanalysts are indirectly resting their views upon evidence from other disciplines. And this opens psychoanalysis to a new challenge to its scientific status, resulting from the dangers of interdisciplinary work. A mark of scientific enquiry, as Popper noted, is to amend one's theory in the light of new evidence. Where the evidence comes from a discipline other than one's own, it is easy to fail to keep up with advances and to overestimate the strength of the evidence, as one is not party to the contin- ual debate. For example, the pleasure principle, as Freud formulated it throughout his life, depends upon the reflex model of the nervous system: pleasure consists in the nervous sys- tem divesting itself of energy. In 1895, the model was defensible in neurology, but by 1940, it was not. Even by 1906, Sherrington had argued that there were severe difficulties facing the model. Yet no trace of this uncertainty appears in its adoption by psychoanalysis. Later psychoanalysts, e.g., Fenichel (1945), took their neurophysiology straight from Freud, and hence from 1895, and not from contemporary developments.

Of course, the significance of this particular example can be debated, given the develop- ment of psychoanalysis away from the economic model (though I doubt that contemporary psychoanalytic models of the pleasure principle have truly freed it from the influence of its original form). But given Freud's extensive borrowing from multiple disciplines, other examples may take its place, e.g., recapitulationism continues to affect psychoanalytic think- ing about mental illness as the re-emergence of earlier forms of mental functioning (Westen 1990). The central point cannot be argued away: As gaps open up between the contemporary developments in a discipline and its historically frozen representation in psychoanalysis, so psychoanalysis is made to "appear to rest on more and more outmoded, simplistic, and spec- ulative ideas" (Kitcher 1992, p. 163). If the disciplines on which Freud drew have moved on, rejecting ideas that psychoanalysis has embedded, those ideas need to be revisited within psychoanalytic theory as well. Evidence is being generated in other areas of psychology that is directly relevant to the truth of psychoanalytic claims.

Kitcher is critical of psychoanalysis for its failure to engage appropriately with the disci- plines from which evidence was borrowed. But in discussing Freud alone, she can, in turn, be criticized for failing to keep up with developments in psychoanalysis which seek to make good this error. It is noteworthy that she is equally critical of contemporary cognitive sci- ence, which she diagnoses as making the same mistakes in interdisciplinary theory con- struction as Freud. Her argument is not to object to interdisciplinary work, nor to argue that it is unscientific, but to advise caution. The interdisciplinary approach taken by Freud and advocated here strengthens the claim of psychoanalysis to be scientific, but avoiding the pit- falls that go with that approach will require careful attention.

Psychoanalysis cannot avoid this challenge as it cannot avoid interdisciplinary work if it is both to be a science and involved in defending a psychological theory that seeks to give an account of the structure and development of (aspects of) the mind. I have argued not only that these are appropriate ambitions of psychoanalysis (see §1.3), but that contemporary developments in the methodology of psychoanalysis are sufficient to secure the scientific status of claims regarding the motivational structure and complex mental processes involved in defense. In principle, these developments meet the challenges of suggestion, bias, and causal inference leveled against psychoanalysis in the historical debate. Even here, an awareness of relevant evidence in other fields is important. But a wider evidential base is crucial for metapsychological, etiological, and developmental claims, not only because the method of inference from clinical data is insufficient to establish such claims, but also because a historically dated evidential base is already implicated in psychoanalytic theory and requires constant revisiting and updating. I conclude that psychoanalysis—the form and method of generating a psychoanalytic model of the mind—can become, and is becoming, a science.

Acknowledgments

Thanks to Richard Gipps, Louise Braddock, and Constantine Sandis for their very helpful comments and support. Thanks especially to my research assistant, Maarten Steenhagen, for the very considerable administrative help and philosophical feedback he has given on this chapter, and to Heythrop College for providing the funding to enable this.

References

Abrams, S., Appy, G., Aslan, C. M., Goldberg, A., Guen, C. L., and Nunes, E. P. (1989). Pre-published statements for the 36th International Psychoanalytical Congress in Rome 30th July to 4th August 1989. *International Journal of Psycho-Analysis, 70*, 3–28.

Ainsworth, M. D., Blehar, M. C., Waters, E., and Wall, S. (1978). *Patterns of Attachment: A Psychological Study of the Strange Situation.* Hillsdale, NJ: Lawrence Erlbaum Associates.

Becker, H. S. (1970). *Sociological Work: Method and Substance.* Chicago, IL: Aldine.

Cassidy, J. and Shaver, P. R. (1999). *Handbook of Attachment: Theory, Research, and Clinical Applications.* New York, NY: Guilford Press.

Dahl, H. (1972). A quantitative study of a psychoanalysis. *Psychoanalysis and Contemporary Science, 1*(1), 237–57.

Dancy, J. (2000). *Practical Reality.* Oxford: Oxford University Press.

Davidson, D. (1963). Actions, reasons, and causes. *The Journal of Philosophy, 23*, 685–700.

Eagle, M. (1997). Attachment and psychoanalysis. *British Journal of Medical Psychology, 70*(3), 217–29.

Erwin, E. (1996). *A Final Accounting: Philosophical and Empirical Issues in Freudian Psychology.* Cambridge, MA: MIT.

Fenichel, O. (1945). *The Psychoanalytic Theory of Neurosis.* New York, NY: W. W. Norton.

Fisher, S. and Greenberg, R. P. (1977). *The Scientific Credibility of Freud's Theories and Therapy.* New York, NY: Basic Books.

Fletcher, G. J. O. (1995). *The Scientific Credibility of Folk Psychology.* Mahwah, NJ: Lawrence Erlbaum Associates.

Flew, A. (1949). Psycho-analytic explanation. *Analysis, 10*(1), 8–15.

Fonagy, P. (2001). *Attachment Theory and Psychoanalysis*. London: Other Press.

Fonagy, P., Roth, A., and Higgitt, A. (2005). The outcome of psychodynamic psychotherapy for psychological disorders. *Clinical Neuroscience Research*, 4(5–6), 367–77.

Fonagy, P. and Target, M. (2003). *Psychoanalytic Theories: Perspectives from Developmental Psychopathology*. London: Whurr.

Freud, S. (1895). Project for a scientific psychology. In J. Strachey (Ed.), *Standard Edition of the Complete Psychological Works of Sigmund Freud* (Vol. I), pp. 281–391. London: Hogarth Press.

Freud, S. (1914a). On narcissism: An introduction. In J. Strachey (Ed.), *Standard Edition* (Vol. XIV), pp. 67–102. London: Hogarth Press.

Freud, S. (1914b). On the history of the psycho-analytic movement. In J. Strachey (Ed.), *Standard Edition* (Vol. XIV), pp. 1–66. London: Hogarth Press.

Freud, S. (1917). Mourning and melancholia. In J. Strachey (Ed.), *Standard Edition* (Vol. XIV), pp. 237–258. London: Hogarth Press.

Freud, S. (1924). The economic problem of masochism. In J. Strachey (Ed.) *Standard Edition* (Vol. XIX), pp. 155–70. London: Hogarth Press.

Freud, S. (1933). New introductory lectures on psycho-analysis. In J. Strachey (Ed.) *Standard Edition* (Vol. XXII), pp. 1–182. London: Hogarth Press.

Freud, S. (1954). *The Origins of Psychoanalysis* (M. Bonaparte, A. Freud, and E. Kris, Eds). New York, NY: Basic Books.

Gawronski, B. (2004). Theory-based bias correction in dispositional inference: the fundamental attribution error is dead, long live the correspondence bias. *European Review of Social Psychology*, 15(1), 183–217.

Gill, M. M. (1982). *Analysis of Transference Vol. 1: Theory and Technique*. New York, NY: International Universities Press.

Gill, M. M. and Hoffman, I. Z. (1982). *Analysis of Transference Vol. 2: Studies of Nine Audio-Recorded Psychoanalytic Sessions*. New York, NY: International Universities Press.

Goldie, P. (2000). *The Emotions*. Oxford: Clarendon Press.

Grünbaum, A. (1984). *The Foundations of Psychoanalysis: A Philosophical Critique*. Berkeley, CA: University of California Press.

Grünbaum, A. (2004). The hermeneutic versus the scientific conception of psychoanalysis. In J. Mills (Ed.), *Psychoanalysis at the Limit: Epistemology, Mind, and the Question of Science*, pp. 139–60. Albany, NY: State University of New York Press.

Habermas, J. (1972). *Knowledge and Human Interests*. London: Heinemann.

Hirt, E. R. and Markman, K. D. (1995). Multiple explanation: A consider-an-alternative strategy for debiasing judgments. *Journal of Personality and Social Psychology*, 69(6), 1069–89.

Hobson, J. A. (1988). Psychoanalytic dream theory. In P. Clark and C. Wright (Eds), *Psychoanalysis, Mind and Science*, pp. 277–308. Oxford: Basil Blackwell.

Holmes, J. (2000). Attachment theory and psychoanalysis: a rapprochement. *British Journal of Psychotherapy*, 17(2), 157–72.

Holt, R. R. (1965). A review of some of Freud's biological assumptions and their influence on his theories. In N. S. Greenfield and W. C. Lewis (Eds), *Psychoanalysis and Current Biological Thought*, pp. 93–124. Madison, WI: University of Wisconsin Press.

Holt, R. R. (2002). Quantitative research on the primary process: method and findings. *Journal of the American Psychoanalytic Association*, 50(2), 457–82.

Holt, R. R. (2009). *Primary Process Thinking: Theory, Measurement, and Research*. Lanham, MD: Jason Aronson.

Hopkins, J. (1988). Epistemology and depth psychology: critical notes on *The Foundations of Psychoanalysis*. In P. Clark and C. Wright (Eds), *Mind, Psychoanalysis and Science*, pp. 33–60. Oxford: Blackwell Publishing.

Kächele, H., Schachter, J., and Thomä, H. (2008). *From Psychoanalytic Narrative to Empirical Single Case Research*. London: Routledge.

Kazdin, A. E. (1981). Drawing valid inferences from case studies. *Journal of Consulting and Clinical Psychology*, *49*(2), 183–92.

Kernberg, O. F. (2000). A concerned critique of psychoanalytic education. *International Journal of Psycho-Analysis*, *81*(1), 97–120.

Kernberg, O. F. (2006). The coming changes in psychoanalytic education: Part I. *International Journal of Psycho-Analysis*, *87*(6), 1650–73.

Kernberg, O. F. (2007). The coming changes in psychoanalytic education: Part II. *International Journal of Psycho-Analysis*, *88*(1), 183–202.

Kernberg, O. F. (2010). A new organization of psychoanalytic education. *Psychoanalytic Review*, *97*(6), 997–1020.

Kitcher, P. (1992). *Freud's Dream: A Complete Interdisciplinary Science of Mind*. Cambridge, MA: MIT.

Klein, G. S. (1976). *Psychoanalytic Theory: An Exploration of Essentials*. New York, NY: International Universities Press.

Knekt, P., Lindfors, O., Härkänen, T., Välikoski, M., Virtala, E., Laaksonen, M. A., *et al.* (2008). Randomized trial on the effectiveness of long- and short-term psychodynamic psychotherapy and solution-focused therapy on psychiatric symptoms during a 3-year follow-up. *Psychological Medicine*, *38*, 689–703.

Knekt, P., Lindfors, O., Laaksonen, M. A., Renlund, C., Haaramo, P., Härkänen, T., *et al.* (2011). Quasi-experimental study on the effectiveness of psychoanalysis, long-term and short-term psychotherapy on psychiatric symptoms, work ability and functional capacity during a 5-year follow-up. *Journal of Affective Disorders*, *132*, 37–47.

Lacewing, M. (2012). Inferring motives in psychology and psychoanalysis. *Philosophy, Psychiatry & Psychology*, *19*, 197–212.

Lacewing, M. (2013). The problem of suggestion in psychoanalysis: an analysis and solution. *Philosophical Psychology*. DOI:10.1080/09515089.2012.725533.

Lakatos, I. (1978). *The Methodology of Scientific Research Programmes*. Cambridge: Cambridge University Press.

Leichsenring, F. (2005). Are psychodynamic and psychoanalytic therapies effective?: a review of empirical data. *International Journal of Psycho-Analysis*, *86*(3), 841–68.

Leichsenring, F. (2011). Long-term psychodynamic psychotherapy in complex mental disorders: update of a meta-analysis. *British Journal of Psychiatry*, *199*, 15–22.

Leichsenring, F. and Rabung, S. (2008). Effectiveness of long-term psychodynamic psychotherapy. *Journal of the American Medical Association*, *300*(13), 1551–65.

Lipton, P. (2004). *Inference to the Best Explanation*. London: Routledge.

Lord, C. G., Lepper, M. R., and Preston, E. (1984). Considering the opposite: a corrective strategy for social judgment. *Journal of Personality and Social Psychology*, *47*(6), 1231–43.

Luborsky, L. (1977). Measuring a pervasive psychic structure in psychotherapy: the core conflictual relationship theme. In N. Freedman and S. Grand (Eds), *Communicative Structures and Psychic Structures*, pp. 367–395. New York, NY: Plenum.

Luborsky, L. (2001). The only clinical and quantitative study since Freud of the preconditions for recurrent symptoms during psychotherapy and psychoanalysis. *International Journal of Psycho-Analysis*, *82*(6), 1133–54.

de Maat, S., de Jonghe, F., Schoevers, R., and Dekker, J. (2009). The effectiveness of long-term psychoanalytic therapy: a systematic review of empirical studies. *Harvard Review of Psychiatry*, 17(1), 1–23.

Maier, N. R. F. (1931). Reasoning in humans II: the solution of a problem and its appearance in consciousness. *Journal of Comparative Psychology*, 12(2), 181–94.

Main, M. and Goldwyn, R. (1985). *Adult Attachment Interview: Scoring and Classification manual*. Unpublished manuscript, University of California at Berkeley.

Marmor, J. (1962). Psychoanalytic therapy as an educational process. In J. Messerman (Ed.) *Psychoanalytic Education Science Series*, pp. 286–99. New York, NY: Grune & Stratton.

Masling, J. M. and Bornstein, R. F. (1983–1998). *Empirical Studies of Psychoanalytic Theories* (Vols I–VIII). Hillsdale, NJ: The Analytic Press.

Maxwell, J. A. (2009). Designing a qualitative study. In L. Bickman and D. J. Rog (Eds), *The SAGE Handbook of Applied Social Research Methods*, pp. 69–100. Thousand Oaks, CA: Sage.

Mill, J. S. (1904). *A System of Logic, Ratiocinative and Inductive*. London: Harper.

Milrod, B., Leon, A. C., Busch, F., Rudden, M., Schwalberg, M., Clarkin, J., *et al.* (2007). A randomized controlled clinical trial of psychoanalytic psychotherapy for panic disorder. *American Journal of Psychiatry*, 164(2), 265–72.

Nickerson, R. S. (1998). Confirmation bias: A ubiquitous phenomenon in many guises. *Review of General Psychology*, 2(2), 175–220.

Nisbett, R. E. and Wilson, T. D. (1977). Telling more than we can know: Verbal reports on mental processes. *Psychological Review*, 84(3), 231–59.

Nisbett, R. E. and Ross, L. (1980). *Human Inference: Strategies and Shortcomings of Social Judgment*. Englewood Cliffs NJ: Prentice-Hall.

O' Connor, T. and Sandis, C. (Eds) (2010). *A Companion to the Philosophy of Action*. Oxford: Blackwell Publishing.

Patton, M. Q. (2000). *Qualitative Evaluation and Research Methods* (3rd edn.). Thousand Oaks, CA: Sage.

Peters, R. (1950). Cure, cause and motive: two brief notes. *Analysis*, 11, 148–54.

Popper, K. (1963). *Conjectures and Refutations*. London: Routledge & Kegan Paul.

Popper, K. (1983). *Realism and the Aim of Science*. London: Hutchinson.

Popper, K. (1995). *The Open Society and its Enemies*. London: Routledge & Kegan Paul.

Ricoeur, P. (1970). *Freud and Philosophy: An Essay on Interpretation*. New Haven, CT: Yale University Press.

Rosenblatt, A. D. (1989). Reinspecting the foundations of psychoanalysis: a rejoinder to Adolph Grünbaum. *Psychoanalysis and Contemporary Thought*, 12(1), 73–96.

Rosenthal, R. (1997). *Interpersonal expectancy effects: a forty year perspective*. Paper presented at American Psychological Association Convention, Chicago.

Rosenthal, R. (2000). Expectancy effects. In A. E. Kazdin (Ed.), *Encyclopedia of Psychology* (Vol. 3), pp. 294–6. Washington, DC: American Psychological Association.

Rosenthal, R. and Rosnow, R. L. (2009). *Artifacts in Behavioral Research: Robert Rosenthal and Ralph L. Rosnow's Classic Books*. Oxford: Oxford University Press.

Rosenthal, R. and Rubin, D. B. (1978). Interpersonal expectancy effects: the first 345 studies. *Behavioral and Brain Sciences*, 1(3), 377–86.

Ross, L. (1977). The intuitive psychologist and his shortcomings: distortions in the attribution process. In L. Berkowitz (Ed.), *Advances in Experiments Social Psychology*, pp. 173–214. New York, NY: Academic Press.

Rubinstein, B. B. (1976). On the possibility of a strictly clinical psychoanalytic theory: an essay in the philosophy of psychoanalysis. *Psychological Issues*, 9(4), 229–64.

Shedler, J. (2010). The efficacy of psychodynamic psychotherapy. *American Psychologist*, 65(2), 98–109.

Solms, M. and Turnbull, O. (2002). *The Brain and the Inner World*. New York, NY: Other Press.

Taylor, C. (1964). *The Explanation of Behaviour*. London: Routledge & Kegan Paul.

Toulmin, S. (1948). The logical status of psycho-analysis. *Analysis*, 9(2), 23–9.

Tuckett, D. (1994). The conceptualisation and communication of clinical facts in psychoanalysis. *International Journal of Psycho-Analysis*, 75, 865–70.

Wallerstein, R. S. (1990). Psychoanalysis: the common ground. *International Journal of Psycho-Analysis*, 71, 3–20.

Wallerstein, R. S. (2005). Psychoanalytic controversies: will psychoanalytic pluralism be an enduring state of our discipline? *International Journal of Psycho-Analysis*, 86(3), 623–38.

Westen, D. (1990). Towards a revised theory of borderline object relations: contributions of empirical research. *International Journal of Psycho-Analysis*, 71, 661–93.

Westen, D. (1998). The scientific legacy of Sigmund Freud: Toward a psychodynamically informed psychological science. *Psychological Bulletin*, 124(3), 333–71.

Westen, D. (1999). The scientific status of unconscious processes: Is Freud really dead? *Journal of the American Psychoanalytic Association*, 47(4), 1061–106.

Westen, D. and Bradley, R. (2005). Empirically supported complexity: rethinking evidence-based practice in psychotherapy. *Current Directions in Psychological Science*, 14(5), 266–71.

Wilson, T. (2002). *Strangers to Ourselves: Discovering the Adaptive Unconscious*. Cambridge: Belknap.

CURE AND CARE

CHAPTER 65

....

INTRODUCTION: CURE
AND CARE

....

This section examines several moral dilemmas and epistemological aporias in clinical practice and shows how clinicians can benefit from the introduction of philosophical methods
and discourse. The authors develop these issues having in mind emblematic mental disorders (e.g., depression, personality disorders, schizophrenia) and typical clinical situations
(e.g., how to establish an effective therapeutic relationship with borderline persons, dream
interpretation, cognitive behavioral therapy (CBT)). One important claim shared by the
authors and made explicit by Foddy et al., is that a great effort has been made to ground
psychiatry on evidence-based science, and to tie it to our growing understanding of the
human brain. This is obviously an exceedingly important project, but it would be a mistake
to assume that the central questions of psychiatry can be completely resolved through scientific inquiry. Science offers guidance for clinical practice only in light of our concepts and
normative judgments.

In Chapter 66, Pickard focuses on a philosophical and clinical conundrum: the combination of responsibility and blame as related to people with "disorders of agency" as severe
personality disorder, addiction, and eating disorders. Clinicians know well that blame is a
common emotion kindled by these patients, and that this is highly detrimental since it may
trigger feelings of rejection and self-blame in them, which bring heightened risk of disengagement from treatment, distrust and breach of the therapeutic alliance, and potentially
self-harm. Clinicians should hold these persons responsible and accountable for behavior
and at the same time compassion and empathy should be maintained. To do so, two sorts
of blame should be sorted out: "detached" and "affective." Detached blame consists in judgments of blameworthiness, and involves accountability and answerability. It encourages
responsible agency. Affective blame consists in negative reactions and emotions, whether
rational or not, which the blamer feels entitled to have. Effective treatment requires responsibility without affective blame: without a sense of entitlement to any negative reactive attitudes and emotions one might experience.

What is autonomy is the focus of Rodoilska's contribution (Chapter 67). Defining "autonomy" is a crucial topic in practical neuropsychiatric ethics since patients with severe mental
disorders, and especially schizophrenic and manic–depressive ("bipolar") psychoses, often
refuse treatment, and it can be especially difficult to establish if such refusals are made by
completely autonomous agents, given the effects that mental disorders can have on a person's

mental capacities. Autonomy can be defined from at least four major philosophical angles. The first relates autonomy to agency and free will, and defines it in terms of motivational states, such as identification, endorsement, or acceptance. A second approach explores it as related to particular values, such as self-respect. A third one sees autonomy in terms of rational agency and moral responsibility and concentrates on the links between responsiveness to reasons and effective control over one's life. Finally, autonomy as a central topic in bioethics is examined in connection to informed consent and decisional capacity. Rodoilska endorses a view of autonomy as primarily an agency concept and applies it to some paradoxes of depression.

The "medicalization" and extensive use of psychiatric drugs to treat a growing list of psychopathological conditions claimed to afflict people who would have been considered normal even in the recent past is one of the biggest changes in first-world lifestyles since the 1970s. Foddy et al. (Chapter 69) argue that this raises serious ethical and epistemological problems: Are "new" illnesses "invented" merely to promote the interests of pharmaceutical companies? Are these new clinical diagnoses in effect value judgments disguised as objective scientific categories? And, if psychotropic drugs threaten to disrupt a person's identity, or disconnect emotion from circumstance and self, will these extensive use of medical treatments in subclinical population affect our sense of being a person and the very philosophical concept of "person"?

A closely related topic is the main focus of Chapter 68 by Svenaeus: How do antidepressant drugs affect the self? The author begins with distinguishing the groups of traits that belong to personality (temperaments, ways of acting, habits, skills, emotional dispositions, enduring preferences and values, and character traits) from the different layers of selfhood (pre-reflective embodied self, reflective self, and narrative self) and then argues that if personality disorders and neuropsychiatric disorders (developmental disorders) are clearly related to personality traits of the self (the person), there are other mental disorders that seem rather to be disorders, not of personality, but of the self itself. The effects of the new antidepressants must be thought of in terms of changes in self-feeling or, more precisely, of "self-vibration of embodiment." Some patients go through the experience of "becoming themselves" while on Prozac, whereas others have the experience of "losing themselves," despite feeling better on the drug. Antidepressant medication represents a way to change this mood profile in a way that is more direct than the ways of psychotherapy, and the effect in question is not limited to alleviating the suffering. It will also have some effects on self and personality, since the temperament and emotional dispositions of the person are, indeed, basic to selfhood.

Similar worries about the ways drugs (including placebos) may affect identity and the self are discussed by Jopling in Chapter 70, which debunks some of the myths surrounding placebo effects through a survey of some of the discoveries that have been made in the last fifty years about placebo effects in medicine. It then looks at how placebo effects make an appearance in psychiatry and psychotherapy, particularly in the case of treatments of depression that involve psychoactive medication and/or talk therapy. Following this is a survey of some of the leading definitions of the placebo effect, as well as a survey of some of the leading explanatory theories. The chapter concludes with a discussion of some new directions in placebo research: namely, open-label placebos and the evolutionary origins of placebo effects.

The last three chapters are focused on "psychological" issues. The concept of care is closely linked to that of the unconscious. Heidegger and Freud, arguably the two greatest "meta-physicians" of the twentieth century, sought to develop a comprehensive account of the human condition and its affliction of the contemporary human situation. Challenging the science of their time, both sought to develop a new science of the human being to serve as the theoretical foundation for psychotherapeutic practice and its application. Heidegger inspired the development of various forms of existential analysis while Freud generated his immensely influential theory/practice of psychoanalysis. Askay and Farquhar (Chapter 71) show that, beyond differences, there is an intimate belonging together of Freud's and Heidegger's views since both have grasped concealment—the unconscious dimension—as a fundamentally important realm of human existence. Heidegger offers a unified account of the hidden ontological dimension of human existence, while Freud offers an account of those hidden conditions through our bodily being. Taken together, they afford a considerably complete account of the human condition, and its relation with meaning, freedom, and autonomy.

In Chapter 72, Gipps discusses four objections to CBT: (1) various CBT formulations conflate the formal relations between different aspects of the same state with causal relations between discrete inner states; (2) some CBT models construe emotionally laden perspectives too much as occurrent inner processes, and too little as a subject's attitudes; (3) such attitudes can sometimes be misdescribed in CBT models as beliefs—when what we really have to deal with here are feelings; (4) CBT models can underplay the significance of changes in the form of (a subject's ownership of) such attitudes when they focus instead on changing their content. Gipps explains that his purpose is not to critique the CBTs en bloc, but instead to scrutinize some ways in which some CBT theories may be inflected in ways that go against what it means to be an emotionally alive human subject. The CBT practitioner is perhaps not aware of what she is really doing with the patient. By helping the patient to give articulate structure to his fears, to think, to be nourished by reality contact, and to distinguish fearful fantasy from genuinely representational belief, the CBT practitioner can be understood as doing far more than helping the patient to regulate his emotions and test out his cognitions: she is perhaps helping to restore her patient's subjectivity.

In Chapter 73, the final chapter of the section, Hopkins brings together psychoanalysis and neurobiology through evolutionary and attachment theories. Psychiatry is liable to tension between a clinical approach that concentrates on the lived experience of mental disorder and a neurobiological one that focuses on the brain in which such experience is realized. Accounts of mental disorder provided by Freud and his successors should not be taken as alternatives to a more adequate neurobiology of mental disorder. Building on clinical as well as anthropological and biological evidence, he puts conflict at the heart of human life. Human beings belong to an astonishingly social but also lethally group-aggressive species. Hopkins sorts out two basic kinds of conflicts: between incompatible emotions and desires, felt toward one and the same person, and between parts or aspects of the self. These emotional conflicts, in turn, seem rooted in evolution, together with the "moral" emotions that go awry in mental disorder as well. Our brain is equipped to deal with conflicts: it has a conflict-mitigating function. It regulates our own emotion by internal representations of ourselves as in relation to members of our own species. Important forms of mental disorder seem rooted in conflicts, and in the fictive experiences by which the brain tries to regulate it.

CHAPTER 66

RESPONSIBILITY WITHOUT BLAME: PHILOSOPHICAL REFLECTIONS ON CLINICAL PRACTICE

HANNA PICKARD

My first experience as a clinician was in a Therapeutic Community for service users with personality disorder.[1] As well as having personality disorder, many of the Community members also suffered from related conditions, such as addiction and eating disorders. Broadly speaking, these conditions are what we might call "disorders of agency." Core diagnostic symptoms or maintaining factors of disorders of agency are actions and omissions: patterns of behavior central to the nature or maintenance of the condition. For instance, borderline personality disorder is diagnosed in part via deliberate self-harm and attempted suicide, reckless and impulsive behavior, substance use, violence, and outbursts of anger; addiction is diagnosed via maladaptive patterns of drug consumption; eating disorders involve eating too much or too little. If a service user is to improve let alone recover from these disorders, they must change the diagnostic or maintaining pattern of behavior.[2] For instance, service users with borderline personality disorder must stop self-harming; addicts need to quit using drugs or alcohol; anorexics must eat. There are, no doubt, equally central cognitive and affective components to these disorders. Borderline personality disorder involves instability of self-image and emotional volatility; addicts may use drugs and alcohol to deal with psychological distress; anorexics may have over-valued ideas about low body weight and express anger and achieve a sense of control by refusing to eat. Nonetheless, actions and omissions are diagnostically central to disorders of agency: effective treatment must address these patterns of behavior, even if outcome is improved by an integrative approach that treats behavior alongside cognition and affect.

Service users with personality disorder are notoriously difficult to treat. Within psychiatry they are stigmatized as the service users "no one likes." In his landmark study of staff

---

[1] For further information on the nature and treatment of personality disorder see Box 66.1.
[2] Cf. Pearce and Pickard (2010).

attitudes to service users with personality disorder in three High Security Hospitals in the UK, Len Bowers suggests the following explanation:

> The generally hopeless, pessimistic attitudes of carers can be seen to originate in the difficult behaviours of PD [personality disorder] patients. They bully, con, capitalize, divide, condition, and corrupt those around them. They make complaints over inconsequential or non-existent issues in order to manipulate staff. They can be seriously violent over unpredictable and objectively trivial events, or may harm and disfigure themselves in ways that have an intense emotional impact on staff. If this were not enough, they also behave in the same way towards each other, provoking serious problems that the staff have to manage and contain. (Bowers 2002, p. 65)

This description is in many ways accurate. Within the Therapeutic Community where I worked, Community members regularly behaved in ways that were harmful to staff and other members, even if physical violence was very unusual. They could be emotionally cruel, or extremely angry and threatening without just cause; they might self-harm or disengage from the Community without explanation, provoking high levels of anxiety in others concerned for their well-being; they might shirk their Community tasks and responsibilities, leaving others to pick up the work. But the staff attitude towards this behavior was not as Bower describes. Rather, the staff were very clear about what their attitude as clinicians should be, and usually, although not invariably, succeeded in achieving it. Service users were responsible for their actions and omissions and accountable to the Community for them, but an attitude of compassion and empathy prevailed, and they were not blamed. As a novice clinician, this stance of responsibility without blame struck me forcefully. It is very different from our ordinary, non-clinical reactive attitudes, where behavior of the sort described typically evokes blame, no doubt alongside related attitudes such as dislike and rejection. And, if I am honest, I initially had no idea how this stance was possible to achieve: when a service user, who was not psychotic and knew what they were doing, was angry and threatening toward me for no reason, and made me feel angry and scared, how was I to hold them responsible for this behavior without blaming them for it? I could make sense of the idea that, despite appearances, they might not be responsible because their disorder excused them, and hence not to be blamed. And I could make sense of the idea that, despite their disorder, they were responsible, and hence to be blamed. But the combination of responsibility without blame for wrongdoing struck me as a philosophical and clinical conundrum.

This chapter offers a solution to this conundrum. Appropriate clinical engagement with the actions and omissions that are the core symptoms or maintaining factors of disorders of agency is central to effective treatment. Clinicians must hold service users responsible and accountable for behavior if they are to improve and recover.[3] But blame, in contrast, is highly detrimental.[4] Blaming service users may trigger feelings of rejection, anger, and self-blame, which bring heightened risk of disengagement from treatment, distrust and breach of the therapeutic alliance, relapse, and, with service users with personality disorder, potentially even self-harm or attempts at suicide: it is essential that compassion and empathy be maintained. So how is this combination possible: How is it possible for clinicians to

---

[3] Cf. Pearce and Pickard (2010) and Pickard (2011).

[4] Cf. Gilbert (2010). For an ex-service user perspective on the role of blame in impeding recovery see Lisa Ward's commentary on this chapter.

hold service users responsible for actions and omissions that are central to their disorder and cause harm and suffering, without blaming them for them? This chapter has five parts. First, I describe the conundrum in more detail. I suggest that clinicians can often find themselves trapped between a desire to rescue and a desire to blame, despite neither response being clinically effective. The key to avoiding this trap is to link responsibility fundamentally to the idea of agency, and to distinguish it clearly from ideas of blameworthiness and blame. So, second, I offer a conceptual framework that clearly distinguishes ideas of responsibility, blameworthiness, and blame. I suggest that these distinctions have not always been sufficiently marked within philosophy, and I argue that clinical practice illustrates the need to do so. Third, within this framework, I distinguish two sorts of blame, which I respectively call "detached" and "affective." Affective, not detached, blame is detrimental to effective treatment. I sketch an account of what affective blame is. This overall framework is central to understanding how the stance of holding a person responsible for harm but not blaming them is conceptually possible. Fourth, I turn to the question of how clinicians can effectively keep affective blame at bay. It is one thing for the appropriate clinical stance to be conceptually possible, but quite another for it to be achieved in practice. I suggest that the key to striking this balance, and avoiding the rescue/blame trap, is an understanding of each individual service user's past history, and that history's power to directly evoke compassion and empathy. Finally, I conclude with some brief reflections on whether or not the clinical stance of responsibility without blame is an appropriate ideal to which we should aspire in ordinary, non-clinical interpersonal contexts.

THE CLINICAL TRAP

Bowers found that staff working with service users with personality disorders believe that, unless the service users are also psychotic or otherwise cognitively impaired, they are responsible for their behavior because they act deliberately and "know what they are doing" (2002, p. 85). When the behavior causes harm, they are therefore "to blame" for the harm caused. We can express this line of thought thus:

1. Service users with personality disorder have control and conscious knowledge[5] of their behavior.
2. Therefore they are responsible for their behavior.
3. The behavior causes harm.
4. Therefore they are to blame for the harm.

---

[5] Throughout this chapter, I use the term "conscious knowledge" of behavior to refer to the way we normally know what we are doing when we do it. It is not straightforward to say what this way is. Normally, we have some knowledge of why we are acting, some knowledge of how we are acting, some knowledge of what we intend in acting, and some knowledge of what effects our actions have on the world. All of this can be part of what we mean when we say we know what we are doing when we act. I do not develop a nuanced account of 'conscious knowledge' in this chapter, but rely on our intuitive understanding.

(1) and (2) embody our common sense conception of agency and responsibility. Our common sense conception of agency draws a basic distinction between actions and mere bodily movements, such as automatic reflexes. What makes a piece of behavior an action, as opposed to a mere bodily movement, is that it is voluntary, where this means that the agent can exercise choice and at least a degree of control over the behavior. This conception of agency and action is traditionally linked, within philosophy, to the idea of free will.[6] On this view, agency and action require two capacities. First, the capacity to choose from a range of possible actions, at least in the minimal sense that, on any particular occasion, one can choose either to act, or to refrain from so acting. Second, the capacity to execute this choice: to do as one chooses, given normal circumstances.[7] This common sense conception of agency naturally grounds judgments of responsibility: one is responsible for actions, as opposed to automatic reflexes, because it is up to one whether and how one acts. So long as one knows what one is doing, one is responsible for one's behavior to the degree that one can exercise choice and control over it.

Core symptoms and maintaining factors of disorders of agency are not mere bodily movements. They are kinds of actions and omissions: the kinds of behavior over which we have choice and control. On the whole, service users possess both relevant capacities with respect to these behaviors. On at least most if not all occasions, service users diagnosed with disorders of agency could, for example, choose not to self-harm or be violent, drink or take drugs, binge or refuse to eat. The evidence for this claim is relatively straightforward: service users routinely do choose to behave otherwise and alter entrenched patterns of behavior, when they have incentive, motivation, and genuinely want to do so.[8] Indeed, this is presupposed by most standard forms of effective psychological treatment for disorders of agency. Cognitive behavioral therapy, motivational interviewing, stop-and-think training, exposure therapy, emotional intelligence, mentalization-based therapy, group therapy for addiction, and Therapeutic Communities, are all united in presuming that service users have the capacity for choice and control over maladaptive behavior, and that the clinical aim is, at least in part, to engage this capacity and support the service user to do things differently and alter entrenched maladaptive patterns. These therapies differ only in the extent to which this presumption is explicitly part of how the clinician engages the service user. For instance, in motivational interviewing, the clinician adopts a non-challenging stance, simply expressing empathy and encouraging the service user to see the unwanted consequences of their behavior. In contrast, the language of agency and responsibility permeates the culture of Therapeutic Communities: the Community is explicit that members are expected to see themselves and others in this light. But in all cases, it is a presumption of treatment that service users have choice and control over their behavior and can therefore be asked to take responsibility for it, as we naturally say.

However, it is important to note two caveats. First, service users with disorders of agency may not always have full conscious knowledge of why they are behaving as they do, or what

---

[6] Steward (2009, 2012) offers a contemporary defence of the view and argues that it is found in philosophers as diverse as Aristotle (1984), Hobbes (1999), Hume (1975), Kant (1960), and Reid (1994). See too Alvarez (2009) for further defence and Bobzien (1998) for historical discussion.

[7] Cf. Holton (2010); for an important analysis of the nature of such capacities, see M. Smith (2003).

[8] Cf. Pickard (2012), Pickard (2013), and Pickard and Pearce (in press). For an ex-service user perspective on the role of choice in recovery see Lisa Ward's commentary on this chapter.

the full effects of their behavior on others may be. Of course, in this, they are not unique: this is a predicament we all face to some extent. But it is possible that some kinds of disorders, most obviously borderline personality disorder, will be associated with reduced capacity for such conscious knowledge: the possibility of mentalization deficits (Fonagy et al. 2004) and high levels of emotional arousal associated with borderline personality disorder may have this effect. Second, it is important to recognize that, on the common sense conception of agency presented earlier, control is a graded notion, and the degree of control possessed by service users with disorders of agency may sometimes be diminished compared to the norm. Patterns of behavior associated with these disorders may be habitual and strongly desired. In so far as these patterns are ways of coping with psychological distress, service users may lack alternative coping mechanisms. Without these alternatives, alongside the hope of a better life, they may also lack the will or motivation to change their behavior, to kick a habitual pattern, and find another way of behaving that is less harmful to self and others. For these reasons, control may be diminished relative to the norm, and with it, responsibility.[9] But reduction is not extinction. The core symptoms and maintaining factors of disorders of agency include actions and omissions: there is at least a degree, and often a significant one, of choice and control.

(1) and (2) thus not only reflect our common sense conception of agency and responsibility. With the earlier mentioned caveats, they are also correctly applicable to service users with disorders of agency. Nonetheless, clinicians working with such service users recognize, at least to some extent, the effect blame can have on care, and struggle not to blame service users for the harm they cause. To this end, so as not to blame service users, they may swing to the opposite pole, and deny (1) and (2). They instead try to rescue service users from blame by denying their agency and absolving them of responsibility. This alternative response may be bolstered by the obvious fact that service users with disorders of agency suffer extreme degrees of distress and dysfunction, which they may have no clear sense how to alleviate or manage, together with the fact that it is a clinician's duty to help and to care. In this mindset, staff may hold that service users "cannot help" behaving as they do. Indeed, this idea is in keeping with popular conceptions of pathological compulsion, whereby the disorder forces service users to engage in the maladaptive behavior, by-passing their capacity for choice and control.[10]

But this alternative response is not viable. First, and most simply, it flouts the evidence regularly and forcefully presented to clinicians who work with service users with disorders of agency. Core symptoms and maintaining factors are actions and omissions over which service users have choice and at least a degree of control, which they routinely exercise when they have incentive, motivation, and genuinely want to do so. Second, it precludes offering clinical treatment that directly addresses the problematic patterns of behavior, whether implicitly or explicitly. For, if clinicians give up the belief that service users have choice and control over their behavior, they cannot rationally decide to work with service users to engage this dual capacity. Indeed, if service users themselves come to believe that they

---

[9] For more detailed discussion of how to explain diminished control particularly in addiction, see Pickard (2012) and Pickard and Pearce (in press).

[10] Cf. accounts of addiction that treat it as compulsive such as Charland (2002), Hyman (2005), Leshner (1997); for dissenting accounts see Foddy and Savulescu (2006), Pickard (2012), Pickard and Pearce (in press).

genuinely have no choice or control over their behavior, they cannot rationally decide to try to change. For one cannot rationally resolve to change that which one believes one is powerless to change.[11] Effective treatment for disorders of agency depends on clinician and service user alike believing that the service user has choice and at least a degree of control over their behavior: they are to that degree responsible agents. The cost of avoiding blame by denying service users agency and thus absolving them from responsibility is high: it precludes both clinician and service user alike from rationally pursuing psychological treatment, leaving only medication as an option.

Clinicians are often trapped between a desire to rescue and a desire to blame. They may cleave to (1) and (2) given the evidence available to them and the demands of effective treatment. But then when harm is caused (3) they find themselves blaming service users (4). Or, recoiling from blame and hoping to rescue instead, they may respond to (3) by denying (1) and (2). But this is not viable: it flouts the evidence available and precludes many forms of effective treatment. The solution is to challenge the inference to (4). It is possible to hold someone responsible for actions and omissions that knowingly cause harm but not to blame them for the harm. To appreciate this possibility we need to better distinguish and understand responsibility, blameworthiness, and blame.

A CONCEPTUAL FRAMEWORK FOR
RESPONSIBILITY WITHOUT BLAME

Within philosophy, there is a tendency to link the idea of responsibility to morality. This link can be weak or strong. Weakly, philosophers often use "moral responsibility" and "responsibility" as if they were interchangeable, suggesting, if sometimes unintentionally, that all responsibility is moral. More strongly, philosophers sometimes argue that the idea of responsibility should be understood by appeal to our practice of holding others responsible via what are called our "reactive attitudes" or "moral emotions" (Strawson 1962). These consist in various responses we can have to the good or ill will that others display towards us, such as forgiveness and gratitude, indignation and resentment, and praise and blame. At its most radical, this link between responsibility and the reactive attitudes is thought to be constitutive. As Watson puts this view: "to regard oneself or another as responsible just is the proneness to react to them in these kinds of ways" (2004, p. 220). Slightly more modestly, Wallace has argued that to hold another responsible is to believe that reactive attitudes are

---

[11] Note that this claim posits only a minimal connection between resolution or intention and belief, in contrast to alternative formulations in the literature. For discussion, see Holton (2009). Note too that the success of twelve-step programmes such as Alcoholics Anonymous (AA) may initially seem striking in relation to this claim, as addicts are asked to admit they are powerless and to turn to God, or a personally chosen higher power, for help in order to change. One natural thought is that resolutions formed in this way are not rational but faith-based: the claim is only that it is not rational to form an intention if one believes one is powerless to effect it, not that it is impossible. Another thought is that AA members are not really asked to admit they are powerless, but rather, asked to admit they are powerless without the help of God or their higher power. Having embraced God or it, it is then possible for them to believe they can change, and so to rationally resolve to do so.

appropriate or fitting responses to their behavior, even if one does not actually feel anything oneself (1994).

Both weak and strong versions of this link between responsibility and morality obscure the possibility of responsibility without blame. With respect to the weaker, linguistic link, it is extremely important that clinicians are able to speak plainly to service users of their responsibility for problematic behaviors without implying that the behaviors even might be morally wrong or the person bad. Compare:

1. If you decide to self-harm/abuse substances/clean obsessively, you are responsible for that.
2. If you decide to self-harm/abuse substances/clean obsessively, you are morally responsible for that.

Note that (2) carries an implication that (1) does not. It suggests moral fault. But behaviors like self-harm, substance abuse, and obsessive rituals, can be damaging to the person without necessarily damaging others.[12] They are not sins, or unequivocally and inherently morally wrong. Whatever responsibility service users have for such behavior, it is neither clinically helpful nor obviously correct to view it as moral. We are responsible for behavior that is morally neutral as well as morally good or bad, and, in clinical and other contexts that support change and reflection, there is point in emphasizing this.

Relatedly, the weaker, linguistic link obscures that fact that service users can be responsible for harm, but not blameworthy, because they have an excuse. Compare:

1. Service users may be responsible for verbal aggression towards clinicians but not blameworthy, because they are acting to relieve high levels of psychological distress, and lack alternative coping mechanisms.
2. *Service users may be morally responsible for verbal aggression towards clinicians but not blameworthy, because they are acting to relieve high levels of psychological distress, and lack alternative coping mechanisms.

Note that (2) does not ring true to native ears. And for good reason. How can it make sense to be morally responsible for behavior but not blameworthy for it? For both moral responsibility and blameworthiness imply moral fault. This is what the explanation appealing to psychological distress and lack of coping mechanisms excuses, despite the fact that responsibility for the aggression yet remains.

Turn now to the stronger link. On this view, the idea of responsibility is constitutively connected, via our practices of holding others responsible, either to the reactive attitudes themselves, or to a belief about their aptness. This link makes the possibility of responsibility without blame not simply obscured, but nearly incoherent. If holding someone responsible for harm just is responding with a reactive attitude like blame, then it is not possible to hold service users responsible for harm without blaming them. Similarly, if holding someone responsible for harm just is believing that blame would be an appropriate or fitting response, then, although one may not oneself be blaming them, one is hardly adopting the blame-free non-judgmental stance which is necessary for effective clinical treatment. In practice, one

---

[12]   If this is not obvious, imagine that the behavior is entirely private, all effects kept hidden from view.

might as well be blaming them: for without further qualifications, it seems one believes that one should. In essence, a view of responsibility that links it so closely to the reactive attitudes is not adequate to account for the clinical practice of holding service users responsible for behavior that causes harm, without blaming them for it. For, according to such a view, blaming is too much a part of what it means to hold another responsible for there to be sufficient room to maneuver between them. On this account of responsibility, clinical practice should be nearly incoherent, never mind practically impossible.

The moral of this discussion is that a conceptual framework that is adequate to account for clinical practice must clearly distinguish between ideas of responsibility, blameworthiness, and blame.[13] Let us begin with responsibility.

Effective clinical treatment presupposes that service users are responsible for their behavior in so far as they have conscious knowledge of what they are doing, and can exercise choice and at least a degree of control over the behavior. As we saw earlier, this is a traditional and common sense conception about what it means to be responsible, applicable not only to service users, but to us all.[14] This idea of responsibility is essentially linked, not to morality and the reactive attitudes, but to agency. Crucially, on this view, we are responsible for all our actions, whether or not they are right, wrong, or neutral from a moral point of view. We are responsible for our actions because we are their agents: insofar as we know what we are doing, and can exercise choice and control our behavior, what we do is up to us.

With this idea of responsibility in mind, it is then possible to understand what, minimally, is involved in holding a person responsible. Most stringently, holding a person responsible may consist simply in judging that they are responsible, that is, that they have conscious knowledge, choice, and a degree of control of their behavior. Usually, however, the idea of "holding responsible" means more than judging others to be responsible, but actually treating them thus: treating them as accountable or answerable for their behavior. What accountability or answerability consists in will vary widely, depending on the context. Within clinical practice, holding a service user responsible for their behavior may involve asking them to explain why they made the choices they did, and encouraging them to behave differently in the future. Alternatively, it may involve the agreed imposition of negative consequences, to increase motivation, and show that the behavior, and the harm it causes, is taken seriously.

But, as the discussion of reactive attitudes makes clear, the idea of holding another responsible can involve more. It can involve judging a person not only to be responsible and therefore accountable for the behavior, but to be blameworthy, and indeed blaming them. So, let us turn now to blameworthiness.

---

[13] A. Smith (2007a) draws these and other distinctions very clearly, and offers a helpful discussion of the ambiguity in the meaning of "holding responsible" together with an account of what she calls "active blame" which is similar to my "affective blame." Her discussion differs from mine in three important respects. First, she is content to maintain the linguistic link that I believe to be misleading, and to view all responsibility as moral responsibility, since she holds that the point of responsibility is that it makes moral appraisal appropriate. Second, she offers a 'rationalist' account of the conditions of responsibility as opposed to the more 'volitional' one suggested here. See A. Smith (2007a, 2007b, 2008). Third, she does not offer an account of what unifies all instances of 'active blame' as blame, nor does she attend to irrational blame (see later).

[14] Readers who are concerned about the threat of determinism or who believe for other reasons that responsibility is not linked to the dual capacities of choice and control can potentially substitute an alternative account of responsibility, such as reasons-responsiveness (Fischer and Ravizza 1998), into the conceptual framework offered here without undermining its basic structure.

We judge a person to be blameworthy when they are responsible for harm, and have no excuse. Excuses come in various kinds, such as bad luck, justifiable ignorace, limited choices, and the intention or quality of will behind the action. As suggested earlier, service users who are responsible, at least to a degree, for harm to self or others may not be judged blameworthy, because they have an excuse, such as limited choices, or levels of psychological distress that we do not expect people to tolerate without taking action to alleviate it. However, sometimes they do not have an excuse.[15] Clinicians may turn a blind eye to this, but equally, they may not: they may recognize that a service user is not only responsible, but blameworthy. Yet, they may still manage to avoid blame and maintain an effective clinical stance.

Distinguishing responsibility and blameworthiness is important to solving the conundrum. For it allows us to see both how it is possible to be responsible, and treated thus, for actions that are not morally wrong; and how it is possible to be responsible, and treated thus, for actions that are morally wrong but for which one is not blameworthy, because one has an excuse. But we are yet left with the problem of how it is possible for clinicians to hold service users responsible for harm for which they are recognized to be blameworthy, and yet not to blame them. To resolve this, we need to understand what blame is.

BLAME

Philosophical accounts of blame are surprisingly few and surprisingly diverse, but they tend to agree on one thing. Blame carries a characteristic "sting." Being the object of another's blame hurts. Capturing the "sting" of blame is thus a constraint on any adequate account of what blame is. The "sting" is also the reason why blame is so clinically counterproductive. Effective treatment is not possible if the service user feels judged, shamed, berated, rejected, attacked, or hurt.

But talk of blame is often ambiguous. When we say that another is "to blame" we may mean one of three things:

1. They are blameworthy.
2. We should blame them.
3. We actually do blame them.

These three propositions are distinct. (1) is a judgment about another. Whatever the conditions of blameworthiness ultimately are, they meet them. It is possible to make such a judgment about another, without also judging that we should blame them, let alone judging that we actually do. For instance, we might judge a historical figure from the distant past

---

[15] Note that the mere fact that a service user has a disorder of agency is not in itself an excuse. There is no reason why any psychiatric disorder should offer a sweeping, across the board excuse, if the service user retains the capacity for conscious knowledge, choice, and control of their behavior. Rather, different disorders point to probable incapacities or deficits, which may offer excuses on examination case-by-case of behavioral problems.

blameworthy for harm perpetrated, but we neither blame them, nor judge that we should—the harm is too far removed.

(2) is about us and what we should do. In this kind of context, "should" can have three different meanings. First, we may be saying nothing more than that blame is *warranted* or *justified*: we should blame another, because they are blameworthy. If so, (2) collapses into (1). Second, we may be saying that blame is *appropriate*, relative to various norms governed by the nature of our relationship with the other and the circumstances. For instance, it may be appropriate for victims to blame perpetrators for harm, when it is not appropriate for legal advocates to do so. Third, we may be saying that blame is *desirable* relative to a given end: whether or not blame is warranted or appropriate to our relationship and the circumstances, perhaps it would do us psychological good to vent, or perhaps it would serve an instrumental purpose, such as deterrence. In all three senses, it may be true that we should blame another, and yet we find that we don't. Perhaps we are simply too weary of battling or teaching this person, or fighting for social good: we are beyond caring at this stage to muster the energy to blame.

Finally, (3) is about us and what we actually do. Often enough, we feel blame towards others when we both judge them blameworthy and judge blame appropriate and desirable. But not always. Blame, like nearly all emotions, can be irrational. Although irrational emotions are often particularly prevalent in clinical contexts, a moment's reflection on the vicissitudes of ordinary personal and family relationships should be sufficient to establish this. When things go wrong for us, especially within long-standing personal relationships, but elsewhere, too, we often look for someone to blame, whether as a way of avoiding responsibility ourselves, or simply as a way of venting our frustrations. We sometimes blame others even when we know that the person we are blaming is not at fault, and that we shouldn't: "I know it's unfair, they don't deserve it, but I can't help blaming them. I'm just so angry!"

In this respect, it may be helpful to compare blame and fear. It is one thing to judge a situation dangerous. It is another to judge that fear is warranted, appropriate, or desirable. And it is another again actually to feel it. The brave soldier judges a situation dangerous, so that they can respond rationally and effectively in battle. But they do not feel fear. Nor do they judge it appropriate or desirable that they should: given their role and aim, better they should not. In contrast, the well-informed British arachnophobe feels fear even when they judge there is no objective danger or reason that they should: it is neither warranted, appropriate, nor desirable to be pathologically afraid of UK spiders. Blame is like fear. It can fly in the face of considered judgments about what is true of the blamed object, and what should be true of the blaming subject.

Past philosophical accounts of blame have tended to draw on one of two ideas. Either blame is a form of punishment (Smart 1961). Or it is a sort of mental ledger or record of a person's behavior, of use in assessing character or predicting behavior (Feinberg 1970; Glover 1970). Neither idea suffices to account for blame. As has often been remarked, blame is a mental state, and punishment is an action (Boyd 2007). It is perfectly possible to blame someone but not show it at all, let alone act so as to punish them. Similarly, it is unclear what a mental ledger or record of a person's behavior is supposed to be, other than a memory that they did it. Moreover, we can blame people for actions we consider one-off, and would not use to assess their character or predict future behavior.

Partially in response to these deficiencies, more recent philosophical accounts of blame have focused instead on the idea that blame is essentially if not exclusively cognitive: a form of consciously accessible, personal-level judgment or belief. For instance, Hieronymi (2004) suggests that blame is the judgment that a person has shown disregard or ill will towards another. Or again, Sher (2006) suggests that blame is the belief that a person has acted badly or has a bad character, in conjunction with a desire or wish that this were not the case. Finally, Scanlon (2008) suggests that blame is the judgment that a person is blameworthy, and so has shown impaired interpersonal attitudes, which renders appropriate the rational revision of one's own attitudes towards them, especially one's intentions.

Such cognitive accounts struggle to capture both the "sting" and the irrationality of blame. Consider first its irrationality. As we saw earlier, blame, like most reactive attitudes and emotions, can fly in the face of judgments or beliefs that a person is blameworthy.[16] If irrational blame is possible, these cannot be necessary, let alone sufficient, conditions of blame. This is not to deny that blame, like fear and other occasionally irrational emotions, can clearly involve subpersonal representations, potentially of threat, harm, slight, or ill will, at some level of information-processing. The cognitive psychology of emotional information-processing is not yet unified and advanced, but theories are developing that aim to explain the varieties of rationality and irrationality, consciousness and unconsciousness, that characterize emotions.[17] But, crucially, the representations posited to accommodate these aspects of emotions are not consciously accessible, personal-level judgments and beliefs.

Consider next blame's characteristic "sting." One complicating factor is that individual differences in temperament and values mean that there can be no universal claims about what does and does not "sting." Some people are more sensitive than others, and some people care more about interpersonal relationships, rights, and wrongs, than others. This point is especially important with respect to differences between service users. For instance, a service user with low self-esteem and a critical superego may be easily "stung" by blame, while a service user with narcissistic and psychopathic tendencies may be more immune. Assessing the extent to which an account of blame captures its "sting" is thus the task of assessing the extent to which an account of blame captures what commonly or prototypically "stings." Disagreements are clearly possible. Nonetheless, there is good reason to hold that personal-level cognitive accounts will not adequately capture this. For judgment and belief are commonly, indeed arguably prototypically, "detached."

Note first that, as discussed earlier, we can judge or believe that a person, such as a historical figure, is blameworthy, even if we neither do feel anything nor judge that we should. Furthermore, the addition of a desire or wish that this not be so need not make the attitude any less detached. But, even when the judgment or belief is about a person with whom one is presently in relation, they may not "sting." For, they may be formed and expressed in a way that does not hurt or harm. For instance, good parenting routinely involves pointing out when a child has shown disregard or ill will towards a sibling, and indeed imposing negative consequences for it. That is part of bringing up children to treat others, including rivals, with regard and respect. Sometimes, no doubt, parents do this in such a way that the child feels bad and blamed. But a loving parent can often help a child understand that their behavior

---

[16] For ease of exposition, I shall ignore the differences in precise content of the various judgments and beliefs suggested, and refer to them all as judgments of blameworthiness.

[17] For a review of the relevant science see Dalgleish and Power (1999), Lane and Nadel (2000); for discussion connecting the science to more standard philosophical concerns, see Prinz (2004).

towards a sibling is neither decent nor permitted, without the child feeling "stung." Further, this "detached" mode of forming and expressing judgments of blameworthiness can be maintained even in face of revision of interpersonal attitudes and intentions. For instance, one can rationally and politely decide to stop socializing with an acquaintance who routinely offends, because one judges them blameworthy and no longer wishes to see them, without either party minding very much. This is importantly different from a situation where one party acts out of anger, writing the other off, whether justifiably or not, without due thought or consideration. There is no doubt that judgments and beliefs of blameworthiness, and the changes in relationship they license, can "sting." The point is that they can also be "detached." Presence or absence of "sting" often depends, not only on the temperament and values of the blamed, but also on the exact nature of the change in attitude and intention of the blamer, and, moreover, how this change is experienced and expressed.

Irrationality and "sting" are both secured by the same thing. The reason why blame can be irrational, and the reason why it hurts, is that it is a reactive attitude, a kind of emotion. Call blame which has these features "affective blame."[18] We need not deny that we sometimes speak of blame in a more "detached" mode. As we saw earlier, judgments that another is "to blame" are ambiguous. Call this non-stinging sort of attitude "detached blame." Detached blame can consist in a judgment or belief of blameworthiness. It can be accompanied by a revision of attitudes or intentions, or a further belief that such revision would be appropriate. It can also be accompanied by the imposition of negative consequences for the action, or a just demand for accountability or answerability. The point is that it need not have any of blame's characteristic "sting." "Sting" is commonly and prototypically secured by negative affect and the potential it has to be expressed and acted on. It is affective blame that really hurts.

But there is a challenge facing this suggestion. Grant that the "sting" of blame is affective. We now face the question: *What kind* of affect? For, it seems that affective blame can consist in a range of different emotions. Most obviously, these include hate, anger, and resentment. But the range can plausibly be extended to include certain other states that have an affective dimension without being uncontroversially identifiable as types of emotion, for instance, disapproval, dislike, disappointment, indignation and contempt. Moreover, as expected given this range, blame's expression can be equally various: for instance, alongside punishing, blame can also be manifest in berating, attacking, humiliating, writing off, rejecting, shunning, abandoning, and criticizing, to name but a few behaviors. The challenge is thus to unite these various emotions and manifestations thereof into a single account of blame. For each kind of reaction can occur without counting as an instance of blame. So we must explain what makes these various reactions count, when they do, as instances of blame.

It is natural to be tempted by the idea that they are united in virtue of being caused by the judgment or belief that a person is blameworthy. But this cannot be right. For, as we saw earlier, blame can be irrational: one can blame someone in absence of such a judgment or belief. Instead, I want to suggest that the phenomenology of affective blame provides a cue. Part of what is distinctive about blame is that, when in its grip, one feels entitled to one's blaming response, because of what the other has done: it feels as if they deserve it, even if one does not judge or believe that they do. This feeling of entitlement—of being in the right, in relation to another's wrong—is the key to unifying affective blame. What makes

---

[18] Cf. A. Smith (2007a, 2007b) on "active blame" and Wolf (2011) on "angry blame."

a negative emotion in reaction to another count as blame is the second-order response the blamer has to their first-order emotion: their feeling of entitlement. This feeling of entitlement places the responsibility for the blaming response on the blamed: the blamer feels entitled to their first-order emotion because of what the blamed has done. It thereby gives the blamer a (defeasible and resistible but nonetheless genuine) feeling of freedom to express blame, to vent, to act out of whatever negative emotion they are experiencing. The blamer acts as if, because of what the other has done, the first-order emotional reaction is *deserved*. In this way, although blame is not an action and so not a form of punishment, it is a *punishing* mental state: in reacting negatively, one feels oneself to be in the right, in relation to another's wrong.

It is important to recognize that this feeling of entitlement is not a judgment: we must eschew a consciously accessible, personal-level cognitive account of emotion at the second-order as well as the first. Rather, whatever the mature, agreed theory of the information-processing underlying first-order emotions turns out to be, we need to import this understanding to the account of blame offered here. This is important, if we are to account not only for the "sting" of blame but also for its potential irrationality. For, just as one can judge that spiders are not dangerous and yet feel fear, so too one can judge that another is not blameworthy and yet not only feel anger, but also feel entitled to this anger. One can feel this, even though one knows one shouldn't.

Of course, if the blamer views their blame as irrational and exercises their capacity for rational reflection, they may try to suppress the first-order emotion, and control their behavioral tendencies. Or, alternatively, in the grip of the feeling, they may not. But what makes an instance, say, of anger towards another into blame, is that the blamer cannot lose the feeling that they are entitled to be angry, even if they judge that this anger is not ultimately deserved.

With the distinction between detached and affective blame in hand, we can now complete the conceptual framework, and solve the conceptual part of the conundrum. Clinicians are able to hold service users with disorders of agency responsible, indeed blameworthy, for harm, without blaming them, because blame comes in two forms: detached and affective. Detached blame consists in judgments of blameworthiness, and may further involve correspondingly appropriate revisions of intentions, the imposition of negative consequences, and accountability and answerability. These can have a place within effective clinical treatment, and, in so far as they encourage responsible agency, may be essential to it. Affective blame consists in negative reactions and emotions, whether rational or not, which the blamer feels entitled to have. Effective treatment requires clinicians to avoid affective blame. Responsibility without blame is responsibility without affective blame: without a sense of entitlement to any negative reactive attitudes and emotions one might experience, no matter what the service user has done.

IMPOVERISHMENT AND EMPATHY

Part of the solution to the clinical conundrum is conceptual: we need a framework that clearly distinguishes responsibility, blameworthiness, and blame, in order to understand how it is conceptually possible to hold service users with disorders of agency responsible for harm without blaming them. But part of the solution is practical: it is not sufficient that it is possible to avoid affective blame, clinicians must actually manage to do so.

Clinical training and experience provide some skills that help with this task. Clinicians learn a way of speaking, which involves both a repertoire of phrases, and an attitude of calm respect, that helps them both think and talk with service users about their responsibility for harmful behavior, without blaming them. Clinicians also develop their own capacity to take responsibility for their own emotions: to reflect deeply on whether their response to a service user is warranted or necessary or even natural, and to "own" their part in interpersonal engagements. Bearing in mind the nature of their relationship with service users, and the inherent power imbalance between them, no doubt further aids this task: compare again, in this respect, the non-judgmental attitude loving parents show children. Finally, when all else fails, clinicians need a good poker face—a commitment and capacity to mask their emotions, and refrain from acting out of any blame they may feel.

But, alongside these various skills, clinicians must cultivate compassion and empathy for service users.[19] Quite generally, compassion and empathy are central to good therapeutic care (Gilbert 2010). They are essential when working with service users where the core symptoms and maintaining factors of the disorder typically cause harm. The reason is simple: a compassionate, empathetic stance is at odds with a blaming stance. Compassion and empathy push the negative emotions constitutive of affective blame aside. They simply cannot comfortably coexist.

One central way that clinicians can achieve compassion and empathy towards service users is simple: proper attention to service users' past history. As is well known, psychiatric disorders in general are associated with impoverished early childhood environments, and, of course, the ensuing psychosocial adversity, interpersonal and occupational problems, and stigma that is consequent upon poor mental health. In particular, personality and related disorders are associated with dysfunctional families, where there is breakdown, death, institutional care, and parental psychopathology; traumatic childhood experiences, with high levels of sexual, emotional, and physical abuse or neglect; and social stressors, such as war, poverty, and migration (Paris 2001). Service users often come from harrowing backgrounds, impoverished of all goods, to an extent that can be unimaginable to people who have not experienced these kinds of conditions. Effective treatment can involve helping service users to explore their past and recognize its effects on their personality and their present experiences and behaviors, both as a way of coming to terms with the past, and as a way of developing skills needed to better manage the present. But, in attending to service users' past history, clinicians and service users together gain understanding of why the service users are as they are. A fuller life story or narrative comes into view, in which the service user is seen not only as one who harms, but as one who has been harmed.[20] As Watson has put this point in relation to the psychopath Robert Harris: "The sympathy towards the boy he was is at odds with outrage towards the man he is" (2004, p. 244). Attention to service users' past history is not only part of effective treatment. It also has the power to help clinicians strike a balance between rescue and blame. It requires clinicians to keep in mind the whole of the person and the whole of their story, which undercuts a single, reactive stance, forcing

---

[19] Cf. Potter (2009).

[20] For information on a first-person narrative account that emphasises this Janus-faced aspect of personality disorder see Box 66.1.

Box 66.1 Further Reading and Resources

For further reading on the nature of personality disorder, see the Special Issue of *Philosophy, Psychiatry, Psychology* (2011, volume 18, number 2) on Personality Disorders, edited by Hanna Pickard. The Special Issue is a multidisciplinary effort to further understanding of personality disorder, drawing on scientific, clinical, philosophical, social, and legal perspectives. It also includes a first-person narrative of an ex-service user's experience of living with personality disorder: "The chasm within: my battle with personality disorder" by Jessica Gray. For a comprehensive collection that focuses more exclusively on scientific and clinical dimensions of personality disorder, see *The Handbook of Personality Disorders: Theory, Research, and Treatment*, edited by W. John Livesley (NY, The Guilford Press, 2001). In addition, two valuable internet resources are The UK National Personality Disorder Website available at http://www.personalitydisorder.org.uk/ and the Emergence Website which is service user-led and available at http://www.emergenceplus.org.uk/.

affective blame to exist alongside compassion and empathy, and thereby at least reducing, if not outright extinguishing, its force.

It is important to recognize that this appeal to past history does not eliminate responsibility or blameworthiness.[21] It may reduce responsibility, insofar as certain kinds of background impede the development of skills that, for instance, facilitate emotional regulation and, correspondingly, behavioral control. Equally, extreme impoverishment can limit choices, which can sometimes excuse bad decisions and the harm they cause. But such reduction is not global, and would depend on the particular kind of background, skills, choices, and harm, in question. Rather, the compassion and empathy that consciousness of past harm arouses directly quells and tempers affective blame. It acts as an antidote.

RESPONSIBILITY WITHOUT BLAME IN
NON-CLINICAL CONTEXTS

When I present the conceptual framework developed in this chapter to friends and family of service users with disorders of agency, they invariably ask whether they too should aim to adopt the clinical stance of holding service users responsible for harm caused by maladaptive behavior without blaming them for it. Friends and family of service users often bear the brunt of this behavior: unlike clinicians and indeed all but crisis services, they are available at all hours, and often a natural target for negative feelings and difficult behavior. But in principle, this is a question that applies not just to friends and family, but to society at large. What sort of attitude should we adopt to service users with disorders of agency who do harm?[22]

---

[21] Cf. Watson (2004).

[22] If the maladaptive behavior is also criminal, this question is also relevant to legal issues of liability and the purpose or intent in sentencing and imprisonment. For discussion of the theoretical value and practical possibility of taking the clinical model of responsibility without blame into a criminal justice context, see Lacey and Pickard (2012). For information on the development of a prison officer training based on this model see Box 66.2.

Box 66.2 Responsibility without Blame Training

The UK Department of Health and Ministry of Justice are currently engaged in a joint initiative to develop a *Knowledge and Understanding Framework for Personality Disorder.* The framework offers different levels of training to support people to work more effectively with personality disorder in a variety of roles and contexts. Hanna Pickard is developing a 'Responsibility without Blame' training as part of a strand of this framework dedicated to promoting psychologically informed and rehabilitative environments within prisons. Information on the *Knowledge and Understanding Framework* is available at http://www.personalitydisorder.org.uk/training/kuf/.

One lesson that clearly can be learned from clinical contexts is this: we do not help service users with disorders of agency by denying their agency and absolving them from responsibility. In so far as we aim to help service users improve or recover, their agency and responsibility should be upheld. Moreover, apart from this aim, agency and responsibility are goods. As Angela Smith elegantly points out: "being held responsible is as much a privilege as it is a burden. It signals that we are a full participant in the moral community" (2007b, p. 269). In other words, in holding service users with disorders of agency responsible, we treat them as *one of us*—as belonging with us, as equals.

Affective blame can, of course, undercut that belonging, by expressing hate, anger, resentment, disapproval, dislike, contempt, rejection, and any number of other negative reactive attitudes and expressions. So it might appear that, in so far as we aim to help, we should adopt the clinical stance: we should avoid affective blame so far as possible when holding service users responsible. I want to conclude by suggesting that such a blanket adoption of the clinical stance is not obviously correct.

First, and most obviously, although the clinical aim is to care and to help, that is not the only aim of friends, family, or others in society at large. Their aims will likely be different and various. For instance, at least one typical and significant aim of friends and family is to have real and genuine relationships. Blame for wrongdoing is ordinarily a natural part of such relationships in our society. Hence the possibility of real and genuine relationships, and of equal standing between service users and others, may be lost if the latter are too careful to act in the former's interest at the expense of how they naturally feel.[23] Outside of clinical contexts, equality, respect, and belongingness may best be expressed through ordinary as opposed to special treatment.

Second, even when we have a primary aim to help, withholding affective blame may not always further that aim. Affective blame is one way of holding people responsible for their behavior in so far as it itself counts as the imposition of negative consequences: it is an affective form of accountability. It may be that, in many non-clinical and clinical contexts alike, other forms of accountability are more effective as instrumental means to helping service users take responsibility. But the desire to avoid the affective blame of friends, family, and society at large, may be a powerful motivating force. There may be occasions where blame is not only natural, but also helpful, in the long-term, to the person blamed.

Hence there is no easy, blanket answer to the question of whether or when we should adopt the clinical stance of responsibility without blame. It is often complicated to

---

[23] Cf. Kennett (2007).

determine whether or not, in a particular context, affective blame is instrumentally effective relative to desired ends. It is equally complicated to determine whether, over and above its instrumental use, affective blame is appropriate, given the nature of the relationship between the parties, the kind of harm caused, and how and why it occurred. Cultural conventions to do with roles and relationships, alongside interpersonal histories and dynamics, affect what is and is not appropriate between people. For this reason, there is no ubiquitous, standardized, rational norm governing when affective blame is and is not appropriate. Working out when it is, and when it is not, is part of the meat of having real, genuine relationships.[24] In the face of this complexity, one thing remains clear: clinicians, family, friends, and others need to hold service users with disorders of agency responsible for their behavior, and ask that they change it, when it causes harm to self or others.

But given this complexity, a second lesson that can perhaps be learned from clinical contexts is this: We should all question, more often than we typically do, whether or not our inclination to affectively blame others is warranted, appropriate, and desirable, given the particular context. As mentioned earlier, clinicians must develop their own capacity to take responsibility for their own emotions: to reflect deeply on whether their response to a service user is warranted, appropriate, or even natural (let alone desirable given their aim to help) and to "own" their part in interpersonal engagements. That is something that, arguably, we all fail to do as much as we ideally should, in relationships with service users and non-service users alike. When we are harmed, deliberately or not, we often look for someone to blame, as a way of venting our anger, hurt, and frustration. Possibly, if we do have a part to play in what has happened to us, we look for someone to blame as a way of avoiding our own responsibility. If we hold others responsible for their behavior, it is incumbent on us to hold ourselves equally responsible, and that may include holding ourselves responsible for our inclination to affectively blame, by questioning our sense of entitlement to our negative reactions, even if we ultimately judge those reactions warranted, appropriate and desirable. If we do blame, we need to do so responsibly.

ACKNOWLEDGMENTS

This research was funded through a Wellcome Trust Biomedical Ethics Clinical Research Fellowship. Versions of this chapter have been given at the Oxford, Edinburgh, and London philosophy departments, the 2010 Royal College of Psychiatry AGM, various psychiatric teams within my own and other NHS Trusts, and the 2010 Oxfordshire Friends and Family of Personality Disorder Annual Conference. I am grateful to all these audiences for their questions, ideas, and criticism. Thanks also to Bennett Foddy and Paula Boddington for helpful comments. Finally, special thanks are due to Steve Pearce and especially Ian Phillips for long-standing and ongoing discussion of these issues.

[24] This is another reason why philosophical accounts of responsibility that constitutively link it to our actual reactive attitudes or our beliefs about their aptness are problematic. The norms that govern our reactive attitudes may be far more complicated, various, and indeed on occasion arational, than the conditions required for ascriptions of responsibility.

REFERENCES

Alvarez, M. (2009). Actions, thought-experiments and the "Principle of alternate possibilities." *Australasian Journal of Philosophy*, *87*(1), 61–81.

Aristotle (1984). Eudemian ethics. In J. Solomon (Trans.) and J. Barnes (Ed.), *The Complete Works of Aristotle, Volume 2*, pp. 1922–81. Oxford: Oxford University Press.

Bobzien, S. (1998). The inadvertent conception and late birth of the free-will problem. *Phronesis*, *43*(2), 133–75.

Bowers, L. (2002). *Dangerous and Severe Personality Disorder: Response and Role of the Team*. London: Routledge.

Boyd, J. (2007). *Blame and Blameworthiness*. PhD thesis, Princeton University, MA.

Charland, L. (2002). Cythnthia's dilemma: Consenting to heroin prescription. *American Journal of Bioethics*, *2*(2), 37–47.

Dalgleish, T. and Power, M. (Eds) (1999). *Handbook of Cognition and Emotion*. New York, NY: Wiley & Sons.

Feinberg, J. (1970). Action and responsibility. In *Doing and Deserving: Essays in the Theory of Responsibility*, pp. 119–151. Princeton, NJ: Princeton University Press.

Fischer, J. M. and Ravizza, M. (1998). *Responsibility and Control*. Cambridge: Cambridge University Press.

Foddy, B. and Savulescu, J. (2006). Addiction and autonomy: Can addicted people consent to the prescription of their drug of addiction? *Bioethics*, *20*(1), 1–15.

Fonagy, P., Gergely, G., Jurist, E. L., and Target, M. (2004). *Affect Regulation, Mentalization, and the Development of the Self*. London: Karnac.

Gilbert, P. (2010). *Compassion Focused Therapy*. London: Routledge.

Glover, J. (1970). *Responsibility*. London: Routledge & Kegan Paul.

Hieronymi, P. (2004). The force and fairness of blame. *Philosophical Perspectives*, *18*, 115–48.

Hobbes, T. (1999). Treatise: Of liberty and necessity. In V. Chappell (Ed.) *Hobbes and Bramhall on Liberty and Necessity*, pp. 15–42. Cambridge: Cambridge University Press.

Holton, R. (2009). *Willing, Wanting, Waiting*. Oxford: Oxford University Press.

Holton, R. (2010). Disentangling the will. In R. Baumeister, A. Mele, and K. Vohs (Eds), *Free Will and Consciousness: How Might They Work?*, pp. 82–100. New York, NY: Oxford University Press.

Hume, D. (1975). *Enquiry Concerning Human Understanding* (L. A. Selby-Bigge, Ed.). Oxford: Oxford University Press.

Hyman, S. E. (2005) Addiction: A disease of learning and memory. *American Journal of Psychiatry*, *162*, 1414–22.

Kant, I. (1960). *Religion within the Bounds of Reason Alone* (T. Greene and H. Hudson, Trans.). New York, NY: Harper and Row.

Kennett, J. (2007). Mental disorder, moral agency, and the self. In B. Steinbock (Ed.), *The Oxford Handbook of Bioethics*, pp. 90–113. Oxford: Oxford University Press.

Lacey, N. and Pickard, H. (2012). From the consulting room to the court room? Taking the clinical model of responsibility without blame into the legal realm. *Oxford Journal of Legal Studies*. First published online Nov 19, 2012. DOI: 10.1093/ojls/gqs028.

Lane, R. and Nadel, L. (Eds) (2000). *Cognitive Neuroscience of Emotion*. Oxford: Oxford University Press.

Leshner, A. I. (1997). Addiction is a brain disease, and it matters. *Science*, *278*(5335), 45–47.

Paris, J. (2001). Psychosocial adversity. In *Handbook of personality disorders* (W. J. Livesley, Ed.), pp. 231–241. New York, NY: Guildford Press.

Pearce, S, and Pickard, H. (2010). Finding the will to recover: philosophical perspectives on agency and the sick role. *Journal of Medical Ethics,* online pub July 31.

Pickard, H. (2011). Responsibility without blame: empathy and the effective treatment of personality disorder. *Philosophy, Psychiatry, Psychology*, 18, 209–23.

Pickard, H. (2012). The purpose in chronic addiction. *American Journal of Bioethics Neuroscience* 3(2): 40–49.

Pickard, H. (2013). Pscyhopathology and the ability to do otherwise. *Philosophy and Phenomenological Research.* First published online April 8, 2013. DOI:10.1111/phpr.12025.

Pickard, H., and Pearce, S. (in press). Addiction in context: philosophical lessons from a personality disorder clinic. In N Levy (Ed.), *Addiction and Self-control.* New York: Oxford University Press.

Potter, N. (2009). *Mapping the Edges and In-Between: A Critical Analysis of Borderline Personality Disorder.* Oxford: Oxford University Press.

Prinz, J. (2004). *Gut Reactions.* Oxford: Oxford University Press.

Reid, T. (1994). *The Works of Thomas Reid Vol. 2* (W. Hamilton, Ed.). Bristol: Thoemmes Press.

Scanlon, T. M. (2008). *Moral Dimensions.* Cambridge, MA: Harvard University Press.

Sher, G. (2006). *In Praise of Blame.* Oxford: Oxford University Press.

Smart, J. J. C. (1961). Free will, praise, and blame. *Mind, 70*, 291–306.

Smith, A. (2007a). On being responsible and holding responsible. *Journal of Ethics*, 11, 465–84.

Smith, A. (2007b). Responsibility for attitudes: activity and passivity in mental life. *Ethics, 115,* 236–71.

Smith, A. (2008). Control, responsibility, and moral assessment. *Philosophical Studies, 138,* 367–92.

Smith, M. (2003). Rational capacities, or: How to distinguish recklessness, weakness, and compulsion. In S. Stroud and C. Tappolet (Eds), *Weakness of Will and Varieties of Practical Irrationality*, pp. 17–38. Oxford: Oxford University Press.

Steward, H. (2009). Fairness, agency, and the flicker of freedom. *Nous, 43,* 64–93.

Steward, H. (2012). *A Metaphysics for Freedom.* Oxford: Oxford University Press.

Strawson, P. F. (1962). Freedom and resentment. *Proceedings of the British Academy, 48,* 1–25.

Wallace, R. J. (1994). *Responsibility and the moral sentiments.* Cambridge MA: Harvard University Press.

Watson, G. (2004). Responsibility and the limits of evil. In *Agency and answerability: selected essays*, pp. 219–59. Oxford: Oxford University Press.

Wolf, S. (2011). Blame, Italian style. In J. Wallace, R. Kumar, and S. Freeman (Eds), *Reasons and Recognition: Essays on the Philosophy of T. M. Scanlon*, pp. 332–47. Oxford: Oxford University Press.

COMMENTARY: ENABLING CHOICE
IN A THERAPEUTIC ENVIRONMENT

LISA WARD

The frustration that must come for clinicians working with people with personality disorder and disorders of agency when the client is still engaging in counterproductive coping mechanisms is understandable. How is it possible to continue to want to help someone who repeatedly injures themselves or others, but seemingly without awareness of the impact of this on themselves and those around them? How is it possible not to blame, or judge, or recoil from a desire to work with the client? And yet at the same time, imagine the frustration at being filled with emotions so intense that they almost freeze you with their power. Particularly at the start of a therapeutic journey, this sense of being flooded by emotions can lead to a sense of impotence, an inability to express emotions in words. More often than not this ends up being expressed through very physical means, such as self-injury, self-starvation or binge-eating, reckless drinking, fighting with others, or even isolating oneself entirely to avoid all physical contact. In short, it can become frustrating, and perhaps even tedious, for clinician and client alike. The person diagnosed with personality disorder may not be able to fathom how the intensity of their emotions cannot be understood, and instead feel like their behavior is judged or criticized by the clinician, who may pressure them to change, or withdraw from the relationship. The clinician, in contrast, may be struggling to comprehend why the client persists in counterproductive coping mechanisms and does not seem to see or care about the impact that their behavior has, both on themselves and on others.

It is often said that those diagnosed with personality disorder typically lack empathy. But, in these kinds of situations, I would argue that both sides lack empathy, which often has negative consequences for quality of care and possibility of recovery. As someone who frequently self-injured, this type of frustration in clinicians often led to feeling blamed, both by them and by myself, that in turn fed into a cycle of guilt. Although to outsiders it may have looked as though I had no awareness of my behavior's impact on myself and others, this was generally not the case. When in the grip of such intense and powerful emotions, I felt forcefully driven to take action to manage these feelings and make them abate, often in a very physical, almost primitive way. The option of self-harming provided relief which I needed, despite the guilt I knew I would face later. Now, imagine coping in the best way you can (in my case self-injury) and being met with blame. Blame, when someone is already feeling guilty, compounds a cycle, and in my case, made me want to self-injure more to punish myself for the impact of my behavior on myself and others. Of course, with hindsight, self-injury was not my only choice to manage my emotions, but until I was supported in a blame-free environment to think about alternatives, it certainly felt like it was.

A clinical approach emphasizing responsibility but grounded in compassion and empathy not only ends the cycle of blame and guilt. It also begins to open up the sense of agency. It is in this state that alternative choices can be explored, and a sense of belief that there is a better way to cope can be instilled. Sitting with, thinking about, and finding new ways to cope with emotions, as well as finding ways to express them in words, were things I'd always longed for, yet never accomplished. Blame-free therapeutic environments work because they provide a place to learn—a place where it is safe to try out new behaviors, to make mistakes without feeling a complete failure, and even, sometimes, to find some spontaneity and a sense of play. Given that so many of the coping mechanisms utilized by people with personality disorder or disorders of agency are physical and so, in a sense, childlike (akin to a child who is not yet able to speak, and so communicates by very physical means) it seems likely that they have not had the opportunity to learn to cope with emotions in an environment which is caring, safe and free from blame.

For me, this approach removed the continued sense of blame and guilt for the ways in which I was coping, which had left me believing that all I was ever going to amount to was a continued disappointment. This in turn filled me with a sense of control: I felt that every action (or reaction) was a choice. This allowed me to see that I had the power to take responsibility and make more helpful choices, and to learn to communicate my emotions verbally and find ways to manage them without causing such harm or distress to myself and others. By being able to view every action as a choice, it felt less like I was being pressured by others to give up old coping mechanisms, and instead that I was willingly choosing to change how I behaved. In turn, this has enabled me to manage my emotional reactions in healthier ways, leading to a fulfilled life, with focus firmly placed on the positive choices I can and have made.

Lisa Ward

CHAPTER 67

....

DEPRESSION, DECISIONAL CAPACITY, AND PERSONAL AUTONOMY

....

LUBOMIRA RADOILSKA

INTRODUCTION

....

Autonomy is the focus of at least four major philosophical inquiries. One of them aims to establish the defining features of autonomous motivational states, such as identification, endorsement, or acceptance (Frankfurt 1998). It relates autonomy to the concepts of agency and freedom of will. Another approach explores the question of whether autonomous choices ought to accord with particular values, such as self-respect (Hill 1991). It identifies covert forms of oppression and elaborates on corrective initiatives. A third inquiry concentrates on the links between responsiveness to reasons and effective control over one's life (Korsgaard 1996). It looks at rational agency and its interrelation with moral responsibility. Finally, autonomy is a central topic in bioethics. It is critically examined in connection to informed consent and decisional capacity (O'Neill 2002).

Arguably, the ensuing proliferation of autonomy conceptions points to the significance of the underlying concept. However, it may also prompt skepticism about its unity and theoretical appeal. From this latter perspective, the lines of inquiries mentioned are deemed not to explore different conceptions of the same concept, but to sketch separate concepts with no necessary interconnections. If this view is correct, we should either replace "autonomy" with narrower, qualified autonomy-concepts, such as autonomy as independence of mind, autonomy as responsiveness to reasons, etc., or abandon "autonomy" altogether, for it has become an overworked and misleading term (Arpaly 2003, p. 118).

In this chapter, I shall not address this kind of general skepticism about autonomy, but aim to respond to a challenge faced by a specific conception of autonomy as an independent, though limited in scope, source of justification. In doing so, I shall make two related assumptions: firstly, that autonomy is primarily an agency concept and, secondly, that the conception I defend is central to it.[1] The challenge I shall address here questions the feasibility of a reliable distinction between autonomous and non-autonomous choices. This challenge is significant because, in the absence of such a distinction, a conception of autonomy as independent source of justification will run into various paradoxes, such as upholding non-autonomous choices in the name of autonomy. This line of inquiry is equally relevant to outlining a plausible conception of decisional capacity, for, as we shall see later, decisional capacity would not be able to fulfil its designated purpose—to protect certain self-regarding initiatives from interference—unless it points to an independent source of justification applicable to such initiatives. Depression offers a promising focal point for the discussion because it credibly substantiates the challenge faced by both decisional capacity and the related autonomy conception.

The argument proceeds as follows. In the next section, I outline two paradoxes about depression and dismiss an initially plausible solution to each of them. In the middle section, I sketch a logical reconstruction of the challenge stating that, in light of the earlier paradoxes about depression, decisional capacity and the related autonomy conception cannot be consistently defined in either value-neutral or value-laden terms. In the penultimate section, I propose a revised value-neutral solution, according to which depression hinders decisional capacity, viz., personal autonomy in so far as it leads to paradoxical identification and thwarts the relationship to one's motives that typically conveys autonomy to ensuing initiatives. In the final section, I anticipate a possible objection suggesting that the account I propose has unacceptable consequences, such as being at odds with respect for depression sufferers as persons.

Two Paradoxes about Depression

Depression poses two important challenges to philosophical reflection about intentional agency. The first relates to a classical conception, according to which we always act under the guise of the good. The underlying claim is that, whenever we engage freely in some kind of pursuit, we do so because we conceive it as valuable in some respect. Immediate examples include finding an activity enjoyable or appreciating its effects. Although this conception has recently come under attack, it would be a mistake to underestimate its intuitive appeal.[2] For it offers a plausible way of explaining core, everyday cases of voluntary actions as opposed to coerced ones. Following this line of thought, voluntary actions could be fully accounted for by an agent acknowledging: "I did φ because I wanted to φ," insofar as this means:

"I did φ because I like/ care about φ-ing," or:
"I did φ because, by φ-ing, I get [closer to] x, y, z that I like/care about."

---

[1] I have argued for both claims in Radoilska (2012). In distinguishing a concept from its conceptions, I draw on Gallie (1956).

[2] Critical approaches include Stocker (1979), Velleman (1992), and, more recently, Setiya (2010).

In contrast, coerced actions are not accurately explained by pointing to the fact that the agent consented to perform them. Even a first-person account, such as "I did φ because I wanted to φ" remains insufficient. In instances of coercion, this statement stands for:

"I did φ because I was made to [want to] φ," or:
"Unless I φ-ed, x, y, z that I like/care about, would have been lost or damaged. So, I did φ."

The distinction between these two categories of actions is central to our thinking about intentional agency. In particular, this contrast helps to pin down the idea of an agent as the ultimate source of actions, which are free, intentional, and uncompelled.[3] A straightforward link between motivation and evaluation is the distinctive feature of such paradigm cases. Conversely, in coerced actions, this link becomes complicated. As a result, the agent cannot be seen as the ultimate source of such actions, for the relationship between motivation and evaluation that they substantiate is conditioned from outside. Hence, the intuition that we always act under the guise of the good enables us to achieve two related goals. The first is to appreciate the distinction between actions proper and actions performed under various degrees of undue influence or coercion. The second is to, nevertheless, conceive the latter category as something partly done *by* the coerced agent rather than merely done *to* her. Thus, intentional actions imply a robust, though not always direct link between motivation and evaluation.

This conception of intentional agency seems at odds with depression, which typically involves mental states where the underlying connection between motivation and evaluation is apparently severed. As Michael Stocker points out:

> Through spiritual or physical tiredness, through accidie, through weakness of body, through illness, through general apathy, through despair, through inability to concentrate, through a feeling of uselessness or futility, and so on, one may feel less and less motivated to seek what is good. One's lessened desire need not signal, much less be the product of, the fact that, or one's belief that, there is less good to be obtained or produced, as in the case of a universal Weltschmertz. Indeed, a frequent added defect of being in such 'depressions' is that one sees all the good to be won or saved and one lacks the will, interest, desire, or strength. (1979, p. 744)[4]

At first sight, the underlying difficulty seems easy to resolve. Arguably, the preceding outline of intentional agency only requires that the motives for an action can be traced back to the agent's appraisal of this action as good under the description, under which it was undertaken (Anscombe 1963). Thus, considering a course of action as worthwhile does not have to be immediately motivating. However, the challenge from depression reappears as soon as we take into consideration that, in depression, the course of action deemed to be worthwhile is typically not abandoned because of some interference from outside, making it, for instance,

---

[3] The proposed sketch of intentional agency draws on Aristotle's account of voluntary actions as opposed to the so-called mixed actions from *Nicomachean Ethics* 3.1–5; see also Radoilska (2007, pp. 191–231). On the notion of a free, intentional, and uncompelled action, see Mele (1987).

[4] Arguably, this outline matches the clinical description of depression proposed by the tenth revision of the International Classification of Disease (ICD-10) and the fourth edition of the *Diagnostic and Statistical Manual of Mental Disorders* (DSM-IV), listing, on the one hand, loss of interest and enjoyment and, on the other, a bleak and pessimistic view of the future as central diagnostic criteria.

less likely to succeed. Instead, the root of the problem seems to be that commitments, the agent still considers as worthwhile, no longer motivate her to act one way or the other. The distinctive paradox brought by depression here is that the desirable is not desired and the choiceworthy does not get chosen.

The second challenge posed by depression calls into question our ability to reliably distinguish autonomous from non-autonomous choices. This affects primarily a key function of attributing autonomy to substantively self-regarding initiatives, which is to protect them from interference.[5] Here, the category of substantively self-regarding is best understood negatively, in the sense that related initiatives require no further justification on moral or prudential grounds. Instead, their permissibility depends entirely on the issue whether a person autonomously commits to them or not. Since autonomy, in this context, stands for an independent source of justification, it seems natural to opt for purely procedural, value-neutral criteria when ascertaining whether an initiative should be protected from interference because it is autonomously undertaken rather than because it is morally commendable or prudentially required. The so-called hierarchical or higher-order accounts of personal autonomy provide a plausible way of identifying autonomous versus non-autonomous choices, which does not implicitly rely on further moral or prudential reasons.[6]

This function of autonomy is particularly relevant to medical contexts. For treatment refusal looks like a central, if not *the* central case of a substantively self-regarding initiative: compared to a person's interest in her life and welfare, the interest of others in the matter can only be secondary.[7] Moreover, the idea of autonomy as a justificatory alternative to moral and prudential reasons, applicable to this particular cluster of choices, often underpins current legal thinking about decisional capacity. The following excerpt of a recent UK High Court ruling is an example:

> A mentally competent patient has an absolute right to refuse to consent to medical treatment for any reason, rational or irrational, or for no reason at all, even where that decision may lead to his or her own death. (*Re MB* 1997)

Depression creates a major difficulty for the underlying approach to decisional capacity and personal autonomy. For recognized symptoms, such as low self-esteem and suicidality, arguably motivate treatment refusal by people who suffer from depression, especially in cases where this is very likely to lead to their own death.[8] The plausible causal link from symptoms

---

[5] In this chapter, I shall employ 'initiatives' as a general term, covering choices, decisions, and actions. The notion of substantively self-regarding as opposed to self-regarding initiatives that are equally other-regarding will be further clarified in the following section. See also Feinberg (1986, chapter 17) and Scoccia (2008).

[6] See Frankfurt (1998, 1999) and Dworkin (1988). For an informative survey of both developments and critiques of hierarchical conceptions of personal autonomy, see Christman (1988) and Taylor (2005).

[7] See however the notion of 'garrison threshold' in Feinberg (1986, pp. 21–23) specifying the conditions under which this is not the case.

[8] It is helpful to distinguish this kind of treatment refusal from others, where a causal path between depressive symptoms and effective motivation is rather doubtful. Examples are cases where a person objects to a particular treatment, e.g., a course of antidepressants rather than to treatment per se. Moreover, not all treatment refusals per se could be plausibly linked back to depression. For instance, a person may be unwilling to undergo any kind of medical treatment for depression because she takes depressive episodes to offer her an opportunity to further her self-knowledge and resolve the underlying conflicts by introspection.

to motives for action casts the related decisions as clear-cut cases of non-autonomous initiatives, on a par with coerced actions, since undue influence onto the agent is present in both kinds of instances. Yet, if we follow the criteria proposed by the hierarchical accounts of autonomy, we seem compelled to acknowledge such depression-induced treatment refusals as autonomous. The paradox comes from the fact that a depressed person could not only identify with this kind of decisions, but also endorse them on reflection.[9] For instance, she may still consider that her life is no longer worth living, whilst being aware that this kind of attitude toward oneself is often interpreted as a symptom of a particular mental disorder. In so doing, she would satisfy both weaker and stronger versions of a hierarchical conception of autonomy. This outcome seems counterintuitive, for, in the context of depression, it requires that we uphold some apparently non-autonomous choices in the name of autonomy.

It is tempting to try and resolve this second paradox about depression by abandoning the underlying, value-neutral approach to decisional capacity, viz., personal autonomy in favor of a substantive or value-laden strategy. The latter strategy suggests that, in order to be autonomous, individual choices ought to accord with particular values, in addition to fulfilling purely procedural constraints.[10] This additional requirement would enable us to accommodate the compelling intuition that symptom-related initiatives cannot be considered as autonomous. In particular, we would be in a position to override depression-induced treatment refusals as non-autonomous on grounds that they are at odds with the crucial value of self-respect.[11] This tempting solution, however, comes at a price, for substantive or value-laden accounts of autonomy seem to undermine its possible function as a sufficient rationale for substantively self-regarding initiatives. This is because they tie up the issue of personal autonomy to that of whether a person effectively commits to worthwhile or rational projects.[12] As a result, autonomy can hardly provide a justificatory alternative. Instead, it appears as a mere appendage to the moral or prudential reasons in favor of a particular self-regarding initiative.

The Challenge to Decisional Capacity:
A Logical Reconstruction

A promising way forward is to bring together the two paradoxes about depression so that we are able to sketch out an account of depression clarifying its impact on both autonomous and broader intentional agency. As a first step in this direction, let us consider the following

---

[9] In Frankfurt (2002) the notions of identification and endorsement are both clarified in terms of acceptance that involves neither evaluative judgment, nor a cognitive process, such as deliberation. In contrast, Dworkin (1988) insists on the role of second-order reflection in order to ensure that the first-order motivations under scrutiny are the agent's own in the required sense, that is, independent from undue influence.

[10] See Charland (2008) and Culver and Gert (2004) arguing in favor of such a move. Both papers take instances of depression-induced treatment refusals in the sense specified earlier as decisive counterexamples to a purely procedural understanding of decisional capacity.

[11] See Hill (1991, pp. 4–18). In the following, I shall use the terms self-respect and self-esteem interchangingly. This is consistent with the contrast between self-respect, on the one hand, and both deference and servility, on the other, which is central to Hill's thesis.

[12] Culver and Gert (2004) provides an example of the latter strategy.

logical reconstruction of the challenge to convincingly define decisional capacity in either value-neutral or value-laden terms.

1. An important function of attributing autonomy to substantively self-regarding initiatives is to protect them from interference. The primary aim is to shield individuals from unwarranted uses of authority, such as the tyranny of majority. This function is associated with and often assimilated to the principle of respect for personal autonomy in bioethics.
   1.1. The distinctive feature of substantively self-regarding initiatives is that, ex hypothesi, they could be solely justified by virtue of being autonomously chosen. If this condition is satisfied, such initiatives should be recognized as permissible in their own right, independently of further values or principles.[13]
   1.2. Notwithstanding, the scope of substantively self-regarding initiatives is, to some degree, context-dependent. The relatively recent decriminalization of suicide attempts is an example. Whilst earlier this kind of self-regarding initiative was not deemed eligible for protection from interference, it is now accepted as substantively self-regarding, independently of its foreseeably detrimental impact on others.
2. Tests of decisional capacity are meant to fulfill a function, relevantly similar to that described in the earlier premise.
   2.1. The choices to which these tests apply, e.g., treatment refusals are presumed substantively self-regarding. What is at stake is whether a person is capable to make such a choice in a particular context so that this choice is worthy of protection from interference independently of further values or principles.
3. A reliable way of distinguishing both autonomous from non-autonomous and capacious from incapacious decisions is crucial to fulfilling the central function as outlined in premise 1.
   3.1. Although treating relevant autonomous choices as non-autonomous often attracts criticisms for being paternalistic, the opposite mistake is just as pernicious because it condones various forms of unfreedom, including coercion, manipulation, and compulsion.
4. The two divides described should overlap so that decisions, acknowledged as autonomous in the sense specified in subsection 1.1, are also deemed capacious as stipulated in 2.1, and vice versa.
   4.1. If the preceding condition is not fulfilled, some substantively self-regarding initiatives will have to be both protected and overruled.
   4.2. Hierarchical accounts of autonomy offer a prima facie plausible way to draw the distinction at issue.
       4.2.1. For they take as relevant only the question of whether the agent endorses the choice under scrutiny at the moment of choice; the suggested procedural constraints are minimal and aim to eliminate only patent mistakes about facts and practical contradictions (Frankfurt 1998, pp. 159–176, 1999, pp. 129–141).

---

[13] This intuition is reflected in the distinction between separate principles of bioethics, where respect for autonomy is contrasted with considerations based on nonmaleficence, beneficence, and justice, see Beauchamp and Childress (1979).

4.2.2. This seems to be an intuitive means to avoid the imposition of evaluative commitments from outside, which is the central aim of both autonomy and capacity attribution in the context of substantively self-regarding initiatives.

4.3. The conditions set out in the Mental Capacity Act 2005 (Office of Public Sector Information 2007) are sometimes interpreted as aligned to a hierarchical understanding of autonomy. These conditions include: the ability to understand the information relevant to the decision; to retain that information; to use or weigh that information as part of the process of making the decision; and to communicate a final decision.

4.3.1. The Wooltorton case is an example of such an interpretation, especially as presented in McLean (2009), on which the following description is based. Kerrie Wooltorton, a twenty-six-year-old woman has ingested antifreeze on nine previous occasions but had accepted lifesaving treatment afterward. She was deemed to have an untreatable emotionally unstable personality disorder and, possibly, to be depressed. In 2007, days before her death, she had drafted an advance statement indicating that she did not wish to be treated should the same circumstances arise in the future, even if she called for an ambulance. Rather than being treated, she wanted to die in a situation where she was not alone and where comfort care was provided. A document containing a rejection of treatment was presented by her on admission to hospital, after ingesting antifreeze for a tenth time. This document was accepted as valid. In addition, she made a contemporaneous refusal of treatment and was considered to satisfy the criteria for decisional capacity. The medical professionals involved did not give lifesaving treatment. A subsequent coroner's ruling upheld their decision as lawful.

5. The claim that this decision was incorrect could be based on the following grounds:

5.1. Treatment refusal after a suicide attempt is ineligible for protection under the principle of respect for autonomy because it is not self-regarding in the required sense (see subsection 1.2);

5.2. Although both substantively self-regarding and capacious, Wooltorton's treatment refusal should have been overridden on grounds of beneficence.

5.3. Wooltorton's treatment refusal was not capacious. Hence, either the underlying procedural interpretation was not adequately applied or this interpretation is itself inadequate.

6. Leaving the first two hypotheses aside, both options identified in subsection 5.3. could be supported by the idea that depression involves a significant impairment and even a breakdown of intentional agency. According to the ICD-10, a considerable difficulty in continuing with ordinary activities is typical of moderate depression, whereas severe depression leads to inability to continue with any, except very limited activities. Related symptoms include:

6.1. Indecisiveness and diminished ability to concentrate and think; and

6.2. General loss of interest and pleasure, sense of worthlessness, hopelessness and suicidality.

7. The symptoms listed in 6.1. could be easily accounted for by a hierarchical interpretation of capacity (see 4.2–4.3); however, the symptoms listed in 6.2. remain unaddressed.

8. Yet, with respect to establishing whether a possible breakdown or severe impairment of intentional agency has taken place, the distinction between the two groups of symptoms is arbitrary. Consider the following excerpts from a memoir of depression:

> I can remember lying frozen in bed, crying because I was too frightened to take a shower and at the same time knowing that showers are not scary. I ran through the individual steps in my mind: You sit up, turn and put your feet on the floor, stand, walk to the bathroom, open the bathroom door, go to the edge of the tub … I divided it into fourteen steps as onerous as the Stations of the Cross. I knew that for years I had taken a shower every day. Hoping that someone else could open the bathroom door, I would, with all the force of my body, sit up; turn and put my feet on the floor; and then feel so incapacitated and frightened that I would roll over and lie face down. I would cry again, weeping because the fact that I could not do it seemed so idiotic to me. (Solomon 1998, pp. 48–49)

> During the worst of my depression, when I could hardly eat, I could not have done myself real harm. In this emerging period, I was feeling well enough for suicide. I could push myself to do pretty much all of what I had always been able to do, but I was unable to experience pleasure. Now I had the energy to wonder *why* I was pushing myself and could find no good reasons. (Solomon 1998, p. 52)

8.1. The first quote offers a plausible description of a breakdown of intentional agency. Although it involves both groups of symptoms as listed in 6.1 and 6.2, the defining feature amounts to a double rift between evaluation and motivation: on the one hand, the agent is not motivated by his evaluative judgments, e.g., "showers are not scary"; on the other, he finds himself acting upon motives that he cannot comprehend, let alone value, e.g., "it seemed so idiotic to me."

8.2. The second quote offers a plausible description of a severe impairment of intentional agency. Similarly to the previous one, it involves both groups of symptoms as listed in 6.1. and 6.2, and the underlying mental state points to a mismatch between evaluation and motivation. The agent does not find his evaluative judgments worthy of acting upon and, with respect to motivation, aggression toward the self takes over.[14]

9. In light of premises 1 and 4, both decisional capacity and the related autonomy conception are incompatible with either a breakdown or a severe impairment of intentional agency as described in subdivisions 8.1. and 8.2. The reason is that respect for choices, made under either of these conditions, would promote a particular kind of unfreedom, whereby the agent lacks either effective control or authority over her motives. This kind of unfreedom is compatible with *autocracy*, whereby I mean a state, in which the agent is unconstrained by undue influence

---

[14] This may not be fully explicit in the excerpt I refer to, however, the proposed account is clearly confirmed by the follow-up episodes in the memoir, where the agent stops short of committing suicide, then engages in various kinds of reckless behaviour, which he abandons only because he realises that this could harm not only him, but also third parties. Similarly, Solomon's change of heart about suicide is essentially motivated by other-regarding concerns: "it would be sad for my father to have worked so hard at saving me and not to have succeeded" (Solomon 1998, p. 52).

from outside; yet, although left on her own, she does not manage to attain successful self-government.[15]

9.1. Autocracy is one way in which personal autonomy may become unstuck.

10. Together with premise 3 and in particular 3.1, the preceding conclusion supports the idea that with respect to depression, the underlying procedural approach may lead to paradoxical decisions to uphold non-autonomous but autocratic choices in the name of autonomy, as in the Wooltorton case.

11. In order to avoid this unwelcome upshot, it may seem natural to opt for a value-laden account of both decisional capacity and the related autonomy conception. However, in light of subsections 1.1 and 4.2.2, this move is apparently blocked. For this kind of solution undermines the crucial intuition, according to which personal autonomy is an independent source of justification for substantively self-regarding initiatives. This becomes clear if we consider in some detail a promising value-laden alternative.

11.1. For instance, if we take it that substantively self-regarding initiatives, set out in a state of mind relevantly similar to 8.1 and 8.2, are non-autonomous by virtue of being patently irrational, this would mean that, whenever we respect this kind of initiatives as autonomously chosen, we effectively respect their putative rationality. In so doing, we implicitly endorse *orthonomy* (Pettit and Smith 1996) as an ideal of intentional agency. In contrast to personal autonomy as inner consistency or self-integration that we achieve by acting only upon motives that we are able to identify with, orthonomy essentially requires that we adjust our motives to independent norms. The core intuition is that we are unfree whenever we choose to engage in pursuits that we would disavow as unworthy, if we were to adopt an ideal observer's perspective. This kind of unfreedom is relevantly similar to constraints that false beliefs impose on our thinking. Arguably, our freedom of thought is undermined, if we are allowed to believe anything we like, regardless of logic and evidence. On this ground, it is plausible to infer that our freedom of action is equally undermined, if we are allowed to pursue any project we like, independently of its worth. Following this line of reasoning, the issue whether a substantively self-regarding initiative is worthy of protection from interference boils down to whether the initiative accords with some independent norm, such as rationality. Hence, the focus of protection clearly shifts from *self*-determination, viz., *auto*nomy to *correct* determination, viz., *ortho*nomy of the will.

11.2. Orthonomy is compatible with a loss of personal autonomy, as in cases where the correct determination of the will is extraneous to the will so determined.[16]

11.3. The trouble does not go away, if we conceive correct determination as a prerequisite for genuine self-determination since this conceptualization implies that self-determination should always be kept in check by further principles or values. It cannot provide an independent rationale for any initiatives, substantively self-regarding or otherwise.

---

[15] On the idea of autonomy as an actual state of self-government, see Feinberg (1986, chapter 18, esp. pp. 31–44).

[16] Berlin's critique of positive freedom (2002, pp. 178–200) could be seen as an expression of this concern.

11.4. The difficulty at issue—finding a reliable way to distinguish autonomous from non-autonomous choices vis-à-vis substantively self-regarding initiatives—is effectively dismissed rather than offered a solution.

12. Hence, decisional capacity and the related autonomy conception cannot be consistently defined in either value-neutral or value-laden terms.

A Possible Solution: Loss of Self-Esteem as Paradoxical Identification

The outcome of the preceding reconstruction is not entirely aporetic, for it helps outline the contours of a satisfactory solution. In essence, this should be a formal rather than a substantive approach to both decisional capacity and the related autonomy conception, the exclusive focus of which is a person's relationship to her motives, as in higher-order accounts. This conclusion follows directly from the earlier observation that the problem posed by depression comes down to a kind of deficit of authority or control over one's motives rather than a conflict with particular evaluative judgments. By focusing on the person's relationship to her motives, we are able to integrate the compelling intuition, according to which there is a close link between autonomy and self-respect. However, unlike substantive conceptions, which take the accord with the value of self-respect as an extra test applicable to the content of initiatives that have already satisfied the procedural conditions for being autonomously chosen, self-respect would be inbuilt in the formal constraints on the kind of relationship to one's motives that is compatible with personal autonomy.

This difference in strategy is significant. If this revised formal account is successful, it will offer a way of distinguishing substantively self-regarding initiatives that should be protected from interference from those that should not, which is both principled and reliable. By being principled, I mean that the criteria will be solely autonomy-based instead of falling back onto further considerations on an ad hoc basis, whenever an apparently autonomous self-regarding initiative seems too striking or counterintuitive to be granted protection. This is a clear advantage vis-à-vis value-laden accounts. In contrast, the improvement with respect to standard higher-order accounts lies in the ability to reliably distinguish autonomous from non-autonomous initiatives and avoid the kind of paradoxical decision to uphold non-autonomous but autocratic choices in the name of autonomy.

Key to the proposed solution is the claim that identification, the kind of relationship to one's motives that typically conveys autonomy to ensuing initiatives, becomes paradoxical in depression. Crucially, depressive identification is self-alienating: it leads to ambivalence, inner conflict and, ultimately, loss of self-esteem, which I take to involve both enmity toward the self and a sense of worthlessness based on a perception of the self as an inadequate source of actions.

This central claim draws on Freud's account of melancholia (1957) and, in particular, the idea that melancholia stems from a person's identification with someone or something that she should not or can no longer care about. According to Freud, the underlying process becomes intelligible by comparison with mourning, for in both cases the objective is coming to terms with a significant loss. However, the loss associated with melancholia is rarely as clear-cut as that conducive to mourning. One reason is that what is experienced as lost in melancholia may not only be a beloved person, but also an abstract idea, such as friendship, inspiration, one's very raison d'être. Another reason is that, unlike most cases of bereavement, the affliction suffered by the melancholic person can effectively be attributed to the object of her loss.

This becomes clear if we look at cases, which Freud considers as central. In such cases, a person gets hurt, disappointed, or abandoned by an intimate relation. Ambivalence, Freud considers, is key to the experience conducive to melancholia. For one and the same person becomes an appropriate target for contradictory attitudes. She is still a friend or a lover that one trusts and is fond of; yet, she also appears as someone that one should be wary of and resent.

A further layer of ambivalence adds up with the fact that the person wronged does not face this interpersonal problem so that it can be resolved by means of either reconciliation or revision of the prior relationship as valueless, deceitful or, perhaps, just over. Instead, the prospective melancholic redirects the resulting frustration toward the self. A possible explanation is that she avoids articulating the problem in such terms out of fear that neither of these options is really available to her. Thus, she takes herself to be unable to either mend the relationship at stake or let it go for good. This contributes to the paradoxical identification with the object of one's frustrations and disappointments, which is at the heart of the phenomenon. The person wronged is now able to shift the blame for what was inflicted upon her onto herself and, consequently, to perceive herself as a wrongdoer rather than a victim. In so doing, she gets the chance to maintain her former attachment and resist the need for change. This, however, comes at the price of internalizing the interpersonal conflict at the root of the problem. To give an example, a woman who discovers that her husband has been cheating on her may be reluctant to confront him because she fears that this could precipitate the end of their marriage. Yet, having chosen to pretend that she is unaware of his infidelity, the cheated wife needs to work out a plausible story about why she would want to continue living with someone who obviously disrespects her. In this story, she is likely to portray herself as the ultimate culprit who has drawn away the kind and loving husband of hers by becoming, say, increasingly plain and boring. The identification with the unpleasant character that she has invented for herself enables the unfortunate wife to maintain her esteem and affection for the husband, whom, according to her story, she does not deserve.

We can now see why the process of paradoxical identification eventually ends up with a loss of self-esteem, understood as a phenomenon whose complementary sides are sense of worthlessness and hostility toward the self. Both follow directly from the fact that the melancholic takes inappropriate responsibility for her misfortune. To return to the preceding example, the cheated wife reinvents herself as undeserving so that she may exculpate her husband. In her eyes, he now appears right to disrespect her, for, allegedly, she is unworthy of respect. Moreover, since the cheated wife casts herself as the one to blame for the failing marriage, her sense of worthlessness ties directly in with hostility toward herself. Having paradoxically identified with the husband who has wronged her, she becomes the target of her original desire to make him pay for this.[17]

[17] Freud (1957, p. 251): "the patients usually still succeed, by the circuitous path of self-punishment, in taking revenge on the original object and in tormenting their loved one through their illness, having resorted to it in order to avoid the need to express hostility to him openly. After all, the person who has occasioned the patient's emotional disorder, and on whom his illness is centred, is usually to be found in his immediate environment."

Building on this model, it is possible to integrate various kinds of abstract ideas as eligible objects, whose perceived loss may be similarly compensated for by paradoxical identification. For instance, an ambitious professional may be unwilling to acknowledge his disappointment with a career move that he carefully planned and worked hard for. Like the cheated wife from the earlier example, he may wish to keep up the pretense that his current position is truly rewarding. In order to do so, he would have to assume that only his own inadequacy prevents him from flourishing at the new workplace. The ensuing paradoxical identification with an organization that he finds frustrating would enable him to resist bringing up the discrepancies between the conditions offered and the opportunities in place. In turn, this could save the ambitious professional both a potentially costly interpersonal conflict and a radical revision of his career plan. However, as in the unfortunate marriage scenario, the avoidance of a would-be professional disaster comes at the price of greatly diminished self-esteem.

To recap the argument of the current section, the notion of paradoxical identification helps explain the lack of authority over substantively self-regarding initiatives that, as shown in the previous section, is typical of depression.[18] These initiatives cannot be considered as autonomous in so far as they substantiate a conflicting relationship to one's motives. This is because the paradoxical identification with something or someone that the agent implicitly loathes, naturally leads to internalized ambivalence. In essence, the agent remains irresolute and fails to take control over her motives. Instead of making up her mind, she absorbs a practical contradiction that she faces. Initiatives that could be traced back to this process are non-autonomous, for they are not actively determined by the agent: she merely goes along with them. Moreover, she cannot be recognized as the ultimate source of such initiatives, whether she is willing to endorse them ex post factum or not.[19] This analysis points to a necessary formal condition that any process of identification should fulfill in order to effectively convey autonomy to related initiatives. In order to be authoritative in this respect, identification with one's motives should be undertaken under the guise of the good.

A related implication is that some initiatives at issue, such as treatment refusals with foreseeably fatal consequences may turn out not to be self-regarding in the required sense. For they could be pinned down as misplaced reactions of either hostility toward identifiable others or generalized resentment. In both instances, apparently self-regarding initiatives become open to reinterpretation as fundamentally other-regarding and, for this reason, ineligible for protection under the principle of respect for autonomy that was specified earlier.

Personal Autonomy and the Guise of the Good

It may be tempting to challenge the proposed solution as leading to unacceptable consequences. The challenge is as follows. If, as I argued, paradoxical identification is

---

[18] See especially steps 8 to10 of the reconstruction.

[19] See Radden (2008) for a comparative analysis of two strategies whereby personal identity is conceived in depression memoirs: "symptom alienating" and "symptom integrating." An important conclusion is that both strategies could be equally self-alienating: either by refusing to acknowledge one's mental states as one's own or by internalising a ready-made, extraneous perspective toward one's experiences.

incompatible with personal autonomy in the relevant sense, protection from interference should be removed from many substantively self-regarding initiatives that some depression sufferers effectively identify with. This move would substantially shrink, if not eliminate the scope for self-determination they are left with. It would equally be at odds with respect for depression sufferers as persons.

This challenge builds on two related assumptions. According to the first, respect for persons is inseparable from respect for their autonomous agency. According to the second, respect for personal autonomy is inseparable from respect for substantively self-regarding initiatives. Jointly, the two assumptions support the idea that the only way to respect a person in the grips of depression is to condone her depression-induced initiatives and, for instance, let her die, if she attempts suicide, as was implied by the Wooltorton case.[20]

To understand the underlying dialectic and successfully take on the challenge, let us consider the concept of practical identity introduced by Christine Korsgaard. According to Korsgaard, practical identity is "a description under which you value yourself, a description under which you find your life worth living and your actions to be worth undertaking" (1996, p. 101). For instance, the fact that I am committed to a particular profession gives me a cluster of reasons for action that I would otherwise not have. In a similar vein, defining myself as a theatre enthusiast, a good friend, or a keen cyclist would each speak in favor of certain projects to the exclusion of others. Following this line of thought, Korsgaard concludes:

> It is necessary to have *some* conception of your practical identity, for without it you cannot have reasons to act. We endorse or reject our impulses by determining whether they are consistent with the ways in which we identify ourselves … For unless you are committed to some conception of your practical identity, you will lose your grip on yourself as having any reason to do one thing rather than another—and with it, your grip on yourself as having any reason to live and act at all. (1996, pp. 120–121)

In light of these observations, depression appears as a distinct impediment to any practical identity that a depressed person could possibly undertake rather than a separate practical identity. This is not to say that depression may lead to an unreasonable or objectionable practical identity, providing the depressed person with reasons for action that do not make sense from an observer's perspective. Instead, the thought is that reasons for actions, recognized as valid from the agent's perspective, get overridden or suspended because of depression and this seems idiotic to the agent herself (Solomon 1998). We are finally able to resolve the initial paradox posed by depression: the perplexing gap between evaluation and motivation can now be explained as a result of the agent's paradoxical identification with something that she implicitly loathes. Related initiatives could be compared with the so-called mixed actions, whereby the original link between evaluation and motivation is thwarted by various kinds of undue influence, such as credible threats. Paradoxical identification has a similar effect. Like coercion, the behavior it affects cannot be considered as fully intentional.

This analogy could remain unnoticed because, in cases of paradoxical identification, the voluntariness of the resulting behavior is impeded by the agent herself rather than another person. This aspect, however, is neither paradoxical, nor of consequence to the analogy between depression and coercion, which was alluded to earlier in terms of autocracy. In fact, there is nothing astonishing in the idea that an agent can incapacitate herself. It suffices

---

[20] See step 4.3.1 of the argument scheme in the section "The challenge to decisional capacity".

that I take myself to be an inadequate source of actions in order to make myself so. This follows directly from the intuitive understanding of intentional action as trying to achieve certain objective. Clearly, I cannot undertake such an action, unless I implicitly believe that the objective is not unattainable for me. Hence, it is rather the mechanism underlying the impediment or breakdown of agency brought about by a depressed self that stands in need of explanation.

Drawing on the preceding analysis, this mechanism becomes intelligible in terms of suspended commitment to many, if not all eligible practical identities. As a result, judgments about projects worth undertaking could be seen as merely entertained rather than endorsed by a person in the grips of severe depression. The lack of motivation to act one way or the other that is so striking from both agent's and observer's perspectives, turns out to be better accounted for as a hindrance to the depressed person's capacity to value rather than as a severed link between evaluation proper and motivation.[21]

This development is fully consistent with the idea that an agent can authoritatively identify only with what she cares about. Whenever this formal constraint is not met, the agent's relationship to her motives becomes paradoxical. This could to lead to a volitional halt to the extent that some of her own aspirations correctly appear to her as impossible to satisfy. For the intrinsic ambivalence of a paradoxical relationship to one's motives translates into inconsistent volitions, whereby the same outcome is both wished for and abhorred. Since these kinds of volitions are bound to end in frustration, they sustain the depressed person's sense that any endeavor is futile and her life is no longer worth living (Solomon 1998).

Returning to the challenge from unacceptable consequences, we are now in a position to critically examine the two premises, on which it depends. For instance, the analogy between paradoxical identification and coercion points to a flaw in the first premise, according to which we can only respect a person in so far as we recognize her to be an autonomous agent. The thought is that respect for persons who have been subject to coercion clearly departs from respect for the choices, they made under duress. In fact, giving credence to the latter would amount to taking sides with the coercers and disregarding the coercees even further. Following this line of thought, it becomes compelling to separate respect for persons from respect for autonomous agency so that instances of forced or improper self-determination do not undermine the possibility for genuine self-determination in the future. In this respect, firm constraints on what a person can authoritatively decide about herself appear to be a prerequisite for rather than an obstacle to her self-determination. The notion of inalienable rights or dignity expresses well this intuition. For only by making certain self-regarding choices ineligible for protection from interference could a society effectively shield individuals from particularly grave kinds of intrusion. The rejection of a right to sell oneself into slavery is a classic example (Mill 1859). Thus, a person may be at liberty to feel and behave as another person's slave, however, she is not at liberty to require that third parties respect this arrangement and treat her as another's slave (Shiffrin 2000).

---

[21] An advantage of this solution is that it does not commit us to a particular account of the nature of either evaluation or motivation. For it is compatible with both a Humean account of valuing as a kind of desire (Roberts 2001), and a scholastic view of desires as subjective conceptions of the good (Tenenbaum 2007, pp. 283–298).

The preceding example helps articulate the significance of disentangling respect for persons from respect for autonomous agency. For it suggests that self-respect is not a necessary condition for being respected as a person.[22] Just as the would-be slave's subservience does not provide us with a reason to treat her as a being of lesser worth, a depressed person's sense of worthlessness does not provide us with a reason to let her die if she attempts to commit suicide.

Furthermore, this observation points to a flaw in the second premise of the challenge from unacceptable consequences, according to which it is exclusively by respecting self-regarding initiatives that we respect personal autonomy. This is consistent with the earlier argument that depression should be understood as an obstacle to having a practical identity rather than an alternative practical identity. As indicated by the two thought experiments in the previous section, both the cheated wife and the frustrated professional end up with diminished self-esteem because of a paradoxical identification with a problem that was imposed on them rather than with a solution of their own. Respect for initiatives motivated by reduced self-esteem can only amplify the initial paradox and curtail the scope for self-determination proper even further. Drawing on this analysis, it becomes clear that respect for personal autonomy is incompatible with respect for depression-induced self-regarding initiatives. This is good reason to doubt the objection from unacceptable consequences, for neither of the assumptions on which it depends could survive critical examination.

REFERENCES

American Psychiatric Association (2001). *Diagnostic and Statistical Manual of Mental Disorders, Fourth Edition, Text Revision*. Washington, DC: American Psychiatric Association.

Anscombe, G. E. M. (1963). *Intention* (2nd edn). Oxford: Blackwell.

Arpaly, N. (2003). *Unprincipled Virtue: An Inquiry into Moral Agency*. New York, NY: Oxford University Press.

Beauchamp, T. L. and Childress, J. F. (1979). *Principles of Biomedical Ethics*. New York, NY: Oxford University Press.

Berlin, I. (2002). *Liberty* (H. Hardy, Ed). Oxford: Oxford University Press.

Charland, L. (2008). Decision-making capacity. In E. N. Zalta (Ed.), *The Stanford Encyclopedia of Philosophy* (Winter 2008 Edition). [Online.] Available at: <http://plato.stanford.edu/entries/decision-capacity/>.

Christman, J. (1988). Constructing the inner citadel: Recent work on autonomy. *Ethics*, 99(1), 109–24.

Culver, C. M. and Gert, B. (2004). Competence. In J. Radden (Ed.), *The Philosophy of Psychiatry: A Companion*, pp. 258–70. New York, NY: Oxford University Press.

Dworkin, G. (1988). *The Theory and Practice of Autonomy*. Cambridge: Cambridge University Press.

Feinberg, J. (1986). *Harm to Self*. New York, NY: Oxford University Press.

Frankfurt, H. (1998). *The Importance of What We Care About: Philosophical Essays*. Cambridge: Cambridge University Press.

[22] See Langton (2007) for a related argument, according to which the value of persons is best understood as unconditional and, therefore, independent of whether a person happens to value herself at a particular moment in time or not.

Frankfurt, H. (1999). *Necessity, Volition, and Love*. Cambridge: Cambridge University Press.

Frankfurt, H. (2002). Reply to Gary Watson. In S. Buss and L. Overton (Eds), *Contours of Agency: Essays from Themes from Harry Frankfurt*, pp. 160–3. Cambridge, MA: MIT Press.

Freud, S. (1957). *Mourning and Melancholia*. In J. Strachey (Ed. and Trans.) *The Complete Psychological Works of Sigmund Freud* (Vol. 14), pp. 243–58. London: Hogarth Press and the Institute for Psychoanalysis. (Original work published 1915.)

Gallie, W.B. (1956). Essentially contested concepts. *Proceedings of the Aristotelian Society, 56*, 167–98.

Hill, Jr, T. (1991). *Autonomy and Self-Respect*. Cambridge: Cambridge University Press.

Korsgaard, C. M. with Cohen, G. A. (1996). *Sources of Normativity*. Cambridge: Cambridge University Press.

Langton, R. (2007). Objective and unconditioned value. *Philosophical Review, 116*(2), 157–85.

McLean, S. (2009). Live and let die. *British Medical Journal, 339*, b4112.

Mele, A. (1987). *Irrationality: An Essay of Akrasia, Self-Deception, and Self-Control*. New York, NY: Oxford University Press.

Mill, J.S. (1959). *On Liberty*. Indianapolis IN: Bobbs Merrill. (Original work published 1859.)

Office of Public Sector Information (2007). *Mental Capacity Act 2005*. London: Office of Public Sector Information. Available at: <http://www.opsi.gov.uk/acts/acts2005/ukpga_20050009_en_1>.

O'Neill, O. (2002). *Autonomy and Trust in Bioethics*. Cambridge: Cambridge: University Press

Pettit, P. and Smith, M. (1996). Freedom in belief and desire. *Journal of Philosophy, 93*(9), 429–49.

Radden, J. (2008). My symptoms, myself: Reading mental illness memoirs for identity assumptions. In H. Clark (Ed.), *Depression and Narrative: Telling the Dark*, pp. 15–28. Albany, NY: State University of New York Press.

Radoilska, L. (2007). *L'Actualité d'Aristote en morale*. Paris: Presses Universitaires de France.

Radoilska, L. (2012). Autonomy and Ulysses arrangements. In Radoilska, L. (Ed.), *Autonomy and Mental Disorder*, pp. 252–80. Oxford: Oxford University Press.

Re MB [1997] 2 FLR 426. Available at: <http://www.bailii.org/ew/cases/EWCA/Civ/1997/3093.html>

Roberts, J. R. (2001). Mental illness, motivation, and moral commitment. *The Philosophical Quarterly, 51*(202), 41–59.

Scoccia, D. (2008). In defense of hard paternalism. *Law and Philosophy, 27*, 351–81.

Setiya, K. (2010). Sympathy for the Devil. In S. Tenenbaum (Ed.), *Desire, Practical Reason, and the Good*, pp. 82–110. New York, NY: Oxford University Press.

Shiffrin, S.V. (2000). Paternalism, unconscionability doctrine, and accommodation. *Philosophy & Public Affairs, 29*(3), 205–50.

Solomon, A. (1998). Anatomy of melancholy. *The New Yorker*, January 12, 46–61.

Stocker, M. (1979). Desiring the bad: An essay in moral psychology. *Journal of Philosophy, 76*(12), 738–53.

Taylor, J. S. (2005). Introduction. In J. S. Taylor (Ed.), *Personal Autonomy: New Essays on Personal Autonomy and Its Role in Contemporary Moral Philosophy*, pp. 1–29. Cambridge: Cambridge University Press.

Tenenbaum, S. (2007). *Appearances of the Good: An Essay on the Nature of Practical Reason*. Cambridge: Cambridge University Press.

Velleman, D. (1992). The guise of the good. *Noûs, 26*(1), 3–26.

World Health Organization (1992). *The ICD-10 Classification of Mental and Behavioural Disorders*. Geneva: World Health Organization.

CHAPTER 68

PSYCHOPHARMACOLOGY AND THE SELF

FREDRIK SVENAEUS

INTRODUCTION

In this chapter an attempt will be made to answer the question of whether psychopharmacological drugs have effects on the self. The answer will be provided by a conceptual analysis discussing what we mean by self, and by considering reports and research on how psychopharmacological drugs actually work and have effects on persons and their brains. Psychotropics raise many more philosophical issues than I will be able to deal with here (for an overview, see Stein 2008), but I think the questions about effects on the self are central to the philosophy of psychopharmacology, since they touch upon not only ontological but also epistemological and ethical issues of vital importance for psychiatry.

Questions about psychopharmacological effects on abilities that belong to the self are often found in bioethical debates on so-called enhancement, that is, medical interventions which go beyond the mission of treating diseases. Psychopharmacology, in these debates, seems to offer us a glimpse of types of changes that we will perhaps attain in the future—some hope and some fear—by means of genetic manipulations, which will offer more solid and stable effects on selfhood. Focused issues in these debates are, for instance, effects on emotional stability, memory, intelligence, and even moral goodness (Gordijn and Chadwick 2008).

Phenomenology will be the main theoretical approach to the questions of psychopharmacology and selfhood in this chapter, but this does not mean that I will favor a subjective or psychological view and sacrifice the objective and biological perspective in psychiatry. Psychiatry is a mixed discipline, and phenomenology, in my view, offers a kind of neutral ground on which it is possible to relate and connect the many different approaches to mental disorders and the treatments of them that we find in the field.

An important issue on the way to answering the question about psychotropic changes to the self is whether different mental disorders include changes in selfhood as a part of the pathologies. If they do, the effects of psychopharmacological drugs in curing or alleviating the disorders must be regarded in relationship to these pathological changes in selfhood. I will give some examples of mental disorders in which the self is likely to have been affected by the pathology and in which the question of psychopharmacological effects on the self will accordingly concern a re-establishment of the healthy self rather than any enhancement to a state that is "better than well" (Elliott 2003).

In order to settle the issue of whether some mental disorders include selfhood changes as part of their diagnoses, we need a rudimentary answer to what we are to mean by self. After providing this through a turn to phenomenology, we will also need to enter into the discussion of what mental disorders are, not to settle the issue, surely, but to relate the methodology of the DSM (I will use *Diagnostic and Statistical Manual of Mental Disorders, Fourth Edition, Text Revision* (DSM-IV-TR) from 2000), in which we find definitions of different mental disorders, to the methodology of phenomenology, by which we will have developed our definition of selfhood. Are mental disorders something that persons (selves) develop and carry like somatic diseases, or are they rather to be thought of as personality changes so severe that we deem them appropriate to treat by medical means? Are some mental disorders disorders *of* a basic layer of selfhood itself, while other are more like changes in vital *dimensions* of selfhood? Perhaps mental disorders can be a bit of all these things, depending on which mental disorders we are discussing, and this will then have implications for our understanding of possible psychotropic effects on the self.

PHENOMENOLOGY AND THE SELF

Phenomenology might be described as the attempt to address all kinds of ontological and epistemological issues by way of exploring and analyzing lived experience. The starting point for the phenomenologist is life, viewed and investigated from a certain perspective: the phenomenological attitude, in which a systematic reflection on the meaning *of* experience is exercised. Human experience is typically intentional in the sense of presenting things in the world *as* such and such things carrying different meaning. Phenomenology, which started out as a philosophical movement about a century ago—its most famous adherents were Edmund Husserl, Martin Heidegger, Maurice Merleau-Ponty, Jean-Paul Sartre, Paul Ricoeur, and Hans-Georg Gadamer—quickly won converts within other disciplines, including aesthetics, psychology, sociology, ethnography, and pedagogy, and developed into a vast interdisciplinary network of research programs. During the past three decades, phenomenology has also gained some attention within the discipline of medicine (Toombs 2001), and particularly within psychiatry (Sass et al. 2011). We can also see the influence of phenomenology on psychiatry at an earlier date, in the work of psychoanalysts and psychotherapists who relied on phenomenological thinkers in developing their theories about mental illness and its treatment (for example, Jacques Lacan, Ludwig Binswanger, and Medard Boss) (Spiegelberg 1972).

The basic methodological exhortation of phenomenology is the need to start from a position free of various scientific claims (about what mental disorders are, for example), but it also strives by way of this non-prejudged starting point to establish a basic ontology (and not only a myriad of subjective views) of the world: a philosophical theory developed from the first- and second-person perspective (I include hermeneutics in my characterization of phenomenology) in which the third-person perspective investigations of science can then attain a proper place and significance (Svenaeus 2006). Phenomenology is neither a materialist theory, since it does not believe that ontological and epistemological issues are settled by way of science only, nor an idealistic theory, since it does not proceed from any soul or psyche freed from the forces of nature. To understand the structure of human experience we need to acknowledge that experience is always embodied and world dependent, but also an ongoing creative effort of bringing meaning into the world by way of intentionality.

But in what way, then, does the self present itself to the phenomenologist when she is conducting her analysis of lived experience as being about different things in the world? The often-quoted remark by David Hume that nowhere in his experience has he come upon any entity which could be referred to as his self, should not fool us into assuming that the self is either a fiction or something we will have to leave to the brain scientists to determine if we really have (Zahavi 2005, p. 101). The self is clearly no homunculus sitting somewhere in the brain, and the "hard" problem of the explanatory "gap" will likely not be solved by identifying *a* brain structure that is the conscious self. Most brain scientists still believe that some way of picking out complex patterns of brain processes (probably spanning many different areas of the brain) will give us the self, at least in its minimal form (e.g., Damasio 1999, p. 323). The phenomenologist will be skeptical of such solutions for the simple reason that they misunderstand what a third-person, in contrast to a first-person, approach is able to accomplish. Our primary access to selfhood is via experience *itself* (the first-person perspective) and not via science (the third-person perspective), argues the phenomenologist. If we investigate human life through the phenomenological approach we will find that all experiences of things in the world *belong* to someone (a self), and this is also the main clue in our endeavors to understand selfhood.

I will argue that identity (selfhood), in the case of persons, is provided through several constituting *layers of processes*. The identity-forming processes of the self (person) include processes of the *body*, processes of the *mind*, and processes of *social and cultural* origin and nature. The processes of selfhood start with meaning formation that takes place on pre-conscious embodied levels, but the processes in question attain a different quality on the conscious level of self-reflection. This happens when I understand, and not only feel, that I am a *something* which, in the experiences I am having, is encountering *other* things. This type of self-understanding means that I become able to attain an epistemological stance in which I direct my explicit attention to my very self in having the experiences, a procedure that allows several ontological as well as existential questions to set in. The processes of self-constitution, through yet another layer, also extend into the cultural world of language in which the person's identity, her personality, is shaped by being related to narrative life plots: stories. Theories about the "narrative self" are very popular in contemporary cultural theory, and some authors even seem to claim that the self essentially *consists* in a story (Jopling 2000). These narrative theories certainly pinpoint an important aspect of selfhood, but they nevertheless often disregard the importance of the two other layers of selfhood I have identified. To be a self hardly means just being a story; it means being a creature who can *tell* stories because it is situated in a meaningful world together with other persons.

Dan Zahavi, in several impressive phenomenological studies, has defended the idea that selfhood is basically the subjective aspect of what it means to be conscious of something *überhaupt* (he calls this the minimal self) (2005, p. 106). This awareness of self is pre-reflective in the sense that the self is not conscious of itself through an act of reflection—looking back upon itself, so to speak—but rather through the *quality* of the experience in question, it being an experience *of* something (a tree, a hat, another human being, a piece of mathematics, or whatever) as an intentional process. Every experience is owned by someone in the sense that it belongs to someone by appearing in a particular stream of consciousness: when I write this text, for example, this is my experience, not yours. There might exist anonymous, or even alien, forms of experiences in which a person has the sense of an experience not belonging to her, or even belonging to somebody else (such as in schizophrenia), but these are not the primary modes of experiences. They are, rather, transformed modes of self-experience that presuppose a basic belonging, a "selfishness" of every stream of consciousness from which the anonymity or alienation can appear (how would the self otherwise be able to character-ize the experiences in question *as* anonymous or alien?) (Zahavi 2005, p. 144). Theories of pre-reflective self-awareness can be found in the work of many phenomenologists. Zahavi's main point of departure is the theories on inner time-consciousness and passive synthesis in Husserl, but, as he shows, similar points are made by Heidegger and Sartre in using the con-cepts of "Jemeinigkeit" and "pour-soi" (Zahavi 2010).

The multilayered makeup of the self should not be understood in an evolutionary or developmental way only. It is certainly true that the pre-conscious level of self-awareness preceded the phenomenon of reflective self-awareness in the evolutionary process of life on earth, and it is also true that it does so in the individual life of a child, but the crucial point is that the different layers (when they have all been put in place) coexist and interact with each other (Zahavi 2005). The narrative-social self never leaves the embodied (or the self-reflective) self behind, since they are all constituents of the *same* self: they are different layers of selfhood. The fact that I depict the self in terms of several layers of *processes* in this chapter is not meant to reify the self (a process could perhaps be understood as a kind of thing), since these processes are designated exactly as being *constitutive* in character. The processes make something appear (the self and a whole world with it). Some phenomenolo-gists would prefer to talk about such processes as transcendental in contrast to empirical in character, but I will not go into that issue here.

Despite the claim that it is the basic belongingness to somebody of every experience in the streaming life of consciousness that is the ground of selfhood, it should be pointed out that this pre-reflectively embodied self is in a way exactly *anonymous* in character, since we do not control it but are, rather, constituted *by* it. The body to a large extent organizes my experiences on a pre-conscious level. Proprioceptively, it makes me present in my own body, and kinesthetically, it allows me to experience the things that are not me: the things of the world that show up to my sensing, moving body in different activities through which they attain their place and significance (Gallagher 2005). To the ways of the lived body also belong the autonomous processes of my biological organism: breath, digestion, blood flow, etc., which are mostly absent from my awareness but nevertheless provide the backdrop for my intentionality when I become conscious of things (Leder 1990).

If the self is to be understood as constituted by a multilayered set of interactive proc-esses, these processes do not only include the experience of being me in doing this or that (pre-consciously as well as reflectively); they also include a being *disposed* to have a certain type of experiences and to display certain types of behaviors and actions in certain situa-tions. Every human self has a *personality* that makes it unique, and this personality consists in different traits, of which many are dispositions: characteristics that are not experienced or displayed constantly by the self but which have developed into a stable pattern over time and which can be exposed by offering the right circumstances. Personalities are heavily dependent upon the narrative layers of selfhood, which provide the person with a plot that is vital to her identity. But they are also dependent upon dispositions to experience, behave, and act, which are not invented by the person herself or other storytellers, but rather put in place by nature and nurture as the self develops.

Peter Goldie, in his book *On Personality*, distinguishes seven classes of such traits that the self exhibits, or is disposed to exhibit, by way of its personality: temperaments, ways of acting, habits, skills, emotional dispositions, enduring preferences and values, and character traits (2004, pp. 11–13). The different forms (classes) of personality traits that Goldie identifies contain various forms of dispositions to not only experience but also *take action* in a certain way. As we have seen, phenomenology reveals a preference for the *experienced* perspective, but this does not mean, as will have become obvious already from the brief introduction to the phenomenology of selfhood given earlier, that the focus of phenomenology is only consciousness in any narrow sense. The embodied ways of inhabiting the world, as a horizon of meaning for the self, necessarily introduce the realm of action. To be conscious of something demands not only a pre-conscious, bodily presence of the self, but also horizons of human projects and stories in which things can stand out and be experienced *as* such-and-such things: a hammer to be used in building a house, to take the most famous example from Heidegger in *Being and Time* when he introduces the concept of "being-in-the-world," which is central to this hermeneutic approach in phenomenology (1986).

Mental Disorders and the Self

I will remain neutral in the extensive debate on what mental disorders are (biological abnormalities, psychological suffering, human disabilities, or cultural constructs) but, just as in the case of selfhood, I believe a multilayered approach to be the most fruitful. Rather than developing this issue further, I will try to give some examples of mental disorders from the DSM that appear to have a close connection with changes in selfhood as defined above. Remember that the claim of the DSM is to be ontologically neutral regarding the questions of what mental disorders are, how they develop, and how they can be treated. This notwithstanding, we find the following quote in the introduction to the manual:

> A common misconception is that a classification of mental disorders classifies people, when actually what are being classified are disorders that people have. For this reason, the text of DSM-IV (as did the text of DSM-III-R) avoids the use of such expressions as "a schizophrenic" or "an alcoholic" and instead uses the more accurate but admittedly more cumbersome, "an individual with Schizophrenia" or "an individual with Alcohol Dependence." (American Psychiatric Association 2000, p. xxxi)

If this were true, there would probably be no point in including the issue of mental disorder in my analysis of how psychopharmacological drugs have effects on the self. But it is obviously not true, at least not if self and personality are interpreted in the way we have done above. Many diagnoses in the DSM are established by checking symptoms and behaviors that are very clearly related to issues of selfhood and personality. And, as many critiques of the new diagnostic psychiatry have pointed out, most diagnoses in the manual do *not* rest on the identification of disorders in the sense of something simply *had* by the individual, which it would be possible to detect without judgments about *who* she is (her life history) (Horowitz and Wakefield 2007). The interpretation of life-world matters is a necessary part of psychiatry to a much larger extent than in the somatic medicine of diseases, a field which the authors of the DSM, in the earlier quote, are clearly trying to gain credibility from by way of analogy.

Now, while the authors of the DSM want to claim that the concept of disorder with which they are working—"a clinically significant behavioral or psychological syndrome or pattern that occurs in an individual and that is associated with present distress (e.g., a painful symptom) or disability (i.e., impairment in one or more important areas of functioning) or with a significantly increased risk of suffering death, pain, disability, or an important loss of freedom" (American Psychiatric Association 2000, p. xxxi)—is *categorical* in nature, a study of the different diagnoses in the manual clearly brings out that the way in which disorders are approached is instead *dimensional* in nature: the disorders overlap by degrees with unwanted or despised, yet still normal, experiences and behaviors of people which are to a large extent personality dependent. The most striking example of this is perhaps the personality disorders, of which it would be very strange indeed to claim that they have nothing to do with personality. That they are special is acknowledged by the DSM authors by putting them on a different "axis"—Axis II—separate from the other disorders in the manual, thereby indicating that personality disorders have more enduring patterns than other mental disorders and that they are therefore easy for doctors to miss if they look upon mental disorders as something that more or less suddenly hit people.

Personality disorders, in their different types, are hard to treat. Some forms of psychotherapy might be effective, but at present there exists no effective pharmacological treatment for personality disorders (some drugs are used to treat patients with personality disorders, but most often either off-label or by indication of other mental disorders on Axis I in the DSM that the patients simultaneously suffer from). This probably has less to do with personality disorders being culturally, rather than biologically, constituted, and more to do with the ingrainment of the disorders in the personality of the persons who are having them. Surveying the diagnostic features of antisocial, borderline, histrionic, or narcissistic personality disorder, we find peculiarities in many of the seven different traits of personality listed by Goldie (American Psychiatric Association 2000, pp. 701–717). Indeed, we often find loathsome features of *character*, and this is also the reason why having a personality disorder does not afford access to the kinds of excuses and freedom from responsibility that we allow perpetrators of crimes who are suffering from, for instance, a sudden outbreak of psychosis that makes them unable to understand what they are actually doing.

There are mental disorders of another type found in the DSM, however, that display features of personality which are deemed to be pathological, and which seem to respond to medication, namely what are most often referred to as neuropsychiatric, or developmental, disorders: attention-deficit/hyperactivity disorder (ADHD), and, in some cases, Asperger's disorder. ADHD is found in the DSM under the heading "Disorders Usually First Diagnosed in Infancy, Childhood, or Adolescence," and it is increasingly treated with methylphenidate, which has a normalizing effect on the difficulties in concentrating and in controlling sudden impulses that are typical for the diagnosis (Wigal 2009). ADHD, like Asperger's disorder, probably gradually overlaps by degrees with normal personality traits, traits that belong primarily to the groups Goldie names: "ways of acting," "habits," "and emotional disposi-tions." That the neuropsychiatric disorders are not called personality disorders is in large part a historical coincidence having to do with the development of different schools in psy-chiatry, but the distinction also reflects the fact that they can normally be diagnosed much earlier in life than the personality disorders (thus the name "developmental disorders"). They are therefore often assumed to arise from deficiencies in brain chemistry (to be "neuropsy-chiatric") rather than being deviations that are the result of a difficult childhood, a claim that is taken to be vindicated by their response to drugs. However, this is very much a matter of speculations rather than facts; maybe ADHD is to a considerable extent a cultural construct, while antisocial personality disorder can be tracked down to a set of genes regulating brain chemistry. Or, perhaps, and very likely, both disorders will be found in the future to display features that can be analyzed by way of biology, but they are nevertheless picked out today as disorders because they stand out as behavioral patterns that we find troublesome in our contemporary Western culture.

If personality disorders and neuropsychiatric disorders (developmental disorders) are clearly related to personality traits of the self (the person), there are other mental disorders that seem rather to be disorders, not of personality, but of the self itself. What do I mean by this? Recall Zahavi's analysis of what he calls the minimal self: pre-reflective, embodied self-awareness in which the experience of selfhood is tied not to reflection but to the felt quality of the flow of experience as such. In schizophrenia and other psychotic disorders, we find experiences of hyper-reflexivity and diminished self-affection, meaning that the flow of the processes of the pre-reflective self is either intensified and interrupted in various ways or flattened out, resulting in feelings of non-existence (Sass et al. 2011). Hyper-reflexivity will be experienced as a basic form of *alienation* of selfhood, the flow of experience being constantly interrupted by thoughts and voices which feel foreign in origin, leading to hal-lucinations (mainly auditory), delusions, and disorganized thoughts on part of the patient. Diminished self-affection is correlated with the so-called negative symptoms of schizophre-nia, the patient feeling non-present and *anonymous*, unable to take initiatives and see the possibility of doing anything. Speech and communication in both cases are severely affected, leading to "word-salad" and being cut off from contact with others (American Psychiatric Association 2000, p. 312).

Schizophrenia and other psychotic disorders respond to antipsychotic (neuroleptic) med-ication, which, in spite of severe side effects, appears to alleviate the basic disturbances of selfhood in many cases. Antipsychotics are also used off-label to treat cases of developmen-tal disorders and dementia in which disturbances of selfhood similar to those in psychosis may be present. Although both methylphenidate and antipsychotics have been the subject of bioethical debates, the most intensive discussions about effects of psychopharmacologi-cal drugs on self have concerned the expanding use of new antidepressants: the SSRIs (selec-tive serotonin reuptake inhibitors, made famous by the brand name of Prozac). SSRIs are used by hundreds of millions of people over the whole world today, and their prescription is most often called for by the diagnosis of depression or an anxiety disorder (though they are also used to treat chronic pain and eating disorders and, off-label, probably many other things as well). Since the use of SSRIs provokes questions that are central to the question of psychopharmacological effects on the self, I will devote a separate section of this chapter to an analysis of how the effects of the new antidepressants are to be understood.

ANTIDEPRESSANTS AND THE SELF

A lingering suspicion, ever since the first reports of the success of Prozac in the late 1980s, has been that the new antidepressants, in addition to relieving the symptoms of depression and anxiety disorders, also have other effects that help explain their popularity. Do the SSRIs have effects on the self in the way Peter Kramer illustrates by way of clinical examples in his well-known book, *Listening to Prozac* (1993)? According to Kramer, some of his patients went through the experience of "becoming themselves" while on Prozac, whereas others had the experience of "losing themselves," despite feeling better on the drug. What might "becoming oneself" or "losing oneself" possibly mean in these cases? By developing some aspects of the groups of personality traits Goldie names "temperaments" and "emotional dispositions," and relating them to the multilayered model of selfhood found in Zahavi, I think we can begin to answer these questions.

The distinguishing characteristic of depressive disorders is the presence of what is called "a major depressive episode" (American Psychiatric Association 2000, p. 356). This condition is adjudged to be present if a depressed mood (sadness, emptiness) and a loss of interest or pleasure have been present most of the day, nearly every day, for at least two weeks, and if, in addition, at least three of the following seven criteria have also been fulfilled during this period: significant weight change; insomnia or hypersomnia; psychomotor agitation or retardation; fatigue or loss of energy; feelings of worthlessness or excessive or inappropriate guilt; diminished ability to think or concentrate; and recurrent thoughts of death. These symptoms must also have resulted in "clinically significant distress or impairment in social, occupational, or other important areas of functioning," and they should not have been directly caused by medication or bereavement (the loss of a loved one).

If we turn to how anxiety disorders are described in the DSM, we find a similar litany of deviant feelings—of problems involving altered embodiment and estranged engagement with the world. Here, the common characteristic of the disorders that are treated with SSRIs is the panic attack—an excess of anxiety triggered by an alarming situation. A panic attack is specified as "a discrete period of intense fear or discomfort," in which symptoms like pounding heart, sweating, trembling, shortness of breath, chest pain, nausea, fear of losing control, going crazy, or dying are developed abruptly and reach a peak within ten minutes (American Psychiatric Association 2000, p. 432). The panic attacks are typically recurrent, and they are often associated with being in a special type of situation (meeting or speaking to strangers in social phobia, for instance). The sufferer not only experiences anxiety while *having* the attacks, he is also in many cases constantly *anxious about* having them.

The type of phenomena we should concentrate on in understanding the effects of antidepressants on depression and anxiety disorders is made fairly clear by the lists of criteria presented in the DSM: central to each diagnostic scheme is the presence of painful *feelings* and of problems involving altered *embodiment* and estranged *engagement* with the *world*. In the recently published paper—"Do Antidepressants Affect the Self?" (Svenaeus 2007)—I tried to show, with the aid of phenomenologists such as Martin Heidegger (1927/1986) and Thomas Fuchs (2000), that the effects of the new antidepressants must be thought of in terms of changes in self-feeling or, more precisely, of "self-vibration of embodiment." These concepts come close to the ancient notions of temperament—a basic disposition of the self to develop characteristic moods—the most famous of the four classic temperaments being the melancholic personality type (Radden 2000), and also to what Goldie terms "emotional dispositions," being more or less disposed by way of the bodily vibration profile to develop certain feelings when being put under stress in certain situations.

In the paper I presented the idea of a spectrum of bodily resonances, which extends from the normal resonance of the lived body, in which the body is able to pick up a wide range of different moods, to various kinds of sensitivities, preferences, and idiosyncrasies, in which certain moods are favored over others, to cases that we unreservedly label pathologies because the body is severely out of tune, or even devoid of tune, and thus useless as a tool of resonance. Different cultures and societies favor slightly differently attuned self-styles as paradigmatic of the normal and of the good life, and the popularity of the SSRIs can therefore be explained not only by defects of embodiment (biology) but also by the presence of certain cultural norms in our contemporary society (Elliott and Chambers 2004). My attempt to understand the effects of antidepressants in the paper was very much in line with the idea that mental disorders overlap by degree with normal profiles of personality traits, in this case in the dimension of embodied self-feelings (what Goldie refers to as temperament and emotional dispositions).

Feelings in the form of moods are, indeed, essential to our self-formation: they are not merely free-floating atmospheres that we add on top of thoughts; rather, moods are world-*constitutive* phenomena (Heidegger 1927/1986, pp. 134ff.). Moods open up a world to human beings in which things *matter* to them in different ways. Feelings, especially in the form of moods, are basic to our being-in-the-world, in Heidegger's phenomenology, since they open up the world as meaningful, as having significance. They are the basic strata of what Heidegger refers to as *facticity*, our being thrown into the world prior to having made any thoughts or choices about it. We find ourselves *there*, in the world, always already busy with different things that matter to us, together with other people. And this "mattering to" rests on an attunement, a mood quality which the being-in-the-world always already has. Indeed, we do not choose our moods; they come to us and cannot easily be changed.

Heidegger's understanding of mood as a world-opening dimension for the self, supplemented by Fuchs's idea of bodily resonance, fits well with Zahavi's idea of the minimal self. Pre-conscious, embodied self-experience is exactly a letting things of the world appear by way of an attunement (mood) which is neither self-instituted nor normally reflected upon. By means of phenomenological analysis it is possible to focus upon the mood and reflect upon how it makes the being-in-the-world of the self possible. It is also possible to analyze different moods and the peculiarities they might harbor. The three basic moods that are characteristic of anxiety disorders and depression, considering the diagnoses from the DSM that we surveyed above, are *anxiety*, *boredom*, and *grief*. What is peculiar about these moods is that they simultaneously open up *and block* the possibility of being-in-the-world—the possibility of engaging with things and other human beings in a way that makes sense to us. They do this in distinct ways, however. Anxiety has a paralyzing quality to it, whereas boredom, rather, puts us to sleep. Grief, in depression at least, reflects a losing and longing, not only of other persons, but actually of the depressed person herself, experienced as a form of self-hate, as Freud (1957) pointed out. In anxiety, the world breaks apart; in boredom, it withers; and in grief, it shrinks (Svenaeus 2007).

To be anxious, bored, or in grief are *unhomelike* experiences. They make settling in the world and being at home in the world hard, since, for people afflicted with any one of these moods, the world resists meaningfulness. What Heidegger calls *authentic* understanding is achieved by nurturing this homesickness to fruition, at which point it becomes possible to exploit the moods for philosophical purposes (1927/1986, 295ff.). The problem from the point of view of psychiatry, however, is that anxiety, boredom, and grief can become destructive, rather than productive, life experiences: they can be so overwhelming that a return to homelikeness becomes impossible. Unhomelikeness is a necessary ingredient of life; it can be very rewarding insofar as it allows us to see things in novel, more nuanced ways. It must be balanced by homelikeness, however, lest we fall into a bottomless pit of darkness. Anxiety, boredom, and, particularly, grief have at their core a feeling of loneliness, which no doubt fascinated Heidegger as it has fascinated philosophers since the time of the Greeks. But this unwilled loneliness, the result of an attunement that blocks engagement with a world shared with others, is not only a philosophical posture; it is also, potentially, a pathological state.

The effects of the SSRIs, and other similar antidepressants, appear to consist in a change of the mood profile of the patient. The general increase of serotonin (and other neurotransmitters) in the synapses of the brain makes people feel less miserable and enhances their sense of self-worth (Knutson et al. 1998). This is not the same thing as making them feel happy or euphoric—Prozac is not a "happy pill"—but it means that the spectrum of moods in which the person lives becomes altered in a characteristic way. The mood spectrum becomes richer as the person is no longer stuck in sad moods and thus becomes more able to enjoy other attunements than the dark ones. The world opens up in more multifaceted ways and allows the self to become at home with itself and in the world. However, the mood spectrum also becomes poorer in that the steep ups and downs of intense moods such as sadness and joy are cut off. The sine curve of life is characteristically flattened out by antidepressants, something that can be both praised and lamented by patients (Knudsen et al. 2002, 2003).

When antidepressants make people feel more at home in the world, this can mean that they feel more at home with themselves, as Kramer pointed out (1993). But it can also mean that they feel less at home with themselves, in spite of being less anxious, bored, and grieving, since they do not recognize their new mood profile—the changed temperament and emotional dispositions—to be their *own* (a mood profile of their distinctive personality). Sometimes the two alternatives will fuse into the claim that the patient for the first time in her life feels at home with herself; that is, she has never really been herself before being on the antidepressant. The last claim makes it hard to defend the idea that antidepressants have effects only on disorders and not on the self, although one might try to fit these cases into the categories of dysthymia (American Psychiatric Association 2000, p. 376) or some type of generalized anxiety disorder (American Psychiatric Association 2000, p. 472), as more or less chronic, long-lasting disorders, in the same way that personality and developmental disorders will often be lifelong. A more probable way to account for the claim made by these patients, however, is that the mood profile of the embodied self is central not only to understanding disorders but also to understanding what it means to be a self with a distinct personality. Antidepressant medication represents a way to change this mood profile in a way that is more direct than the ways of psychotherapy (Svenaeus 2009), and the effect in question is not limited to alleviating the suffering of disorders in the mood spectrum; it will also have some effects on self and personality (in most cases, maybe not in the dramatic way Kramer describes), since the temperament and emotional dispositions of the person are, indeed, basic to selfhood.

CONCLUSION

Psychopharmacological drugs have effects on selfhood in ways that often overlap with the treatment of mental disorders, but the effects also go beyond the domain of disorder in some cases. In this way the drugs can be used for enhancement of the self in addition to treating mental disorders. It is likely that we will see more of such use in the future, though perhaps not so much by way of off-label treatment as through the continued expansion of the realm of mental disorders into what many take to be painful, unwanted, and despised, but nevertheless normal, aspects of human life. The critique of contemporary diagnostic psychiatry has many voices, and it is likely to continue when DSM-5 is published (two well-informed and philosophically reflective examples of the critique are Horwitz (2002), and Kutchins and Kirk (1997)). If the critiques are right, many of the persons who are diagnosed with mental disorders are unhappy or ill-behaved rather than unhealthy. This does not mean that psychopharmacological drugs could not be of help for these people (or for the ones who have to live with them), but one should remember that the positive effects of drugs are likely to be exaggerated in all possible ways by the companies that sell them (Healy 2004).

The psychotropic effects on selfhood can be understood by distinguishing the groups of traits that belong to personality according to Goldie (temperaments, ways of acting, habits, skills, emotional dispositions, enduring preferences and values, and character traits) and that form *dimensions* of selfhood, but they can also be distinguished by acknowledging the different *layers* of selfhood we found with Zahavi (pre-reflective embodied self, reflective self, and narrative self). (To use a topographic image we could think of the layers of selfhood being put on top of each other in a horizontal way, whereas the dimensions of selfhood would stretch through the layers in a vertical way.) The effects of the drugs sometimes normalize the alienating experiences of the breakdown of minimal selfhood (antipsychotic medication); sometimes, rather, they bring about changes in basic dimensions of selfhood and personality: temperaments and emotional dispositions in the case of SSRIs, and ways of acting, habits, and emotional dispositions in the case of methylphenidate. The effects in both of the latter cases can probably be seen in additional groups of the traits distinguished by Goldie, since the groups are in some cases conceptually, as well as causally, tied to each other. Emotional dispositions, for example, are hard to separate from character traits in many cases, and even if a distinction between emotional *reactions* and considered *decisions* to act in certain ways can be maintained on the conceptual level, living with certain emotional dispositions will make it much harder to embody certain character traits (being friendly to people in stressful situations if you easily become anxious and annoyed, for example).

What do I mean by claiming that the drugs have effects in more *basic* dimensions of selfhood in the case of SSRIs and methylphenidate? Some of the groups of traits that Goldie distinguishes have more to do with the layers of selfhood involving self-reflection and culture than with pre-reflective experiences, since it makes little or no sense to talk about the dimensions as being present already at the layer of the minimal self. I am thinking primarily about character traits, but also about ways of acting, and perhaps also skills and enduring preferences and values. To influence these dimensions of selfhood probably takes more than consuming drugs; maybe it takes psychotherapy, or, at least, conscious decisions and plans to change oneself in certain ways. A drug like Prozac, which has become famous in our culture and society, could indeed achieve effects for the people consuming it in the dimensions of more reflective aspects of personality, but it would do so, then, because the persons *identify* with the drug and find their values and self-worth through it (Crossley 2003). The narrative layers of selfhood are very clearly involved when one of Kramer's patients calls herself "Ms. Prozac" (Kramer 1993).

What about the distinction between psychopharmacological drugs and alcohol and narcotics? Do the latter not affect selfhood in some of the dimensions we have pinpointed? Yes, they do, but in contrast to most psychopharmacological drugs, alcohol and narcotics have a rather temporary effect, and in the case of longer use—abuse—they have a destructive rather than enhancing effect on personality as well as somatic health. The idea that narcotics could mean a liberation of the self was popular in the 1960s (Huxley 1962; Jünger 1970), but is rather frowned upon today. This notwithstanding, the borderline between medical drugs and narcotic drugs is far from sharp.

One last question remains: Does not my analysis of selfhood as consisting in different layers and dimensions, where some go deeper and are more basic than others, support an understanding of mental disorders as being *based* in biological dysfunctions but nevertheless admitting psychological and cultural filling, so to speak? If this were true, I would not be neutral in the debate on what mental disorders are, as I claimed to be above. To start with, the layer of minimal selfhood and the dimension of temperament (to pick one of the dimensions which appear to be basic) are not biological entities in the sense of something identified by means of biological analysis; they are phenomena found by way of analyzing the structure of lived experience. It is true that the minimal self is primary since there can be no reflective or narrative self which is not also a pre-conscious, embodied self. Some creatures on earth (babies, non-human animals) probably only have pre-reflective selfhood. But the crucial point about selfhood is that the different layers (when they have all been put in place) coexist and interact with each other, since they are all constituents of the *same* entity (the same self).

There is, of course, nothing conceptually wrong in assuming that some mental disorders could in the future be identified by way of biological investigations, whereas other would still require a diagnosis based on the world of human feelings, thoughts, and actions. But the parallel with selfhood is not a necessary one, since the deepest layers of self and mental disorder (if we assume a biological grounding of mental disorders) do not map onto each other as being of the same type. Every mental disorder will certainly be amenable to some kind of physiological or biochemical analysis (as any type of experiences a person has will be), but the questions of whether it will be possible to find the borderline between mental illness and health, as well as the nature and limits of individual mental disorders, by way of such analyses remain open. Psychotropic effects do not prove the reality of mental disorders to be exclusively biological, any more than effects of psychotherapy would prove them to be non-biological. As I stated earlier, mental disorder, just like selfhood, is probably a multilayered and multidemensional phenomenon, but what layers are most basic in the case of (different) mental disorder(s) remains, to a very large extent, to be determined.

References

American Psychiatric Association (2000). *Diagnostic and Statistical Manual of Mental Disorders, 4th Edition, Text Revision.* Washington, DC: American Psychiatric Association.

Crossley, N. (2003). Prozac nation and the biochemical self: A critique. In S. Williams, L. Birke, and G. Bendelow (Eds), *Debating Biology: Sociological Reflections on Health, Medicine and Society*, pp. 245–58. London: Routledge.

Damasio, A. R. (1999). *The Feeling of What Happens: Body and Emotion in the Making of Consciousness.* New York, NY: Harcourt Brace.

Elliott, C. (2003). *Better Than Well: American Medicine Meets the American Dream.* New York, NY: Norton.

Elliott, C. and Chambers, T. (Eds) (2004). *Prozac as a Way of Life.* Chapel Hill, NC: University of North Carolina Press.

Freud, S. (1957). Mourning and melancholia. In *The Standard Edition of the Complete Psychological Works of Sigmund Freud, Volume 14.* London: Hogarth.

Fuchs, T. (2000). *Psychopathologie von Leib und Raum: Phänomenologisch-empirische Untersuchungen zu depressiven und paranoiden Erkrankungen.* Darmstadt: Steinkopff.

Gallagher, S. (2005). *How the Body Shapes the Mind.* Oxford: Oxford University Press.

Goldie, P. (2004). *On Personality.* London: Routledge.

Gordijn, B. and Chadwick, R. (Eds) (2008). *Medical Enhancement and Posthumanity.* Dordrecht: Springer.

Healy, D. (2004). *Let them Eat Prozac: The Unhealthy Relationship Between the Pharmaceutical Industry and Depression.* New York, NY: New York University Press.

Heidegger, M. (1986). *Sein und Zeit* (16th edn.). Tübingen: Max Niemeyer Verlag. (Original work published 1927.)

Horwitz, A. V. (2002). *Creating Mental Illness.* Chicago, IL: University of Chicago Press.

Horwitz, A. V. and Wakefield, J. C. (2007). *The Loss of Sadness: How Psychiatry Transformed Normal Sorrow into Depressive Disorder.* New York, NY: Oxford University Press.

Huxley, A. (1962). *Island.* New York, NY: HarperCollins Publishers.

Jopling, D. A. (2000). *Self-Knowledge and the Self.* London: Routledge.

Jünger, E. (1970). *Annäherungen: Drogen und Rausch.* Stuttgart : Ernst Klett Verlag.

Knudsen, P., Hansen, E. H., and Eskildsen, K. (2003). Leading ordinary lives: A qualitative study of younger women's perceived functions of antidepressants. *Pharmacology World Science*, 25(4), 162–7.

Knudsen, P., Holme Hansen, E., Morgall Traulsen, J., and Eskildsen, K. (2002). Changes in self-concept while using SSRI antidepressants. *Qualitative Health Research*, 12(7), 932–44.

Knutson, B., Wolkowitz, O. M., Cole, S. W., Chan, T., Moore, E. A., Johnson, R. C., *et al.* (1998). Selective alteration of personality and social behavior by serotonergic intervention. *American Journal of Psychiatry*, 155(3), 373–9.

Kramer, P. (1993). *Listening to Prozac: A Psychiatrist Explores Antidepressant Drugs and the Remaking of the Self.* London: Fourth Estate.

Kutchins, H. and Kirk, S. A. (1997). *Making Us Crazy: DSM, the Psychiatric Bible and the Creation of Mental Disorders.* New York, NY: Free Press.

Leder, D. (1990). *The Absent Body.* Chicago, IL: University of Chicago Press.

Radden, J. (Ed.) (2000). *The Nature of Melancholy: From Aristotle to Kristeva.* Oxford: Oxford University Press.

Sass, L., Parnas, J., and Zahavi, D. (2011). Phenomenological psychopathology and schizophrenia: Contemporary approaches and misunderstandings. *Philosophy, Psychiatry and Psychology*, *18*(1), 1–23.

Spiegelberg, H. (1972). *Phenomenology in Psychology and Psychiatry*. Evanston, IL: Northwestern University Press.

Stein, D. J. (2008). *The Philosophy of Psychopharmacology: Smart Pills, Happy Pills, and Pep Pills*. New York, NY: Cambridge University Press.

Svenaeus, F. (2006). Medicine. In H. Dreyfus and M. Wrathall (Eds), *A Companion to Phenomenology and Existentialism*, pp. 412–24. London: Blackwell Publishing.

Svenaeus, F. (2007). Do antidepressants affect the self? A phenomenological approach. *Medicine, Health Care and Philosophy*, *10*(2), 153–66.

Svenaeus, F. (2009). The ethics of self-change: Becoming oneself by way of antidepressants or psychotherapy? *Medicine, Health Care and Philosophy*, *12*(2), 169–78.

Toombs, S. K. (2001). *Handbook of Phenomenology and Medicine*. Dordrecht: Kluwer Academic Publishers.

Wigal, S. B. (2009). Efficacy and safety limitations of attention-deficit hyperactivity disorder pharmacotherapy in children and adults. *CNS Drugs*, *23*(Suppl 1), 21–31.

Zahavi, D. (2005). *Subjectivity and Selfhood: Investigating the First-Person Perspective*. Cambridge, MA: MIT Press.

Zahavi, D. (2010). Is the self a social construct? *Inquiry*, *52*(6), 551–73.

....

CHAPTER 69

PRACTICAL NEUROPSYCHIATRIC ETHICS

....

BENNETT FODDY, GUY KAHANE, AND JULIAN SAVULESCU

INTRODUCTION

Moral philosophers have long been involved in the pursuit of a goal shared by researchers in psychiatry and the cognitive sciences: understanding the relationship between the functioning of the human mind and human well-being. For this reason there is a considerable overlap between ethical and psychiatric concerns. The overlap is particularly significant in the domain of *practical ethics*, which is concerned with understanding the moral dimension of policies and actions in the real world.

One familiar point of intersection relates to the ethics of psychiatric practice. Psychiatric practice can raise ethical problems relating to autonomy, consent, and paternalism. For example, psychiatric patients often refuse treatment, and it can be especially difficult to establish if such refusals are made by completely autonomous agents, given the effects that psychiatric conditions can have on a person's mental capacities (Radden 2002). These and similar issues have been much discussed. Our aim in this chapter is not to add to that discussion, but to draw attention to other important points of contact between psychiatry and practical ethics—to new philosophical and ethical questions that are emerging out of recent advances in neuropsychiatric research and related scientific developments.

Some of these advances have been recently discussed in the emerging discipline of *neuroethics*, frequently defined as the "ethics of neuroscience and the neuroscience of ethics" (Roskies 2002), and part of what we wish to discuss here falls under that banner, applied to psychiatry. "Practical neuropsychiatric ethics" concerns not only neuroscience but cognitive science more generally applied to ethical issues arising in or derived from psychiatry and psychology, as well as the normative dimensions of mental illness, health, and personality.

In this chapter, we review several areas which illustrate the significance that philosophy and philosophical ethics have for psychiatry and psychology, and vice versa, viewed through the lens of advances in the cognitive sciences. We shall consider areas in which psychiatric research has presented new practical problems for ethical analysis, and cases where the study of psychiatric disorders may lead to new progress in longstanding moral and philosophical puzzles. But there are also cases in which the important developments and methods in philosophy might be used to stimulate progress in psychiatry and psychology.

Psychopharmacology and Practical Ethics

One of the biggest changes in lifestyles in developed countries since the 1970s has been the widespread use of psychiatric drugs—not only to treat extreme forms of mental illness but also, increasingly, to treat a growing list of psychiatric conditions claimed to afflict people who would have been considered normal even in the recent past. Unlike other medicines, these drugs influence not just our bodies but also our psychology—they can alter our memories and desires, even our personalities. Some believe that as the power of such drugs grows, they might even have the capacity to change basic human nature. And for this reason, progress in psychiatric pharmacology has generated an ever-expanding set of new problems in practical ethics: challenges that arise both within the psychiatric clinic and in the wider world, as psychopharmacology takes a stronger grip even on those of us who have never been to see a psychiatrist.

One debate about psychopharmacology in psychiatry has focused on the worry that psychiatry is increasingly "medicalizing" normal human traits, thereby removing them from the scope of moral assessment and turning them into biological conditions to be treated using pills (Conrad 2007; Rose 2006). Some worry that this represents the "invention" of disease merely to promote the interests of pharmaceutical companies (Baughman 2006). Others worry that this trend is displacing deeper forms of therapy (Manninen 2006). Still others that it presents what are in effect value judgments in the misleading guise of objective scientific assessments (Hawthorne 2007).

But this debate has taken a different form in practical ethics. Several ethicists have argued that there is no deep or morally important distinction between therapy (treating disease) and enhancement (making people better) (Kahane and Savulescu 2009; Kamm 2005; Savulescu and Kahane 2009). On this view, our central aim should be to promote human well-being and flourishing, not to cure scientifically identified biological disorders and dysfunctions, independently of how and whether they affect human well-being. To the extent that psychopharmacology can be used to promote human well-being, we have a prima facie moral reason to encourage its use, so long as it is safe and effective. Whether the person taking the drug could be said to be afflicted by a mental disease or disorder matters little if we adopt such a "welfarist" approach (Kahane and Savulescu 2009).

This view is controversial, but if it is correct, then some of the fiercest debates within psychiatry may be less significant and intractable than they appear. Once we reject the assumption that it is appropriate to use biomedical means only in the context of disease and disorder, then many current worries about "medicalization" may turn out to be misguided. Nor should we worry that the development and use of psychopharmacology is guided by value judgments, or assume that such judgments must be merely "subjective." Instead, we should openly debate the relevant questions of value, and worry whether current psychopharmacology is guided by *mistaken* value judgments. And we should also rethink the role of science. Its role is not to identify which psychological traits or dispositions are mental disorders we ought to cure. Rather, we should openly discuss questions about the nature of human well-being (Griffin 1986; Parfit 1984) and then use science to identify which means of promoting human well-being are most effective and safe, as well as broadly ethically acceptable.

The debate about pills versus "talking" therapy has also taken a somewhat different form in recent practical ethics. Here the main worry has been that enhancing human psychology using pills will rob the resulting change of its value by making it inauthentic, or too effortless to count as a genuine achievement (President's Council on Bioethics 2003; Singh 2005). And, as we shall see next, our approach to these problems will depend on how we answer a deeper philosophical question: the question of what constitutes a person's identity.

Antidepressants, mood enhancement, and identity

One of the biggest revolutions in psychiatric medicine has been the emergence and overwhelming adoption of modern antidepressant medications. Since their introduction in 1987, selective serotonin reuptake inhibitors (SSRIs) have become the most often-prescribed class of drugs in the USA and the most popular class of psychiatric drugs in the world (Ludwig et al. 2009).

But the rise of the modern antidepressants has been accompanied by growing concern about their use, overuse, and abuse. The major moral objection to the use of antidepressants emerges from the fact that depression can be seen as an expression, or even an aspect, of a person's personality. When a person takes an antidepressant, supposing that the drug is effective, we expect to see significant changes occur over a relatively short space of time in her mood and, some would say, in her personality.

To understand why this might be of moral significance, we might look at the famous case of Phineas Gage. Gage was a railway worker whose left frontal lobe was obliterated in a railway construction accident when an iron spike pierced his skull. Miraculously, he survived the accident, but his friends noticed that his mood and personality had changed. Though he had previously been known as an affable, calm person, he had become irritable and impulsive as a result of the accident. In the eyes of his friends and family, Mr Gage was no longer himself—he was now a new person who bore little in common with the man who existed prior to the accident (Damasio 1994).

It is natural for human personality and mood to shift gradually as a person grows older. Yet even when a person's personality changes suddenly, or significantly, we do not always regard the change in the same way as Gage's family regarded his transformation. If someone "turns over a new leaf" or has an epiphany, we would rarely say that she has turned into another person. But if, for example, a previously cheerful and confident person becomes chronically anxious and irritable after a traumatic car accident, we are often tempted to view that as a fundamental (and unwelcome) change in their identity.

Carl Elliott has claimed that regular users of antidepressants display personality characteristics that do not truly belong to them, in the sense that they are inconsistent with their past characteristics, behavior, and goals (Elliott 1998). Their un-depressed personalities do not fit in neatly with the overall narrative of their lives. If a person has a real set of reasons to be depressed (whether these are material or even just existential) then, Elliott argues, antidepressants would do little more than change her into a different person. The new, happier version would be an inauthentic copy, a fake. Worse, this inauthentic copy won't even appropriately match the person's circumstances: the person on pills would be happy when it is *appropriate* to be sad.

David DeGrazia, on the other side, has argued that taking antidepressants is often an expression of a sincere desire for change which a depressed person enacts in an effort to change their personality, or to reclaim their previous, pre-depressed personality (Degrazia 2000). In DeGrazia's eyes, the choice to take antidepressants can be a paradigm example of an authentic choice, as it moves a person closer to their own understanding of who they are.

The line between authenticity and inauthenticity is contentious. Some changes in a person's personality will clearly count as inauthentic, as in the case of dramatic and immediate changes that result from traumatic brain injury, tumor, or other pathology. At the other end of the spectrum there will be changes that appear clearly authentic, such as epiphanies and life-altering decisions. What is unclear is whether patients who take antidepressants are more like Phineas Gage or more like a wrongdoer who has finally seen the light. To complicate things, antidepressants are an artificial, exogenous cause of change like the railway spike that impaled Gage's head. Yet unlike the railway spike, they are often voluntarily chosen by depressed patients in a deliberate attempt to modify their personalities in specific ways.

This debate around authenticity cannot be resolved by further scientific investigation. It can only be resolved by a philosophical analysis of the concepts of identity and authenticity, which will indicate how these concepts are best defined and why they matter.[1] For example, it could be that the real me is the person I want to be, or it could be that I am defined by my behavior or by some account of my intrinsic nature. It might also be that I am better off being happy in an inauthentic way than miserable in a way that is genuinely representative of my identity. Our attitude to the growing use of psychopharmacological drugs will be determined by how we approach these still unresolved philosophical puzzles.[2]

One of us, however, has recently argued that the issue of authenticity, and thus these difficult philosophically questions about identity, can be largely side-stepped (Kahane 2011a). The most difficult question about the use of mood enhancing drugs isn't about authenticity or identity, but about the appropriateness of certain emotions. It is inappropriate to feel cheerful at a funeral, or to respond with growing despair to one's successes. In these ways, our emotions may fail to be appropriate to our circumstances—may fail to correspond to

---

[1] It is important to keep in mind here the philosophical distinction between "numerical" and "narrative" senses of identity (DeGrazia 2005). Questions about numerical identity are metaphysical questions: questions about the conditions for the persistence of some entity over time. Questions about narrative identity are rather concerned with the conditions under it is appropriate to attribute various psychological traits and experiences to a person—a looser notion of identity that is closer to the everyday use of this term. On most views of numerical identity, taking a mood-altering drug is very unlikely to turn you into what is literally another person—so that you literally no longer exist; but if its effects are strong enough, it may well radically transform your identity in the second, narrative sense.

[2] In addition, the very act of taking antidepressants might also raise issues of authenticity, quite independently of the actual effect of the drug. For example, the practice of taking pills might reinforce the passivity often associated with depression.

what we ought to feel. One central worry about antidepressants is that they similarly lead to a mismatch between our emotions and our circumstances: they might prevent us from appropriately responding to the negative aspects of our lives. Peter Strawson famously described "reactive attitudes" such as resentment and blame as representing the way in which we hold other people morally responsible for their actions (Strawson 1974). But just as certain attitudes may be appropriate in our reactions to others, certain emotions may be appropriate reactions to our own behaviors and to the situations we find ourselves during the course of our lives.

In this way, drugs like antidepressants might erode essential aspects of our social and emotional functioning. Whether this worry has genuine force, however, depends on how antidepressants change mood. Critics sometimes assume that psychopharmacological drugs directly affect mood, regardless of circumstances. But they might also affect mood in more benign ways, by making it easier for us to appreciate what it is appropriate to feel—by making it easier, for example, to respond to the positive dimensions of our lives. Future scientific research may shed further light on this issue. But, once again, the question of how we *ought* to feel is a deep question that cannot be resolved by science alone.

These ethical problems are not limited to the use of antidepressants. Attention-modulating drugs like methylphenidate or amphetamine also change basic aspects of a patient's mood and personality. Furthermore, the use of mood-altering psychiatric drugs is not limited to people who have a psychiatric condition that they wish to remedy. Some mood states, like euphoria, are simply more pleasurable than others, and for this reason SSRIs, anxiolytics, and attention-increasing drugs are increasingly used in non-therapeutic ways. If the psychiatric use of these drugs threatens to disrupt a person's identity, or disconnect emotion from circumstance and self, then off-label use will raise similar ethical concerns. In this way, the emergence of drugs for psychiatric conditions has generated ethical issues that affect everybody.

The ethics of placebos

Recently, another kind of moral dilemma has been brewing regarding the use of antidepressants. Modern antidepressants, as well as being an unprecedented commercial success story, have been an enormous clinical success. In dozens (if not hundreds) of published trials, it has been shown that depressed patients improve significantly better than untreated patients (Kirsch and Sapirstein 1998)—this marks an unprecedented success in treating a mental illness with a drug. Since the drugs are apparently so effective, and since depression is so widespread and so debilitating, ethical debate has so far been focused on the effects of antidepressant use on people with only mild or even no depression at all, as we discussed in the "Antidepressants, mood enhancement, and identity" section.

However, new ethical dilemmas emerge when we compare the effectiveness of these drugs not to untreated patients but to those receiving placebo. In 2008, Irving Kirsch published the results of a meta-analysis that for the first time included unpublished trials of modern antidepressant drugs that were logged with the US Food and Drug Administration. Across forty-seven clinical trials, these antidepressants failed to perform significantly better than placebo in mildly depressed patients and performed only somewhat better than placebo in severely depressed patients. Furthermore, Kirsch points out that while the drugs did perform better than placebo for severely depressed patients, the data clearly show that as patients become more severely depressed, the group who are given the drug do not fare any better; rather, members of the control group who are taking placebo fare worse (Kirsch et al. 2008). If these findings are correct, it would seem that severely depressed patients do not respond as strongly to the placebo effect. Consequently, although there is a larger difference between the drug group and the placebo group among severely depressed patients, the drug is no more effective.

In other words, in one of the very few currently available meta-analyses which include results from unpublished trials, results raise the possibility that these enormously popular and effective drugs might work no better than placebo. Needless to say, this suggestion is highly controversial. What we now want to briefly explore is not whether it is correct—a question for science to resolve—but what ethical difficulties it would generate for the prescribing psychiatrist if it proved to be correct.

In the first place, doctors in the USA and elsewhere are forbidden from knowingly prescribing a placebo to a patient without revealing its nature, since deception in treatment is countermanded by the requirement of fully informed consent (American Medical Association 2007). The American Medical Association has argued that placebos *could* be given to patients openly, and at least one study suggests that this would work, but it would likely be less effective than placebo prescribed under the cover of deception, and more seriously, it would tend to undermine the effectiveness of regular, non-placebo drugs (Foddy et al. 2011b; Kaptchuk et al. 2010; Kolber 2007). Thus, the revelation that antidepressants work primarily through the placebo effect—if correct—suggests that doctors cannot continue to use these drugs without compromising either the drugs' effectiveness or their own professional standing. But the conundrum runs deeper than law and professional policy.

The underlying causes of depression are not well understood. All we have in order to define it as a disease are its symptoms. Six of the nine diagnostic symptoms for depression relate to a patient's subjective experiences, while the other three relate to his or her behavior (American Psychiatric Association 2000). The evidence seems to indicate that modern antidepressants can elicit a real change in both the felt experience of depression and in its behavioral correlates. If the diagnostic symptoms were alleviated by the placebo effect, then it is hard to see that as anything but an effective treatment, so long as the disease is defined in terms of its symptoms. Even if it turned out that the symptoms of depression reflect some underlying neurological or endocrinological condition, it is arguable that it is the behavior and the experienced feelings of depression that we primarily seek to treat when we aim to try to alleviate or cure depression, not the (currently unidentified) underlying biological condition.[3]

This argument can be extended to other disorders. For example, pain—like depression—is a condition which may have a certain neurobiological cause but which is defined mainly in terms of its subjective experience. According to the International Association for

---

[3] There may be deeper psychological issues that undergird many cases of depression: for example, suppressed anger, or unresolved interpersonal conflict. And it is true that a placebo cannot resolve these real problems on its own. Though placebo treatments cannot replace therapy, for this reason, a purely symptomatic relief of the mental anguish associated depression would still be of great value. Moreover, depression is characteristically self-sustaining since its affective symptoms make it difficult for sufferers to address their real problems. Symptomatic relief using placebo (or non-placebo antidepressants) could help depressed patients to escape this downward spiral.

the Study of Pain, "pain is always subjective" (Merskey 1991). Now clearly, malingerers or hypochondriacs might misrepresent the amount of pain they are in, so we cannot use patient self-report as a reliable measure of pain, as McCaffery claims ("pain is whatever the experiencing person says it is, existing whenever he says it does"; McCaffery 1968). But whether or not we can rely on patients to report it accurately, if a patient genuinely experiences pain, there can be no neurological or psychological test which shows that they are pain-free.

And pain, like depression, is responsive to placebo treatments. If we can justify prescribing placebo for depression, why not also prescribe placebo for chronic or untreatable pain? (Foddy 2011b). At present, many doctors are forbidden by law or by professional codes of ethics from prescribing placebos without revealing them to their patients (Shah and Goold 2009) but the moral status quo is under pressure as evidence mounts showing that placebos have substantial subjective benefits and that they may even form a larger component of existing, popular therapies than was previously thought. This echoes a point we made earlier: what ultimately matters is whether some intervention makes people better, not whether it works by this or that causal mechanism.

Cognitive enhancers

Psychiatric drugs are also posing new ethical challenges in cases where remedial psychiatric medications can be repurposed by healthy individuals, not only to enhance their mood or produce pleasurable experiences, but also to enhance their cognitive capacities. Methylphenidate, which is often prescribed as a treatment for attention deficit disorder, is now reportedly widely used as an attention-promoting drug by university students studying for exams (Sahakian and Morein-Zamir 2007). Beta-blockers, prescribed for hypertension, are repurposed by professional musicians and archers to quell the trembling associated with stage fright (Foddy 2011a). And the wakefulness-promoting drug modafinil can be used to promote cognitive function (Myrick et al. 2004) (see Box 69.1).

This repurposing of psychiatric drugs presents us with a prototypical example of what philosophers call a "dual-use problem" (Miller and Selgelid 2007). The broad availability of these drugs is clearly beneficial when considering their on-label use, but it is inevitable that, despite our tightly-controlled prescription system, the drugs will be used off-label as well.

Box 69.1 One Person's Experience Using Modafinil for Cognitive Enhancement

I use modafinil two to three times per month to have a sharp and energetic day. Typically I take a pill in in the morning, go back to bed, and then wake up making plans for the day. I tend to space usage in order to avoid habituation and to avoid wearing myself out. My subjective experience of the drug is as if there was a small electric motor quietly running at the back of my head: a constant, subliminal activation. There is an obvious stimulant effect that allows me to get going at tasks, but also a more subtle feeling of a wider mental range and higher precision in thought. Maybe this is due to extended working memory space, maybe it is purely a placebo effect due to the ritual aspect of taking the pill. I find the drug a useful way of controlling my mind and getting things done, but it does have limitations. While it helps work, it does not make me wiser: I will have energy and enjoyment in solving problems, but I have learned that I must take care so I do not spend my effort on the wrong ones.

Indeed, some ethicists argue that, if these drugs can enhance cognitive capacity in normal people, they should be made available for such use (Bostrom and Sandberg 2009).

There are, however, a number of ethical worries about the use of psychiatric drugs for cognitive enhancement. Martha Farah, for one, has suggested that the widespread use of cognitive enhancers may lead to a situation in which employees are required to use cognitive enhancers (Farah et al. 2004). Indeed, it may already be the case that in certain settings—in trucking, in the military or even in professional baseball—cognitive enhancers are already needed to perform at a competitive level (Foddy 2008).

Of course, performing at a competitive level in sports or even in employment often requires us to do things we would rather not do; to be unethical these requirements need to be unreasonable, for example, because they are dangerous or illegal or bad in some other way. A number of commentators argue that the widespread use of cognitive enhancers would have pernicious effects. Michael Sandel, perhaps most famously, argues that we are morally bound to accept the gifts given to us by nature, and should avoid tampering with our defining characteristics. We should be grateful for whatever cognitive abilities we were born with, and not try to transcend our given nature through cognitive enhancers. Such enhancement, Sandel argues, expresses a hubristic drive to mastery (Sandel 2007). Carol Freedman has similarly argued that the off-label use of psychiatric drugs as enhancers may tempt us to see our brains as mere biological machines that can be souped up with the appropriate pill (Freedman 1998).

We doubt, however, that there is anything inherently problematic in seeing our cognitive capacities as based in manipulable biological systems, or in trying to transcend our given natural limitations (Kahane 2011b). Our cognitive capacities really *are* based in manipulable biological systems. And nobody objects when we treat our physical organs and traits in purely mechanistic terms. When athletes perform sit-ups to improve abdominal strength, or when they train at high altitude in order to increase their red blood cell count, we applaud their commitment to peak physical performance, even though intense training can be a risky or even harmful endeavor. It is far from obvious that there is a deep, morally relevant distinction between exercise and cognitive enhancement. But even if there were, this distinction is surely blurred by the fact that exercise also temporarily enhances a person's cognitive ability (Tomporowski 2003). Perhaps we will come to see cognitive enhancement as the embodiment of a laudable commitment to improving human performance, rather than as a repudiation of the value of our biological gifts.

One of us has argued that cognitive enhancement does indeed raise serious worries—but not because it is in any way morally problematic in itself, but because radical forms of cognitive enhancement could be used in the service of highly pernicious ends (Persson and Savulescu 2008). Cognitive enhancement will make us smarter, but it won't, on its own, make us morally better, and this asymmetry may dramatically amplify the dangers we impose on each other. This, however, is not an argument against enhancement, but an argument in favor of forms of enhancement that would also improve our moral motivation and behavior.

A Broader Neuroethics

There is a burgeoning interest in the study of "neuroethics." To date, much of what has been written under the banner of neuroethics has been limited to the ethical analysis of emerging neuroscientific technologies, such as the debate about psychopharmacology we discussed earlier (Farah 2011). However, we see neuroethics as a much bigger tent, encompassing the psychological and neuroscientific study of moral decision-making and also the philosophical and ethical analysis of psychiatry and cognitive science. In the next two subsections, we will explore two of the ways in which neuroethics can expand by marrying philosophy, psychiatry, psychology, and neuroscience.

The ethics of addiction, compulsion, and moral responsibility

One area where we believe that psychiatry has suffered for a lack of philosophical input is the problem of addiction and compulsion. As Stephen Morse points out, the concept of "compulsion or something like it" is essential to a psychiatric conception of addiction, since it is compulsion that distinguishes addiction as a disordered state rather than a mere bad habit (Morse 2011). And sure enough, compulsion is one of the most widely-cited symptoms of addiction in the psychiatric literature.

Although older revisions of the psychiatric diagnostic manuals included the concept of "compulsion" or "compulsive use" in their definitions of alcohol and drug dependence, the newest revisions are increasingly vague about the question of whether or not addictions involve compulsive drug use. The tenth revision of the International Statistical Classification of Diseases and Related Health Problems (ICD-10), for example, suggests that addicted people feel "a strong desire or *sense of compulsion* to take the substance," while the draft version of the fifth edition of the *Diagnostic and Statistical Manual of Mental Disorders* (DSM-5) omits the word entirely, referring instead to "strong desires" or "urges" that lead to "unsuccessful efforts" to control drug use.

For all of that, the language of compulsion remains at the heart of contemporary psychiatric discourse around addictive drug use.

In a widely-cited paper by Lubman et al., the preamble suggests what may seem obvious: "Addiction has been conceptualized as a shift from controlled experimentation to uncontrolled, compulsive patterns of use" (Lubman et al. 2004). More recently, in "The 10 most important things known about addiction," Sellman writes:

> 1. Addiction is fundamentally about compulsive behavior.
> 2. Compulsive drug seeking is initiated outside of consciousness. (Sellman, 2010)

Like much of the psychiatric literature, both Sellman and Lubman never define what it means for behavior to be compulsive, but they allude toward a certain vague picture of automatism in the behavior of addicts. Sellman refers to drug users becoming "dehumanized" as they become incapable of "normal flexibility" in their drug-seeking behavior. Lubman, echoing the ICD-10, uses the phrase "a strong desire or sense of compulsion" as though the two concepts are interchangeable.

The term is not clearly defined anywhere in the literature, and it seems to enter the psychiatric discourse by way of an accident rather than by any particular empirical finding. Two widely-cited papers from 1965, by Eddy et al. (1965) and Jaffe (1965), seemed to introduce the concept out of the blue. Jaffe equates compulsion with "craving" while Eddy uses the term interchangeably with "overpowering desire."

The question of whether overpoweringly strong desires are really enough to render a behavior compulsive is complicated and extremely difficult one, as is the question of whether free, non-compulsive behavior must always be generated by a flexible behavioral system. But these difficult, important questions are often brushed aside in the psychiatric literature. Dissenting views, while present, have been unable to shift the orthodoxy away from the view that substance abusers come to use their drugs in a compulsive way (Davies 1997; Peele and Brodsky 1976).

Defining compulsion

What is compulsion? In the most abstract terms, it is easy to find an acceptable definition: compulsion is an irresistible pressure to perform some behavior. The difficulty lies in determining what it means for a pressure to be irresistible. Consider that most researchers in the cognitive science adopt a *deterministic* model of human behavior which suggests that our behaviors are entirely determined by the precise arrangement of our biological and electrical states and the configuration of the environment around us. If this model is correct, then strictly speaking *every* behavior is caused by some irresistible pressure—yet it cannot be correct that every behavior is compulsive.

It is certainly the case that laypeople equate the identification of neurological causation with compulsion and a lack of responsibility (De Brigard et al. 2009). And there was once a live philosophical debate over the question of whether behaviors with causes could be free behaviors. After millennia of discussion, however, many philosophers subscribe to the view known as *compatibilism*, which holds that our behaviors can be free despite having identifiable and deterministic biological causes (Watson 1987). On a compatibilist view, all of our behaviors are caused by environmental and biological processes which may be irresistible, but only certain kinds of causes will make a person perform actions that are characteristically compulsive. How then are we to draw the line between freedom and compulsion? What, indeed, would it mean to act in a way that is free (i.e., not compulsive) yet fully nevertheless determined by physical systems?

A handful of candidates are gestured at, though not discussed, in the psychiatric papers cited earlier. When Sellman suggests that a compulsive person lacks the "normal flexibility," this gestures toward one influential solution to the problem. In this solution, a non-compulsive actor is one whose behaviors are determined by a system that can change course in the face of appropriate counterincentives. Clearly even the most disciplined person will ignore certain kinds of counterincentives, so we need some means to identify what kinds of counterincentives a person ought to be sensitive to. In Fischer and Ravizza's account, for example, a non-compulsive person must be able to respond to a set of counterincentives that is "well-structured and sane" (Fischer and Ravizza 1998).

In the psychiatric literature it is frequently mentioned that drug users do not respond to the rising health costs of chronic drug use; indeed, this is one of the diagnostic criteria built into both the DSM and ICD definitions of drug dependence. Along similar lines, it is often reported that drug-dependent animals are insensitive to changes in the "cost" of their drug (Ahmed and Koob 2005; Everitt and Robbins 2005). These things form part of a justification of the claim that addictive drug use is compulsive. We can see them as an attempt to show that addicts are incapable of responding to a "well-structured and sane" set of counterincentives. But do they show this? It is not obvious to us that a person must respond to any particular set of health-related counterincentives to drug use by limiting or halting their drug use, and it seems entirely possible that a reasonable person might be prepared to gradually pay more for a drug as they gradually grew to enjoy it more and to desire it more strongly. Indeed, Fischer and Ravizza allow that a person might be in complete control of themselves despite entirely disregarding the value of their health. The question of how we should measure the flexibility of a person's motivational structures is an extremely deep philosophical problem that is nowhere near being solved decisively. In the meantime, the attitudes of addicts toward costs are not decisive evidence for the claim that they seek drugs compulsively.

The ICD-10, as we mentioned earlier, seems to equate compulsion (or at least a *sense* of compulsion) with strong desires or cravings. In the psychiatric literature it is very frequently suggested that strong desires might constitute an irresistible force. But this too is at the heart of a very longstanding and unsettled philosophical debate. Can we resist very strong desires? Opinions among philosophers run the gamut of possibilities: Velleman argues that our strongest desires *always* determine our behaviors, while Feinberg argues that no desire is irresistible, since we have a capacity to override our desires with willpower (Feinberg 1970; Velleman 1992).

In the end, it is not clear from the available evidence that addicts are any less flexible in their behavior than anybody else who strongly wishes to perform some behavior, nor is it clear that strong desires or wishes are enough to compel a person to pursue them (Foddy and Savulescu 2010). Various philosophers have settled on the idea that addictive drug use might be voluntary but not completely *free*, either because the addict becomes irrational in making valuations of the drug (Wallace 1999), because an unsatisfied desire is unreasonably aversive or unpleasant (Morse 2000), or because our capacity for exerting willpower becomes exhausted in the face of persistent strong desires (Levy 2006, 2009). Each of these things might undermine a person's *autonomy*—their capacity for self-government. Importantly, however, none of these philosophers claims that addictive drug use is *compulsive*.

Finally, the psychiatric literature has often appealed to irresistible *biological* forces to establish that drug use is compulsive. Since the early 1990s, an ever-increasing body of neuroscientific evidence has shown that the brains of addicts change in certain ways over their drug-taking careers (Koob and Nestler 1997; Leshner 1997; Volkow and Li 2004). But there is no clear or well-evidenced biological model of compulsion that is free of the familiar philosophical objections (Morse 2011). As we outlined earlier, it is not enough to show that a behavior has a biological cause or a neurological correlate. According to the dominant view, every human behavior is caused by some change in the human brain in conjunction with changes in the external environment. In order to be able to say whether the changes in an addict's brain are enough to constitute compulsion, we would need to be able to say exactly which kinds of irresistible causes are compulsive. Since there is no clearly dominant philosophical account of compulsion, and since no satisfactory account of compulsion has yet been offered by the neuroscientific or psychiatric literature, it is unlikely that an magnetic resonance imaging scanner can reveal that a drug addict is prone to behave compulsively. This is not a question, we believe, that can be solved without conceptual input from philosophy.

Thus, although according to Sellman the most important thing we know about addiction is that "addiction is fundamentally about compulsive behavior," this is a claim we are currently far from being able to substantiate, in part because it depends on answers to several difficult questions in moral philosophy and philosophy of mind.

The modern scientific method can be characterized by restraint. Scientific progress isn't just about learning new things—sometimes progress consists of getting clear about what we don't know. If psychiatrists and neuroscientists were more clearly aware of what we don't know about the nature and characterization of compulsion, nobody would ever have claimed, as Sellman did, that we know that addiction is about compulsive behavior. In cases such as this, psychiatry and psychology can clearly benefit from the introduction of philosophical methods philosophical discourse.[4]

Compulsion is a phenomenon of real practical and moral significance, especially when it is involved in a behavior that is illegal and/or dangerous, as drug taking so often is. If we act compulsively, we are deemed to lack full moral—and possibly legal—responsibility for our actions. This also means that we can be justifiably forced into treatment, and the choices we make can be overruled by doctors or families or police officers. Clarifying the relation between addiction and compulsion is thus not merely an academic question. It may depend on rather abstract philosophical issues, but it has profound moral and legal implications.

Autism, empathy, and moral psychology

When psychologists use the term "moral psychology," they are referring to the scientific study of moral behavior and moral development. Philosophers have used the term in a different way, to denote the conceptual analysis of the relationship between the mind and moral action. Moral psychology, in this second sense, represents an area in which psychiatric research is suggesting new ways to think about longstanding philosophical problems.

One of the thorniest problems in moral psychology concerns the respective roles of reason and emotion in moral behavior. On one extreme we find the rationalist view associated with Immanuel Kant, on which morality is grounded in reason itself and must be independent of our contingent motivations and emotions (Kant 2005). At the other extreme is the "sentimentalist" view associated with David Hume, on which reason alone can never motivate us to act—moral behavior must be based in our emotions or "passions" (Hume 2000). In one influential version of the sentimentalist view, which also has its roots in Hume's work, morality is ultimately based in the natural human capacity for sympathetic concern for other people.

In some of its forms, this longstanding debate may relate to purely conceptual questions about morality and the sources of normativity. But it can also be understood as a question about the basis of actual human moral behavior, and about the psychological capacities that moral behavior requires. Several philosophers have recently drawn attention to important ways in which experimental evidence from psychiatry might bear on this second, partly empirical question. After all, individuals with disorders such as autism, psychopathy, and damage to the prefrontal cortex suffer from deficits in social emotion. If such individuals also exhibit parallel deficiencies in moral behavior, this would seem to support the view that sympathetic concern plays a key role in moral motivation.

---

[4] Of course there have been dissenting voices from the cognitive sciences on the question of compulsion in addiction. Stanton Peele, for example, has been arguing against the disease model of addiction for decades. And Gene Heyman has more recently argued that addiction is a "disorder of choice." However, even skeptical writing by scientists has made little use of the available philosophy.

But here the psychiatric science has thrown up a puzzle for philosophers. Both autistic people and people with psychopathy or antisocial personality disorder (APSD) suffer from severe deficits in their ability to relate to other people. But whereas psychopaths exhibit parallel deficits in moral behavior, autistic people are able—and are motivated—to follow moral rules (Kennett 2003).

Jeanette Kennett takes the asymmetry between autism and psychopathy to suggest one solution to the old debate. On reviewing the psychiatric evidence, Kennett observes that psychopaths, unlike autistic people, are self-destructive: they don't always understand interests (even their own) as giving them reasons for actions. Since autistic people do not have this defect, in her view, they can understand that moral principles give a reason to act. Indeed, she takes the fact that autistic people often attempt to act morally as evidence in favor of Kant's view, at least to the extent that it suggests that it is *possible* to arrive at moral action through purely cognitive, non-emotional means.

Other authors have viewed this interpretation of the evidence with skepticism. McGeer takes note of the example of an autistic piano lover who thinks everyone should be compelled by law to own a piano. She concludes that when autistic people behave morally, they do it because they have an abnormal need for rules and order that motivates them to follow moral rules simply as one rule among many (McGeer 2008). Batson, along similar lines, argues that the kind of rule-following altruism manifested by autistic people is not expressive of genuine moral motivation but merely mimics it (Batson 1997).

Although the analysis of psychiatric cases has not yet succeeded in settling the issue, this is partly because the science currently has only a limited grasp of the reasons why autistic people and psychopaths behave the way they do. But future advances in the scientific understanding of empathy, social emotion and moral behavior, and of the bases of psychiatric deficits in these capacities, are also certain to offer new perspectives on such central questions in moral philosophy, forcing philosophers to better distinguish purely conceptual claims about moral judgment and motivation from what are in fact empirical claims about our moral psychology that are open to scientific testing and falsification.

Conclusion

In this chapter, we have explored areas in which psychiatry and the cognitive sciences have been employed in the philosophical discourse, but we have discussed no cases in which philosophical research has been fruitfully employed by psychiatric scientists. That is altogether unfortunate but unavoidable. The psychiatric sciences stake out a territory which concerns a wide range of phenomena and concepts which are in some ways still only poorly understood: identity, depression, compulsion, and even pain. The science will be hamstrung if it does not engage more fully with the philosophical progress that is being made in understanding these notions. By the same token, we think it is reasonable to hope that a philosophy that is better informed by advances in psychiatry will be more likely to make progress on some of the most intractable philosophical problems.

Over the past few decades, a great effort has been made to try to base psychiatry on rigorous, evidence-based science, and to tie it to our growing understanding of the human brain. This is an exceedingly important and still ongoing project. But it would be a mistake to assume that the central questions of psychiatry can be completely resolved through scientific inquiry. As we have tried to highlight in this chapter, science offers guidance for clinical practice only as interpreted through our concepts and classifications, and only in light of our normative judgments—judgments about what matters, and about what we have most reason to do. Science on its own cannot tell us whether we should be concerned about the level of serotonin in someone's brain, and whether that level should be raised or decreased and by what means. We can only answer such questions by tying such scientific data to concepts such as self, suffering, and well-being, and by seeking agreement on core values and moral principles. These are questions that some may prefer to avoid, or to conceal behind scientific jargon, but they are unavoidable—and they cannot be answered without input from philosophy and practical ethics.

References

Ahmed, S. H. and Koob, G. F. (2005). Transition to drug addiction: a negative reinforcement model based on an allostatic decrease in reward function. *Psychopharmacology (Berl), 180,* 473–90.

American Medical Association (2007). *Code of Medical Ethics: Current Opinions with Annotations, 2006–2007.* Chicago, IL: American Medical Association.

American Psychiatric Association (2000). *Diagnostic and Statistical Manual of Mental Disorders, Fourth Edition, Text Revision.* Washington, DC: American Psychiatric Association.

Batson, M. (1997). Self–other merging and the empathy–altruism hypothesis: Reply to Neuberg et al. *Journal of Personality and Social Psychology, 73,* 517–22.

Baughman, F. (2006). There is no such thing as a psychiatric disorder/disease/chemical imbalance. *PLoS Medicine, 3*(7), 318.

Bostrom, N. and Sandberg, A. (2009). Cognitive enhancement: Methods, ethics, regulatory challenges. *Science and Engineering Ethics, 15,* 311–41.

Conrad, P. (2007). *The Medicalization of Society: On the Transformation of Human Conditions into Treatable Disorders.* Baltimore, MD: Johns Hopkins University Press.

Damasio, A. (1994). *Descartes' Error: Emotion, Reason, and the Human Brain.* New York, NY: Putnam Publishing.

Davies, J. B. (1997). *The Myth of Addiction,* Amsterdam: Harwood Academic.

De Brigard, F., Mandelbaum, E., and Ripley, D. (2009). Responsibility and the brain Sciences. *Ethical Theory and Moral Practice, 12,* 511–24.

Degrazia, D. (2000). Prozac, enhancement, and self-creation. *The Hastings Center Report, 30,* 34–40.

Degrazia, D. (2005). *Human Identity and Bioethics.* Cambridge: Cambridge University Press.

Eddy, N. B., Halbach, H., Isbell, H. and Seevers, M. H. (1965). Drug dependence: Its significance and characteristics. *Bulletin of the World Health Organanization, 32,* 721–33.

Elliott, C. (1998). The tyranny of happiness: Ethics and cosmetic psychopharmacology. In E. Parens (Ed.), *Enhancing Human Traits: Ethical and Social Implications,* pp. 177–88. Washington, DC: Georgetown University Press.

Everitt, B. J. and Robbins, T. W. (2005). Neural systems of reinforcement for drug addiction: from actions to habits to compulsion. *Nature Neurosciences, 8,* 1481–9.

Farah, M. J. (Ed.) (2011). *Neuroethics: An Introduction with Readings.* Cambridge, MA: MIT Press.

Farah, M. J., Illes, J., Cook-Deegan, R., Gardner, H., Kandel, E., King, P., et al. (2004). Neurocognitive enhancement: What can we do and what should we do? *Nature Review Neurosciences*, 5, 421–5.

Feinberg, J. (1970). *Doing and Deserving*. Princeton, NJ: Princeton University Press.

Fischer, J. M. and Ravizza, M. (1998). *Responsibility and Control: A Theory of Moral Responsibility*. Cambridge: Cambridge University Press.

Foddy, B. (2008). Risks and asterisks: Neurological enhancements in baseball. In D. Gordon (Ed.), *Your Brain on Cubs: Inside the Heads of Players and Fans*. New York, NY: Dana Press.

Foddy, B. (2011a). Enhancing skill. In J. Savulescu, R. Ter Meulen, and G. Kahane (Eds), *Enhancing Human Capacities*, pp. 313–25. Oxford: Wiley-Blackwell.

Foddy, B. (2011b). The ethical placebo. *Journal of Mind-Body Regulation*, 1(2), 53–62.

Foddy, B. and Savulescu, J. (2010). A liberal account of addiction. *Philosophy, Psychiatry and Psychology*, 17, 1–22.

Freedman, C. (1998). Aspirin for the mind: Some ethical worries about psychopharmacology. In E. Parens (Ed.), *Enhancing Human Traits: Ethical and Social Implications*, pp. 135–50. Washington, DC: Georgetown University Press.

Griffin, J. (1986). *Well-Being*. Oxford: Clarendon Press.

Hawthorne, S. (2007). ADHD drugs: Values that drive the debates and decisions. *Medicine, Health Care, and Philosophy*, 10, 129–40.

Hume, D. (2000). *A Treatise of Human Nature*. Oxford: Oxford University Press.

Jaffe, J. (1965). Drug addiction and drug abuse. In L. Goodman and A. Gilman (Eds), *The Pharmacological Basis of Therapeutics: A Textbook of Pharmacology* (3rd edn), pp. 285–311. New York, NY: Macmillan.

Kahane, G. (2011a). Reasons to feel, reasons to take pills. In J. Savulescu, R. ter Meulen, and G. Kahane (Eds), *Enhancing Human Capacities*, pp. 166–78. Oxford: Wiley-Blackwell.

Kahane, G. (2011b). Mastery without mystery: Why there is no Promethean sin in enhancement. *Journal of Applied Philosophy*, 28(4), 355–68.

Kahane G. and Savulescu, J. (2009). The welfarist account of disability. In A. Cureton and K. Brownlee (Eds), *Disability and Disadvantage*, pp. 14–53. Oxford: Oxford University Press.

Kamm, F. M. (2005). Is there a problem with enhancement? *American Journal of Bioethics*, 5(3), 5–14.

Kant, I. (2005). *The Moral Law: Groundwork of the Metaphysic of Morals*. London: Routledge.

Kaptchuk, T. J., Friedlander, E., Kelley, J. M., Sanchez, M. N., Kokkotou, E., Singer, J. P., et al. (2010). Placebos without deception: a randomized controlled trial in irritable bowel syndrome. *PLoS ONE*, 5(12), e15591.

Kennett, J. (2003). Autism, empathy and moral agency. *The Philosophical Quarterly*, 52, 340–57.

Kirsch, I., Deacon, B. J., Huedo-Medina, T. B., Scoboria, A., Moore, T. J. and Johnson, B. T. (2008). Initial severity and antidepressant benefits: a meta-analysis of data submitted to the Food and Drug Administration. *PLoS Medicine*, 5, e45.

Kirsch, I. and Sapirstein, G. (1998). Listening to Prozac but hearing placebo: A meta-analysis of antidepressant medication. *Prevention & Treatment*, 1, Art. 0002a.

Kolber, A. (2007). A limited defense of clinical placebo deception. *Yale Law & Policy Review*, 26(1), 75–134

Koob, G. F. and Nestler, E. J. (1997). The neurobiology of drug addiction. *Journal of Neuropsychiatry and Clinical Neurosciences*, 9, 482–97.

Leshner, A. I. (1997). Addiction is a brain disease, and it matters. *Science*, 278, 45–7.

Levy, N. (2006). Autonomy and addiction. *Canadian Journal of Philosophy*, 36, 427.

Levy, N. (2009). Addiction, responsibility and ego depletion. In G. Graham and J. Poland (Eds), *Addiction and Responsibility*, pp. 89–112. Cambridge, MA: MIT Press.

Lubman, D. I., Yucel, M., and Pantelis, C. (2004). Addiction, a condition of compulsive behaviour? Neuroimaging and neuropsychological evidence of inhibitory dysregulation. *Addiction*, 99, 1491–502.

Ludwig, J., Marcotte, D. E. and Norberg, K. (2009). Anti-depressants and suicide. *Journal of Health Economics*, 28, 659–76.

Manninen, B. A. (2006). Medicating the mind: A Kantian analysis of overprescribing psychoactive drugs. *Journal of Medical Ethics*, 32, 100–5.

McCaffery, M. (1968). *Nursing Practice Theories Related to Cognition, Bodily Pain, and Man-Environment Interactions*. Los Angeles, CA: University of California.

McGeer, V. (2008). Varieties of moral agency: Lessons from autism and psychopathy. In W. Sinnott-Armstrong (Ed.), *Moral Psychology, Volume 3: The Neuroscience of Morality: Emotion, Brain Disorders, and Development*, pp. 227–96. Cambridge, MA: MIT Press.

Merskey, H. (1991). The definition of pain. *European Journal of Psychiatry*, 6, 153–9.

Miller, S. and Selgelid, M. J. (2007). Ethical and philosophical consideration of the dual-use dilemma in the biological sciences. *Science and Engineering Ethics*, 13, 523–80.

Morse, S. (2000). Hooked on hype: Addiction and responsibility. *Law and Philosophy*, 19, 3–49.

Morse, S. (2011). Addiction and criminal responsibility. In J. Poland and G. Graham (Eds), *Addiction and Responsibility*, pp. 159–200. Cambridge, MA: MIT Press.

Myrick, H., Malcolm, R., Taylor, B. and Larowe, S. (2004). Modafinil: Preclinical, clinical, and post-marketing surveillance—a review of abuse liability issues. *Annals of Clinical Psychiatry*, 16, 101–9.

Parfit, D. (1984). *Reasons and Persons*. Oxford: Oxford University Press.

Peele, S. and Brodsky, A. (1976). Addiction as a social disease. *Addictions*, Winter, 2–21.

Persson, I. and Savulescu, J. (2008). The perils of cognitive enhancement and the urgent imperative to enhance the moral character of humanity. *Journal of Applied Philosophy*, 25, 162–77.

President's Council on Bioethics (2003). *Beyond Therapy: Biotechnology and the Pursuit of Happiness*. Washington, DC: President's Council on Bioethics.

Radden, J. (2002). Psychiatric ethics. *Bioethics*, 16, 397–411.

Rose, N. (2006). Disorders without borders? The expanding scope of psychiatric practice. *BioSocieties*, 1, 465–84.

Roskies, A. (2002). Neuroethics for the new millenium. *Neuron*, 35, 21–3.

Sahakian, B. and Morein-Zamir, S. (2007). Professor's little helper. *Nature*, 450, 1157–9.

Sandel, M. (2007). *The Case Against Perfection: Ethics in the Age of Genetic Engineering*. Cambridge, MA: Harvard University Press.

Savulescu, J. and Kahane, G. (2009). The moral obligation to create children with the best chance of the best life. *Bioethics*, 23, 274–90.

Sellman, D. (2010). The 10 most important things known about addiction. *Addiction*, 105, 6–13.

Shah, K. R., and Goold, S. D. (2009). The primacy of autonomy, honesty, and disclosure—Council on Ethical and Judicial Affairs' placebo opinions. *American Journal of Bioethices*, 9(12), 15–17.

Singh, I. (2005). Will the "real boy" please behave: Dosing dilemmas for parents of boys with ADHD. *The American Journal of Bioethics: AJOB*, 5, 34–47.

Strawson, P. F. (1974). *Freedom and Resentment and other Essays*. London: Methuen.

Tomporowski, P. D. (2003). Effects of acute bouts of exercise on cognition. *Acta Psychologica, (Amst)*, *112*, 297–324.

Velleman, J. D. (1992). What happens when someone acts? *Mind*, *101*, 461–81.

Volkow, N. D. and Li, T. K. (2004). Drug addiction: the neurobiology of behaviour gone awry. *Nature Reviews Neuroscience*, *5*, 963–70.

Wallace, R. (1999). Addiction as a defect of the will. *Law and Philosophy*, *18*, 621–54.

Watson, G. (1987). Free action and free will. *Mind*, *382*, 145–72.

CHAPTER 70

··

PLACEBO EFFECTS
IN PSYCHIATRY AND
PSYCHOTHERAPY

··

DAVID A. JOPLING

Why do doctors begin by practising on the credulity of their patients with so many false promises of a cure, if not to call the powers of the imagination to the aid of their fraudulent concoctions? They know … that there are men on whom the mere sight of medicine is operative.

de Montaigne "On the power of the imagination" (1574/1958, pp. 36–48)

THE NOTHING TREATMENT

··

The nothing treatment. A pious fraud. A treatment calculated to amuse for a time. A sham treatment. A nuisance variable. Given more to please than to benefit the patient. A commonplace method in medicine. A humble humbug. A make-believe medication. The medical equivalent of an urban myth. Something from nothing. The cheapest medicine in the world. Much ado about nothing.

Placebos, it seems, get no respect. Clinicians have looked upon them as the bane of clinical medicine—located somewhere between long-debunked treatments and pseudo-treatments. Medical ethicists have judged the use of placebos to be morally impermissible, on the grounds that administering placebos to patients invariably involves duping them, misinforming them, or intentionally keeping them in the dark. Medical scientists have dismissed placebo effects as fake or unreal, because (so it is said) placebos fail to have anything more than transient psychological effects on patients. And the designers of clinical trials have regarded placebo effects as little more than the troublesome statistical background noise that needs to be factored out in order to determine the effectiveness of new medications. As Kirsch and Sapirstein (1998) observe, "although almost everyone controls for placebo effects, almost no one evaluates them."

Despite the disrespect, however, the history of medicine and psychiatry from prehistory to present times is rife with placebos and their curious effects. They have put in appearances in everything from the most routine clinical check-ups to the most sophisticated of clinical trials; from the lowliest home remedies administered at the mother's knee to the most elite experimental laboratories; and from the exotic world of alternative medicine (Bausell 2007; Kaptchuk 2002) to the high-stakes world of sports medicine (Benedetti 2009). Even the so-called "gold standard" of medical evidence, the double-blind placebo-controlled clinical trial, could not exist without carefully designed placebos.

Placebos have even made appearances in literature and popular culture. Writers as diverse as Michel de Montaigne (1574/1958), Fyodor Dostoevsky (1880/1981, vol. II, p. 3), Mark Twain (Ober 2003), Jerome K. Jerome (1889/1964), George Bernard Shaw (1911/1941), Sinclair Lewis (1980), and Patrick O'Brian (1998) have provided literary accounts—as often comical as not—of placebos, nocebos (inert procedures or substances that have negative effects on health), sham cures, and symbolic healing rituals, as well as of the colorful physicians and patients who have encountered them (Marshall 2004).

It should come as no surprise that a large proportion of current clinical practice involves the use, inadvertent or otherwise, of placebos. In one survey conducted in the USA (Sherman and Hickner 2008), 45% of academic physicians admitted to having used placebos in their clinical practice. Of those polled, 96% believed that placebos had therapeutic effects, and 40% believed that placebos had physiological benefits. In another survey, 86% of Danish general practitioners admitted that they had used placebo treatments at least once in the past year, and 48% had used them ten times or more (Hrobjartsson and Norup 2003). Thirty percent of those polled believed that placebos had effects on objective outcomes, and 46% regarded their use as ethically acceptable. The frequency and range of placebo use in psychiatry and psychotherapy, however, is still very much a mystery: as it is often said, "more research is required."

Where then to begin this research? Some of the questions calling out for answers are obvious: What *is* a placebo? What is a placebo effect? What mechanisms could explain placebo effects? More pertinently, what relevance, if any, do placebos and their effects have for psychotherapy and psychiatry? But before tackling some of these questions, however, some ground clearing and debunking is in order.

Myths and Misconceptions

Adding to the dismal reputation of placebos are a number of persistent myths and misconceptions circulating in medicine and psychiatry, some of which have acquired the status of truisms. These include the following:

1. Because placebos are physiologically inert, they can exert no effect on physiological function or pathophysiology.
2. Placebos can only affect psychological symptoms (or, conversely, if they relieve symptoms, then the symptoms must have been unreal or imaginary).
3. Almost any medical condition can respond to placebo.

4. Once patients know that their treatment is a placebo, the treatment will be ineffective.
5. Placebos have only transient effects.
6. Giving placebos to patients is unethical, because it always involves tricking them into believing that they are receiving active medications.

However obvious they may be, claims (1) to (5) do not stand up to the emerging clinical and experimental evidence; and claim (6) calls for substantial rethinking in light of new research on open-label placebos. Consider the following highly selective sampling of this evidence, a sampling that is only a small fraction of the discoveries that have been made since the 1950s, the time when the placebo effect became a subject of scientific inquiry in its own right.

- A number of diseases and disorders are responsive to placebo treatment, including: allergies, angina, anxiety, asthma, colitis, cough, depression, dyspepsia, fever, gastric dysfunction, headache, insomnia, irritable bowel syndrome, movement disorders, nausea, Parkinson's disease, rheumatoid arthritis, sexual dysfunction, skin conditions, and ulcers.
- Placebo administration shows a clear dose–response relationship, with four placebo pills a day more effective than two (DeCraen et al. 1999).
- Placebo injections are more effective than placebo pills (DeCraen et al. 2000), and placebo surgeries are more effective than both placebo pills and placebo injections (Moseley et al. 2002).
- The magnitude of placebo response is correlated with the color of placebo pills (Blackwell et al. 1972), as well as with the type of presentation and the type of information given to patients about the pills.
- High-priced placebos are more effective than low-priced placebos (Kirsch 2010), and branded placebos are more effective than unbranded placebos (Braithwaite and Cooper 1981).
- Nocebos have been shown to have adverse effects on health (Hahn 1997; Barksy et al. 2002), and have triggered such reactions as headaches, bronchial constriction, and skin rashes.
- Patients who adhere strictly to a regimen of placebo pills (placebo adherence) tend to show greater therapeutic improvement than patients whose adherence is inconsistent.
- Physiologically inert placebos can generate multiple side effects, some of which mimic the side effects of active medications (Benedetti 2009; Kirsch 2010).
- Placebos can affect galvanic skin temperature, pulse, temperature, cholesterol and cortisol levels, systolic and diastolic blood pressure, mean arterial pressure, and blood sugar level.
- Placebo responsiveness and placebo response magnitude are subject to wide cultural variation (Moerman 2000, 2002), with, e.g., placebo injections more effective than placebo pills in the USA but not in Europe (DeCraen et al. 2000), and higher placebo healing rates for ulcer in Germany than elsewhere in Europe.
- Placebo effects are subject to sequencing effects, with placebos given to patients after they have been treated with drugs (such as two previous administrations of a painkiller) proving more effective than placebos given for the first time (Amanzio and Benedetti 1999).

- Placebo responsiveness is linked with genetic variants, with placebo-induced anxiety relief correlated with genetically controlled serotonergic modulation of amygdala activity (Furmark et al. 2008).
- Both pharmacologically active and pharmacologically inert placebos can be effective, although the former (which produce side effects because they contain chemically active ingredients) tend to display an enhanced placebo effect compared to the latter (Kirsch 2010).
- Patients who have been told they are receiving placebo treatment often exhibit placebo effects (Kaptchuk et al. 2010; Park and Covi 1965).
- Many pain conditions are responsive to placebo, including headache (DeCraen et al. 2000), postoperative pain (Bausell 2007; Benedetti 2009, 2011), molar extraction pain, experimentally induced pain (Kirsch and Sapirstein 1998), and phantom limb pain (Wager 2005). There is also wide variation in the magnitude of placebo analgesia, depending on the interaction of cultural, individual, and disease variables.

This is a telling list of discoveries, and it grows longer each year. What it suggests, among other things, is that placebo effects are not merely in the minds of patients, mere subjective phenomena that float on the surface of physiology like oil on water (Harrington 1997); nor are they merely phony interventions devised to placate obstreperous patients, a "pious fraud," as Thomas Jefferson described them. The view emerging in the medical, behavioral, and neurosciences is that placebo effects are functions of the human organism's intricately evolved and innate capacity to heal itself, to restore itself to equilibrium, and to repair damage (Bausell 2007; Benedetti 2009, 2011; Guess et al. 2002; Harrington 1997; Humphrey 2002; Kirsch 2010; Meissner et al. 2011). Placebo effects, in other words, are real, powerful, and measurable, and in addition to a powerful subjective presence they often have objective effects on physiological function and pathophysiology (for a dissenting view see Hróbjartsson and Gøtzsche 2001).

It would be a mistake, however, to conclude from this list of discoveries that *all* medical conditions are responsive to placebo. There is no current evidence that conditions such as infertility, bones fractures, diabetes, and cancer respond to placebos, even though the pain associated with some of these conditions often does. It would also be a mistake to conclude that *all* medical conditions have approximately the same number of placebo responders, as Beecher suggested in his seminal (1955) paper "The powerful placebo." Beecher's estimate, now considered a "vintage number" (Kaptchuk 1988), was 30%. In fact, however, the range of placebo response is between 0% and 100%.

Finally, it would be a mistake to conclude that the growing body of evidence that this list represents points unmistakably to the conclusion that placebos only influence illness, but not physical disease itself: that is, that they have no effect on the underlying physiological causes of disease, but only on the experienced symptoms. This view has been defended by some (Miller et al. 2009), but it is a view that rests largely on conceptual grounds, and it stands or falls accordingly. According to this view, it is the organism—the object of biomedicine—that is affected by the disease; and it is the person as a whole—the object of the hermeneutics and phenomenology of medicine—that is affected by the illness. Given this distinction, placebos can occasion symptomatic relief, but they have no significant impact on underlying pathophysiology and progression of disease processes. This distinction between illness and disease seems to be intuitively plausible, but the boundaries it marks out are subject to a problematic degree of fuzziness. Some diseases, for example, do not manifest as illnesses (e.g., asymptomatic diseases), and some illnesses are not diagnosable diseases. Moreover, it is unclear, in light of the emerging evidence, how placebos could *not* affect the organism. The distinction between illness and disease rests on the broader distinction between the body as physical object and the body as lived and experienced, the latter marking out a terrain that is the subject of intense investigation from the cognitive and neurosciences, and phenomenology. Ultimately, the usefulness of this way of understanding placebo effects will depend on the explanatory advantages to be had from keeping a double set of books.

Placebo Effects in Psychiatry
and Psychotherapy

Many disorders and diseases responsive to placebos are in the field of somatic medicine. But are placebo effects also found in psychiatry and psychotherapy? Do common psychological disorders such as depression, anxiety, and phobia respond to placebo? Do psychological treatments, like some somatic treatments, trade—perhaps unknowingly—in placebos? Do they outperform, match, or underperform placebos in head to head comparisons, if such comparisons are even possible?

Many of these questions do not yet have answers. Some researchers have thrown down the gauntlet to the psychological treatments (especially the psychotherapies), asking them for proof that they are effective *at all*—and finding them wanting (Eysenck 1965). Some have suggested that the available meta-analytic evidence shows that most psychotherapies are no more effective than credible placebos—which themselves can be quite effective with certain disorders (Erwin 1997; Prioleau et al. 1983). Some have suggested that the psychotherapies are nothing more than placebos (Frank 1983). Some have suggested that the very idea of transposing the concept of placebo in medical and pharmaceutical research to psychotherapy outcome studies is just plain misguided and ought to be abandoned (Parloff 1986a, 1986b). And some have suggested that the terms placebo and psychotherapy are synonyms, and the phrase "placebo psychotherapy" an outright oxymoron (Kirsch 2005).

There is, clearly, more than a fair share of controversy and confusion here. So what is to be done? Among the several workable strategies for sorting out the mess and developing some tentative answers to the questions about placebo effects in psychiatry and psychotherapy are the following: (a) defining placebos and placebo effects; (b) looking for evidence of placebo effects in clinical case histories; (c) looking at the effectiveness of placebos in controlled clinical trials of medications for psychiatric conditions, to see how they perform against active medications; and (d) looking for evidence of placebos in the history of psychiatry and psychological treatments.

Definitions

What is a placebo? And what is the placebo effect? As the following sample shows, there is wide disagreement about how to define both terms; and with the proliferation of definitions come definitions that are too vague, too wide, too narrow, or guilty of smuggling in theories of causation and mechanism, thereby conflating explanation with definition. Still, when handled with care, definitions can be useful for guiding inquiry.

1. A placebo is a procedure that is without specific activity for the condition being evaluated (Shapiro 1964; Shapiro 1971).
2. A placebo is a condition for which there is "no currently supported theoretical reason why ... [it] would influence the behavior under question" (O'Leary and Borkovec 1978).
3. A placebo is a factor that is common to most types of therapy, such as expectancy of improvement, credibility of rationale, and perceived belief by therapists in their treatment procedures (Critelli and Newman 1984).
4. A placebo is a pharmacologically inactive substance that can have a therapeutic effect if administered to a patient who believes that he or she is receiving an effective treatment (Bausell 2007).
5. The placebo effect is a meaning response, which is the psychological and physiological effect of meaning in the origin and treatment of illness (Moerman 2002).
6. The placebo effect is a dynamic, unpredictable, and constantly changing variable that covaries with other psychological and physical variables in the therapeutic process (Bootzin and Caspi 2002).
7. The placebo effect is a set of related causal processes within interpersonal healing, by means of which the context of the clinical encounter and the relationship between a healer and a patient produce therapeutic benefit (Kaptchuk et al. 2010).
8. The placebo is a sham, fake, inert, or empty treatment, and the placebo effect is what is produced by the self-confirming nature of response expectancies (Kirsch 1985, 2005; Montgomery and Kirsch 1988).
9. A placebo is a therapy for which none of the characteristic factors of the treatment are remedial for the specified target disorders, but the disorders are improved because of the effect of the therapy's incidental factors (Grünbaum 1986).

Consider two of the more well-known of these definitions. Shapiro's definition of placebo (1964, 1971) captures some of the prototypical features of placebo phenomena. At the same time, it sets up a puzzling distinction. A placebo he defines as "any therapeutic procedure (or a component of any therapeutic procedure) which is given (a) deliberately to have an effect, or (b) unknowingly and has an effect on a symptom, syndrome, disease, or patient but which is objectively without specific activity for the condition being treated ... The placebo effect is defined as the changes produced by placebos." According to Shapiro's definition, then, the specific activity of acetylsalicylic acid (ASA) in aspirin pills produces specific effects on a specific target disorder, whereas the arousal of hope, or the expectation of cure, produces nonspecific, placebo effects, on the target disorder.

As with all definitions, one definition calls for another and then another: What is specific activity, and where does it end and non-specific activity begin? And just how specific is specific activity? Shapiro's answer is not especially helpful. Specific activity is defined as the therapeutic influence that is attributable solely to the contents or processes of the therapies rendered, the criterion for which is based on scientifically controlled studies (1977; Shapiro and Shapiro 1997). But this further definition raises more questions: What *precisely* is the therapeutic influence attributable solely to the therapy, and how is it to be distinguished from influence that is not? How does this definition do justice to the fact that some placebos have effects that are as specific as those of non-placebo treatments? And what scientifically controlled studies serve as criteria, and why?

Grünbaum's (1986) definition advances the discussion by replacing Shapiro's intuitive but vague distinction between specific and non-specific activity with a less problematic one between "characteristic" and "incidental" factors of a treatment. A placebo he defines as a therapy for which none of the "characteristic factors" of the treatment are remedial for the specified target disorders, but the target disorders are nonetheless improved because of the effect of the therapy's "incidental factors." What does Grünbaum mean by the "characteristic factors" of a treatment? These he defines as the components of the treatment that are thought to be (or theorized to be) remedial for the target disorder: for instance, ASA for the treatment of pain. The incidental factors, by contrast, are those components of a treatment that are not thought to be (or theorized to be) remedial for the disorder: for instance, the particular color, shape, or smell of the pill that contains ASA, or the physician's level of confidence about the effectiveness of ASA. The difference between a placebo and a non-placebo, then, is not based on the distinction between nonspecific and specific activity, but on whether or not the treatment's characteristic factors play a therapeutic role for the target disorders.

From this it should be clear that Grünbaum's definition relativizes placebos and placebo effects to therapeutic theories. The only way that some therapeutic effect counts as a placebo effect is in terms of an overarching therapeutic theory which hypothesizes that certain therapeutic factors count as characteristic, and others as incidental. Treatment gains count as placebo effects only in light of the therapeutic theory, and only when the therapeutic effect is caused by treatment factors other than those which the overarching theory hypothesizes as remedial for the disorder. Thus some factor X might be characteristic under one theory and incidental under another theory: one and the same thing might count as a placebo and a non-placebo, depending on how it is theorized. One of the shortcomings with Grünbaum's definition, however, is that does not define two crucial terms—namely, "remedial" and "placebo effect."

Two Case Histories

Are psychological disorders responsive to placebo treatments? Are placebos deployed in psychological treatments, either intentionally or inadvertently? The evidence from clinical case histories is useful in helping to decide the question—at least to a degree. This is not only because clinical case histories tend to be reported through the lens of particular psychotherapeutic theories, with the attendant bias from theory-mediated descriptions of salient psychological and behavioral facts; nor is it only because they sometimes rely on anecdotal reports, such as uncorroborated reports that therapeutic improvement has taken place (Kazdin 1981). The main obstacle is that they typically report on individuals, or case series covering a number of individuals—a slim empirical base from which to generalize about wider populations. With these caveats in mind, however, consider the following two case histories.

Patient A is a forty-six-year-old woman with major depressive disorder (Greenberg 2003). Psychoactive medications have proven to be ineffective for her. After extensive screening and consent procedures A enrolls in a double blind clinical trial of a new antidepressant drug. She does not know whether the pills she is given are placebos or the drug, but her depression begins to alleviate, and with the appearance of side effects consistent with those of antidepressant medications she guesses that she is assigned to the verum group. Her improved mood is confirmed by a battery of psychological and neurological tests during and after the trial.

Patient B, a young married mother suffering from depression, is treated with brief psychodynamic psychotherapy over a period of several weeks (Frank and Frank 1991, pp. 205–210). The patient, who had a difficult childhood, is facing large-scale life changes, including marriage and motherhood. Jerome Frank, her psychotherapist, learns that when B was a young child, her mother committed suicide, not long after which her father remarried and was posted overseas. At an early stage in the treatment, at a point when he had had little time to assemble a sufficient amount of clinical material to develop a clear picture of B's past and her difficulties, Frank offers a psychodynamic interpretation. Tying together themes from her childhood and her current marital conflicts, the interpretation "goes off like a gong." It triggers in B a number of insights, which in turn lead to positive changes in behavior and mood, which in turn advances the progress of the treatment.

What, if anything, is common in these cases? First, both patients suffered from similar psychological disorders that were severe enough to require treatment. Second, both patients showed clear signs of therapeutic improvement following treatment. Third, both patients were treated with placebos, and, most likely, improved as a result. But how? What could there be in common here to justify calling such different things placebos?

The placebo given to patient A was a conventional physical placebo: that is, a pill containing none of the active pharmacologic agents (the characteristic factors) hypothesized by the overarching therapeutic theory to target depression, but disguised and presented as an active medication. To make it a more credible placebo, and to help minimize the chances of A breaking the blind, the pill contained ingredients that triggered some of the same kinds of side effects of antidepressant medications. There is good reason for designing credible placebos: breaking the blind introduces into trials such as A's a number of confounds that skew inferences about the pharmacologic effectiveness of the active medications and placebos. For example, had A guessed that she had been assigned to the placebo group, she might have concluded that her depression would not have been helped by a "mere" placebo, and this might have exacerbated her feelings of hopelessness and helplessness. But since she guessed (incorrectly) that she had been assigned to the verum group, she had heightened expectations of improvement, which generated a kind of self-fulfilling prophecy. And had she been assigned to the verum group, and guessed that she had been, she might have improved even more on the active drug than on the placebo simply because she believed that she was taking an active drug rather than an inert pill, thereby giving a false impression of therapeutic efficacy of the medication. A patient's knowledge that he or she is taking an active drug enhances the effectiveness of the drug significantly more than it would if the patient were not aware of it (Bausell 2007; Kirsch 2010).

The placebo given to patient B was of a much different type from that given to patient A: rather than a discrete physical entity, it was a complex and multiply staged procedure that pressed in to service words, symbols, rhetoric, subtext, gesture, and weighty authority.

Placebos that fit this profile—procedural placebos—include practices ranging from sham surgeries (Moseley et al. 2002) to elaborate ceremonies involving narratives, rituals, and the manipulation of religio-magical healing symbols.

In B's case the procedural placebo involved the presentation and exploration of a psychodynamic interpretation, one of the high points of the talking cures, and considered by many to be a trigger of catharsis, insight, and psychological healing. The interpretation given to B seemed to work, and it seemed to work because it seemed to have precisely delineated and non-suggestive effects on the disorder to which it was applied. In fact, however, it was an interpretation placebo, the psychological analogue of a sugar pill. It lacked some of the main ingredients of bona fide interpretations: namely, correctness, exactness, fit to the facts, and genuine explanatory power. Frank could not have known if the interpretation was historically and psychologically accurate, as he presented it at an early stage of the treatment, with only a slim base of clinical material from which to work. He knew little about the patient and her history. What the interpretation contained, however, and what assured its status as a credible placebo, were a number of incidental or surrounding factors, including a passable degree of psychological plausibility and coherence. The interpretation proved to be reassuring to B, it enabled her to re-label her feelings as normal, and it enhanced her sense of mastery (Frank and Frank 1991, p. 207). But it was an inexact, vague, and one-size-fits-all interpretation, so much so that it could have been replaced by a number of other loose-fitting and minimally credible interpretations; and it could have been true of any number of people (thus illustrating the so-called "Barnum effect"). Frank acknowledged much of this, without explicitly conceding that the interpretation was a placebo: "The healing power of my interpretations seemed to lie more in the general attitude they conveyed than in their precise content" (1991, p. 210). Elsewhere Frank writes: "An effectively reassuring explanation simultaneously promotes patients' feelings of mastery and offers hopes of recovery" (1991, p. 128). "Therapists ... who believe that only 'correct' interpretations will lead patients to change, find it hard to accept that the attitude their words convey may contribute more to therapy than the words' precise content" (Frank and Frank 1991, p. 210).

Interpretations, and the client's insights that follow them, are hypothesized to be among the active ingredients (or the characteristic factors) of the talking cures, particularly those with psychodynamic and psychoanalytic orientations. With interpretations and insights, it is claimed, the patterns of unruly forces that govern lives and derail relationships, that make people strangers to themselves, finally come to be named, understood, and rendered more subject to conscious control (Jopling 2008). Interpretations and insights, in other words, are as central to the treatment and relief of psychic pain, and just as precisely targeted, as active chemicals like ASA are to the relief of somatic pain. With the exception of certain post-modern and narrativist variants, most of the talking cures work on the assumption that only "correct" or true interpretations and insights can be therapeutically efficacious. The talking cures after all do not trade in fictions, confabulations or illusions: one of their primary goals is to put clients in touch with who they *really* are.

Underlying this view of the therapeutic efficacy of interpretations and insights is what might be called the principle of therapeutic specificity (Jopling 2008), a principle adopted and adapted by psychological treatments from somatic medicine. According to this principle, psychological treatment methods have exact, precisely delineated, and non-suggestive effects on the disorders to which they are applied. Like their analogues in somatic medicine, psychological treatments are not merely a motley assemblage of amorphous techniques that succeed by hit and miss, or by placebo effect, or by suggestion. Rather, they target disorders in ways that are precise, uniform, measurable, and replicable; and the disorders they target cannot be adequately accessed by any more appropriate means. Those treatments that satisfy the principle of therapeutic specificity are characterized by a precisely specifiable set of mechanisms (or characteristic factors) that engage the target disorders like keys engaging locks. Just as the edges of keys fit precisely onto the tumblers of locks, so the unique mechanisms of treatment methods fit precisely onto the target disorders. One of these keys is the interpretation; another is the client's insight.

Criticisms, Cautions, Caveats

The narrativist criticism

One criticism of the claim that placebo effects are at play in psychological treatments comes from the direction of narrativist psychology, a branch of the hermeneutic approach to the social and clinical sciences. According to narrativist approaches, patient B's response to her psychotherapist's interpretation was not a response to placebo, and her insights—those that "went off like a gong"—were not insight placebos. What really happened was that she responded to a meaningful narrative that was, in some sense, true. Interpretations and insights may not neatly fit historical and psychological facts, but this does not mean that they are merely fictional; nor does it mean that they are bogus or sham elements of a treatment, in the way that inert sugar pills are. They are true, insofar as they are coherent, internally consistent, and plausible; and this kind of truth is one of the central therapeutically active ingredients (or characteristic factors) of treatment, no different in principle from therapeutically active ingredients such as ASA.

Narrativist approaches typically distinguish between different kinds of truth, different types of evidence, different methods of getting at truth, and different contexts in which different truths matter (Schafer 1981, 1992; Spence 1982). They typically view "historical truth" (the correspondence of an interpretation or insight with extra-linguistic facts) as less important in matters psychotherapeutic than "narrative truth" (the internal coherence of the interpretation, in terms of which extra-linguistic facts are organized and given meaning). And they view narrative truths as flexible enough to accommodate factual errors, factually incorrect (or false) memories, and psychologically incorrect descriptions, all of which inconveniences are tolerated as relatively insignificant noise with respect to the broader effort to create meaning.

The problem with this criticism, however, is that it is not clear how it can distinguish between narratives that are mere fictional stories, and narratives that are truth-tracking; or between sham or confabulated narratives (placebo interpretations and insights) that display some of the marks of coherence and plausibility, and bona fide narratives. Freed from the constraints of objective historical and psychological fact, the risk is that narratives start the slide down the slope of confabulation, moral convenience, illusion, or self-deception (Held 1995; Jopling 2008).

Real and apparent placebo effects

Another criticism of the claim that placebo effects are at work in the psychological treatments comes from the direction of the logic and methodology of the clinical sciences. Perhaps placebos can affect some conditions, and can bring about powerful effects. Nonetheless, they are also sometimes mistakenly credited with therapeutic effects they did not cause. Caution is therefore in order. The mere fact that patients such as A and B show clinically significant responses after administration of placebo is not, by itself, sufficient to establish that the improvement was the effect of placebo; to assume that it is, is to commit the *post hoc ergo propter hoc* fallacy. A number of other factors that can give the appearance of a placebo effect—the natural history of the disease or disorder, natural fluctuation of symptoms, regression to the mean, and patient bias—first have to be ruled out before concluding that placebos caused the therapeutic effects.

Some psychological disorders, for instance, are self-limiting. Just as the progress of a common cold in an otherwise healthy host in a normal environment tends to follow a broadly predictable course, with more or less delineable patterns of onset, course, duration, and symptom remission, so some psychological disorders follow natural courses if left untreated (Bausell 2007). If a placebo is given while a disorder is on the wane, then the changes following the placebo intervention might have occurred anyways, and any conclusions about a powerful placebo effect would be doubtful. Perhaps this is what happened to patients A and B. One way to control for natural history would be to put patients in a controlled clinical trial with three arms, with one arm designed to observe a group that receives no treatment at all. This way, the natural history of the disorder can be compared to its progress in the verum and placebo groups. But comparisons like these are not possible with single case histories, or with case series with small numbers of patients.

Another confounding factor that would have to be ruled out before concluding that A and B's disorders had responded to placebo treatment is regression to the mean—the "phenomenon that a variable extreme on its first measurement will tend to be closer to the center of the distribution for a later measurement" (Davis 1976, 2002). In some cases, what appears to be therapeutic change following the administration of placebo is an artifact of the *measurement* of therapeutic change. Patients typically seek help when symptoms are increasing in severity, and they tend not to seek help when symptoms are decreasing. This means that the first tests or measurements of their conditions will tend to pick up extreme symptoms, and later tests will tend to pick up less extreme symptoms. What might seem to be a case of therapeutic change due to placebo is in some cases a function of how and when the disorder is measured.

Adding to the list of potential confounds is patient and psychiatrist bias. Patients are subject to measurement reactivity biases, one of the variants of the Hawthorne effect (Adair 1984): that is, their awareness that they are the subjects of measurement and clinical observation (following the administration of placebo) influences the reports they provide about their conditions. Some patients, for instance, will exaggerate their symptoms in order to be chosen for inclusion in a clinical trial, or to get treatment; and some will exaggerate their improvement at the end of a trial or course of treatment in order to be rewarded as good patients, with the improvement then being falsely credited to the placebo effect. Physicians, psychiatrists, and psychotherapists, moreover, are subject to a number of potent cognitive biases (Dawes 1989; Dawes et al. 1989; Faust 1986; Meehl 1953) which inadvertently influence their selection and treatment of patients, and their interpretation of clinical results.

In addition to these culprits, a number of other confounding factors may create the false impression of powerful placebo effects in psychiatry and psychotherapy (Ernst and Resch 1995; Kiene 1993a, 1993b; Kienle and Kiene 1997), including: random fluctuation of symptoms, additional or parallel treatment, subsiding toxic effects of previous medication, patient bias (e.g., answers of politeness and experimental subordination), conditioned answers, and time effects (e.g., improved investigator skills from one measurement to the next, and decreases in "white coat hypertension" in patients).

False transposition of the placebo concept

A third criticism of the claim that placebos and placebo effects are found in psychological treatments focuses on the very idea of transposing the placebo concept from medicine to psychology. Some critics reject the idea that there are such things as psychological placebos: there are, they claim, no plausible theoretical, clinical, and experimental analogies between the pill placebos used in clinical trials in medical and pharmaceutical research, and the psychological placebos used in psychotherapy and psychotherapy effectiveness studies (Parloff 1986a, 1986b; Shapiro 1971). If successful, this objection would call into question the fifty-year long research tradition in psychotherapy and psychiatry that relies on placebo controls to test the efficacy of psychological treatments. It would also have the consequence of undermining criticisms of the effectiveness of psychotherapy which claim that psychotherapy is no more effective than placebo (Eysenck 1965).

Parloff (1986a, 1986b), for example, argues that the very concept of placebo controls in psychotherapy effectiveness studies is incoherent, because the specific components of psychological treatments cannot, in principle, be factored out from the nonspecific components. It is not only practically impossible to design a placebo control that is identical in all relevant respects to the psychological treatment, with the sole exception that it is missing the ingredients that are theorized to be therapeutically specific; the very idea of such a control is incoherent. Parloff observes that there is no consensus among the many different theoretical approaches to psychological treatments about what constitutes specific and nonspecific components; nothing, that is, is recognized as a standardized placebo control. It is not uncommon, for instance, for a treatment component that is designated as therapeutically specific in one approach to be designated as nonspecific in another. This situation is not found in medical and pharmacological clinical trials, where there is a large degree of consensus about the specific—nonspecific distinction, and about what counts as a standardized placebo control. "Because each placebo must be carefully designed and described to contrast with the particular experimental treatment for which it is to serve as a control, the hope of developing a standard placebo applicable to all treatments loosely identified as psychotherapy cannot be realized. Any placebo whose rationale was so ingenious as to elicit and sustain a high degree of credibility in patients would not long be considered theoretically inert" (Parloff 1986b, p. 83).

What this means is that the putative placebo controls in psychotherapy effectiveness studies are simply alternative forms of active psychological treatment, rather than genuine placebos. "If the placebo includes ingredients hypothesized by any formal psychosocial treatment as specific for the treatment of specified problems, then the intended placebo, when applied to the same problems, must be considered an alternative treatment form rather than a placebo." (Parloff 1986b, p. 84) To illustrate his point, Parloff cites the large 1985 US National Institute of Mental Health depression study (Treatment of Depression Collaborative Research Program; Elkin et al. 1985), which aimed to compare two forms of psychotherapy (cognitive behavior therapy and interpersonal therapy), an antidepressant drug (imipramine) plus clinical management, and a drug–placebo condition (pill placebo plus clinical management). The problem with the study was that the researchers were unable to design genuine placebo controls for psychotherapy: "Placebo conditions proposed were judged to be either too fanciful, implausible, unethical, or simply an attenuated version of an existing form of treatment" (Parloff 1986b, p. 84).

Once Parloff's main assumption is granted—namely, that placebo controls must be identical in every respect except one (viz., the treatment's specific factors) to the treatment against which they are compared, in order to establish a fair and informative comparison—then the conclusion seems to follow: namely, that there are no such things as psychotherapy placebo controls, since what remains once specific factors are removed is itself an alternative form of treatment which, from the viewpoint of other psychotherapeutic theories, contains specific factors. The problem, however, is that Parloff's criticism demands too much. A fair comparison in controlled clinical trials or outcome studies does not require the *identity* between the placebo (less the specific factors) and the treatment in question, but only the relative therapeutic *credibility* of the placebo (Jopling 2008). That is, the placebo only needs to be as credible as a treatment to the volunteers in the study or trial as the treatment for which it serves as a control, while lacking the specific factors of the treatment. Therapeutic credibility, unlike identity, is a matter of more or less rather than all or none. If the placebo was incredible, significantly less credible, or plainly implausible in relation to the treatment against which it was to be measured, then it would be easy to show that the treatment outperformed the placebo.

Kirsch (2005) approaches the question of the extension of the placebo concept from medical research to the psychotherapeutic setting from a different angle than Parloff's, but arrives at similar conclusions. He argues, first, that it is *practically* impossible to design a psychological placebo that is both identical in appearance to the active treatment *and* devoid of the relevant active ingredients. The match-and-replace strategy is unproblematic in medical and pharmaceutical research, where the relevant properties that need to be controlled are physical and isolable, but it does not work in psychotherapy research, where the relevant properties to be controlled are all psychological. "If a psychological treatment contained the same psychological properties as the real treatment (i.e., if the therapist used the same words and procedures), it would no longer be a placebo or a control condition of any other kind. Instead, it would be the treatment. As a result, procedures used as placebos in psychotherapy research are usually very different from the psychotherapies to which they are being compared" (Kirsch 2005, p. 796). But these so-called placebos, which include such things as listening to stories, reading books, attending language classes, viewing films, playing with puzzles, sitting quietly with a silent therapist, and discussing current events (Kirsch 2005, p. 796), are not genuine placebos in the sense of being sham, fake, empty, or inert. None of them can therefore ensure a fair comparison.

Second, Kirsch argues that if placebos are characterized as fake, sham, inert, or empty treatments, as they ought to be, then it is *logically* impossible to extend the placebo concept from medical research to the psychotherapeutic setting. Psychological treatments trade in words and meanings, and there is no such thing as fake, sham, or inert meanings (Kirsch 2005, p. 797); and, by implication, there is no such thing as fake or sham psychotherapies which can be contrasted with bona fide psychotherapies. For Kirsch, then, the terms placebo and psychotherapy are synonymous, or definitionally equivalent; *and*, the phrase placebo psychotherapy is an oxymoron. The problem with Kirsch's argument, however, is that it lumps together indiscriminately all of the factors of psychological treatments, thereby ruling out the very possibility of designing psychological placebos that omit the characteristic factors of a treatment. Every property of every psychological treatment is on a par with every other—so much so that "it does not matter what those [psychologically] active ingredients are" (Kirsch 2005, p. 800). "In principle, these [factors such as hope, faith, response expectancy] are no different from any other psychological factor than [*sic*] can alleviate distress" (Kirsch 2005, p. 800). However, the multiple factors at play in psychotherapies are not all of a piece: they differ from one another in terms of relative causal powers, mechanisms of action, patient receptivity, epistemic status, degree of credibility, and theoretical centrality, among other things (Jopling 2008). One of the central goals of psychotherapy outcome research is to identify, isolate, test, and control for these factors. Without this, psychological treatments would be no more than inscrutable black box procedures, and the scientific validation of competing psychological explanations of therapeutic change would be rendered irrelevant.

Depression

As the two case histories seem to suggest, depression is sometimes responsive to placebo treatment. In fact, some psychiatrists have recommended placebo as a first line of treatment for depression (Brown 1994, 1998a, 1998b). Others have observed that placebo treatments have proven to be surprisingly effective in treating depression, at least in clinical trial settings. The placebo response rate in double-blind controlled clinical trials for antidepressant medication is statistically and clinically significant, in some cases rivaling that of pharmacologically active antidepressants, and in some cases outperforming it (Kirsch 2010; Kirsch et al. 2002). In a series of meta-analytic studies, Kirsch and Sapirstein (1998) found that improvement in patients who had received placebo was about 75% of the response to the antidepressant medication. That is, only 25% of the benefit of the antidepressant treatment was due to the chemical effects of the medication, and 50% of the improvement was a placebo effect. The placebo effect, in other words, was twice as large as the drug effect. Kirsch et al. (2002) also found that when antidepressants are compared to active placebos such as atropine (which is used to treat gastric dysfunctions rather than depression, but nonetheless has side effects that mimic those of antidepressants), the differences in outcome are hard to find; and that when differences in side effects are controlled for, the differences between antidepressant drugs and placebos are not statistically significant. Kirsch and Sapirstein (1998) and Kirsch et al. (2002) credit response expectancies rather than pharmacologic action with a significant degree of the effect produced by antidepressant medications.

Critics have argued against these conclusions on a number of grounds: the studies used in the meta-analyses have limited generalizability (Klein 1998); the logic of using simple post-treatment minus pre-treatment differences in an outcome variable for a treatment or placebo group does not indicate a treatment or placebo effect (Dawes 1998); the trials were too short to show the real effects of antidepressants; the people recruited in to the trials were not depressed enough (Rush and Ryan 2002); the trials did not study people with severe depression (Editorial 2008); the patients in clinical trials, unlike those in clinical practice, know that they might be receiving a placebo, thereby reducing the antidepressant effects of the active drug; and, clinical practice shows clearly that antidepressants work (Werner 2008).

Explanatory Theories of
the Placebo Effect

What could explain placebo effects, especially those that show up in psychological treatments? What mechanisms are involved? The two leading theoretical contenders in placebo research are expectancy theory and conditioning theory, but there are a number of other contenders as well, and their theoretical compatibility and inter-theoretic reducibility is the subject of ongoing discussion. These theories include placebo responder theory, neurobiological theories, social-cognition theory, interpersonal healing theory, meaning-making theory, and evolutionary theory.

Expectancy theory holds that placebo effects can be explained in terms of patients' expectations for relief (or, in the case of nocebo effects, their expectations for further deterioration or pain) (Kirsch 1985, 1997, 1999, 2010; Kirsch et al. 2002; Montgomery and Kirsch 1996). Patients improve because they expect to improve when given treatments, and in many cases their expectations produce the improvement that they are expecting as a kind of self-fulfilling prophecy—even if the treatments contain no physiologically active ingredients. Expectations are enhanced or diminished by physicians' attitudes and the type of information they convey to patients, as well as by cultural conceptions of the effectiveness of medications and procedures, and even differences in the *materia medica* (such as the size and color of the pills, or the use of injections rather than pills). The expectancy theory places a great deal of emphasis on the forward-looking attitudes of patients, especially their expectations of future outcomes and future responses. Patients typically have expectations about their own emotional and physiological responses to health-related events and procedures, and these expectations, coupled with other cognitive factors such as memory, motivation, and hope, influence their behaviors. Forward-looking attitudes are a function of a deeper and much harder to explain fact—perhaps a brute fact—about human beings, namely, that they care for their future and their future selves *at all*.

Another leading explanatory theory of the placebo effect is conditioning theory, according to which placebo effects can be explained in terms of classical conditioning theory, as the response of an organism to a conditioned stimulus (Ader 1997; Ader and Cohen 1975; Voudouris et al. 1985). Under the right conditions, patients (or their psycho-neuro-immunological systems) learn to associate a new stimulus, such as an inert substance or procedure (the conditioned stimulus), with a pre-existing stimulus, such as an active treatment (the unconditioned stimulus), and eventually they respond to the conditioned stimulus as if it were actually the unconditioned stimulus. For example, repeated exposure to pills of a certain size, color, and shape, together with the elaborate preparations of drug administration and the repertoire of contextual cues, leads to associations being made with the pharmacological effects of those pills (the unconditional stimulus). Much of the associative machinery is unconscious, and need not involve interpersonal interaction. The immune system, for example, has proven to be particularly susceptible to conditioning. Some of the first evidence for immune conditioning (when the conditioned response is immune activity) was demonstrated in Ader and Cohen's (1975) experiments on learned taste aversion, which showed that rats could learn to suppress their own immune responses. Evidence for human variants of conditioned immunosuppression is seen in chemotherapy patients who start to feel nauseous even before treatment begins. However, not all conditioned responses are placebo effects, and, by implication, not all placebo effects are conditioned stimuli. The evidence suggests that immune conditioning is a much wider category than the placebo effect.

The placebo responder theory explains placebo effects in terms of enduring personality traits or personality types, including suggestibility, optimism and pessimism, neuroticism, and hypochondriasis. This theory first made its appearance in the 1950s, but after numerous attempts it appeared that there were no consistent correlations between response to placebo and personality traits and types, and the theory fell out of favor. Only recently has it been revived, with new experimental evidence suggesting a correlation between personality type and placebo responsiveness. De Pascalis et al. (2002), for example, found that individual differences in suggestibility play a role in the magnitude of placebo analgesia, and Geers et al. (2005) found that the personality variable optimism-pessimism, with appropriate situational variables, interacts with placebo responsiveness.

One of the rapidly emerging explanatory approaches to placebo effects is neurobiology, a field which is advancing hand in hand with developments in functional imaging techniques, positron emission tomography, and functional magnetic resonance imaging. Placebo effects have been shown to involve the activation and increased correlation between a variety of neural regions, including the anterior cingulated, prefrontal, orbitofrontal and insular cortices (Benedetti 2009, 2011). This is particularly evident in the analgesic placebo response (Benedetti et al. 2005; Fields and Price 1997; Levine et al. 1978), which involves the activation of endorphins, the brain's own natural painkillers.

Interpersonal healing theory holds that placebo effects are explained in terms of the complex interpersonal dynamics of the healer–patient relationship, which generates intense interpersonal emotions such as hope, trust, care, and compassion. Physicians and psychiatrists are themselves walking and talking placebos (or, as the case may be, walking and talking nocebos), independently of the specific treatments they provide to patients (Frank and Frank 1991; Miller et al. 2009; Strupp 1972, 1979): that is, they heal by their mere presence, by the confidence they display in their diagnoses and treatments, by their prestige, by the air of safety and confidentiality they exude, and by their socially sanctioned authority. Psychodynamically inclined interpersonal theories have characterized the healer–patient relationship as a version of the parent–child relationship.

According to the meaning response theory, placebo effects can be explained in terms of culturally-situated meaning responses, which are the psychological and physiological effects of meaning in the treatment of illness (Brody 1997; Frank and Frank 1991; Moerman 2000, 2002). Therapeutic improvement is a function of patients receiving treatments that are rich in healing symbols and metaphors, and that exert powerful effects on imagination, belief, and emotion. One of the factors common to all healing modalities, from the most ancient shamanistic ritual to the most technologically advanced cancer treatment, is that patients are supplied with a rationale, conceptual scheme, or myth that offers a meaningful explanation for otherwise puzzling and frightening symptoms.

NEW DIRECTIONS IN PLACEBO RESEARCH

Much is still to be learned about placebo effects, their role in psychiatry and psychotherapy, and their potential for being harnessed in ethically permissible ways. Two potentially important future directions for research are open-label placebos and the evolutionary origins of placebo effects.

Open-label placebos

One of the persistent misconceptions about placebos is that they are ineffective if patients know that they are receiving them. If placebos are to work, then patients have to believe they are receiving "real" treatments with active ingredients (Bausell 2007). Hence the commonly accepted view that placebos are "lies that heal" (Brody 1982), and the commonly-heard criticism that administering placebos is unethical because it involves deceiving patients and thereby violating their autonomy (Bok 1974, 1975, 2002).

These assumptions are problematic. At least for some patients, for some conditions, and for some healer–patient relationships, open-label placebos have been proven to be therapeutically effective, sometimes to the point where they match proven active treatments (Aulas and Rosner 2003; Brown 1994, 1998a, 1998b; Kaptchuk et al. 2010; Park and Covi 1965; Vogel et al. 1980). One study conducted in 1965 (Park and Covi) followed fifteen adult outpatients presenting with symptoms of moderate to high anxiety and diagnosed as "neurotic." The patients were seen twice over the course of one week, and the prescription of placebo in the first visit was accompanied by a carefully designed script informing them that they were being given placebo pills that contained no medication. The results were surprising. Fourteen of the fifteen patients completed the study, at the end of which eight patients still believed that the pills were placebos, and six patients believed that the pills contained an active drug (because of the side effects they had experienced). Thirteen of the fourteen patients showed improvement on the symptom checklist, fourteen patients improved on the target symptoms measures, thirteen patients improved on the patient overall change measures, and twelve patients improved on the pathology measures. The study has not been replicated, and because of design flaws (e.g., small sample, short study duration, and absence of a no-treatment control group), it is possible that therapeutic improvement was a function of other factors that were not controlled for (e.g., regression to the mean, the natural history of the disorder, the random fluctuation of symptoms, or observer and selection bias).

More recently, a more methodologically rigorous study with open-label placebos was conducted with a group of patients diagnosed with irritable bowel syndrome (IBS) (Kaptchuk et al. 2010). The three-week study followed eighty patients with IBS who were randomized to an open-label placebo group or a no-treatment control group, both groups receiving the same amount of interaction with clinicians. Those given the placebos were informed they were being given inert pills that contained no medication, and they were told, crucially, that placebo pills "have been shown in rigorous clinical testing to produce significant mind-body self-healing processes."

Again, the results were surprising. It was found that open-label placebo treatment significantly influenced subjective symptoms compared to no treatment, occasioning significantly higher mean global improvement scores, reduced symptom severity scores, and adequate relief scores (at the midpoint and the endpoint of the study). There was also a trend favoring open-label placebo for quality of life at the endpoint. Crucially, no deception or concealment was required to produce these results.

Open-label placebos may prove to have beneficial clinical uses, particularly as front line psychiatric treatments. In addition to being cost-effective and free from the long-term side effects of psychoactive medications, they may offer some patients a degree of freedom from pharmaceutical dependence, especially for patients who suffer from high levels of anxiety about side effects, addiction, or dependence, or who are at risk of addiction or deleterious side effects (Vogel et al. 1980). They may also be effective in strategies of graduated medication reduction for patients who are at risk of toxic side effects (Brown 1994; Vogel et al. 1980). With the right contextual cues, physician support, and informed consent procedures, and the right script informing patients about the nature of placebos, psychoactive medications could be reduced and eventually replaced with placebo, while maintaining the same dosaging regimen. Patients would know that they are gradually receiving more placebo, without knowing when it had started; and they would know that what they are putting in motion is a conditioned drug response, which is one of the physiological bases of the placebo response. However, more research is required to determine which conditions might be responsive to open-label placebos, and how they are responsive. Moreover, regulatory guidelines are needed in order to address the ethical concerns of using treatments that may require temporarily withholding from patients the "best" available medical care.

Evolutionary origins of the placebo effect

Most explanatory theories of the placebo effect have focused on the proximate causes of placebo effects, with a view to explaining *how* they occur. Few have addressed the issue of the evolutionary causes of placebo effects—that is, questions of why humans are capable of placebo responses at all, why natural selection has favored rather than eliminated the genes that make them possible, what design features make humans susceptible to disease as well as capable of self-repair (Nesse and Williams 1994), whether placebo responsiveness is evolutionarily advantageous, and whether it is a byproduct of evolution (i.e., an exaptation, or a trait that evolved to serve one function but was later co-opted to serve another) or a direct product of adaptive selection. Proximate explanations and evolutionary explanations go hand in hand, the former answering the "What?" and "How?" questions of structure and mechanism, the latter answering the "Why?" questions of function and origin.

If placebo responsiveness is a direct product of adaptive selection, then whatever neural and physiological mechanisms that subserve it must have yielded some evolutionary advantage: the immediate ancestors of modern humans, or perhaps even more distant ancestors in the hominidae family, that had these mechanisms survived and reproduced more efficiently than those that did not have them. If it is not a direct product, then the mechanisms that subserve it evolved to perform other functions, and it might be an evolutionary accident that they also enabled humans to respond to placebo. Evans (2004), for instance, defends the former view: the placebo effect is a specific adaptation that has evolved to allow humans to respond to the provision of medical care. The forces of natural selection wired the pain generating circuits in the brain to inputs from the brain regions that are sensitive to social support, because there are evolutionary advantages to mechanisms that shut down pain when help from others is provided. The neural and physiological mechanisms responsible for suppressing the acute phase of infection (pain, swelling, fever, lethargy) can be activated by the arrival of social help, and the placebo response is a way to accelerate the normal process of termination.

Humphrey (2002) also proposes that the placebo effect needs to be understood in an evolutionary framework, as well as in terms of a cost–benefit analytic approach that looks at how living organisms manage their own valuable immune resources in the most cost-efficient and adaptive manner in a hostile environment. An organism's "natural health care service" evolved to deal with multiple and constant threats to its well-being. But the system is not always *self*-triggered and it is not always operative at full force: sometimes, it allows illness to prevail and actively inhibits the mechanisms for self-cure and self-repair, and sometimes it allows only third parties such as doctors or shamans to activate it. The full weight of the body's immune resources are not thrown at all incoming threats, because sometimes there are greater benefits than costs to remaining sick, and greater costs than benefits to premature cure. The endogenous health care system deploys a globalized cost–benefit resource strategy to optimize the organism's responses. For example, prolonged pain and fever serve as reminders to organisms to seek shelter and rest. Full-fledged immune responses to deal with pain or fever are energy-consuming and risky; not only do they leave the organism depleted and vulnerable at later times when it might need precious immune resources even more; they can also result in costly side effects, such as autoimmune disorders. The evolutionary advantages of this strategy are clear. Sick organisms that deployed their endogenous resources stingily probably survived and reproduced more efficiently than those that did not. At some point in the distant evolutionary past, placebo effects made their first appearance. Healers are the external variables that trigger the endogenous mechanisms of self-cure, allowing patients to be more generous with their otherwise carefully managed resources. Once treatment becomes available, the endogenous health care system can fully unleash its internal resources for self-cure without having to be concerned about the costs of conservation.

Placebos in the History of Medicine and Psychiatry

Finally, it is worth noting the role of placebos in the history of medicine and psychiatry. From ancient times to the present, medicine has been witness to a passing parade of strange etiologies and nosologies, dramatic and often dangerous treatments, curious pharmacopeia and *medica materia*, and ineffective reasoning strategies based on a priori speculation, unquestioning respect for authority, superstition, and blind dogma. Very few medical treatments in the distant and not so distant past actually worked: most were useless, some dangerous, and some even fatal.

Despite the history of failure, medicine has flourished. Many treatments had enough *apparent* therapeutic effects that patients were convinced of their efficacy and physicians were convinced of their own medical prowess. But incautious conclusions and false clinical judgments are commonplace in medicine (Dawes et al. 1989; Meehl 1953), due in no small part to the systemic cognitive biases that pervade all forms of human reasoning (e.g., confirmatory biases, illusory correlations, baseline neglect, availability and representativeness biases, attributional errors, and faulty probabilistic judgments; Dawes 1994; Dawes et al. 1989; Kahneman 2011). In many cases, whatever efficacy medical treatments displayed was not owing to their putatively active ingredients, which failed to accurately target the relevant pathogens or disease processes; it was because of self-limiting disease processes, the natural fluctuation of symptoms, or the incidental factors of the treatments, which triggered placebo effects.

Is the situation any different in the history of psychological treatments? It seems not. First, there are close parallels between the diagnostic and treatment failures of somatic medicine and those of the psychological treatments. Psychiatry and psychotherapy have deep roots in ancient soul doctoring, shamanism, religio-magical practices, hypnotism, quackery, mesmerism, and suggestion therapy (Frank and Frank 1991; Radden 2000; Torrey 1986), most of which treatments, like their medical analogues, were useless or dangerous, or merely disguises for unrecognized placebo effects. Second, like the history of medicine, the history of psychological treatments is a history marked by deep and ongoing uncertainty about the very idea of therapeutic efficacy, the very idea of clinical evidence, and the very standards of clinical reasoning. Not only is there wide (and healthy) disagreement about what counts as a successful treatment for any particular psychological disorder; there is wide (and healthy) disagreement about what counts as a treatment *at all*—and how to distinguish treatment from placebo treatment. Third, just as many of the theories of human physiology and pathology across the history of medicine have rested on a slim empirical base, and have questionable logical and conceptual credentials, so too have many of the psychological theories of personality, behavior, and psychopathology been supported by limited empirical, clinical, and experimental evidence. Finally, just as physicians of the past have more often than not claimed to be possessed of a certain expertise in healing, and have claimed to be guardians of esoteric knowledge about physical maladies, despite a long history of explanatory and treatment failures, so psychotherapists have claimed to be expert healers of minds, and guardians of esoteric knowledge about psychological maladies—despite an equally long history of explanatory and treatment failures (Erwin 1997). John Ayrton Paris' (1843) warning about the dangers of medical hubris is as true today as it was in the 1800s: "What pledge can be afforded that the boasted remedies of the present day will not, like their predecessors, fall into disrepute, and in their turn serve only as a humiliating memorial of the credulity and infatuation of the physicians who recommended and prescribed them?" (pp. 4–5).

Far from a humble humbug or a nothing treatment or a pious fraud, the history of medicine and psychiatry *is* the history of the placebo effect (Shapiro and Shapiro 1997).

References

Adair, J. G. (1984). The Hawthorne effect: A reconsideration of the methodological artifact. *Journal of Applied Psychology*, 69, 334–45.

Ader, R. A. (1997). The role of conditioning in pharmacotherapy. In A. Harrington (Ed.), *The Placebo Effect: An Interdisciplinary Exploration*, pp. 138–65. Cambridge, MA: Harvard University Press.

Ader, R. A. and Cohen, N. (1975). Behaviorally conditioned immunosuppression. *Psychosomatic Medicine*, 37, 333–40.

Amanzio, M. and Benedetti, F. (1999). Neuropharmacological dissection of placebo analgesia: Expectation-activated opioid systems versus conditioning-activated specific subsystems. *Journal of Neuroscience*, 19, 484–94.

Aulas, J. J. and Rosner, I. (2003). Effets de la prescription d'un placebo annoncé. *L'Encéphale: Revue de psychiatrie clinique, biologique, et therapeutique*, 29, 68–71.

Barksy, A., Saintfort, R., Rogers, M. P., and Borus, J. F. (2002). Nonspecific medication side effects and the nocebo phenomenon. *Journal of the American Medical Association*, 287(5), 622–7.

Bausell, R. B. (2007). *Snake oil science: The Truth about Complementary and Alternative Medicine*. New York, NY: Oxford University Press.

Beecher, H. (1955). The powerful placebo. *Journal of the American Medical Association*, 159, 1602–6.

Benedetti, F., Mayberg, H. S., Wager, T. D., Stohler, C. S., and Zubieta, J.-K. (2005). Neurobiological mechanisms of the placebo effect. *Journal of Neuroscience*, 25(45), 10390–402.

Benedetti, F. (2009). *Placebo Effects: Understanding the Mechanisms in Health and Disease*. Oxford: Oxford University Press.

Benedetti, F. (2011). *The Patient's Brain: The Neuroscience Behind the Doctor-Patient Relationship*. Oxford: Oxford University Press.

Blackwell, B., Bloomfield, S. S., and Buncher, C. R. (1972). Demonstration to medical students of placebo responses and non-drug factors. *Lancet*, 1(763), 1279–82.

Bok, S. (1974). The ethics of giving placebos. *Scientific American*, 231, 17–23.

Bok, S. (1975). Paternalistic deception in medicine and rational choice: The use of placebos. In M. Black (Ed.), *Problems of choice and decision*, pp. 73–107. Ithaca, NY: Cornell University Press.

Bok, S. (2002). Ethical issues in the use of placebos in medical practice and clinical trials. In H. A. Guess, A. Kleinman, J. W. Kusek and L. Engel (Eds), *The Science of the Placebo: Towards an Interdisciplinary Research Agenda*, pp. 53–74. London: BMJ Books.

Bootzin, R. R. and Caspi, O. (2002). Explanatory mechanisms for placebo effects: cognition, personality and social learning. In H. A. Guess, A. Kleinman, J. W. Kusek, and L. Engel (Eds), *The Science of the Placebo: Towards an Interdisciplinary Research Agenda*, pp. 108–132. London: BMJ Books.

Braithwaite, A. and Cooper, P. (1981). Analgesic effects of branding in treatment of headaches. *British Medical Journal (Clinical Research Edition)*, 282, 1576–8.

Brody, H. (1982). The lie that heals: The ethics of giving placebos. *Annals of Internal Medicine*, 97, 112–18.

Brody, H. (1997). The doctor as therapeutic agent: A placebo effect research agenda. In A Harrington (Ed.), *The Placebo Effect: An Interdisciplinary Exploration*, pp. 77–92. Cambridge, MA: Harvard University Press.

Brown, W.A. (1994). Placebo as a treatment for depression. *Neuropsychopharmacology, 10,* 265–9.

Brown, W. A. (1998a). The placebo effect. *Scientific American,* (Jan.), 90–95.

Brown, W. A. (1998b). Harnessing the placebo effect. *Hospital Practice, 33*(7), 107–16.

Critelli, J. W. and Newman, K. F. (1984). The placebo: Conceptual analysis of a construct in transition. *American Psychologist, 39,* 32–9.

Davis, C. E. (1976). The effect of regression to the mean in epidemiologic and clinical studies. *American Journal of Epidemiology, 5,* 493–8.

Davis, C. E. (2002). Regression to the mean or placebo effect? In H. A. Guess, A. Kleinman, J. W. Kusek, and L. Engel (Eds), *The Science of the Placebo: Towards an Interdisciplinary Research Agenda,* pp. 158–166. London: BMJ Books.

Dawes, R. (1994). *House of Cards: Psychology and Psychotherapy Built on Myth.* New York, NY: Free Press.

Dawes, R. M. (1998). Listening to Prozac but hearing placebo: Commentary on Kirsch and Sapirstein. *Prevention and Treatment, 1*(2). Art. 5c.

Dawes, R., Faust, D., and Meehl, P. E. (1989). Clinical versus actuarial judgment. *Science, 243,* 1668–74.

DeCraen, A. J., Moerman, D. E., Heisterkamp, S. H., Tytgat, G. N., Tijssen, J. G., and Kleijnen, J. (1999). Placebo effect in the treatment of duodenal ulcer. *British Journal of Clinical Pharmacology, 48*(6), 853–60.

DeCraen, A. J., Tijssen, J. G., de Gans, J., and Kleijnen, J. (2000). Placebo effect in the acute treatment of migraine: Subcutaneous placebos are better than oral placebos. *Journal of Neurology, 247*(3), 183–8.

de Montaigne, M. (1574/1958). On the power of the imagination. In *Essays* (J. M. Cohen, Trans.), pp. 36–47. Harmondsworth: Penguin.

De Pascalis V., Chiaradia, C., and Carotenuto, E. (2002). The contribution of suggestibility and expectation to placebo analgesia phenomenon in an experimental setting. *Pain, 96,* 393–402.

Dostoevsky, F. (1981). *The Brothers Karamazov* (A. H. MacAndrew, Trans.). New York, NY: Bantam Books. (Original work published 1880.)

Editorial (2008). A double edged sword. *Nature Reviews Drug Discovery, 7,* 275.

Elkin, I., Parloff, M. B., Hadley, S., and Autry, J. H. (1985). NIMH treatment of depression collaborative research program. *Archives of General Psychiatry, 42,* 305–16.

Ernst, E. and Resch, K. L. (1995). Concept of true and perceived placebo effects. *British Medical Journal, 311,* 551–3.

Erwin, E. (1994). The effectiveness of psychotherapy: Epistemological issues. In G. Graham and G. L.. Stevens (Eds), *Philosophical Psychopathology,* pp. 261–84. Cambridge, MA: MIT Press.

Erwin, E. (1997). *Philosophy and Psychotherapy: Razing the Troubles of the Brain.* Thousand Oaks, CA: Sage.

Evans, D. (2004). *Placebo: Mind over Matter in Modern Medicine.* New York, NY: Oxford University Press.

Eysenck, H. (1965). The effects of psychotherapy. *International Journal of Psychiatry, 1,* 97–168.

Faust, D. (1986). Research on human judgment and its application to clinical practice. *Professional Psychology: Research and Practice, 17,* 420–30.

Fields, H. L. and Price, D. D. (1997). Toward a neurobiology of placebo analgesia. In A Harrington (Ed.), *The Placebo Effect: An Interdisciplinary Exploration,* pp. 593–16. Cambridge, MA: Harvard University Press.

Frank, J. D. (1983). The placebo is psychotherapy. *Behavioral and Brain Sciences, 6*, 291–2.

Frank, J. D. and Frank, J. B. (1991). *Persuasion and Healing* (3rd edn). Baltimore, MD: Johns Hopkins University Press.

Furmark, T., Appel, L., Henningsson, S., Ahs, F., Faria, V., Linnman, C., *et al.* (2008). A link between serotonin-related gene polymorphisms, amygdala activity, and placebo-induced relief from social anxiety. *Journal of Neuroscience, 28*, 13066–77.

Geers, A. L., Helfer, S. G., Kosbab, K., Weiland, P. E., and Landry, S. J. (2005). Reconsidering the role of personality in placebo effects: dispositional optimism, situational expectations, and the placebo response. *Journal of Psychosomatic Research, 62*, 563–70.

Greenberg, G. (2003). Is it Prozac? Or placebo? *Mother Jones, November/December*, 78–81.

Grünbaum, A. (1986). The placebo concept in medicine and psychiatry. *Psychological Medicine, 16*, 19–38.

Guess, H. A., Kleinman, A., Kusek, J. W., and Engel, L. (Eds) (2002). *The Science of the Placebo: Towards an Interdisciplinary Research Agenda*. London: BMJ Books.

Hahn, R. A. (1997). The nocebo phenomenon: Scope and foundations. In A. Harrington (Ed.), *The Placebo Effect: An Interdisciplinary Exploration*, pp. 56–76. Cambridge, MA: Harvard University Press.

Harrington, A. (Ed.) (1997). *The placebo effect: An Interdisciplinary Exploration*. Cambridge, MA: Harvard University Press.

Harrington, A. (2002). Seeing the placebo effect: Historical legacies and present opportunities. In H. A. Guess, A. Kleinman, J. W. Kusek, and L. Engel (Eds), *The Science of the Placebo: Towards an Interdisciplinary Research Agenda*, pp. 35–52. London: BMJ Books.

Held, B. (1995). *Back to Reality: A Critique of Post-Modern Theory in Psychotherapy*. New York, NY: Norton.

Hróbjartsson, A. and Gøtzsche, P. (2001). Is the placebo powerless? An analysis of clinical trials comparing placebo with no-treatment. *New England Journal of Medicine, 344*, 1594–602.

Hróbjartsson, A. and Norup, M. (2003). The use of placebo interventions in medical practice—a national questionnaire survey of Danish clinicians. *Evaluation and the Health Professions, 26*, 153–65.

Humphrey, N. (2002). Great expectations: The evolutionary psychology of faith healing and the placebo effect. In N. Humphrey (Ed.), *The Mind Made Flesh*, pp. 255–85. New York, NY: Oxford University Press.

Jerome, J. K. (1964). *Three Men in a Boat (To Say Nothing of the Dog)*. New York, NY: Time Incorporated. (Original work published 1889.)

Jopling, D. A. (2008). *Talking Cures and Placebo Effects*. New York, NY: Oxford University Press.

Kahneman, D. (2011). *Thinking, Fast and Slow*. New York, NY: Farrar, Strauss, and Geroux.

Kaptchuk, T. J. (1998). Powerful placebo: The dark side of the randomized controlled trial. *Lancet, 351*, 1722–5.

Kaptchuk, T. J. (2002). The placebo effect in alternative medicine: Can the performance of a healing ritual have clinical significance? *Annals of Internal Medicine, 136*, 817–25.

Kaptchuk, T. J., Friedlander, E., Kelley, J. M., Sanchez, M. N., Kokkotou, E., Singer, J. P., *et al.* (2010). Placebos without deception: A randomized controlled trial in irritable bowel syndrome. *PloS One, 5*(12), e15591.

Kazdin, A. (1981). Drawing valid inference from case studies. *Journal of Consulting and Clinical Psychology, 49*, 183–92.

Kiene, H. (1993a). A critique of the double-blind clinical trial: Part 1. *Alternative Therapies, 2*(1), 74–80.

Kiene, H. (1993b). A critique of the double-blind clinical trial: Part 2. *Alternative Therapies, 2*(2), 59–64.

Kienle, G. S. and Kiene, H. (1997). The powerful placebo effect: Fact or fiction? *Journal of Clinical Epidemiology, 50*, 1311–18.

Kirsch, I. (1985). Response expectancy as a determinant of experience and behavior. *American Psychologist, 40*, 1189–202.

Kirsch, I. (1997). Specifying nonspecifics: Psychological mechanisms of placebo effects. In A. Harrington (Ed.), *The Placebo Effect: An Interdisciplinary Exploration*, pp. 166–186. Cambridge, MA: Harvard University Press.

Kirsch, I. (Ed.) (1999). *How Expectancies Shape Experience*. Washington, DC: American Psychological Association.

Kirsch, I. (2005). Placebo psychotherapy: Synonym or oxymoron? *Journal of Clinical Psychology, 61*, 791–803.

Kirsch, I. (2010). *The Emperor's New Drugs: Exploding the Antidepressant Myth*. New York, NY: Basic Books.

Kirsch, I., Moore, T. J., Scoboria, A., and Nicholls, S. S. (2002). The emperor's new drugs: An analysis of antidepressant medication data submitted to the U.S. Food and Drug Administration. *Prevention and Treatment, 5*, Art. 23.

Kirsch, I. and Sapirstein, G. (1998). Listening to Prozac but hearing placebo: A meta-analysis of antidepressant medication. *Prevention and Treatment, 1*, Art. 0002a. Available at: <http://www.journals.apa.org/prevention/volume1/pre0010002a.html#c22>.

Klein, D. F. (1998). Listening to meta-analysis but hearing bias. *Prevention and Treatment, 1*(2) Art. 6c.

Levine, J. D., Gordon, N. C., and Fields, H. L. (1978). The mechanism of placebo analgesia. *Lancet, 2*, 654–7.

Lewis, S. (1980). *Arrowsmith*. Scarborough, ON: New American Library.

Marshall, M. F. (2004). The placebo effect in popular culture. *Science and Engineering Ethics, 10*, 37–42.

Meehl, P. (1953). *Clinical versus statistical prediction: A theoretical analysis and a review of the evidence*. Minneapolis, MN: University of Minnesota Press.

Meissner, K., Kohls, N., and Colloca, L. (Eds) (2011). Placebo effects in medicine: mechanisms and clinical implications. *Philosophical Transactions of the Royal Society B: Biological Sciences, 366*, 1572.

Miller, F. G., Colloca, L., and Kaptchuk, T. (2009). The placebo effect: Illness and interpersonal healing. *Perspectives in Biological Medicine, 52*(4), 518.

Moerman, D. E. (2000). Cultural variations in the placebo effect: Ulcers, anxiety, and blood pressure. *Medical Anthropology Quarterly, 14*(1), 51–72.

Moerman, D. E. (2002). *Meaning, Medicine and the "Placebo Effect."* Cambridge, MA: Cambridge University Press.

Montgomery, G. and Kirsch, I. (1996). Mechanisms of placebo pain reduction: An empirical investigation. *Psychological Science, 7*, 174–6.

Moseley, J. B., O'Malley, K., Petersen, N. J., Menke, T. J., Brody, B. A., Kuykendall, D. H., *et al.* (2002). A controlled trial of arthroscopic surgery for osteoarthritis of the knee. *New England Journal of Medicine, 347*, 81–8.

Nesse, R. M. and Williams, G. C. (1994). *Why We Get Sick: The New Science of Darwinian Medicine*. New York, NY: Vintage.

Ober, K. P. (2003). *Mark Twain and Medicine: Any Mummery Will Cure*. Columbia, MO: University of Missouri Press.

O'Brian, P. (1998). *The Hundred Days*. New York, NY: W. W. Norton.

O'Leary, K. D. and Borkovec, T. D. (1978). Conceptual, methodological, and ethical problems of placebo groups in psychotherapy research. *American Psychologist, 33*, 821–30.

Paris, J. A. (1843). *Pharmacologia: Being An Extended Inquiry into the Operations of Medicinal Bodies, Upon Which are Founded the theory and Art of Prescribing* (9th edn). London: Samuel Highley.

Parloff, M. B. (1986a). Frank's "common elements" in psychotherapy: Nonspecific factors and placebos. *American Journal of Orthopsychiatry, 56*, 521–30.

Parloff, M. B. (1986b). Placebo controls in psychotherapy research: A sine qua non or a placebo for research problems? *Journal of Consulting and Clinical Psychology, 54*, 79–87.

Park, L. C. and Covi, L. (1965). Nonblind placebo trial: An exploration of neurotic outpatients' response to placebo when its inert content is disclosed. *Archives of General Psychiatry, 12*, 336–45.

Prioleau, L., Murdock, M., and Brody, N. (1983). An analysis of psychotherapy versus placebo studies. *Behavioral and Brain Sciences, 6*, 275–310.

Radden, J. (2000). From melancholic states to clinical depression. In J. Radden (Ed), *The Nature of Melancholy*, pp. 3–51. Oxford University Press, Oxford.

Rush, A. J. and Ryan, N. D. (2002). Current and emerging therapeutics for depression. In K. L. Davis, D. Charney, J. T. Coyle and C. Nemeroff (Eds), *Neuropsychopharmacology: The Fifth Generation of Progress*, pp. 1081–95. New York, NY: Lippincott, Williams & Wilkins.

Shapiro, A. K. (1964). Etiological factors in placebo effect. *Journal of the American Medical Association, 187*, 712–15.

Shapiro, A. K. (1971). Placebo effects in medicine, psychotherapy, and psychoanalysis. In A. E. Bergin and S. L. Garfield (Eds), *Handbook of Psychotherapy and Behavior Change: An Empirical Analysis*, pp. 439–73. New York, NY: Wiley.

Shapiro, A. K. and Shapiro, E. (1997). *The Powerful Placebo: From Ancient Priest to Modern Physician*. Baltimore, MD: Johns Hopkins University Press.

Shaw, G. B. (1941). *The Doctor's Dilemma*. New York, NY: Dodd, Meed. (Original work published 1911.)

Sherman, R. and Hickner, J. (2008). Academic physicians use placebos in clinical practice and believe in the mind-body connection. *Journal of General Internal Medicine, 23*, 7–10.

Schafer, R. (1981). *Narrative Actions in Psychoanalysis*. Worcester, MA: Clark University Press.

Schafer, R. (1992). *Retelling a Life: Narration and Dialogue in Psychoanalysis*. New York, NY: Basic Books.

Spence, D. (1982). *Narrative Truth and Historical Truth: Meaning and Interpretation in Psychoanalysis*. New York, NY: W. W. Norton.

Strupp, H. H. (1972). Needed: A reformulation of the psychotherapeutic influence. *International Journal of Psychiatry, 10*, 114–20.

Strupp, H. H. (1979). Specific versus non-specific factors in psychotherapy. *Archives of General Psychiatry, 36*, 1125–36.

Torrey, E. F. (1986). *Witch Doctors and Psychiatrists: The Common Roots of Psychiatry and its Future*. New York, NY: Harper and Row.

Vogel, A. V., Goodwin, J. S., and Goodwin, J. M. (1980). The therapeutics of placebo. *American Family Physician, 22*, 105–9.

Voudouris, N. J., Peck, C. L., and Coleman, G. (1985). Conditioned placebo responses. *Journal of Personality and Social Psychology, 48*, 47–53.

Wager, T. (2005). The neural bases of placebo effects in pain. *Current Directions in Psychological Science, 14*(4), 175–9.

Werner, R. (2008). Losing the point. *PLoS Medicine*, February 28. Available at: <http://medicine.plosjournals.org/perlserv/?request-read-response&doi-10/journal.pmed.0050045>

CHAPTER 71

....

BEING UNCONSCIOUS:
HEIDEGGER AND FREUD

....

RICHARD ASKAY AND JENSEN FARQUHAR

"I hardly know anymore who and where I am." None of us knows that, as soon as
we stop fooling ourselves.

Martin Heidegger, *Country Path Conversations* (2010, p. 71)

The moment a man questions the meaning and value of life, he is sick, since objectively neither has any existence.

Sigmund Freud (Jones 1955, p. 465)

Martin Heidegger and Sigmund Freud were arguably the two greatest "meta-*physicians*" of
the twentieth century. Both sought to develop a comprehensive, unified, holistic account
of the human condition, and proposed a diagnosis of and solution for the affliction of the
contemporary human situation. Both endeavored to decipher life's hidden meaning while
accepting that there is ultimately no deep unifying meaning underlying human existence.
And both proposed concrete therapeutic means for assisting individuals who are having
difficulty coping so that they could adjust and, to some extent, be at home in the world.
Finally, both challenged the science of their time, and sought to develop a new "science of
the human being" (Heidegger 2001, pp. 136, 140, 222) to serve as the theoretical foundation for psychotherapeutic practice and its application. As a result, Heidegger inspired the
development of various forms of existential analysis while Freud generated his immensely
influential theory/practice of psychoanalysis.

However, despite their mutual interests, neither thinker was open to the other's perspective. Historically, Freud rejected Heidegger's ideas based on what little exposure he had
through Binswanger (Needleman 1963, p. 4) while Heidegger experienced severe ontological dyspepsia in reaction to Freud's metapsychological theory (Hoeller 1988, p. 9). Hence,
both have typically been viewed as holding incommensurable theoretical paradigms
(Hoeller 1988). This is ironic, especially in light of the fact that Heidegger's hermeneutical
phenomenological ontology has served as the primary historical impetus around the globe
for the actual engagement of phenomenology with psychoanalysis and psychology (Askay
and Farquhar 2011).

In the face of this, some crucial questions emerge: Given that the two have made truly substantial contributions to our understanding of the human condition, are the two so utterly incompatible after all (as Heidegger clearly believed)? Or are they potentially reconcilable? Those arguing for compatibility on the philosophical side include Needleman (1963) and Richardson (1965), and on the psychoanalytic side include Binswanger, Boss, Federn, Leavy, Loewald, Chessick, Frie, Mills, and Thompson. Interestingly, Heidegger (2001, p. 266) opened the door to such attempts through his insight: "Intimate interrelatedness does not mean a merging and effacing of differences. Intimate interrelatedness means the belonging together of the unfamiliar ..." We shall argue that, despite what would clearly be Heidegger's expostulations to the contrary, there is an "intimate belonging together" of Being and the unconscious. What makes such a rapprochement possible is the fact that Heidegger moved from an extreme holism (i.e., in *Being and Time*, the network of relationships is all we are—our exclusive relatedness to "the world," others, and ourselves) to a more moderate holism that allows other considerations along with these relations to matter. In doing so, we will contend that Heidegger's position permits a merger with Freud's to offer a more complete and unified account of the human condition (Askay and Farquhar 2006, pp. 332–338). While doing so both offer mutually reinforcing positions which can facilitate the cessation of pandemic human suffering by showing how it involves forms of fragmentation and constriction of the above unity. For both, the goal of therapy was to liberate clients from their pathologically constricted ways of relating by restoring to them the fullness of their potentialities of existence. Indeed both were convinced that their respective approaches should lead to the self-transformation of therapists and clients.

HEIDEGGER'S PHILOSOPHY AND THERAPY

Heidegger's general attitude toward Freud's psychoanalysis was uniformly antipathetic. He saw it as an especially dangerous version of the scientist worldview uncritically spreading across Europe. What was at stake? For Heidegger, it was the potential loss of our very humanity. In an attempt to stem this tide, he sought to combat it directly by agreeing to convene the Zollikon seminars (1959–1969) to break the hold of "the dictatorship of scientific thinking" (Heidegger 2001, pp. 260, 274). These were delivered in two-day doses to large groups of psychiatrists, psychoanalysts, psychotherapists, and so forth, (most of whom were trained exclusively in the sciences with little or no philosophical training) in the home of his most loyal psychoanalytic adherent—Medard Boss. Given his interest in "the problems of psychopathology and psychotherapy regarding their principles," Heidegger (2001, p. 237) called into question their most basic presuppositions regarding what it means to be human. His goal was to make his philosophical insights available to therapists and clients in need of help, while providing therapists with a sound philosophical foundation for their therapeutic practice—to enable them to think in a new way.

One of Heidegger's most basic insights toward a new way of thinking was to point out that it is where one begins one's inquiry that sets the horizon for what can be disclosed. To appreciate this in Heidegger's case it is helpful to begin with a brief account of his hermeneutical phenomenological ontology (Askay and Farquhar 2006, pp. 190–210). A natural place to start is with what Heidegger described as "the fundamental characteristic of being human," the primordial condition that makes it possible for humans to experience (disclose) any meaning or significance whatsoever: *Being-open*.

First, for Heidegger there is an open clearing (a Free realm) which makes it possible for any being to *be*, part of which Dasein (i.e., beings such as us who are always situated in a relational context of meaning and have an understanding of what it means to be) "stands out into." Our general mode as Dasein (as a self) is such that each of us is a process of openness: the self is a "happening" in the process of realizing itself (Heidegger 1984, p. 139). To exist as Dasein is to "sustain a realm of openness," a "clearing," "the Free"; Dasein *is* its Being-in-the-world *existingly*. We, as the unique clearing of being make the appearance of beings of any kind possible; we are the event of "letting-be" ("receiving-perceiving") what emerges into the openness of the world. Within this situatedness, persons decide their existence in the way in which they seize or neglect their possibilities in life: "a human being who adjusts to the limits of a given situation is at home with himself, is *Himself*" (Heidegger 2001, p. 188). Reciprocally, Being is the generative ground of beings (i.e., it serves as the universal and necessary condition for the emergence of any possible being), and yet itself is a "groundless ground" (i.e., not a being, "nothing"; there is "nothing" to ground being (Heidegger 1962, pp. 221–222)). Being and Dasein are regarded as equiprimordial—each requires the other in order to be, since any ontological occurrence of meaning at all depends upon the presencing of beings to us.

Heidegger directly applied this insight to the helping professions: therapists cannot use therapy to cure their clients without first restoring their relation to Being—therapists must help clients with their understanding of what it means to be, to enable them "to be at home" with themselves, by being free for themselves in their authentic existence. Authentic existence is actualized when clients are able to be autonomous and take hold of their own possibilities. In order to accomplish this, therapists must take-in/listen-to the ways of being of their clients: how their clients "take-in/listen-in" and "interrogate" whatever presences or discloses itself to them so as to uncover what is hidden (i.e., being), and then actively uncover what is hidden in their clients' being-in-the-world.

One important dimension of this is the emergence of stress in our lives as essentially belonging to our very constitution (Boss 1979, pp. 207–211; Heidegger 2001, p. 137). It involves being "burdened" by having a claim made on us as we are addressed by the presencing beings. For some clients existence itself is a burden (or, in this case, called into question) during the experience of existential anxiety or boredom. The significance of our very existence (once understood as groundless) is shattered into a profound crisis of meaning, which can serve as the initial step toward subsequent authenticity and joyful serenity (Heidegger 2001, p. 166, 1962, p. 173). Furthermore, in their openness to the world, therapists encounter their clients as sites of self-disclosure of their openness to the world, as historical "selves" (i.e., always already existing as situated, contextual beings) (Heidegger 2001, p. 175). Persons are in need of help because they are in danger of losing or not facing themselves and hence the goal is to show how "each illness is a loss of freedom, a constriction of the possibility for living" (Heidegger 2001, p. 157), and how this can be opened up by the therapists' own openness so that the former can become authentic, responsible selves (Boss 1963, p. 254).

How specifically does Dasein sustain this realm of openness? As being-in-the-world—as a unified field of meaning which presupposes universal and necessary transcendental structures (Richardson 1967, p. 179) which make it possible for each of us to relate to other human beings (Being-with), objects (in-the-world), and ourselves (Being-in). While doing so, various structures of disclosedness (or unconcealment) are presupposed as necessary conditions for us to experience the world. First, to be ontologically attuned to the world makes possible the actual state in which we find ourselves, and hence for anything to matter to us as it is a given, actual presencing as part of our situation. (Situations matter to us because we always find ourselves disposed at a certain "pitch" within them, e.g., in joyfulness. It shows *how* one finds oneself in ones way of being attuned to the world.) Second, understanding makes it possible for us to be aware of our possibilities as we assign meaning in our relational context. Third, the structure of discourse enables us to articulate the intelligibility of the world, most typically in the way of a common public interpretive mode (one which an individual has not chosen but is uncritically expected to adopt from this public mentality), which results in the alienation of ourselves from our genuine selves. For Heidegger (2001), one common task of therapy is to treat this very condition in therapists and clients alike. These structures are all unified in what Heidegger terms Care—we care about our actualities, possibilities, and what "they" (i.e., the public mentality) care about. Finally, it is our intrinsic mode of being as temporality—as "been already" (past), "alongside the world" (present), and "ahead of itself" (future)—which primordially makes all of these possible, indeed, any experience of meaning and significance at all. It is because temporality is primordially intrinsic to one's Being (2001, p. 38) that we are ecstatic beings (i.e., ones that can "stand out into being" (2001, p. 121) and reclaim one's past memories, project one's future possibilities, and unify them in the presencing of the moment) that we are able to stand out and experience Being-in-the-world at all (Heidegger 1962, pp. 277, 375–376, 2001, p. 96).

Heidegger (1962, p. 225) disclosed the very possibility of a client's being-in-the-world as having a structure—it is primordially and constantly whole and unified in time. This is why Heidegger himself insisted that the issue of how the human being stands and lives in relationship to time must be of especial interest to therapists and clients alike (2001, p. 58). This understanding of human existence enables therapists to describe and understand the multifarious neuroses/psychoses, moods versus affects, and so forth as specific modifications of the a priori structure of human existence. This is why Heidegger (2001, p. 191) suggested that there is a "regional ontology of psychiatry" (as grounded in fundamental ontology). To understand any pathological phenomena, the three temporal ecstases and their particular modifications must be taken into consideration (Boss 1979, pp. 213–214; Heidegger 1962, pp. 377–378). For example, disturbed relationships to time itself occur in some forms of mental illness (Heidegger 2001, p. 44). Clients can enable themselves to be entirely unreflectively absorbed in their present concrete situations. "In contrast to the small child, the old person has having-been-ness, but conceals itself" (Boss 1979, p. 214; Heidegger 2001, p. 883). They may be utterly oblivious to their pasts and take themselves to be hopping from one instant to the next without finding any unity to their existence as they simply drift along. Or again, the dominant mode of attunement or temporality at any given time serves as the condition of our openness for perceiving and dealing with what we encounter. A specific mode of attunement may powerfully dominate (i.e., narrow) a client's existence without his or her awareness at any given time. Particularly important modes open us up to our whole situation (e.g., existential anxiety, boredom, and joy) while others narrow, distort, or close us off to our situation (e.g., fear, anger, jealousy). Proceeding to this level of understanding means to have moved from a merely implicit understanding of what it means to be, to a clear, explicit, holistic ontological understanding. For Heidegger, it is vital that therapists acquire this else the therapeutic process would be arbitrary, "free-floating," and insufficiently grounded, (i.e., therapists would have no alternative but to merely "grope in the dark" (Boss 1979, p. 280)).

Heidegger offers therapists a way to understand the modifications of the fundamental structures, which permits the uniqueness of each client to manifest as they presence themselves to their therapists and to themselves. In addition, his analysis enables therapists to understand more clearly the fundamental roles that truth as unconcealment, concealment, fleeing, temporality, openness, the constriction of possibilities, the honest acceptance of the "givens" of the world, and so forth play in the therapeutic context. For Heidegger, the end result should be that therapists and clients are freed from any constriction of their possibilities in their respective roles in this context.

HEIDEGGER'S CRITICISM OF FREUD'S
METAPSYCHOLOGY AND THE UNCONSCIOUS

Heidegger's alternative way of approaching human existence appears contrary to Freud's (SE XIV, pp. 78, 105, 222n) metapsychology which is designed to "provide a stable theoretical foundation for psychoanalysis"—a grounding for all of its ideas, techniques, and approaches. The doctrine of psychoanalysis was understood, by Freud (SE XIV, p. 78), as a superstructure that would eventually have as its foundation an organic infrastructure described in his metapsychological theory. Human meaning, then, would ultimately be grounded in bodily processes. According to Heidegger (2001, p. 282), such an approach was inherently oblivious to the ontological characteristics of what it means to be human—in other words, Freud simply failed to see the "clearing" (Heidegger 2001, p. 228). In its place, Freud uncritically adopted the fundamental presuppositions of the metaphysical/epistemological tradition out of which he emerged—Cartesianism/Kantianism. The most important of which was to reify the mind into a thing, an encapsulated object that contained consciousness and the unconscious. The ultimate result was that Freud, as a major representative of scientism, concealed Being.

Freud (SE XVIII, p. 247), on the other hand, considered the unconscious to be an indispensable cornerstone for the foundation of psychoanalytic theory. Freud found the assumption of the unconscious necessary because else we could not intelligibly make sense of the huge number of gaps in our everyday consciousness. As evidence of these he mentions parapraxes, dreams, thoughts that suddenly emerge without our knowing their sources, intellectual conclusions arrived at we do not know how, and so forth. According to Freud, such occurrences are only rendered intelligible once we interpolate between them unconscious acts. In addition, all of that which is accessible in consciousness is currently in a state of latency as memories. Given these phenomena, Freud (SE XIV, p. 167) asserted, "A gain in meaning is a perfectly justifiable ground for going beyond the limits of direct experience."

Freud's psychoanalytic technique was a method for retracing the immediately experienced conscious thoughts back to their previously inaccessible origins. Such a process intrinsically involved what Freud (SE XIV, p. 147) designated as one of the other cornerstone concepts of psychoanalysis—"repression": "its essence lies simply in turning something away, and keeping it at a distance." For example, Freud (SE IX, p. 22) held that "no one forgets anything without some secret reason or hidden motive," and that forgetting is "determined by unconscious purposes" (SE VI p. 169). One goal of psychoanalytic therapy, then, was to unmask these when they occurred in order to "free" the analysand (see Askay and Farquhar 2006, pp. 27–39, 316–32). The success of his psychoanalytic procedure, in Freud's opinion, further confirmed the existence of the unconscious.

Heidegger (2001, pp. 207–208) predominantly viewed Freud's creation of the unconscious as a natural outcome of scientism. In the spirit of scientific thinking, Freud simply postulated "the complete explanation of psychical life" (the "psychoanalytic case history"), that is, "the continuity of causal connections" in mental life. Since there are "gaps" in consciousness, Freud found it necessary "to invent the unconscious" as "a construct" to account for this continuity. Heidegger (2001, p. 254) referred to Freud's bifurcation of consciousness and the unconscious as a "fatal distinction": "This fateful, modern, metaphysical concept" (Heidegger 1996, p. 91) had disastrous ramifications for Heidegger. It created a hidden "psychic black box" beneath consciousness thereby fragmenting Dasein's being-in-the-world into a psyche, body, and external world. Heidegger (2001, p. 245) also thereby repudiated Freud's claim that dreams are "the royal road to the unconscious": "Dreams are not symptoms and consequences of something lying hidden behind them" (see Askay and Farquhar 2006, pp. 220–223; Heidegger 2001, pp. 308–312).

From this discussion it is clear that Heidegger utterly rejected Freud's formulation of the unconscious. But does it follow that there is simply no room for an "unconscious" in Heidegger's philosophy?

Existential Analysis:
Binswanger and Boss

Binswanger was the first to undertake the task of trying to synthesize Heidegger's phenomenological ontology (from which he argued existential analysis received its primary historical impetus) and Freudian psychoanalysis. Indeed, he both knew personally and formed a life-long friendship with Freud. He argued that existential analysis (as the attempt to reconstruct the world of the client's experience) gained its philosophical foundation/justification and methodological guidelines from *Being and Time* (1962). However, he observed that Freud's concept of the unconscious always remained absolutely essential to the conduct of psychotherapeutic practice, and it was only when he turned to phenomenology/existential analysis that he conceived of the unconscious as intrinsic to hidden givenness, as the "transcendental horizon" (Needleman 1963, p. 99) of the body. Binswanger (1957, p. 64) emphasized, "bodily existence as the epitome of various 'veiled forms' of being-with-self" which involved forgetting and repression (Binswanger 1963, p. 171). Indeed, Binswanger (1958, p. 277) stressed that, "the body represents the identity of worldly condition, *my* body, and of inner body-awareness, '*existence-in-the-body.*'" As part of Binswanger's analysis, he investigated the biological world (in deference to Freud, though he rejected Freud's tendency to reduce everything in terms of it) as intrinsic to Dasein's givenness. Hence, in line with the thesis of this chapter, Binswanger suggested that "human existence never goes forth exclusively as spirit or instinct, it is always both … we have attempted to show the degree to which spirituality extends its reach down to the deepest valleys of 'vitality'" (Needleman 1963, p. 3) into the unconscious as bodily existence as thrown, situational attunement (Binswanger 1963, p. 212). Indeed, Freud himself agreed: "Man has always known he possessed spirit: I had to show him that there was such a thing as instinct" (Binswanger 1957, p. 183).

Using *Being and Time* as a basis and seeking to "improve" upon it, Binswanger proceeded to develop a "phenomenological anthropology" of the fundamental forms of human existence that focused on Dasein's immediate everyday experience. While doing so, he investigated the world-design (the all-encompassing pattern of an individual's modification of being-in-the-world which is occasionally dominated by one category) a client developed which made possible various pathological experiences. He saw the task of therapy to be the opening up of new structural possibilities for such altered processes. In general, Binswanger's primary objection to Heidegger's work was that it was too individualistic, and neglected to offer a sufficient account of the primordial social dimension of love in human existence that was more fundamental than Heidegger's concept of being-with others: that love had been abandoned by Heidegger to freeze outside of his projection of being. In love, Binswanger thought, we transcend the cares of everyday existence and participate in an "eternal now."

Heidegger (2001) vehemently disregarded the "psychiatric Daseinsanalysis" of Binswanger because among other things: Binswanger did not see the ontological dimension of human beings (p. 115), or the understanding of being (p. 192), he conflated the ontological with the everyday level of existence (p. 203) thereby missing the ontological difference, and he developed a kind of philosophical anthropology (p. 122) on a merely ontical (everyday level) (p. 207) and subjective level (p. 227). Binswanger subsequently conceded these points as his "creative misunderstanding" of *Being and Time* (Heidegger 2001, pp. 303–307). Nonetheless, Needleman (1963, p. ix) argued that despite this, Binswanger's analysis "still stands a valid, necessary, and remarkably far-seeing supplementation of Heidegger's thought."

Dissatisfied with his own therapeutic approach, Medard Boss contacted Heidegger to solicit help in providing a proper philosophical foundation for therapy in 1947 after which they developed a lifelong friendship. It was in Boss' home in Zollikon that the aforementioned seminars were delivered by Heidegger. Boss' form of Daseinsanalysis enjoyed the full support of Heidegger—Heidegger (2001, p. 307) proofread and corrected Boss' major texts, and argued that Boss' magnum opus, *Existential Foundations in Medicine and Psychology* articulated the crucial response to scientistic thinking within the discipline of psychology (Heidegger 2001, p. 269). The primary reason was that Heidegger saw Boss as fully appreciating (i.e., adhering to) the basics of his fundamental ontology, especially that humans are "receptive-perceptive world-openness" and "world-disclosing" beings. He endorsed Boss' notion of "world-relations," some of which get blocked as one's own modes of being human. Boss also adopted Heidegger's notion of a constriction by neurotic/psychotic clients of their world-openness. Boss endeavored to determine what specific modifications of normal being-in-the-world accounted for the occurrence of such constrictions.

Initially influenced by Binswanger, and an analysand of Freud's in training, Boss (1963, p. 237) conceded that Freud's concrete suggestions concerning psychoanalytic technique had been unsurpassed, though he rejected Freud's metapsychological idea of the unconscious. Boss (1963, pp. 61–74) attempted to salvage Freud's "original insights" by essentially arguing that Freud had a philosophically split personality—Freud the clinician (therapist), and Freud the metapsychologist (theorist)—and that it was the philosophical presuppositions of the former that were at least compatible with Heidegger's hermeneutical ontology. His fundamental claim was that all of Freud's therapeutic techniques were designed to enable the client "to unveil himself and to unfold into his utmost openness" (Boss 1963, p. 62). Indeed, Boss claimed that Heidegger himself recognized this disparity (Hoeller 1988, pp. 9–10). Boss felt that Freud obnubilated his own insights by attempting to conceptualize his discoveries (e.g., the unconscious) within a scientific paradigm, and that by applying Heidegger's philosophy to psychoanalysis he could extend the scope of Freud's insights.

However, Boss' case is unconvincing for two primary reasons. First, the evidence he adduced is sparse, and shows Freud as operating on only the everyday and/or existential level of human existence, and never on the ontological level of understanding. For example, offering only three references (which are more than open to alternative interpretation), Boss (1963, p. 67) suggested that Freud and Heidegger shared a recognition of the significance of existential freedom while ignoring Heidegger's insistence that such freedom cannot be truly understood independently of ontological openness (i.e., "the Free") (Heidegger 1992, p. 149), and makes possible all other forms of freedom, including existential freedom (Heidegger 1962, p. 232, 1977, p. 125). Second, Freud (SE XXII, p. 138) would have unhesitatingly rejected Boss' claim by pointing out that for him, psychoanalysis as a whole was a unified science—a research procedure, and therapeutic method—which were interrelated and grounded in his metapsychological theory; a theory of mental life that is ultimately rooted in physical, bodily processes (Freud SE XIV, p. 78). Hence, any talk of fundamental philosophical differences between his two approaches would have been utterly unacceptable to him. We argue on Freud's behalf that, though it has unresolved tensions, it is indissolubly unified (Askay and Farquhar 2006, pp. 328–336).

Contemporary Efforts

at Reconciliation

Richardson (1965, p. 177) was the first contemporary philosopher to try to find a way to situate "the unconscious" in Heidegger's philosophy. (He later makes an entirely different attempt by trying to reconcile Heidegger's thought with the unconscious in Lacan's form of psychoanalysis (Richardson 1993).) Two decades before the publication of *Zollikoner Seminare* (1987), he noted a "remarkable consonance" between Freud's (SE IV, p. 262) and Heidegger's (1959, pp. 90–91) descriptions of Sophocle's play, *Oedipus Rex*. According to Richardson (1965) both Freud and Heidegger interpreted it as a metaphor for the process of revelation in the whole human condition. Both saw the need to uncover what is hidden in our existence so that we can fulfill our possibilities as whole beings. Freud likened this process to that of psychoanalysis while Heidegger identified it with the realization of authenticity. In light of this, Richardson (1965, p. 187) suggested that the place of unconscious processes in Heidegger's thought is in "the onto-conscious-self" conceived as the ontological dimension of the conscious subject as conscious, which is not conscious—hence "unconscious." As this dimension the human being is open to Being as a process of transcendence. As a condition of knowledge we discover it as a pre-cognitional intimacy of Dasein with its Being-structure (Richardson 1967, pp. 97–103). We first dwell "unthematically" (i.e., unaware of any particular meanings) as being-in-the-world, hence "a human being's limited belonging to the realm of the unconcealed [situation] constitutes his being a self" (Heidegger 2001, p. 188) and it is out of this, that the self conceived on the everyday level as an "ego," as "consciousness," and "unconsciousness" emerge. The publication of the *Zollikoner Seminare* confirmed Richardson's interpretation as consistent with Heidegger who clearly spoke about two levels of dwelling "unthematically" as being-in-the-world: (1) on the ontological level as having a pre-thematic implicit awareness of Being (Heidegger 2001, p. 121), the most general characteristics of our being, temporality, care, and so forth (Heidegger 2001, p. 32), and (2) on the everyday level (Heidegger 2001, p. 170), oneself or objects as being "unthematically" present in our environment (Heidegger 2001, p. 32). We should be careful to note that this notion of the unconscious is, of course, not Freud's since Heidegger's "unconscious" operates on both levels.

To extend Richardson's hypothesis, the two thinkers recognized the hidden unity and antagonism of being and appearance (Heidegger 1959, p. 90). Our everyday lives consist of an appearance, a self-manifestation, a presencing, a "happeningness," and within it is concealed the reality of who we really are (in our very Being). Appearance involves concealment and distortion while reality involves unconcealment. For Heidegger, it is Being that serves as the necessary condition for that which appears. For both, we can potentially move from an understanding of who we appear to be to a disclosedness of who we really are. However, in our everyday being we most typically cloak the latter and thereby deceive ourselves. We are "forgetful" (i.e., are unconscious) of Being and its structures.

In line with Richardson's interpretation, Needleman (1963, p. 88) described the "Existential *A Priori*" (the horizonal manifestation of the universal and necessary structures of Heidegger's "being-in-the-world") as a specific "meaning-context" that includes the unconscious as part of the givenness of the human condition. We typically have only a pre-cognitive awareness of those categories through which we construct our everyday individual world-design.

BEYOND RICHARDSON

We now want to extend Richardson's analysis to show that this notion of "the unconscious" not only does not exclude Freud's notions of consciousness/"the unconscious," but that it makes these modes of being possible. Indeed, we shall show why Heidegger himself can embrace a reinterpreted notion of the unconscious on the everyday level.

First, not only did Heidegger (2001, pp. 158, 207) *not* deny the existence of consciousness/unconscious, he simply argued that they are presupposed by the "clearing" and our pre-cognitive immersion in the openness of the world of meaning. He conceded that this kind of epistemological account has its place; it is just not primordial. Second, concealment includes (but is not identical with) the unconscious. For Heidegger (2001, p. 183), it is the openness (i.e., the clearing) that makes possible the presencing of being and beings—Dasein conceals/unconceals that which *is* in the clearing. There is that which presences and that which simultaneously discloses/covers-up that which presences. Hence, even the hidden manifests itself. This is why Heidegger claimed that we are both in the truth and the untruth. Given the tradition from which we emerge, it is tempting to equate that which is unconcealment with consciousness (Heidegger 2001, p. 182) and, reciprocally, identifying that which conceals as unconsciousness. This, however, would be a mistake since concealing/unconcealing something must not be represented as an event somehow "immanent in the subject" (as Heidegger claims it was for Freud). Instead, concealing/unconcealing belong to the clearing. This is why Heidegger held that concealment is not to be identified with the kind of hiding that occurs in what he interpreted as Freud's notion of repression, (i.e., as necessarily involving a mechanistically hiding of a representation within an encapsulated ego). A better account, Heidegger suggested, is that it is the *phenomenon* itself that is hidden, (i.e., it withdraws itself from the domain of the clearing and is inaccessible). Yet what conceals itself remains what it is. This is why Heidegger (2001, p. 183) claimed that "hiding [as repression] is a special way and manner of being in the clearing." Heidegger, then, did not deny the existence of repression as a possible occurrence; he held that it is a special mode of being that is not equitable with concealment. By holding that that which conceals itself remains what it is, it must do so in some dimension of being of which we are not thematically aware. Heidegger further developed this point while discussing the phenomenon of "forgetting." A person can avoid ones' self as one who is continuously afflicted by a painful event, (i.e., "forget it"). While doing so, one is present to oneself in an unthematic way; one is entirely absorbed in this avoidance in a non-reflective way. Heidegger (2001, pp. 170–171) wrote that "Being absorbed by forgetting refers to concealment, which withdraws itself" (see also Boss 1979, pp. 115–117).

We contend that it is this that makes it plausible for Heidegger (2001, p. 287) to claim that "repression shows itself as one of the possible modes of human comportment." Through it we can refuse to face ("flee from") things which address and afflict us. Boss (1963, pp. 120–121) offered a similar description. As such, it engages other originary modes of being, in other words, its temporality, as an ecstatic-intentional relationship (i.e., as a standing outside of itself) to the world of things, living beings, and fellow human beings. As such, repression is understood as a phenomenon of existence (Boss 1979, pp. 244–247). Boss (1963, pp. 62, 69, 100–101) himself supports our argument that in his quest for the unconscious, Freud too must have grasped concealment as a fundamentally important realm of human existence— for without it we could not be the uncovering kind of being that we are or be openness as well. Furthermore, Heidegger (2001, pp. 163–165) implicitly acknowledged unconscious comportments that we "divert/avert" in ourselves while seeing them in others in his reinterpretation of Freud's "projection," "introjection," and "transference." Boss (1963, pp. 117, 120–121, 235, 1979, p. 263), too, could not help himself as a therapist in appealing to an unconscious repeatedly, which "testifies to Freud's deep understanding of man" (Boss 1963, pp. 78–79). These are clearly places Heidegger and Boss make room for the unconscious. As such, in Heideggerian terms, an unconscious is a part of the clearing as a potentiality-to-be, even as hidden, as part of concealment.

Here we think it is important to note an important analogical similarity between Heidegger and Freud's accounts. Just as the clearing is a greater openness that includes Dasein as standing-out into part of it, so too is Freud's (SE XIV, p. 166) unconscious a wider compass than that which is repressed in it. The difference is that Freud's unconscious as grounded in somatic sources must be seen as intrinsic to Dasein's being in order for it to be a condition for its field of meaning.

To prevent their analysis of the unconscious from seeming merely free-floating, however, it will be important for us to see how it is grounded in their analysis of bodily being.

HEIDEGGER ON BODILY BEING

Heidegger claimed that Freud failed to see the ontological dimension of human existence as extending to the sphere of the body. This is especially true since Freud saw the unconscious as grounded in the physical body. Heidegger (2001, p. 170) saw Freud's analysis of the body as reducing it to a mere mechanistic system (a thing ontology), which was "already beforehand to have destroyed the body as body." (This is mitigated by the fact that Heidegger (2001, p. 202) and Boss (1963, pp. 111, 140) do not deny the importance of understanding the physical processes of the brain as one major aspect of bodying forth.) Yet, Heidegger (2001, p. 184) insisted that we must avoid the propensity to view the body merely as a corporeal, self-contained being. Doing so led to Cartesian dualism in Freud's metapsychology. Once Freud did this, his metapsychology was stuck with the intractable traditional problems of how to account for the ostensibly incommensurable relationship between the psyche (the level of meaning) and the physicalistic processes of the body (Heidegger 2001, p. 233).

Yet, conventional wisdom argues that Heidegger himself neglected the body. Did he? Well, yes and no.

No: Heidegger (2001, p. 234) acknowledged that it is an important aspect of the givenness of Dasein: "how immediately and limitlessly all bodily nature belongs to the human way of existing" Heidegger (1962, pp. 75, 143, 151) even went so far as to suggest that bodily being has a regional ontology, which would be well worth investigating as a part of philosophical anthropology, although this was not his project since it "hides a whole problematic of its own" (Heidegger 2001, p. 80). Furthermore, Heidegger advocated a "metontology" as a metaphysics of the primal phenomenon of human existence. Heidegger (1984, pp. 155–158) wrote:

> *metaphysica naturalis* in Dasein itself … the possibility that being is there in the understanding presupposes the factical existence of Dasein, and this in turn presupposes the factual extantness of nature … In their unity, fundamental ontology and metontology constitute the concept of metaphysics.

This makes room for a metontology of the body in its presencing, for example, its sexuality (Kisiel 2007, p. 291). In the therapeutic context, Heidegger (2001, p. 96) emphasized that "silence" and "hearing is a being-with-the-theme in a bodily way," and "every feeling is a bodying forth tuned" (Heidegger 1979, vol. I, p. 100).

Furthermore, Heidegger (2001, p. 202) and Boss (1979, p. 200) both argued that modes of illnesses show impairment of the bodily sphere of human existence and that hence it is important to pay attention to the bodily being. It is Daseinsanalysis that shows not only how the afflicted bodily sphere is disturbed, but also what way of relating is disturbed. For example, concealment can occur on the bodily level when various world-relations get closed-off (Boss 1963, p. 145). Hence, Boss (1979, p. 259) insisted that the therapist pay close attention to the meaning of how the patient relates bodily at each moment of therapy.

Yes: Heidegger denied that a body belongs to Dasein's primordial structure. While acknowledging that factically existing Dasein always has a body, Heidegger (1984, pp. 136–137) pointed out the interpretation of Dasein's being precedes "every factual concretion." Heidegger (2001, p. 158) seemed to merely take it for granted that the body is "alive," and then simply ignored the nature which "runs through us," focusing on the body's "outside" relatedness in nature. Heidegger (2001, p. 73) stated that "The pervasive way of all being-open is our immediate being with things that affect us physically." We contend that by doing so Heidegger (1962, p. 186) failed to follow his own dictum, "to allow beings to be seen as beings in their being." Eugen Fink attempted to nudge Heidegger (1993, p. 145) in this direction, trying to get him to see the dark ground and forces that we share with animals, but Heidegger would have none of it. Heidegger (1993, p. 145, 1977, p. 204) stated, "The bodily in the human is not something animalistic." This is why Heidegger (1995, pp. 236–237) restricted his extensive analysis of instincts, urges, and so forth to animals, and never considered them in human beings. Transcending Heidegger, Boss (1963, p. 144) recognized the importance for human beings of "the dark, mute spheres of existence … in the somatic realm" as an important condition for the emergence of meaning. Dasein needs to be understood as "including the body as organically connected to a material nature that we share with other beings" (Boss 1963, p. 140).

To understand the reason for Heidegger's ambivalence here, it is important to see what he took to be the nature of the relationship of bodily being and existence. Heidegger (2001, p. 233) claimed that Dasein's openness, as being-in-the-world (i.e., existence) and as a receptive/perceptive relatedness to something which address us from out of it, is ontologically more primordial than bodily being. Bodily being is the necessary yet insufficient condition for Dasein's being-in-the-world (Heidegger 2001, p. 186). Bodily being belongs essentially to, is not as comprehensive as, and yet presupposes being-in-the-world. While bodily being is necessary for us to be related to the world in any situation (i.e., it plays a pivotal role in one's openness), being-in-the-world is necessary for there to be any relations at all. Hence, being-in-the-world is the ontological precondition for the possibility of bodily being (Askay and Farquhar 2006, pp. 346–348) with its concrete attributes such as sexuality (Heidegger 1984, pp. 136–137). And since temporality is the transcendental condition for being-in-the-world, it is prior to bodily being as well (Heidegger 1982, p. 325).

A CRITIQUE OF HEIDEGGER ON THE BODY

Heidegger (2001, p. 157) lamented, "So far a sufficiently useful description of the phenomenon of the body has not emerged, that is, one viewed from the perspective of the being-in-the-world." However, it was Merleau-Ponty (1962, pp. 164–166) who first recognized Heidegger's (2001, p. 200) error in claiming that "presencing itself is not a body-forth." Merleau-Ponty emphasized that it is the body that *actualizes* existence, "runs through me," thereby providing the *thrown* possibility for my presencing in the world. Merleau-Ponty (1962, p. 148) asserted that "The body is pure presence to the world and openness to its possibilities." My body is an intrinsic aspect of my presencing in the world as I engage that which presences itself to me and as such is ontologically primordial. Hence, the lived-body and existence are mutually implicatory; each alone is a necessary yet insufficient condition for the ontological relationship of the world. What is particularly strange here is the fact that Heidegger's phenomenological analysis of bodily being actually closely mirrors Merleau-Ponty's, viz., gesture and expression, spatiality, phantom limb, and so forth (Askay and Farquhar 2006, p. 440, n. 33). Boss (1979, p. 202) too made similar observations to Merleau-Ponty's (1962, pp. 103ff) regarding how brain-injury impairs human ways of relating to the world. Yet, Heidegger rejected Merleau-Ponty's conclusion that bodily being and Being are equiprimordial (i.e., indissolubly fundamental).

Binswanger pointed out that embodiment is intrinsic to Heidegger's being-in-the-world as thrown, factical attunement. Indeed, Heidegger (1984, pp. 136–137; 1979, vol. 1, p. 100) acknowledged this, and that "bodying forth … is a mode of Dasein's being" (Heidegger 2001, p. 86). The problem is, however, that being-in-the-world cannot be both ontologically prior to bodily being *and* intrinsically include embodiment within its very ontological structure. Heidegger failed to take seriously the idea that not only does Dasein transcend nature and is surrounded by it, but nature runs through Dasein's very being as it is embodied. Hence, Heidegger refused to recognize the natural sources of embodied desire, passion, and sexuality. We argue that such are a manifestation of *physis* (as the Greeks understood it) as the unaided bringing forth of something, as a blossom bursts forth into bloom (Heidegger 1977, p. 129) by an overwhelmingly powerful, mysterious force (Heidegger 1959, p. 150). Nature radiates to and through us as embodied. The idea is to "let what is coming arrive" by following the "Origin" (Heidegger 1977, p. 149). Nevertheless, the therapist can aid this bringing forth in their clients (i.e., *techne* (Heidegger 1977, p. 294)).

Hence, it is clear that the body is the key as the necessary condition for both a more holistic account of human being and the emergence of meaning in the first place. It is here that Heidegger and Freud's accounts complement one another. While Heidegger focuses on how the body engages its natural environment, Freud focuses on what emerges through the body itself.

FREUD'S BODY-EGO

This takes us to the question of how our existence emerges through our body. Freud (SE XIX, p. 26) was certainly aware that the psyche is indissolubly unified with the body: "The ego is first and foremost a body-ego." And it is the unconscious Id—the original "core of our being"—from which the ego evolves (Freud SE XIV, p. 78). On the deepest level, as the "dark, inaccessible" "core of our being," Freud (SE XXII, p. 73; SE XIV, p. 78) described the Id as "a cauldron full of seething excitations," within which the organic, somatic instincts operate. As purely unconscious, Id lacks organization, temporality, and strives for the satisfaction of instinctual needs in accordance with the pleasure principle. In it, contrary and conflicting impulses exist proximally, the law of contradiction does not apply, and as pure internality it is cut off from the external world. It is not until body and brain develop in the infant that the ego is formed and the "reality principle" gains priority. In other words, Id knows of no external world and has no meaning. Rather the instinctual strivings of unconscious bodily being are the condition for what is yet to come—meaning and an awareness of what it means to be.

One of Heidegger's (2001, p. 173) criticisms of Freud was based upon the former's misunderstanding that the instincts cause (in the traditional, deterministic sense) us to do/think what we do/think. Here instincts are conceived as material processes. To the contrary, we argue that a very plausible alternative way to interpret Freud is that the instincts do not *cause* in a material sense—rather instincts are an aspect of the transcendental condition for the possibility that meaning x occurs and manifests as a series of conditional states (2006, pp. 334–335; SE, XIV, p. 171). As such, the unconscious Id is the source (in bodily being) of all human motivation which is free in being and thought, but not in action (see Askay and Farquhar 2006, pp. 136–152 where we argue that Freudian psychoanalysis is properly grounded in Schopenhauerian metaphysics). Hence, for Freud we are the very stirring of our instincts, and this stirring precedes meaning. Heidegger (2001, p. 173) insisted, however, that one cannot construct being-in-the-world from willing and urges. Rather, the structure of Care and being-in-the-world form the primordial basis of willing (Heidegger 1979, vol. 1, p. 315, 2001, p. 274); willing and urge are ways of enacting being-in-the-world as structural modifications of Care (Heidegger 2001, p. 172).

What is strange is that manifesting his romanticist rootedness, Heidegger (2010, p. 146) wrote that the goal of all our striving, whether we understand it or not is the "unification of ourselves with nature, with the One infinite totality," "the original all-unifying One." Heidegger (1979, vol. II, pp. 222–312) rejected Freud on this score while acknowledging in a positive way Schelling's "Willing is primal being." This would not be strange, given Heidegger's perception of Freud as representative of the traditional metaphysics that he repudiates, but Schelling was a member of the very same tradition. Here Heidegger is ostensibly oblivious to what Freud's analysis of the unconscious Id and the ego-body has to offer his own account—one of the clearest accounts of our bodily being as it manifests itself through our sexuality, instincts, and unconscious processes (Askay and Farquhar 2006, pp. 126–136). Hence, such an analysis could help explicate Heidegger's metontology (the body's regional ontology) described earlier.

Our claim is that it is precisely our bodily being which can shine its own radiance (i.e., bodily being is a necessary condition that makes it possible for us to experience any presencing by beings at all, including bodily being). It is a crucial aspect of our "dwelling," which, in Heidegger's (1977, p. 329) words "means to remain at peace within the free sphere that cares for each thing in its own nature." We need to truly care-for bodily being in its own nature, to "set something free in its own presencing," (1977, p. 328) to enable it to come into its full being. This is an essential condition for being-at-home in the world. It is *Gelassenheit* (letting be free) that releases clients from their entrapment in homelessness and any constriction in Being-in-the-world and from the pandemic suffering intrinsic to the human condition. Furthermore, it is through our embodiment that we let ourselves into (*Gelassenheit*) our way of existing in the first place.

THE IMPORTANCE OF *GELASSENHEIT*

Heidegger (2001, p. 211) emphatically held that therapists must stand back and let their clients be. Therapists must attempt to be attuned to the worldviews of their clients as they presence themselves, in other words, let clients manifest and unconceal themselves as they are to the therapists. For example, Heidegger (1995, p. 68) wrote, "Awakening means letting an attunement be." This is why Heidegger and Boss insisted that this is most effectively achieved through the phenomenological method. Freud too recognized that this was essential to the therapeutic process by his advocacy of "free association" as the primary principle of psychoanalytic method.

There are several important facets of this insight. First, for Heidegger (2010, pp. 72–73), *Gelassenheit* conveys a sense of "calm composure"—a non-willing way of thoughtfully dwelling in the open-region of being (through a profound existential experience of letting go, or letting oneself into, or letting be)—a fundamental attunement to Being in "resolute openness." This applies to both therapist and client when it comes to letting into, letting-go, and letting-be, or accepting/surrendering to whatever manifests itself in life which might seem ominous or threatening. This could free clients for their basic openness to the world. Second, by "letting clients be," both the therapists and clients are freed from imposing any preconceived, dogmatic psychological constructions (especially those presupposing the scientific Weltanschauung) on the therapeutic process. Heidegger (1962, p. 158, 1995, p. 91) described this as an inauthentic intervening mode whereby, for example, the therapists may leap into the clients' existence in such a way as to dominate and encourage dependency. Heidegger (1962, p. 158) and Boss (1963, p. 73) both concurred that the authentic mode would be for therapists to leap ahead of clients and help them explore their possibilities with them in a greater openness while not imposing therapists' interpretations on clients. Instead, therapists should help clients keep their eyes open to what their own phenomenological experiences are showing them about their situation so that they may better understand them. (Indeed, this is what Heidegger took himself to be doing while conducting "group therapy" during the Zollikon seminars.) Therapists would then help to "free the ['client'] in his freedom for himself" (Heidegger 1962, p. 343).

Finally, we argue that one essential aspect of letting clients be (i.e., accepting the clients as they show themselves) is to let their bodily being be, which requires that it be regarded as equiprimordial as their being-in-the-world. And just as Heidegger (2001 p. 224) emphasized that "ontological (genuine) phenomena cannot be "seen" immediately in the same way as ontic appearances can," we argue that bodily being (which includes the unconscious) cannot in the same way. Heidegger's (1962, p. 59) words apply equally well to bodily being:

Manifestly, it is something that proximally and for the most part does *not* show itself at all: it is something that lies *hidden* … but at the same time it is something that belongs to what thus shows itself, and it belongs to it so essentially as to constitute its meaning and its ground.

Indeed, while discussing the body, Heidegger (1962, p. 52) himself confirmed our point that in the "symptoms of a disease" the body simultaneously shows itself and also "indicates" something which does not show itself. Ironically, Heidegger (1962, p. 57) then wrote, "The Being of entities … can be covered so extensively that it becomes forgotten." It appears that Heidegger himself forgot the being of the body. By insisting on conceiving of Freud's notion of the unconscious as a "black box" while remaining oblivious to the power of his clinical insights which disclose its basis in bodily being, Heidegger (1962, p. 60) himself has "stubbornly" fallen prey to a kind of covering-up. Hence, far from "neglecting to determine the human being's character of being" as Heidegger contended, Freud did just that on precisely the one ontological aspect of Dasein's being Heidegger neglected.

HEIDEGGER'S DIAGNOSIS

Heidegger (1977, p. 134) thought that we are all caught up in the fateful epochal history of the West, what is sent: destiny, it conceals the true meaning of Being, As such, we are prisoners of our technological *Zeitgeist* in the age of the absolutization of the technological disclosedness of Being (Heidegger 2001, p. 58, Boss 1979, p. 287). Hence, scientism has assumed the throne of knowledge. As Heidegger (2001, p. 95) put it, science dogmatically claims that it exclusively offers "*the* truth about genuine reality." For Heidegger (2001, pp. 228, 241), as a "contrived psychological theory," Freudian psychoanalysis, as a major representative of scientism, concealed being itself by uncritically getting us to focus exclusively on beings conceived as things. It thereby constricted our horizon of disclosure. According to Heidegger (2001, p. 132), Freud fell prey to the uncritical application of scientific thinking to human beings. He thereby reinforced our "oblivion to Being." Also, individuals are "already deranged" because they are caught up in a technology which takes itself to be the only valid approach, whereby they frame whatever they uncritically think in terms of its unrecognized presuppositions (Heidegger 2001, p. 51). We are dominated by a nearly exclusive dogmatic technical-calculative mode of thinking (Heidegger 2001, pp. 141, 258). We interpret everything in terms of its usefulness, for instance, human resources (Heidegger 1977, p. 288) or try to control it with instrumental reason (Heidegger 1977, p. 288). In doing so, Heidegger (2001, p. 160) claimed that we try to fill the emptiness left by the meaninglessness of modern life.

Heidegger's (and Boss') Solution

Our task is to recover the ground, the origin of our being by "recollecting" Being (Heidegger 1977, p. 136), "the original all-unifying One" (Heidegger 2010, p. 146); recollecting, that is, that human beings never construct their own horizons of disclosure. Boss (1979, p. 292) suggested that modern ailments ultimately originate in the ill person's comportment to modern industrial society (the "dis-ease in civilization"), and that Heidegger's (2001, p. 296) philosophy can serve to treat effectively pathogenic behaviors, the feeling of homelessness, and the various other forms of spiritual sickness which have resulted from it, by responsibly appropriating all one's possible world-disclosing relationships as extensively as possible (Boss 1963, p. 47). It is when a person fails to do so that she or he experiences existential "guilt" (Boss 1963, p. 270) or through the devastating idea that "nothing matters." Therapists assist their clients in becoming aware of and acknowledging all of their life possibilities as possibilities, and thereby enable them to achieve authentic self-knowledge (Boss 1963, p. 254). In doing so, one exists engrossed as who one genuinely is in one's task of living while at the same time being explicitly aware that there is no deep unifying meaning to life. Freud completely agreed (Jones 1955, p. 345).

Heidegger's Hermeneutical Realism

We now want to show how it is Heidegger's adoption of a hermeneutical realism that makes for a truly holistic account of the human condition. Heidegger (2001, p. 178) claimed that the clearing as the openness is more encompassing than Dasein; Dasein stands out in the clearing. It is Being (as the generative ground of being) and Dasein's being as disclosedness (i.e., the "hermeneutic") which make it possible for anything to presence itself (Heidegger 1969, p. 19), to show up for us in the clearing; hence Being and human being are mutually implicatory and primordial. Dasein is necessary for the presencing of Being (Heidegger 2001, p. 176). Dasein is therefore the server and guardian of the clearing (Heidegger 1977, p. 210).

However, even Heidegger acknowledged that there might be other generative grounds for being (which he leaves room for). Heidegger (1962, pp. 228, 255, 269, 1977, p. 105, 1982, pp. 168, 220, 1984, p. 153, 2001, p. 140) clearly held that nature *is*, as it is metaphysically, independently of us, and hence is a "minimal hermeneutic realist" (Dreyfus 1991, p. 253). Heidegger's (1962, p. 100) position was that Dasein engages a nature that surrounds it: "the nature which "stirs and strives," which assails us and enthralls us as landscape." We contend that since nature manifests itself through our thrown bodily being and our attunement occurs through it, this opens room for the unconscious on the bodily level. This would be to render Heidegger's position consistent with Freud's unconscious. For example, as with Freud, Heidegger (1982, p. 262) held that "there is no nature-time."

More significantly, Heidegger (1977, pp. 302–303) held that there are a multiplicity of ways of understanding nature, and that different theories can disclose different aspects of nature on different levels. For instance, Heidegger (2010, p. 71) wrote, "our world disclosure is but the side facing us of an openness which surrounds us; an openness which is filled with many views." Indeed, while discussing the Being of beings as Will, Heidegger (1979, vol. I, p. 36) asserted, "all great thinkers think the same. Yet this "same" is so essential and so rich that no single thinker exhausts it." Heidegger (2001, pp. 18, 110, 123) took science to be one of the primary ways of understanding nature as long as it truly recognized its limitations and did not claim exclusivity to the truth. Since, for Heidegger, no one way of disclosing is exclusively correct, accepting one, such as Heidegger's fundamental ontology, does not commit us a priori to rejecting others, but rather opens the door to such theories as Freud's metapsychology.

In the end, Heidegger found himself on the horns of a dilemma: either he must concede that there is a dualism intrinsic to reality (Dasein versus non-Dasein, e.g., nature)—one which he spent his entire philosophical career arguing against—or he must acknowledge that humans are nature as well in order to have a cogent holistic account of human reality. Since Heidegger unequivocally rejected the notion that humans share animalistic characteristics as part of nature, Heidegger was forced to renounce a holistic account and found himself entrapped in a dualism, which his philosophy was designed to overcome.

To summarize, what does each orientation have to offer the other in order to gain a truly holistic account of human existence? Heidegger offers a unified account of the human sphere of meaning and its hidden ontological dimension, while Freud offers an account of those hidden conditions through our bodily being that both serve as conditions for, and are presupposed by, that very sphere of meaning. Taken together they afford a considerably more unified and complete account of the human condition.

REFERENCES

Askay, R. and Farquhar, J. (2006). *Apprehending the Inaccessible: Freudian Psychoanalysis and Existential Phenomenology*. Evanston, IL: Northwestern University Press.

Askay, R. and Farquhar, J. (2011). Psychoanalysis. In S. Luft and S. Overgaard (Eds), *The Routledge Companion to Phenomenology*, pp. 596–610. London: Routledge.

Binswanger, L. (1957). *Sigmund Freud: Reminiscences of a Friendship*. New York, NY: Grune and Stratton.

Binswanger, L. (1958). The case of Ellen West. In R. May (Ed.), *Existence: A New Dimension in Psychiatry and Psychology*, pp. 237–364. New York, NY: Basic Books.

Binswanger, L. (1963). *Being-in-the-World: Selected Papers of Ludwig Binswanger*. New York, NY: Harper and Row.

Boss, M. (1963). *Psychoanalysis and Daseinsanalysis*. New York, NY: Basic Books Publishing Company.

Boss, M. (1979). *Existential Foundations of Medicine and Psychology*. New York, NY: Aronson.

Dreyfus, H. (1991). *Being-in-the-World: A Commentary on Heidegger's Being and Time*. Cambridge, MA: MIT.

Freud, S. (1960). *The Standard Edition of the Complete Psychological Works of Sigmund Freud* (Vols. I–XXIV) (J. Strachey, Ed. and Trans.). London: Hogarth.

Heidegger, M. (1959). *An Introduction to Metaphysics*. New York, NY: Anchor Books.

Heidegger, M. (1962). *Being and Time*. New York, NY: Harper and Row.

Heidegger, M. (1969). *Identity and Difference*. New York, NY: Harper and Row.

Heidegger, M. (1977). *Basic Writings*. New York, NY: Harper and Row.

Heidegger, M. (1979). *Nietzsche* (Vols I and II). San Francisco, CA: Harper Publishers.

Heidegger, M. (1982). *The Basic Problems of Phenomenology*. Bloomington, IN: Indiana University Press.

Heidegger, M. (1984). *The Metaphysical Foundations of Logic*. Bloomington, IN: Indiana University Press.

Heidegger, M. (1992). *Parmenides*. Bloomington, IN: Indiana University Press.

Heidegger, M. (1995). *The Fundamental Concepts of Metaphysics: World, Finitude, Solitude*. Bloomington, IN: Indiana University Press.

Heidegger, M. (1996). *Holderlin's Hymn "The Ister" (Studies in Continental Thought)* (W. McNeill and J. Davis, Trans.). Bloomington, IN: Indiana University Press.

Heidegger, M. (2001). *Zollikon Seminars: Protocols, Conversations, Letters*. Evanston, IL: Northwestern University Press.

Heidegger, M. (2010). *Country Path Conversations*. Bloomington, IN: Indiana University Press.

Heidegger, M. and Fink, E. (1993). *Heraclitus Seminar*. Evanston, IL: Northwestern University Press.

Hoeller, K. (Ed.) (1988). *Heidegger and Psychology*. Seattle, WA: Review of Existential Psychology and Psychiatry.

Jones, E. (1955). *The Life and Works of Sigmund Freud* (Vol. 3). New York, NY: Basic Books.

Kisiel, T. (2007). *Becoming Heidegger: On the Trail of His Early Occasional Writings, 1910–1927*. Evanston, IL: Northwestern University Press.

Merleau-Ponty, M. (1962). *Phenomenology of Perception*. New York, NY: The Humanities Press.

Needleman, J. (1963). *Being-in-the-World: Selected Papers of Ludwig Binswanger*. New York, NY: Harper and Row.

Richardson, W. (1965). The place of the unconscious in Heidegger. *Review of Existential Psychology & Psychiatry*, 5(3), 265–90.

Richardson, W. (1967). *Heidegger: Through Phenomenology to Thought*. The Hague: M. Nijhoff.

Richardson, W. (1993). Heidegger among the doctors. In J. Sallis (Ed.), *Reading Heidegger: Commemorations*, pp. 49–66. Bloomington, IN: Indiana University Press.

....

CHAPTER 72

COGNITIVE BEHAVIOR THERAPY: A PHILOSOPHICAL APPRAISAL

....

RICHARD G. T. GIPPS

INTRODUCTION: COGNITIVE BEHAVIOR THERAPY AND PHILOSOPHY

....

Cognitive behavior therapy (CBT) is a broad church embracing many theories, models, and techniques, often now held in conjunction with other approaches to the mind in health and distress (e.g., compassion, mindfulness, dialectics, psychodynamics, etc.). Within this church there are denominations that complement, but also those that compete, with one another, both in their empirical claims and also in some of their underlying theoretical principles (Hofmann and Asmundson 2008).

There are, for example, those who treat the "cognitive" aspect of CBT theory as referring specifically to maladaptive *thoughts and beliefs* (e.g., Beck 1979). These psychological states are considered distinct from what members of this congregation would stipulate as the *non-cognitive* states and processes of perception, emotion, and behavior. The causal-explanatory force of appeals to cognition should now be clear: disorders of behavior and feeling are to be explained by reference to disturbances in underlying, ontologically distinct, cognitive states and processes. Other theorists, however, tie what is "cognitive" not specifically to thought and belief, but rather to the processing of *meaning* (e.g., Teasdale 1997). They do not assume that meaning is an exclusive function of thought or belief, and instead allow it to already belong properly to emotion, behavior, and perception. In such cases the explanatory force of a cognitive model may derive from its identification of the distinct structures of meaning immanent within emotion and behavior themselves, rather than from showing how antecedent thoughts allegedly give rise to such disturbed emotion and behavior.

Because there are such different versions not only of the "C" (Dobson and Dozois 2010), but also of the "B" (Hayes and Brownstein 1986) in versions of what are still often described as "CBT" it makes little sense to offer a philosophical critique "of CBT" per se, and such a wide-ranging critique is not attempted in this chapter. Nevertheless, underlying several popular CBT models and treatments (henceforth "CBTs") are, I shall suggest, several questionable assumptions about the significance of cognitive factors in psychopathology. In this chapter I add to previous critique (McEachrane 2009; Lacewing 2004; Whiting 2007) in specifying four related philosophical misunderstandings regarding the nature of the mind in health and distress that, I claim, can sometimes affect CBT's understanding both of psychopathology and of therapeutic action.

Before I begin I think it might be helpful if I set out, using some examples, what makes for a distinctly *philosophical* critique of a particular CBT theory. Consider first the following questions that can, and have, been asked of the CBTs:

1. For what range of difficulties, experienced by what kinds of populations, are CBTs effective?
2. Are CBTs more or less effective than other therapies (e.g., psychodynamic, narrative, person-centered or drug therapies) and practical interventions (e.g., employment and dating advice, social sport, and gardening)?
3. How durable are the effects of CBTs compared with other treatments?
4. When a CBT is effective, can this be explained using typical CBT models of psychopathology and therapeutic action, or must we account for it using ideas taken from other cognitive, systemic, or psychodynamic theories of therapeutic action?
5. When a CBT is found to be more or less effective than another therapy, is this to be accounted for:
   a. ideologically (i.e., because of treatment effects due to the convictions of investigators, therapists or patients), or because of
   b. differential treatment efficacy, or because
   c. measures are being used which are tailored to what one but not another therapy would view as meaningful or valuable change (e.g., is it characterological or symptomatic changes that are being measured)?

These are all important questions for therapists, patients, and public health policymakers. Yet there is, I suggest, little that is distinctly philosophical about them. Part of what it means to say this is that they are not answerable through reflection alone, but must instead be answered by empirical investigation. The exception is the last (5c): reflection on what *counts* as efficacy is a form of theoretical reflection on conceptual matters of meaning, rather than discernment of empirical matters of fact. Even so, such theoretical reflection is not, in the sense in which I shall use the term here, itself particularly philosophical. For whilst all theoretical thought concerns itself with matters of meaning, what I have in mind by distinctly philosophical thought instead concerns itself with whether what is said can genuinely be understood in the way its author seems to hope for it. Philosophical reflection in this sense concerns itself not simply with meaning but more particularly with meaningfulness; not with how, but rather with whether, something can really be understood in the way it invites us to understand it.[1]

---

[1] In making this distinction I am not intending to be understood as suggesting that a hard and sharp distinction can *everywhere and always* be drawn between matters empirical and theoretical, or between matters theoretical and philosophical.

In what follows I articulate four ways in which CBTs can sometimes invite the psychological theorist to construe ourselves to ourselves, both in our healthy functioning and in our emotional distress, in ways that, it seems to me, go against what it means to be a human subject. More particularly, I shall consider certain conceptions, tacitly present within the psychopathological theories offered by various CBTs, of what it is to think, feel, and meaningfully respond. My claim will be that whilst these conceptions appear to motivate the practice, conceptually dovetail with the theory, and validate the distinctive scientific self-conception, of various CBTs, they nevertheless simply do not tally with what reflective understanding reveals as the character of human mental and emotional life. Such reflection reveals that our mindedness has a character and richness not always aptly captured by the concepts and theories employed in certain CBT theories. Therapists guided more by such theories than by their own humanity may accordingly run the risk of embodying or offering to their patients a distorted or impoverished understanding of emotional distress and therapeutic action. Given that such CBTs can nevertheless prove helpful to some patients, it follows that they must sometimes do so for reasons other than those they themselves suggest.

Aspects Versus Causes

The CBTs, along with other cognitive approaches in psychology, often present their understanding of psychopathology in a "box and arrow" format. The arrows are intended to represent causal relations; the boxes represent what are intended to be understood as isolable cognitive, behavioral or emotional factors. Such schematic models are appealing because they are clear-cut and appear to offer a cogent rationale for investigation and intervention. Consider the highly condensed summaries of typical cognitive models shown in Box 72.1.

Such models are, I find, often useful in clinical practice since they clearly depict what may be the main meanings and maintaining factors in the various difficulties with which patients present; they also immediately suggest strategies for intervention. They may also attempt to do justice to the complex, dynamic (non-linear) causality operative in the mind. My objection at this stage is not to their clinical or heuristic utility, and neither am I alleging any excessive simplicity or linearity in their causal schematics; it is instead a rather modest demurral to a quite different aspect of their implicit causal theorization of the mind. The objection could be summarized by saying that such models tend to encourage us to mistake: (a) a fact about our representations of the mind for (b) a fact about what is represented. The (a) fact about our representations that I have in mind is that we can *separately depict* various aspects of (say) a depressive state, such as our behavioral dispositions, thoughts, motivation, mood, affects, etc. My objection here is that this cannot by itself be taken to indicate a (b) fact about what is represented: that there are *separately existing* assumptions and perceptions and moods and motivational states—states "in us," as we can hardly now but put it—linked by causal connections (the arrows in the diagrams (Box 72.1)).

Take the case of panic. The CBT model separates out a stimulus, a perception of it as threatening, a state of apprehension, and bodily sensations, and places these separated phenomena into a causal sequence. Yet whilst all these ingredients are clearly present in a panic attack, and whilst we can separate them for formal (descriptive) purposes, it is not obvious that they really are, in the normal run of things, best conceived of as separate states within

Box 72.1 CBT formulation summaries

One aspect of contemporary CBT models of panic can be elaborated as follows: A patient experiences a bodily sensation. They catastrophically misinterpret this as a sign of danger (e.g., that they are fainting or having a heart attack). This leads to a further perception of threat, giving rise to further fear, which in turn gives rise to further sensations that are in turn catastrophically misinterpreted. The patient is left in a rapidly cycling, self-fuelling anxiety state (cf. Clark 1989) (Fig. 72.1).

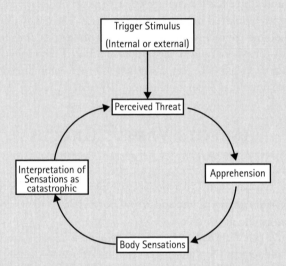

FIGURE 72.1 CBT panic model. Reprinted from *Behaviour Research and Therapy*, 24 (4), David M. Clark, A cognitive approach to panic, Pages No. 461–70, Copyright (1986), with permission from Elsevier.

The depressed patient as encountered by the CBT therapist is an individual with underlying pessimistic assumptions that organize his or her experience of the world. When activated by critical incidents these assumptions are thought to lead to the development of negative automatic thoughts (e.g., gloomy and non-deliberative thoughts about the current situation, self, or future). These then give rise to negative emotions (e.g., guilt or fear), a lowering in mood, and consequently to a reduction in motivation and activity and engagement. A vicious cycle of depressed thoughts and depressed mood results (cf. Beck 1979; Fennell 1989).

The patient with social anxiety often carries underlying assumptions (e.g., "unless someone shows they like me, they dislike me"). The CBT model describes how these can be activated in social situations, resulting in a belief that they are in "social danger" (e.g., believing that others will treat me badly) (Fig. 72.2). Such beliefs may then cause anxiety, which in turn can cause various somatic and cognitive symptoms (sweating, mind going blank, shaking). These in turn can heighten a self-conscious mode of attention in which the patient considers that they are, for example, likely to make fools out of themselves (cf. Clark and Wells 1995).

(*continued*)

Box 72.1 (Continued)

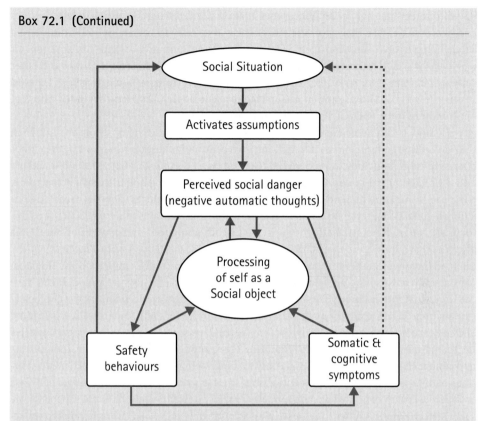

FIGURE 72.2 CBT social phobia model. Reproduced from Clark, D.M. and Wells, A. A Cognitive model of social phobia. In R. Heimberg, M. Liebowitz, D.A. Hope, and F.R. Scheier (Eds), *Social Phobia: Diagnosis, assessment, and treatment*, pp. 69–93 © 1995 Guilford Press, with permission.

a person which causally trigger one another. A better description of them may accordingly be as different *aspects* of the same (anxiety) state. We are "stirred up"—in both our action-readiness and in a somatosensory way—by fearful stimuli, and our being stirred up in this way is itself *of a piece* with our registering of that stimulus as fearful. The components of our fear response are not in any obvious way isolable and several causally related *states in us*, but may rather be more naturally understood as merely notionally separable aspects of *the* state which *we are in*.

Much the same can be said about the CBT conceptions of depression and social anxiety outlined earlier. It can almost seem as if something of the passive and objectifying voice of depressive anxiety has found its way into the CBT conceptualization of the nature of our mental life per se. Thus we now have assumptions that can be "activated"; meanings become reified into occurrent processes and states to be known as "cognitions"; the agent become a locus of "behaviors." Everywhere we have to do with nouns, and nowhere with verbs: to do with nouns that bolster an appearance that we are referring to several isolable entities and processes, rather than with their root verbs that refer to the action and attitude of a single living entity. The living agent who makes assumptions, understands his experience a particular way, and undertakes actions becomes instead a locus of separate inner and outer states which causally trigger one another. The concept of a unitary living person as featured in our everyday emotional and moral discourse accordingly risks being degraded into that of a bundle of inner and outer states and processes.

CBT models can be useful as heuristics for thinking about psychopathology, and when they do outline genuine causal interactions (two genuinely causal interactions in the earlier discussed models include those between fear and bodily sensations in panic, and inactivity and depressed mood in depression) they significantly help to guide therapy. Furthermore, their use of mechanistic and objectivizing rhetoric which reduces diverse (causal, dispositional, constitutive, etc.) relations to causal relations is not in itself a mortal sin; the CBT theorist is after all not pretending to provide us with a nuanced metaphysics of mind. It is also true that a spuriously mechanistic model of the mind need not lead to a mechanistically pursued therapy; whether that risk obtains in fact would need to be empirically investigated. My criticism at this juncture is instead as follows. First, that the cognitive models can have the somewhat misleading appearance of providing more by way of a scientific psychological explanation than is really available; they are therefore potentially scientifically misleading and may accordingly impede CBT research. Second, they often appear to possess a greater degree of scientific precision than found in other models of therapy—even though this appearance may be partly or solely due only to their having misleadingly dressed up descriptions of different aspects of the patient's disturbance as a causal-explanatory model of it. For, to repeat, as often as not, what such models are really describing are different aspects of the same state we are in, rather than describing scientifically teased out, causally linked, interruptible, states and processes within us.

ATTITUDES VERSUS COGITATIONS

Whilst all CBT theorists adhere to the centrality of *cognition* in emotional disturbance, not all theorists appear to agree on the meaning of the term, a term that in any case is most often left undefined. As described in the introduction, for some the term appears to refer to any aspect of psychological performance (e.g., in perception, action, emotion, judgment, etc.) that involves the conscious or preconscious *processing or discrimination of meaning*. Under consideration may be enduring attitudes—dispositions of thought, feeling and behavior which may become sedimented in character—or passing emotions, perceptions, cogitations, and imaginings. For others, including the founding fathers of CBT, the term refers more exclusively to our *thinking*, which in itself is understood as realized in the words and images that pass across our minds. Such thinking is conceived of as the second or third tier of a hierarchy of cognitive elements which move from the most subconscious and dispositional (the underlying schemata) level, through to more readily avowable maladaptive beliefs, up to occurrent automatic thoughts passing across the mind. What follows in this section concerns only the latter sense of cognition (as occurrent thoughts passing across the mind—what I henceforth call "cogitation"), and draws in part on the thoughtful critique of McEachrane (2009).

Here are some examples of the idea that it is either the content of (in traditional CBT), or the patient's fused relationship with (in "third-wave" CBTs such as acceptance and commitment therapy—"ACT"), inner representational events that maintain and mediate emotional disturbance:

> CBT therapists encourage [patients] to become aware of their thoughts and thought processes. Cognitions are generally classified into negative automatic thoughts and dysfunctional or irrational beliefs. Negative automatic thoughts are thoughts or images that occur in specific situations when an individual feels threatened in some way. (Hofman and Asmundson 2008, p. 4)
>
> When a person is able to fill in the gap between an activating event and the emotional consequences, the puzzling reaction becomes understandable. With training, people are able to catch the rapid thoughts or images that occur between an event and an emotional response. (Beck 1979, p. 26)
>
> ACT aims to alter the context in which thoughts occur so as to decrease the impact and importance of difficult private events.... Clinically we want to teach clients to see thoughts as thoughts, feelings as feelings, memories as memories, and physical sensations as physical sensations. None of these private events are inherently toxic to human welfare when experienced for what they are. (Hayes et al. 2004, p. 8)
>
> [In] cognitive fusion ... the event and one's thinking about it become so fused as to be inseparable and that creates the impression that verbal construal is not present at all.... A worry about the future is seemingly about the actual future, not merely an immediate process of construing the future. The thought "Life is not worth living" is seemingly a conclusion about life and its quality, not a verbal evaluative process going on now. (Hayes et al. 2004, p. 25)

In these examples we see clearly an idea that crops up not infrequently in the CBT literature: that to think something is to have a thought pass across one's mind. We are, it is said, often oblivious to such inner events even occurring, perhaps (in the case of ACT) because we are overidentified or "fused" with them. The therapist's job is accordingly to help us notice and either simply de-fuse from, or more aggressively challenge, these events that supposedly mediate between outer events and our feelings (on which more in the "Feeling and believing" section). But as McEachrane (2009) suggests:

> To say of someone that they 'thought that p' does not imply that they 'thought of p' or 'thought about p' or formulated p or that p occurred to them or was in their thoughts.... [If] a client says that in a particular situation they thought that, say, 'I'll never be like them' or ... 'I'm not a likeable person', then this does not necessarily mean that the client in that situation thought *of* these things, formulated these things to herself, that these things occurred to her or were in her thoughts.' If you ask me what I think about the economic situation I need not wait on inner mental events to occur which I can then report. Instead I simply tell you how the situation seems to me, and in this telling I express what we could call my "attitudes" rather than report on my occurrent "cogitations." (p. 86)

It is important to be clear about the scope of this criticism. It is the aim of many psychological therapies to help the patient to take a more flexible, reflective, or "ironic" stance toward their own attitudes (Lear 2003). Psychodynamic therapies, for example, may aim to help a patient develop in their "mentalizing," to become aware that theirs is but one among many possible ways of thinking about things, and to increase their inner playfulness or psychological flexibility (Holmes 2009). Further, it is true that the depressed person can indeed become ruminatively lost in an inner world of depressed and depressing cogitations; in this case, talk of "thoughts" can indeed often be taken as talk of inner musings or imagery. Helping the patient become aware that this is going on, and encouraging them to instead harness their attentional resources to, and increase their physical engagement with, the external world are well known to be therapeutically valuable. But treating thoughts as if they are *typically* inner events leaves a therapist at risk of talking past the patient. Consider the following:

> Therapist:Now I'd like to spend a few minutes talking about the connection between thoughts and feelings. Can you think of some times this week when you felt upset?
> Patient:Yeah. Walking to class this morning.
> T:What emotion were you feeling: sad? anxious? angry?
> P:Sad.
> T:What was going through your mind?
> P:I was looking at these other students, talking or playing Frisbee, hanging out on the lawn.
> T:What was going through your mind when you saw them?
> P:I'll never be like them.
> T:Okay. You just identified what we call an *automatic thought*. Everyone has them. They're thoughts that just seem to pop into our heads. We're not deliberately trying to think about them; that's why we call them automatic. Most of the time, they're real quick and we're much more aware of the emotion—in this case, sadness—than we are of the thoughts. Lots of times the thoughts are distorted in some way. But we react *as if* they're true.
> P:Hmmm. (Beck, 1995, p. 78; quoted by McEachrane 2009, p. 85)

Here the therapist is interested in the patient's cogitations, and takes the patient's reply ("I'll never be like them") as literally describing something going through the mind. But nothing in what the patient says confirms the correctness of the idea that they are experiencing "automatic thoughts"; instead they may simply be describing their beliefs. The possible discrepancy is even clearer with some of the reported thoughts described by Hayes et al. (2004) ("A worry about the future is seemingly about the actual future, not merely an immediate process of construing the future. The thought "Life is not worth living" is seemingly a conclusion about life and its quality, not a verbal evaluative process going on now.") You ask me: "Why are you troubled?" and I say "I'm worried about being made redundant, and the possible effect of this on my family life." Whilst it may indeed be possible for me to be overly worried and lose perspective, it is not at all clear that this is best described as a matter of fusion with "immediate processes of construing" or with "verbal evaluative processes going on now." By contrast with what Hayes suggests, we can and indeed should say that a thought that life is not worth living is indeed a judgment about life and its quality, regardless of whether the judgment is expressed in inner speech; and we also can and indeed should say that a worry about the future is indeed about the future, regardless of whether it manifests in a current episode of worrying.

The risks of misconstruing the phenomenology of thought do not include merely that of the therapist and patient talking past one another. An oft discussed concern in therapeutic circles is when we can count externalization—the capacity to develop a noticing, more distant and reflective, attitude toward one's own thoughts—as a healthy, and when as an unhealthy, procedure. Externalization can, for example, be a healthy strategy for the patient who has become swept along by ruminative cycles of cogitations—as typified by certain cases of depression. It can also be helpful when the patient is unable to appreciate that they do have one amongst other possible attitudinal stances toward the world—as typified by certain cases of borderline personality disorder. But it can be unhelpful when the therapeutic task is that of helping a patient take ownership of her attitudes, stand behind them as her own, live from and embody them, count herself as their true subject—rather than, say, using irony or intellectualization or projection (attributing them elsewhere) as a defense, or seeing them as unwanted foreign intrusions. And so one risk in misconstruing all thought as cogitation which the patient can relate to, rather than live from, may be that of encouraging an unhealthy form of externalization or self-alienation. For some of our thoughts—in particular certain emotionally painful ones which register personal losses—precisely do need to be engaged with and suffered, rather than reflectively noticed, if the patient is ever to be able to acknowledge and thereby move past their painful experiences.

Another risk is that of underestimating the therapeutic task. By misconstruing thought as thinking—by conflating attitudes with cogitations—the CBT therapist may start to attempt to help their patient change what he thinks (his attitudes) through changing his relation to, or the content of, his thinking (his cogitations). Yet it is surely natural to suppose that our cogitations are often enough a function of our attitudes and not, on the whole, vice versa. If, that is, my attitude is that my life is not worth living then, when I am invited to attend only to my own cogitation, I shall most likely be attending to it—say to my occurrent thought of "this is all hopeless"—from just this attitude. In such a case my challenging of, or distancing myself from, cogitations that reflect my attitudes risks becoming little more than a strategy promoting bad faith or self-alienation. What is really required is, rather, a change of attitude, a change which may at times be facilitated by attention to one's cogitations but which is unlikely to proceed solely from such a change. In CBT terms what may be required is not work on "automatic thoughts" but rather deeper work on "core beliefs" or "schemata"; the risk of misconstruing attitudes as cogitations is that this requirement gets overlooked. The patient may of course benefit in all sorts of ways by being able to attend to their occurrent ruminations which can often go unnoticed. First, however, they need to possess a healthy standpoint from which to assess their own mental contents and processes—and this can itself take significant therapeutic work.

Feeling and Believing

Perhaps the central claim of much CBT is that disturbances of emotion arise from disturbances of cognition. This is often presented as a modern-day form of the Stoic principle that "men are disturbed, not by things, but by the principles and notions which they form concerning things" (Epictetus 2004, section V; Robertson 2010). As discussed earlier, much will turn on the question of whether we are to understand cognition as (a) referencing any meaningful uptake or information processing of "things," or (b) whether we are to understand it as referring instead to cognitive items such as acts of interpretation, the application or formation of "principles and notions," or to those of our attitudes which are most aptly described as "underlying beliefs." I shall return to (a) in the conclusion; in this section I shall consider this more restricted latter sense (b) of cognition, and ask whether emotional disturbance is aptly theorized as consequent upon it.

Within the CBTs it is the "ABC" model of emotional disorder, imported from Albert Ellis's Rational Emotive Behaviour Therapy (Ellis 1991; Wilson and Branch 2005), that most explicitly embodies the notion of cognitions as thoughts or beliefs. "A" here stands for the *activating* events or situations experienced; "Bs" are the subject's *beliefs* about or interpretations of these events; "Cs" are the emotional or behavioral *consequences*. The ABC model accordingly construes the cognitive state of belief as a determining intermediary between experience and emotional response. The viability of conceiving of the "C" in CBT along the lines of the "B" in ABC has been questioned by CBT theorists on both theoretical and empirical grounds (Kohlenberg and Tsai 1994; Teasdale 1997; Rachman 1997). One rather obvious empirical objection to the Stoic claim that we are affected not by things but by the notions we form regarding them comes from medical and conditioning approaches to anxiety: I may be made mildly anxious directly by very strong coffee (even if I mistakenly believe it to be decaffeinated); I may be directly emotionally affected by hormonal changes or head injuries; I may feel compelled to perform compulsions to reduce obsessional anxiety even whilst knowing there is no rational basis for this; and I can be afraid of stimuli, such as spiders or birds, which I believe to be perfectly safe (Whiting 2007, p. 239)—hence the continued relevance of simple behavioral therapies for certain phobic or compulsive behaviors. Another objection comes from the observation that, whilst certain thoughts and beliefs may be depressogenic or anxiogenic, this may only occur for people who are already caught up in a particular frame of mind, perhaps driven by certain unconscious desires and emotions (Whiting 2006, p. 241). This, in fact, is an objection anticipated by a key founder of CBT, Aaron Beck, who claimed only to identify the maintaining factors, and not the underlying causes, of depression (Beck et al. 1979; Clark and Steer 1996). The question to be answered in this chapter, however, asks whether there are distinctly philosophical grounds for questioning the idea that disturbed emotions are typically driven by beliefs. My claim is that this idea can sometimes be seen to arise from a misunderstanding, inscribed in certain CBT theories, of what it means to be an emotionally reactive human subject.

A standard cognitive model of depression has it that aversive early experience can lead to the formation of dysfunctional assumptions which, when activated by a critical incident, lead to cycles of negative automatic thoughts and other behavioral, motivational, affective, cognitive, and somatic symptoms (Fennell 1989, p. 171). These assumptions or beliefs are said to take such forms as "If someone thinks badly of me, I cannot be happy," or "I must do well at everything I undertake," "I am inferior as a person," "My worth depends on what other people think of me" (Fennell 1989, pp. 171–178). Therapy then consists in strategies such as teaching the patient to become aware of depressing thoughts as they occur, or undertaking tasks to test the truth of fixed negative beliefs (Williams 1997, p. 265). The first thing to be said about such propositions is that, whilst the therapist probing for core *beliefs* may well elicit them, they are often far more naturally taken to express a patient's *feelings*. McEachrane (2009 p. 92) quotes Ellis (1994, pp. 32–33) attempting to convince a patient of the opposite of this:

> "I know I'm doing better of course, and I'm sure it's because of what's gone on here in these sessions. And I'm pleased and grateful to you. But I still feel basically the same way—that there's something really rotten about me, something I can't do anything about, and that the others are able to see. And I don't know what to do about this feeling."
> "But this 'feeling', as you call it, is largely your *belief*—do you see that?"

"How can my feeling be a belief? I really—uh—*feel* it. That's all I can describe it as, a feeling?"

"Yes, but you feel it *because* you believe it. If you believed, for example, really believed you were a fine person, in spite of all the mistakes you have made and may still make in life, and in spite of anyone else, such as your parents, thinking that you were not so fine; if you really *believed* this, would you then feel fundamentally rotten?"

"Oh, Hmm. No, I guess you're right; I guess I then wouldn't feel that way."

However the logical error here seems to be Ellis's rather than his patient's. Ellis appears to be assuming that, since I am unlikely to feel rotten about myself if I truly believe I am a good and fine person, then it must be the case that my feeling rotten about myself is a product of my believing myself to be rotten. But what, we might ask, if we start with the idea that beliefs are often products of feelings rather than vice versa—might we not expect to arrive at the same state of affairs? That is to say: If I felt bad about myself then may I not, as a consequence, be disposed to form negative beliefs about myself? And then again isn't it also true that sometimes we feel that there is something rotten about us without forming any associated belief—just as, say, a phobic person may find herself feeling that spiders or birds are dangerous without believing anything of the sort? It may be hard to imagine truly believing that one is a fine person whilst feeling one is rotten, but this may reflect nothing more than the powerfully constraining impact of feeling on believing.

One way in which a CBT theorist might try to salvage the idea that it is maladaptive beliefs that drive emotional disturbance could be as follows. Beliefs, they may say, possess intentionality and carry mental content (they are *about this or that*). Feelings, on the other hand, are merely "positive" or "negative" ("hot" or "cold") emotions, sensations, or states of being. Feelings therefore need to be driven by beliefs before they can properly be said to be about anything or to express any kind of understanding. The reply to this is that it is hard to understand why we should accept such an impoverished conception of our feelings as *merely* aversive or hedonic sensations. For feelings often precisely are about something: I feel furious *that* he has wasted my time; she is sad *about* his departure. And since our feelings are very naturally taken to be already about states of affairs, it is hard to see what help they need from intermediary beliefs. Taking "cognitive" in sense (a) from earlier—as referring to any meaningful uptake of things—emotions and feelings can be understood as already cognitive, i.e., as constituted by cognition rather than obtaining in any kind of simple or complex causal relation with separable non-affective cognitive states (cf. Lacewing 2004). Helping the patient understand that their unwanted feelings are not simply free-floating meaningless sensations, but have a meaningful content which situates them in an intentional context, is in fact, and of course, the work of pretty much all non-behavioral therapy. One risk, then, of cleaving to a model which divorces our feelings from their intrinsic intentional contents, only to attempt to causally glue them back on to other meaningful states, is that of colluding with an unhelpful aspect of the patient's self-understanding. Another risk is of not adequately theorizing what, in various CBTs, as well as in the psychodynamic and person-centered therapies, is seen as the centrality of emotionally-charged experiential changes for meaningful therapeutic change (Samoilov and Goldfried 2000).

To consider further the relationship between emotion and belief: imagine that I always dreamed of being a psychologist but then fail my exams and become morose. This emotional state of mine worsens and I start to believe that I cannot be happy unless I am a psychologist. A CBT therapist who becomes wedded to the idea that intermediary beliefs or adherence to rules underpins emotional distress may propose that it is precisely this belief of mine that is driving my despondency. It is indeed surely possible that such additional beliefs may serve to maintain or worsen depression. What isn't clear though is why much of my sadness may not be thought of as arising simply because I have not realized my life's ambition. What is significant here is not an intervening *belief* about what I need to be happy, but more generally how I *see* my life, my *outlook* on, *felt sense* about, or *evaluative perception* of, my self, my situation, and my future (cf. McEachrane 2009, pp. 94–95). In a depressive frame of mind I may arrive at beliefs such as "I cannot be happy unless I am a psychologist," but such beliefs are, I suggest, in the run of things more likely to result from my sense of my situation rather than vice versa.

What, then, are we to make of the not infrequent CBT insistence that beliefs have a key pathogenic role to play in depression and other emotional disorders? My own belief is that, whilst certain CBT therapists may sometimes be driven by an overly intellectual (belief- or rule-mediated) conception of our emotional perception of our worlds, what has more often happened is that they have stretched the meaning of "belief" to fit the phenomenology and save the theory. For example, I once asked my CBT supervisor what she meant by her talk of her patients' "beliefs," and she replied that you knew that what you had to do with was a belief when a patient cried in articulating it. This clearly has little to do with the normal notion of belief, given that the infinity of our everyday beliefs (that it is not raining, that most people have legs, that the next symbol is an ellipsis …) hardly provokes an infinity of tears. What instead we have to do with here may rather be the result of a common enough situation in psychiatry and psychotherapy generally: that the practical meanings of clinical terms become constituted more by their actual clinical uses than by associated theory, where such clinical uses are themselves a product of a distinctive lexicon being forced to carry *whatever* are the communicative and therapeutic burdens of the clinical encounter. The result is an implicit and unacknowledged argot, the non-standard meanings of which are implicitly known to the practitioners in question.

This explanation should not, of course, be mistaken for exculpation. CBT theorists have as much a professional duty to communicate clearly and accurately as all psychologists, and misusing ordinary terms ("belief," "thought") may be no less unhelpful than deploying the language of science when it adds nothing to what is better stated in everyday language.[2] And the fact remains that we do ordinarily distinguish between beliefs and feelings, and use the distinction to mark situations in which, say, we feel scared of a cat even whilst believing it to be safe. The person who is scared of the cat may have all sorts of inarticulate feelings about cats which could helpfully be made more explicit in therapy, but it isn't clear what—other than saving an exclusively "cognitive" (in sense (b)) model—is to be gained from describing these as implicit beliefs. Furthermore cognitive neuroscience has now provided several models outlining different streams of information processing for propositional and embodied understandings (cf. Power and Dalgleish 1999; Teasdale 1997). Rather than think of the emotionally significant meanings which arise as a patient experiences their world as encoded in propositionally structured interpretations or beliefs, such theorists instead invite us to consider the prime significance of non-linguistic and somatosensory forms of

---

[2] For an example of the latter, Mollon (2007, p. 13) complains of the scientistic rhetoric of the CBT literature, where "facing your fears is called 'exposure', refraining from an activity is called 'response prevention', learning to relax is called 'stress inoculation', and revising your thoughts is called 'cognitive restructuring.'"

meaning. The clinical upshot is that therapy must aim at helping a patient change their way of being in the world through changing such non-belief-based meanings.

In this section I have added to such empirical critique by providing philosophical reasons for thinking that an "ABC"-style model falsifies what it actually means to be an emotionally reactive, meaning sensitive, human subject. *If*, when a CBT theorist tells us that emotional reactions are shaped by our "cognitions" they mean by "cognitions" something like our *beliefs*, and if by our "beliefs" they mean something other than how we *feel about or see* our situations, *then* the CBT theorist appears to run the risk of radically misconstruing the foundations of our affectivity by putting the cart of our belief before the already-meaningful horse of our emotion.

ON ARTICULATING OUR ASSUMPTIONS

In this section I inquire into the relation between (a) a patient's verbal articulations in therapy of their underlying self-understandings, and (b) the nature of such underlying self-understandings. Typical CBT models expound something like the following: (a) that the first, rather preliminary, step of cognitive therapy is to help the patient clearly *identify* their emotionally problematic core beliefs, rules and assumptions. And (b) that the second task is to encourage them to quasi-scientifically *test out* these assumptions, either through rational engagement (e.g., Kuehlwein 2002) leading to what is sometimes called "cognitive restructuring," or more practically through "behavioral experiments" (e.g., Bennett-Levy 2004).

In what follows I will challenge such a conception of what is happening in therapy when assumptions are articulated, questioned, or put to the test. My aim is not to question the CBT practice, but rather to question the conception of self-understanding that it encourages for the theorist: that articulation of one's own self-understanding in therapy is a rather preliminary stage occurring prior to the genuine transformations that can occur only when such self-understandings are challenged and healthier alternatives considered and embraced. The criticism offered here will be that those CBTs operating according to the above mentioned description risk underplaying both (a) the intrinsically transformative nature of the acknowledgment of one's deepest fears, and (b) the way in which verbal, behavioral, and experiential therapeutic techniques function not merely to test hypotheses, but rather to effect a more fundamental change in the form of the patient's thought. A more fundamental change, that is, that first of all enables it to become penetrable by the light that experience and rational enquiry can shine into the fearful recesses of the mind.

To start to explore what this means, consider first what happens when an underlying dysfunctional assumption gets put into words, perhaps through the application of the "downward arrow" technique. (This technique has the therapist repeatedly ask of, say, a patient voicing self-critical thoughts, questions such as "and if that were true, what would that say about you?" until a definitive underlying negative fear is articulated.) Here is how Fennell (1989) articulates the therapeutic strategy:

> Rather than challenging the thoughts themselves, the therapist asks: "Supposing that was true, what would that mean about you?" This and similar questions ... are repeated until

it is possible to formulate a statement general enough to encompass not only the original problem-situation, but also other situations where the same rule is operating.... Once a dysfunctional assumption has been identified, questioning and behavioural experimentation are used to find a new, more moderate and realistic rule. (pp. 204–205)

Fennell's own assumption is that dysfunctional assumptions can be hard to unearth because, "rather than [being] discrete events occurring in consciousness, they are generalized rules which may never have been formulated in so many words" (1989, p. 204). Why such assumptions should not have been put into words is not considered by her, nor is the emotional experience of the patient who articulates them—which, in my clinical experience at least, typically involves a quite particular mixture of distress and relief.[3] This empirical issue is not, however, our key concern here—which is instead philosophical and concerns what *happens* to such tacit assumptions when they are voiced. Fennell's presentation, which is quite standard in the CBT literature, encourages the view that their voicing involves merely their being put into words. But reflection on what is meant by the voicing of our deepest troubling thoughts—reflection that is philosophical in so far as it concerns itself with how the objects of psychological investigation ought to be characterized, rather than itself depending on the results of empirical enquiry—reveals something far richer. The articulation of one's previously unarticulated fears involves, that is, not merely voicing but also *acknowledgment* (Finkelstein 1999), a correlative *increase in self-understanding*, an *emancipation* which comes from making visible or thinkable those assumptions which otherwise continue to invisibly constrain our meaningful experience and, so long as the resultant fears can be contained until they dissipate, an *increased capacity to tolerate reality*.

To take up the last of these: the patient who presents under the influence of a dysfunctional assumption which they have not yet articulated to themselves can often be seen to be failing to fully distinguish between fear (or wish) and belief. Whether they always really *believe*, for example, that others laugh at them as they walk down the street, or whether this is simply what they fearfully *imagine or think*, is not always entirely clear. An important reason for this is that they can be presenting in a state of mind which somewhat ablates the very distinction between fearing and believing.[4] Their "safety behaviors" (which they perform to prevent (what they imagine will be) the experienced realization of their fears—e.g., never meeting the gaze of others for fear of meeting a hostile look, or never failing to grip onto the shopping trolley for fear that they would collapse) similarly keep in place the constitutive lack of clarity of the anxious state. However when the CBT therapist encourages them to test out their fears by surveying the beliefs of others, or by undertaking a behavioral experiment (which may involve seeing if matters really do deteriorate if they don't perform their safety behaviors), what happens is not merely that the truth of an assumption is evaluated, nor that they simply become more reflectively aware of what they already thought, but that a clear distinction between fear and genuine belief begins to be instated in the mind. A fearful state of mind that demotes reality contact becomes displaced by an empirical hypothesis.

---

[3] The psychodynamic theorist has a ready explanation of such phenomenology: that the articulation of such assumptions involves the patient coming to acknowledge that which has previously been defended against as too emotionally painful.

[4] In psychodynamic terms, their thinking is more a matter of "primary" than "secondary process."

Or perhaps the patient is invited to put a probability figure to their fear: what is the actual likelihood that you will be scoffed at if you show your face in the town center? Ninety percent? Twenty percent? Once again the CBT strategy invites the transformation of what would once have been called a "neurotic" state (in which an avoidance of reality has conspired with and inspired a fusion of fear, belief, and experience—a state which may sometimes be compensated for by structurally similar fusions of wish, belief, and experience) into an empirical hypothesis. Various CBT strategies have the clarifying effect of helping the patient shape up their fearful state so that it can be brought into contact with reality, first expressing it in the necessary bivalent (true/false) or probabilistic form of a genuinely reality-oriented proposition. They have this effect, that is, despite often understanding themselves as merely being in the business of promoting the voicing and then the testing of beliefs. What is significant, however, is not so much the disproving, but the emotional shift of rendering such fears provable or disprovable: reality testing (i.e., becoming able to distinguish between thought and fantasy) is a precondition of, and not a synonym for or consequence of, hypothesis testing.

In this section I have suggested that whether we are dealing with the verbal articulation, or with the testing, of a patient's deepest dysfunctional assumptions, what is principally significant is a change in the form of the patient's fears. For what renders such assumptions dysfunctional is not simply their content but also their neurotic form—their insulation from empirical testing and rational thought, their fusion with wish or fear. What I am suggesting is that mere reflection on the phenomenology of the patient's experience in therapy shows that it is a change in such form that ultimately makes for the possibility of a change in unhelpful content. The CBT therapist's armory of tools for unearthing and engaging with such assumptions has the effect of shining the light of reason into the darker recesses of the patient's mind, encouraging their thought to be governed not by fearful fancy but rather by (what psychoanalysts would call) "the reality principle." In the process their thought becomes articulated—which is to say, not merely voiced but structured—so that it now more clearly embeds a distinction between appearance and reality, is less insulated from reality testing, and is less a hostage of their deepest fears and wishes.

A much debated concern in the scientific CBT literature is whether the benefits of CBT are mediated by cognitive changes in the patient, whether such benefits may occur before cognitive techniques have even been applied, and whether cognitive techniques really add much to behavioral therapy (Longmore and Worrell 2007). One way of putting the philosophical point I am making here is that expressive and behavioral techniques can already be seen to be cognitive—insofar as they involve a change in the form of the patient's fearful or depressive preoccupations (cf. Carey and Mansell 2009). The various techniques of CBT serve to free the patient from those inchoate fears which have hitherto not found adequate, clearly delineated, expression. Making the fears less inchoate and more thinkable risks making them feel more real, and the avoidance of this scary possibility often seems to have been a significant part of the patient's difficulties. Therapy, however, provides an emotionally "containing" environment in which the therapist's clarity regarding, say, the relatively benign and possibly even nourishing nature of social reality—by contrast with what the patient fearfully imagines to be the case—can become internalized by the patient. It is for this reason that a good therapeutic relationship must not merely be collaborative (Leahy 2008) but also be containing, and an effective CBT therapist's containing manner shows itself in such trans-model common factors as her confidence in her methods, her clarity, reality orientation, compassion, and warmth.

Conclusion

To summarize the four objections: The first proposed that various CBT formulations conflate the formal relations between different aspects of the same state with causal relations between discrete inner states. The second had it that some CBT models construe emotionally laden perspectives too much as occurrent inner processes, and too little as a subject's attitudes. The third considered that such attitudes can sometimes be misdescribed in CBT models as beliefs—when what we really have to do with here are feelings that are themselves already about the events and situations that arouse them. The fourth argued that CBT models can underplay the significance of changes in the form of (a subject's ownership of) such attitudes when they focus instead on changing their content. In these concluding paragraphs I first consider whether a unifying diagnosis can be given of these diverse tendencies to distort what it means to be a living human subject before going on to ask what can be done about it.

My suggestion here is that what unifies these disturbances of vision is their being expressive of what could be called an "alienated" conception of human subjectivity. Imagine that the self were no longer an expressive bodily being located immanently by its feelings within a meaningful intersubjective world—but had retreated inward, away from the world, the body, and even the mind, becoming instead a disengaged inner spectator trying to make sense of the intersubjective world from without. Perhaps such a self is a prototype of a scientist-observer who is in the business of trying to control and predict the world by constructing inner representations or interpretations of it.[5] The effects of such a retreated conception of the self would be several. The mind and body, having been denuded of subjectivity, will now more naturally appear as a domain of merely causally (rather than meaningfully) inter-related, objectified states and processes. Mind becomes a domain of inner states and processes rather than a matter of how we are embedded in our intentional worlds. The self will no longer speak *from* its attitudes, but will rather be reduced to speaking *about* them. Our minds and bodies become not so much what we could call the flesh of the self, but instead show up as domains of inner and outer processes that require to be controlled from within. Therapy, accordingly, would get theorized as no longer in the business of self-transformation, but instead becomes a technology—grounded in what will appear to be, amongst the therapies, uniquely scientific causal models of inter-related inner processes—for helping us manage our feelings. Our relationships too will be reduced to a merely external form—which is to say, that they will become theorized not as constitutive of who we are, but rather seen merely to causally connect us to that which is essentially other. So too the being of the patient will no longer be thought of as partly immanent in the emotional flux of the therapeutic relationship; that relationship will instead risk being reduced in the theorist's vision to something which is merely a collaboration between distinct relata.

---

[5] George Kelly, psychologist of "personal constructs," proposed just such a scientist-observer conception of the human subject (Kelly 1955). His work significantly influenced the early CBT theorist Albert Ellis.

Precisely such a mechanistic and self-alienated conception of the mind can, it seems to me, be what we often find in the patient who presents wanting to know how to better "control their anxiety," "change their thoughts" or "manage their minds". Such a patient has, we could say, become alienated from their own inner life which, accordingly, is seen as an independent domain painfully afflicting them and requiring management or excision. Now it bears recollection that in this chapter I have not been concerned to critique the CBTs en bloc, nor on the whole to question the cogency of CBT therapy, but instead to scrutinize some ways in which some CBT theories may be inflected in ways that go against what it means to be an emotionally alive human subject. The risk for the CBTs that I have identified may now be described as one of being encouraged by an infelicitous theoretical model of joining the earlier-described patient in such a de-subjectivized vision of their psyche. But by helping the patient to give articulate structure to his fears, to think, to be nourished by reality contact, and to distinguish fearful fantasy from genuinely representational belief, the CBT practitioner can be understood as doing far more than, say, helping the patient to test out his hypotheses: she is helping to restore her patient's subjectivity.

The final question is: What can the CBTs do about all of this? The answer, I think, is already possessed by many CBT theorists, and has already been mentioned. It is to considerably broaden the conception of what counts as "cognitive"—to include not only a patient's thoughts, interpretations, and beliefs, but also any aspect of her meaningful engagement with her world. Cognition now becomes the name for an inherent property of perception, emotion, action readiness, interaction, etc., and we can drop the intellectualist consideration that perception, say, must be supplemented by acts of interpretation before it can be said to disclose a meaningful world for us. An example of this broadening of the domain of the cognitive was provided for me at a recent teaching session on treating childhood trauma by a well-known CBT author at a well-known UK cognitive therapy training center. A model of self-disturbances in trauma was outlined that stressed the priority of emotion, the central role of emotional and interpersonal avoidance (read: defenses) in the maintenance of psychopathology, and the therapist's use of self in therapy. The presenter then commented that this approach could still be counted as "cognitive" since it concerned itself with the *meaning* of the patient's experience. The obvious question to ask at this point, however, is: What therapy would now *not* be properly called "cognitive"?

At present it is fair to say that various features tend to characterize the therapeutic practice of those who consider themselves "cognitive" in orientation. These include a readiness to use information-sharing and instruction ("psycho-education"), an active and structured encouragement of within- and between-session behavior change, and a focus on collaboration rather than containment in the therapeutic relationship.[6] My suspicion is that, as for other therapies too, being "cognitive" means, in practice, to be identified with the interests, blindspots, and those fairly subtle helpful and unhelpful habits of mind and action tacitly

---

[6] One common misunderstanding that ought to be cleared up is the suggestions that in CBT—unlike, say, psychodynamic therapy—the focus is on the present rather than the past. This misconstrues both CBT and psychodynamic therapy. On the one hand, both psychodynamic therapy *and* the CBT for, say, depressive and personality difficulties, pay considerable initial, and to some degree an ongoing, attention to the patient's childhood. On the other hand, contemporary psychodynamic therapy typically pays a good deal *more* attention than CBT does to the immediate here-and-now interaction, in both its real and its transference dimensions, between patient and therapist; CBT's focus, by contrast, is often on the more distant emotional experiences of the patient's past week.

embedded in particular psychological communities. The clinician's temptation may often be to attempt to justify their unique orientation with reference to the empirical or theoretical credentials of their model. But if we read "cognitive" in its most theoretically plausible sense—i.e., as referring generally to structures and processes of meaning rather than merely to thoughts and beliefs—the impossibility of distinguishing CBT from, say, psychodynamic therapy by referring to the former's focus on cognition should now be clear.

ACKNOWLEDGMENTS

This chapter has benefitted considerably from the thoughtful comments of Louise Braddock, Michael Lacewing, and Rebecca Murphy.

REFERENCES

Beck, A. T. (1976). *Cognitive Therapy and the Emotional Disorders*. New York, NY: Meridian.

Beck, A. T., Rush, A. J., Shaw, B. G., and Emery, G. (1979). *Cognitive Therapy of Depression*. New York, NY: Guilford.

Bennett-Levy, J., Butler, G., Fennell, M., Hackmann, A., Mueller, M., and Westbrook, D. (2004). *Oxford Guide to Behavioural Experiments in Cognitive Therapy*. Oxford: Oxford University Press.

Carey, T. A., and Mansell, W. (2009). Show us a behaviour without a cognition and we'll show you a rock rolling down a hill. *The Cognitive Behaviour Therapist*, 2, 123–33.

Clark, D. M. (1989). Anxiety states: Panic and generalized anxiety. In K. Hawton, P. Salkovskis, J. Kirk, and D. Clark (Eds), *Cognitive Behaviour Therapy for Psychiatric Problems: A Practical Guide*, pp. 52–96. Oxford: Oxford University Press.

Clark, D. M. and Steer, R. A. (1996). Empirical status of the cognitive model of anxiety and depression. In P. M. Salkovskis (Ed.), *Frontiers of Cognitive Therapy*, pp. 75–96. New York, NY: Guilford.

Clark, D. M. and Wells, A. (1995). A cognitive model of social phobia. In R. G. Heimberg, M. R. Liebowitz, D. A. Hope, and F. R. Schneier (Eds), *Social Phobia: Diagnosis, Assessment, and Treatment*, pp. 69–93. New York, NY: Guilford.

Dobson, K. S. and Dozois, D. J. A. (2010). Historical and philosophical bases of the cognitive-behavioral therapies. In K. S. Dobson, (Ed.) *Handbook of Cognitive-Behavioral Therapies* (3rd edn), pp. 3–38. New York, NY: Guildford Press.

Ellis, A. (1991). The revised ABC's of rational-emotive therapy (RET). *Journal of Rational Emotive and Cognitive Behavior Therapy*, 9(3), 139–72.

Ellis, A. (1994). *Reason and Emotion in Psychotherapy. Revised and Updated*. Toronto: Carol Publishing Group.

Epictetus (2004). *Enchiridion*. New York, NY: Dover.

Fennell, M. J. V. (1989). Depression. In K. Hawton, P. M. Salkovskis, J. Kirk, and D. M. Clark (Eds), *Cognitive Behaviour Therapy for Psychiatric Problems*, pp. 169–234. Oxford: Oxford University Press.

Finkelstein, D. H. (1999). On the distinction between conscious and unconscious states of mind. *American Philosophical Quarterly*, 36(2), 79–100.

Hayes, S., Strosahl, K., Bunting, K., Twohig, M., and Wilson, K. (2004). What is acceptance and commitment therapy? In S. Hayes and K. Strosahl (Eds), *A Practical Guide to Acceptance and Commitment Therapy*, pp. 1–30. New York, NY: Springer.

Hofmann, S. G. and Asmundson, G. J. (2008). Acceptance and mindfulness-based therapy: new wave or old hat? *Clinical Psychology Review*, 28(1), 1–16.

Holmes, J. (2009). *Exploring in Security: Towards an Attachment-Informed Psychoanalytic Psychotherapy*. Hove: Routledge.

Kelly, G. (1955). *The Psychology of Personal Constructs*. New York, NY: W. W. Norton & Co.

Kohlenberg, R. J. and Tsai, M. (1994). Improving cognitive therapy for depression with functional analytic psychotherapy: theory and case study. *The Behavior Analyst*, 17, 305–19.

Kuehlwein, K. T. (2002). The cognitive treatment of depression. In Simos, G. (Ed.), *Cognitive Behaviour Therapy: A Guide for the Practising Clinician*, p. 3–48. Hove: Brunner-Routledge.

Lacewing, M. (2004). Emotion and cognition: Recent developments and therapeutic practice. *Philosophy, Psychiatry, & Psychology*, 11, 175–86.

Leahy, R. (2008). The therapeutic relationship in cognitive-behavioural therapy. *Behavioural and Cognitive Psychotherapy*, 36, 769–77.

Lear, J. (2003). *Therapeutic Action: An Earnest Plea for Irony*. New York, NY: Other Press.

Longmore, R. J. and Worrell, M. W. (2007). Do we need to challenge thoughts in cognitive behavior therapy? *Clinical Psychology Review*, 27, 173–87.

McEachrane, M. (2009). Capturing emotional thoughts: The philosophy of cognitive-behavioral therapy. In Y. Gustafsson, C. Kronqvist, and M. McEachrane (Eds), *Emotions and Understanding: Wittgensteinian Perspectives*, pp. 81–101. London: Palgrave Macmillan.

Mollon, P. (2007). Debunking the 'pseudoscience' debunkers. *Clinical Psychology Forum*, 174, 13–16.

Power, M. J. and Dalgleish, T. (1999). Two routes to emotion: some implications of multi-level theories of emotion for therapeutic practice. *Behavioural and Cognitive Psychotherapy*, 27, 129–41.

Robertson, D. (2010). *The Philosophy of Cognitive-Behavioural Therapy (CBT): Stoic Philosophy as Rational and Cognitive Psychotherapy*. London: Karnac Books.

Samoilov, A. and Goldfried, M. R. (2000). Role of emotion in cognitive-behavior therapy. *Clinical Psychology: Science and Practice*, 7(4), 373–85.

Teasdale, J. (1997). The relationship between cognition and emotion: the mind-in-place in mood disorders. In D. Clark and C. Fairburn (Eds), *Science and Practice of Cognitive Behaviour Therapy*, pp. 67–93. Oxford: Oxford University Press.

Whiting, D. (2007). Why treating problems in emotion may not require altering eliciting cognitions. *Philosophy, Psychiatry, & Psychology*, 13, 237–46.

Williams, J. M. G. (1997). Depression. In D. M. Clark and C. G. Fairburn (Eds), *Science and Practice of Cognitive Behaviour Therapy*, pp. 259–83. Oxford: Oxford University Press.

Wilson, R. and Branch, R. (2005). *Cognitive Behavioural Therapy for Dummies*. Chichester: John Wiley & Sons.

CHAPTER 73

UNDERSTANDING AND HEALING: PSYCHIATRY AND PSYCHOANALYSIS IN THE ERA OF NEUROSCIENCE

JIM HOPKINS

PSYCHIATRY AND THE PROBLEMS OF MIND

Psychiatry encounters the philosophical problems of mind and body in a particularly urgent, poignant, and intractable form. For psychiatrists have characteristically sought to treat the sufferings and disabilities of *mental* disorder as disturbances of the *physical* brain. The reasons for this are unimpeachable. We have come fully to appreciate that the processes we experience *as mental* are in fact physical ones, centered in the brain. In light of this we accept, as the tradition of Hippocrates has long maintained, that we "ought to know that from the brain and nothing else but the brain ... we become mad and delirious, and fears and terrors assail us ... and dreams, and untimely wanderings, and cares that are not suitable, and ignorance of present circumstances."[1]

But of course acknowledging the role of the brain has no effect at all on the way we actually think when we engage with persons and other objects in the world. Whatever their scientific orientation human beings alike experience perceiving, feeling, thinking, deciding, etc. as *mental phenomena*—things that are registered *in their minds*—and that they distinguish from the *physical phenomena* that they can see and touch, observe in an X-ray or brain scan, etc. This deep sense of difference persists alongside the acknowledgment of sameness

---

[1] Hippocrates, "On the Sacred Disease" (F. Adams, Trans.), available at: <http://classics.mit.edHippocrates/sacred.html>. Throughout this essay I assume that physicalism holds true for token events, and that linguistically specified psychological types, while themselves types of the physical, resist strict reduction to any other form.

because the sense of difference is rooted not in the things themselves but in the ways we think about them.[2]

Reality is one thing, the ways we think about it another. These are many and diverse; and we cannot readily alter or reduce them one to another. So our rightly holding that mental causes like desires can also be regarded as physiological mechanisms centered in the brain does not resolve the problems of mental versus physical, but rather restates them as limitations of scientific understanding.

THE ROLE OF EVOLUTION

We can understand this as part of our evolutionary heritage. Roughly, it seems that natural selection has equipped human beings (like other sexually reproducing species) with specialized neural mechanisms for relating to conspecifics. In the case of our ultra-social species these adaptations are particularly numerous and highly developed. They apparently include, in our expanded cerebral cortices, the representational resources required for language and, interwoven with this, for thinking of ourselves as agents who perceive, feel, think, and seek to communicate and satisfy our desires in concert with others of our kind.[3] This, in turn, is a main component of our ability to cooperate and coordinate our activities in groups of all sizes, including, of course, the episodes of ferocious group-on-group aggression and violence that have punctuated our history, and now marshal sufficient power to put a stop to it.

Engagement in this framework apparently begins with attachment—the infantile establishing of basic emotional bonds with parents or carers—and thus with the formation of the first and most basic of our social groups, the family. This process is sufficiently advanced by the fourth postnatal month for careful observation to yield predictions about the nature of the bonds then in formation (see Beebe et al. 2010). Stable and typical patterns of attachment, which apparently influence emotional relations throughout life, are often achieved by the end of the first year (see Cassidy and Shaver 2008). Hence in a recent neuroscientific study of depression Douglas Watt and Jaak Panksepp (2009, p. 93) describe attachment as establishing "the massive regulatory-lynchpin system of the human brain," which exercises a "primary influence" on the "multiple prototype emotional regulatory systems" that we share with other mammals.

Clearly this social and psychological framework ramifies deeply into our neurological being. But since its evolutionary function is to facilitate reproductive success via the communication of purpose and the coordination of action, we apprehend its deliverances in the language- and motive-ready categories of our everyday psychology of belief, desire, and emotion, as opposed to the neurobiological categories we have labored to devise during the short scientific period of our history.

---

[2] My own account of these modes is related to the problem of consciousness in Hopkins (2007) and to the representational role of conceptual metaphor and psychoanalytic symbolism in Hopkins (2000).

[3] The evolution of this framework is discussed in Hopkins (2000b). Both it and psychoanalysis more generally are related to neuroscience in Hopkins (2012).

LINGUISTIC AND PSYCHOLOGICAL
UNDERSTANDING

In using this evolved fusion of natural language and psychological understanding we specify the (representational or intentional) contents of motives such as desire, belief, hope, fear, etc., by appending to the appropriate psychological verb a phrase or sentence specifying the object or situation desired, believed, hoped, feared, etc. Thus we may say, e.g., that someone *desires [that she gets] a drink of water from that glass in front of her,* and likewise we can say that a person believes, hopes, fears, etc. *that P,* where "P" can be replaced by any sentence serving to specify the relevant state of mind.

This provides us with a potentially infinite, and hence endlessly flexible, set of shared descriptions for representing our mental states and the worldly (or imaginary) objects and situations that would render them true, satisfied, fulfilled, etc. The ability thus to frame the shared ideas and goals of our collaborative efforts is crucial to our attaining them. But from the point of view of neuroscience, this same flexibility appears as a descriptive variability so radically sensitive to each individual and situation as to render systematic translation into alternative scientific forms of description technically impossible.

Thus we can readily regard a desire or other mental state described in this way as realized by a behavior-governing neurological mechanism that operates from within the subject's body and brain. But at the same time we must also acknowledge that the terms in which we naturally conceive such mechanisms—via sentences like "[that she gets] a drink of water from the glass in front of her"—have no near scientific neighbor. Such ascriptions of psychological content mark a complex representational and causal relation that connects the neural mechanisms that we describe as a person's desires and other motives with the functional targets of these mechanisms external to that person's body, such as the glass, water, and world- and self-altering act of moving and drinking that we describe in the same breath as we specify the internal mechanism itself. Evolution has evidently compacted reference to these mechanisms into our concepts of desire, belief, etc., and bridged the relation of the mechanisms to the environment, and thence to related mechanisms in other communicating brains, with the natural-language sentences we use to specify what we feel, think, and want. What evolution has here woven together, science has scarcely begun to unravel.

So we encounter an enduring gap, as between our natural understanding of the mind (that is, of the mechanisms in the brain that we conceptualize as desires, beliefs, and other content-bearing motives and mental states), and our scientific understanding of the brain and body as the kind of biological and physical entities they are. This gap, however, is particularly important for the understanding of mental disorder. For such disorder mainly consists in disruption of the paradigmatic *mentally described* phenomena—perceptions, thoughts, feelings, desires, emotions—that our natural linguistically informed mode of psychological understanding has apparently evolved to articulate, coordinate, and regulate.

From this it follows, as we observe, that our approaches to mental disorder are subject to constant conceptual tension. In a clinical perspective it seems we must seek to understand disorder in terms of the evolutionarily preformed mental/linguistic categories in which it arises and in which we naturally experience and communicate about it. In the perspective of research, by contrast, we seem required to seek deeper understanding via the radically disparate categories of neuroscience, psychopharmacology, and other scientific disciplines. Hence the stance continually forced on psychiatry: one foothold in natural understanding; but always stretching towards other ground, surprisingly hard to reach, in sciences related to the brain—and often across gaps of incommensurability that render categorical synthesis a hopeless task.

THIS TENSION AND THE WORK OF FREUD

As is well known, such tension was formative for the work of Freud. He approached psychiatry as a neuroscientist who had written numerous papers based on bench research, as well as a monograph on aphasia that synthesized and extended current thinking. His neurological background enabled him to observe that hysterical neuralgias and paralyses (e.g. "glove paralysis") occurred within boundaries set by everyday thinking, as opposed to the nervous system itself. ("Hysteria knows nothing of anatomy.") Such knowledge, however, provided no means for actually treating the patients concerned. So on learning from Joseph Breuer of a therapeutic success achieved with a patient who remembered and relived emotionally significant incidents from her past related to her symptoms—a procedure the patient called a "talking cure"—Freud began trying to treat his patients in the same way.[4]

Breuer had enquired into this patient's symptoms, memories, and imaginings in great detail. "Her life" as he said, "had become known to me to an extent to which one person's life is seldom known to another" (Breuer and Freud, 1957, 21). Freud tried to treat his patients by an even deeper and more encompassing understanding, and so met with them frequently and pressed them for memories related to their symptoms. Shortly, however, it became clear that such memories, while sometimes veridical, were also liable to be distorted or replaced by fantasy.[5]

---

[4] Breuer's treatment of the patient described as Anna O has itself become a locus of historical imagining, much of it, as usual, aimed at discrediting Freud. This has recently been subjected to a careful and clarifying discussion in Skues (2006). This allows Breuer's modest but apparently genuine therapeutic success to be discerned.

[5] This lesson had to be relearned nearly a hundred years later, when thousands of women in the USA began to report recovered memories of childhood sexual abuse of the kind that Freud had elicited from his early patients. As the *Guardian* reported on December 3, 1993: " Across the United States, thousands of adults are recovering memories of having been sexually abused in childhood, memories they never knew they had. Sometimes they appear in a flashback, triggered by an event in their adult lives. But often the memories begin to emerge in therapy—even though the person may have sought therapy with little hint that his or her emotional problems stemmed from childhood abuse ... Psychiatrists, psychologists, and other mental-health professionals have split into warring camps over whether the sudden surge in recovered memories stems from better therapeutic techniques or a horrible abuse of therapeutic power ... What no one can say is how many of these memories are true, an uncertainty that has plunged the psychological-psychiatric community into a crisis."

As this indicates, a first response was to accept the claims of abuse, and criticize Freud or Freudians for claiming that some people were prone to imagine abuse that had not occurred. A second was to hold that the claims were often false, but to criticize Freud or Freudians for having elicited them by suggestion. Few reflected that the whole episode—the excited proliferation of the claims, as well as the intensity and tenacity with which they were maintained—was in accord with Freud's view that on this score memory was particularly liable to be distorted by fantasy and could not be trusted.

To avoid this Freud stopped pressing his patients for memories and asked them instead to cooperate in treatment by engaging in free association—that is, by describing the rapidly changing contents of their own conscious states of mind in as much detail as possible, and without omission or censorship. Such full and collaborative self-disclosure was without precedent in previous psychological investigation, and remains without parallel even today. It proved a singularly rich and valuable source of data, since over time it enabled Freud to learn as much about his patients' experiences, memories, thoughts, and feelings as they were able to put into words. In addition he was able to observe how these expressions were related to one another, to daily actions, and to dreams and symptoms. And here he was able to observe that repeatedly instantiated kinds of connections—interpretively detectable correlations[6]—held among the contents of associative memories, significant motives and emotions, dreams and symptoms, and intentional actions.

These correlations enabled Freud to reach conclusions about the symptoms of mental disorder (as well as dreams, slips, and other phenomena) that were fundamentally different from, but also provided an explanation of, those he had previously drawn on the basis of recovered memories. He came to see that his patients' ability to put their own mental states into words—the extent of their first-person authority in respect of their own minds and motives (Gertler 2011)—had striking and systematic limitations, which were explicable together with the symptoms of disorder in thinking and feeling that had impelled them to seek therapy. In particular, he now saw that there was often good and repeated reason to ascribe to patients, as to human beings more generally, unconscious activations of powerful but contradictory emotions—e.g. forms of admiration, gratitude, and love on the one hand, and contempt, anger, fear, and hatred on the other—that were directed both towards themselves and towards the persons most significant in their lives.

Such present-day conflicts, in turn, could be seen as repeating similar and more powerful conflicts experienced earlier and in relation to their parents. These were rooted in disparate images of the parents—the "earliest parental imagos" (1933, p. 54)—who during infancy were apparently liable to be felt both as very good and nurturing, and also as very bad and moralistically cruel, even from before articulate autobiographical memory. These early representations of the parents, moreover, seemed to play a deep regulatory role in the personalities of those he analyzed, particularly as regards the direction of aggression. In his analysis of the personality in terms of ego, superego, and id, he described how these imagos served to direct moralistic aggression against the self, as he had observed in (introjective) depression, and how this same aggression could also be externalized, as in paranoia.

Apparently psychological coherence in the individual and harmony in the family had required that images in which the parents were represented as good (or good enough for family cooperation) became dominant in the governance of behavior, whereas those in which they were represented as malicious or bad became recessive. This was achieved via the exclusion of the "bad" from consciousness, and so from a full role in thought and choice. Still, as it seemed, the excluded (and hence unthinkable) feelings and images remained causally active, and so were expressed in formations that were unchosen and irrational. Their influence could be seen in dreams and bungled actions, and again in distortions of consciousness and motivation characteristic of mental disorder. Thus aggression rooted in split-off images from the past might be felt in the present, and directed towards others in a

---

[6] This topic is discussed more fully in Hopkins (1999).

way that sabotaged projects and relationships; or again as directed towards the self, as in the ferocious self-criticism of depression and suicide.

A Psychiatric Illustration

As just indicated, the conflicts Freud described and sought to lessen were of two related kinds. There were, first, conflicts between incompatible emotions and desires, felt towards one and the same person—such as a parent who provided care but also aroused a high degree of anger and fear, or again a sibling with whom a deep family connection went with serious rivalry. Secondly, there were conflicts between parts or aspects of the self that had, as it were, crystallized around the early imagos of the parents, and now served in the regulation of emotion, e.g. *by turning moralistic aggression against the self.* Thus as Freud remarked, in certain kinds of depression: "We see how in [the depressed person] one part of the ego [*das Ich*] sets itself over against the other, judges it critically, and, as it were, takes it as its object."

Those who are depressed often direct ferocious moralistic anger towards themselves, regarding themselves as "worthless" and "morally despicable" (Freud 1957d, pp. 246–247). In this, Freud came to hold, they are identifying themselves with—taking as part of their selves or egos—the "earliest parental imagos" mentioned earlier. They are criticizing themselves with a ferocity, or from an idealized moralistic perspective, derived from early (and perhaps imaginary) experience. On Freud's account we all do this, and we will consider some normal examples below. But in those who are liable to mental disorder, these criticisms have an absoluteness and ferocity that makes them particularly difficult to knit into any kind of moral or psychological unity. Mental disorder is thus disorder in the kind of psychological functioning common to all people, but in psychological conditions so extreme that malfunction is much more likely.

Thus consider Elyn Saks' recent account of her own breakdown into depression and schizophrenia (Saks 2008). As she began to get depressed, Saks reports, her thoughts started to run along such intensely self-critical lines as: "I am not sick. I'm just a bad, defective, and evil person. Maybe if I would talk less I wouldn't spread my evil around" (Saks 2008, p. 58).

As time passed her self-reproaches became more constant, violent, and repetitive: "I am a piece of shit and I deserve to die. I am a piece of shit and I deserve to die. I am a piece of shit and I deserve to die" (Saks 2008, p. 61).

Saks' friends witnessed her deterioration and persuaded her to enter a psychiatric hospital, where she was diagnosed as depressed and given antidepressant medication. As the depression temporarily lessened, she told her doctor *that she felt less angry*, and remarked on "how much rage I had felt, directed mostly at myself" (Saks 2008, p. 69). We can see this as the phenomenon that Freud described earlier, in which one part of the self—the superego, or ego-ideal—sets itself over and above the other, and takes it as object of moralistic anger and hatred. And after Saks was discharged her self-reproaches resumed, so that she had to be admitted again, hating herself more than ever.

Despite constant and helpful attention from doctors and nurses her condition worsened, and she began to lose her sense of agency in relation to her own self-condemnation. The reproaches now: "crashed into my mind like a fullisade of rocks someone or something was hurling at me—fierce, jagged, and uncontrollable" (Saks 2008, p. 83). At this stage Saks still felt the reproaches as her own thoughts, albeit thoughts that came into her as concrete entities hurled aggressively by another. Shortly later she lost her sense of agency in this entirely. She no longer felt that *she* was engaged in self-reproach, nor that *her own* thoughts were involved. Rather she was "receiving commands" from "shapeless powerful beings that controlled me with thoughts (not voices) that had been placed in my head." Thus she was commanded: "Walk through the tunnels and repent. Now lie down and don't move. You are evil" (Saks 2008, p. 84).

As was appropriate to her evil, she also received commands to injure herself, which she obeyed by burning herself with cigarette lighters, electric heaters, or boiling water. Finally she spent most of her time: "alone in the music room or in the bathroom, burning my body, or moaning and rocking, holding myself as protection from unseen forces that might harm me" (Saks 2008, p. 86).

Thus Saks passed from a diagnosis of depression to one of paranoid schizophrenia. This trajectory had often been traced in psychoanalytic writings, beginning with Freud's account as to how, in schizophrenia, "the voices, as well as the undefined multitude [of potentially critical psychological presences embodied in the superego/ego-ideal] are brought into the foreground again by the disease" so that the sufferer's superego/ego-ideal "confronts him in a regressive form as a hostile influence from without" (Freud 1914/1957c)[7]—For this is what we see in Saks' reporting that "the commanding influence" responsible for her own self-directed moralistic cruelty "came from within my own head, but was not mine. It was someone else commanding me" (Saks 2008, p. 85).

In this we also see that Saks' diagnostic transition—and hence both the categories of depression and schizophrenia as applied in her particular case—fit Freud's overall description of mental disorder as rooted in emotional conflict. Her psychotic transition consisted in a kind of disintegration—together with an externalization or projection—of what had formerly been her depression-inflicting superego/ego-ideal. In this she (or her ego or brain) in effect substituted one form of emotional conflict for another: she (ego, brain) substituted *conflict with imaginary punishing others that constituted a kind of paranoia*, for *the unendurably painful conflict with an unrelentingly critical and cruel part of herself that had constituted her depression*.

As closely as this fits Freud's description, there is nothing yet in it to suggest any connection between the figures Saks felt menaced or controlled by and her parents as she saw them in infancy. Still some of the events she reports might be understood in this way. For example she describes her first experience of schizophrenic breakdown, at age seven or eight, as follows:

> My heart sinks at the tone of [her father's] voice: I've disappointed him. And then something odd happens: My awareness (of myself, of him, of the room, of the physical reality around and beyond us) instantly grows fuzzy ... I think I am dissolving ... like a sand castle with all the sand sliding away in the receding surf. *This is scary, please let it be over!* ... Most people know what it's like to be seriously afraid ... "disorganization" is a different matter altogether ... One's centre gives way ...
>
> Of course, my dad didn't notice what had happened, since it was all happening inside me. And frightened as I was at the moment, I intuitively knew that this was something I needed to hide from him, and from anyone else as well. (Saks 2008, pp. 12–13)

Saks first experienced terrifying schizophrenic disorganization in response to a moral reprimand from her father. This is consistent with the idea that the reprimand activated an

---

[7] For some recent discussion of partly similar examples see, e.g., Maltsberger (2008) and Bell (2008).

image of her father linked with deep fear from early in her life, so evoking the disintegrating terror she then felt. Although this is only a theoretical speculation about her particular case, the hypothesis would cohere with psychoanalytic findings in other cases.

For example, Freud's patient known as the Rat Man experienced his breakdown into obsessional neurosis when he was told—by the "Cruel Captain" who was "obviously fond of physical punishment"—of a torture in which hungry rats ate into the anuses of their victims, causing a painful death. At that moment he felt—as in a kind of waking nightmare—that the same torture was somehow being applied both to the girl he hoped to marry, and to his father, who was long dead. Overcome with anxiety and guilt, he started to try to prevent or preclude such torture by a series of obsessional actions.

This patient knew that he had been anxiously preoccupied with his father's death since early childhood. In his analysis he imagined Freud as a punitive "beast of prey" who would "fall on him to search out what was evil in him"—again the kind of image that Freud was later to relate to the superego/ego-ideal, and comparable both with the punitive figures imagined by Saks, and the way she was to imagine her own analyst in the course of her therapy. At the same time he remembered how his father's punishing him as a child had made him fear for his own life.

In experiencing Freud and remembering his father in this way, he could see—and with great relief—that both his present experience of Freud and his past experience of his father were illusory. This in turn made it possible to understand his breakdown (as well as the unconscious anger shown in his imagining his father being tortured) via the hypothesis that the cruel captain had unconsciously reminded him of his father as he had imagined him as a little child.[8] Saks' analysis concentrated on her present experience, and she had no such memories as Freud's Rat Man. Sill it is possible that a similar unconscious arousal of a past *imago* was responsible for her responding to her father's admonition with such disintegrative terror; and in the absence of some such account, her terror would remain inexplicable.

THEORETICAL DESCRIPTION

Previously we described Saks (or her ego or brain) in terms of a kind of *alteration in her conscious experience*. In place of *consciously and moralistically condemning and hating herself*, she came to imagine herself as *enslaved by moralistic condemning others who ensured that she was punished*. That is: the alterations in which her mental disorder was expressed (and in which it changed from depression to schizophrenia) we *alterations in her experience of herself*, or again *of herself as in relation to others*.

This is the kind of description facilitated by Freud's tripartite analysis of the personality as consisting of ego, superego/ego-ideal, and id. Although this account is now regarded as limited in various ways, it will be useful for exegetical purposes here. The Freudian Id was the hypothetical locus of the drives, or the "endogenous stimuli" that "gave rise to the major needs" (1950, 297a). We can now take these to be realized by the homeostatic and "multiple prototype emotional regulatory systems" mentioned earlier, which are shared across

---

[8] See "Notes upon a case of obsessional neurosis" and "Addendum: original record of the case" in Freud (1909/1957). This episode is discussed in the context of an account of the superego, ego, and id in terms of Bayesian neuroscience in Hopkins (2012).

mammalian species, and whose role has recently been elucidated by the work of Panksepp, Damasio, and other affective neuroscientists.[9]

Likewise we can take Freudian ego (*das Ich*) as the self, but conceived as in recent cognitive science, that is, not just as the subject of person-level states such as desire and belief, but also as the coordinator of a range of subpersonal functions. In Freud's conception one of the most important of these "executive functions" is that of regulating the basic drives and emotions, and in particular in managing conflicts among them, such as we see in Saks' and other examples of mental disorder. And as recently argued by Richard Carhart-Harris and Karl Friston, a functional conception of this kind, together with Freud's notion of primary and secondary processes, accords with a wide range of observations drawn from neuropsychology, neuroimaging, and psychopharmacology.[10]

The Freudian superego/ego-ideal is also conceived as a functional part of the self, but one whose work is discharged via (the ego's) representations of *persons,* or more fully, via *representations of the self,* or *of the self as in relation to others.* The representations we have taken this way so far include the representations of herself as morally hateful that were active in Saks' depression; those of herself as condemned and punished by others that were active in her paranoia; and the Rat Man's (paranoid) image of himself as in danger of punishment by a figure who would search out what was evil in him.

These are all examples of images in which moralistic aggression is directed towards, or turned against, the self. In light of them we can see that Freud's account of the functional role of the superego/ego-ideal contains an insight that has been lost in more recent and explicitly mechanical or computational discussions. This is, that *in our ultra-social species much of the mind's (or brain's) internal governance of its own motivation and emotion is effected by internal representations of our selves as in relation to members of our own species.* For, of course, it is natural that our brains should regulate our own emotions, as well as our relations with the individuals who are objects of these emotions, by images derived from, and representing, such individuals—and starting, as Freud held, with images of the parents, who are the first objects, as well as the first regulators, of the emotions in question.

Having seen something of the role of such imaginary images in mental disorder, it may be useful to compare an example from a normal dream. In this case the example is only illustrative, but we will come to better data later.

A Normal Comparison

Barack Obama's (1995) *Dreams from My Father* describes, among other things, his youthful attempts to come to terms with his emotional inheritance from the distant and authoritarian father who he had seen in person only for two short periods—the second marred by his

---

[9] For recent discussion—and for the important and closely related idea that both motivated behaviour and the conscious experience that accompanies and regulates it originate in the same subcortical regions and via the same or closely coordinated mechanisms—see Damasio et al. (2012) and Solms and Panksepp (2012). The consequences of this for psychoanalysis are considered in detail in Solms (in press) together with commentaries including Hopkins (in press).

[10] See Carhart-Harris and Friston (2010/2012). While these authors discuss ego-functions they lay no emphasis on emotional conflict.

resentment at his father's forbidding him (contrary to the practice of the grandparents who actually took care of him) to waste time watching television. (This intervention seems to have made a deep impression on Obama: in the presidential debates he described the role of the father in terms of telling the children to turn off the television to get on with their homework.)

An important episode in Obama's search for identity occurred when his aunt told him about his grandfather, supposedly the only man his father feared, and with whom, as she said, "the problems in this family all started" (1995, pp. 370ff). As she recalled: "A man came to the edge of our compound with a goat on a leash. He wanted to pass."

Obama's grandfather refused this reasonable request on the grounds that the goat might eat his plants. After pleading and assurance he agreed, but with a strict condition: "You can pass with your goat. But if even one leaf is harmed—if even *one half* of one leaf ... then I will cut down your goat also."

And in the event he enforced this condition remorselessly: "We had walked maybe twenty steps when the goat stuck out its head and started nibbling a leaf. Then—whoosh! My dad cut one side of the goat's head clean through ... The man had been warned."

After hearing this Obama had the following dream:

> I was walking along a village road ... I heard the growl of a leopard and started to run into the forest, tripping over roots and stumps and vines until at last I couldn't run any further ... I turned around to see the day turned to night, and a giant figure looming tall as the trees, wearing only a loincloth and a ghostly mask. The lifeless eyes bored into me, and I heard a thunderous voice saying only that it was time, and my entire body began to shake violently with the sound, as if I were breaking apart ... I jerked up in a sweat ... I couldn't get back to sleep again. (p. 372)

The figure that Obama imagined in his dream was clearly different from the "shadowy beings" imagined by Saks, or again the bestial figure imagined by Freud's patient. But like these the figure was a fearful one, and one in which, again, what we can see as moralistic aggression is directed towards, or turned against, the self. For Obama clearly saw this figure as personifying the harsh moral exactitude of the paternal line in which he was now seeking to locate himself, as this had been shown towards the little goat in the story he had been told. Also, it seems, he recognized the dream as articulating his own uneasy sense that he might be wasting his own lifetime, in travelling in Africa in search of a sense of identity and vocation that might enable him to fulfill the vague but apparently intense ambitions instilled in him by his parents (cf. his mother's waking him regularly early in the morning to go over his homework for the coming day: on the question of work for the future both parental figures were in agreement.)

So like Saks' depression and paranoia, or the Rat Man's obsessional neurosis, such a dream admits description in terms of Freud's account of the superego/ego-ideal. For as is made clear throughout his autobiography, the young Obama, like the little goat whose fate prompted his dream—and like Adam and Eve expelled from Eden—was not destined to waste time nibbling forbidden leaves.[11] In this perspective the terror that disrupted Obama's

---

[11] At pp. 377–378 Obama (1995) describes what seems a linked incident, in which his grandfather recues a little goat, abducted by a terrifying night runner, which seems the kind of figure depicted in the dream. So I am inclined to guess that this story may also have entered into the formation of this dream, although Obama describes hearing it afterwards.

sleep—"as if I was breaking apart"—may have been similar in nature to that experienced by Saks in her schizophrenic disintegration. Both these instances of mental disturbance apparently involved the arousal of overwhelming fear, in the context of emotional conflict; and the same holds for Freud's patient's breakdown into obsessional neurosis and his terrified imaginings about Freud.

Further evidence (were we able to collect it) might well support the claim that in all of these instances the fear involved was derived from the early images of the parents that Freud took to be embodied in the superego/ego-ideal. And although we cannot collect further evidence in these cases, we can compare them with others in which more evidence is available, and in a usefully illustrative way.

THE REGULATION OF EMOTION BY IMAGINARY FIGURES AND FICTIVE EXPERIENCE IN DREAMS

The kinds of figure we have been discussing are often described in post-Freudian psychoanalysis as *internal objects*. The particular emotion-regulating personifications that Freud gathered under the head of the superego/ego-ideal are now seen as just the clinically first-discovered of a *range* of figures that play comparable regulatory roles. This shift of attention facilitates more detailed clinical focus on the particular constellations of imaginary figures that are to be found in each individual case. (A similar development has taken place in respect of the personified archetypal figures described by Jung.) So we can ask: How do such imaginary figures serve to regulate emotion? Here part of the answer seems both simpler and deeper than might first appear. We can start to describe it by considering the causal role of desire together with two simple dreams.

In human beings as well as other animals desire operates in accord with a regular causal pattern. Both motivation and consciousness seem to have their sources deep in subcortical systems that we have taken as the locus of the Freudian drives; for, as we are now discovering, motivation and consciousness are systematically related to one another, since motor behavior is regulated via its sensory consequences, including immediate sensory feedback. In animals in which this regulatory neural input takes the form of *conscious experience of the causes of input*[12] this is a particularly important aspect of ongoing (external and internal) sensory experience.

We are concerned with an aspect of such regulation of motor behavior, namely the way experience regulates the motives that give rise to purposive action. To examine this in a general way we can take the paradigmatic case of thirst and drinking: for this is both a basic aspect of homeostatic regulation and one whose working is clearly marked in conscious experience. Let us refer to the subcortical mechanisms that govern the arousal of thirst,

---

[12] Hence the significance, in this context, of the Bayesian slogan that (in conscious animals) *the brain represents neural input as conscious experience of the causes of the input*. This is the point at which the conception of the Bayesian brain, as described in Hopkins (2012) dovetails with the claim by Damasio, Panksepp, and others that the mechanisms that produce motives also produce the conscious experience that regulates motivation. On this see also Hopkins (in press).

and hence the subsequent motor behavior of drinking, simply as desire-producing mechanisms.[13] Then representing the agent by "A" and the appropriate causal relations by "→," we can trace a sequence from the subcortical activation of motivation and consciousness through the production of conscious desire (conscious thirst, or a conscious desire to get a drink) and then through the production of desire-satisfying intentional action (the action of getting a drink) to the sensory feedback (the experience of drinking) that pacifies desire—presumably by inhibiting both the experiential and motivational role of thirst at the subcortical level at which it originates. This gives:

> Desire-producing mechanisms in A → A desires that A drinks → A drinks → A experiences, believes A drinks → A's desire that A drinks is pacified (ceases to operate).

This pattern can readily be generalized and abbreviated to cover the arousal of desires of all kinds:

> Desire-producing mechanisms in A → A desires P → P → A exps, bels P → A des P pacified.

Here "P" can be replaced by any suitable sentence specifying an agent's desire that he or she act in a certain way, so (if successful) bringing about the satisfaction of that desire, and then the experience of having acted successfully that terminates its operation. This indicates the pattern in accord with which desire-producing mechanisms operate to cause an action-producing conscious desire, and how the regulation of that desire in action is effected by sensory feedback from the action itself—in particular by what Freud called the *experience of satisfaction*—whose role we have abbreviated in the "A exps, bels P" in the earlier schema. This desire-regulating experience was also a key component of Freud's clinical psychology, and of the neuroscientific hypotheses that he framed to take account of his clinical findings; and it played a central role in his understanding of dreams as well.

We can illustrate this via the role of thirst in dreams. Freud observed that when he had eaten anchovies or other salty foods, he was liable to dream *that he was drinking delicious cool water.* He would have this dream several times, until finally he awoke and got a drink. (There is, of course, a parallel dream concerning urination. In this case, having dreamt several times of having a satisfying pee, the dreamer awakes to experience sensations of a full bladder, and empties it for real.)

Dreams produce genuine, if fictitious, conscious experience; and this dream shows the same pattern of the control of motivation by an experience of satisfaction as we saw in the case of desire in action earlier. In the case of dreaming of drinking we have:

> Desire-producing mechanisms in A → A des A drinks → A *dream-exps, bels* A drinks → A's des A drinks pacified.

Here, and by contrast with the case of waking action, the experience of satisfaction that pacifies the nascent desire occurs as part of a dream, and so is not actually produced by

---

[13] This is meant to integrate the present discussion with Ruth Garret Millikan's descriptions of the role of representation-producing mechanisms (including desire- and belief-producing mechanisms) in her account of intentionality. This is briefly discussed in connection with neuroscience in Hopkins (2012).

the satisfaction of the desire in question. Rather *this experience is a fiction produced by the brain*, presumably (as Freud hypothesized) *to prolong sleep by pacifying the nascent desire that might interrupt it*. This is another instance of conflict, and among basic homeostatic mechanisms; for waking would perturb the homeostatic functions of sleep, which the brain at this juncture seems to be working to continue.[14] So such simple examples indicate how *the brain works to regulate its own motivational functioning in situations of conflict by providing fictitious sensory input that has a comparable effect (here in the pacification of desire) to that which real experience would have.*

Freud called such use of the desire-pacifying role of the experience of satisfaction *wishfulfilment*, and his first distinctively psychoanalytic discoveries often consisted in detecting the role of wishfulfilment in various forms of motivational conflict: in slips, dreams, symptoms, and other formations where the brain apparently used this mechanism to pacify one or another desire involved in conflict. This appears to be a form of neurobiological regulation that links Freudian psychology with psychiatry and neuroscience. For the cases involving the superego/ego-ideal that we have been considering also apparently involve the regulatory use of fictitious experience, but in more complex ways.

As we have seen, the provision by Saks' brain (or her ego) of a fictive experience of punitive moralistic external presences served to mitigate the internal conflict—moralistic anger directed by herself at herself—that constituted her depression. As noted, we have very little evidence bearing on Obama's dream. But it, too, seems an example of his own brain producing a fictive experience of a presence directing anger against the self; and we can recognize that the question of *it being time* may well have been particularly significant for the ambitious and self-controlled and so far not particularly successful young man who had it. And while we lack further data that might help us understand Obama's dream, we can find much fuller and more detailed examples in those of Freud.

The first dream Freud analyzed—the "Specimen Dream" of Irma's injection—was prompted by his colleague Otto's mentioning to him that his former patient Irma (whose family Otto had just visited) seemed "better, but not yet well."[15] For reasons Freud's associations make clearer, he felt this as some sort of reproof, and began writing up Irma's case history in order to justify himself. That night he dreamt that Irma had a serious organic illness, caused, as it transpired in the dream, by Otto's having thoughtlessly given her an injection that was toxic, and with a dirty syringe. Freud construed this as a wishfulfilment, on the same model as the dream of drinking earlier, and we can see why he did so. The dream represented Irma's distress as organic, so that his psychotherapy could not be at fault; and it represented her distress as the responsibility of Otto as opposed to himself.[16]

Freud's early account of dreaming as wishfulfilment left the matters with which we have been concerned—the superego/ego-ideal and its relations to depression, externalization in the form of paranoia, etc.—out of account. Still if we look at Freud's early associations in

---

[14] This again is discussed in Hopkins (2012). Since that article Hobson and Friston (2012) have produced a comprehensive Bayesian account of dreaming that indicates a role for neural homeostasis consistent with that discussion, and also with the present account of the role of imaginary experience in regulating emotion.

[15] The quotations in the following paragraphs are from Freud's "Analysis of a specimen dream" (1900/1957a).

[16] For an account that spells this out in detail see Hopkins (1999).

light of the later development of his theories, we can see how they fit with the account of the regulation of emotion by fictive experience that we have been considering. For as Freud records, his association turned to a series of his own medical failures and derelictions. These included his advocacy of cocaine ("which had brought serious reproaches down on me"), and two cases involving injection: one in which a patient he had injected had died as a result, and another in which a "dear friend" whom he had encouraged in the use of cocaine had died from injecting it. These were clearly matters of potential self-reproach, and they were particularly transformed in the dream: for it was Otto as opposed to Freud who gave a toxic injection, and Freud who condemned him for it, by saying "one does not give such injections so thoughtlessly; and probably the syringe was not clean."

As he recorded his associations about his own derelictions, Freud remarked: "It seemed as if I had been collecting all the occasions I could bring up against myself as evidence of lack of medical conscientiousness." And indeed the part or aspect of himself that was collecting and bringing such things against himself seemed also to threaten him with a primitive form of moral retribution.

> [the patient who succumbed to his toxic injection] had the same name as my eldest daughter. It had never occurred to me before, but it struck me now almost like an act of retribution on the part of destiny. It was as though the replacement of one person by another [in his dream] was to be continued in another sense: this Mathilde for that Mathilde, an eye for an eye and a tooth for a tooth.

So in Freud's associations to the first dream he analyzed, we find that he spontaneously recorded *how a part or aspect of his self was collecting instances of his own medical dereliction to set against him*; or, as he was to put the same idea in the context of psychotic depression many years later, how a part or aspect of his ego "set itself over against the other, judged it critically, and as it were took it as its object." And this part of his self seemed to the early Freud somehow to threaten him with retribution in the form of the death of his own daughter, taking "this Mathilde for that Mathilde, an eye for an eye and a tooth for a tooth."

We could scarcely hope to find a more precise description of the working of the moralistic and ruthlessly self-critical part of the self that Freud was later to describe in terms of the superego/ego-ideal. Freud's associations here enable us to see him detecting the nocturnal working of his superego/ego-ideal without recognizing that he was doing so. His overall response, however, was strikingly different from that of Saks. The fictive experience provided by his brain—of Otto's having carelessly given Irma a toxic injection—*enabled him to regard Otto, as opposed to himself, as the source of such derelictions as his superego/ego-ideal had been collecting to bring against him.* So in the dream he could turn the tables on Otto, and assume the role of superego/ego-ideal himself—as he did in ending the dream by saying "One does not make injections of that kind so thoughtlessly."[17]

---

[17] As this indicates, the dream Freud first analyzed as an instance of wishfulfilment is better seen as an instance of projection, in which Freud represents himself as better and Otto as worse by locating in Otto the characteristics he would condemn in himself, the better to condemn them in Otto. This can be seen as wishfulfilling, because it represented things as Freud would have wished them to be; but in general projection should be distinguished from wishfulfilment: as in Saks, Schreber, and countless other examples, the projection of badness into other persons of groups can lead directly to forms of paranoia.

We can thus regard the various examples we have considered—the symptoms of Saks' depression and schizophrenia, Obama's dream, the Rat Man's symptom, Freud's simple dream of drinking and the comparable dream of urination, and Freud's more complex dream of Irma's injection—as instances of the working of the same sort of neurobiological mechanism. The mechanism is *the brain's management of motivational or emotional conflict, by the presentation to the self of fictitious conscious sensory experience.* There seems little doubt that there is such a mechanism—it is too clearly in play in the simple dreams to be dismissed—and it is a very intelligible development of the deep and pervasive role of the regulation of motive by conscious experience that seems to hold for all mammals, and probably for other animals as well. So let us consider the possible explanatory scope of this mechanism in more detail.

FORMS OF CONFLICT AND FORMS OF DISORDER

We saw earlier how Saks could be described as having projected aspects of the superego/ego-ideal that had animated her own depressing moralistic self-hatred. Another conflict-mitigating alternative, in Freudian terms, would have been for her to *identify herself* with her superego/ego-ideal, and thereby represent all morally censurable faults as located elsewhere than in her self. This is in effect what Freud did in his dream of Irma's injection, and he later took this mode of defense to be characteristic of mania.

Freud's concept of the superego/ego-ideal thus involves a "choice of illness" for the main mental disorders, as related to the role of the imagos the he took to be derived from the parents. The alternatives are: (a) suffering the persecuting self-denigrating superego/ego-ideal in depression (b) relieving the depressive conflict by imagining oneself to embody the superego/ego-ideal (and hence unrealistically overvaluing the self and undervaluing others), as in mania (with oscillations between these positions constituting bipolar disorder). And (c) relieving the depressive conflict by projecting and fragmenting the superego/ego-ideal in various paranoid formations, as apparent in Saks and many comparable cases, including that of Schreber as described by Freud.[18]

EVOLUTION, EMOTION, AND GROUP CONFLICT

The roles that we can discern here in individuals also accord with those Freud assigned to the same psychological structures in the emotional regulation of groups. He took human groups to achieve the common moral and ideological stance required for ingroup cooperation by taking leaders and/or creeds (ideologies, norms) as constitutive of their superegos/ego-ideals. This entailed that within-group deviations from these—disloyalty to the leader, failure to adhere to patriotic or other norms—would be grounds for individual guilt and shame and social punishment. Hence also, as Freud stressed, such ingroup cohesion went

---

[18] See "Autobiographical notes on a case of paranoia" in Freud (1911/1957b).

with hatred and violence towards outgroups. For ingroup idealization of a group-defining creed or leader was liable to represent outgroups defined by dissociation from these as morally reprehensible, and hence as potential objects of morally mandated outgroup violence.[19]

This illustrates how internal conflicts of the kind suffered by Saks (as well, if Freud is right, as everybody else) are externalized in groups and relations among them. The group mindset of *good us against bad them* produced by the group equivalent of antidepressive mania—ingroup identification with the superego/ego-ideal entailing the location of depressing badness elsewhere—seems a common feature of human group conflict. It has animated countless religious conflicts and wars, and can be seen in the facilitation of the holocaust by the idealization of Hitler, the current demonization of Muslims and idealization of militarism in the United States, and so on *ad finem nostrum*. Also there is a strong case for holding that this same mindset—and hence the Freudian mechanisms that underpin it—should itself be regarded as a product of evolution.

Darwin originally sought to explain "the moral and social qualities of man"—including our capacities for self-sacrifice and cooperation—by the fact that "at all times throughout the world tribes have supplanted other tribes." The key to success in this process, he thought, was ingroup cooperation for outgroup conflict. This entailed the selection of ingroup self-sacrifice, patriotism, and other distinctive human adaptations, as opposed to the "selfishness and treachery" that "the survival of the fittest" might otherwise be expected to yield. Such a process, we may note, might also promote the evolution of language, emotions like guilt and shame, institutions of social punishment, and that ability to understand one another in commonsense terms with which we began. Each of these seems apt to improve the ingroup cooperation and cohesion that Darwin had in mind; and evolutionary theorists have recently produced convincing accounts of the co-evolution of genes and culture in which ingroup cooperation for outgroup competition plays a central role (see, e.g., Richerson and Boyd 2006).

Such accounts can also be taken to predict the kind of internalization of norms and punishment that suppress aggression so as to yield cooperation within ingroups while directing aggression towards outgroups that we see in the Freudian account of the superego/ego-ideal.[20] If so then, as Freud envisaged, we might regard the kinds of conflict that give rise to mental disorder as rooted in evolution. The kinds of mental disorder we have been considering would then be explicable in a still wider context. They would be expectable form of malfunctioning, in the complex task set the ego (or the brain) in the management of aggression in our astonishingly social but also lethally group-aggressive species.

We cooperate in multiple ingroups, in which we inhibit aggression towards others, and take it as cause for ingroup guilt, shame, and punishment; and this can at least partly be seen as controlling aggression by turning aggression against ourselves. At the same time this cooperation is characteristically in the service of competing with outgroups, and so often involves directing aggression against them. In this case the role of guilt, shame, and punishment is no longer that of inhibiting aggression: patriotism puts these emotions into the service of amplifying aggression against the outgroup, via the stance of *good us/bad them* discussed earlier.

---

[19] For a recent and more up-to-date treatment of this topic see Kernberg (2003).

[20] The relation between Freudian and Darwinian theories touched on here is discussed further in Hopkins (2003, 2004).

The basic parameters for this remarkably complex system—involving the constant determination and re-determination of in- and out-groups and the direction of aggression among them—seem again to be set in early childhood, and also via the use of the early imagos Freud described in terms of the superego/ego-ideal. This in turn seems part of the reason that the paradigmatic mental disorders involve excesses of aggression-inhibiting guilt, forms of overvaluing the self as opposed to others, and paranoid fear, all of which play essential roles in ingroup cohesion for outgroup aggression that parallel their roles in individual disorder. Deeper understanding of mental disorder should clarify these links as well.[21]

Emotional Conflict Within Psychoanalytic Therapy

Engrossed in her fictive experience, Saks continued to deteriorate, until the doctors caring for her arranged for a consultation with a psychiatrist who was also a psychoanalyst. On meeting him she felt, for the first time, that despite her confusion she might be understood by another, and so might be able to understand herself. Encouraged by this she arranged to begin full-time treatment with a non-medical analyst outside her mental hospital. Although her prognosis was thought poor, she left hospital for this purpose. And as was to be expected, in this setting her emotional conflicts began to take new and equally powerful forms.

As her analysis progressed her psychotic thoughts grew more violent during her sessions. Her relationship to her analyst became suffused with three partly contradictory currents of imagination and feeling—intense anger and fear, intense dependent affection, and intense anxiety and dread at separation. So, e.g. she associated to her analyst: "You are an evil monster … a witch … you are trying to kill me … Don't cross me. I've killed hundreds of thousands of people with my thoughts" (Saks 2008, p. 97). Or again she thought to herself: "She is evil and dangerous … She is a monster. I must kill her, or threaten her, to stop her doing evil things to me" (p. 98).

The closer she felt to her analyst the more terrified she became. So she perused shops for weapons, and for period brought a box-cutter or serrated knife to her sessions (which of course she never had occasion to use). But also:

> At the very same time as I was terrified of Mrs. Jones, I was equally terrified that I was going to lose her, so much so that I could barely tolerate weekends when I would not see her for two days. I would start to unravel on Thursday and be nearly inconsolable until Tuesday. In the intervening time it took everything I had to protect myself … all the while plotting ways to keep Mrs. Jones from abandoning me. *I will kidnap her and keep her tied up in my closet. I will take good care of her … She will always be there to give me psychoanalysis …* her steady and calm presence contained me, as if she were the glue that held me together. I was falling apart, flying apart, exploding—and she gathered my pieces and held me. (Saks 2008, pp. 97–98)

Violent and contradictory as her feelings and phantasies were, expressing and discussing them, and testing them against what she actually experienced in her relationship with her

---

[21] The discussion of ego, superego and id in Hopkins (2012) is supplement by consideration of recent advancements in affective neuroscience in Hopkins (in press).

analyst, gradually had an effect. Although she remained liable to hallucinatory presences, she found that as she:

> became accustomed [in analysis] to spooling out the strange products of my mind my paranoia began to shift … the actual daily people in my comings and goings seemed less scary and more approachable … slowly I made one friend, then two … I began to move back into the world again … Blinking and shaky (as though I'd been in a cave, and the light, as welcome as it was, was something I had to get used to) I began to move back into the world again. (Saks 2008, pp. 93–94)

Again, Saks' phantasies provide clear examples of conflicting motives directed at one and the same person. Also they exemplify the state of mind that Melanie Klein described as the paranoid-schizoid position, in which the same person (originally, in Klein's account, the mother, or the part of her that was the most important early sensory focus, her breast) is felt either as extremely bad and threatening or as extremely helpful and good. So on their hypotheses—as indicated by Freud's remarks on the regressive fragmentation of the super-ego/ego-ideal in schizophrenia—the passage from depression to schizophrenia considered earlier would represent a reversal of the process by which the self-condemning part of herself manifest in her depression was originally formed.

On this kind of account the gathering together of her fragmenting self that Saks gratefully ascribed to her analyst would represent a partial reworking in the present of basic processes of integrating the self that take place in the interaction of an infant with its mother (and other carers) from early in life. Likewise the pain of separation that Saks found so intolerable at weekends, and the grief and phantasies of control that it evoked, would partly repeat those of an infantile self, threatened by separation with loss of the parental presence that seemed the source life and coherence for the self.

As this indicates, Saks' analysis was felt by her to be healing and revelatory, and enabled her to resume work and to relate to people, and to start to build for herself what was to prove an intellectually distinguished and emotionally satisfying life. This does not, of course, mean that it was a cure for her schizophrenia. Remarkable as her analysis was at sustaining and helping her in the absence of medication, when she sought to terminate it she broke down. After her last session she had to be torn from a radiator to which she had attached herself, and was persuaded to leave her analyst's house only when she realized that the alternative was removal by the police. She was to rely on chemical as well as psychoanalytic help for many years to come.

Still her treatment remains an impressive example of psychiatric help that came from being deeply understood, and that was life-changing in relation to a serious psychotic condition. This accords with recent clinical and neuroscientific studies indicating that psychoanalytic therapy has demonstrable therapeutic effect; and there is some evidence that this turns on its effect on images of the parents, as these have been independently investigated in attachment-based developmental psychology (see Buchheim 2012; Schedler, 2010). Also it underlines a point that may prove important in psychiatry. What appears as comorbidity among distinct diagnostic categories (and at times Saks was obsessional and anorexic as well) may in a deeper psychological perspective be seen as different forms of the same underlying—and universal—human emotional conflicts, as these are mediated by a provision of fictive experience that may have evolved for this purpose.

Moral Conflict and Its
Emotional and Genetic Roots

Why did Saks think she was so evil that she was a piece of shit who deserved to die? Her account does not fully explain this. In the case of the Rat Man we can see clearly how the guilt he suffered stemmed directly from his aggressive phantasies—for he would become anxious and guilty, and think he deserved to die, as a result of imagining his father tortured. Saks also had powerful aggressive phantasies, sometimes related to guilt. As she claimed during one of her breakdowns: "*There will be raging fires, and hundreds, maybe thousands of people lying dead in the streets. And it will all—all of it—be my fault*" (Saks 2008, p. 4).

Her dialogues show how she constantly imagined killing the analyst upon whom, at the same time, she felt utterly dependent, and even as she was feeling relief, hope, and gratitude for the treatment she was receiving. But in addition she had another and particularly striking set of imaginings, that might well have been linked with guilt. She constantly imagined killing fetuses and babies. Indeed she found her thoughts about this particularly hard to control, as she supposed that others might agree with her:

> There were whole parts of myself I tried desperately to keep hidden. I knew, for instance, not to share my ongoing delusions of evil ... but as hard as I tried, I'd sometimes find the wrong words coming to my lips—for example the memorable night we all sat on the roof and I casually mentioned having killed many children.
>
> "It's a joke!" I quipped ... noting with alarm the expressions on their faces—uncertainty at first, and then, slowly, a hint of horror. "A stupid joke! Oh come on, everybody wants to kill kids once in a while, don't they." (Saks 2008, p. 95)

In her analysis these phantasies were understood as expressions of *sibling rivalry*. From the time he wrote *The Interpretation of Dreams* Freud held that analysis indicated that everyday rivalries between brothers and sisters were underlain by deeper unconscious hostilities. This was later borne out in Melanie Klein's analyses of children, who often played out hostile phantasies towards siblings or parents in detail.[22] More recently biologists have come to recognize that aggression towards siblings, and even towards parents, may be predicted by evolutionary theory. This is discussed in terms of the interrelated notions of *parental investment, sexual conflict*, and *parent–offspring conflict*.[23] Some relations among these are depicted in Fig. 73.1, which is based on that at p. 41 of Mock and Parker (1997), *The Evolution of Sibling Rivalry*. The developmental arrow at the right has been added for discussion here.

At first pass the notions of sexual conflict and parent–offspring conflict concern only probabilities for the replications of genes. But evolutionary theorists take these to yield

---

[22] For a recent discussion see Mitchell (2003).

[23] Robert Trivers' pioneering essays on these topics are in Trivers (2002): see particularly "Parental investment and reproductive success" and "Parent–offspring conflict." The latter is linked in detail with sexual conflict in Mock and Parker (1997) and both are illuminatingly discussed in Hrdy (2000). The linked topics of parental investment and parent-offspring conflict related briefly to psychoanalysis in Hopkins (2003, 2004) as well as to neuroscience and attachment in Hopkins (2012).

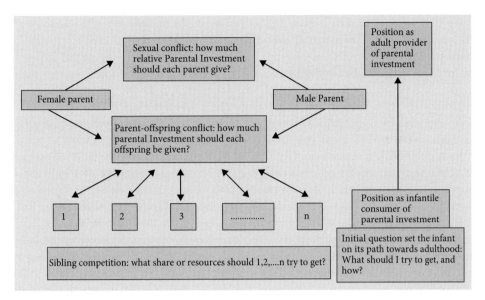

FIGURE 73.1 Relationships between parental investment, sexual conflict, and parent–offspring conflict. Adapted from Mock, D. and Parker, A. (1997). *The Evolution of Sibling Rivalry*, p. 41 © 1997, Oxford University Press, with permission.

co-evolving patterns of adaptation and counter-adaptation that encompass both physiology and psychology.[24] The notion of *parental investment* is intended to encompass the provision by parents of anything that contributes to the thriving of a particular offspring, where this is done at a cost to the parent in contributing to the thriving of other offspring (or at cost to the parent's fitness more generally). Such an abstract notion is difficult to apply in practice, but reasonable comparisons and judgments can still be made. Thus the physiological and emotional investment (or cost) incurred a female who conceives an offspring, carries it for months in her womb, gives birth to it, and feeds it from her breast for some months afterwards, can clearly be regarded as more significant than that incurred by a male who participates for a few minutes in its conception and looks after (and plays with it, etc.) for some hours a week after it is born. (And of course the investment of a father who opts out of post-coital participation is infinitesimal even by comparison with this).

[24] Thus the working of these conflicts can apparently be observed from conception, in the invasion of the mother's body by the placenta. This organ is constructed via the activity of the father's genome, to extract maternal investment on behalf of the fetus, and discounting, in accord with the father's ability to invest elsewhere, other children the mother might have. Accordingly the placenta develops as "a ruthless parasitic organ existing solely for the maintenance and protection of the fetus, perhaps too often to the disregard of the maternal organism" (quoted in Hrdy 2000). In this it bores into the mother's blood vessels, secreting hormones that raise her blood pressure and sugars in ways that may injure her but benefit the fetus. The mother's body responds by producing hormones that counteract these; and so on. Here we can see how sexual conflict between the genes of the parents, as carried forward in countervailing physiological adaptations over countless generation, is also physiological conflict between a pregnant mother and her unborn child. (And the sexual conflict embodied in the placenta may be involved in sibling rivalry more directly, as when one of a potentially multiple birth aborts others.) For further discussion see Haig (1993).

As this suggests, among human beings (as among mammals generally) females are the greater providers of parental investment—so much so that women's capacity for child-bearing sets a limit to men's reproductive success. But where the nature of parental investment systematically differs as between reproductive partners, so too must many aspects of reproductive functioning and behavior related to it—the parents' strategies in courting and choice of mates (and so the conditions in which the seek or avoid intercourse), their responses to conception and pregnancy, their behavior in rearing offspring once they are born, and so on.

Such differences generate *sexual conflict*, for they entail that radically different motives or conflicting patterns of behavior will result in successful replication of a mother's as opposed to a father's genes (see Gegestand 2007). Thus if female fecundity limits male reproductive success we should expect males to compete for access to females, and to work hard to gain it, as is observed for many species. And if females must incur much larger costs than males in investing in an offspring, they have far more to lose by fast and indiscriminate mating, and correspondingly more to gain by exercising careful choice (e.g. in the genes or capacity for investment of those they mate with). So as in many other species, human females copulate more selectively than males. This pits female selectivity against male opportunism, in the forms of sexual conflict that are still referred to as the battle of the sexes.

Part of this battle stems from the fact that there are many circumstances in which it is in the genetic interests of either parent to shift the burden of investment to the other, or again to reproduce elsewhere. Men regularly abandon partners, leaving them to bring up children on their own, sometimes to start another family elsewhere; and women occasionally do the same. A woman can sometimes secure investment by establishing or feigning paternity, as a man can avoid it by denial or simply refusing to participate. These are familiar sources of infidelity, deceit, betrayal, and other sources of domestic discord. As they indicate, both men and women can also shift investment from present to future offspring, where the future can include alternative reproductive partners. The means for this include abortion, infanticide, adoption, orphanage, and many forms of selective neglect.

These are sometimes employed with offspring that seem bad or costly bets: burdensome, unviable, unrewarding, socially inconvenient, or just less likely than others to carry on the line. But in hard times abandoning one or more children may be the only means of securing the survival of others. So the notions of parental investment and sexual conflict carry that of parent–offspring conflict—conflict between the interests of the genes of parents as opposed to those of their offspring—in their wake. This in turn sets the stage for sibling rivalry, as we see even in domestic pets. Puppies or kittens often die because they cannot get access to milk; and this is not simple misfortune, but the effect of sibling competition as mediated by parental investment.

So in other circumstances some pigs are born with tusks to slash their sibs, young birds regularly peck weaker sibs to death, bird parents intervene to kill superfluous nestlings, and so on and on.[25] Sharks are particularly striking in this respect. The female sand tiger has two uteruses, and the fetuses in each devour one another until only a separated pair remains. This compression of development and learning enables her selected brood to enter the sea as well-nourished, natural-born, and practiced killers (Eilperin 2012). The corresponding

---

[25] For examples and discussion see Mock (2005) and Mock and Parker (1997).

psychoanalytic claim—that human infants have hostile impulses towards parents and siblings that are repressed within the family, in such a way as to be channeled into outgroup competition—seems mild and sociable by comparison.

The links between parental investment and sexual and parent–offspring conflict have led evolutionary theorists to argue that the genetic interests of offspring would best be served by what they describe as "true monogamy" (Mock and Parker 1997, esp. p. 222) which corresponds to the human moral ideal of lifelong faithful marriage centered on the rearing of children. It is remarkable that biological and moral concepts should coincide in this way, and suggests that we should see the imagos produced by the superego/ego-ideal as regulating sexual and parent–offspring conflict. For, which emotions work to limit infidelity, deception, and betrayal of partners, or again against neglect, infanticide, or abandonment of children? Of course there are forms of love, attachment, and empathic concern. But also, and crucially, there is guilt, shame, and fear of punishment or censure—the so-called moral emotions—and the internalization of these in the superego/ego ideal. As our addition to Mock and Parker's diagram is meant to illustrate, the infant's brain and mind first come to address the basic practical/moral question of life—What shall I try to get, and how?—as powerless dependent consumers of parental investment. A significant part of maturation apparently consists in moving from this initial position to that of a competent provider of such investment, and one who is perforce in potential sexual conflict with his or her partner or partners. From the perspective of evolution, this seems one of the most significant of human psychological developments.

Unlike sharks human infants are born neurologically premature and physically uncoordinated. Their individual shortcomings, however, are more than offset by their social connections. The subcortical homeostatic and "multiple prototype emotional regulatory systems" are operative at birth, and wired for expression in their faces, voices, and movements. Their automatic engagement enables infants to begin life-sustaining emotional relationships with others even before they start the related task of using their experience of these relationships to build the *representations* of their selves in relation to others that will later subject the same emotions to cortical and cognitive regulation. For since the basic sub-cortical mechanisms of motivation also produce the conscious experience of the consequences of movement that regulates the working of motive, the scope of infantile consciousness and infantile action develop together, and towards the setting of the "regulatory lynch-pin" of attachment that is achieved by the end of the first year.

Infants are also born into parent–offspring conflict. For while we should expect evolution to prepare offspring to secure a maximum of parental investment for themselves, it should prepare parents to apportion investment over more than one offspring—so fating offspring to seek more than parents are prepared to give, and at the expense of siblings, whether actual or potential. (Parents themselves, moreover, are liable to conflict over provision, even from relatively soon after birth: a father's genes might be best served by rapid re-impregnation of the mother, but hers by waiting to ensure that infant she has labored to bring to term is well established, and her body recovered, before starting again.) In such conflicts human babies can exercise few powers apart from their expressions of emotion.

Speaking very roughly, babies can express emotion in their own genetic interests in two main ways. They can use the circuits that Panksepp describes in terms RAGE, FEAR, and separation distress/PANIC/GRIEF. These tend to operate together, as they seem to do in babies' uniquely penetrating, guilt-inducing, and compelling cries. In this they serve as babies' main means of coercing what they most urgently need. (And in light of parent–offspring conflict we can see that an infant's expressions of rage at shortcomings in maternal care are continuous with the evolutionary function of anger in conflict over resources more generally.) Alternately, however, babies can exercise the systems that Panksepp describes in terms of SEEKING, LUST, and PLAY. These are ingredients of cooperative and affectionate attachment, and the "good" early imagos of the parents, as Freud stressed (and as research in attachment seems to be bearing out) apparently serve as lifelong prototypes for relationships of affection and love.

Sara Blaffer Hrdy has long stressed the evolutionary importance for babies of being able to evoke love and care (see Hrdy 2000, 2009). It seems a direct consequence of the concepts we have been considering that babies stand to increase their share of parental investment by using their abilities to evoke love and care—as well as their anger, distress, etc.—in a particular way: that is, *in any emotional or other manipulation that impedes their parents in conceiving another child.* And this obstruction of alternative lives is not some remote theoretical possibility: rather it is what babies naturally and affectionately do in feeding at the breast. Infants often show every sign of regarding this as a particularly significant, valuable, and pleasurable relationship; and something similar may hold for mothers as well. But since the infant's activity at the breast is contraceptive, it can also be seen as part of an alliance between mother and infant—saving the former from the wear and tear of fast-repeated pregnancy, and enabling the latter better to thrive—as against the genetic interests (and in some cases the overt jealousy) of the father.

The infant's first sensual and affectionate relationship at the breast is also its first engagement in parent–offspring and sexual conflict. This may be the neurobiological inception of the developments that Freud described in terms of the Oedipus complex—and it also involves the regulation of aggression by the development of guilt, concern, and other moral emotions that (as I have sketched elsewhere) we can partly trace over the course of the first year.[26] In this we see evolutionary and emotional conflict at work together, for human infants are bound in the network of conflict we have been considering *to feel and express powerful but conflicting emotions towards one and the same person—particularly the mother—from shortly after birth.* This seems to constitute a natural liability in our species to the kind of emotional conflict that in some appears as disorder of the mind.

As long as infants do not recognize that their mothers or other carers are single and unique individuals the direction of radically conflicting emotions towards them need present no psychological difficulties. The conflicts become important for infants themselves only as they start to apply the concept of numerical identity, and so to regard themselves and others as individuals who are enduring and unique in space and time. This development coincides with what Melanie Klein regarded as the transition from the paranoid-schizoid to the depressive position, and there is some reason to suppose, as she held, that it starts to take hold during the fourth month of life.[27] This might well also be the time at which imaginary attacks on the mother, or again on siblings, would start to be felt by infants themselves as potential

[26] The regulation of anger in infancy is discussed in terms of Bayesian neuroscience and attachment in Hopkins (2012, in press). Emotional development and conflict are also discussed in relation to the infant's recognition of the mother as a single enduring object in Hopkins (1987).

[27] On this developments see the readings cited in footnote 27, particularly the last. As discussed there and also briefly in Hopkins (2003, 2004) one experiment seems particularly relevant. Bower (1977)

causes of grief and distress at separation, and so would engage with aggression-punishing images produced via the superego/ego-ideal. Hence we might finally speculate that this development took place in Saks' individual case in a way that was incomplete,[28] and so left her with a disposition to imaginary aggression (particularly as regards the killing of babies) that remained a source of guilt in later life.

In any cases we can see that human infants steadily learn to regulate their anger over the course of the first year, and in accord with the images of themselves as in relation to others that experience builds in their cortices. At four months, for example, infants angered by an experimenter's impeding hand direct their anger at the hand itself. They apparently still conceive even the persons around them (and hence the mother and her breast) as part-objects, as psychoanalysis has held. By seven months, however, they direct their anger at an offender's face, and their history of experience with an offender determines the kind of anger they feel. Infants of this age are especially angry if their mothers annoy them after a stranger has already done so, for by now they apparently expect her comfort in such a situation and regard her joining the stranger in annoying them as a betrayal. Overall it appears that infants' recognition of their carers and themselves as unique individuals leads to an increase in separation distress and also to a fear of strangers, as if the consolidation of mother and infant as a first *good us* led also to a first *bad them* in the form of fearful strangers.

This would bring our evolutionary speculations about infancy into line with those about group competition and the role of the superego/ego-ideal considered earlier. The overall structure is registered in a familiar proverb.

Myself against my brother
My brother and I against the family
My family against the clan
All of us against the foreigner.

describes: "A simple optical arrangement that allows one to present infants with multiple images of a single object ... If one presents the infant with multiple images of its mother — say three 'mothers'" — the infant of less than five months is not disturbed at all but will in fact interact with all three 'mothers' in turn. If the setup provides one mother and two strangers, the infant will preferentially interact with its mother and still show no signs of disturbance. However, past the age of five months (after the coordination of place and movement) the sight of three 'mothers' becomes very disturbing to the infant. At this same age a setup of one mother and two strangers has no effect. I would contend that this in fact shows that the young infant (less than five months old) thinks it has a multiplicity of mothers, whereas the older infant knows it has only one" (p. 217). This experiment does seem to admit interpretation as evidence that while at four months the infant takes its mother as a psychological other to whom it relates, it does not yet regard her as a single enduring person, as opposed to a potential multiplicity of presences whose spatiotemporal dimensions are as yet indeterminate. By five months, however, the baby apparently opposes uniqueness to episodic multiplicity, and starts to represent the mother (and by implication/identification its own self) as individual, continuous, and lasting. If this is correct, then the four- to five-month consolidation of the mother's image via the concept of spatiotemporal numerical identity represents a synthesis in the imagination by which the baby integrates the major parameters of its internal and external worlds. We should regard this as a momentous event, particularly in light of the considerations about motivational conflict advanced here. As such it deserves fuller experimental investigation.

[28] Contemporary neurobiological accounts of schizophrenia, such as the "Dysconnection" hypothesis advanced by Friston and others, are consistent with the idea that that the disorder should involve biologically based failures in the resolution and management of conflict. See, e.g., Stephan et al. (2009).

This represents sibling rivalry and parent–offspring conflict as part of a larger pattern of cooperating to compete that channels aggression via successively larger groups. Even such a schematic account brings to the fore a consequence that we seem actually to face. Insofar as we cooperate in groups to compete in groups we cannot manage to cooperate as a single group even when important common interests require it. Rather we are liable to regress to competition against the foreigner instead.

Psychiatry, Psychoanalysis, and Neuroscience

At the outset we observed that psychiatry is liable to tension between a clinical approach that concentrates on the lived experience of mental disorder and a neurobiological one that focuses on the brain in which such experience is realized. This tension caused Freud to abandon neuroscience,[29] and in recent times—as registered in the history of the *Diagnostic and Statistical Manual of Mental Disorders* (DSM)—it has caused psychiatry to abandon Freud.

In this chapter I have tried to argue that this tension, large as it now looms, may be liable to at least a partial intellectual dissolution. The ideas that we have considered suggest that the accounts of mental disorder provided by Freud and his successors should not be taken as alternatives to a more adequate neurobiology of mental disorder, but rather as indicating paths we might take towards attaining one. Our circumstances of life entail that our basic emotional systems are liable to conflict; and important forms of disorder seem rooted in conflict of this kind, and the fictive experiences by which the brain seems to regulate it. These emotional conflicts, in turn, seem rooted in evolution, together with the "moral" emotions that go awry in mental disorder as well.

These claims are speculative, but increasingly sustained by evidence. Insofar as they prove to be correct, psychoanalysis and our future accounts of the neurobiology of mental disorder should converge, at least within the limits set by the differences in their categories. It is a further question whether such convergence would help us to regulate our use of group-on-group

---

[29] As his clinical work progressed, Freud at first sought to combine it with neuroscience. Following Fechner, he hypothesized that the nervous system worked to minimize a kind of energy, and so to regulate "free energy" produced by external perception and inner instinctual demands. In this he represented learning as modifying connections ("facilitations") between neural cells correlated in their activations, and "psychic acquisition" as embodied in such connections—two ideas which have remained central to computational neuroscience. He conceived lack of satisfaction of instinctual needs as activating motor expressions of frustration, which became associated with memories of satisfaction provided by carers, which could be activated in a kind of primary process in response to need. Sensory and motor learning produced a neural organization—an "ego"—which could inhibit this primary process so as to integrate motor activity along lines which had proven successful in achieving satisfaction.In all this Freud was prescient. In a contemporary Bayesian "free energy" approach to neuroscience, as indicated in Carhart-Harris and Friston (2010/2012), the processes he described would appear as he described them, that is, as basic processes in the minimizing of free energy, which is seen as the fundamental task of the brain. But as the burden of recasting his psychological discoveries in neurobiological terms became too great he abandoned this attempt, and contented himself with structuring his later psychological accounts to fit around the skeleton of the sketch he had begun.

violence, or to cooperate in the absence of human enemies whom we can demonize to our own satisfaction. But understanding mental disorder in this way is of a piece with understanding the irrationalities that are part of human nature; and we may hope to progress in both together.

References

Beebe, B., Jaffe, J., Markese, S., Buck, K., Chen, H., Cohen, P., *et al.* (2010). The origins of 12-month attachment: A microanalysis of 4-month mother-infant interaction. *Attachment and Human Development, 12*(1), 3–141.

Bell, D. (2008). Who is killing what or whom? In S. Briggs, A. Lemma, and W. Crouch (Eds), *Relating to Self-Harm and Suicide: Psychoanalytic Perspectives on Practice, Theory and Prevention*, pp. 45–60. London: Routledge.

Bower, T. (1977) *Development in Infancy*. San Francisco, CA: W. H. Freeman.

Breuer, J. and Freud, S. Studies on Hysteria. In J. Strachey (Ed.) *The Standard Edition of the Complete Psychological Works of Sigmund Freud , Vol II*, p. 21, London: Hogarth Press (Original work published 1895).

Buchheim, A., Viviani, R., Kessler, H., Kachele, H., Cierpka, M., Roth, G., *et al.* (2012). Changes in prefrontal-limbic function in major depression after 15 months of long-term psychotherapy. *PLoS One, 7*(3), e33745. doi:10.1371/journal.pone.0033745

Carhart-Harris, R. and Friston, K. (2010). The default-mode, ego-functions and free-energy: A neurobiological account of Freudian ideas. *Brain, 133*, 1265–83. (Revised and reprinted in Fotopolu, A., Pfaff, D., and Conway, M. (Eds) (2012). *From the Couch to the Lab: Psychoanalysis, Neuroscience and Cognitive Psychology in Dialogue*, pp. 219–29. Oxford: Oxford University Press.)

Cassidy, J. and Shaver, P. (2008). *Handbook of Attachment*. London: Guildford Press.

Damasio, A., Damasio, H., and Traniel, D. (2012). Persistence of feelings and sentience after bilateral damage of the insula. *Cerebral Cortex*, doi:10.1093/cercor/bhs077.

Eilperin, J. (2012). *Demon Fish: Travels through the Hidden World of Sharks*. London: Duckworth.

Freud, S. (1950) Project for a Scientific Psychology. In J. Strachey (Ed.), *The Standard Edition of the Complete Psychological Works of Sigmund Freud, Vol I*, p. 275a, London: Hogarth Press.

Freud, S. (1957a). The interpretation of dreams. In J. Strachey (Ed.), *The Standard Edition of the Complete Psychological Works of Sigmund Freud, Volume V*, pp. 96–121. London: Hogarth Press. (Original work published 1900.)

Freud, S. (1957b). Autobiographical notes on a case of paranoia. In J. Strachey (Ed.), *The Standard Edition of the Complete Psychological Works of Sigmund Freud, Volume XII*, p. 9–82. London: Hogarth Press. (Original work published 1911.)

Freud, S. (1957c). On narcissism. In J. Strachey (Ed.), *The Standard Edition of the Complete Psychological Works of Sigmund Freud, Volume X*, pp. 78–102. London: Hogarth Press. (Original work published 1914.)

Freud, S. (1957d). Mourning and Melancholia. In J. Strachey (Ed.), *The Standard Edition of the Complete Psychological Works of Sigmund Freud, Volume XIV*, p.237-58. London: Hogarth Press (Original work published 1917).

Gegestand, S. (2007). Reproductive strategies and tactics. In R. Dunbar and L. Barrett (Eds), *Oxford Handbook of Evolutionary Psychology*, pp. 321–32. Oxford: Oxford University Press.

Gertler, B. (2011). Self-knowledge. In E. N. Zalta (Ed.), *The Stanford Encyclopedia of Philosophy* (Spring 2011 Edition). [Online.] Available at: <http://plato.stanford.edu/archives/spr2011/entries/self-knowledge/>.

Haig, D. (1993). Genetic conflicts in human pregnancy. *Quarterly Review of Biology, 68*, 495–532.

Hobson, J. and Friston, K. (2012). Waking and dreaming consciousness: Neurobiological and functional considerations. *Progress in Neurobiology, 98*, 82–98.

Hopkins, J. (1987). Synthesis in the imagination: Psychoanalysis, infantile experience, and the concept of an object. In J. Russell (Ed.), *Philosophical Perspectives on Developmental Psychology*, pp. 140–70. Oxford: Basil Blackwell.

Hopkins, J. (1999). Patterns of interpretation: Speech, action, and dream. In L. Marcus (Ed.), *Cultural Documents: The Interpretation of Dreams*, pp. 123–59. Manchester: Manchester University Press.

Hopkins, J. (2000a). Psychoanalysis, metaphor, and the concept of mind. In M. Levine (Ed.), *The Analytic Freud. Philosophy and Psychoanalysis*, pp. 11–35. London: Routledge.

Hopkins, J. (2000b). Evolution, consciousness, and the internality of mind. In P. Carruthers and A. Chamberlin (Eds), *Evolution and the Human Mind*, pp. 276–98. Cambridge: Cambridge University Press.

Hopkins, J. (2003). Evolution, emotion, and conflict. In M. Chung (Ed.), *Psychoanalytic Knowledge*, pp. 132–56. London: Macmillan/Palgrave Press.

Hopkins, J. (2004). Conscience and conflict: Darwin, Freud, and the origins of human aggression. In D. Evans and P. Cruse (Eds), *Emotion, Evolution, and Rationality*, pp. 225–48. Oxford: Oxford University Press.

Hopkins, J. (2007). The problem of consciousness and the innerness of the mind. In M. M. McCabe and M. Textor (Eds), *Perspectives on Perception*, pp. 19–46. Frankfurt: Lancaster Publishers.

Hopkins, J. (2012). Psychoanalysis representation and neuroscience: The Freudian unconscious and the Bayesian brain. In A. Fotopolu, D. Pfaff, and M. Conway, M. (Eds), *From the Couch to the Lab: Psychoanalysis, Neuroscience and Cognitive Psychology in Dialogue*, pp. 230–65. Oxford: Oxford University Press.

Hopkins, J. (in press). Conflict creates an unconscious id. *Neuropsychoanalysis.*

Hrdy, S. (2000). *Mother Nature*. London: Vintage.

Hrdy, S. (2009). *Mothers and Others*. Cambridge, MA: Harvard University Press.

Kernberg, O. (2003). Sanctioned social violence: A psychoanalytic view. Pt I. *International Journal of Psycho-Analysis, 84*, 683–698; Pt II: 953–68.

Maltsberger, J. T. (2008). Self break-up and the descent into suicide. In S. Briggs, A. Lemma, and W. Crouch (Eds), *Relating to Self-Harm and Suicide: Psychoanalytic Perspectives on Practice, Theory and Prevention*, pp. 38–44. London: Routledge.

Mitchell, J. (2003). *Siblings*. Cambridge: Polity Press.

Mock, D. (2005). *More than Kind and Less than Kind*. Cambridge, MA: Harvard University Press.

Mock, D. and Parker, A. (1997). *The Evolution of Sibling Rivalry*. Oxford: Oxford University Press.

Obama, B. (1995). *Dreams from My Father: A Story of Race and Inheritance*. New York, NY: Random House.

Richerson, P. and Boyd, R. (2006). *Not by Genes Alone: How Culture Transformed Human Evolution*. Chicago, IL: University of Chicago Press.

Saks, E. (2008). *The Center Cannot Hold: My Journey Through Madness*. New York, NY: Hyperion.

Schedler, J. (2010). The efficacy of psychodynamic psychotherapy. *American Psychologist*, 65(2), 98–109.

Skues, R. (2006). *Sigmund Freud and the History of Anna O: Reopening a Closed Case.* London: Palgrave, Macmillan.

Solms, M. (in press) The conscious id. *Neuropsychoanalysis.*

Solms, M. and Panksepp, J. (2012). The "id" knows more than the "ego" admits: Neuropsychoanalytic and primal consciousness perspectives on the interface between affective and cognitive neuroscience. *Brain Sciences, 2,* 147–75.

Stephan, K., Friston, K., and Frith, C. (2009). Dysconnection in schizophrenia: From abnormal synaptic plasticity to failures of self-monitoring. *Schizophrenia Bulletin, 35*(3), 509–27

Trivers, R. (2002). *Natural Selection and Social Theory.* Oxford: Oxford University Press.

Watt, D. and Panksepp, J. (2009). Depression: An evolutionarily conserved mechanism to terminate separation distress? A review of aminergic, peptidergic, and neural network perspectives. *Neuropsychoanalysis, 11,* 7–51.

AUTHOR INDEX

Subject Index